CANCER   1

A COMPREHENSIVE TREATISE

SECOND EDITION

ETIOLOGY: Chemical and Physical Carcinogenesis

CANCER 1

A COMPREHENSIVE TREATISE

SECOND EDITION

ETIOLOGY: Chemical and Physical Carcinogenesis

FREDERICK F. BECKER, EDITOR

University of Texas System Cancer Center
M.D. Anderson Hospital and Tumor Institute
Houston, Texas

PLENUM PRESS • NEW YORK AND LONDON

Library of Congress Cataloging in Publication Data

Main entry under title:

Cancer: a comprehensive treatise.

Includes bibliographies and indexes.
Contents: v. 1. Etiology, chemical and physical carcinogenesis.
1. Cancer — Collected works. I. Becker, Frederick F. [DNLM: 1. Neoplasms.
QZ 200 C2143]
RC261.C263 1982   616.99′4   81-21050
ISBN 0-306-40701-9   AACR2

©1982 Plenum Press, New York
A Division of Plenum Publishing Corporation
233 Spring Street, New York, N.Y. 10013

Printed in the United States of America

To Mary Ellen Becker

without whose encouragement and support
this treatise would not have been completed.

Contributors

to Volume 1

ROBERT W. BALDWIN, Cancer Research Campaign Laboratories, University of Nottingham, Nottingham, England

FREDERICK F. BECKER, Department of Anatomic and Research Pathology, M. D. Anderson Hospital and Tumor Institute, University of Texas System Cancer Center, Houston, Texas

ISAAC BERENBLUM, The Weizmann Institute of Science, Rehovot, Israel

K. GERHARD BRAND, Department of Microbiology, University of Minnesota Medical School, Minneapolis, Minnesota

EMMANUEL FARBER, Departments of Pathology and Biochemistry, University of Toronto, Toronto, Ontario, Canada

JACOB FURTH, Institute of Cancer Research and Department of Pathology, Columbia University College of Physicians and Surgeons, New York, New York

VINCENT F. GUINEE, Department of Epidemiology, The University of Texas System Cancer Center, M. D. Anderson Hospital and Tumor Institute, Houston, Texas

W. E. HESTON, Laboratory of Biology, National Cancer Institute, National Institutes of Health, Bethesda, Maryland

ALBRECHT M. KELLERER, Institut für Medizinische Strahlenkunde, University of Würzburg, Würzburg, Federal Republic of Germany

ALFRED G. KNUDSON, JR., The University of Texas Health Science Center at Houston, Graduate School of Biomedical Sciences, Houston, Texas

CORNELIS J. M. MELIEF, Hematology Service, New England Medical Center Hospital, and Department of Medicine, Tufts University School of Medicine, Boston, Massachusetts

PETER C. NOWELL, Department of Pathology, School of Medicine, University of Pennsylvania, Philadelphia, Pennsylvania

viii
CONTRIBUTORS

MICHAEL POTTER, National Cancer Institute, Laboratory of Cell Biology, Bethesda, Maryland

MICHAEL R. PRICE, Cancer Research Campaign Laboratories, University of Nottingham, Nottingham, England

S. RAJALAKSHMI, Department of Pathology, University of Toronto, Toronto, Ontario, Canada

PREMA M. RAO, Department of Pathology, University of Toronto, Toronto, Ontario, Canada

JANARDAN K. REDDY, Department of Pathology, Northwestern University Medical School, Chicago, Illinois

HARALD H. ROSSI, Radiological Research Laboratory, Department of Radiology, Cancer Center/Institute of Cancer Research, Columbia University College of Physicians and Surgeons, New York, New York

D. S. R. SARMA, Department of Pathology, University of Toronto, Toronto, Ontario, Canada

ROBERT S. SCHWARTZ, Hematology Service, New England Medical Center Hospital, and Department of Medicine, Tufts University School of Medicine, Boston, Massachusetts

JOHN B. STORER, Biology Division, Oak Ridge National Laboratory, Oak Ridge, Tennessee

DONALD J. SVOBODA, Department of Pathology and Oncology, University of Kansas College of Health Sciences, Kansas City, Kansas

ARTHUR C. UPTON, Health Sciences Center, State University of New York at Stony Brook, Stony Brook, New York

FREDERICK URBACH, Temple University School of Medicine, Skin and Cancer Hospital, Philadelphia, Pennsylvania

J. H. WEISBURGER, American Health Foundation, Naylor Dana Institute for Disease Prevention, Valhalla, New York

G. M. WILLIAMS, American Health Foundation, Naylor Dana Institute for Disease Prevention, Valhalla, New York

Preface

Six years ago when the first edition of this volume appeared as the first of the series, questions were posed in its preface that are as valid today as they were then. In that preface, I proposed the following challenges:

> (1) We must identify carcinogenic agents, and by an analysis of their "nature," e.g., structure and physical characteristics, we may better understand their mechanism of action. (2) We must identify crucial interactions between these carcinogens and important macromolecules within the cell, distinguishing those which relate to carcinogenesis from those which are extraneous. (3) We must examine the alterations of cell function induced by these reactions, for it is with an understanding of phenotypic variation that we may know why malignant cells escape from normal homeostatic control. (4) Last, and perhaps of greatest importance, we must define malignancy—define those characteristics of cellular activity that permit the malignant cell to compete so effectively with the normal constituent, which ultimately leads to such destructive events.

Although great strides have been made toward those goals, as evidenced by a number of new chapters and the new information gathered into others, and although the achievement of those goals sometimes appears but a tantalizing experiment away, none have been achieved. For example, several chapters include descriptions of the progress that has been made toward the development of "quick assays." The aggregate of methods they describe is aimed at making available a test or cascade of tests that, in a short time and for reasonable cost, will indicate with a high probability of accuracy whether a given chemical agent would be carcinogenic for man. The socioeconomic implications of such tests should be all too familiar to the reader. In the main, these tests extrapolate from mutation or other cellular alteration to carcinogenicity. By implication, they can cause chemicals of value to be proscribed or they can justify the persistence of a carcinogen in our environment. Additionally, these tests, which utilize organisms ranging from the lowest forms of prokaryotes to human cells in aggregate, may yield information about the type of basic alteration responsible for the initiation (in the broadest sense) of the carcinogenic process.

The overlap of these findings with those described by Rajalakshmi and others is evident. An enormous amount of information has emerged concerning the nature and specificity of intracellular macromolecular interactions by these agents. Their "imprinting" on the cell's genome, the balance of repair and misrepair, the magnification of the alteration by cell division, and other cellular phenomena are becoming more apparent. Yet all these findings, as well as those of the quick assays, have not answered the pertinent questions: Is DNA alteration obligate in the process? What is the nature of that change induced by agents totally different in their macromolecular interaction that results in malignancy? How is that change induced?

Berenblum, Farber, and others elaborate on the sequences of cellular alteration required for the development of the carcinogenic process. These presentations demonstrate great progress in our attempts to learn the sequence of carcinogenesis. But they also elucidate the second great question in this field, the nature of the cellular alterations induced by the initial changes that evoke malignant behavior. We have come far since Warburg's hypothesis on the nature of the underlying cellular metabolic alterations, and indeed, interest in that hypothesis has appeared again. Still, the obligate cellular alterations remain unknown.

Thus, it should be no surprise that the most important of all the questions that remain unanswered is, what is malignancy?

It has been proposed that if we could identify all the environmental causes of cancer and remove them or modify their effects (with the so-called chemoprotective agents), we could eliminate malignancy. However, we have become increasingly aware that problems in the environment are not simply due to contamination by chemicals (see Becker), and even the most optimistic enthusiast does not envision agents to protect us totally against our environment. The cancer therapist puts forth the thesis that once a "general" cure is found, concern, and indeed experimentation, in the field can cease. However, if we have learned any single lesson in the last half decade, it has been that these studies have enormous potential beyond understanding cancer. Aging, genetic diseases, and many other problems apparently overlap in cause and potential remedies.

More important is the strong possibility that the basic experiments to which I referred above will lead to the final eradication of this dread condition. The cure will be *knowledge*! Thus, while the optimism in each approach can help sustain its protagonists, we must not let this surety place us in adversarial roles. The most certain contribution to the future, to cancer's elimination and to our general understanding of disease, is an understanding of the processes that establish and maintain the normal function and health of the cell.

F.F.B.

Houston

Contents

General Concepts

Genetics: Animal Tumors   2

W. E. HESTON

Genetic Influences in Human Tumors   3

ALFRED G. KNUDSON, JR.

Hormones as Etiological Agents in Neoplasia 4

JACOB FURTH

Pathogenesis of Plasmacytomas in Mice 5

MICHAEL POTTER

Immunocompetence and Malignancy   6

Cornelis J. M. Melief and Robert S. Schwartz

Epidemiologic Approach to Cancer   7

Vincent F. Guinee

Chemical Carcinogenesis

Chemical Agents, the Environment, and the History of Carcinogenesis   8

FREDERICK F. BECKER

Metabolism of Chemical Carcinogens   9

J. H. WEISBURGER AND G. M. WILLIAMS

Chemical Carcinogenesis: Interactions of Carcinogens with Nucleic Acids 10

S. Rajalakshmi, Prema M. Rao, and D. S. R. Sarma

Some Effects of Carcinogens on Cell Organelles   11

DONALD J. SVOBODA AND JANARDAN K. REDDY

Sequential Aspects of Chemical Carcinogenesis: Skin 12

Isaac Berenblum

Sequential Events in Chemical Carcinogenesis 13

Emmanuel Farber

Neoantigen Expression in Chemical Carcinogenesis 14

Robert W. Baldwin and Michael R. Price

Physical Carcinogenesis

Physical Carcinogenesis:
Radiation—History and Sources   15

ARTHUR C. UPTON

Biophysical Aspects of Radiation
Carcinogenesis   16

ALBRECHT M. KELLERER AND HARALD H. ROSSI

Ultraviolet Radiation: Interaction with Biological Molecules   17

FREDERICK URBACH

Radiation Carcinogenesis   18

JOHN B. STORER

Cancer Associated with Asbestosis, Schistosomiasis, Foreign Bodies, and Scars   19

K. Gerhard Brand

General Concepts

Cytogenetics

Peter C. Nowell

1. Introduction

The relationship between chromosome abnormalities and neoplasia has been the subject of investigation and speculation for many years. It was noted very early that mitotic irregularities were common in routine sections prepared from many human tumors, and these observations were extended by workers such as von Hansemann (1890) and Boveri (1914) to suggest a causal relationship between chromosome alterations and cancer. With the development of modern techniques of mammalian cytogenetics in the late 1950s (Hsu and Pomerat, 1953; Tjio and Levan, 1956; Moorhead et al., 1960), interest in chromosome studies of tumors was reawakened, and subsequently a wide variety of human and animal neoplasms were studied. This work has received additional impetus in the past few years from the introduction of "banding" methods that permit the identification of individual chromosomes and of alterations in smaller segments of chromosomes than was possible by previous techniques (Caspersson et al., 1968; Seabright, 1971). Although these newer methods have not yet been fully exploited, it must also be recognized that even with the banding procedures, there may still remain significant genetic alterations in neoplastic cells that are below the level of detection with the light microscope.

Nonetheless, the data that have been accumulated on chromosome alterations in tumor cells do provide significant evidence on the role of genetic change in neoplasia and also have proved to be of some practical clinical value. It is the purpose of this chapter to summarize present knowledge in the field and to speculate briefly on its significance. No attempt has been made to present an exhaustive review; rather, the purpose is to illustrate with pertinent data such generalizations as can be made and to emphasize those findings that appear to have the greatest theoretical or practical interest.

PETER C. NOWELL ● Department of Pathology, School of Medicine, University of Pennsylvania, Philadelphia, Pennsylvania.

In the light of present knowledge, the following three general statements appear warranted at this time.

1. Most tumors are chromosomally abnormal. This is particularly true of solid malignancies, and only in a few tumors, such as the acute leukemias of man, is there a significant proportion of cases with no demonstrable chromosome change. Furthermore, it is usual that the more aggressive or "malignant" a neoplasm, the greater the degree of cytogenetic abnormality. This latter observation has led to the suggestion that sequential genetic changes in the neoplastic cell population underlie the phenomenon of biological and clinical tumor progression.

2. Chromosome alterations are often the same in all cells of a given tumor. Where there is a spectrum of karyotypic changes, these are often demonstrably related. This represents one body of evidence that tumors are clones, i.e., they originate from a single cell. Even in highly malignant neoplasms with much karyotypic variation, characteristic marker chromosomes recognizable in all cells of a given tumor lend support to this clonal concept.

3. Neoplasms of a particular type do not show a consistent cytogenetic alteration from one tumor to another. A specific change occurring in nearly every tumor of a given type, such as the Philadelphia chromosome in human chronic granulocytic leukemia (Section 2.1), is the exception rather than the rule. Banding studies have clearly demonstrated, however, that certain alterations in specific chromosome segments do occur nonrandomly in many tumors, indicating specific sites where genes significant in the development of neoplasia are apparently located.

1.1. Technical Considerations

Before discussing the findings that support these generalizations, it is appropriate to comment on some of the technical problems associated with these studies, as they significantly influence the quality and quantity of data available. First, it must be reiterated that the chromosome alterations under consideration are limited to the neoplastic cells and, with rare exceptions, do not represent constitutional changes affecting all the tissues of the individual. Hence, dividing *tumor* cells must be obtained, and the usual sources of normal cells for chromosome study, lymphocytes from peripheral blood cultures and fibroblasts from skin cultures, are not appropriate. For investigation of the cytogenetic changes in the leukemias, both in man and in animals, suspensions of proliferating neoplastic cells frequently have been available from blood or bone marrow. With solid tumors, however, it has been necessary to apply various mechanical and chemical means of disaggregation in order to prepare suspensions of cells suitable for chromosome study. With small early tumors and precancerous lesions in which mitoses are few, it has been particularly difficult to obtain preparations with adequate numbers of mitotic figures.

Improved techniques have recently been developed for obtaining metaphases from solid tumors, such as growing the cells in soft agar (Hamburger *et al.*,

1978), but debate remains concerning the relative merits of direct versus tissue culture methods. Opponents of the use of short-term culture as a source of dividing cells, both with the solid tumors and with leukemias, have shown that under some circumstances the cells that proliferate *in vitro* are not representative of those dividing *in vivo*. On the other hand, if direct preparative techniques are used, many of the abnormal metaphases observed may represent cells incapable of completing mitosis successfully in the body, and the normal metaphases seen may be proliferating inflammatory cells rather than tumor cells.

With respect to the last possibility, it has been generally recognized, both with the leukemias and with solid neoplasms, that many tumor chromosome preparations contain a mixture of normal and neoplastic cells, and, more importantly, that the tumor metaphases are often of much poorer technical quality than the normal cells (Nowell and Hungerford, 1964; Sandberg, 1966). Individual chromosomes are fuzzy and overlapping with poorly defined centromeres, and the neoplastic metaphases can easily be overlooked in favor of the technically more satisfactory chromosomes present in the normal cells. The tumor metaphases also frequently do not band as well as do nonneoplastic cells, and since preparations must be of good quality for the recognition of alterations in small segments of individual chromosomes, one should be aware of these special problems in assessing reports of cytogenetic studies on neoplastic material (Levan and Mitelman, 1976; Whang-Peng, 1977).

Two additional methodological approaches have recently been described that may well provide additional important data on tumor chromosomes if the technical limitations of the neoplastic material can be overcome. Yunis *et al.* (1978) have developed a method of "prophasic banding" that results in more than 1000 individual bands being recognizable in the haploid set of human chromosomes. This technique has already been utilized to demonstrate small constitutional chromosome deletions that were not identifiable by the usual banding techniques. Hittelman and Rao (1978) have been able to force interphase cells from various sources, including human bone marrow, into mitosis through virus-induced fusion with mitotic cells from tissue culture lines. By this approach, termed "premature chromosome condensation," chromosome preparations for study occasionally can be obtained from cell populations that normally would not be proliferating.

Other techniques, such as flow cytophotometry, are also proving increasingly valuable for the identification and characterization of non-dividing aneuploid tumor cell populations, but as these methods do not involve the direct study of chromosomes, they are beyond the scope of this chapter.

2. Human Leukemias

These neoplasms have been more extensively studied cytogenetically than any other group of tumors, and so provide much of the data upon which the generalizations given earlier are based. It has often been possible to follow patients by means of sequential chromosome studies, and, as indicated above, dividing neoplastic cells (from blood or bone marrow) are usually much more readily obtainable than from solid tumors. The following subsections summarize the cytogenetic information available on these neoplasms, emphasizing both the theoretical considerations and the clinical applications that have resulted from these studies. Chronic granulocytic leukemia has provided the most data in both respects, and so is considered first. This is followed by largely recent, and corroborative, evidence from the acute leukemias and from related "pre-leukemic" myeloid dyscrasias. Lymphoproliferative disorders (chronic lymphocytic leukemia and the solid lymphomas), for which generally less information is available, are considered last.

2.1. Chronic Granulocytic Leukemia and the Philadelphia Chromosome

Chronic granulocytic leukemia (CGL) is the best documented example of a neoplasm in which nearly every typical case is characterized by the same chromo-

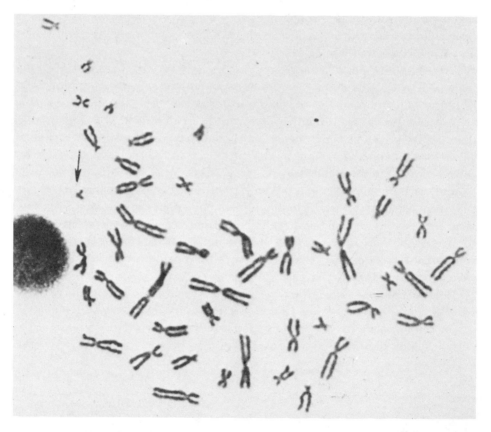

FIGURE 1. Dividing marrow cell arrested in metaphase from a patient with chronic granulocytic leukemia. The smallest of the 46 chromosomes is the abnormal Philadelphia chromosome (arrow), found in the neoplastic cells in nearly every typical case of chronic granulocytic leukemia.

some change (Nowell and Hungerford, 1960). This characteristic abnormality, the Philadelphia chromosome (Ph), is a small acrocentric chromosome derived from chromosome 22 by the loss of approximately one-half of its long arm (Fig. 1). Banding studies by Rowley (1973) and others have demonstrated that the missing chromosome segment is not lost from the cell but is typically translocated onto the long arm of chromosome 9. In perhaps 10–15% of the cases, the missing segment of chromosome 22 is translocated to another chromosome in the complement or even involved in a complex three-way rearrangement. These variants appear to have no significance with respect to the clinical characteristics of the disease, and so it appears that it is the displacement of the segment of chromosome 22 that is of major importance, rather than the site to which it goes (Sonta and Sandberg, 1977).

There is considerable evidence that the Ph abnormality is an acquired phenomenon rather than an inborn defect. It is apparently limited to the neoplastic hemic cells of affected individuals, including megakaryocytic, erythroid, monocytic, and lymphoid elements, as well as those of the myeloid series, but it is not found in nonhemic tissues, such as cells cultured from the skin (Trujillo and Ohno, 1963; Whang *et al.*, 1963; Mitelman, 1975). In addition, the Ph chromosome has been found to be absent in the monozygotic twin of six patients with Ph-positive GCL, and it is also not observed in children whose parents have the disease (Woodliff, 1971).

These data have led to the suggestion that CGL is induced by the production, in a totipotential marrow stem cell, of this specific aberration by one or another of the mutagenic agents known to break chromosomes. The fact that ionizing radiation has been shown to produce a similar chromosome change in occasional cells of otherwise normal individuals lends support to this hypothesis.

It seems a reasonable assumption that the presence of a Ph chromosome confers a selective advantage on the mutant stem cell, and that this results in leukemia. Proliferation of the mutant cell leads to a clone of Ph^+ hematopoietic elements that overgrow the normal marrow and produce the clinical disease. (The term "clone," as used here and elsewhere in this chapter, only indicates a population of cells derived from a single cell. It does not imply complete homogeneity, as subpopulations may coexist within the clone). Recent studies, using the enzyme glucose-6-phosphate dehydrogenase as a marker, have supported the view that essentially all of the lymphohematopoietic elements in a patient with CGL do indeed constitute a clone, with the possible exception of a proportion of the T lymphocytes (Fialkow, 1979).

While the foregoing process has not been explained in terms of a specific advantageous metabolic alteration in the leukemic cells, it is noteworthy that CGL is characterized by an unusually constant biochemical change, markedly reduced levels of alkaline phosphatase in the neoplastic granulocytes. This observation suggests that there may be a genetic locus on chromosome 22 that influences, in some fashion, the quantity of this enzyme in the leukemic cells (Pedersen and Hayhoe, 1971). There is, however, no obvious association between this demonstrable enzyme change (which is useful diagnostically) and the undefined alteration that provides the leukemic cells with their neoplastic growth characteristics.

With successful treatment of CGL, immature cells normally disappear from the peripheral blood; but even in clinical remission, the abnormal clone persists in the marrow, and chromosome studies on dividing marrow cells usually show the Ph chromosome in all, or nearly all, metaphases. There have been occasional case reports of unusual sensitivity to chemotherapy, with marked marrow depression and a concomitant marked reduction in the size of the neoplastic clone as judged by the percentage of Ph$^+$ cells. In several instances, this sensitivity to conventional therapy has been associated with prolonged remission, but thus far, attempts to eliminate the Ph$^+$ clone by more vigorous treatment of those responding normally to standard therapy have been largely unsuccessful (Finney *et al.*, 1972; Gee *et al.*, 1978).

When CGL progresses to the accelerated "blast" phase, which usually characterizes the terminal stages of the disease, chromosome studies have shown that in the neoplastic cells of approximately 75% of the cases, there are cytogenetic abnormalities in addition to the Ph chromosome (Fig. 2). In nearly every instance, these additional alterations involve one or more of the following: A second Ph

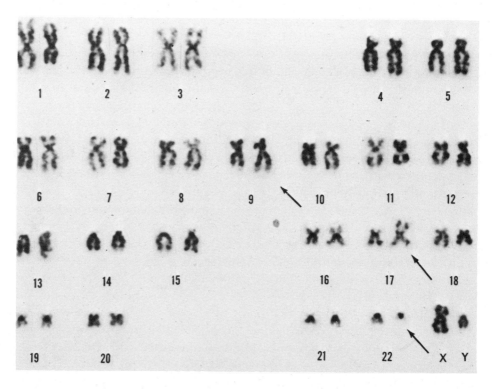

FIGURE 2. Banded karyotype from a patient with chronic granulocytic leukemia in the terminal accelerated phase. In addition to the typical translocation from chromosome 22 to chromosome 9, t(9q;22q), producing the Philadelphia chromosome, there is an isochromosome for the long arm of 17, iso-17q, replacing a normal 17. This additional abnormality occurs nonrandomly in the blast phase of chronic granulocytic leukemia.

chromosome, an isochromosome for the long arm of 17 (iso-17q),* and trisomy for chromosome 8 (Alimena *et al.*, 1979). It has been suggested that these additional, nonrandom, abnormalities constitute further significant genetic change in the neoplastic clone, producing greater deviation from the normal balance between proliferation and differentiation (Pedersen, 1973; Nowell, 1976). The additional selective advantage conferred by these new patterns of growth permits the cells with supplementary chromosome changes to overgrow not only the normal elements, but also the original Ph^+ clone, producing the more aggressive, terminal stage of the leukemia. This association between genetic evolution within the neoplastic clone (recognized cytogenetically) and clinical progression of the disease has been best documented for human tumors in studies of CGL, but such "clonal evolution" may have general significance, and it will be considered in more detail later.

The recognition of additional cytogenetic changes in CGL during the course of the disease is therefore usually a grave prognostic sign, but interestingly, a different nonrandom alteration, absence of the Y chromosome from a Ph^+ clone, has in a number of instances been associated with unusually long survival (Berger and Bernheim, 1979).

The Ph chromosome is not present in 10–15% of adult hemic disorders diagnosed as CGL. There is general agreement that Ph^- CGL usually occurs in patients over 60, and frequently one or more aspects of the disease are clinically atypical. These individuals generally do not respond well to therapy and have a survival time significantly shorter than that of patients with Ph^+ CGL (Canellos *et al.*, 1976).

Two forms of CGL occur in childhood. The "adult" form is very similar to the typical disease in the adult. The Ph chromosome is present, and the response to therapy is usually good. In the "infantile" or "juvenile" form, there is usually a more subacute clinical picture. The Ph chromosome is absent (although there may be other chromosome changes), and the response to therapy is usually not favorable. Since the "adult" form can occur in children as young as 2 years, chromosome studies may be prognostically valuable, particularly so because leukocyte alkaline phosphatase levels may be low in both of the childhood forms of CGL (Nowell, 1967; Brodeur *et al.*, 1979).

This last point illustrates the occasional lack of correlation between the presence of the Ph chromosome and reduced leukocyte alkaline phosphatase, which can occur both in children and in adults. There are also instances in which the Ph chromosome has been present in hemic disorders other than CGL, and these have been both myeloid and lymphoid. The Ph^+ nonlymphocytic dyscrasias have ranged from acute leukemia to chronic myeloproliferative disorders such as polycythemia vera and megakaryocytic myelosis. Cases have also been reported of Ph^+ acute lymphocytic leukemia, in both children and adults, as well as the appearance of lymphoid blasts in the late stages of previously typical Ph^+ CGL (Bloomfield *et al.*, 1978). These phenomena are now well documented by banding

* In standard nomenclature, the short and long arms of a chromosome are designated p and q, respectively (Paris Conference, 1971).

studies as involving the typical 9;22 translocation; and thus it appears that in some instances, either early or late in the disease, the cells of a Ph^+ clone, derived from a mutant totipotential hemic stem cell, may differentiate predominantly along a lymphoid or other pathway rather than in the usual myeloid direction. These variants have not been characterized by any specific cytogenetic alteration other than the Ph chromosome, but Ph^+ acute leukemia does not usually respond well to standard therapy, and so the recognition of this entity is of some value in prognosis (Bloomfield *et al.*, 1978).

Despite these occasional exceptional circumstances, the cytogenetics of CGL provides the clearest example in man of the role that chromosome changes may play in both the initiation and the progression of neoplasia.

2.2. Acute Leukemias

Cytogenetic studies of human acute leukemias have been of particular interest because in approximately half of all cases, no demonstrable chromosome abnormality is present, a phenomenon not observed with any other major type of human neoplasm. Banding studies have not altered this conclusion, but they have revealed, in those cases that have cytogenetic changes, nonrandom patterns of both theoretical and practical significance (Rowley, 1978). It is convenient to consider these disorders in two subgroups, acute nonlymphocytic leukemia (ANLL) and acute lymphocytic leukemia (ALL).

2.2.1. ANLL

Those cases of ANLL with cytogenetic alterations show considerable variation in karyotype, ranging from translocations within the diploid chromosome set to extensive departures from normal chromosome number and morphology. Typically, all the dividing leukemic cells examined from the blood and marrow of a given patient show the same karyotypic alteration, or related changes, indicating that the entire neoplastic population has derived from a single progenitor stem cell. Unlike CGL, however, the abnormal chromosome pattern observed in one patient has generally been different from that observed in others with the same disease. With banding, however, it has become clear that certain patterns tend to occur with a nonrandom frequency, particularly gain of a chromosome 8, loss of a No. 7, and abnormalities of No. 21, including an 8;21 translocation (Mitelman *et al.*, 1976; Rowley, 1978).

The abnormal karyotype in ANLL is often quite stable, with the same aberration persisting in a given individual throughout the course of the disease. During remissions, dividing cells with the abnormal pattern may not be demonstrable either in the peripheral blood or in the bone marrow; however, this does not represent the reversion of leukemic cells to normal, but simply reduction of the neoplastic clone to such small size as to be undetectable among regenerating normal elements. With subsequent exacerbation of the disease and recurrence of large numbers of neoplastic cells in the marrow and peripheral blood, cells with the same aberrant karyotype are again readily demonstrable.

In patients with acute leukemia treated by bone marrow transplantation, such relapse can usually be shown, by cytogenetics, to represent the original tumor; but in occasional cases, involving transplantation from a sib of opposite sex, sex chromosome differences have indicated that the presumed "recurrence" was in fact a new neoplasm, arising in cells of donor origin (Thomas *et al.*, 1972).

In some cases of ANLL, the cells at the time of relapse may show additional chromosome alterations, and this evidence of karyotypic evolution may be associated with new biological characteristics of the disease, including resistance to therapy (Testa and Rowley, 1978). Although such cytogenetic evolution is less common in ANLL than in CGL, it frequently involves the acquisition of an extra chromosome 8 in both disorders.

In a rare form of ANLL, acute promyelocytic leukemia, a translocation involving the long arms of chromosomes 15 and 17 has been observed in a high proportion of cases. In at least one series (Rowley *et al.*, 1977) it has been sufficiently consistent to be of diagnostic value.

Another small group of patients with ANLL of particular interest are those developing leukemia subsequent to treatment of another neoplasm with radiation or with chemotherapeutic drugs, particularly alkylating agents. In most of these patients, the leukemic clone shows extensive chromosome rearrangements, presumably reflecting the mutagenic effects of the previous therapy (Dahlke and Nowell, 1975; Foucar *et al.*, 1979). In some instances, such clones may be detectable in the bone marrow of these patients during a cytopenic phase preceding the development of frank leukemia. The diagnostic value of chromosome studies in such "preleukemic" patients will be discussed later.

2.2.2. ALL

This disorder, more common in children than adults, has been less extensively studied cytogenetically than ANLL, but the same generalizations appear applicable. Approximately half of all cases, both childhood and adult, do not have visible chromosome changes. In those with alterations, the changes are variable, clonal in nature, and in some cases show evolution over time in association with the clinical course. The abnormalities are again nonrandom to some degree, with certain differences from ANLL. Frequently observed changes include deletion of the long arm of chromosome 6 ($6q^-$) and gains of chromosomes 8, 21, and X (Oshimura and Sandberg, 1977; Rowley, 1978). The occasional occurrence of Ph^+ ALL and its poor prognosis have already been mentioned.

It is apparent that from a practical diagnostic standpoint, the absence of chromosome change in a suspected case of either ANLL or ALL does not rule out the disease, but the presence of karyotypic alteration in a hemic clone may help to establish the diagnosis. The particular chromosome abnormalities observed in these disorders, although nonrandom, do not appear to be of clear prognostic significance with respect to the course of the disease, except for the

Ph^+ cases already noted. Several studies do suggest that the proportion of chromosomally abnormal cells in the bone marrow at the time of diagnosis of acute leukemia may provide some indication of response to treatment. In both children and adults, those with a normal karyotype in the leukemic cells appear to survive longer than those having abnormal patterns; and in the latter case, the prognosis is better if some normal cells are still demonstrable in the marrow (Golomb et al., 1978; Benedict et al., 1979; Hossfeld et al., 1979). These conclusions are not yet fully substantiated, and the ultimate role of chromosome studies in decisions concerning patient management in acute leukemia remains to be determined.

2.3. Preleukemic Disorders: Myeloproliferative and Cytopenic

There are a number of poorly defined blood dyscrasias that are not generally considered neoplasms but that carry an increased risk for the subsequent development of ANLL. To better classify these disorders, they have been subdivided into two major groups: myeloproliferative disorders [including polycythemia vera, myelofibrosis, undifferentiated myeloproliferative disorders, and essential thrombocythemia (Lazlo, 1975)] and the so-called "preleukemic syndrome," which encompasses various unexplained anemias and cytopenias (Linman and Bagby, 1976). The myeloproliferative disorders carry perhaps a 10% risk of subsequent development of leukemia, and the preleukemic cytopenias have a much higher risk, perhaps 50–75%. Chromosome studies have been carried out on a number of these patients in an attempt to understand the relationship of these disorders to leukemia and to determine if such investigations might be of prognostic value.

In both the myeloproliferative and the cytopenic groups, clones of chromosomally abnormal cells have been found in the bone marrow of 20–40% of the patients studied. No completely specific alterations have been demonstrated for a particular dyscrasia, but various nonrandom abnormalities have been observed, often identical with those noted in the leukemias and other tumors (Fig. 3). In addition to the monosomy 7, trisomy 8, and iso-17q previously mentioned, these have included trisomy for the long arm of chromosome 1 and deletion of the long arm of chromosome 20 ($20q^-$), particularly in the myeloproliferative disorders, and deletion of a portion of the long arm of chromosome 5 ($5q^-$) in the cytopenias (Sokal et al., 1975; Whang-Peng et al., 1977; Nowell and Finan, 1978).

Progression of these dyscrasias to frank leukemia has, in some instances, been associated with either the initial appearance of a karyotypic change in the hemic clone or evidence of additional chromosome change, as previously described in the progression of CGL and some acute leukemias (Pierre, 1975). These similarities have led to the suggestion that the only fundamental difference between acute leukemia, chronic leukemia, and the so-called "preleukemic states" is the rate at which the abnormal hemic clone is expanding. In this view, progression from chronic to acute leukemia or from preleukemia to clinical

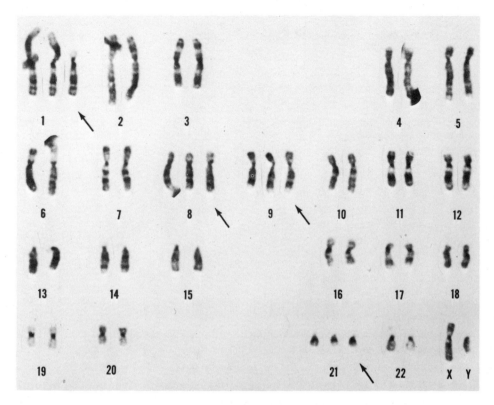

FIGURE 3. Representative karyotype of 50 chromosomes from an abnormal hemic clone of a patient with myelofibrosis (agnogenic myeloid metaplasia). Extra chromosomes include 8, 9, 21, and an abnormal No. 1 (1q⁻). All represent nonrandom changes reported in a number of neoplastic and preneoplastic disorders. From Nowell and Finan (1978) with permission.

leukemia results from an increased rate of clonal expansion, due often to additional genetic change in the clone that may be recognizable cytogenetically (Nowell, 1977).

Some effort has been made to determine to what degree the presence or absence of a marrow chromosome abnormality is of predictive value in "preleukemic" patients with respect to the subsequent development of frank leukemia. Our own investigation, which has extended over a number of years (Nowell and Finan, 1978), is summarized in Table 1. We have followed 140 patients with either myeloproliferative or cytopenic disorders for at least 1 year or until death. In each group, approximately 40% had a chromosomally abnormal hemic clone. It is evident from Table 1 that for the myeloproliferative disorders, this had little predictive value, but in the cytopenias, 77% with a cytogenetic abnormality developed leukemia versus 37% without. Of particular interest is the fact that 12 of 13 cytopenic patients with multiple karyotypic alterations, involving more than two chromosomes, died within 6 months, 9 with leukemia.

Other workers have reported generally similar findings to those summarized in Table 1 (Wurster-Hill *et al.*, 1976; Pierre, 1978*a*; Harousseau *et al.*, 1978;

TABLE 1

Relation of Chromosome Abnormalities to Subsequent Leukemia in 140 Patients with Preleukemic States

Diagnosis	Patients with chromosome abnormalities (leukemia/total)	Patients without chromosome abnormalities (leukemia/total)
Myeloproliferative disorders		
Polycythemia vera	2/8	3/12
Myelofibrosis	1/11	0/8
UMPD[a]	2/4	2/13
Thrombocythemia	0/1	0/6
Total	5/24 (21%)	5/39 (13%)
Cytopenic states		
Refractory anemia		
Sideroblastic	1/1	2/8
Other	4/6	2/4
Pancytopenia		
Sideroblastic	3/3	1/3
Other	16/21	12/31
Total	24/31 (77%)	17/46 (37%)

[a] UMPD, undifferentiated myeloproliferative disorders.

Heimpel *et al.*, 1979). The results suggest that cytogenetic data may be helpful in determining which cytopenic "preleukemic" patients are at particularly high risk for developing leukemia and so might be considered for aggressive therapy, although some will progress to leukemia without any visible karyotypic change.

Thus far, chromosome studies appear to have little predictive value in the myeloproliferative disorders, but the data do indicate that cytogenetically abnormal clones can exist in human tissues for years, in some circumstances, without functioning as clinical neoplasms.

This phenomenon of "nonneoplastic" clones with chromosome aberrations has also been observed following exposure to mutagenic agents (e.g., ionizing radiation) and in patients with evidence of constitutional chromosome fragility (to be discussed later), as well as in the hemic tissues and cultured skin fibroblasts of normal elderly individuals (Nowell, 1969; O'Riordan *et al.*, 1970; Harnden *et al.*, 1976). Usually, the karyotypic alterations in these nonneoplastic clones are relatively minor, involving balanced translocations or loss of a sex chromosome. Such observations demonstrate that somatic genetic change can occasionally produce a cell with sufficient selective growth advantage to generate a recognizable clone, but not with the degree of autonomy necessary for continued expansion and the production of a frank neoplasm.

2.4. Chronic Lymphocytic Leukemia and Solid Lymphomas

These lymphoproliferative disorders have been less extensively studied cytogenetically than the other hemic dyscrasias discussed above, primarily

because of technical difficulties in obtaining dividing neoplastic cells. However,
considerable banding data are currently emerging, particularly on the non-Hodgkin's lymphomas, and these will be considered after the more limited information on chronic lymphocytic leukemia (CLL).

2.4.1. CLL

In 90–95% of all cases, CLL is a B-cell disorder in which a clone of neoplastic B cells is widely dispersed throughout the lymphoid and hematopoietic tissues (Seligman *et al.*, 1976; Siegal and Good, 1977). There is usually not enough mitotic activity of the neoplastic cells in lymph nodes or marrow to provide adequate numbers of leukemic metaphases for chromosome study in biopsy material, and in mitogen-stimulated peripheral blood cultures, it is apparently the nonneoplastic T cells that proliferate, not the neoplastic B cells. Nearly all reports on the chromosomes of CLL have been based on such cultures, and so it is not surprising that the karyotypes have been reported as "normal" in most instances (Fitzgerald and Adams, 1975). There are now a very few reports, with banding, of aberrant chromosomes in B-cell CLL. These include cases with spontaneously proliferating blasts late in the disease, and also data on two CLL cell lines established in culture (Fleischman and Prigogina, 1977; Autio *et al.*, 1979; Hurley *et al.*, 1980). The findings are as yet too few to indicate any specific patterns of chromosome involvement.

There have recently been improvements in methods for polyclonal stimulation of normal human B lymphocytes *in vitro*, and these may ultimately prove useful with the cells of B-cell CLL. Until then, we must consider that the chromosome patterns in this disease are largely unknown rather than "normal."

That the karyotype in B-cell CLL might often be found to be aberrant if adequate material for study could be obtained is suggested by the limited data available on the chronic T-cell leukemias. These constitute a rare and heterogeneous group of chronic disorders, ranging from clinically typical CLL to variants of the Sezary syndrome and mycosis fungoides. As the circulating neoplastic T lymphocytes normally do respond, at least to some degree, to available mitogens, chromosome studies can utilize peripheral blood cultures.

We have investigated nine such patients by banding techniques, and in all instances a chromosomally abnormal clone was identified in the peripheral blood (Nowell *et al.*, 1980). No consistent cytogenetic change was present, but there were nonrandom alterations involving chromosomes 2, 14, and 18, as well as one instance of an iso-17q. In two individuals, there was a translocation to the long arm of chromosome 14, producing a 14q$^+$, with the breakpoint in the terminal portion (Fig. 4), an abnormality that has been observed in a number of other lymphoproliferative disorders (see Section 2.4.2). Sequential studies in several patients revealed clonal evolution of the cytogenetic abnormalities, associated with changes in various clinical or biological aspects of the disease, but there are not yet sufficient data in our work or that of others to indicate whether such evolution has the same grave prognostic significance as has been the case in CGL.

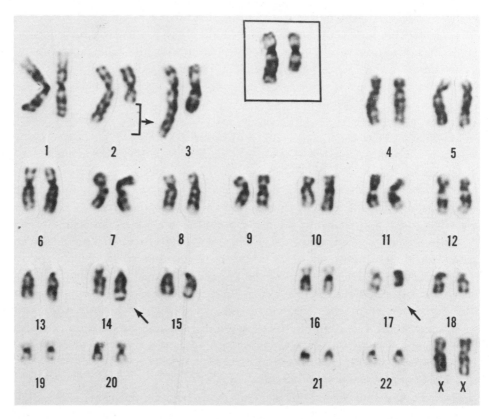

FIGURE 4. Representative karyotype from a neoplastic lymphocyte clone in a patient with T-cell chronic lymphocytic leukemia. Abnormalities include a translocation from the long arm of chromosome 2 to chromosome 3, t(2q;3); translocation from chromosome 18 to the long arm of chromosome 14, t(14;18q), producing a 14q$^+$; and an extra band in the long arm of chromosome 17. The insert illustrates normal and abnormal No. 3 chromosomes from another cell. The 14q$^+$ anomaly is present in many lymphoproliferative disorders. From Nowell *et al.* (1979) with permission.

2.4.2. Solid Lymphomas

Although it has been generally more difficult to obtain cytogenetic data on the solid lymphomas than on most of the leukemias, information is being acquired, both from direct lymph node preparations and from short-term cultures of cells from neoplastic nodes. These lesions are usually of B-cell origin, but T-cell lymphomas, often with skin involvement, also occur. Chromosome changes have been observed in nearly all cases where adequate material has been obtained, and the findings have generally indicated a clonal type of neoplastic growth. In some instances, the presence of an abnormal karyotype has been helpful in distinguishing a well-differentiated lymphoma from nonneoplastic reactive hyperplasia (Pierre, 1978b).

No specific chromosome aberration has been consistently correlated with a particular histologic pattern or clinical course in the lymphomas, although certain of the nonrandom alterations already mentioned have been reported (e.g., trisomy for 1q, 6q⁻, and abnormalities of No. 18) and particularly translocations producing a $14q^+$ chromosome (Lawler *et al.*, 1975; Mark, 1977; Fukuhara *et al.*, 1978; Edelson *et al.*, 1979). It appears that this latter rearrangement involving the terminal portion of the long arm of chromosome 14 includes a site that is particularly associated with abnormal proliferation of lymphocytes, both B cells and T cells. It has been observed in a variety of lymphoproliferative disorders, including solid lymphomas, multiple myeloma, and leukemia, as well as in nonneoplastic T-cell clones occurring in patients with ataxia telangiectasia (see Section 4.1) (McCaw *et al.*, 1975). A $14q^+$ chromosome has rarely been reported in nonlymphocytic tumors, and a 7;14 translocation noted occasionally in cultured normal T lymphocytes involves a different breakpoint on 14q (Kaiser-McCaw *et al.*, 1979).

In most lymphoid neoplasms, the chromosome segment translocated to chromosome 14 is from a variety of locations (e.g., chromosome 11, 18, etc.), but in the Burkitt tumor, the rearrangement characteristically involves translocation from the long arm of chromosome 8 to the long arm of chromosome 14 (Manolov and Manolova, 1971; Pierre, 1978*b*). This 8;14 translocation has been found in American Burkitt tumors, both Epstein–Barr virus positive and negative, as well as in the common African variety, and so its relationship to the putative causative agent of the disease remains unclear (Klein, 1979).

In Hodgkin's disease, cells with abnormal chromosome numbers in the triploid and tetraploid range have been observed, and these presumably represent Sternberg–Reed cells in division. On the other hand, metaphases with chromosome numbers in the diploid range obtained from nodes involved in this disease have usually had a normal karyotype, and these may well represent proliferating nonneoplastic cells involved in a host response rather than actual constituents of the tumor (Lawler *et al.*, 1975; Mark, 1977). There is some evidence that chromosome studies on nodes or effusions may occasionally be useful for detecting Hodgkin's disease which is not apparent histologically (Pierre, 1978*b*; Hossfeld and Schmidt, 1978).

3. Human Solid Tumors

Many of the generalizations concerning the leukemias and lymphomas also apply to nonhematopoietic human tumors. Because of the greater technical difficulties in preparing material for chromosome study, investigations have often been done on mitotically active far-advanced lesions, including cells from malignant effusions. Limited data have been obtained by direct and culture methods on earlier stages of malignancy, and on some benign and "premalignant" lesions of the cervix, bowel, breast, and other organs. With the development of improved techniques for obtaining dividing tumor cells, including culture on a "feeder layer" or in soft agar, as well as transplantation into "nude" mice, the earlier success rate (10–20%) resulting from cytogenetic study of human solid malignancies is being improved upon (Hamburger *et al.*, 1978). As with all methods other than direct preparations, however, the problem of nonrandom selection of the tumor cells still remains.

3.1. Malignant Tumors

Nearly all human malignant solid tumors studied to date have shown chromosome abnormalities; there are only a few cases reported in which the karyotype appeared normal (Sandberg and Hossfeld, 1970; Koller, 1972; Mark, 1977; Kakati and Sandberg, 1978; Van der Riet-Fox *et al.*, 1979). In many instances, particularly in the far-advanced tumors and malignant effusions, extensive alterations have been observed, with chromosome numbers varying widely and major structural rearrangements producing distinctive "marker" chromosomes. There has frequently been, in these cases, correlation between the extent of karyotypic change and the stage of progression of the tumor, the most advanced tumors showing the most extensive cytogenetic alterations.

As with the leukemias, a clonal type of growth is often indicated by a characteristic aberrant karyotype or the presence of a distinctive abnormal marker within all, or nearly all, cells of a particular tumor. In some instances, the same marker chromosome present in cells with different chromosome numbers has suggested the possible sequence of evolutionary events occurring during the development of the neoplasm (Spriggs, 1976; Mark, 1977). However, the cytogenetic evidence for a clonal pattern of growth in human solid malignancies has generally been much less clear than in the leukemias; and particularly in those solid tumors examined by direct preparative techniques, considerable variation in chromosome number and morphology within the same tumor has been common (Koller, 1972; Spriggs, 1976). More than in the leukemias, it appears that instability of the mitotic apparatus permits constant production of additionally aberrant cells within the proliferating population. Most of these presumably do not survive, but some provide the basis for continual selection of more and more deviant subclones superimposed on earlier ones.

Similar conclusions may be drawn from the few chromosome studies that have utilized metastatic tumors. The karyotype of the metastases has generally been similar to that of the primary neoplasm, but frequently with additional superimposed cytogenetic alterations, tending toward higher ploidy, and a greater range in chromosome numbers (Sandberg and Hossfeld, 1970; Kakati and Sandberg, 1978).

With this degree of variability, it is not surprising that specific cytogenetic alterations associated consistently with particular solid neoplasms have been difficult to demonstrate in man. However, as with the hematopoietic disorders, banding studies have indicated nonrandom patterns of chromosome change. For instance, abnormalities of chromosome 1, particularly extra copies of a portion of the long arm (either in the form of trisomy, duplication, or iso-1q), have been observed in a variety of solid malignancies, including carcinomas of the breast, lung, ovary, bladder, and also melanomas (Cruciger *et al.*, 1977; Atkin and Pickthall, 1977; Atkin and Baker, 1978; Kakati and Sandberg, 1978). Other nonrandom alterations, such as trisomies 8 and 9, have also been reported in various solid malignancies, but, as noted above, these generally have not been associated with particular tumor types (Mitelman and Levan, 1978); nor does there seem to be a characteristic association between a specific chromosome change and a particular etiologic agent, as has been suggested for some animal tumors (see Section 6).

Meningiomas represent an exception to these generalizations. Several workers (Zankl and Zang, 1972; Mark, 1977) have demonstrated that a high proportion of these tumors, including some that are clinically benign, show a common cytogenetic alteration, loss of all or part of chromosome 22. When the loss is partial, it is from the long arm ($22q^-$), but unlike the Ph chromosome in CGL, there is no evidence of translocation to another site. It has also been observed that biological and clinical progression of meningiomas to a more malignant stage may be associated with karyotypic evolution of a nonrandom nature, with chromosomes 1, 8, 9, and 15 particularly involved. Interestingly, unlike most other tumors, this evolution has frequently involved loss of chromosome material, resulting in increasingly hypodiploid cell populations. The findings with meningiomas represent both the most consistent cytogenetic alteration and also the best documented chromosome evolution among nonhematopoietic human neoplasms.

Considerable attention has recently been directed to another relatively rare human tumor, neuroblastoma, because of its association with two unusual types of chromosome abnormalities. In the prebanding era, large marker chromosomes were reported in neuroblastoma material, as well as the occasional appearance of multiple, small, doubled fragments, which were termed "double minutes" (DMs) (Sandberg et al., 1972). With the advent of banding methods, particularly banding with Giemsa stain, it was discovered that some of the large neuroblastoma marker chromosomes, as well as similar large markers in several tissue culture lines derived from experimental tumors in animals, contained elongated chromosome segments that were uniformly weakly stained throughout and did not show any banding pattern. These segments were termed "homogeneous staining regions" (HSRs) (Biedler and Spengler, 1976). These workers determined that in certain Chinese hamster cell lines, the presence of an HSR in the karyotype was associated with resistance to antifolates (e.g., methotrexate), apparently as a result of increased levels of the enzyme dihydrofolate reductase. They concluded that the HSR might represent visible evidence of gene amplification, with multiple copies of the gene for dihydrofolate reductase accounting for the increased levels of the enzyme and the consequent selective advantage of the affected cells. Several laboratories have subsequently provided evidence in support of this hypothesis (Dolnick et al., 1979).

HSRs have now been observed in a number of other human and animal tumors, and Miller et al. (1979) have described what they call "differentially stained regions" (DSRs) in a rat hepatoma cell line, apparently representing multiple copies of ribosomal RNA genes. Balaban–Malenbaum and Gilbert (1978) demonstrated, in cultured human neuroblastoma material, the presence of both

HSRs and DMs in the same cell line, but not in the same cell, suggesting that DMs may result from dissociation of HSRs and represent another form of the amplified genetic material.

These exciting observations are currently being explored in a variety of human and experimental systems. It is too early to speculate as to how important this type of alteration, gene amplification, may be in the development of neoplasia, as compared to other types of change in genetic structure and function, including those visible cytogenetically, which may also confer selective advantage on a tumor cell population.

Finally, in this section on human solid malignancies, mention should be made of the few rare circumstances in which individuals with a specific *constitutional* chromosome abnormality are at high risk for a particular malignant neoplasm, with or without other congenital anomalies. Perhaps best documented in this category is the syndrome in children born with a deletion of a portion of the long arm of chromosome 13, characterized by mental retardation, various physical defects, and a 25% incidence of retinoblastoma (Knudson *et al.*, 1976). High-resolution banding studies (Yunis and Ramsey, 1978) of cells from these patients, as well as unbanded data on retinoblastoma cells from otherwise normal individuals, have provided strong evidence of a particular location in 13q (band q14) as being the site of a gene associated with the development of this neoplasm.

A similar phenomenon has been observed in several cases of Wilms' tumor associated with aniridia, where a constitutional deletion in one band of the short arm of chromosome 11 has been demonstrated, pointing to this locus as being important in the etiology of the tumor (Riccardi *et al.*, 1978). Most recently, three generations of a family have been described in which a very high incidence of renal carcinoma, approaching 90%, was limited to those family members with a constitutional balanced translocation involving chromosomes 3 and 8 (Cohen *et al.*, 1979). In this instance, it is not yet clear which of the two chromosomes carries the critical gene locus. These results indicate that constitutional cytogenetic abnormalities, in individuals or families, may occasionally help to indicate the location of genes specific for particular human solid malignancies, but it appears that, at least with present techniques, such associations will be rare; in no other familial tumor studied to date has a related constitutional karyotypic alteration been demonstrable.

3.2. Benign and Precancerous Lesions

As with malignant tumors, chromosome studies of human benign and premalignant lesions have generally revealed a rough correlation between the degree of histological abnormality and the extent of cytogenetic change. Data are relatively sparse, in part because of the scarcity of mitoses available for study in small early lesions and in slow-growing benign tumors, but some results have been obtained from lesions of the colon, cervix, breast, bladder, placenta, and ovary (Auersperg *et al.*, 1967; Enterline and Arvan, 1967; Koller, 1972; Falor and Ward, 1978; Kakati and Sandberg, 1978; Szulman and Surti, 1978). The bowel polyps diagnosed as benign or hyperplastic by the pathologist generally have a normal karyotype or show less alteration than those considered malignant or premalignant. Similarly, dysplasias of the cervix are less abnormal cytogenetically than carcinoma *in situ.* Comparable results have been obtained at the other sites mentioned, but it is also clear that the relationships among the pattern of cytogenetic change, the degree of histological alteration, and subsequent malignant behavior do vary from one organ to another.

Even in very early lesions, marker chromosomes often indicate a clonal type of neoplastic growth, and in a few instances, such as the involvement of chromosomes 8 and 14 in polyps of the colon, nonrandom associations are beginning to emerge (Mitelman *et al.*, 1974). However, in some studies, the few mitoses obtained from small early lesions of various organs have contained a mixture of abnormal and diploid metaphases without a clear clonal pattern and with the possibility that some of the dividing cells represented nonneoplastic elements. These difficulties indicate that laborious collection of additional data will be needed before it can be decided whether the demonstration of aneuploidy or of a particular chromosome alteration in a given human premalignant lesion is of practical value in predicting its subsequent course.

4. Chromosome Breakage and Cancer

Thus far, the discussion has been limited almost exclusively to the karyotypic abnormalities observed in the cells of tumors. However, the relationship between cytogenetic change and neoplasia is also indicated by various circumstances in which there are chromosome breaks and rearrangements in nonneoplastic cells of individuals who also show an increased incidence of cancer. Often this cytogenetic damage is attributable to the action of exogenous agents (e.g., ionizing radiation, "radiomimetic" and other chemicals, infectious viruses), but there are also a number of relatively rare congenital disorders that confer on affected individuals an increased propensity for spontaneous chromosome breakage. Various aspects of these so-called "chromosome breakage syndromes", as well as the effects of exogenous agents, are discussed in more detail elsewhere in this volume, and so they will be considered only briefly here.

4.1. Genetic Disorders

Among genetically determined syndromes in man associated with chromosome instability and increased tumor incidence, four have been most extensively studied: Bloom's syndrome, Faconi's anemia, ataxia telangiectasia, and xeroderma pigmentosum (German, 1977; Hecht and McCaw, 1977; Setlow, 1978). Each of these disorders appears to be determined by a single recessive gene. In the first three instances, chromosome instability has been demonstrated in peripheral blood lymphocyte cultures, where metaphases show various kinds

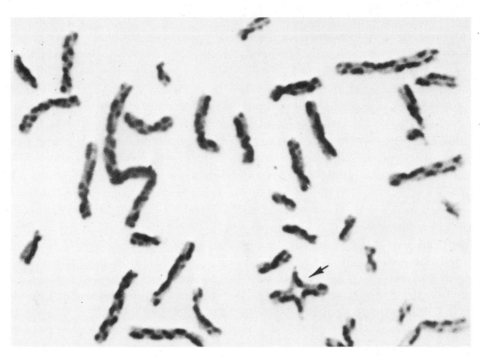

FIGURE 5. Chromosomes of a lymphocyte from a patient with Bloom's syndrome cultured and stained to demonstrate sister chromatid exchanges. These are the alternating light and dark areas in nearly every chromosome; a normal individual would have fewer than 10 sister chromatid exchanges per cell. The arrow indicates a quadriradial configuration resulting from chromatid exchange between two chromosomes, a characteristic finding in Bloom's syndrome. Courtesy of Dr. J. German.

of spontaneous chromatid and chromosome aberrations, including gaps, breaks, and multiradial products of complex exchanges (Fig. 5). The frequency and types of alterations in lymphocyte cultures differ in the different syndromes; for instance, the multiradial lesions occur almost exclusively in Bloom's syndrome (German *et al.*, 1979).

Recently, a new measure of chromosome instability has become feasible through improved techniques for demonstrating the frequency per cell of exchanges of homologous chromatid segments within a chromosome (Latt, 1974). This phenomenon of sister chromatid exchange (SCE) occurs normally in low frequency, and is increased by many mutagenic agents. The spontaneous frequency is unusually high in lymphocyte cultures from patients with Bloom's syndrome, but this is not the case in Fanconi's anemia, ataxia telangiectasia, or xeroderma pigmentosum (Chaganti *et al.*, 1974) (Fig. 5).

Chromosome fragility in all of these syndromes can be accentuated by subjecting cell cultures to agents known to be mutagenic or carcinogenic, such as ultraviolet radiation, X rays, and both chemotherapeutic and carcinogenic chemicals. Again, the individual disorders respond differently to different clastogenic agents, with respect to both chromosome breakage and SCE, presumably reflecting differences in the underlying gene defect (Higurashi and Conen, 1973; Auerbach and Wolman, 1976).

It is assumed that the aberrant cytogenetic findings in these various syndromes reflect a defect in DNA repair (Setlow, 1978), or in some other aspect of DNA "housekeeping," but this has not yet been clearly demonstrated in all of the disorders. Best documented are the abnormalities in xeroderma pigmentosum cells, primarily involving deficient excision repair of ultraviolet-induced damage (Cleaver and Bootsma, 1975). Less firm evidence indicates defective excision repair, in ataxia telangiectasia, of lesions produced by ionizing radiation and certain chemicals; and, in Fanconi's anemia, of DNA damage involving cross-linkage (Paterson et al., 1976; Remsen and Cerutti, 1976; Poon et al., 1974). Work is currently under way in a number of laboratories to define further the specific molecular mechanisms underlying the chromosome instability demonstrable in vitro in all these syndromes.

These patients also give evidence of chromosome instability in vivo. Clones of chromosomally abnormal cells have been demonstrated in hematopoietic tissues and occasionally in skin fibroblasts (German, 1977; Hecht and McCaw, 1977). Perhaps most interesting are reports of families with ataxia telangiectasia in whom nonneoplastic lymphocyte clones with a $14q^+$ marker have been observed in the blood for several years before eventual progression, in some instances, to T-cell leukemia (McCaw et al., 1975; Levitt et al., 1978; Saxon et al., 1979). The involved segment of 14q is the same as that described for the Burkitt tumor and other lymphoid neoplasms (Section 2.4.2). Several of these ataxia telangiectasia cases showed clonal evolution in the karyotype associated with clinical progression; and in other cases, they demonstrated that, in ataxia telangiectasia at least, a rearrangement of 14q may confer sufficient growth advantage to generate a demonstrable T-cell clone without necessarily leading to frank neoplasia.

In general, individuals with these syndromes show an increased incidence of cancer, and this too has been assumed to reflect, in some way, the inherited defect in nucleic acid metabolism. The repair deficiency in xeroderma pigmentosum, for instance, apparently leads to persistent chromosome aberrations, cytogenetically abnormal clones in the skin cell population, and multiple skin cancers (German, 1977; Hecht and McCaw, 1977). In the other three syndromes, the increased incidence of neoplasia most frequently involves the hematopoietic system.

It is possible that factors other than direct chromosome damage contribute to this high frequency of tumors. Each of these disorders is characterized by a somewhat different cluster of clinical abnormalities, but each involves some degree of immunological deficiency, and this could be significant in allowing aberrant clones to emerge as frank neoplasms. Also, it has been shown that in Fanconi's anemia and perhaps in several other of these syndromes, the patient's cells show increased susceptibility to neoplastic "transformation" by an oncogenic virus, SV40, in tissue culture (Todaro et al., 1966; Webb and Harding, 1977).

A few studies have investigated the relatives of patients with the chromosome breakage syndromes to determine if either increased chromosome fragility or increased cancer incidence could be demonstrated in individuals presumed to be heterozygous for the causative gene defect. Most attempts to show increased chromosome damage or SCE *in vitro*, either spontaneously or following exposure to clastogens, have been negative or inconclusive, but there is a report of increased spontaneous chromosome breakage in fibroblast cultures from relatives of ataxia telangiectasia patients (Cohen *et al.*, 1975). Swift and his colleagues (1976) have shown an increased frequency of cancer in blood relatives of both ataxia telangiectasia and Fanconi's anemia patients, but such an association has not been demonstrated for xeroderma pigmentosum.

In addition to these four well-defined disorders, there is limited evidence suggesting that there are other human conditions in which some aspect of DNA replication or repair may be defective and associated with increased cancer incidence. This is perhaps best documented in individuals with constitutional chromosome disorders, particularly Down's syndrome (trisomy 21). Although these patients do not show increased spontaneous chromosome breakage or SCE in standard lymphocyte cultures, they do show increased breakage after exposure to ionizing radiation. The results available to date indicate that virtually any constitutional chromosome abnormality is associated with such increased sensitivity to radiation damage (Seabright, 1976). There are also data demonstrating that individuals with Down's syndrome as well as other constitutional chromosome disorders have an increased probability of developing cancer as compared to appropriate controls (Knudson *et al.*, 1973). Finally, there is a recent report of a family with 12 cases of cancer and 2 cases of leukemia in which slightly increased chromosome fragility was demonstrable in standard leukocyte cultures (Cervenka *et al.*, 1977).

Taken together, these various observations support the concept of a significant relationship between chromosome abnormality *in vivo*, chromosome instability *in vitro*, and neoplasia; and the molecular basis for this association is currently the subject of active investigation in various population groups. In this regard, it may prove necessary to differentiate between these conditions of general chromosome instability, just discussed, and the phenomenon of fragility involving a single chromosome. Recurrent breakage at a specific site on chromosome 2, 10, 11, 16, 20, or X has been reported as a heritable trait in certain families, associated in the latter case with X-linked mental retardation, but to date there has been no related increase in tumor incidence (Sutherland, 1979).

4.2. Exogenous Agents: Radiation, Chemicals, Viruses

In addition to constitutional disorders, there is considerable evidence for a relationship between cytogenetic lesions and neoplasia in studies of the carcinogenic effects of a variety of chromosome-damaging agents, both in man and in experimental animals. Most investigations have been qualitative in nature, largely restricted to the enumeration of those agents that produce damage and the types of aberrations produced (e.g., chromatid vs. chromosome lesions, SCE); but some effort is being made, through both epidemiology and laboratory studies, to obtain quantitative data on the cytogenetic effects produced by exposure to various agents and the relationship to subsequent tumor development.

Ionizing radiation has long been known to produce chromosome breakage (Fig. 6), and it is possible, by enumerating chromosome lesions and/or SCE in cultured lymphocytes from the peripheral blood, to make rough estimates of the radiation dose in some exposed humans (Syed, 1978; Chaudhuri, 1978). Ionizing radiation is also a potent carcinogen, and it has been suggested that tumor induction may often be mediated through direct damage to the genome, as indicated by visible chromosome lesions, although indirect mechanisms, such as viral activation or alteration in hormone levels, may also be important (Cole and Nowell, 1965). There have been few attempts to establish precise quantitative relationships among a given radiation exposure, the resultant chromosome aberration, and the number and kinds of tumors that subsequently occur.

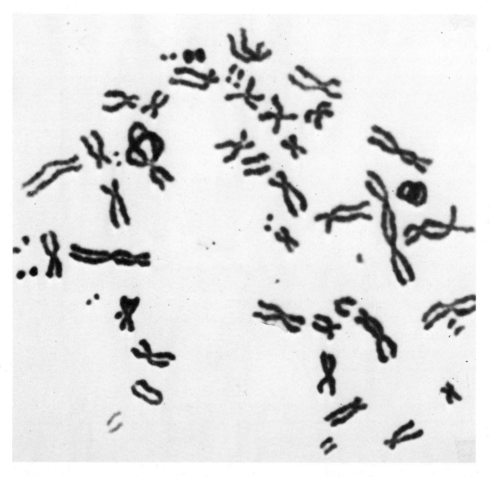

FIGURE 6. Metaphase from a peripheral blood lymphocyte of a monkey exposed to whole-body X-irradiation. Note the radiation-induced chromosome damage: large and small acentric fragments, dicentics, and rings. From Weber and Nowell (1965) with permission.

Interestingly, in one preliminary study in mice (Nowell and Cole, 1965), comparing the effects on the liver of high and low doses of radiation, chromosome aberration was higher and the subsequent incidence of hepatomas lower after exposure to high-dose radiation than after exposure to low-dose radiation. It was postulated that a cell-killing effect of the high-dose radiation, associated with visible chromosome aberrations, may have removed potentially neoplastic cells from the surviving population. Until there is a somewhat better understanding of the specific mechanisms of carcinogenesis in various circumstances, it will remain difficult to relate directly the number or type of radiation-induced chromosome abnormalities observed in a given mammalian system to the incidence or kind of neoplasms that may subsequently appear.

Similar statements can be made concerning those chemicals known to produce mammalian chromosome damage and their potential carcinogenicity. A variety of drugs and chemicals are capable of producing chromosome lesions and/or increased SCE in human and other mammalian cells, both *in vivo* and *in vitro*, with nonrandom distribution of breakpoints in some instances (Shaw, 1970; Schmid, 1977; Roberts, 1978; Meyne *et al.*, 1979). Few of these agents, however, have been clearly shown to be carcinogenic in man, and thus it is difficult to demonstrate a direct relationship (Mitelman *et al.*, 1978). Benzene is perhaps best documented in this regard; it is one of the few chemicals known to produce human tumors (leukemia) as well as chromosome aberrations *in vivo* (Forni and Moreo, 1967; Aksoy, 1977).

Recently, a number of drugs used in cancer chemotherapy, and particularly alkylating agents, have been shown to break chromosomes and to increase SCE in human cells (Schmid, 1977; Nevstad, 1978; Lambert *et al.*, 1978). A small percentage of patients treated with these agents develop acute leukemia several years later, presumably from the mutagenic effects of the drug (Dahlke and Nowell, 1975; Sieber and Adamson, 1975; Harris, 1979; Foucar *et al.*, 1979). The leukemic cells typically show multiple cytogenetic abnormalities. Studies are under way, both *in vivo* and *in vitro*, to determine if individuals who develop such leukemias are unusually susceptible to chromosome damage by these agents.

Similarly, testing programs now being widely utilized to explore the mutagenic or carcinogenic effects of new drugs or compounds to which the general human population will be exposed often include their ability to produce cytogenetic lesions in experimental animals or in tissue culture cell lines (Schmid, 1977). This may provide additional examples of chemical agents in which carcinogenicity and gross genetic damage are related.

Both RNA and DNA viruses can also break chromosomes in mammalian cells. This was first observed with nononcogenic viruses, but has subsequently been demonstrated, both *in vivo* and *in vitro*, with a wide spectrum of oncogenic agents as well (Nichols, 1966; Harnden, 1974). At the present time, no general statement is possible concerning differences between the cytogenetic effects of carcinogenic and noncarcinogenic viruses, but it is of interest that the Schmidt–Ruppin strain of the Rous virus causes chromatid abnormalities in human leukocyte cultures and tumors in experimental animals, while the Bryan strain of the same virus, under similar circumstances, produces neither chromosome changes nor neoplasms (Nichols *et al.*, 1964). Such correlations have not been universal (Harnden, 1974), but they do indicate the need for additional investigation of the possible significance, both for mutagenesis and for carcinogenesis, of virus-induced chromosome abnormalities in mammalian cells.

There is also considerable evidence that some oncogenic viruses can produce malignant tumors that show no demonstrable chromosome change (Mark, 1969; Mitelman, 1971; Harnden, 1974). Here, the oncogenic event presumably does not require actual chromosome breakage, although it may involve other types of direct or indirect interaction of the virus with the host cell genome.

It may be of significance that most of the cytogenetic damage caused by viruses, as well as by the majority of chemical mutagens, involves the *chromatid*, in contrast to the *chromosome* lesions produced by ionizing radiation (Figs. 5 and 6). This indicates that viruses and chemicals usually produce lesions only in the G_2 (postsynthetic) phase of the cell cycle rather than the G_1 (presynthetic) phase or in a noncycling stage (G_0). It is also consistent with the observation that ionizing radiation can produce genetic alterations in a mitotically inactive cell population (G_0) such as the liver, kidney, or circulating lymphocytes, with these alterations expressed as chromosome lesions whenever the cells subsequently proliferate. Although such "resting" cells may repair chromosome damage to varying degrees during the period prior to cell division, these differences between the action of ionizing radiation and most viruses and chemicals must be considered in assessing their carcinogenic potential (Nowell, 1969).

With respect to the involvement of specific chromosome sites by these various exogenous agents, banding studies are now providing considerable information both in man and in various experimental systems. With the exception of certain animal tumors, there is little indication that the nonrandom cytogenetic changes in neoplasia reflect the particular chemical or radiation inducing the tumor (Rowley, 1974; DiPaolo and Popescu, 1976). With viruses, however, there is greater evidence, both *in vivo* and *in vitro*, for the propensity of the causative agent to involve specific chromosome locations. For instance, it appears that successful neoplastic transformation of human cells in tissue culture by the SV40 virus requires incorporation of viral DNA at particular chromosome sites, although these may differ from one cell line to another (Croce, 1977).

Although the exact mechanism of carcinogenesis by any of these agents remains unsolved, there appears generally to be a clear correlation between the capacity to produce chromosome aberrations and the capacity to induce neoplasia. In order to obtain meaningful estimates of the risks of tumor production following exposure to these exogenous agents, either in individuals or in populations, additional quantitative information is needed. Some will be cytogenetic data, but this must be supplemented by the use of more precise methods of assessing the effects of point mutations and other interactions with the genome that are not visible at the chromosome level. For such studies, cells in tissue culture provide a valuable adjunct to cytogenetic investigations in human populations and experimental animals, and this approach is considered in more detail in the following section.

5. *Cytogenetics of Cells in Culture*

Tissue culture cell lines are being used increasingly both to assess the cytogenetic effects of the agents discussed above and their relation to neoplasia, and to discover the location of specific genes involved in carcinogenesis.

In the first instance, the major approach has been through investigations of cellular transformation *in vitro* by oncogenic viruses and by chemical agents. The results generally support the conclusions from *in vivo* studies that chromosome changes are common, but not essential, in tumorigenesis. Viral or chemical transformation of mammalian cells in tissue culture to a malignant state, as indicated by their capacity to form tumors when transplanted into suitable animal hosts, is usually associated with major cytogenetic abnormalities, but not always. Conversely, some aneuploid tissue culture lines do not form tumors in animals; and changes in the neoplastic behavior of cultured cells, both *in vitro* and *in vivo*, are not always accompanied by new karyotypic alterations (Moorhead and Weinstein, 1966; MacPherson, 1970; Bloch-Shtacher and Sachs, 1977; Zuna and Lehman, 1977; Barski, 1978). In any of these studies it is important to distinguish between "transformed" cells defined only in terms of *in vitro* characteristics, and those shown to be malignant *in vivo* (Freeman and Huebner, 1973).

With respect to the role of specific genes in the initiation and maintenance of malignant characteristics in mammalian cells, and their chromosome location, cell hybridization techniques in tissue culture are providing important information. Several experiments have suggested that "malignancy" acts as a recessive trait, with hybrids of malignant and nonmalignant cell lines losing their tumorigenic properties (Harris *et al.*, 1969; Sidebottom, 1976; Stanbridge, 1976). With other cell lines, however, the malignant trait has appeared to be dominant in hybridization experiments (Croce *et al.*, 1979). In a few instances, in rodent cells, control of malignancy has apparently been associated specifically with a particular chromosome (Azumi and Sachs, 1977; Bloch-Shtacher and Sachs, 1977; Jonasson *et al.*, 1977), but in general, it has not yet been possible to identify consistently the acquisition or maintenance of neoplastic characteristics with a particular chromosome site in either the human complement or the complement of other mammalian species (DiPaolo and Popescu, 1976). Further studies utilizing hybridization methods may ultimately permit definite identification and chromosome mapping of one or more gene loci that, when present in the cell, either repress its unlimited growth potential and hence prevent expression of a neoplastic character, or, conversely, produce a gene product that in some way allows the cell to escape from normal growth regulation.

In this regard, as banding techniques have recently permitted recognition of a number of nonrandom chromosome alterations in human tumors, it has been of interest to attempt to correlate these findings with the expanding map of the

human genome being developed through hybridization methods (Ruddle, 1977).
The frequent involvement of the long arm of chromosome 17 in human neoplasms, for instance, has led to the suggestion that the gene for thymidine kinase,
known to be located on 17q (Miller *et al.*, 1971), might be of critical importance
in tumor development through its role in the regulation of DNA synthesis
(Harnden, 1977). Other genes involved in the control of nucleic acid biosynthesis
have been mapped to chromosome sites that are nonrandomly involved in human
tumors (Harnden, 1977; Rowley, 1977). However, 17q is also the location for
the galactokinase gene, perhaps importantly involved in the synthesis of external
membrane receptors important in growth regulation, as well as being a preferential site for incorporation of the oncogenic DNA viruses, adenovirus 12 and
SV40 (Elsevier *et al.*, 1974; Croce, 1977). Without knowing the precise nature
of the genetic alteration and the gene product of critical importance in any
neoplastic "transformation," it is clear that even with banding techniques, the
problem of correlating specific chromosome aberrations with carcinogenic mutations remains formidable. It is also apparent from these *in vitro* studies, as well
as from the *in vivo* data discussed earlier, that significant genetic changes
associated with malignant transformation need not always be visible at the
chromosome level.

6. Animal Tumors

Chromosome studies of tumors in experimental animals have, in some instances,
provided the opportunity to investigate in detail the relationship between
cytogenetic change and various stages of neoplastic development. The results
have generally paralleled the findings in man, but it has been possible with
animal systems to study much more closely the early steps in neoplastic transformation, as well as later stage of tumor progression.

Only in animals can one investigate chromosome patterns in neoplasms
definitely known to be caused by oncogenic viruses. As noted above, it seems
clear that a significant number of virus-induced tumors have no demonstrable
cytogenetic alterations in their early stages. This has been particularly true of
those neoplasms induced by RNA viruses, such as the Rous sarcoma and the
murine leukemias of Moloney, Friend, and Rauscher; but a few studies on tumors
induced by DNA viruses (SV40, polyoma, Shope rabbit papilloma virus) have
also demonstrated a diploid chromosome constitution in a proportion of early
lesions (Mark, 1969; Koller, 1972; Levan and Mitelman, 1976). Several of these
workers have considered the problem of distinguishing between neoplastic and
nonneoplastic diploid metaphases.

When it has been possible to follow such experimental viral tumors over time,
it has been common to find chromosome alterations in the later stages of
neoplastic progression (McMichael *et al.*, 1964; Mark, 1969; Levan and Mitelman,
1976), but it is clear that developing virus-induced tumors have generally had
less karyotypic abnormality than similar tumors induced by radiation or by

chemicals. As discussed earlier, this difference suggests that some mechanisms of viral oncogenesis do not involve visible damage to the host cell genome, and that actual chromosome breakage may be more important in the initiation of neoplasms by ionizing radiation and carcinogenic chemicals.

As with human tumors, it has been rare to find in animal systems a characteristic chromosome abnormality consistently associated with a particular type of primary neoplasm. However, in the prebanding era, several examples of nonrandom abnormalities were observed in both rat and mouse leukemias as well as in certain rat thyroid carcinomas (Wald *et al.*, 1964; Sugiyama *et al.*, 1967; Al-Saadi and Beierwaltes, 1967), and such findings have been confirmed and extended with banding techniques. A number of recent studies of various rumors and related cell lines in different species have demonstrated nonrandom involvement of specific chromosomes, including excess of chromosome 4 in ethylnitrosourea-induced neurogenic tumors of the rat, deletion of chromosome 15 in mouse plasmacytomas, and excess of chromosome 3 in neoplasms derived from SV40-transformed hamster cells (Au *et al.*, 1977; Bloch-Shtacher and Sachs, 1977; Yoshida *et al.*, 1978).

In some instances, the findings in animals have suggested that a particular nonrandom cytogenetic alteration is associated with a particular etiologic agent rather than with a specific neoplasm. Thus, banding studies of rat sarcomas induced by Rous virus have frequently demonstrated trisomy for chromosome 7, while similar sarcomas caused by 7,12-dimethylbenz[α]anthracene often show trisomy for chromosome 2. Rat leukemias and epithelial tumors induced by 7,12-dimethylbenz[α]anthracene have also been trisomic for chromosome 2 (Levan and Mitelman, 1977). This association of cytogenetic change and causative agent has not been demonstrated for human neoplasms, and it is clearly not true for all animal tumors (DiPaolo and Popescu, 1976; Kovi and Morris, 1976). One of the most consistently observed abnormalities, trisomy 15 in murine T-cell lymphomas, appears to be present whether the tumor is induced by virus, X-rays, or chemicals (Chan, 1978). It could be argued that these mouse lymphomas are, in fact, all caused by the same agent, through activation of a latent C-type virus, but recent studies suggest that this is unlikely (Klein, 1979). In any event, it appears that, as in human neoplasms, the nonrandom cytogenetic changes being observed in animal tumors do point to specific sites in the genome where one or more genes important in the development of neoplasia are located.

6.1. Clonal Evolution in Animal Tumors

Cytogenetic studies in animal systems have permitted not only the investigation of early stages of neoplastic growth, but have also provided some of the strongest evidence in support of the concept of clonal evolution in tumor progression. With most human malignancies, there have been only single "snapshots" of what has been interpreted as an evolutionary process of neoplastic development; but with animal tumors, it has been possible to obtain sequential biopsies of individual neoplasms or to study serial generations of a transplantable tumor line, and thus follow in detail the progression of a particular malignant cell population.

As noted earlier, in a number of primary sarcomas induced in mice and rats by the Rous virus, the karyotype was initially normal (Mark, 1969; Levan and Mitelman, 1976). Serial biopsies of individual tumors as they gradually acquired more malignant properties revealed the sequential appearance of predominant cell clones identified by abnormalities in chromosome number and morphology, overgrowing and replacing the original diploid tumor population. In the studies of Rous sarcomas in rats, involving both primary lesions and transplantable tumors derived from them, banding data have indicated a relatively consistent pattern of stepwise karyotypic change, with first the addition of chromosome 7, then 13, and then 12 (Mitelman, 1971; Levan and Mitelman, 1976). These further cytogenetic alterations apparently provided additional selective growth advantages over the earlier tumor cells, both diploid and aneuploid.

There have been similar observations with other induced primary tumors in animals, although, as has already been noted with some human tumors, results have differed from one study to another in terms of both the variation around the modal chromosome number in a particular tumor and the stability of the basic cytogenetic alteration with time (Koller, 1972).

Studies with transplantable tumors have shed additional light on the concept of clonal evolution within neoplastic cell populations. In general, transplanted solid tumors have been aneuploid, with a single stem line predominating in a particular transplant generation (Hsu, 1961; Al-Saadi and Beierwaltes, 1967; Yosida, 1974; Levan and Mitelman, 1976). Frequently, particularly in early passages, it has been possible to demonstrate the appearance over several generations of progressively more abnormal predominant clones, with cytogenetic changes in addition to those first seen. In some cases, very stable chromosome patterns have emerged after a number of passages and subsequently persisted for years; in other tumor lines, variants have continued to appear.

These phenomena have been well illustrated in cytogenetic studies of the Morris hepatomas, a series of transplantable rat liver tumors induced by chemical agents and generally selected for their high degree of differentiation and slow growth. In a few of these neoplasms, the cells were diploid when first studied, and the development of predominant aneuploid clones was not observed until later generations. Most of the tumors were already aneuploid when first investigated, and a number subsequently showed additional chromosome changes, often accompanied by an increase in growth rate and other indications of greater malignancy. Banding studies have suggested nonrandom involvement of chromosome 2 (Nowell et al., 1967; Nowell and Morris, 1969; Kovi and Morris, 1976). The fact that there has been a conscious effort with many of these hepatomas to retard progression by selection for the slowest-growing neoplasms in each generation probably accounts for the relatively high degree of both phenotypic and karyotypic stability in the Morris tumors.

An unusual example of cytogenetic evidence for clonal growth in an animal solid tumor deserves special mention. Canine venereal sarcoma is a malignancy of dogs that occurs with a worldwide distribution. Chromosome studies of this sarcoma from widely separated geographical locations in the United States, Japan, and elsewhere have consistently revealed highly aneuploid but very similar karyotypes (Makino, 1963; Weber *et al.*, 1965; Cohen, 1978). The chromosome number has usually been 59, as compared to the normal 78, with a relatively consistent pattern of rearrangements conserving a near-normal DNA content. It seems highly unlikely that such a constant, very abnormal chromosome pattern would evolve in unrelated primary tumors, and so the findings strongly suggest that the tumors seen in different countries are not separate primary neoplasms. Rather, they appear to be subpopulations of a single malignant clone, with cells that are spontaneously transplanted during venereal contact, and which by this means have spread throughout the world, maintaining a highly aberrant but very stable karyotype over a long period of time.

The chromosome banding studies that are continuing on a variety of primary and transplantable tumors of animals are providing additional evidence of both nonrandom alterations and karyotypic evolution that supplements significantly the findings in man.

7. Conclusions and Speculations

The data summarized in the preceding sections indicate that most mammalian neoplasms have demonstrable cytogenetic abnormalities and that many carcinogenic agents and precancerous conditions are associated with chromosome damage. In attempting to assess the significance of these observations, one may first consider karyotypic alteration in relation to the initiation of neoplasia and next its role in tumor progression.

7.1. Chromosome Changes and Tumor Initiation

Although alterations are present in most tumors, the fact that some mammalian malignancies show no visible cytogenetic abnormalities indicates that chromosome change is not essential for the neoplastic state. This does not rule out the possibility that neoplasia may always involve genetic alteration at some level, but the absence of demonstrable chromosome aberrations in some leukemias and early solid tumors demonstrates that if genetic lesions are present in all neoplasms, they are sometimes submicroscopic. The late appearance of chromosome abnormalities in some animal tumors studied sequentially that were originally diploid further supports the view that many of the cytogenetic alterations seen in fully developed cancers were not present at the outset.

It has also been difficult, until recently, to associate alterations at specific chromosome sites with the initiation of neoplasia, either *in vivo* or *in vitro*, or, for that matter, with any of the metabolic abnormalities observed in neoplastic or transformed cells. There are still only a few circumstances, such as the

TABLE 2

Human Chromosomes Preferentially Engaged in 15 Tumor Types[a]

Tumor type	Chromosomes
Myeloproliferative disorders	
Acute myeloid leukemia	5, 7, 8, 21
Chronic myeloid leukemia	8, 9, 17, 22
Polycythemia vera	1, 8, 9, 20
Various myeloproliferative disorders	1, 5, 7, 8
Lymphoproliferative disorders	
Malignant lymphomas (non-Burkitt)	1, 3, 9, 14
Burkitt's lymphoma	7, 8, 14
Acute lymphocytic leukemia	1, 21, 22
Chronic lymphocytic leukemia	1, 14, 17
Monoclonal gammopathies	1, 3, 14
Solid tumors	
Meningiomas	8, 22
Benign epithelial tumors	8, 14
Carcinomas	1, 3, 5, 7, 8
Malignant melanoma	1, 9
Neurogenic tumors	1, 22
Sarcomas	13, 14

[a] From Mitelman and Levan (1979) with permission.

involvement of chromosome 22 in human (CGL) and meningioma, in which a particular chromosome change is consistently associated with a specific tumor. However, the major contribution of the banding techniques has been to reveal a variety of human and animal neoplasms in which alterations in certain individual chromosomes and chromosome segments clearly occur with greater than random frequency. A number of these have already been mentioned, and Table 2 summarizes the nonrandom relationships between specific human chromosomes and different tumors based on a survey of 856 cases by Mitelman and Levan (1979). (Banding data are currently accumulating so rapidly that any such summary is already incomplete by the time of publication; the careful reader will recognize certain inconsistencies between Table 2 and statements in the text.)

It is also clear from the banding data that involvement of any one of these human chromosomes in neoplasia frequently takes a characteristic form. Thus, chromosome 8 is usually trisomic, while chromosome 7 is often monosomic. Alterations in chromosome 1 commonly involve an extra copy of the long arm, while changes in chromosomes 5 and 20 typically appear as deletions in the long arm. When chromosome 17 is involved, an isochromosome for the long arm usually replaces a normal chromosome 17 (Mitelman and Levan, 1978). The possible significance of such "dosage" phenomena will be considered later.

These nonrandom abnormalities in human tumors seem to indicate the general chromosome location of a finite number of genes that, when altered in one way or another, can confer a selective growth advantage on potentially neoplastic cells and so play a role in tumor initiation. In some instances, the specific karyotypic change apparently favors a particular cell type or pathway of differentiation, resulting in its frequent association with one type of tumor, such as $14q^+$ in lymphoproliferative disorders. In other instances, the cytogenetic alteration (such as trisomy for 1q) may be equally advantageous for all cell types. There is no evidence that the nonrandom abnormalities observed in tumors reflect increased mutability of the involved chromosome sites. These particular alterations are apparently recognized not because they occur more frequently than normal, but because of the selective advantage that they confer on cells bearing them, allowing the progeny of such cells to emerge as neoplastic clones.

These cytogenetic observations obviously do not identify specific "cancer" genes or their products, but cell hybridization techniques in tissue culture are rapidly expanding the map of the human genome, localizing more and more genes to specific chromosome segments, and also defining incorporation sites for oncogenic viral DNA. Eventually, through such techniques, it may be possible to recognize certain genes and their products that are critical to tumor development, either in man or in other species.

As noted earlier, some progress in this direction has been made in tentatively determining chromosome sites of genes controlling the neoplastic state in several rodent tumor systems (Azumi and Sachs, 1977; Bloch-Shtacher and Sachs, 1977; Jonasson *et al.*, 1977), but in no instance has the significant gene product been identified. In man, many of the chromosome segments nonrandomly involved in human neoplasia have already been shown to contain one or more genes controlling some aspect of nucleic acid biosynthesis or other metabolic pathways perhaps critical in growth regulation. For example, it has been mentioned earlier that the long arm of chromosome 17 contains genes regulating thymidine kinase and also galactokinase (perhaps important in membrane synthesis), and that 17q is also a preferential site for incorporation of both adenovirus 12 and SV40 (Harnden, 1977; Rowley, 1977). One certainly cannot yet confidently relate neoplastic behavior *in vivo* to specific genetic loci in the human genome, or to specific gene products, but the banding techniques are indicating a limited number of chromosome segments where such investigations might be focused.

The fact that involvement of chromosome 17 in human tumors usually involves an imbalance of the long and short arms (appearing as an isochromosome for 17q) (Fig. 2) is also of some interest. From the earliest studies of tumor cytogenetics, the difficulty in associating the initiation of neoplasia with a single chromosome change has led some authors to invoke a more nonspecific concept of "chromosome imbalance" to explain carcinogenesis (Rabinowitz and Sachs, 1970). They have suggested that it is not simply the gain or loss of a particular chromosome or gene locus that is critical to the maintenance of the neoplastic state, but rather a matter of imbalance among several genes located on different chromosomes or at different sites on the same chromosome, which control either expression or suppression of malignancy. Preliminary supportive evidence for this hypothesis has been obtained in several systems (Hitotsumachi *et al.*, 1971; Codish and Paul, 1974), but its general applicability remains unproved.

Related to this concept of genetic imbalance is the view that the "dosage" of critical genes may be important in carcinogenesis, particularly increased dosage. Most aneuploid tumors are hyperdiploid rather than hypodiploid, and Ohno (1971) has discussed the deleterious effects of monosomy and the potential advantages to the neoplastic cell, particularly with respect to both lethal and useful mutations, of chromosome duplication. The recently described HSRs and DSRs in the chromosomes of certain tumors, apparently indicating areas of gene amplification, represent another mechanism by which additional copies of a gene beneficial to a neoplasm might be acquired (Dolnick *et al.*, 1979; Miller *et al.*, 1979). It has also been suggested that the chromatid interchanges that occur spontaneously between homologous chromosomes in Bloom's syndrome (Fig. 5) may produce homozygosity at critical gene loci and thus contribute to the increased cancer incidence in these patients (Passarge and Bartram, 1976). Obviously, an actual gain in genetic material is not always necessary, as for the earlier mentioned nonrandom occurrence of monosomy for chromosome 7 in several human tumors; and the key translocations in CGL, involving chromosomes 9 and 22, and in the Burkitt tumor (8;14) may reflect significant "position effects" rather than any net changes in DNA content.

In addition to these attempts to relate specific types of cytogenetic change to the initiation of mammalian tumors, there is considerable evidence that non-specifically relates chromosome damage to the malignant state. The capability of most carcinogenic agents, such as radiation, chemicals, and viruses, to break chromosomes has already been discussed in detail, as well as the increased tumor incidence associated with those congenital disorders in which an inherited defect in DNA repair apparently results in a high frequency of "spontaneous" chromosome breakage *in vivo*.

Taken together, all of these data suggest that direct involvement of the host cell genome is an extremely common, if not essential, factor in the initiation of virtually all forms of neoplasia; and that in many instances, but not all, this involvement is indicated by demonstrable chromosome abnormality. The exact nature of the critical genetic lesion and the resulting initial change in cell function are, of course, not known and remain the key mysteries in defining the primary carcinogenic event. As several kinds of genetic alterations have been demonstrated in different neoplasms, both at the chromosome level (gain and loss of chromosomes, balanced and unbalanced translocation, HSRs) as well as such submicroscopic phenomena as point mutations and incorporation of viral genome, it seems unnecessary to postulate that any one particular type of genetic lesion is necessarily common to all tumors.

7.2. Chromosome Changes and Tumor Progression

With respect to the relationship of karyotypic alterations to the phenomenon of tumor progression (Foulds, 1954), the cytogenetic data again do not lead to definitive answers, but do provide strong supportive evidence for a model of tumor development in which genetic change is of critical importance. This concept of "clonal evolution" (Hauschka, 1961; Nowell, 1976; Spriggs, 1976; Klein, 1979) encompasses two major principles: (1) Tumors are unicellular in origin (clones); and (2) tumors progress on the basis of genetic instability within the neoplastic population, leading to the sequential emergence of mutant subpopulations with increasingly malignant properties (Fig. 7). Demonstrable chromosome changes may appear early or late in this process, but once present, they permit easy identification of the sequential nature of the genetic alterations taking place.

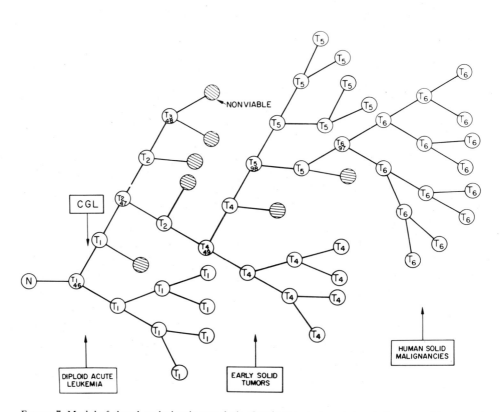

FIGURE 7. Model of clonal evolution in neoplasia. Carcinogen-induced change in progenitor normal cell (N) produces a diploid tumor cell (T_1, 46 chromosomes) with growth advantage permitting clonal expansion to begin. Genetic instability of T_1 cells leads to production of variants (illustrated by changes in chromosome number, T_2 to T_6). Most variants die, due to metabolic or immunologic disadvantage (hatched circles); occasionally one has an additional selective advantage (for example, T_2, 47 chromosomes), and its progeny become the predominant subpopulation until an even more favorable variant appears (for example, T_4). The stepwise sequence in each tumor differs (being partially determined by environmental pressures on selection), and results in a different, aneuploid karyotype predominating in each fully developed malignancy (T_6). Earlier subpopulations (for example, T_1, T_4, T_5) may persist sufficiently to contribute to heterogeneity within the advanced tumor. Biological characteristics of tumor progression (for example, morphological and metabolic loss of differentiation, invasion and metastasis, resistance to therapy) parallel the stages of genetic evolution. Human tumors with minimal chromosome change (diploid acute leukemia, chronic granulocytic leukemia) are considered to be early in clonal evolution; human solid cancers, typically highly aneuploid, are viewed as late in the developmental process. Modified from Nowell (1976).

Supporting evidence for this view of tumor progression comes from cytogenetic studies as well as from several other disciplines. The clonal nature of tumors is indicated by the fact that chromosome abnormalities are often the same throughout all the cells of a given tumor. Where there is a spectrum of cytogenetic changes, these are often demonstrably related. Even in highly malignant solid neoplasms with much karyotypic variation, characteristic marker chromosomes, recognizable in all cells of a given tumor, lend support to the view that the entire neoplastic population is derived from a single cell.

Studies of the distribution of the enzyme glucose-6-phosphate dehydrogenase in many tumors (Fialkow, 1977), and of the monoclonal characteristics of the immunoglobulin produced by a number of lymphoproliferative neoplasms also support this clonal concept. It should be stressed again that the term "clone" is being used here only to indicate the unicellular origin of the tumor and not homogeneity of the neoplastic population. As will be discussed in more detail below, since a malignancy in its later stages, through somatic mutation, may often come to consist of a large number of genetically different subpopulations derived from the original clone, it is not surprising that many tumors prove heterogeneous for whatever phenotypic characteristic is being examined. Also, it should be noted that this clonal hypothesis does not rule out the possibility that application of a carcinogen to an organ or to an area of skin can produce many potentially neoplastic cells; it simply indicates that as a tumor evolves from such an area, the progeny of one or, at most, a very few cells ultimately overgrow the site and account for the macroscopic tumor.

With respect to the second principle of this concept of clonal evolution, that biological and clinical tumor progression results from the sequential emergence of mutant subpopulations within the clone, the cytogenetic data provide most of the supportive evidence. I have already cited the findings in CGL and some other human tumors, as well as data from the Rous sarcoma system in animals, in which biological progression of a neoplasm to more malignant characteristics is associated with the emergence of a new predominant subpopulation of tumor cells having additional genetic alterations, recognizable cytogenetically. As banding techniques are more widely applied to a variety of mammalian neoplasms, this demonstrable relationship between more mutant sublines and biological or clinical tumor progression is being increasingly documented; although, recognizing the relatively crude nature of chromosome studies in exploring genetic change, it is not surprising that the results are not universally consistent.

There is some direct evidence of the genetic instability of tumor cells as a basis for the generation of these mutant sublines. In tissue culture, neoplastic cells have been shown to be more susceptible to chromosome breakage, nondisjunction, SCE, and other genetic alterations than comparable normal cells (Klein, 1963; Weiner et al., 1974; Sokova et al., 1976; Otter et al., 1978). Although the basis for these phenomena is not certain, it has been postulated, with some supportive experimental data, that neoplastic cells in normal individuals might undergo somatic mutation involving a "mutagenic" gene. Through this mechanism they might acquire abnormalities in DNA repair similar to those in the chromosome breakage syndromes or develop other defects in DNA synthesis or in the mitotic apparatus itself, which would make subsequent genetic alterations in the tumor cells more likely (Nichols, 1963; Cairns, 1975; Loeb *et al.*, 1975; Heston, 1977). It is possible, of course, that genetic lability of malignant cell populations *in vivo*, as recognized by sequential chromosome changes, need not always reflect a defect within the neoplastic cells themselves. It could result from the continued presence of a carcinogenic agent (chemical, radiation, or viral) or from other mutagenic factors in the tumor environment, including therapy (Cole and Nowell, 1965; Freed and Schatz, 1969; Harnden, 1974; Adachi and Ingalls, 1976).

Whatever the mechanism, it does appear that chromosome alterations do occur repeatedly in many evolving tumor cell populations, and as one observes this phenomenon sequentially in experimental neoplasms, the trend with respect to chromosome number is usually toward an increase. Commonly, the first demonstrable change may be the gain of a single chromosome. I have already mentioned the discussion by Ohno (1971) of the potential advantages to the tumor cell of chromosome duplication, and this may help to explain why later steps in the progression of many mammalian solid malignancies may be toward a near-triploid or near-tetraploid karyotype as indicated in Fig. 7. It also appears, both from human and from animal studies, that there is something of a "cascade" effect as the tumor evolves, with continually increasing genetic instability, so that the probability of further genetic change is greater in each succeeding cell generation. Evidence of this phenomenon is observable in the high frequency of grossly abnormal mitoses in far-advanced malignancies (Oksala and Therman, 1974).

A significant concern raised by the chromosome findings in advanced human tumors is the indication that neoplastic growth is very often at an irreversible stage when first observed in man. If the aneuploid karyotype that we find in most fully developed cancers is the result of a multistep evolutionary process in which mutants have been repeatedly selected for their increasingly efficient capacity to function as malignant cells, the possibility of restoring this population to normal seems extremely remote. Introducing a normal karyotype, by some trick of genetic engineering, into a proportion of the tumor cells would not be helpful; any remaining aberrant cells, retaining their selective advantages, would once again overgrow the normal elements and reestablish the malignancy. Nor does it seem likely that manipulation of the internal environment of the host might somehow induce highly aneuploid neoplastic cells to differentiate and function normally, even though most, if not all, of the original genetic information presumably remains within the aneuploid genome. Perhaps such alteration of the local environment would have a greater chance of restoring the normal balance between proliferation and differentiation in a diploid or near-diploid tumor population, such as is seen in many of the human leukemias.

There have been a few experiments suggesting that under specialized circumstances, both diploid and aneuploid neoplastic cells can be induced to differentiate *in vivo* (DiBerardino and King, 1965; Braun, 1969; Mintz, 1978). This may be

Wilms' tumor, and teratocarcinoma, that in some respects function as "embryonic
rests," with an inherent propensity for further differentiation and associated loss
of malignant characteristics (O'Hara, 1978). Even for such tumors, however,
experimental studies with teratocarcinoma suggest that success in forcing the
malignancy to differentiate is most likely if the karyotype is diploid or near-
diploid, and it usually requires conditions that are unlikely to be feasible in
treating a primary neoplasm (Mintz, 1978). Nevertheless, this approach certainly
warrants continued investigation, even if it proves impractical for all but a small
minority of human cancers.

7.3. Clinical Applications of Tumor Chromosome Studies

In addition to these theoretical considerations, it is also appropriate to review
the current practical value for diagnosis or prognosis of cytogenetic investigations
in human neoplasms. Some aspects have been considered earlier in the text, as
well as possibilities for further development. The diagnostic use of chromosome
data to aid in the classification of confusing cases of human leukemia and
preleukemia has been mentioned, as well as the occasional elucidation of benign
versus malignant solid lesions and effusions by cytogenetic techniques (Dewald
et al., 1976).

The practical results with respect to prognosis, predicting survival and response
to therapy, have also been limited. In some of the leukemic and preleukemic
states, the presence or absence of chromosome abnormalities, the nature and
extent of the alteration, and the frequency of cytogenetically abnormal cells in
the bone marrow all have been of some predictive value (Canellos *et al.*, 1976;
Golomb *et al.*, 1978; Nowell and Finan, 1978; Benedict *et al.*, 1979). Currently,
a number of large national and international studies are under way to extend
these observations and to determine in what circumstances chromosome studies
should be part of the routine initial workup for patients with various disorders
of the hematopoietic system. Eventually, similar considerations may be warranted
for premalignant and malignant lesions of such organs as the cervix, bowel,
bladder, and skin.

More importantly, however, in considering the general problem of cancer
therapy, one must acknowledge the chromosomal evidence that indicates that
most malignancies, as seen clinically, are highly individual and highly abnormal
from a genetic standpoint. There are a few diploid neoplasms, notably many
cases of acute leukemia, that, because of their less altered genetic makeup, may
prove more consistent in their response to various types of therapeutic manipulation. The vast majority of cancers, however, are aneuploid, and in addition to
having highly individualized genetic patterns, also demonstrate the capacity to
generate new predominant variants if their environment is altered. These characteristics should be recognized by the cancer therapist, and they provide a profound challenge to his or her ingenuity.

8. References

ADACHI, K., AND INGALLS, T., 1976, Ovum aging and pH imbalance as a cause of chromosomal anomalies in the hamster, *Science* **194**:946.

AKSOY, M., 1977, Leukemia in workers due to occupational exposure to benzene, *N. Istanbul Contr. Clin. Sci.* **12**:3.

ALIMENA, G., BRANDT, L., DALLAPICCOLA, B., MITELMAN, F., AND NILSSON, P., 1979, Secondary chromosome changes in chronic myeloid leukemia: Relation to treatment, *Cancer Genet. Cytogenet.* **1**:79.

AL-SAADI, A. A., AND BEIERWALTES, W. H., 1967, Sequential cytogenetic changes in the evolution of transplanted thyroid tumors to metastatic carcinoma in the Fischer rat, *Cancer Res.* **27**:1831.

ATKIN, N., AND BAKER, M., 1978, Abnormal chromosomes and number 1 heterochromatin variants revealed in C-banded preparations from 13 bladder carcinomas, *Cytobios* **18**:101.

ATKIN, N., AND PICKTHALL, V., 1977, Chromosome 1 in 14 ovarian cancers. Heterochromatin variants and structural changes, *Humangenetik* **38**:25.

AU, W., SOUKUP, S., AND MANDYBUR, T., 1977, Excess chromosome 4 in ethylnitrosourea induced neurogenic tumor lines of the rat, *J. Natl. Cancer Inst.* **59**:1709.

AUERBACH, A., AND WOLMAN, S., 1976, Susceptibility of Fanconi's anemia fibroblasts to chromosome damage by carcinogens, *Nature (London)* **261**:494.

AUERSPERG, N., COREY, M. J., AND WORTH, A., 1967, Chromosomes in preinvasive lesions of the human uterine cervix, *Cancer Res.* **27**:1394.

AUTIO, K., TURUNEN, O., PENTTILA, O., ERAMAA, E., DE LA CHAPELLE, A., AND SCHRODER, J., 1979, Human chronic lymphocytic leukemia: Karyotypes in different lymphocyte populations, *Cancer Genet. Cytogenet.* **1**:147.

AZUMI, J., AND SACHS, L., 1977, Chromosome mapping of the genes that control differentiation and malignancy in myeloid leukemic cells, *Proc. Natl. Acad. Sci. USA* **74**:315.

BALABAN-MALENBAUM, G., AND GILBERT, F., 1978, Double minute chromosomes and the homogeneously staining regions in chromosomes of a human neuroblastoma cell line, *Science* **198**:739.

BARSKI, G., 1978, Morphokinetic aspects of cell transformation *in vitro*, *Natl. Cancer Inst. Monogr.* **48**:263.

BENEDICT, W., LANGE, M., GREENE, J., DERENCSENYI, A., AND ALFI, O., 1979, Correlation between prognosis and bone marrow chromosomal patterns in children with acute nonlymphocytic leukemia: Similarities and differences compared to adults, *Blood* **54**:818.

BERGER, R., AND BERNHEIM, A., 1979, Y chromosome loss in leukemias, *Cancer Genet. Cytogenet.* **1**:1.

BIEDLER, J., AND SPENGLER, B., 1976, Metaphase chromosome anomaly: Association with drug resistance and cell-specific products, *Science* **191**:185.

BLOCH-SHTACHER, N., AND SACHS, L., 1977, Identification of a chromosome that controls malignancy in Chinese hamster cells, *J. Cell. Physiol.* **93**:205.

BLOOMFIELD, C., LINDQUIST, L., BRUNNING, R., YUNIS, J., AND COCCIA, P., 1978, The Philadelphia chromosome in acute leukemia, *Virchows Arch. B* **29**:81.

BOVERI, T., 1914, *Zur Frage der Entstehung maligner Tumoren*, Vol. 1, Gustav Fischer Verlag, Jena.

BRAUN, A. C., 1969, *The Cancer Problem*, Columbia University Press, New York.

BRODEUR, G., DOW, L., AND WILLIAMS, D., 1979, Cytogenetic features of juvenile chronic myelogeneous leukemia, *Blood* **53**:812.

CAIRNS, J., 1975, Mutation, selection, and the natural history of cancer, *Nature (London)* **255**:197.

CANELLOS, G., WHANG-PENG, J., AND DEVITA, V., 1976, Chronic granulocytic leukemia without the Philadelphia chromosome, *Am. J. Clin. Pathol.* **65**:467.

CASPERSSON, T., FARBER, S., FOLEY, G. E., KUDYNOWSKI, J., MODEST, E. J., SIMONSSON, E., WAGH, U., AND ZECH, L., 1968, Chemical differentiation along metaphase chromosomes, *Exp. Cell Res.* **49**:219.

CERVENKA, J., ANDERSON, R., NESBIT, M., AND KRIVIT, W., 1977, Familial leukemia and inherited chromosomal aberration, *Int. J. Cancer* **19**:783.

CHAGANTI, R., SCHONBERG, S., AND GERMAN, J., 1974, A manyfold increase in sister chromatid exchanges in Bloom's syndrome lymphocytes, *Proc. Natl. Acad. Sci. USA* **71**:4508.

CHAN, F., 1978, Chromosome studies in induced murine thymomas, *Diss. Abstr. Int. B* **38**:3994.

CHAUDHURI, J., 1978, A cytogenetic schedule to assess multiple parameters from a single preparation applicable to screen populations exposed to environmental mutagens, *Mutat. Res.* **53**:165.

CLEAVER, J., AND BOOTSMA, D., 1975, Xeroderma pigmentosum: Biochemical and genetic characteristics, *Annu. Rev. Genet.* **9:**18.

CODISH, S., AND PAUL, B., 1974, Reversible appearance of a specific chromosome which suppresses malignancy, *Nature (London)* **252:**610.

COHEN, A., LI, F., BERG, S., MARCHETTO, D., TSAI, S., JACOBS, S., AND BROWN, R., 1979, Hereditary renal-cell carcinoma associated with a chromosomal translocation, *N. Engl. J. Med.* **301:**592.

COHEN, D., 1978, The transmissible venereal tumor of the dog: A naturally occurring allograft?, *Isr. J. Med. Sci.* **14:**14.

COHEN, M., SHAHAM, M., DAGAN, J., SHMUELI, E., AND KOHN, G., 1975, Cytogenetic investigations in families with ataxia telangiectasia, *Cytogenet. Cell Genet.* **15:**338.

COLE, L., AND NOWELL, P., 1965, Radiation carcinogenesis: The sequence of events, *Science* **150:**1782.

CROCE, C., 1977, Assignment of the integration site for simian virus 40 to chromosome 17 in GM54VA, a human cell line transformed by simian virus 40, *Proc. Natl. Acad. Sci. USA* **74:**253.

CROCE, C., BARRICK, J., LINNENBACH, A., AND KOPROWSKI, H., 1979, Expression of malignancy in hybrids between normal and malignant cells, *J. Cell. Physiol.* **99:**279.

CRUCIGER, Q., PATHAK, S., AND CAILLEAU, R., 1977, Human breast carcinomas: Marker chromosomes involving lq in 7 cases, *Cytogenet. Cell Genet.* **17:**231.

DAHLKE, M., AND NOWELL, P., 1075, Chromosomal abnormalities and dyserythropoiesis in the preleukemic phase of multiple myeloma, *Br. J. Haematol.* **31:**111.

DEWALD, G., DINES, D., WEILAND, L., AND GORDAN, H., 1976, Usefulness of chromosome examinations in the diagnosis of malignant pleural effusions, *N. Engl. J. Med.* **295:**1494.

DIBERARDINO, M. A., AND KING, T. J., 1965, Transplantation of nuclei from the frog renal adenocarcinoma. II. Chromosomal and histologic analysis of tumor nuclear-transplant embryos, *Dev. Biol.* **11:**217.

DIPAOLO, J., AND POPESCU, N., 1976, Relationship of chromosome changes to neoplastic cell transformation, *Am. J. Pathol.* **85:**709.

DOLNICK, B., BERENSON, R., BERTINO, J., KAUFMAN, R., NUNBERG, J., AND SCHIMKE, R., 1979, Correlation of dihydrofolate reductase elevation with gene amplification in a homogeneously staining chromosomal region in L5178Y cells, *J. Cell Biol.* **83:**394.

EDELSON, R., BERGER, C., RAAFAT, J., AND WARBURTON, D., 1979, Karyotype studies of cutaneous T cell lymphoma: Evidence for clonal origin, *J. Invest. Dermatol.* **73:**548.

ELSEVIER, S., KUCHERLAPATI, R., NICHOLS, E., CREAGAN, R., GILES, R., RUDDLE, F., WILLECKE, K., AND MCDOUGALL, J., 1974, Assignment of the gene for galactokinase to human chromosome 17 and its regional localization to band q 21–22, *Nature (London)* **251:**633.

ENTERLINE, H. T., AND ARVAN, D. A., 1967, Chromosome constitution of adenoma and adenocarcinoma of the colon, *Cancer* **20:**1746.

FALOR, W., AND WARD, R., 1978, Prognosis in early carcinoma of the bladder based on chromosomal analysis, *J. Urol.* **119:**44.

FIALKOW, P., 1977, Clonal origin and stem cell evolution of human tumors, *Prog. Cancer Res. Ther.* **3:**439.

FIALKOW, P., 1979, Clonal origin of human tumors, *Annu. Rev. Med.* **30:**135.

FINNEY, R., MCDONALD, G. A., BAIKIE, A. G., AND DOUGLAS, A. S., 1972, Chronic granulocytic leukemia with Ph negative cells in bone marrow and a ten year remission after Busulphan hypoplasia, *Br. J. Haematol.* **23:**283.

FITZGERALD, P., AND ADAMS, A., 1975, Chromosome studies in chronic lymphocytic leukemia and lymphosarcoma, *J. Natl. Cancer Inst.* **34:**827.

FLEISCHMAN, E., AND PRIGOGINA, E., 1977, Karyotype peculiarities of malignant lymphomas, *Humangenetik* **35:**269.

FORNI, A., AND MOREO, L. 1967, Cytogenetic studies in a case of benzene leukemia, *Eur. J. Cancer* **3:**251.

FOUCAR, K., MCKENNA, R., BLOOMFIELD, C., BOWERS, T., AND BRUNNING, R., 1979, Therapy-related leukemia. A panmyelosis, *Cancer* **43:**1285.

FOULDS, L., 1954, Tumor progression: A review, *Cancer Res.* **14:**327.

FREED, J. J., AND SCHATZ, S. A., 1969, Chromosome aberrations in cultured cells deprived of single essential amino acids, *Exp. Cell Res.* **55:**393.

FREEMAN, A. E., AND HUEBNER, R. J., 1973, Problems in interpretation of experimental evidence of cell transformation, *J. Natl. Cancer Inst.* **50:**303.

FUKUHARA, S., ROWLEY, J., VARIAKOJIS, D., AND SWEET, D., 1978, Banding studies on chromosomes in diffuse "histiocytic" lymphomas: Correlation of 14q⁺ marker chromosome with cytology, *Blood* **52**:989.

GEE, T., CUNNINGHAM, I., DOWLING, M., CHAGHANTI, R., AND CLARKSON, B., 1978, The L-5 protocol: Intensive treatment for patients with chronic myeloid leukemia, *Bull. Inst. Sieroter Milan* **57**:289.

GERMAN, J., 1977, The association of chromosome instability, defective DNA repair, and cancer in some rare human genetic diseases, in: *Human Genetics* (S. Armendares and R. Lisker, eds.), pp. 64–68, Excerpta Medica, Amsterdam.

GERMAN, J., BLOOM, D., AND PASSARGE, E., 1979, Bloom's syndrome. VII. Progress report for 1978, *Clin. Genet.* **15**:361.

GOLOMB, H., VARDIMAN, J., ROWLEY, J., TESTA, J., AND MINTZ, U., 1978, Correlation of clinical findings with quinacrine-banded chromosomes in 90 adults with acute nonlymphocytic leukemia, *N. Engl. J. Med.* **299**:613.

HAMBURGER, A., SALMON, S., KIM, M., TRENT, J., SOEHNLEN, B., ALBERTS, D., AND SCHMIDT, H. J., 1978, Direct cloning of human ovarian carcinoma cells in agar, *Cancer Res.* **38**:3438.

HARNDEN, D., 1974, Viruses, chromosomes, and tumors: The interaction between viruses and chromosomes, in: *Chromosomes and Cancer* (J. German, ed.), pp. 151–190, Wiley, New York.

HARNDEN, D., 1977, The relationship between induced chromosome aberrations and chromosome abnormality in tumor cells, in: *Human Genetics* (S. Armendares and R. Lisker, eds.), pp. 355–366, Excerpta Medica, Amsterdam.

HARNDEN, D., BENN, P., OXFORD, J., TAYLOR, A., AND WEBB, T., 1976, Cytogenetically marked clones in human fibroblasts cultured from normal subjects, *Somat. Cell Genet.* **2**:55.

HAROUSSEAU, J., SMADJA, N., KRULIK, M., AUDEBERT, A., AND DEBRAY, J., 1978, Study of karyotypes in preleukemic states, *Nouv. Presse Med.* **7**:3431.

HARRIS, C., 1979, A delayed complication of cancer therapy—cancer, *J. Natl. Cancer Inst.* **63**:275.

HARRIS, H., MILLER, O. J., KLEIN, G., WORST, P., AND TACHIBANA, T., 1969, Suppression of malignancy by cell fusion, *Nature (London)* **223**:363.

HAUSCHKA, T. S., 1961, The chromosomes in ontogeny and oncogeny, *Cancer Res.* **21**:957.

HECHT, F., AND McCAW, B., 1977, Chromosome instability syndromes, *Prog. Cancer Res. Ther.* **3**:105.

HEIMPEL, H., DRINGS, P., AND QUEISSER, W., 1979, A prospective study on course and prognostic criteria in 'preleukemia,' *Klin. Wochenschr.* **57**:21.

HESTON, L., 1977, Alzheimer's disease, trisomy 21, and myeloproliferative disorders: Associations suggesting a genetic diathesis, *Science* **196**:322.

HIGURASHI, M., AND COHEN, C., 1973, *In vitro* chromosomal radiosensitivity in "chromosomal breakage syndromes," *Cancer* **32**:380.

HITOTSUMACHI, S., RABINOWITZ, Z., AND SACHS, L., 1971, Chromosomal control of reversion in transformed cells, *Nature (London)* **231**:511.

HITTELMAN, W., AND RAO, P., 1978, Predicting response or progression of human leukemia by premature chromosome condensation of bone marrow cells, *Cancer Res.* **38**:416.

HOSSFELD, D., AND SCHMIDT, C., 1978, Chromosome findings in effusions from patients with Hodgkin's disease, *Int. J. Cancer* **21**:147.

HOSSFELD, D., FALTERMEIER, M., AND WENDEHURST, E., 1979, The relationship between chromosomal findings and prognosis in acute nonlymphoblastic leukemia, *Blut* **38**:377.

HSU, T. C., 1961, Chromosomal evolution in cell populations, *Int. Rev. Cytol.* **12**:69.

HSU, T. C., AND POMERAT, C., 1953, Mammalian chromosomes *in vitro*. II. A method for spreading the chromosomes of cells in tissue culture, *J. Hered.* **44**:23.

HURLEY, J., FU, S., KUNKEL, H., CHAGANTI, R., AND GERMAN, J., 1980, Chromosome abnormalities of leukemic B lymphocytes in chronic lymphocytic leukemia, *Nature (London)* **283**:76.

JONASSON, J., POVEY, S., AND HARRIS, H., 1977, The analysis of malignancy by cell fusion. VII. Cytogenetic analysis of hybrids between malignant and diploid cells and of tumors derived from them, *J. Cell Sci.* **24**:217.

KAISER-McCAW, B., PEAKMAN, D., HECHT, F., AND ROBINSON, A., 1979, Recurrent somatic 7;14 translocations in lymphocytes, *Am. J. Hum. Genet.* **31**:99A.

KAKATI, S., AND SANDBERG, A., 1978, Chromosomes in solid tumors, *Virchows Arch. B* **29**:129.

KLEIN, G., 1963, Genetics of somatic cells, in: *Methodology in Mammalian Genetics* (W. Burdette, ed.), pp. 407–468, Holden–Day, San Francisco.

KLEIN, G., 1979, Lymphoma development in mice and humans: Diversity of initiation is followed by convergent cytogenetic evolution, *Proc. Natl. Acad. Sci. USA* **76**:2442.

KNUDSON, A., STRONG, L., AND ANDERSON, D., 1973, Heredity and cancer in man, *Prog. Med. Genet.* **9:**113.

KNUDSON, A., MEADOWS, A., NICHOLS, W., AND HILL, R., 1976, Chromosomal deletion and retinoblastoma, *N. Engl. J. Med.* **295:**1120.

KOLLER, P. C., 1972, *The Role of Chromosomes in Cancer Biology*, Springer, New York.

KOVI, E., AND MORRIS, H., 1976, Chromosome banding studies of several transplantable hepatomas, *Adv. Enzyme Regul.* **14:**139.

LAMBERT, B., RINGBORG, U., HARPER, E., AND LINDBLAD, A., 1978, Sister chromatid exchanges in lymphocyte cultures of patients receiving chemotherapy for malignant disorders, *Cancer Treat. Rep.* **62:**1413.

LATT, S., 1974, Sister chromatid exchanges as indices of human chromosome damage and repair: Detection by fluorescence and induction by mitomycin C., *Proc. Natl. Acad. Sci. USA* **71:**3162.

LAWLER, S., REEVES, B., AND HAMLIN, I., 1975, A comparison of cytogenetics and histopathology in the malignant lymphomata, *Br. J. Cancer* **31:**162.

LAZLO, J., 1975, Myeloproliferative disorders (MPD)—Myelofibrosis, myelosclerosis, extramedullary hematopoiesis, undifferentiated MPD, and hemorrhagic thrombocythemia, *Semin. Hematol.* **12:**409.

LEVAN, G., AND MITELMAN, F., 1976, G-banding in Rous rat sarcomas during serial transfer: Significant chromosome aberrations and incidence of stromal mitoses, *Hereditas* **84:**1.

LEVAN, G., AND MITELMAN, F., 1977, Chromosomes and the etiology of cancer, *Chromosomes Today* **6:**363.

LEVITT, R., PIERRE, R., WHITE, W., AND SICKERT, R., 1978, Atypical lymphoid leukemia in ataxia telangiectasia, *Blood* **52:**1003.

LINMAN, J., AND BAGBY, G., 1976, The preleukemic syndrome: Clinical and laboratory features, natural course, and management, *Blood Cells* **2:**11.

LOEB, L., BATTULA, N., SPRINGGATE, C., AND SEAL, G., 1975, On mutagenic DNA polymerase and malignancy, in: *Fundamental Aspects of Malignancy* (A. Gottlieb, O. Plescia, and D. Bishop, eds.), pp. 243–256, Springer, Berlin.

MACPHERSON, I., 1970, Characteristics of animal cells transformed *in vitro*, *Adv. Cancer Res.* **13:**169.

MAKINO, S., 1963, Some epidemiologic aspects of venereal tumors of dogs as revealed by chromosome and DNA studies, *Ann. N.Y. Acad. Sci.* **108:**1106.

MANOLOV, G., AND MANOLOVA, Y., 1971, A marker band in one chromosome No 14 in biopsies and cultures from Burkitt lymphomas, *Hereditas* **69:**300.

MARK, J., 1969, Rous sarcoma in mice: The chromosomal progression in primary tumors, *Eur. J. Cancer* **5:**307.

MARK, J., 1977, Chromosomal abnormalities and their specificity in human neoplasms: An assessment of recent aberrations by banding techniques, *Adv. Cancer Res.* **24:**165.

McCAW, B., HECHT, F., HARNDEN, D., AND TEPLITZ, R., 1975, Somatic rearrangement of chromosome 14 in human lymphocytes, *Proc. Natl. Acad. Sci. USA* **72:**2071.

McMICHAEL, H., WAGNER, J., NOWELL, P., AND HUNGERFORD, D., 1964, Chromosome studies of virus-induced rabbit papillomas and derived, primary carcinomas, *J. Natl. Cancer Inst.* **31:**1197.

MEYNE, J., LOCKHART, L., AND ARRIGHI, F., 1979, Nonrandom distribution of chromosomal aberrations induced by three chemicals, *Mutat. Res.* **63:**201.

MILLER, O., ALLERDICE, P., MILLER, D., BREG, W., AND MIGEON, B., 1971, Human thymidine kinase gene locus assignment to chromosome 17 in a hybrid of man and mouse cells, *Science* **173:**244.

MILLER, O., TANTRAVAHI, R., MILLER, D., YU, L., SZABO, P., AND PRENSKY, W., 1979, Marked increase in ribosomal RNA gene multiplicity in a rat hepatoma cell line, *Chromosoma* **71:**183.

MINTZ, B., 1978, Genetic mosaicism and *in vivo* analyses of neoplasia and differentiation, *Annu. Symp. Cancer Res.* **30:**27.

MITELMAN, F., 1971, The chromosomes of fifty primary Rous rat sarcomas, *Hereditas* **69:**155.

MITELMAN, F., 1975, Comparative cytogenetic studies of bone marrow and extramedullary tissues in chronic myeloid leukemia, *Ser. Haematol.* **8:**113.

MITELMAN, F., AND LEVAN, G., 1978, Clustering of aberrations to specific chromosomes in human neoplasms. III. Incidence and geographic distribution of chromosome aberrations in 856 cases, *Hereditas* **89:**207.

MITELMAN, F., AND LEVAN, G., 1979, Chromosomes in neoplasia: An appeal for unpublished data, *Cancer Genet. Cytogenet.* **1:**29.

MITELMAN, F., MARK, J., NILSSON, P., DENCKER, H., NORRYD, D., AND TRANBERG, K., 1974, Chromosome banding pattern in human colonic polyps, *Hereditas* **78:**63.

MITELMAN, F., NILSSON, P., LEVAN, G., AND BRANDT, L., 1976, Non-random chromosome changes in acute myeloid leukemia. Chromosome banding examination of 30 cases at diagnosis, *Int. J. Cancer* **18**:31.

MITELMAN, F., BRANDT, L., AND NILSSON, P., 1978, Relation among occupational exposure to potential mutagenic/carcinogenic agents, clinical findings, and bone marrow chromosomes in acute nonlymphocytic leukemia, *Blood* **52**:1229.

MOORHEAD, P. AND WEINSTEIN, D., 1966, Cytogenetic alterations during malignant transformation, in: *Recent Results in Cancer Research*, Vol. VI (W. Kirsten, ed.), pp. 104–111, Springer, New York.

MOORHEAD P., NOWELL, P., MELLMAN, W., BATTIPS, D., AND HUNGERFORD, D., 1960, Chromosome preparations of leukocytes cultured from human peripheral blood, *Exp. Cell Res.* **20**:613.

NEVSTAD, N., 1978, Sister chromatid exchanges and chromosomal aberrations induced in human lymphocytes by the cytostatic drug adriamycin *in vivo* and *in vitro*, *Mutat. Res.* **57**:253.

NICHOLS, W. W., 1963, Relationships of viruses, chromosomes, and carcinogenesis, *Hereditas* **50**:53.

NICHOLS, W. W., 1966, The role of viruses in the etiology of chromosome aberrations, *Am. J. Hum. Genet.* **18**:81.

NICHOLS, W. W., LEVAN, A., CORIELL, L. L., GOLDNER, H., AND AHLSTROM, C. G., 1964, Chromosome abnormalities *in vitro* in human leukocytes associated with Schmidt–Ruppin Rous sarcoma virus, *Science* **146**:248.

NOWELL, P., 1967, Chromosome abnormalities in the childhood leukemias, in: *The Clinical Pathology of Infancy* (F. Sunderman and F. Sunderman, Jr., eds.), pp. 447–482, Thomas, Springfield, Ill.

NOWELL, P., 1969, Biological significance of induced human chromosome aberrations, *Fed. Proc.* **28**:1797.

NOWELL, P., 1976, The clonal evolution of tumor cell populations, *Science* **194**:23.

NOWELL, P., 1977, Preleukemia. Cytogenetic clues in some confusing disorders, *Am. J. Pathol.* **89**:459.

NOWELL, P., AND COLE, L., 1965, Hepatomas in mice: Incidence increased after gamma irradiation at low dose rates, *Science* **148**:96.

NOWELL, P., AND FINAN, J., 1978, Chromosome studies in preleukemic states. IV. Myeloproliferative vs. cytopenic disorders, *Cancer* **42**:2254.

NOWELL, P., AND HUNGERFORD, D., 1960, A minute chromosome in human chronic granulocytic leukemia, *Science* **132**:1497.

NOWELL, P., AND HUNGERFORD, D. A., 1964, Chromosome changes in human leukemia and a tentative assessment of their significance, *J. Natl. Cancer Inst.* **27**:1013.

NOWELL, P., AND MORRIS, H. P., 1969, Chromosomes of "minimal deviation hepatomas": A further report on diploid tumors, *Cancer Res.* **29**:969.

NOWELL, P., MORRIS, H. P., AND POTTER, V. R., 1967, Chromosomes of "minimal deviation" hepatomas and some other transplantable rat tumors, *Cancer Res.* **27**:1565.

NOWELL, P., ROWLANDS, D., DANIELE, R., BERGER, B., AND GUERRY, D., 1979, Changes in membrane markers and chromosome patterns in chronic T cell leukemia, *Clin. Immunol. Immunopathol.* **12**:323.

NOWELL, P. DANIELE, R., ROWLANDS, D., AND FINAN, J., 1980, Cytogenetics of chronic B-cell and T-cell leukemia, *Cancer Genet. Cytogenet.* **1**:273.

O'HARA, M., 1978, Teratomas, neoplasia, and differentiation: A biological overview. I. The natural history of teratomas, *Invest. Cell. Pathol.* **1**:39.

OHNO, S., 1971, Genetic implication of karyological instability of malignant cells, *Physiol. Rev.* **51**:496.

OKSALA, T., AND THERMAN, E., 1974, Mitotic abnormalities and cancer, in: *Chromosomes and Cancer* (J. German, ed.), pp. 239–263, Wiley, New York.

O'RIORDAN, M. L., BERRY, E., AND TOUGH, I., 1970, Chromosome studies on bone marrow from a male control population, *Br. J. Haematol.* **19**:83.

OSHIMURA, M., AND SANDBERG, A., 1977, Chromosomal 6q⁻ anomaly in acute lymphoblastic leukemia, *Lancet* **2**:1405.

OTTER, M., PALMER, C., AND BAEHNER, R., 1978, Elevated sister chromatid exchange rate in childhood lymphoblastic leukemia, *Proc. Am. Assoc. Cancer Res.* **19**:202.

PARIS CONFERENCE, 1971, Standardization in human cytogenetics, *Birth Defects Orig. Artic. Ser.* **8**:7 (1972).

PASSARGE, E., AND BARTRAM, C., 1976, Somatic recombination as possible prelude to malignant transformation, *Birth Defects Orig. Artic. Ser.* **12**:177.

PATERSON, M., SMITH, B., LOHMAN, P., ANDERSON, A., AND FISHMAN, L., 1976, Defective excision repair of gamma-ray damaged DNA in human (ataxia telangiectasia) fibroblasts, *Nature (London)* **260**:444.

PEDERSEN, B., 1973, The blastic crisis of chronic myeloid leukemia: Acute transformation of a preleukemic condition? *Br. J. Haematol.* **25**:141.

PEDERSEN, B., AND HAYHOE, F. G. J., 1971, Cellular changes in chronic myeloid leukemia, *Br. J. Haematol.* **21**:251.

PIERRE, R., 1975, Cytogenetic studies in preleukemia: Studies before and after transition to acute leukemia in 17 subjects, *Blood Cells* **1**:163.

PIERRE, R., 1978a, Preleukemic syndromes, *Virchows Arch. B* **29**:29.

PIERRE, R., 1978b, Cytogenetics of malignant lymphoma, *Virchows Arch. B* **29**:107.

POON, P., O'BRIEN, R., AND PARKER, J., 1974, Defective DNA repair in Fanconi's anemia, *Nature (London)* **250**:223.

RABINOWITZ, Z., AND SACHS, L., 1970, Control of the reversion of properties in transformed cells, *Nature (London)* **225**:136.

REMSEN, J., AND CERUTTI, P., 1976, Deficiency of gamma ray excision repair in skin fibroblasts from patients with Fanconi's anemia, *Proc. Natl. Acad. Sci. USA* **76**:2419.

RICCARDI, V., SUJANSKY, E., SMITH, A., AND FRANCKE, U., 1978, Chromosomal imbalance in the aniridia–Wilms' tumor association: 11p interstitial deletion, *Pediatrics* **61**:604.

ROBERTS, J., 1978, The repair of DNA modified by cytotoxic, mutagenic, and carcinogenic chemicals, *Adv. Radiat. Biol.* **17**:211.

ROWLEY, J., 1973, A new consistent chromosomal abnormality in chronic myelogenous leukemia identified by quinacrine fluorescence and Giemsa staining, *Nature (London)* **243**:290.

ROWLEY, J., 1974, Do human tumors show a chromosome pattern specific for each etiologic agent?, *J. Natl. Cancer Inst.* **52**:315.

ROWLEY, J., 1977, Mapping of human chromosomal regions related to neoplasia, *Proc. Natl. Acad. Sci. USA* **74**:5729.

ROWLEY, J., 1978, Chromosomes in leukemia and lymphoma, *Semin. Hematol.* **15**:301.

ROWLEY, J., GOLOMB, H., AND DOUGHERTY, C., 1977, 15/17 translocation: Consistent abnormality in acute promyelocytic leukemia, *Lancet* **1**:549.

RUDDLE, F., 1977, New approaches to human gene mapping by means of somatic cell genetics, in: *Human Genetics* (S. Armendares and R. Lisker, eds.), pp. 269–283, Excerpta Medica, Amsterdam.

SANDBERG, A., 1966, The chromosomes and causation of human cancer and leukemia, *Cancer Res.* **26**:2064.

SANDBERG, A., AND HOSSFELD, D. K., 1970, Chromosomal abnormalities in human neoplasia, *Annu. Rev. Med.* **21**:379.

SANDBERG, A., SAKURAI, M., AND HOLDSWORTH, C., 1972, Chromosomes and causation of human cancer and leukemia. VIII. DMS chromosomes in a neuroblastoma, *Cancer* **29**:1671.

SAXON, A., STEVENS, R., AND GOLDE, D., 1979, Helper and suppressor T-lymphocyte leukemia in ataxia telangiectasia, *N. Engl. J. Med.* **300**:700.

SCHMID, W., 1977, Mutagen/carcinogen-induced chromosome damage in human and mammalian cells *in vivo* and *in vitro*, in: *Human Genetics* (S. Armendares and R. Lisker, eds.), pp. 53–63, Excerpta Medica, Amsterdam.

SEABRIGHT, M., 1971, A rapid banding technique for human chromosomes, *Lancet* **2**:971.

SEABRIGHT, M., 1976, Patterns of induced aberrations in humans with abnormal autosomal complements, *Chromosomes Today* **5**:293.

SELIGMAN, M., PREUD'HOMME, J., AND BROUET, J., 1976, Surface cell markers in human lymphoid malignancies, *Recent Results Cancer Res.* **56**:91.

SETLOW, R., 1978, Repair deficient human disorders and cancer, *Nature (London)* **271**:713.

SHAW, M. W., 1970, Human chromosome damage by chemical agents, *Annu. Rev. Med.* **21**:409.

SIDEBOTTOM, E., 1976, The contribution of cell fusion studies to the analysis of neoplasia, in: *Scientific Foundations of Oncology* (T. Symington and R. Carter, eds.), pp. 36–44, Heinemann, London.

SIEBER, S., AND ADAMSON, R., 1975, Toxicity of antineoplastic agents in man: Chromosomal aberrations, antifertility effects, congenital malformations and carcinogenic potential, *Adv. Cancer Res.* **22**:57.

SIEGAL, E., AND GOOD, R., 1977, Human lymphocyte differentiation markers and their application to immune deficiency and lymphoproliferative diseases, *Clin. Hematol.* **6**:355.

SOKAL, G., MICHAUX, J., VAN DEN BERGHE, H., CORDIER, A., RODHAIN, J., FERRANT, A., MORIAU, M., DEBRUYERE, M., AND SONNET, J., 1975, A new hematologic syndrome with a distinct karyotype: The 5q chromosome, *Blood* **46**:519.

SOKOVA, O., VOLGAREVA, G., AND POGOSIANTZ, H., 1976, Effect of fluorafur on chromosomes of normal and malignant Djungarian hamster cells, *Genetika* **12**:156.

SONTA, S., AND SANDBERG, A., 1977, Chromosomes and causation of human cancer and leukemia. XXIV. Unusual and complex Ph^1-translocations and their clinical significance, *Blood* **50**:691.

SPRIGGS, A., 1976, Chromosomes in human neoplastic disease, in: *Scientific Foundations of Oncology* (T. Symington and R. Carter, eds.), pp. 147–155, Heinemann, London.

STANBRIDGE, E., 1976, Suppression of malignancy in human cells, *Nature (London)* **260**:17.

SUGIYAMA, T., KURITA, Y., AND NISHIZUKA, Y., 1967, Chromosome abnormality in rat leukemia induced by 7,12-dimethylbenz[α]anthracene, *Science* **158**:1058.

SUTHERLAND, G., 1979, Heritable fragile sites on human chromosomes. II. Distribution, phenotypic effects, and cytogenetics, *Am. J. Hum. Genet.* **31**:136.

SWIFT, M., SHOLMAN, L., PERRY, M., AND CHASE, C., 1976, Malignant neoplasms in the families of patients with ataxia telangiectasia, *Cancer Res.* **36**:209.

SYED, I., 1978, Principles and problems of biological dosimetry, *Appl. Radiol.* **7**:42.

SZULMAN, A., AND SURTI, U., 1978, The syndromes of hydatidiform mole. I. Cytogenetic and morphologic correlations, *Am. J. Obstet. Gynecol.* **131**:665.

TESTA, J., AND ROWLEY, J., 1978, Cytogenetic patterns in acute nonlymphocytic leukemia, *Virchows Arch. B* **29**:65.

THOMAS, E. BRYANT, J., BUCKNER, D., CLIFT, R., FEFER, A., JOHNSON, F., NEIMAN, P., RAMBERG, R., AND STORB, R., 1972, Leukaemic transformation of engrafted human cells *in vivo*, *Lancet* **1**:1310.

TJIO, J., AND LEVAN, A., 1956, The chromosome number of man, *Hereditas* **42**:1.

TODARO, G., GREEN, H., AND SWIFT, M., 1966, Susceptibility of human diploid fibroblast strains to transformation by SV40 virus, *Science* **153**:1252.

TRUJILLO, J. M., AND OHNO, S., 1963, Chromosomal alteration of erythropoietic cells in chronic myeloid leukemia, *Acta Haematol.* **29**:311.

VAN DER RIET-FOX, M., RETIEF, A., AND VAN NIEKERK, W., 1979, Chromosome changes in 17 human neoplasms studied with banding, *Cancer* **44**: 2108.

VON HANSEMANN, D., 1890, Über asymmetrische Zellteilung in Epithelkrebsen und deren biologische Bedeutung, *Virchows Arch. Pathol. Anat. Physiol.* **119**:298.

WALD, N., UPTON, A. C., JENKINS, V. K., AND BORGES, W. H., 1964, Mouse post-irradiation leukemia: Consistent occurrence of an extra and a marker chromosome, *Science* **143**:810.

WEBB, T., AND HARDING, M., 1977, Chromosome complement of SV40 transformation of cells from patients susceptible to malignant disease, *Br. J. Cancer* **36**:583.

WEBER, W., AND NOWELL, P., 1965, Studies on long-lived small lymphocytes in the rhesus monkey and some other mammals, *J. Reticuloendothelial Soc.* **2**:326.

WEBER, W., NOWELL, P., AND HARE, W. C. D., 1965, Chromosome studies of transplanted and a primary canine venereal sarcoma, *J. Natl. Cancer Inst.* **35**:537.

WEINER, F., DALIANIS, T., KLEIN, G., AND HARRIS, H., 1974, Cytogenetic studies on the mechanism of formation of isoantigenic variants in somatic cell hybrids, *J. Natl. Cancer Inst.* **52**:1779.

WHANG, J., FREI, E., TJIO, J. H., CARBONE, P. P., AND BRECHER, G., 1963, The distribution of the Philadelphia chromosome in patients with chronic myelogenous leukemia, *Blood* **22**:664.

WHANG-PENG, J., 1977, Banding in leukemia: Techniques and implications, *J. Natl. Cancer Inst.* **58**:3.

WHANG-PENG, J., GRALNICK, H., KNUTSEN, T., BRERETON, H., CHANG, P., SCHECHTER, G., AND LESSIN, L., 1977, Small F chromosome in myelo- and lymphoproliferative diseases, *Leukemia Res.* **1**:19.

WOODLIFF, H. J., 1971, *Leukemia Cytogenetics*, Lloyd-Luke, London.

WURSTER-HILL, D., WHANG-PENG, J., MCINTYRE, O., HSU, L. F., HIRSCHHORN, K., MODAN, B., PISCIOTTA, A., PIERRE, R., BALCERZAK, S., WEINFIELD, A., AND MURPHY, S., 1976, Cytogenetic studies in polycythemia vera, *Semin. Hematol.* **13**:13.

YOSHIDA, M., MORIWAKI, K., AND MIGITA, S., 1978, Specificity of the deletion of chromosome 15 in mouse plasmacytoma, *J. Natl. Cancer Inst.* **60**:235.

YOSHIDA, T., 1974, Chromosome alteration in the course of serial transplantation of experimental tumors and aging of tumor stemline cells, *Recent Results Cancer Res.* **44**:86.

YUNIS, J., AND RAMSEY, N., 1978, Retinoblastoma and subband deletion of chromosome 13, *Am. J. Dis. Child.* **132**:161.

YUNIS, J., SAWYER, J. R., AND BALL, D. W., 1978, The characterization of high resolution G-banded chromosomes of man, *Chromosoma* **67**:293.

ZANKL, H., AND ZANG, K., 1972, Cytological and cytogenetical studies on brain tumors. IV. Identification of the missing G chromosome in human meningiomas as No. 22 by fluorescence technique, *Humangenetik* **14**:167.

ZUNA, R., AND LEHMAN, J., 1977, Heterogeneity of karyotype and growth potential in simian virus 40-transformed Chinese hamster cell clones, *J. Natl. Cancer Inst.* **58**:1463.

2

Genetics: Animal Tumors

W. E. HESTON

1. Introduction

The development of our knowledge of the role of genes in the physiology and biochemistry of the cell during the past three-quarters of a century has erased any doubt that cancer is in some way genetic. It is inconceivable that anything so closely related to the physiology of the organism and the differentiation of the cell could be otherwise.

During the first decade of the century, Tyzzer, Haaland, Loeb, Murray, and Bashford had individually observed in mice that mammary cancer, the one so easily observed, occurred in certain families more than in others. Bashford (1909) and Murray (1911) kept pedigrees of their mice and noted that females in whose ancestry mammary cancer occurred not further back than grandmothers were more liable to develop cancer than those in whose ancestry it was more remote. During the second decade, Slye (1926) collected extensive pedigree data on her mice. She appears to have been motivated by the hope of demonstrating a simple mode of inheritance and the possibility of eradicating cancer through eugenics. Indeed, she concluded from her early data that cancer was inherited as a simple recessive gene. During subsequent decades, the problem of cancer has not been solved by eugenics, but genetics has had a very significant role in our continuing search for a complete understanding of the disease.

Genetics has given us the inbred strains with which to do cancer research. Genetics has helped us to understand that cancer is not a single disease but a group of different diseases, separate entities genetically. Genetics has contributed to our appreciation of the complexity of the problem, for few cancers are inherited as single genes; in fact, in the mouse most have been shown to behave as threshold characters influenced by multiple genetic and nongenetic factors. Genetics has

W. E. HESTON ● Laboratory of Biology, National Cancer Institute, National Institutes of Health, Bethesda, Maryland.

integrated the approaches to the problem, for each approach has had to take into account the genetic elements. The genetics of cancer has thus evolved as an integral part of all cancer research, helping us to understand the occurrence and nature of cancer, supplying us with the proper genetic material for the research, establishing the foundation for the immunological and immunogenetic studies of cancer, and leading to the identification of some of the cancer viruses. A major role in the immediate future will be in advancing our understanding of the transmission of these viruses.

2. Speciation and Tumor Formation

If the occurrence of cancer, even a specific kind of cancer, is influenced by genes, one would expect that in the course of evolution there would be established certain gene patterns which would tend to produce specific kinds of tumors in the different species. This has occurred. Tumors have been observed in practically all species of multicellular animals. Even plants have neoplasms, as any naturalist can tell you who has walked among the spruce trees on Mt. Desert Island in Maine and observed their huge tumors. It is particularly significant that some form of tumor occurs in the most lowly multicellular organism with little normal cell differentiation. This indicates that the basic neoplastic change involves a very primitive physiological process.

2.1. Invertebrates

Without becoming involved in the question of how far back in phylogeny one can rightfully call disorganized growth a true neoplasm, it can be accepted that such uncontrolled growth does occur, and from it certain basic information on neoplasia can be gained.

Neoplasms have not been described in sponges, possibly because they cannot be recognized in the primitive growth and differentiation of these forms, but abnormal growth structures do occur in the diploblastic coelenterates. Many who have worked with *Hydra* have observed the phenomenon described by Brien (1961). *Hydra pirardi* goes into a sexual phase when cultured at low temperatures, developing testes and ovaries. If the temperature is then raised, the testes involute and in their place sprouts of disorganized heads and other parts of the *Hydra* occur. This has sometimes been compared with teratogenesis in man, where a higher incidence of teratomas has occurred in undescended testes maintained at higher temperatures than that of the testes in the scrotal sac. It is also inconceivable that some of the genes of this primitive animal are not involved in the occurrence of these growths. Could these genetic mechanisms be comparable in some way to those controlling the occurrence of the genetic teratomas of the testes of strain 129 mice studied extensively by Stevens (1970)? If segregating differences could be demonstrated in *Hydra*, they might be analyzed more easily there than in the more complex mammal.

Higher up the evolutionary scale, spontaneous tumors have been described by

Lange (1966) in two species of *Planaria*. These apparently are derived from the
neoplasts, and they grow progressively and lead to lysis of the host. Tumors
induced with carcinogens in other species of *Planaria* are also derived from this
cell type (Foster, 1969), suggesting that in this lower organism any gene action
involved may well be the same for the spontaneous and the induced neoplasms.
Cooper (1969) believes that the earthworm may be an excellent species for
investigating primitive neoplastic processes. Myoblastomas occur in *Lumbricus*
spontaneously. They can be transplanted and studied immunologically. Fontaine
(1969) has described in the echinoderm *Ophiocomina nigra* a pigmental tumor the
growth and invasiveness of which suggest that it may be a true neoplasm.
Neoplasms have been described in mollusks, but as Pauley (1969) points out in his
review of these lesions, it is difficult to distinguish among neoplasia, hyperplasia,
and injury response in them. These and other examples that could be given
indicate that these primitive species of invertebrates can inherit genes that not
only cause abnormal growths that in many cases could be called neoplasms, but
also determine the type of neoplasm and the cell of origin.

It is in the insects where we first encounter significant genetic studies of
neoplasia. Tumors or tumorlike lesions have been observed in crustaceans and
have been studied in the cockroach, but the tumor that has received greatest
genetic attention in the arthropods has been the small melanoma in *Drosophila*.
This is not because it is a highly progressed neoplasm—in fact, there are those who
still doubt that it is a true neoplasm—but it happens to occur in a species long a
model for genetic studies. The tumors appear in the late larvae as rounded masses
of cells that become surrounded by shells of melanin. They are transplantable but
apparently not malignant, since they do not kill the host, probably because
pupation stops their growth.

These tumors in *Drosophila* were first described by Bridges (1916) as being
inherited as sex-linked lethals in a stock designated as $l(1)7$. Russell (1940) later
attributed the lethality in this stock to an accompanying abnormality of the gut
causing complete obliteration of the lumen so that the larvae die of starvation. She
concluded that all the melanotic tumors in *Drosophila* were similar and that none
was malignant. Russell's (1942) genetic analysis showed that the tumor factor in
the *tu-36a* strain was located on chromosome II with modifiers on I and III.
Hartung (1950) in his analysis of the inbred strain *bu tu* confirmed the presence of
a recessive tumor factor on chromosome II and estimated the locus at 83.9. There
was limited penetrance, however, in that his strain although inbred had a tumor
incidence of only 40%. Nongenetic factors such as temperature, nutrition, and
crowding could affect the incidence.

Some investigators have discounted the value of studies on these tumors since it
can be questioned whether they represent true neoplasms. However, Burdette
(1951) has found them of value in his attempted correlation between carcinogenesis and mutagenesis, since tests for both can be made in the same
organism.

An inherited abnormality designated as "tumorous head" has been described in
Drosophila (Gardner and Woolf, 1949; Gardner, 1959). The trait is caused by two

interacting genes, *tu-1* on chromosome I and *tu-3* on chromosome III. Expression is influenced by modifying genes and also by temperature. Reciprocal crosses have revealed a maternal effect controlled by *tu-1*. There is no genetic relationship between tumorous head and the internal malanotic tumors, and there is no evidence that these irregular growths of the head are neoplastic.

2.2. Vertebrates

There is equal evidence among the vertebrates as among the invertebrates that in the evolution of the species certain gene complexes have been sorted out to give rise to specific tumors in specific species. This has been confirmed in the development of the inbred strains of mice and rats, where man has hastened selection of such gene patterns, as will be discussed later. Along with this process, oncogenic viruses have also been selected, and these or at least most of them have undoubtedly been transmitted genetically.

The melanoma of the platyfish–swordtail hybrid offers clear evidence of such selection of tumor genes. This neoplasm results from a complex of genes, some of which are contributed by each of the parent species. The genetics of this tumor will be discussed in a subsequent section along with that of other tumors resulting from hybridization.

Other tumors possibly also of genetic origin occur in fish. Schlumberger (1952) extensively studied a colonly of goldfish in the lily pond in front of the Art Museum on the campus of Case-Western Reserve University in Cleveland, Ohio, because these fish had a high incidence of neurilemomas and neurofibromas. It would appear that these neoplasms were due to genes or oncogenic viruses selected not only in this species but in this specific colony. No exogenous carcinogen could be identified, and bluegills and largemouthed black bass in the pool did not have these neoplasms. Recently, attention has been focused on the epidemic of hepatomas in rainbow trout from fish hatcheries (Halver and Mitchell, 1967). While it is now well established that these hepatomas were caused by aflatoxin contamination in the food, the fact that, in contrast to the highly susceptible rainbow trout, channel catfish were very resistant and coho salmon intermediate indicated the influence of genetic factors (Halver, 1969; Halver *et al.*, 1969).

Among the amphibians, attention has been focused on the Lucké adenocarcinoma of the kidney of leopard frogs, reviewed by Mizell (1969). This occurs naturally in a high proportion of frogs from certain geographical areas. Present evidence indicates that it is caused by a herpes-type virus, but the geographical restriction (McKinnell, 1969) suggests that genes for susceptibility are isolated in animals of those areas. The fact that in man herpes viruses appear to be associated with Burkitt's lymphoma and in chickens with Mareck's disease further suggests the establishment in the leopard frog of a gene complex limiting the neoplastic action of the virus to the kidney. Also, the viral information may yet be shown to be transmitted genetically in this species.

The predominant tumors of the domestic fowl belong to the group of lymphomas and related neoplasms caused by the avian tumor viruses. These neoplasms have been a model for extensive, fruitful genetic studies integrated with studies of the viruses. In his summary of work in this area, Payne (1972) points out that host genes, sometimes single loci, have been identified which control virus infection, neoplastic transformation of the infected cell, and progressive growth of the neoplasm. There is also evidence of integration of this viral genetic material with the genome of the host, a discussion of which is beyond the scope of this chapter.

Schlumberger (1954) reported a large number of spontaneous chromophobe adenomas of the hypophysis in parakeets. No etiological factors were identified. If a virus was involved, it was not transmitted in unsuccessful attempts to transplant the neoplasm. Schlumberger pointed out that he had no evidence of a genetic factor in the induction of the tumors, yet the fact that this appears to be the most frequently occurring tumor in this species and that it occurs in this species probably more frequently that in any other species would certainly suggest that in the evolution of the parakeet a certain genetic complex favoring the development of this neoplasm had been established.

Progressing to mammals, certain tumors characteristic of species stand out. The tumor most often found in cattle surprisingly is not a mammary tumor—neoplasms of the udder are rare—but rather the ocular squamous carcinoma commonly known as "cancer eye." This is of great economic importance for the ranchers of the southwestern states with Hereford herds. From 3 to 10% of the animals must be removed each year because of the disease. Etiological agents include both nongenetic factors, particularly sunlight, and genetic factors. The genetic factors are of two groups, those controlling the amount of pigment of the eyelid—the greater the amount of pigment the less chance for cancer when it involves the eyelid—and those controlling susceptibility (Anderson, 1959). The gene loci for susceptibility and the loci for pigmentation do not appear to be the same. Although the possibility of a viral factor in the etiology is presently stressed in approaches to control of the disease, breeding systems have been outlined which undoubtedly would eliminate it (J. L. Lush, personal communication). However, it has been difficult to get a rancher to follow these breeding systems. He hesitates to eliminate a bull for which he may have paid several thousand dollars.

As the most typical tumor of the rat, one would probably have to name the induced sarcoma, although many other tumors can be induced. *Induced* denotes action of a carcinogen, but the fact that these sarcomas are so easily induced indicates the establishment of certain genetic complexes for susceptibility in this species.

Most striking about guinea pigs is their apparent resistance to neoplasms. Rogers (1951), who kept guinea pigs to very old age, observed a few spontaneous tumors, but they are rare in this species. It is interesting to speculate that this resistance may be the result of artificial genetic drift. From what one can ascertain, laboratory stocks of guinea pigs in this country were derived from European stocks, but it seems highly likely that they were originally derived from a relatively few animals brought from their native South America.

Lung tumors and subcutaneous tumors can be induced with the polycyclic hydrocarbons in guinea pigs, but unlike those in other species most of the induced subcutaneous tumors are liposarcomas (Shimkin and Mider, 1941; Russell and Ortega, 1952; Heston and Deringer, 1952b). This is a genetic characteristic of the guinea pig.

The widest spectrum of tumors outside the human species occurs in the laboratory mouse, undoubtedly because of the multitude of inbred strains in which genes for specific kinds of neoplasms have been purposely or unintentionally selected. This has led to the mouse being used more extensively in cancer research than any other species, which in turn has led to description of more tumors in the species (see Heston, 1960). When all strains are considered, probably leukemia and other reticulum cell neoplasms are the most prevalent tumors of the mouse. It appears now that C-type viruses are involved in the etiology of most of these neoplasms, but they are transmitted vertically, apparently as genes are transmitted, and thus may have become fixed during the evolution of the species much as gene complexes are fixed.

3. Hybridization and Tumor Formation

3.1. Hybridization of Species

Since cancer must be a negative selective factor in the evolution of species, there must have been some selection against certain complexes of genes or genes and viruses favoring the development of cancer which could be restored through hybridization of species. That this has in fact occurred is beautifully illustrated in the melanomas of platyfish–swordtail hybrids extensively studied by Gordon (1958).

The melanomas of these small fish result from stimulation of macromelanophores by certain modifying genes. The neoplasms are so invasive that it is hard to conceive of a species surviving with them. The platyfish (*Xiphophorus maculatus*) that Gordon collected in southeastern Mexico had the macromelanophores, which he showed are controlled by five dominant sex-linked genes, but within this species these cells do not become neoplastic. Of 9000 adults collected, 1879 had macromelanophores but in not one had they progressed to melanoma. The swordtail (*Xiphophorus helleri*) has the modifying genes which could cause the malignant change but they are balanced in this species by the recessive allele of the dominant genes for the macromelanophores. When Gordon hybridized the two species, bringing together the genes for the macromalanophores and the modifying genes in the F_1 hybrid, these large pigment cells developed into melanomas. A recent interpretation by Anders *et al.* (1974) is that the melanomas result from a loss in the hybrids of controller genes on chromosomes other than that with the macromelanophore genes.

Gordon also hybridized geographically distinct populations of the platyfish, but in these hybrids progression of the atypical growth was not as great as in the interspecies hybrids, indicating that the modifiers are not as divergent in the isolated populations of the same species as in the different species.

Alleles of the macromelanophore gene established the site of spotting, e.g., dorsal fin spotting or belly spotting. In the outcross, these alleles thus in turn established the location in which the melanoma would develop.

Melanin itself was not an important factor in the neoplastic process. When platyfish with macromelanophores were outcrossed to albino swordtails, the hybrids developed melanotic melanomas, but when these hybrids with melanomas were backcrossed to the albino swordtail parent, some of the backcross hybrids developed amelanotic melanomas. These had certain cellular characteristics of even a higher degree of malignancy than the pigmented neoplasms.

Diagnosis of malignancy was justified in that these melanomas eventually led to the death of the fish. However, transplantation was not possible because the fish were not inbred. Tissue culture of the melanotic tumors could be maintained, providing systems for biochemical studies of this form of neoplasia (Grand *et al.*, 1941).

Little (1939) recorded an increase in tumors resulting from hybridization of mammalian species. When he crossed the common laboratory mouse, *Mus musculus*, of strain C57BL, with the little Asiatic mouse, *Mus bactrianus*, he observed a higher incidence and greater variety of tumors in the F_1 than in either the C57BL strain or the stock of the small Asiatic species. Whereas nonepithelial tumors occurred in none of the *Mus bactrianus* mice and in only 13% of the C57BL, they occurred in 40% of the F_1 hybrids. Furthermore, multiple tumors were found more frequently in the F_1 hybrids.

3.2. Hybridization of Strains

Anyone who has hybridized inbred strains of mice and observed the F_1 generation for occurrence of tumors generally has found not only a higher incidence of tumors but also a greater variety of tumors in the F_1 than in either parent strain. This can be the result of bringing together more genes favoring tumor development, introduction of specific genes having a general positive effect on tumor development, or even production of new virus–gene combinations that cause tumors. In a cross between strains C3HfB (then called C3Hb) and C57BL, we noted a greater variety of tumors in the F_1 than in either parent strain, including some tumors not found in either strain (Heston and Deringer, 1952a). Yellow F_1 mice resulting from crossing various strains with the low tumor strain YBR usually had more tumors than either parent strain because of the A^y gene introduced from YBR (Heston and Vlahakis, 1961). When one crosses strain BALB/c with a strain having a medium incidence of mammary tumors and having the mammary tumor virus (MTV), the resultant F_1 has a higher mammary tumor incidence than either parent strain because of combining the high genetic susceptibility of BALB/c with the MTV.

Two other reasons, both of which are basically genetic, for an increase of tumors in the F_1 are that F_1 mice tend to grow faster and live longer than either parent strain. Both of these factors tend to increase tumor incidence and a greater variety of tumors.

It is interesting to speculate whether hybridization in the people of the United States, in contrast to the more homogeneous populations of other countries, may have increased the occurrence of certain cancers. While this possibility exists, the degree of hybrid effect in the people of the United States cannot be expected to be comparable to that in a cross between two inbred strains of mice.

4. Inbreeding and Occurrence of Tumors

4.1. Development of Inbred Strains

With the early research on effects of inbreeding, from which Johannsen in 1903 postulated his pure-line theory as background, C. C. Little as early as 1909 could foresee that to make an adequate study of tumors genetically or otherwise it would be necessary to have genetically controlled strains of experimental animals. It was in that year that he started inbreeding strain DBA mice. Inbreeding increases the percentage of gene pairs that are homozygous, the rate of increase depending on the mating system used. An inbred strain has been defined as one in which brother and sister inbreeding has been performed for 20 or more generations. With that number of inbred generations, the percentage of homozygous genes would theoretically exceed 99%.

Origins and relationships of the inbred strains are of importance. In 1921, Little started the C57 strains and strain C58 from mice received from Miss Lathrop. Two females, 57 and 58, were mated to littermate male 52. Offspring from female 57 segregated as black and brown, and these segregants when inbred gave rise to strains C57BL and C57BR. Strain C57L was derived from a leaden mutation that later arose in C57BR. MacDowell inbred the offspring of female 58, developing strain C58.

A second family of strains is that derived from strain DBA that Little had started from a stock with the three coat color mutations dilution (*d*), brown (*b*), and nonagouti (*a*) and from the Bagg albino mice. Dr. Halsey Bagg started the Bagg albinos from some albino mice he obtained in 1913 from a dealer in Ohio. In 1920, Dr. L. C. Strong crossed the Bagg albinos with Little's strain DBA and from the hybrids inbred several strains including the well-known C3H and CBA. In 1921, Strong crossed a Bagg albino mouse with one from an albino stock that Little had and from these hybrids inbred strain A. About a year later, MacDowell started inbreeding some Bagg albinos, giving rise to strain BALB/c.

Other strains have been derived elsewhere such as two originated in Europe, RIII started by Dr. Dobrovolskaia-Zavadskaia and GR inbred more recently by Mühlbock, but the major part of cancer research throughout the world has been done with mice of these two families of strains that were started in the first quarter

of the century by Little and by Strong. Since then, many geneticists have
contributed to the inbreeding of these strains, developing the various sublines we
have today, but the origins of the strains have continued to be of extreme
importance in understanding observations made on them.

55
GENETICS:
ANIMAL
TUMORS

4.2. Tumor Characteristics of Inbred Strains of Mice

Certain of these strains were developed as high tumor strains not as a result of the
inbreeding *per se* but by the selection during inbreeding of susceptibility genes and
related oncogenic viruses. Little selected for mammary tumors in strain DBA, but
the Bagg albinos also must have had susceptibility genes and the mammary tumor
virus (MTV), for strain BAGG was a high mammary tumor strain, as was strain A.
In the process of inbreeding strain BALB/c from the Bagg albinos, the virus must
have been lost, for BALB/c has the susceptibility genes but not the MTV. It was
also from the DBA and Bagg albino source that C3H received susceptibility genes
and the MTV. Probably all lines of MTV have come from this narrow source
except the lines in strains RIII, GR, and DD, which may be a third family of strains.
Although strain DD was developed in Japan, it originally came from Central
Europe, where RIII and GR were derived, and all three have the same coat color
genes and all develop premalignant hormone-responsive plaques from which at
least some of their mammary tumors originate. In contrast, in the American-
derived strains the mammary tumors appear to originate in hyperplastic nodules.

The DBA–Bagg albino family also contains the high lung tumor strains A and
BALB/c and the high hepatoma strains C3H and CBA. Selection for these tumors
was done without anyone being aware of it, for these strains were discovered as
being high lung tumor and high hepatoma strains after they were inbred.

Except for C58, which is a high leukemia strain, the strains in the Lathrop
family of strains have generally been used as low tumor strains. It is interesting,
however, that all the C57 strains related to the high leukemia strain C58 have a
relatively high incidence of other reticulum cell neoplasms.

4.3. Role of Inbred Strains and Their Hybrids in Cancer Research

These inbred strains of mice, and to a lesser degree inbred strains of rats, guinea
pigs, and now rabbits, hamsters, and chickens, have supplied the tumors for basic
cancer research. They also have supplied groups of experimental animals that are
genetically identical in which response is uniform and from which repeatable
results can be obtained with smaller numbers.

Wide use has likewise been made of the F_1 hybrid between two inbred strains.
Like animals of the parent inbred strains, the F_1 hybrids are genetically uniform,
although heterogeneity occurs with any further matings. There are several
advantages offered by the F_1. Deleterious genes tend to be recessive but their
effects are often suppressed in the F_1, resulting in more vigorous, longer-lived
animals than those of either parental inbred strain. Furthermore, by proper

choice of parental strains, one can get many desirable gene–gene, gene–virus, or gene–absence of virus combinations. Today, there are approximately 200 inbred strains of mice, and from 200 one could get 39,800 kinds of reciprocal hybrids. In addition, by systems of backcross matings, as Snell (1958) originally demonstrated, isogenic lines can be developed. These are two lines of an inbred strain that differ only at one gene locus and possibly closely linked loci. If the concept of an oncogene or provirus proves to be a reality with respect to oncogenic viruses, it presumably will be possible through a similar mating system to develop two lines exactly alike except that one has the genetically transmitted virus and the other does not. In all these ways, genetics has amply provided the animal material with which to do cancer research.

5. Genetics of Spontaneous Tumors

5.1. The Threshold Concept in the Inheritance of Cancer

The development of the inbred strains in itself yielded significant data on the inheritance of cancer. The fact that through inbreeding with selection strains were produced that developed specific kinds of cancer of specific incidences generation after generation was good evidence that genes were involved. We have since come to realize that in addition to genes certain viruses also were selected, the most recent concept being that they were selected as a segment of the host genome—the provirus as conceived by Bentvelzen (1972) or the oncogene as conceived by Huebner (see Huebner and Gilden, 1972).

Of special significance was the fact that the incidence of a specific kind of spontaneous tumor in an inbred strain, although relatively constant from generation to generation, usually fell someplace between zero and 100%. At the time, the genetics of lung tumors in the mouse was being studied extensively (Lynch, 1940; Heston, 1942a, b); the incidence in strain A was 90% instead of 100% and the incidence in strains C57BL and C57L was less than 5% but not zero. Yet the incidence in BALB/c was 20% and the incidence in Lynch's SWR was approximately 40%. The same picture prevailed even when a virus was involved, as in mammary tumors in the mouse.

In this regard, tumors fell in line with other so-called threshold characters. In working with otocephaly and polydactyly in inbred strains of guinea pigs, Wright (1934a, b) had first described this kind of character as one influenced by multiple genetic and nongenetic factors, the character appearing when the total effect of these factors surpassed certain physiological thresholds. The factors leading to the occurrence of such a trait can encompass inherited genes, inherited or introduced viruses, endogenous or exogenous hormones, physical or chemical carcinogens, or even ordinary nutritional factors. Deficiencies in one set of factors can be overcome by introduction of others. Time can be a factor, and thus latency as well as incidence can be a measure of response.

But what is this threshold? Obviously, it is the neoplastic change in the cell, and in certain tumors where there are well-defined preneoplastic stages there is more than one threshold. Early attempts to define this change or these changes gave birth to the somatic mutation hypothesis, the concept that the malignant change involves a mutation in the genetic material of the somatic cell. No hypothesis concerning cancer has through the years stimulated more discussion than this one, and in the end resolution depends on just how one defines mutation, but some change in the genetic material of the cell is indicated.

In the past, approaches to confirmation of the hypothesis had to be indirect, because it was not possible to hybridize somatic cells. One approach was to look for a positive correlation between mutagenicity and carcinogenicity, and within certain limits there was a positive correlation. The alkylating agents that were shown to induce mutations in *Drosophila* (Auerbach, 1949) induced lung tumors in mice when injected intravenously or inhaled and induced sarcomas when injected subcutaneously (Heston, 1953). But a detailed review by Burdette (1955) of data on all agents tested for mutagenicity and carcinogenicity did not establish a 100% positive correlation. Burdette tested for both carcinogenicity and mutagenicity in *Drosophila* using the induction of the melanomas as his measure of carcinogenicity and the induction of lethal mutations in the special stocks as his measure of mutagenicity. Even these tests in the same species did not give an absolute answer, and the plaguing question was whether these melanomas in *Drosophila* are true neoplasms. Yet the hypothesis continued to stimulate research. For example, when it was shown that increased oxygen increased the mutation rate in lower organisms, strain A mice were exposed to various oxygen levels. It was found that oxygen concentration greater than that in air increased the number of methylcholanthrene-induced lung tumors and concentrations less than that of air decreased the number (Heston and Pratt, 1959).

Another approach to information relative to the somatic mutation hypothesis has been through an analysis of the dose–response curve in induced tumors. In their analysis of the number of papillomas induced in mice with repeated paintings with benzpyrene, Charles and Luce-Clauson (1942) noted a linear relationship between the square root of the number of papillomas and the elapsed time, which would be proportional to the cumulative dose of carcinogen. This indicates the necessity of two events in the neoplastic change, which would be expected with a recessive gene mutation. In contrast, Heston and Schneiderman (1953) observed a straight-line relationship between the number of induced pulmonary tumors in mice and the dose of the carcinogen dibenz[*a*,*h*]anthracene above a certain low threshold. This indicated the necessity of only a single event, which if a gene mutation would be dominant.

Today the somatic mutation hypothesis is finding supporting evidence in viral carcinogenesis. It is generally assumed that in the cell neoplastically transformed by a DNA virus the viral genetic material has been integrated in the cell genome as a provirus. Furthermore, it now appears that with the recently demonstrated

RNA-dependent DNA polymerase DNA copies of RNA oncornaviruses are made which then serve as a template for further RNA synthesis, resulting in the neoplastic conversion. It is suggested that this synthesized DNA provirus is integrated in the host genome. Bentvelzen and Daams (1972) have pointed out that this would be a form of somatic mutation, a concept suggested earlier but without the present substantiating evidence (Heston, 1963).

6. Genetics of Chemically Induced Tumors

6.1. Pulmonary Tumors in Mice

Chemically induced pulmonary tumors of the mouse offered a great advantage for genetic analysis in that by counting the induced nodules one obtained a quantitative measure of response. Responses measured in this way of susceptible strain A and resistant strain C57L and their hybrids to intravenous injection of dibenz[a,h]anthracene were typical of characters with multiple-factor quantitative inheritance (Heston, 1942a). F_1 hybrids were intermediate between the parent strains, as were the F_2s, but the distribution curve of the F_2 showed a greater spread than that of the F_1, indicating segregation of genes. From a comparison of the variance of the F_2 with that of the F_1, it was estimated that the parent strains differed by at least four pairs of genes controlling susceptibility.

An analysis of the genetics of induced pulmonary tumors was then made using latent period as a measure of response, and again the results indicated multiple gene inheritance. Then the carcinogen was omitted and response was measured in incidence and latent period. The results indicated that spontaneous pulmonary tumors, like the induced tumors, were controlled by multiple genes (Heston, 1942b).

One advantage in working with the induced pulmonary tumors was that the latent period was greatly reduced, which along with the quantitative measure of response has greatly facilitated linkage studies. Lethal yellow (A^y) on chromosome 1 was associated with an increase in lung tumors. Vestigial tail (vt), shaker-2 (sh-2), and waved-2 (w-2) on chromosome 11, obese (ob) on chromosome 6, flexed-tail (f) on chromosome 13, hairless (hr) on chromosome 14, and fused (fu) on chromosome 17 all were associated with a decrease in lung tumors. Dwarf (dw) inhibited lung tumors (Heston, 1957; Burdette, 1952). It would appear, however, that these results represented the effect of the genes themselves rather than true linkage, that they were in some way related to the effect of the genes on normal growth. Each gene affected normal growth in the same direction as it affected the number of induced tumors, or in the case of spontaneous tumors the incidence of tumors.

Tatchell (1961) obtained similar results in her test for linkage with the genes wa-2, sh-2, and vt on chromsome 11. She interpreted her results as indicating true linkage with a tumor gene that she designated as tu. Her observations, however, were based on coupling data and were not confirmed by repulsion data. From results of crosses between strains A and C57BL, Bloom and Falconer (1964) postulated a pulmonary tumor resistant gene *ptr*, but this proposed gene has not been located in a linkage group.

6.2. Subcutaneous Sarcomas in Mice

In general, the genetics of chemically induced subcutaneous sarcomas in mice is similar to that of pulmonary tumors. The fact that the inbred strains differed in their response to subcutaneous injection of a carcinogen indicated the influence of genetic factors. Andervont (1938) mated susceptible strain C3H with resistant strains I and Y and noted that the susceptibility of the F_1 hybrids to induced subcutaneous tumors was intermediate between that of the parent strains. He concluded that if there were genetic factors involved they probably were multiple. Later, Burdette (1943) measured the susceptibility of strains C3H and JK mice and their F_1 hybrids to methylcholanthrene-induced subcutaneous sarcomas and observed that the F_1s were intermediate between the susceptible C3H and the resistant JK. He concluded that these observations were compatible with the existence of more than one gene controlling susceptibility, at least one of which was dominant and at least one recessive.

6.3. Selection of Appropriate Strain for Testing Carcinogens

This concept of multiple-factor inheritance involving a threshold assists in the selection of the genetically appropriate strain for testing a suspected carcinogen. Any population of experimental animals when plotted according to the total genetic and nongenetic susceptibility factors of each would have a bell-shaped distribution, with a few relatively susceptible animals, a few relatively resistant animals, and most of the animals in between these extremes. For the inbred strain with reduced genetic variation, this distribution would be narrowed. With constant nongenetic factors, the genotype of the inbred strain would determine the tumor incidence by determining where this distribution fell with respect to the tumor threshold. The role of the carcinogen could be viewed as that of shifting the distribution of the population to the right, bringing a greater percentage of the individuals beyond the threshold and thus increasing the incidence of tumors. When the genetic susceptibility of the strain is relatively weak so that only the outer edge of the bell-shaped distribution is beyond the threshold, the shift in this distribution by a carcinogen, especially if it is a weak carcinogen, may not bring enough of the whole population beyond the threshold to make a significant increase in incidence. When the genetic susceptibility is very strong so that all except the lower tail of the distribution is above the threshold, the shift in the population by the same carcinogen also may not make a significant change in incidence. However, when the genetic susceptibility of the strain approximately equally distributes the population above and below the threshold the same shift to the right in the population distribution by this carcinogen will bring a much greater portion of the total population beyond the threshold, giving a significant increase in tumor incidence. Thus the appropriate inbred strain for testing whether a substance is carcinogenic is neither one that has a high genetic susceptibility nor one that has a low genetic susceptibility but a strain with an intermediate susceptibility.

Carbon tetrachloride could not be shown to be carcinogenic in C3H mice. In this highly susceptible strain, it did not increase the occurrence of hepatomas above the spontaneous incidence. Its hepatic carcinogenicity was discovered in the less susceptible strain A. Dibenz[a,h]anthracene probably would not have been shown to be carcinogenic for pulmonary tumors had it been tested only in the genetically very resistant strain C57L. Only a very long time after administration of the carcinogen did any pulmonary tumors appear, and then they were so few and so small that they would have been overlooked in a casual examination. Yet the same dose of dibenz[a,h]anthracene induces multiple lung tumors in 100% of the more susceptible strain BALB/c mice.

A carcinogen should not be considered only as a substance that will induce tumors in a strain of mouse that otherwise never gets tumors. Such a strain in which a certain kind of tumor never occurs is probably nonexistent. Furthermore, by selecting very resistant strains one would probably miss many potential carcinogens. The aim in carcinogenic testing is to ascertain whether or not the substance to be tested will cause tumors to arise in any animals that would not have gotten them without the substance.

With the bell-shaped distribution in mind, one can visualize the argument for using an inbred strain rather than a heterogeneous population of test animals. The object is not to duplicate the heterogeneous population of human beings but to get an established, repeatable result. This can be done best by selecting an inbred strain the distribution of which falls in proper relation to the threshold so that an increase in tumors can be noted. Since it is inbred, with a narrower distribution, a significant increase in incidence can be shown with fewer animals, and since the inbred strain is genetically uniform the result is repeatable.

Of course, the results of testing for carcinogenesis in an inbred strain of mice or rats cannot necessarily be applied to a particular human being. Results of testing in one human being might not be applicable to a second human being, for they would probably differ in genetic susceptibility. If a substance can be shown to be carcinogenic in a mammal such as the mouse or rat, it is highly probable that some human beings would have the degree of susceptibility for the substance to induce tumors in them. It is these susceptible individuals about whom we are concerned.

7. Genetics of Hormonally Induced Tumors

7.1. Mammary Tumors

Even before the discovery of the mammary tumor virus, it was known that hormones were influential in the induction of mammary tumors in mice. Castration reduced the occurrence of mammary tumors in female mice, and stilbestrol induced mammary tumors in castrated males. In practically all mouse strains, parity increased the incidence of mammary tumors or lowered the tumor age in proportion to the number of litters born.

This effect of parity was much more noticeable in strains with a median susceptibility than in either the very susceptible or the very resistant strains. Both breeding and virgin females of the highly susceptible strain C3H have a mammary tumor incidence of 100%, but the tumors arise about 2 months later in the virgins than in the breeders. But in strain C3HfB, with a lower mammary tumor incidence because of the absence of the milk-borne MTV, the incidence is significantly higher in breeders than in virgins. In the highly resistant strain C57BL, in which few mammary tumors occur, breeding does not significantly increase their occurrence. Yet in strain A, in which with MTV the incidence in breeders is around 70%, the incidence in virgins is about 5 or 10%.

In reciprocal crosses between the highly susceptible strain C3H, in which the effect of parity was expressed only as a 2-months' difference in tumor age, and strain A, in which parity greatly increased the mammary tumor incidence, both groups of F_1 females had a high mammary tumor incidence (Bittner et al., 1944; Heston and Andervont, 1944). This indicated that the difference in effect of parity of these two strains was basically a genetic difference that could be expressed through control over hormonal production or over response of the mammary cell to hormonal stimulation. The fact that both conditions prevailed was evident from results of Huseby and Bittner (1948), who transplanted ovaries between the parent strains C3H and A and their F_1 hybrids. Spayed (C3H × A)F_1 females bearing C3H and (C3H × A) F_1 transplanted ovaries had a higher tumor incidence than did those F_1 females with A ovaries, suggesting, since the hosts were the same and the ovaries were different, that genic action was controlling amount of hormone produced by the ovary. However, F_1 females bearing A ovaries had a higher tumor incidence than spayed A females bearing transplanted A ovaries, indicating that some genic action was controlling response of the mammary cell to the hormonal stimulation from the ovary since in this case the ovaries were the same but the hosts were different.

7.2. Hypophyseal Tumors

The usual tumor of the hypophysis of the mouse is the chromophobe adenoma, and it occurs rarely except in the C57 strains. In a recent tabulation in this laboratory (Heston et al., 1973) of 151 untreated C57BL virgin females, 49 had chromophobe adenomas of the hypophysis and one had a tumor of the pars intermedia.

Prolonged treatment with estrogenic hormones induces these chromophobe adenomas, particularly in the susceptible C57 strains. In the study referred to above, there were 149 C57BL females continuously fed the antifertility drug Enovid, which contains estrogen, and of these 89 developed chromophobe adenomas, a significant increase over the untreated mice. Yet the Enovid did not produce a significant increase in the other four strains used in the study.

Gardner and Strong (1940) had observed induction of hypophyseal tumors in C57BL mice with prolonged estrogen treatment but not in strains A, C3H, CBA, C12I, N, and JK similarly treated. When Gardner (1954) crossed C57BL with the resistant strains CBA and C3H, he observed a high incidence in the estrogen-treated F_1 hybrids approaching that in the C57BL, and this high incidence was maintained in the backcross generation of the F_1 to the C57BL, but greatly reduced in the backcross to the CBA. Similar results were observed in this laboratory (Heston, unpublished data). The strain differences in occurrence of tumors of the hypophysis suggest the influence of genetic factors on this tumor, and these results from the F_1 and backcross hybrids indicate segregation of such genes.

7.3. Adrenocortical Tumors

Spontaneous adrenocortical tumors occur in the mouse, particularly in certain strains. Accurate incidences were obtained for five strains in a study mentioned above (Heston *et al.*, 1973) in which the adrenals were routinely fixed and sectioned from control virgin females permitted to live their natural life span. Strain BALB/c was the susceptible strain, with these tumors found in 43 of 163 mice. In contrast, one of 55 C3H females and seven of 156 C3HfB females had adrenocortical tumors, but none occurred in 169 strain A and 151 strain C57BL females. Such strain differences indicate the influence of genetic factors.

However, genetic influences have been much more clearly shown in studies by Woolley *et al.* (1941, 1953) on the occurrence of the adrenocortical tumors in various strains of mice by neonatal gonadectomy. The most susceptible strain was CE/Wy, in which all the mice developed adrenocortical carcinomas following early gonadectomy. The adrenal glands of strain DBA/2Wy also responded to early gonadectomy, but the lesion progressed only to hyperplasia of the cortex. With the same treatment, hybrids of the two strains always developed adrenocortical carcinomas, indicating dominance of the carcinoma.

An interesting hybrid effect was noted in some crosses (Dickie, 1954). When strain A/Wy, which showed little change in the adrenal gland following gonadectomy, was crossed with C3H/Di, which responded with nodular hyperplasia, the F_1 hybrids after gonadectomy responded with adrenocortical carcinomas. The same response was also observed in F_1 hybrids between DBA, which responded with nodular hyperplasia, and DE/Wy, which gave little response in the adrenal glands. These results can be compared with those of Gordon (1958) reviewed earlier on the production of melanomas in the platyfish hybrids. It would appear that the neoplastic response of the adrenal gland to neonatal gonadectomy in the mouse was due to multiple genes controlling the degree of response, and in certain crosses genes that were contributed from both parents could result in carcinoma in the hybrid whereas in neither parent strain did progression extend beyond hyperplasia.

8.1. Inheritance of Susceptibility to the Mammary Tumor Virus

Following their development of high and low mammary tumor strains of mice, geneticists made one of the signal discoveries of cancer research—the discovery of the mouse mammary tumor virus. The original observation was made simultaneously by the staff of the Jackson Laboratory (1933), where many of these strains were being inbred, and by Korteweg (1934) at the Netherlands Cancer Institute with strains he had obtained from the Jackson Laboratory. In crossing their high and low strains, both groups had the good fortune to make reciprocal crosses. The observation was that the F_1 females tended to develop mammary cancer when their mothers were of the high tumor strain but not when their fathers were of the high tumor strain. This indicated that some causative factor was being transmitted from the mother, and since the reciprocal F_1 females were genetically identical it had to be some extrachromosomal factor. The sequence of events that followed is well known. Through his foster-nursing experiments, Bittner (1939) showed that this extrachromosomal factor was passed through the milk; he referred to it as the "milk agent." Later, the agent was shown to be filtrable, a particle was seen, and this agent became accepted as a mammary tumor virus which in the mature virion is now referred to as the "B particle."

Evidence that this virus was under genetic control accumulated. It was only in certain strains that this virus replicated and was transmitted well. Strain C3H had the virus and it caused a high mammary tumor incidence, but when the virus was removed by foster-nursing C3H on C57BL, the C3HfB, as it was now designated, had a greatly reduced mammary tumor incidence with an increased latent period, and remained thusly through successive generations. When the virus was reintroduced, the picture in the original C3H was immediately restored. Strain BALB/c did not have the milk-transmitted virus and had a low mammary tumor incidence, but it was obviously genetically susceptible to the virus because when infected with C3H virus BALB/c immediately became a high mammary tumor strain and remained so generation after generation. In contrast, when C3H MTV was introduced into C57BL, although some of the originally infected females developed mammary tumors the virus died out in a generation or two, indicating that C57BL was genetically resistant to it (Andervont, 1945).

Proof that segregating genes did in fact control the replication of the virus came from a hybridization study by Heston *et al.* (1945). High tumor strain C3H females with MTV were mated to low tumor strain C57BL males. The resulting F_1 females, also with MTV which caused a high mammary tumor incidence in them, were then backcrossed on the one hand to strain C3H males and on the other to C57BL males. That the resulting C3H backcross females could replicate and transmit the agent better than the C57BL backcross females was shown by a higher tumor incidence in test females foster-nursed by the C3H backcross females than in the same kind of test females foster-nursed by the C57BL backcross females. This difference in degree of replication and transmission had to be the result of the difference between the C3H genes and the C57BL genes in these two groups of backcross females.

Later studies (Heston *et al.*, 1956) showed that in further backcrosses to the C57BL males the MTV was completely eliminated, and this was done as early as the third backcross generation. This indicated that the virus was controlled by only a few genes and possibly only one. However, a later attempt (Heston, 1960) to show distinct backcross groups segregated as to their ability to transmit MTV failed, indicating that the influencing genes must be multiple.

Another significant observation in these backcross studies was that once the MTV was eliminated by eliminating the susceptibility genes it could not be caused to reappear by then backcrossing to C3H males to reintroduce the susceptibility genes. None of these genes was the more recently described provirus that will be discussed in a later section.

8.2. Inheritance of Susceptibility to Leukemia

In some respects, the genetics of leukemia has paralleled that of mammary tumors. Through selection, high and low leukemia inbred strains of mice were developed. These were then hybridized in attempts to observe patterns of segregation.

Cole and Furth (1941) crossed the high leukemia strain AKR with the low leukemia strain Rf and from the incidences of leukemia in the F_1, F_2, F_3, and backcross generations concluded that leukemia was probably inherited as a multiple-factor character. The common logarithm of the percent leukemia in the various crosses was a simple function of the percent heredity from the AKR strain.

Another attempt to ascertain whether single-gene segregation could be demonstrated in leukemia was carried out by MacDowell *et al.* (1945) in one of the most carefully executed genetic experiments in all of cancer research. The approach was through progeny tests of 50 backcross males that were the progeny of (susceptible C58 × resistant Sto-Li)F_1 females backcrossed to Sto-Li males. The question was whether the incidence of leukemia in the progeny of each of these males would show them to be intrinsically uniform or diverse in regard to the tendency to leukemia. Results showed that the males were diverse. The incidences of leukemia in the 50 backcross families varied from zero to 42.8%, which indicated the segregation of genes. However, instead of the families grouping as would be expected from segregation of a single pair or few pair of genes, the frequency distribution was fairly symmetrical with the modal class as 17–20%. Thus it was apparent that genes were influential in the causation of leukemia but that the number of such genes by which these two strains differed was multiple.

8.3. Genetic Transmission of Tumor Viruses

8.3.1. MuLV

Gross (1951) made cell-free filtrates from leukemic AKR mice and injected them into C3H mice, which later developed leukemia. He then noted that this leukemia

was transmitted from parent to offspring through future generations of the C3H
mice. He referred to this as "vertical" transmission of what experiments later
proved to be a leukemia virus. There was, however, a clear distinction between this
vertical transmission of leukemia and the vertical transmission of the mammary
tumor virus that had been described earlier. The mammary tumor virus known at
that time was transmitted maternally through the milk, but, as Gross rightfully
noted, crosses involving AKR mice had shown that the leukemia was transmitted
by the father as well as by the mother. He therefore considered that this vertical
transmission of leukemia was through the embryo, presumably from the sperm
and egg.

Stimulated by these earlier observations of vertical transmission of leukemia in
mice now recognized as due to C-type RNA virus, Huebner and Todaro (1969)
carried out seroepidemiological and cell culture studies from which they formulated the hypothesis that the cells of most or all vertebrate species have C-type
RNA virus genome. They refer to this viral information as the "virogene," which
would include that portion causing the normal cell to undergo the malignant
transformation which they have termed the "oncogene" (see Huebner and
Gilden, 1972). Physical and chemical carcinogens and other factors associated
with the normal aging process would induce the leukemia through the activation
or derepression of the oncogene. It is this viral information that is inherited,
presumably as an integrated portion of the chromosome. Further discussion of
the genetics of the virus and the mechanisms through which it induces the
neoplasm is found in other chapters of this volume.

Genetic studies of the vertical transmission of the mouse leukemia virus have
been carried out by Rowe and coworkers (Rowe, 1972; Rowe and Hartley, 1972;
Rowe et al., 1972) through hybridization of high and low leukemia mouse strains.
They used the high leukemia strain AKR, in which the virus is normally
transmitted vertically and can be detected readily as appearance of virus infectivity. The bone of the tail was found to be high in virus, providing readily accessible
tissue for viral assay in tissue culture by the technique they describe. The AKR
virus is N-tropic; i.e., it replicates readily in the presence of a gene, $Fv-1^n$ that AKR
carries. Strain AKR was outcrossed to five low leukemia mouse strains, all of which
also carried the $Fv-1^n$ gene so that maximum opportunity should have been
provided for replication of the virus in any hybrids that had inherited the virus
inducing locus or loci which might actually be the viral information. F_1, F_2, and first
and second backcross hybrids were produced and tested for virus in the tails at 2
wk of age and again at 6 wk.

Results with the F_1 hybrids indicated dominant inheritance with high penetrance of the AKR viruses contributed equally well by both sexes. Segregation
ratios of the F_2 and first backcross generations, however, did not show single-gene
or two-gene inheritance, but indicated that the virus resulted from the presence of
either of two independently segregating genes, which initially were labeled V_1 and
V_2. Tests of 19 second backcross generation families indicated that three (or four)
of the first backcross parents carried two virus-inducing loci, 12 (or 13) carried
one, and three carried none. This substantiated the two-locus model indicated by
the F_2 and first backcross generations.

In an attempt to determine if the virus-inducing loci in AKR actually contain MuLV genetic determinants or are genes which promote the expression of the viral information located elsewhere (presumably Huebner's oncogene), strain AKR ($Fv\text{-}1^n$ genotype and with N-tropic virus) was outcrossed to four low leukemia strains of the $Fv\text{-}1^b$ genotype which are sensitive to B-tropic virus and relatively resistant to the N-tropic virus. Since the segregating hybrids could be $Fv\text{-}1^n$, $Fv\text{-}1^{nb}$, and $Fv\text{-}1^b$, one would expect all the hybrids to carry N-tropic AKR MuLV if the virus-inducing loci were genetic elements of the virus itself, whereas virus-positive hybrids should show virus of both parental types if the virus-inducing loci merely promoted the expression of the "oncogene" located elsewhere. The virus identified in the segregating hybrids was almost always of the AKR type, providing evidence that the V_1 and V_2 loci contain MuLV genetic determinants.

By utilization of the markers carried by the various strains, it was demonstrated that one of the virus-inducing loci (V_1) was linked with albinism (c) and the β-chain of hemoglobin locus (Hbb) in linkage group I with the probable gene order V_1–c–Hbb, and with V_1 about 30 units from the c–Hbb region. In a later cross (Rowe *et al.*, 1973) involving the locus for the isozymes of glucose phosphate isomerase ($Gpi\text{-}1$) also in linkage group I, it was established that V_1 is about 12 units from $Gpi\text{-}1$, the order now being V_1–$Gpi\text{-}1$–c–Hbb. Other crosses have now located in linkage group VIII the $Fv\text{-}1$ locus, the major determinant of the sensitivity of mouse cells to infection with naturally occurring MuLV.

8.3.2. MTV

The mouse mammary tumor virus was originally observed to be transmitted through the milk, but over the past 25 years evidence has also been accumulating for genetic transmission of mouse MTV. Strain C3HfB/He, derived in this laboratory in 1945 by foster-nursing caesarean-derived C3H mice on C57BL to remove the milk-transmitted MTV, instead of having no mammary tumors as expected had an incidence among breeding females of approximately 40% (Heston *et al.*, 1950). The tumors in these C3HfB females, however, arose at an average age of 18 months rather than the 7 months observed in the C3H. In contrast to the early crosses between high and low tumor lines in which maternal transmission was demonstrated, when C3HfB was crossed with C57BL no difference in tumor incidence was observed between the reciprocal hybrids, indicating that the factor or factors causing the mammary tumors in C3HfB were transmitted by the male parent as well as by the female parent (Heston and Deringer, 1952*a*).

A line of strain C3HfB was sent to the Cancer Research Genetics Laboratory at Berkeley, and the staff there examined the tumors that arose in the breeding females electron microscopically and in them found B particles indistinguishable from the B particles found in the high tumor strains with milk-transmitted MTV (Pitelka *et al.*, 1964). This indicated that the mammary tumors of C3HfB were also caused by a virus, which was designated as the nodule-inducing virus (NIV) since the C3HfB, like C3H, developed the hyperplastic nodules from which the tumors arose (Nandi, 1966).

Later, another strain, C3H-A^{vy}fB, was developed by foster-nursing a litter of caesarean-derived C3H-A^{vy} mice on C57BL (Vlahakis *et al.*, 1970). Because of the presence of the A^{vy} gene, strain C3H-A^{vy} has a higher susceptibility to mammary tumors than C3H, which is expressed in earlier appearance of the tumors since the incidence in both strains is 100%. Also strain C3H-A^{vy}fB has a higher tumor response than C3HfB, the tumor incidence in C3H-A^{vy}fB being 90% with an average tumor age of 15 months. These C3H-A^{vy}fB tumors also contain B particles.

Although C3H-A^{vy}fB had a relatively high incidence of mammary tumors, its virus was not transmitted through the milk. BALB/c females foster-nursed on C3H-A^{vy}fB females had the same low tumor incidence normally seen in BALB/c. The virus of the C3H-A^{vy}fB was, however, readily transmitted through the germ cells. When reciprocal crosses were made between C3H-A^{vy}fB and BALB/c, both groups of reciprocal hybrid females had a high incidence of mammary tumors like that of C3H-A^{vy}fB. Furthermore, the tumors of these hybrid females also contained B particles. Thus this strain C3H-A^{vy}fB had a high incidence of mammary tumors caused by a virus indistinguishable morphologically from the usual MTV but instead of being transmitted in the milk was transmitted through the sperm and egg.

At the Netherlands Cancer Research Institute, Mühlbock (1965) had developed mouse strain GR that was to make a unique contribution to our understanding of the genetic transmission of the mammary tumor virus. This is a very high mammary tumor strain with an incidence of 100% at an average age of 4 months. Through a series of well-designed experiments, Mühlbock and his staff showed that the virus of this strain, which is also a B particle morphologically not unlike other lines of MTV, was transmitted through the sperm and egg, although it could also be transmitted in the milk. When this GR virus was transmitted to strain 020, it was no longer transmissible through the sperm but was transmitted maternally as the usual MTV. Thus it appeared that this male transmission of the GR virus was not a characteristic of the virus but of the GR strain of mice (for review, see Bentvelzen, 1968).

As a result of his analysis of hybridization studies, Bentvelzen concluded that the high susceptibility of the GR strain to mammary tumors was due to a single Mendelian factor. Furthermore, in an analysis of the male transmission, he concluded that the ability of the male to transmit MTV was also due to a single Mendelian factor, probably the same as the gene for the high susceptibility of the strain. It was from these and other observations that Bentvelzen (1972) formulated his provirus theory for the transmission of the GR mammary tumor virus and possibly other lines of MTV. He postulated that the viral information is transmitted as a provirus incorporated in the host genome, transcription of this DNA viral information to the RNA virus being controlled by a regulator gene and an operator gene.

In certain aspects, Bentvelzen's concept of the provirus parallels Huebner's concept of the oncogene. That the two are not the same is evidenced by the fact that they control different viruses. The virus that presumably arises from the oncogene in its mature form is a C particle. The mammary tumor viruses of the various lines are B particles, and thus far they have been found to produce only mammary tumors.

Proof of the MTV provirus, like proof of the oncogene, will come through segregation studies demonstrating that the viral information segregates as a genetic locus followed by linkage studies locating it on a certain chromosome. Early mammary tumor segregation studies were troubled by the fact that the expression of the MTV was the occurrence of the mammary tumor late in life after possible influence by any of a number of other factors. This difficulty can now be overcome by identification of the virus early in the life of the mouse. Van Nie *et al.* (1972) in Amsterdam have identified the presence of the virus by hormonal induction of early small mammary tumors in the GR strain. She can identify these approximately 3 wk after introduction of the first hormonal pellet. Ratios in hybrids resulting from their outcrossing strain GR to low tumor strains have indicated segregation of a single locus controlling production of the virus.

Using originally the immunofluorescent test and later the radioimmune test, Hilgers, also of the Amsterdam group, has likewise obtained evidence of single Mendelian segregation of the viral antigen. It is hoped that both observations can be extended and confirmed by establishing this gene, presumably the provirus in a linkage group.

These observations on the genetic transmission of mouse tumor viruses may be of significance in understanding the transmission of human cancer. Early studies on breast cancer in women showed that something transmitted from parent to daughter influenced the probability that breast cancer later would occur. Yet whatever was being transmitted was transmitted from the father as readily as from the mother. If there are human tumor viruses, as we suspect there are, they too will probably be found to be transmitted genetically.

9. References

ANDERS, A., ANDERS, F., and KLINKE, K., 1974, Regulation of gene expression in the Gordon–Kosswig melanoma system. I. The distribution of the controlling genes in the genome of the Xiphophorin fish, *Platypoecilus maculatus* and *Platypoecilus variatus*, in: *Genetics and Mutagenesis of Fish* (J. H. Schröder, ed.), pp. 34–52, Springer-Verlag, Berlin-Heidelberg-New York.

ANDERSON, D. E., 1959, Genetic aspects of bovine ocular carcinoma, in: *Genetics and Cancer* (Staff of University of Texas, M. D. Anderson Hospital and Tumor Institute, eds.), pp. 364–374, University of Texas Press, Austin.

ANDERVONT, H. B., 1938, The incidence of induced subcutaneous and pulmonary tumors and spontaneous mammary tumors in hybrid mice, *Publ Health Rep.* **53:**1665.

ANDERVONT, H. B., 1945, Fate of the C3H milk influence in mice of strains C and C57 black, *J. Natl. Cancer Inst.* **5:**383.

AUERBACH, C., 1949, Chemical mutagenesis, *Biol. Rev.* **24:**355.

BASHFORD, E. F., 1909, The influence of heredity on disease, with special reference to tuberculosis, cancer and diseases of the nervous system, *Proc. Roy. Soc. Med.* **2:**63.

BENTVELZEN, P., 1968, *Genetical Control of the Vertical Transmission of the Mühlbock Mammary Tumor Virus in the GR Mouse Strain*, pp. 35–40, Hollandia, Amsterdam.

BENTVELZEN, P., 1972, Hereditary infections with mammary tumor viruses in mice, in: *RNA Viruses and Host Genome in Oncogenesis* (P. Emmelot and P. Bentvelzen, eds.), pp. 309–337, North-Holland, Amsterdam and London.

BENTVELZEN, P., and DAAMS, J. H., 1972, Oncornaviruses and their proviruses, *Rev. Europ. Etudes Clin. Biol.* **17:** 245.

BITTNER, J. J., 1939, Relation of nursing to the extra-chromosome theory of breast cancer in mice, *Am. J. Cancer* **97:** 90.

BITTNER, J. J., HUSEBY, R. A., VISSCHER, M. B., BALL, Z. B., and SMITH, F., 1944, Mammary cancer and mammary structure in inbred stocks of mice and their hybrids, *Science* **99:** 83.

BLOOM, J. L., and FALCONER, D. S., 1964, A gene with major effect on susceptibility to induced lung tumors in mice, *J. Natl. Cancer Inst.* **33:** 607.

BRIDGES, C. B., 1916, Non-disjunction as proof of chromosome theory of heredity, *Genetics* **1:** 1.

BRIEN, P., 1961, Étude d'*Hydra pirardi*. Origine et repartition des nematacystes. Gamétogènese. Involution postgamétique. Evolution reversible des cellules interstitielles, *Bull. Biol. France Belg.* **95:** 301.

BURDETTE, W. J., 1943, The inheritance of susceptibility to tumors induced in mice. II. Tumors induced by methylcholanthrene in the progeny of C3H and JK mice, *Cancer Res.* **3:** 318.

BURDETTE, W. J., 1951, A method for determining mutation rate and tumor incidence simultaneously, *Cancer Res.* **11:** 552.

BURDETTE, W. J., 1952, Induced pulmonary tumors, *J. Thoracic Surg.* **24:** 427.

BURDETTE, W. J., 1955, The significance of mutation in relation to the origin of tumors: A review, *Cancer Res.* **15:** 201.

CHARLES, D. R., and LUCE-CLAUSEN, E. M., 1942, The kinetics of papilloma formation in benzpyrene-treated mice, *Cancer Res.* **2:** 261.

COLE, R. K., and FURTH, J., 1941, Experimental studies on the genetics of spontaneous leukemia in mice, *Cancer Res.* **1:** 957.

COOPER, E. L., 1969, Neoplasia and transplantation immunity in annelids, *J. Natl. Cancer Inst. Monogr.* **31:** 655.

DICKIE, M. M., 1954, The use of F_1 hybrid and backcross generations to reveal new and/or uncommon tumor types, *J. Natl. Cancer Inst.* **15:** 791.

FONTAINE, A. R., 1969, Pigmented tumor-like lesions in an ophiuroid echinoderm, *Natl. Cancer Inst. Monogr.* **31:** 255.

FOSTER, J. A., 1969, Malformation and lethal growths in *Planaria* treated with carcinogens, *Natl. Cancer Inst. Monogr.* **31:** 683.

GARDNER, E. J., 1959, Genetic mechanism of maternal effect for tumorous head in *Drosophila melanogaster*, *Genetics* **44:** 471.

GARDNER, E. J., and WOOLF, C. M., 1949, Maternal effect involved in the inheritance of abnormal growths in the head region of *Drosophila melanogaster*, *Genetics* **34:** 573.

GARDNER, W. U., 1954, Studies on ovarian and pituitary tumorigenesis, *J. Natl. Cancer Inst.* **15:** 693.

GARDNER, W. U., and STRONG, L. C., 1940, The strain-limited development of tumors of the pituitary gland in mice receiving estrogens, *Yale J. Biol. Med.* **12:** 543.

GORDON, M., 1858, A genetic concept for the origin of melanomas, *Ann. N.Y. Acad. Sci.* **71:** 1213.

GRAND, C. G., GORDON, M., and CAMERON, G., 1941, Neoplasm studies. VIII. Cell types in tissue culture of fish melanotic tumors compared with mammalian melanomas, *Cancer Res.* **1:** 660.

GROSS, L., 1951, Pathogenic properties, and vertical transmission of the mouse leukemia agent, *Proc. Soc. Exp. Biol. Med.* **78:** 343.

HALVER, J. E., 1969, Aflatoxicosis and trout hepatoma, in *Aflatoxin—Scientific Background, Control, and Implications* (L. A. Goldblatt, ed.), pp. 265–306, Academic Press, New York.

HALVER, J. E., and MITCHELL, I. A. (eds.), 1967, Trout Hepatoma Research Conference Papers, Research Report no. 70, Bureau of Sport Fisheries and Wildlife, Government Printing Office, Washington, D.C.

HALVER, J. E., ASHLEY, L. M., and SMITH, R. R., 1969, Aflatoxicosis in coho salmon, *Natl. Cancer Inst. Monogr.* **31:** 141.

HARTUNG, E. W., 1950, The inheritance of a tumor in *Drosophila melanogaster*, *J. Hered.* **41:** 269,

HESTON, W. E., 1942a, Genetic analysis of susceptibility to induced pulmonary tumors in mice, *J. Natl. Cancer Inst.* **3:** 69.

HESTON, W. E., 1942b, Inheritance of susceptibility to spontaneous pulmonary tumors in mice, *J. Natl. Cancer Inst.* **3**:79.

HESTON, W. E., 1953, Occurrence of tumors in mice injected subcutaneously with sulfur mustard and nitrogen mustard, *J. Natl. Cancer Inst.* **14**:131.

HESTON, W. E., 1957, Effects of genes located on chromosomes III, V, VII, IX, and XIV on the occurrence of pulmonary tumors in the mouse, in: *Proceedings of International Genetics Symposia, 1956, Cytologia,* Suppl. Vol. 219.

HESTON, W. E., 1960, The genetic concept of the etiology of cancer, in: *Proceedings of the 4th National Cancer Conference,* Lippincott, Philadelphia.

HESTON, W. E., 1963, Genetics of neoplasia, in: *Methodology in Mammalian Genetics* (W. J. Burdette, ed.), pp. 247–264, Holden-Day, San Francisco.

HESTON, W. E., and ANDERVONT, H. B., 1944, Importance of genetic influence on the occurrence of mammary tumors in virgin female mice, *J. Natl. Cancer Inst.* **4**:403.

HESTON, W. E., and DERINGER, M. K., 1952a, Test for a maternal influence in the development of mammary gland tumors in agent-free strain C3Hb mice, *J. Natl. Cancer Inst.* **13**:167.

HESTON, W. E., and DERINGER, M. K., 1952b, Induction of pulmonary tumors in guinea pigs by intravenous injection of methylcholanthrene and dibenzanthracene, *J. Natl. Cancer Inst,* **13**:705.

HESTON, W. E., and PRATT, A. W., 1959, Effect of concentration of oxygen on occurrence of pulmonary tumors in strain A mice, *J. Natl. Cancer Inst.* **22**:707.

HESTON, W. E., and SCHNEIDERMAN, M. A., 1953, Analysis of dose response in relation to mechanism of pulmonary tumor induction in mice, *Science* **117**:109.

HESTON, W. E., AND VLAHAKIS, G., 1961, Influence of the A^{vy} gene on mammary-gland tumors, hepatomas, and normal growth in mice, *J. Natl. Cancer Inst.* **26**:969.

HESTON, W. E., DERINGER, M. K., AND ANDERVONT, H. B., 1945, Gene–milk agent relationship in mammary-tumor development, *J. Natl. Cancer Inst.* **5**:289.

HESTON, W. E., DERINGER, M. K., DUNN, T. B., AND LEVILLAIN, W. D., 1950, Factors in the development of spontaneous mammary gland tumors in agent-free strain C3Hb mice, *J. Natl. Cancer Inst.* **10**:1139.

HESTON, W. E., DERINGER, M. K., AND DUNN, T. P., 1956, Further studies on the relationship between the genotype and the mammary tumor agent in mice, *J. Natl. Cancer Inst.* **16**:1309.

HESTON, W. E., VLAHAKIS, G., AND DERINGER, M. K., 1960, Delayed effect of genetic segregation on the transmission of the mammary tumor agent in mice, *J. Natl. Cancer Inst.* **24**:721.

HESTON, W. E., VLAHAKIS, G., AND DESMUKES, B., 1973, Effects of the antifertility drug Enovid in five strains of mice, with particular regard to carcinogenesis, *J. Natl. Cancer Inst.* **51**:209.

HUEBNER, R. J., AND GILDEN, R. V., 1972, Inherited RNA viral genomes (virogenes and oncogenes) in the etiology of cancer, in: *RNA Viruses and Host Genome in Oncogenesis* (P. Emmelot and P. Bentvelzen, eds.), pp. 197–219, North-Holland, Amsterdam and London.

HUEBNER, R. J., AND TODARO, G. J., 1969, Oncogenes of RNA tumor viruses as determinants of cancer, *Proc. Natl. Acad. Sci.* **64**:1087.

HUSEBY, R. A., AND BITTNER, J. J., 1948, Studies on the inherited hormonal influence, *Acta Unio Int. Contra Cancrum* **6**:197.

JACKSON LABORATORY STAFF, 1933, The existence of nonchromosomal influence in the incidence of mammary tumors in mice, *Science* **78**:465.

KORTWEG, R., 1934, Proefondervindelijke onderzoekingen Aangaande Erfelijkhéid von Kanker, *Nederl. Tijdschr. Geneesk.* **78**:240.

LANGE, C. S., 1966, Observations on some tumors found in two species of planaria: *Dugesia etrusca* and *D. ilvana, J. Embryol. Exp. Morphol.* **15**:125.

LITTLE, C. C., 1939, Hybridization and tumor formation in mice, *Proc. Natl. Acad. Sci.* **25**:452.

LYNCH, C. J., 1940, Influence of heredity and environment upon the number of tumor nodules occurring in lungs of mice, *Proc. Soc. Exp. Biol. Med.* **43**:186.

MACDOWELL, E. C., POTTER, J. S., AND TAYLOR, M. J., 1945, Mouse leukemia. XII. The role of genes in spontaneous cases, *Cancer Res.* **5**:65.

MCKINNELL, R. G., 1969, Lucké renal adenocarcinoma: Epidemiological aspects, in: *Recent Results in Cancer Research,* Special Suppl.: *Biology of Amphibian Tumors* (M. Mizell, ed.), pp. 254–260, Springer, New York, Heidelberg, and Berlin.

MIZELL, M., 1969, State of the art: Lucké renal adenocarcinoma, in: *Recent Results in Cancer Research,* Special Suppl.: *Biology of Amphibian Tumors* (M. Mizell, ed.), pp. 1–25, Springer, New York, Heidelberg, and Berlin.

MÜHLBOCK, O., 1965, Note on a new inbred mouse strain GR/A, *Europ. J. Cancer* **1**:123.

MURRAY, J. A., 1911, Cancerous ancestry and the incidence in mice, *Proc. Roy. Soc. Lond.* **84**:42.

NANDI, S., 1966, Interactions among hormonal, viral, and genetic factors in mouse mammary tumorigenesis, *Canad. Cancer Conf.* **6**:69.

PAULEY, G. B., 1969, A critical review of neoplasia and tumor-like lesions in mollusks, *Natl. Cancer Inst. Monogr.* **31**:509.

PAYNE, L. N., 1972, Interaction between host genome and avian RNA tumor viruses, in: *RNA viruses and Host Genome in Oncogenesis* (P. E. Emmelot and P. Bentvelzen, eds.), pp. 93–115, North-Holland, Amsterdam and London.

PITELKA, D. R., BERN, H. A., NANDI, S., AND DE OME, K. B., 1964, On the significance of virus-like particles in mammary tissues of C3Hf mice, *J. Natl. Cancer Inst.* **33**:867.

ROGERS, J. B., 1951, Spontaneous tumors of senile guinea pigs, *J. Gerontol.* **6**(Supplement to No. 3): 142.

ROWE, W. P., 1972, Studies of genetic transmission of murine leukemia virus by AKR mice. I. Crosses with $Fv-1^n$ strains of mice, *J. Exp. Med.* **136**:1272.

ROWE, W. P., AND HARTLEY, J. W., 1972, Studies of genetic transmission of murine leukemia virus by AKR mice. II. Crosses with $Fv-1^b$ strains of mice, *J. Exp. Med.* **136**:1286.

ROWE, W. P., HARTLEY, J. W., AND BREMNAR, T., 1972, Genetic mapping of a murine leukemia virus–inducing locus of AKR mice, *Science*, **178**:860.

ROWE, W. P., HUMPHREY, J. B., AND LILLY, F., 1973, A major genetic locus affecting resistance to infection with murine leukemia viruses. III. Assignment of the *Fv-1* locus to linkage group VIII of the mouse, *J. Exp. Med.* **137**:850.

RUSSELL, E. S., 1940, A comparison of benign and "malignant" tumors in *Drosophila melanogaster, J. Exp. Zool.* **84**:363.

RUSSELL, E. S., 1942, The inheritance of tumors in *Drosophila melanogaster*, with special reference to an isogenic strain of *st sr* tumor 36a, *Genetics* **27**:612.

RUSSELL, W. O., AND ORTEGA, L. R., 1952, Methylcholanthrene induced tumors in guinea pigs, a review of the literature on tumors induced with polycyclic carcinogenic hydrocarbons in this species, *Arch. Pathol.* **53**:301.

SCHLUMBERGER, H. G., 1952, Nerve sheath tumors in an isolated goldfish population, *Cancer Res.* **12**:890.

SCHLUMBERGER, H. G., 1954, Neoplasia in the parakeet. I. Spontaneous chromophobe pituitary tumors, *Cancer Res.* **14**:237.

SHIMKIN, M. B., AND MIDER, G. B., 1941, Induction of tumors in guinea pigs with subcutaneously injected methylcholanthrene, *J. Natl. Cancer Inst.* **1**:707.

SLYE, M., 1926, The inheritance behavior of cancer as a simple mendelian recessive, *J. Cancer Res.* **10**:15.

SNELL, G. D., 1958, Histocompatability genes of the mouse. II. Production and analysis of isogenic resistant lines, *J. Natl. Cancer Inst.* **21**:843.

STEVENS, L. C., 1970, Experimental production of testicular teratomas in mice of strains 129, A/He, and their F_1 hybrids, *J. Natl. Cancer Inst.* **44**:923.

TATCHELL, J. A. H., 1961, Pulmonary tumors, group VII and sex in the house mouse, *Nature (Lond.)* **190**:837.

VAN NIE, R., HILGERS, J., AND LENSELINK, M., 1972, Genetical analysis of mammary tumor development and mammary tumor virus expression in the GR mouse strain, in: *Recherches Fondamentales sur les Tumeurs Mammaires*, pp. 21–29, Ministere de la Santa Publique, Paris.

VLAHAKIS, G., HESTON, W. E., AND SMITH, G. H., 1970, Strain C3H-A^{vy}fB mice: Ninety percent incidence of mammary tumors transmitted by either parent, *Science* **170**:185.

WOOLLEY, G. W., FEKETE, E., AND LITTLE, C. C., 1941, Effect of castration in the dilute brown strain of mice, *Endocrinology* **28**:341.

WOOLLEY, G. W., DICKIE, M. M., AND LITTLE, C. C., 1953, Adrenal tumors and other pathological changes in reciprocal crosses in mice. II. An introduction to results of four reciprocal crosses, *Cancer Res.* **13**:231.

WRIGHT, S., 1934a, The results of crosses between inbred strains of guinea pigs, differing in number of digits, *Genetics* **19**:537.

WRIGHT, S., 1934b, On the genetics of subnormal development of the head (otocephaly) in the guinea pig, *Genetics* **19**:471.

3

Genetic Influences in Human Tumors

Alfred G. Knudson, Jr.

1. Introduction

Although the genetic analysis of cancer in animals has played a major role in the development of knowledge and new ideas about the etiology and pathogenesis of cancer, the genetic study of human cancer has played a very minor role. Part of this difference is attributable to the fact animal data have been provided to a great extent by experimental manipulation of selected species and genetic strains, whereas human data have been largely descriptive and not related either to animal data or to critical etiological hypotheses. Genetic analyses of human cancer have consisted primarily of population, family, and twin studies of tumor occurrence and cytogenetic analyses. The results of cytogenetic analyses of human tumors are thoroughly discussed elsewhere in this volume, and reference to them in this chapter will be confined largely to discussion of genetically predisposing conditions which involve chromosomal abnormality. It is the study of the occurrence of tumors that has contributed most significantly to the understanding of etiology.

The study of cancer in populations is of course not necessarily a study of the genetics of cancer. It has been repeatedly observed that population or subpopulation (e.g., occupational) differences are attributable to differences in environmental exposure. Nevertheless, it is still not known whether the gross ethnic differences in incidence of many specific cancers, such as those occurring in breast, stomach, and colon, are due to genetic or environmental factors. Support for a genetic basis for ethnic difference could be provided by evidence of correlation of

Alfred G. Knudson, Jr. • The University of Texas Health Science Center at Houston, Graduate School of Biomedical Sciences, Houston, Texas. Supported in part by Medical Genetics Center Grant GM 19513 from the National Institute of General Medical Sciences.

cancer incidence with a specific genetic marker, as has been provided by the finding within the Caucasian population that cancer of the stomach shows some association with blood group A. Evidence may also be provided by comparing the incidence of a particular tumor in populations genetically alike but living in different environmental conditions. However, at present there is no conclusive evidence that any ethnic differences in cancer incidence are attributable to genetic difference.

Study of the families of cancer patients has revealed that most forms of cancer display an increased familial incidence, suggesting a genetic component to susceptibility. The patterns of inheritance are not generally those of single Mendelian genes, and broad surveys have therefore not shed any light on the origin of human cancer. On the other hand, detailed analysis of selected families in which there is a concentration of similar cases has clearly shown that cancer in some instances is inherited in Mendelian fashion. These examples will be discussed in further detail.

A unique category of family study is that of twins. Comparison of concordance in identical and in fraternal twins has often been employed as a measure for assessing the relative roles of heredity and environment in the causation of disease. For most cancers, the concordance is very low for both kinds of twins, suggesting that heredity plays a minor role. Exceptions include cancer of the breast, childhood cancer, and the tumors which demonstrate a Mendelian form of predisposition.

With these general observations in mind, it can only be concluded that the informative cancers of man are those in which predisposition occurs in individuals with well-defined genetic states or in which the tumor is inherited in Mendelian fashion.

2. Genetic States Predisposing to Cancer

2.1. Chromosomal Disorders

In Down's syndrome, or mongoloid idiocy, there is an extra chromosome 21. In most cases this appears in the form of trisomy 21, but in some it appears as an equivalent translocation. In both forms there is an increased risk of leukemia, estimated to be 10–20 times the risk in normal children (Miller, 1970). An increased susceptibility to solid tumors has also been reported (Young, 1971). Leukemia is found in children with Down's syndrome 2–3 yr earlier on the average than it is in normal children. An increased incidence of leukemia has also been observed in trisomy D and in Klinefelter's syndrome (Fraumeni, 1969). *In vitro* oncogenic transformation by the tumor virus SV40 is also increased in fibroblasts from trisomic individuals.

The enhanced risk of leukemia in these aneuploid states may not be attributable to the aneuploidy *per se*. There has also been reported an increased risk for leukemia in the sibs of subjects with Down's syndrome, raising the possibility that some causative factor may be common to both (Miller, 1963). Hecht *et al.* (1964) mention several possible mechanisms, including (1) underlying chromosomal rearrangement, (2) an autoimmune process, as has been suggested by Fialkow (1966) for aneuploidy, and (3) latent virus infection.

No other such highly significant relationship is known between aneuploidy and cancer. As far as structural abnormality and cancer are concerned, there is the very important example of the Philadelphia chromosome and chronic myeloid leukemia (Nowell and Hungerford, 1960, 1961). This is a deleted chromosome 22 (Caspersson *et al.*, 1970), which has been demonstrated to be associated with an apparently balanced translocation to chromosome 9 (Rowley, 1973). But the Philadelphia chromosome is found only in the hematopoietic system and is clearly a somatic rather than germinal change. This reduces any assurance that it *precedes* the development of leukemia. The problem of the relationship of cytogenetic change in somatic cells to the origin of cancer is discussed elsewhere in this volume.

One deletion which is definitely prezygotic and predisposing to a specific form of cancer is a deletion in the long arm of a D chromosome, chromosome 13 in verified cases. This deletion is often associated with a clinical syndrome of congenital defects known as the D deletion syndrome. Nine of some 40 affected individuals have also suffered from retinoblastoma, seven of these bilaterally (Wilson *et al.*, 1973). However, retinoblastoma is not usually accompanied by this deletion; in 12 cases, seven bilateral, no D chromosome deletion was found (Ladda *et al.*, 1973).

Although newer techniques for disclosing subtle chromosomal abnormality may yet prove the opposite, present evidence suggests that very few cases of cancer occur in individuals with visible chromosomal abnormalities in any significant number of noncancerous cells.

2.2. Mendelian Conditions

The syndromes of Fanconi and Bloom are both autosomal recessive disorders, both predispose to leukemia and cancer, and both are associated with increased rates of chromosome breakage *in vitro* and *in vivo* (German, 1972). Cells from patients with Fanconi's syndrome are also abnormal in their response to various environmental carcinogens; there is a greatly increased sensitivity to X-ray-induced chromosome breakage (Higurashi and Conen, 1971), an increased incidence of endoreduplication and tetraploidy *in vitro* in response to benzpyrene (Hirschhorn and Bloch-Shtacher, 1970), and a greatly increased rate of *in vitro* neoplastic transformation of fibroblasts in response to the tumor virus SV40 (Miller and Todaro, 1969).

Although leukemia is the only neoplastic condition reported excessively in patients with Fanconi's syndrome, it is not the only one in Bloom's syndrome. Three patients with the latter condition who have attained the age of 30 yr have each developed at least one cancer of the digestive tract (German, 1972). Since

Fanconi's syndrome is so often lethal, it should not be eliminated as a more generally predisposing disorder. Quite possibly the transformation of normal cells to cancer cells occurs at an increased rate in all tissues in these two diseases. Knowledge of the mechanisms which are defective in these diseases could obviously illuminate early steps in neoplastic transformation, possibly relating molecular change to the chromosomal changes so ubiquitous in cancer cells.

Ataxia-telangiectasia is another autosomal recessive disease associated with chromosomal abnormality and a strong predisposition to cancer, in this instance lymphoid neoplasia. In the majority of reported cases, lymphocytes respond poorly to mitogens *in vitro*, but the cells which do divide show increased rates of spontaneous chromosome breakage. The manner in which leukemia might develop in this disease has been suggested by Hecht *et al.* (1973), who studied the development of a clone of chromosomally abnormal cells in a patient over a 4-yr period. A population of cells containing a translocation, involving both chromosomes 14, grew from 1–2% to 56–78% of the patient's peripheral lymphocyte population. Although the patient died without leukemia, two of his sibs with the disease did die of leukemia. These authors report two other patients with ataxia–telangiectasia with translocation clones, one between chromosomes 7 and 14 and one between 14 and 1. The break occurred at the same point on chromosome 14 in all three cases.

Patients with ataxia-telangiectasia also commonly have a deficiency in the immune system, most often involving immunoglobulins A and E. The cause for this and its relation to chromosome breakage and leukemia are not known. Conceivably the immune deficiency could result from the emergence of a defective clone of lymphocytes, as noted above, suggesting that immune deficiency and leukemia are different end points of the same process.

Lymphoreticular neoplasms are also much more common than expected by chance among patients with any of several recessively inherited immune deficiency diseases. Gatti and Good (1971) have classified these according to autosomal or X-linked inheritance and to impairment of humoral and/or cellular immunity. The detailed features of these conditions will not be noted, except to observe that chromosomal abnormality and SV40 transformability are not features of cells from affected individuals (Kersey *et al.*, 1972). Predisposition to cancer in this case seems not to involve the process of transformation of a normal cell to a cancer cell but rather failure of the immunological surveillance mechanism which normally operates to interfere with cell proliferation. In this respect these conditions seem to differ from ataxia-telangiectasia.

Another recessively inherited disease which predisposes to cancer is also the one whose basic defect is best understood, namely, xeroderma pigmentosum. Photosensitivity and skin cancer are major features of this condition, an inborn error of metabolism in which there is a deficiency of an enzyme necessary for the repair of ultraviolet light-induced damage to DNA (Cleaver, 1968, 1969; Setlow *et al.*, 1969). Defective repair of damage induced by the chemical carcinogen *N*-acetoxy-2-acetylaminofluorene has also been observed (Setlow and Regan, 1972). Chromosomal abnormality is not a feature of the condition *in vivo*, but cultured fibroblasts show occasional pseudodiploid clones (German, 1972) and there is a great increase in ultraviolet light-induced chromosomal aberrations *in vitro* (Parrington *et al.*, 1971). On the other hand, SV40-induced transformation is not increased (Aaronson and Lytle, 1970; Parrington *et al.*, 1971). It is apparent that xeroderma pigmentosum is a genetic state which predisposes to environmentally induced skin cancer. This effect may be mediated via chromosome damage.

Some general conclusions emerge from a consideration of genetic states which predispose to cancer. None of these states invariably leads to cancer, with the exception of xeroderma pigmentosum. Several conditions are chromosomal abnormalities and some others predispose to the generation of chromosomal abnormality in somatic tissues. This observation, combined with the knowledge that most cancers have abnormal karyotypes, suggests that chromosomal damage may be a mediating event in the initiation of cancer cells. A different kind of predisposition is evidently provided by the immune deficiency diseases, in which initiation is not enhanced but tumor cell growth after initiation is.

3. Dominantly Inherited Tumors

As a group, the dominantly inherited tumors differ sharply from the genetic conditions discussed above in that tumor is a critical phenotypic feature and occurs with high penetrance. In some instances, a tumor is part of a syndrome, other manifestations of which are other kinds of tumors or nonneoplastic signs. In other instances, tumor occurs in just one tissue, although it may be multiple in that tissue.

3.1. Tumor Syndromes

3.1.1. Polyposis of the Colon

Perhaps the best known and clinically most important dominant cancer syndrome is polyposis of the colon. Multiple benign polyps of the colon are an invariant feature in gene carriers by adulthood. What makes the disease serious is the also invariant occurrence of one or more adenocarcinomas, nearly always by the age of 50 yr. The average age at death is 40 yr (Neel, 1971); in contrast is the much later age at death for patients with carcinoma of the colon generally. Polyposis thus displays two features typical of dominantly inherited tumors: earlier onset than their nongenetic counterparts and multiplicity.

Some patients with polyposis develop tumors at other sites. The most common site is connective tissue, with such tumors as fibroma, fibrosarcoma, and osteoma. In some families, these tumors have so high an incidence that the name "Gardner's syndrome" is applied (Gardner and Richards, 1953). Whether such diversity of polyposis cases is attributable to alleles at the same genetic locus is not known.

3.1.2. Cancer Family Syndrome

Another dominant syndrome associated with cancer of the colon is the cancer family syndrome, or hereditary adenocarcinomatosis, made famous by the early report by Warthin (1913) of a large pedigree which has since been extended by Lynch and Krush (1971). In this family and similar ones, cancer has been reported at several sites, but two, colon and endometrium, are particularly common (Anderson, 1970). More than one tumor may occur in an organ, especially colon. Tumors frequently occur before the age of 40 yr, so this syndrome resembles polyposis with respect to both multiplicity in a given organ and early onset. Each syndrome accounts for only a small fraction of all cases of colon cancer, probably of the order of magnitude of 1% or less.

3.1.3. Basal Cell Nevus Syndrome

The basal cell nevus syndrome consists of a complex which includes multiple basal cell carcinomas of the skin, epidermoid cysts of the jaw, ectopic calcification of soft tissues, and various congenital skeletal anomalies. The jaw cysts are usually evident by adulthood and the carcinomas often by then, which is much earlier than these tumors appear in the population generally. Again, multiplicity and early onset characterize a dominant syndrome (Anderson, 1970).

As noted above, various cystic tumors appear excessively in this syndrome. In addition, there is a significant incidence of a very uncommon tumor, medulloblastoma, which has an incidence of less than one per 10,000 in the normal childhood population. All these syndromes noted so far therefore predispose to tumors in more than one tissue.

3.1.4. Multiple Endocrine Tumor Syndromes

There are two distinct multiple endocrine tumor syndromes. One of these, usually called "multiple endocrine adenomatosis," is very complex because so many tissues may be involved. These tissues include anterior pituitary, parathyroid, thyroid, pancreas (islet cells), and adrenal cortex. Carcinoid tumors of the bronchus and digestive tract have also been observed. The clinical expression of this syndrome is therefore understandably varied, depending on tumor site. In one instance, at least, the symptoms have given rise to the creation of a separate syndrome, the Zollinger–Ellison syndrome of peptic ulcer, excessive gastric secretion, and non-insulin-producing islet cell tumors. Penetrance for expression of some feature of the parent multiple endocrine syndrome is very high in early adulthood (Anderson, 1970), expression occurring at a much earlier age than when solitary tumors of these tissues occur in the general population.

The second syndrome has a narrower spectrum, producing two tumors, pheochromocytoma of the adrenal medulla and medullary carcinoma of the thyroid, with high penetrance, and parathyroid adenomas, with intermediate penetrance. A number of cases of the syndrome have been reported in children. Nearly all gene carriers attaining the age of 50 yr have developed at least one of

each of the first two tumor types, the mean number of tumors at each site being
estimated at four (Knudson and Strong, 1972a). When pheochromocytoma is found, it is bilateral in 75–80% of cases.

A significant fraction of patients with the syndrome of pheochromocytoma and medullary carcinoma of the thyroid do not have a family history of the disease. However, the offspring of such individuals are at a 50% risk, indicating that these sporadic cases result in fact from new mutations. Tumor multiplicity and age at expression are similar whether the family history is positive or not (Knudson and Strong, 1972a).

A variant of this syndrome involves other lesions, notably neuromas of the buccal mucosa and other selected areas. Known as the "mucosal neuroma syndrome," it displays the same features with respect to pheochromocytoma and medullary carcinoma of the thyroid. It may represent a different allele at the same genetic locus. The presence of *café-au-lait* spots has caused it to be confused with neurofibromatosis, from which it should be distinctly separated (Williams and Pollock, 1966; Gorlin *et al.*, 1968).

Although these syndromes involve more than one endocrine tissue, they have readily separable specificities. Thus pheochromocytoma and medullary carcinoma of the thyroid are not found in the first syndrome. Both syndromes resemble other dominantly inherited syndromes in that only specific tissues are affected, tumor multiplicity is common, and age at onset is earlier than usual for solitary sporadic tumors.

3.1.5. Neurofibromatosis

Pheochromocytoma is also found in about 10% of cases of the syndrome of neurofibromatosis, the principal manifestations of which are *café-au-lait* spots and neurofibromas. The pheochromocytomas do not occur multiply in one patient, nor do they occur earlier than in unselected cases (Knudson and Strong, 1972a). The incidence of pheochromocytoma is not concentrated in certain pedigrees.

Neurofibromatosis is one of a group of dominant syndromes categorized as phacomatoses. Other entities are the von Hippel–Lindau syndrome and tuberous sclerosis. Each is associated with unusual tumors which in some respects resemble hyperplasia more than neoplasia. In this regard the phacomatoses depart from the other dominant tumor syndromes.

3.2. Specific Tumors

3.2.1. Childhood Tumors

The best-known example of a dominantly inherited tumor which is not a feature of a syndrome is retinoblastoma, a malignant eye tumor of young children with an incidence of more than one per 20,000,000 children in the United States. Since surgery and radiotherapy have been partially effective weapons for some time, a substantial number of patients have survived to reproduce, permitting the demonstration of dominant genetic transmission. However, a puzzling result was that, while essentially 50% of the offspring of bilaterally affected persons were also affected, only 10–15% of the offspring of unilaterally affected persons were also affected. Furthermore, while approximately 25–30% of all cases are bilateral, the frequency of bilaterality in the affected offspring of affected individuals, whether unilateral or bilateral, is approximately 70%. The conclusion has been reached that only some (about 40%) of all cases are germinal, or hereditary, and that the remainder are nonhereditary. Many of the hereditary cases result from new mutations and do not involve a family history. About 5% of those who carry the responsible mutation develop no tumor at all, about 30% develop tumor unilaterally, and the remainder have bilateral tumors. These observations fit the hypothesis that tumor development in gene carriers is a matter of chance, with a mean number of tumors of three per carrier (Knudson, 1971). Those who do not carry the gene have a probability of about one in 30,000 of developing one tumor and therefore a vanishingly small prospect of having bilateral disease.

The transformation of a retinoblast into a tumor cell is a rare event even in the gene carrier. The number of retinoblasts during early development can probably be numbered in the millions, suggesting that the rate of transformation is of the same order of magnitude as mutation itself. The hypothesis has been developed therefore that transformation is a mutational event occurring in somatic cells (Knudson, 1971). The initiation, or formation of the first tumor cell, of retinoblastoma is visualized as a two-step process in gene carriers; both are regarded as mutational, the first in germinal cells, the second in somatic cells. Nonhereditary cases presumably result from the same process, except that both mutations occur in somatic cells; since both of these events must occur postzygotically, it is anticipated that the age at onset would be later. It is not surprising then that hereditary and nonhereditary cases occur at mean ages of 15 and 30 months, respectively.

Retinoblastoma has been an uncommon disease because the incidence has been limited by mutation rates and because the disease until this century was probably always lethal. It should become more common as gene carriers survive and reproduce. It would also increase if mutation rates generally were increased.

Although most patients with germinal, or hereditary, retinoblastoma do not have an affected parent or other antecedent relative, a few percent have an affected sibling. This event is too frequent to be attributed to lack of penetrance, which is very high (95%) once the mutation is expressed in a pedigree. Some of these sibling cases probably result from mutation in early stages of gametogenesis and the subsequent gonadal mosaicism it produces. Others may be examples of "premutation" (Auerbach, 1956; Neel, 1962). In rare instances, the affected sibling is a twin. From the above considerations, an expectation can be created: the probability that a fraternal twin of an affected child would also be affected is slightly less than 0.5 if they have an affected parent and about 0.02 if they do not, giving an overall expectation for concordance of the order of magnitude of 0.05. Unfortunately, there have not been enough reports to test this expectation. On the other hand, since approximately 40% of all cases are germinal, the probability that the identical twin of an affected child would be a gene carrier is 0.4, which taken together with a penetrance of 0.95 leads to an expected probability of 0.38. The observed data, which are too sparse to be very reliable, suggest a fraction of 0.40–0.45.

Two other childhood tumors, Wilms' tumor of the kidney and neuroblastoma, have been examined for compatibility with this model (Knudson and Strong, 1972a,b). Again multiplicity of tumor and earlier age of patient are associated with hereditary cases. It is estimated that approximately 38% of Wilms' tumor cases and 22% of neuroblastoma cases are of the hereditary, or germinal, type. These tumors have not previously been regarded as similar in etiology to retinoblastoma because so few examples of generation-to-generation transmission exist. However, there are numerous cases of sib involvement. These results are presumed to be an expression of the fact that until very recently the mortality rates for Wilm's tumor and for neuroblastoma were far higher than for retinoblastoma. In addition, some survivors have undoubtedly been sterilized by irradiation. As survival and fertility increase, an increase in the number of examples of vertical transmission and an increasing resemblance to retinoblastoma can be expected. A survey of other childhood tumors suggests that other types exist in germinal and somatic forms, too, and that the phenomenon is a general one for childhood cancer.

3.2.2. Pheochromocytoma

Although pheochromocytoma is primarily an adult tumor, it also displays the main features of the childhood tumors. A number of pedigrees showing dominant inheritance have been presented. These are pedigrees that contain no cases of medullary carcinoma of the thyroid, so the two mutations are obviously different. They differ in other ways, too; pheochromocytoma alone may occur in any part of the sympathetic nervous system, it is often associated with sustained hypertension, and the principal amine produced is norepinephrine. In syndrome cases, pheochromocytoma is found only in the adrenal, sustained hypertension is not found, and the principal amine is epinephrine. In familial cases of simple pheochromocytoma, tumor is multiple in 50%, whereas only 12% of all cases are multiple. The modal age in multiple cases is approximately 20 yr, whether they are familial or not, while the modal age in nonfamilial cases is 35–40 yr. Again, familial cases are multiple and earlier in onset. The hereditary, or germinal, form of this tumor is estimated to comprise 22% of all cases (Knudson and Strong, 1972a). Approximately 90% of gene carriers will have at least one tumor by the age of 50 yr, the mean number per gene carrier being between two and three.

Syndrome cases of pheochromocytoma with medullary carcinoma of the thyroid account for about 30% of all familial cases of pheochromocytoma. Presumably the two familial forms result from mutation at two different genetic loci. It is visualized that tumor initiation proceeds by two steps in both, just as with the childhood tumors. In both forms, the first step can be a germinal mutation and produce a dominantly inherited tumor. All cases of the syndrome with medullary carcinoma of the thyroid are of this type because the probability that both of these tissues would have both steps occur in them is vanishingly small, just as is the probability of two tumors arising in one tissue by somatic change alone. Nonhereditary, or somatic, cases of pheochromocytoma could therefore represent first-step mutations at either locus.

Retrospective examination of the syndrome of multiple endocrine adenomatosis suggests that here too a mutation is inherited which affects a multiplicity of tissues. In any one of those tissues in which further change takes place a tumor cell will be initiated. Thus different affected members of the same pedigree may be affected in quite different ways, which are dependent on the tissue site of the second stochastic process (Knudson *et al.*, 1973).

3.2.3. Common Cancers

Although there are other accepted examples of dominantly inherited tumors and tumor syndromes, not enough details are available to complete the kind of analysis that has been performed on the examples above. Qualitatively, however, these heritable, or prezygotic, forms do show the pattern of multiplicity and earlier onset, in contrast to nonheritable, or postzygotic, forms. The difference between the syndromes and single tissue tumors is also maintained. The syndromes are always heritable, presumably because the probability of mimicry by somatic mutations is so small, while the single-tissue tumors exist in both heritable and nonheritable forms. The dualism of dominant (syndrome or single-tissue) and somatic forms appears to hold for childhood tumors, endocrine tumors, cancer of the colon, and basal cell carcinoma of the skin. Question then arises whether this is a general phenomenon for all cancers.

For the two most common forms of cancer, skin and colon, it is already apparent that dominant forms exist. For colon cancer, there are at least two, polyposis and the cancer family syndrome. For skin cancer, there is at least one, the basal cell nevus syndrome, and a dominant form of melanoma also probably exists (Anderson, 1971). The chief difference between these common cancers and the childhood cancers is that the dominant forms comprise a much smaller fraction, probably about 1–2%, of total cases of the former, and 20–40% of the latter.

Another of the common cancers, carcinoma of the breast, may also exist in a dominant form (Anderson, 1972). Numerous pedigrees displaying vertical transmission of the disease have been reported. Concordance in identical and fraternal twins is estimated to be 28 and 12%, respectively (Knudson *et al.*, 1973), again suggesting a strong genetic effect. Familial cases of breast cancer occur at significantly younger ages and are much more frequently bilateral. The hereditary form is primarily a premenopausal disease.

The small contribution of the cancer family syndrome to endometrial carcinoma has already been noted. In addition, this cancer frequently occurs alone in a familial, possibly dominant, form (Lynch *et al.*, 1966). This latter form is estimated by these investigators to contribute at least 13% of all endometrial cancer. Numerous examples of what may be dominantly inherited cancers of other sites in

the gastrointestinal and genitourinary systems have been reported (Knudson *et*
al., 1973).

One tumor which does not follow this pattern with any measurable frequency is
bronchogenic carcinoma. Perhaps this is a result of environmental influences
which have greatly expanded any nonhereditary component in this century.
Heredity in some way does seem to be important, and evidently interacts with
cigarette smoking to produce a synergistic effect (Tokuhata, 1964). Further
details of the interaction of heredity and environment in this disease will be
discussed below.

It is quite clear that leukemia and lymphoma are associated with several
chromosomal abnormalities and recessively inherited disorders, but it is less clear
whether a dominant contribution exists. There are pedigrees with as many as four
generations of affected individuals. Concordance in twins is estimated to be
approximately 25% (MacMahon and Levy, 1964; Miller, 1968), which is too high
to be explained by the contribution of known predisposing recessive conditions. It
has been surmised on the basis of familial patterns and earlier onset of familial
cases that a dominant subgroup exists, although its contributions to the total
cannot be estimated (Knudson *et al.*, 1973).

Consideration of the common cancers leads then to the conclusion that it is
highly probable that all human cancers contain at least one dominantly inherited
subgroup of cases, even though its contribution to the total may vary from as high
as 40% for some childhood tumors to as low as 1% or less for some adult tumors.
Features that the dominant forms invariably share are earlier onset and tendency
to multiplicity,

4. A Mutation Model for Human Cancer

4.1. Initiation in Two or More Steps

A two-step mutation model has been created for retinoblastoma in which it is
assumed that initiation of cancer occurs by the transformation of a normal cell into
a cancer cell in two steps. The first step is thought to be a mutation because it can be
inherited; in nonhereditary, or postzygotic, cases it is thought to occur in somatic
cells. The second step always occurs in somatic cells and may also be a mutation.
The process is considered to be essentially the same in all cases. Tumor
development then proceeds by the proliferation of these initiated cells.

The possibility that all forms of cancer have a dominantly inherited subgroup
suggests that such a model may serve for cancer generally. Both two-stage and
multistage models have been constructed previously (Armitage and Doll, 1954,
1957; Ashley, 1969*a*). These models are based on consideration of the age-specific
incidence or mortality. A steep rise in incidence or mortality with age would
indicate more stages, or "hits." So many assumptions must go into these
estimates that they are very hazardous. In any case, however, more than one hit is
visualized. These hits have been considered as somatic mutations. Burch (1962,
1965) has surmised that one or more hits could be inherited, thus reducing the

necessary number of somatic mutations. A comparison has been made by Ashley (1969*b*) between colon cancer generally and polyposis of the colon in particular on this basis. It is concluded that the total number of hits is reduced by one or two in the latter. If mutant cells exhibit higher growth rates, the number would be placed at one. Since polyposis results from the heritable mutation, this may indeed be the case. A good possibility is that carcinoma of the colon arises in two or more steps and that in polyposis the number is reduced by one.

If, then, a model of two or more steps is tenable, question arises whether the second step is mutational. No direct evidence is available on this point, although support for the idea has been presented on the basis of an increased incidence of connective tissue tumors in hereditary cases of retinoblastoma and a still further increase in response to irradiation (Strong and Knudson, 1972; Knudson, 1973).

4.2. Genetic Consequences

A genetic initiation of cancer implies that individual cancers originate from a single cell. This prediction has been tested by the study of tumor-bearing females heterozygous for variant alleles at the X-linked locus for glucose-6-phosphate dehydrogenase. The evidence reviewed by Fialkow (1972) clearly supports the conclusion that cancer generally arises by clonal growth from a single cell. Contrary evidence is found in the case of neurofibromatosis and hereditary multiple trichoepitheliomas. Whether these tumors are relevant to cancer generally is not certain. If they are, this evidence argues against a second step being mutational. If hereditary tumors generally are derived clonally, then strong support is offered for the notion that any step beyond the first is also mutational. In any case, the available evidence gives strong support to the idea that the first step in nonhereditary tumors is a somatic mutation, even in viral-induced warts and in a tumor such as Burkitt's lymphoma, which is thought to be induced by a virus.

The initiation of cancer in two or more steps, at least one of which is mutational, creates no requirement for chromosomal change, yet the latter can be clearly associated with cancer. It was noted that in retinoblastoma visible chromosomal deletion can be associated, but is usually not. The term "mutation" should be used broadly here to signify heritable chromosomal change, be it deletion, rearrangement, point mutation, or other change. What relationship this mutation may have to the subsequent chromosomal abnormalities which characterize most cancers is not apparent. It is possible that these are only secondary changes having nothing to do with the process of initiation.

One consequence of this mutation hypothesis is that the mutational change in the first step is tissue(s) specific. All of the dominant tumors and tumor syndromes characteristically affect one or a few tissues and do not predispose to cancer generally. This may provide a clue to the physiological nature of the gene which is the site of the mutation. The most obvious type of candidate is a genetically specified cell-surface component, since cell surfaces are known to harbor tissue specificity and to play a role in the normal cell-to-cell interactions which are disturbed in cancer.

4.3. Role of Environmental Carcinogens

If mutation, either germinal or somatic, is an invariant phenomenon in the initiation of cancer, then what is the mechanism whereby environmental carcinogens act? Do they act as mutagens or do they operate in some basically different manner? A survey of principal carcinogens—viruses, radiation, and chemicals—suggests that all operate by changing the host genome, or, in the broadest sense, by acting as mutagens. Major sections of this volume are devoted to each of these environmental agents, so only those aspects related to the present discussion will be considered here.

Although there is no direct proof that viruses can cause cancer in man, it seems improbable that so many animal tumors could be caused by viruses without any human cancers being so caused. All that is known about mechanism must, however, come from animal tumor viruses. Tumor viruses in general, whether DNA- or RNA-containing, seem to interact with the host genome. Integration into host DNA is achieved by viral DNA, or, in the case of RNA viruses, a DNA transcript of viral RNA. Chromosomal breakage is characteristic of many tumor virus infections, and one, SV40, produces many more breaks in cells from individuals with Down's and Fanconi's syndromes than in normal cells (Miller and Todaro, 1969). Integrated tumor virus genomes can also be transmitted vertically and so resemble germinal mutations.

Point mutations and chromosome breaks could conceivably lead to cancer by providing tumor viruses with opportunity for integration; in this scheme, the viral genome might be considered as a necessary but not sufficient condition. Second, mutations or breaks might be caused by tumor viruses as well as by other agents; viruses would be sufficient but not necessary. Third, cancer mutations and integrated viral genomes—oncogenes (Todaro and Huebner, 1972)—or integrated precursors of viral genomes—protoviruses (Temin, 1972)—might be identical.

It has been repeatedly demonstrated that radiation can be a carcinogen in man. As noted above, recessively inherited xeroderma pigmentosum provides direct evidence that ultraviolet light is carcinogenic via damage to DNA. Increased sensitivity to X-ray-induced chromosome breakage occurs in Fanconi's syndrome (Higurashi and Conen, 1971), although the mechanism is not known. Such mutations do not provide tissue specificity in the sense that dominant mutations can, but are predisposing to damage by irradiation.

Xeroderma pigmentosum cells also exhibit defective repair of DNA lesions produced by a chemical carcinogen, N-acetoxy-2-acetylaminofluorene (Setlow and Regan, 1972). The carcinogenic metabolic derivatives of several polycyclic hydrocarbons have been shown to be mutagenic in a bacterial system (Ames *et al.*, 1973), making it now highly probable that the effects of chemical carcinogens are mediated via mutation. Of even greater consequence for human oncology is the observation that genetic predisposition to lung cancer is associated with a variant of an enzyme involved in the metabolic conversion of polycyclic hydrocarbons (of the type found in tobacco smoke) to active carcinogens. Kellermann *et al.* (1973) have studied the enzyme aryl hydrocarbon hydroxylase, an enzyme whose activity is greatly increased by various inducing agents. Approximately 50% of the population of the United states is homozygous for an allele associated with low inducibility. Among heavy smokers, these individuals are evidently less susceptible to lung cancer than are those who are homozygous for a "high inducibility" allele or those who are heterozygous for the two alleles. Among 50 patients with bronchogenic carcinoma, all heavy smokers, only two were found to be homozygous for low inducibility.

For all three classes of carcinogens evidence is mounting that their effects are produced by "mutation," using that term to include any transmissible change in the host genome.

5. Conclusions

The dominantly inherited tumors and tumor syndromes of man occur in all categories of cancer, where they comprise an estimated 1–40% of the total, depending on the tumor in question. More importantly, they suggest that a common mechanism, mutation in a tissue-specific gene, is a first step in the initiation of cancer. This step is not sufficient alone to produce cancer, and at least one more event must occur. Such another event may also be a mutation, although no direct evidence is available on that point.

Genetic predisposition to cancer is imparted by several chromosomal and recessively inherited conditions. The mechanisms whereby these genetic changes induce susceptibility are probably several, but for only one disease, xeroderma pigmentosum, is the mechanism known. There the genetic damage produced by ultraviolet light cannot be repaired, and it is reasonable to assume that mutations of the type found in the dominantly heritable tumors occur at an increased rate.

Environmental carcinogens seem to produce their effects via alterations in the host genome and are, in a broad sense, mutagenic. Tumor viruses present a special case in that integrated viral genomes or integrated precursors of viral genomes may be indistinguishable from mutations of the type which are dominantly inherited.

6. References

AARONSON, S. A., AND LYTLE, C. D., 1970, Decreased host cell reactivation of irradiated SV40 virus in xeroderma pigmentosum, *Nature (Lond.)* **228**:359.

AMES, B. N., DURSTON, W. E., YAMASAKI, E., AND LEE, F. D., 1973, Carcinogens are mutagens: A simple test system combining liver homogenates for activation and bacteria for detection, *Proc. Natl. Acad. Sci.* **70**:2281.

ANDERSON, D. E., 1970, Genetic varieties of neoplasia, in: *Genetic Concepts and Neoplasia* (M. D. Anderson Hospital Symposium), pp. 85–109, Williams and Wilkins, Baltimore.

ANDERSON, D. E., 1971, Clinical characteristics of the genetic variety of cutaneous melanoma in man, *Cancer* **28:**721.

ANDERSON, D. E., 1972, A genetic study of human breast cancer, *J. Natl. Cancer Inst.* **48:**1029.

ARMITAGE, P., AND DOLL, R., 1954, The age distribution of cancer and a multi-stage theory of carcinogenesis, *Brit. J. Cancer* **8:**1.

ARMITAGE, P., AND DOLL, R., 1957, A two-stage theory of carcinogenesis in relation to the age distribution of human cancer, *Brit. J. Cancer* **11:**161.

ASHLEY, D. J. B., 1969a, The two "hit" and multiple "hit" theories of carcinogenesis, *Brit. J. Cancer* **23:**313.

ASHLEY, D. J. B., 1969b, Colonic cancer arising in polyposis coli, *J. Med. Genet.* **6:**376.

AUERBACH, C., 1956, A possible case of delayed mutation in man. *Ann. Hum. Genet.* **20:**266.

BURCH, P. R. J., 1962, A biological principle and its converse: Some implications for carcinogenesis, *Nature (Lond.)* **195:**241.

BURCH, P. R. J., 1965, Natural and radiation carcinogenesis in man. II. Natural leukemogenesis: initiation, *Proc. Roy. Soc. Lond. Ser. B* **162:**240.

CASPERSSON, T., GAHRTON, G., LINDSTEN, J., AND ZECH, L., 1970, Identification of the Philadelphia chromosome as a number 22 by quinacrine mustard fluorescence analysis, *Exp. Cell Res.* **63:**238.

CLEAVER, J. E., 1968, Defective repair replication of DNA in xeroderma pigmentosum, *Nature (Lond.)* **218:**652.

CLEAVER, J. E., 1969, Xeroderma pigmentosum: A human disease in which an initial stage of DNA repair is defective, *Proc. Natl. Acad. Sci.* **63:**428.

FIALKOW, P. J., 1966, Autoimmunity and chromosomal aberrations, *Am. J. Hum. Genet.* **18:**93.

FIALKOW, P. J., 1972, Use of genetic markers to study cellular origin and development of tumors in human females, *Advan. Cancer Res.* **15:**191.

FRAUMENI, J. F., 1969, Constitutional disorders of man predisposing to leukemia and lymphoma, *Natl. Cancer Inst. Monogr.* **32:**221.

GARDNER, E. J., AND RICHARDS, R. C., 1953, Multiple cutaneous and subcutaneous lesions occurring simultaneously with hereditary polyposis and osteomatosis, *Am. J. Hum. Genet.* **5:**139.

GATTI, R. A., AND GOOD, R. A., 1971, Occurrence of malignancy in immunodeficiency diseases: A literature review, *Cancer* **28:**89.

GERMAN, J., 1972, Genes which increase chromosomal instability in somatic cells and predispose to cancer, *Prog. Med. Genet.* **8:**61.

GORLIN, R. J., SEDANO, H. O., VICKERS, R. A., AND CERVENKA, J., 1968, Multiple mucosal neuromas, pheochromocytoma and medullary carcinoma of the thyroid—A syndrome, *Cancer* **22;**293.

HECHT, F., BRYANT, J. S., GRUBER, D., AND TOWNES, P. L., 1964, The nonrandomness of chromosomal abnormalities: Association of trisomy 18 and Down's syndrome, *New Engl. J. Med.* **271:**1081.

HECHT, F., McCAW, B. K., AND KOLER, R. D., 1973, Ataxia-telangiectasia—Clonal growth of translocation lymphocytes, *New Engl. J. Med.* **289:**286.

HIGURASHI, M., AND CONEN, P. E., 1971, *In vitro* chromosomal radiosensitivity in Fanconi's anemia, *Blood* **38:**336.

HIRSCHHORN, K., AND BLOCH-SHTACHER, N., 1970, Transformation of genetically abnormal cells, in: *Genetic Concepts and Neoplasia* (M. D., Anderson Hospital Symposium), pp. 191–202, Williams and Wilkins, Baltimore.

KELLERMANN, G., SHAW, C. R., AND LUYTEN-KELLERMANN, M., 1973, Aryl hydrocarbon hydroxylase inducibility and bronchogenic carcinoma, *New Engl. J. Med.* **289:**934.

KERSEY, J. H., GATTI, R. A., GOOD, R. A., AARONSON, S. A., AND TODARO, G. J., 1972, Susceptibility of cells from patients with primary immunodeficiency diseases to transformation by simian virus 40, *Proc. Natl. Acad. Sci.* **69:**980.

KNUDSON, A. G., 1971, Mutation and cancer: Statistical study of retinoblastoma, *Proc. Natl. Acad. Sci.* **68:**820.

KNUDSON, A. G., 1973, Mutation and human cancer, *Advan. Cancer Res.* **17:**317.

KNUDSON, A. G., AND STRONG, L. C., 1972a, Mutation and cancer: Neuroblastoma and pheochromocytoma, *Am. J. Hum. Genet.* **24:**514.

KNUDSON, A. G., AND STRONG, L. C., 1972b, Mutation and cancer: A model for Wilms' tumor of the kidney, *J. Natl. Cancer Inst.* **48:**313.

KNUDSON, A. G., STRONG, L. C., AND ANDERSON, D. E., 1973, Heredity and cancer in man, *Prog. Med. Genet.* **9**:113.

LADDA, R., ATKINS, L., LITTLEFIELD, J., AND PRUETT, R., 1973, Retinoblastoma: Chromosome banding in patients with heritable tumor, *Lancet* **2**:506.

LYNCH, H. T., AND KRUSH, A. J., 1971, Cancer family "G" revisited: 1895–1970, *Cancer* **27**:1505.

LYNCH, H. T., KRUSH, A. J., LARSEN, A. L., AND MAGNUSON, C. W., 1966, Endometrial carcinoma: Multiple primary malignancies, constitutional factors, and hereditary, *Am. J. Med. Sci.* **252**:381.

MACMAHON, B., AND LEVY, M. A., 1964, Prenatal origin of childhood leukemia: Evidence from twins, *New Engl. J. Med.* **270**:1082.

MILLER, R. W., 1963, Down's syndrome (mongolism), other congenital malformations and cancer among the sibs of leukemic children, *New Engl. J. Med.* **268**:393.

MILLER, R. W., 1968, Deaths from childhood cancer in sibs, *New Engl. J. Med.* **279**:122.

MILLER, R. W., 1970, Neoplasia and Down's syndrome, *Ann. N.Y. Acad. Sci.* **171**:637.

MILLER, R. W., AND TODARO, G. J., 1969, Viral transformation of cells from persons at high risk of cancer, *Lancet* **1**:81.

NEEL, J. V., 1962, Mutations in the human population, in: *Methodology in Human Genetics* (W. J. Burdette, ed.), pp. 203–224, Holden-Day, San Francisco.

NEEL, J. V., 1971, Familial factors in adenocarcinoma of the colon, *Cancer* **28**:46.

NOWELL, P. C., AND HUNGERFORD, D. A., 1960, A minute chromosome in human chronic granulocytic leukemia, *Science* **132**:1497.

NOWELL, P. C., AND HUNGERFORD, D. A., 1961, Chromosome studies in human leukemia. ii. Chronic granulocytic leukemia, *J. Natl. Cancer Inst.* **27**:1013.

PARRINGTON, J. M., DELHANTY, J. D. A., AND BADEN, H. P., 1971, Unscheduled DNA synthesis, u.v.-induced chromosome aberrations and SV40 transformation in cultured cells from xeroderma pigmentosum, *Ann. Hum. Genet.* **35**:149.

ROWLEY, J. D., 1973, A new consistent chromosomal abnormality in chronic myelogenous leukemia identified by quinacrine fluorescence and Giemsa staining, *Nature (Lond.)* **243**:290.

SETLOW, R. B., AND REGAN, J. D., 1972, Defective repair of N-acetoxy-2-acetylaminofluorene-induced lesions in the DNA of xeroderma pigmentosum cells, *Biochem. Biophys. Res. Commun.* **46**:1019.

SETLOW, R. B., REGAN, J. D., GERMAN, J., AND CARRIER, W. L., 1969, Evidence that xeroderma pigmentosum cells do not perform the first step in the repair of ultraviolet damage to their DNA, *Proc. Natl. Acad. Sci.* **64**:1035.

STRONG, L. C., AND KNUDSON, A. G., 1972, Mutation and childhood cancer: A model and its implications, *Am. J. Hum. Genet.* **24**:48a.

TEMIN, H. M., 1972, The RNA tumor viruses—Background and foreground, *Proc. Natl. Acad. Sci.* **69**:1016.

TODARO, G. J., AND HUEBNER, R. J., 1972, The viral oncogene hypothesis: New evidence, *Proc. Natl. Acad. Sci.* **69**:1009.

TOKUHATA, G. K., 1964, Familial factors in human lung cancer and smoking, *Am. J. Pub. Health* **54**:24.

WARTHIN, A. S., 1913, Heredity with reference to carcinoma: As shown by the study of the cases examined in the pathological laboratory of the University of Michigan, 1895–1913, *Arch. Int. Med.* **12**:546.

WILLIAMS, E. D., AND POLLOCK, D. J., 1966, Multiple mucosal neuromata with endocrine tumours: A syndrome allied to von Recklinghausen's disease, *J. Pathol. Bacteriol.* **91**:71.

WILSON, M. G., TOWNER, J. W., AND FUJIMOTO, 1973, Retinoblastoma and D-chromosome deletions, *Am. J. Hum. Genet.* **25**:57.

YOUNG, D., 1971, The susceptibility to SV40 virus transformation of fibroblasts obtained from patients with Down's syndrome, *Europ. J. Cancer* **7**:337.

4

Hormones as Etiological Agents in Neoplasia

JACOB FURTH

1. General Considerations

1.1. Historical

The hormonal concept of carcinogenesis was initiated by the intuitive studies of Beatson (1896) on the relation of breast cancer to the ovary. Epidemiological studies of mammary tumors of highly inbred strains of mice led Bittner and his associates (Bittner, 1946–1947) to the recognition of genetic, viral, and hormonal components in the development of breast cancer. Independently, Rous and Kidd (1941), on the basis of experimental studies on induction of skin cancers with carcinogens, advanced the multifactorial concept of tumorigenesis and postulated the existence of latent cancer cells. The recognition of "progression" during the course of neoplastic disease was best conceived by Foulds (*cf.* 1969). Finally, the recognition of immunosurveillance (Burnet, 1970; Jerne, 1973; Klein, 1973–1974) and of immunological and hormonal factors capable of restraining or enhancing tumor growth completed the picture of the complexity of forces involved in initiation and growth of tumors. The last of these—hormones—is reviewed here in light of all other forces.

1.2. Nomenclature and Abbreviations

Table 1 presents a simplified nomenclature (Furth *et al.*, 1973*d*), slightly modified, with the many synonyms which are still widely used. Our nomenclature utilizes

JACOB FURTH ● Institute of Cancer Research and Department of Pathology, Columbia University College of Physicians and Surgeons, New York, New York. Supported by USPHS grant CA-02332 from the National Cancer Institute. Prepared with the technical and editorial assistance of Mrs. Judith Grauman.

TABLE 1

Nomenclature and Abbreviations

Pituitary cell type		Old nomen- clature	Hormone	Class of Li (1972)	Pitui- tary tumor	End- organ tumor
Name	Abbrevi- ation					
Adrenotrope	At	Basophil (?)	AtH (ACTH)	I	AtT	AT
Mammotrope	Mt	Acidophil	MtH (prolactin, P[a], LtH[b])	II	MtT	MT
Somatotrope	St	Acidophil	StH(growth hormone, GH[a])	II	StT	
Thyrotrope	Tt	Basophil	TtH (TSH)	III	TtT	TT
Gonadotrope[c]	Gt	Basophil	GtH	III	GtT	OT, etc.[d]
Luteotrope	Lt	Basophil	LH[e]	III	LtT	
Folliculotrope	Ft	Basophil	FtH (FSH)	III	FtT	

[a] Abbreviations such as these are helpful, but when first used they should be accompanied by the generally accepted synonym.

[b] The synonym LtH, for MtH (prolactin), is widely and, in my opinion, incorrectly used. Prolactin, as Li (1972) states, is involved in "growth, development and lactation of the mammary gland . . . ." Hence MtH is preferable.

[c] Recent studies favor the view that one cell, the gonadotrope, secretes both FtH and LH. Those who hold the opposite view can express it by the use of Ft and Lt.

[d] Since the gonads are composed of several different types of hormone-secreting cells, names of their tumors should be given in full and indicated according to the author's concept. For example, the ovarian tumors (OT) can be composed of granulosa cells secreting estrogens, lutein cells secreting predominantly progestins, and so on.

[e] The still common usage of LtH for prolactin made it inadvisable to adopt LtH for the luteinizing hormone.

three letters. The first is the initial of the target organ of the hormone; the second, a small "t," is for tropin (*tropos* = turning to; stimulating); the third is either H (hormone) or T (tumor). For example, TtH stands for thyrotropic hormone, TtT for thyrotropic tumor, and TT for thyroid tumor.

In historical sequence, the nomenclature of pituitary cells was first tinctorial, then morphological, and then "Greek lettered," combining the former two features. This terminology was rendered obsolete by great differences in staining properties of the same cell in different species and in different physiological states within a species, as well as by changes in techniques used. I recommend that the pituitary cells be named after the type of hormone they secrete. Presently, this scheme cannot be rigidly applied, as indicated in footnotes to Table 1. It remains for an international committee to arrive at a standard nomenclature based not on perpetuating the historical confusion but rather on sound current knowledge.

As to hypothalamic hormones, I recommend the suffix .RH (releasing) or .IH (inhibiting), preceded by the initial of the pituitary hormone, when the hormones have been isolated (or synthesized). When their existence is based on circumstantial evidence, the suffix .RF or .IF (F, factor) is preferable. Hormone release is probably a stimulus of hormone production, by virtue of hormonal homeostasis.

Hence the hypothalamic releasing hormones are analogous to the pituitary tropic (or stimulating) hormones.

1.3. Neoplasia: Basic Defect and Types

Neoplasia is a multitude of diseases with one common denominator: failure of homeostatic control to limit the number of differentiated cells. The neoplastic cells are either hyperreactive to their physiological stimulant(s) or tardy in responding to their physiological inhibitor(s), thus gaining a proliferative advantage in their hosts. If the defect is complete, that is, if a cell fails to recognize its specific restraining influences—hormones, in the broad sense—the resulting tumorous growth is fully *autonomous*. If the defect is incomplete, the cell can be stimulated or inhibited, but not fully arrested, by its specific regulators, and is best called hormone *responsive*. The widely used mammary tumors (MT) induced in rats by chemical carcinogens, as described by Huggins *et al.* (1959), belong in the latter category. They are usually incorrectly labeled as hormone *dependent*. They grow progressively in the presence of the ovary and normal prolactin levels (Nagasawa *et al.*, 1973). Hence they are correctly labeled hormone responsive. Kim and Furth (1960*a,b*) found that regression of these tumors following ablation of the pituitary or ovaries (*cf.* Huggins and Yang, 1962) was incomplete and that the tumors could be resuscitated by high levels of MtH (Kim *et al.*, 1960*a*) (Fig. 1). This was done by grafting on these rats isologous, highly functional MtT, even several months after apparently "complete" regression. Further, after such treatment many new tumors appeared which can be considered hormone *dependent*. These studies were confirmed by some (first by Sterental *et al.*, 1963) and challenged by others. The controversy over the primacy of estrogens vs. proclactin is discussed in Section 3.

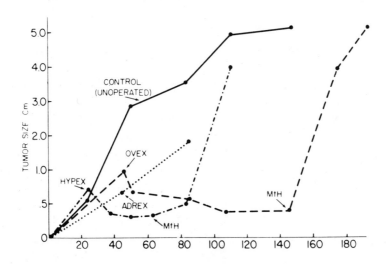

FIGURE 1. Induction, "extinction," and resuscitation of mammary tumors. From Kim *et al.* (1960*a*).

In man, about one-third of all MT are hormone responsive, and hormone-dependent tumors are unknown. In rats, all three types are known, but among the spontaneous tumors the benign fibroadenomas represent the majority. In mice, most MT are autonomous; few are hormone responsive and fibroadenomas are extremely rare. Most, if not all, murine mammary carcinomas (autonomous or responsive) carry a virus (MTV of Bittner). This virus is homologous to that found in MT of other species, including man (*cf.* Spiegelman and Schlom, 1972; Schlom and Spiegelman, 1973). Some leukemia viruses bear a similar relation to thymic hormones.

Different species and different inbred strains of the same species have a characteristic range of spontaneous tumors and sensitivity to diverse inducing agents. For example, thyrotropic pituitary tumors can be induced in all mice by thyroid hormone (TH) deficiency, but not in any other species.

1.3.1. Inducers and Promoters

The popular two- or multistage concept of carcinogenesis was initiated by the work of Rous and Kidd (1941) and expanded by Berenblum and associates (Berenblum, 1947). The changes produced by inducers (initiators) are irreversible, while those produced by promoters are reversible. We conceive of initiation as akin to mutation, modifying the reproductive apparatus of somatic differentiated cells (DNA-protein). The three classes of inducers—chemicals, ionizing radiations, and viruses— can alone induce neoplastic transformation and do it more efficiently in cells stimulated to proliferation. In contrast, evanescence is a basic feature of the effect of hormonal promoters.

The three classes of carcinogens are essentially alike in their basic mode of action, all being chromatinophilic, but there are marked differences among them. Electromagnetic radiation can affect resting cells instantaneously; particulate irradiations are more slow acting. Chemicals differ widely in their mode of action. The nucleic acid of viruses can persist and multiply in the cytoplasm or become incorporated in the DNA of the host's cell in latent form until some secondary "factor" brings about neoplastic transformation of a host cell. By and large, the causative chemicals, unlike the viruses, are absent when the tumors are detected.

As a generalization, dividing the components of carcinogenesis into two categories, inducers and promoters, is didactically useful but not absolutely correct. There is suggestive evidence that sustained proliferation of cells, as induced by persisting hormonal derangement, is conducive to spontaneous mutations, even without the aid of a conventional carcinogen (see Section 6).

A unique feature of carcinogen-induced tumors is that they are usually autonomous at the start, while those initiated by homeostatic derangements are initially hormone responsive and then go through sequential transformation (mutation) toward autonomy. Notable exceptions are Huggin's dimethyl-benz[a]anthracene (DMBA) induced MT of rats (Huggins *et al.*, 1961), which begin as hormone-dependent tumors.

TABLE 2
*Breast Cancer Induction with Subcarcinogenic Doses
of Carcinogens Aided by Hormones*

Carcinogen:	Radiation	Chemical[a]	Virus
Dose:	50 R	10 mg	0.1 ml milk[b]
Species:	Rat	Rat	Mouse
Carcinogen alone:	0	0	0
MtH alone:	0	0	0
Carcinogen + MtH:	58%	85%	40%

[a] 3-Methylcholanthrene.
[b] Containing MTV.

Sustained, uninterrupted stimulation of a cell can be the determinant of whether a cell transformed by a carcinogen will develop into a tumor. This is illustrated in Table 2 (*cf.* Yokoro *et al.*, 1961; Yokoro and Furth, 1962; Kim and Furth, 1960*c*). The three classes of carcinogens were applied in subcarcinogenic doses. No tumors developed when either hormone or carcinogen alone was applied. The combination of the two caused many tumors.

Hormones promote carcinogenesis by enhancing cell replication. The consequences of enhanced replication of cells are (1) increasing the chance of error of DNA copying, (2) enhancing code-breaking action of subthreshold doses of mutagens (virus, chemicals, radiation), (3) unmasking latent DNA changes caused earlier by mutagens. (In this manner, hormones are procarcinogens.) Cell replication is enhanced *in vivo* by regenerative hyperplasia and in cell cultures by the absence of the cell-specific homeostatic inhibitors or by the addition of nonspecific growth factors. In cell cultures, neoplastic and nonneoplastic transformations are inevitable without a carcinogen. This can be explained as resulting from frantic replication of cells unchecked by homeostatic inhibitors and pushed by diverse growth factors.

The significance of the events sketched in Table 2 is apparent when one considers that small doses of carcinogens are invariably present in the human body and in its environment. The inducers can hit many cells and create mutants of various kinds (lethal or viable latent or overtly transformed cells). We propose to subdivide the mutants into metabolic and neoplastic types. The former are related to aging, the latter to neoplasia.

1.3.2. Progression

Foulds (*cf.* 1969) was the first to emphasize the concept of "progression" in neoplasia. The hormone-induced experimental cancers are the best models for demonstration of progression. Behind it lies the surveillance mechanism of the host (Burnet, 1970), which can act as a brake in progression, but it rarely brings about complete spontaneous arrest of spontaneous (unlike grafted) tumors.

Recent developments in knowledge of immunological deviations in spontaneous tumors promise significant therapeutic advancements.

1.3.3. Phanerosis

A rarely considered mode of hormonal action which can bring about expression of latent cancer may be termed "phanerosis." This has been best demonstrated by subjecting DMBA-treated, ovariectomized rats to large doses of MtH. It should be recalled that fully hormone-dependent MT grow only in MtH-enriched hosts. This is the mildest form of neoplastic transformation. It may explain the very late manifestation of some neoplasms due to changing hormonal environment with age—for example, MT of women in menopause or radiation-induced OT of mice.

1.4. Homeostasis (Cybernetics) and Neoplasia

The term "homeostasis," meaning the maintenance of the internal environment to attain a steady state, was introduced by Cannon (1932) following the ideas of Claude Bernard.

Hormones, in common usage, are substances produced by one type of cell that regulate the growth or function of another cell, which they reach by way of the bloodstream. Increase or decrease in function of cells regulated by hormones proceeds incessantly, as by a thermostat, without cytogenetic changes. Most hormones are pituitary related (hence the expression "master gland"). Until recently, neoplasia could be dealt with as a disturbance of feedback mechanisms (positive or negative) between a pituitary cell and its target organ. Neoplasia is now viewed as a derangement of a highly ordered communication system which limits the number of each cell type, assigning a quota to each, adjusting this quota to the shifting need (cf. Wiener, 1948; Furth, 1969). Mutation-like transformation of a cell is accepted as a common, but not the sole, event that can lead to neoplastic growth. Interruption of the communication system is another. Wiener (1948) pointed out that life in a pluricellular organism exists through a delicate integration of many regulatory centers possessing specialized functions. Integration is achieved by systems of communication, termed by him "cybernetics."

Recent developments have led to the recognition of four levels of communications—I, cerebral; II, hypothalamic; III, pituitary; and IV, visceral—the derangements of which play a major role in the origin and growth of neoplasms (Figs. 2 and 3). The basic defect can reside in either the regulating or the regulated cell or merely in disruption of their communication. Superimposed on this system are numerous nonspecific growth modulators. (For details on intercellular communications leading to loss of contact inhibition, see Lowenstein, 1968, and for details on the hypothetical substances acting by contact, named "chalones," see Iversen, 1970.)

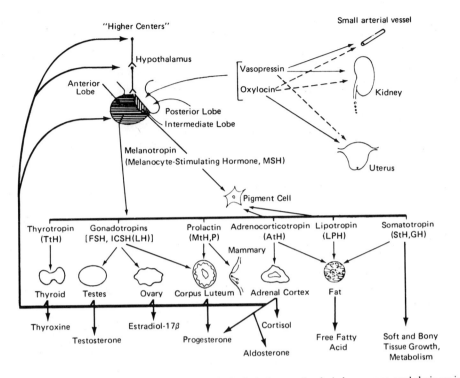

FIGURE 2. The classic scheme of Lyons and Li of pituitary cells, their hormones, and their major target organs, updated by Li (1972) and modified slightly by us.

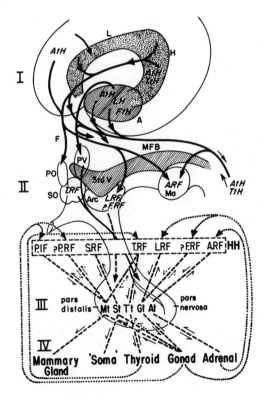

FIGURE 3. A cybernetic sketch indicating with arrows the four levels of communications. I. Cerebral and limbic; II, hypothalamic; III, pituitary; IV, peripheral target organs. Abbreviations: L, limbic system; H, hippocampus; A, amygdala; F, fornix; MFB, medial forebrain bundle; Ma, mammillary body; PV, paraventricular nucleus; PO, preoptic nucleus; SO, supraoptic nucleus; Arc, arcuate nucleus; HH, hypothalamic hormones. From Furth *et al.* (1973*d*).

1.5. Tumorigenesis by Hormonal Derangement

The efficiency of procedures to induce tumorigenesis by hormonal derangement varies with different tumors. In general, the tumors so induced are benign, and there is a "fluid" transition between hyperplasia, conditioned neoplasia, and autonomous neoplasia. This is best exemplified by induction of TtT, in which events proceed in "slow motion." Neoplasms experimentally induced by carcinogens are often autonomous at the start. This may be a matter of the dose and may not hold for spontaneous neoplasms.

1.5.1. Ablation of an Endocrine Gland

Ablation of an endocrine gland, thereby removing the specific inhibitor of a pituitary tropic cell, is illustrated by induction of TtT by thyroidectomy (tumorigenesis by exaggeration of negative feedback) (Fig. 4) (*cf.* Furth *et al.,* 1973*a*). The induction of "basophilic" tumors of the anterior pituitary, estrogen-secreting adrenocortical tumors, and MT in neonatally gonadectomized mice was

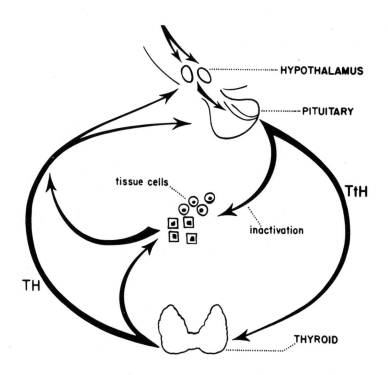

FIGURE 4. The original feedback scheme of the thyroid–thyrotrope axis. Disruption of TH pathway yields TtT by negative feedback; TtH excess yields TT by positive feedback. The routes of TH to peripheral (somatic) organs and the modulating routes of TH to the hypothalamic centers are indicated. From Furth (1969).

reported by Dickie and Woolley (1949) and Dickie and Lane (1956). Houssay *et al.*
(1953, 1954) confirmed the induction of similar AT and pituitary tumors in
gonadectomized rats and described the latter as GtT. Following similar procedures, Iglesias *et al.* (1969, 1972) reported the isolation of a GtT with very low
potency. These observations are good examples of Claude Bernard's principle of
determinism, illustrating how a single event (gonadectomy) sets in motion a
sequence of changes: compensation by adrenal cortical cells for loss of ovarian
estrogen secretion, formation of adrenal adenomas, and, finally, development of
MT and pituitary adenomas of yet to be determined character (*cf.* Furth and
Clifton, 1958).

1.5.2. Sustained Administration of a Specific Stimulant

Sustained administration of a specific stimulant, as induction of MtT with
estrogens and of TT with TtH (Fig. 4), is an example of the reverse type of
procedure: exaggeration of positive feedback (*cf.* Furth and Clifton, 1966). The
induction of a pituitary tumor with estrogens was discovered almost simultaneously by several investigators in 1936. By 1953, Gardner *et al.* listed 24 articles on
induction of pituitary tumors in animals by steroid hormones. The functional
character and histological types of these tumors were disputed until transplantation studies, analysis of the secondary changes, and bioassays established that they
have mammary gland stimulating and growth-promoting activities (*cf.* Furth and
Clifton, 1966).

The convenient way to induce MtT in rats and mice is by administration of
diethylstilbestrol (DES) pellets. The latency period of tumor development is in
direct relation to the dose. Pellets of 5–10 mg are toxic in rats, causing early death
of the animals with or without macroscopic MtT. Estradiol is more effective than
estrone; estriol is ineffective. Androgens and progestins are antitumorigenic.
Elevation of plasma MtH values is progressive during the course of estrogen
treatment. Mammary gland hyperplasia with milk secretion documents the
functional character of the primary tumors. On transplantation, MtH activity
tends to decline; StH activity rises and occasionally becomes dominant.

MtT is the most common pituitary tumor in old rats of both sexes (*cf.* Ito *et al.*,
1972*a*). The high incidence of spontaneous MtT in male rats is puzzling.

Sustained hyperstimulation of GtH can be attained by grating ovaries in spleens
of castrates. The gonadal hormones are inactivated in the liver, thereby raising the
circulating GtH levels, as illustrated in Fig. 5 (more fully described in Section
2.3.1.).

Prolonged administration of StH (reported by Moon *et al.*, 1950*a,b,c*, 1951)
causes an increase in development of several types of tumors.

1.5.3. Blocking Hormone Synthesis

Blocking hormone synthesis, as blocking TH synthesis by antithyroidal substances, can produce hyperstimulation of TtH, resulting in TtT and/or TT.

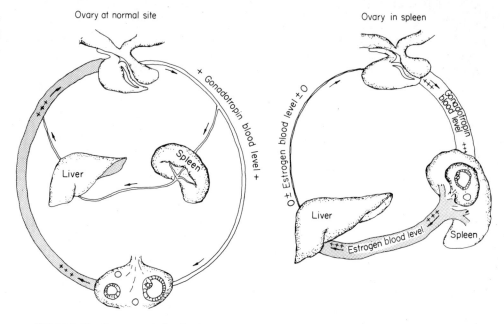

FIGURE 5. Ovarian tumor induction by intrasplenic grafts of ovaries in castrates, an example of neoplasia induction by misplacement of an organ. From Furth (1969).

1.5.4. Isografts of the Pituitary

Isografts of the pituitary (introduced by Loeb and Kirtz, 1939) in extrasellar locations result first in excessive discharge of MtH, causing MT and later MtT at the site of the graft. These and other related events have been reviewed elsewhere (Furth *et al.*, 1973*d,e*), including more recent studies with rats and the use of radioimmunoassays.

Hormone-responsive transplantable MT are best obtained by a *combination* of subthreshold doses of a carcinogen and high levels of MtH (Kim and Furth, 1960*b*).

1.5.5. Problems

The idea that low-dose irradiations and other carcinogens may lead to a technique for induction of as many types of transplantable pituitary tumors as there are hormone-producing pituitary cells has thus far not been adequately explored.

Although most findings reported are well documented the character and pathogenesis of the various tumors induced, notably pituitary tumors following gonadectomy and AtT induced by ionizing radiations, remain to be elucidated.

Tumorigenesis can probably be modified (promoted or inhibited), possibly even initiated, by drugs acting via the hypothalamus. This is another area yet to be fully explored.

For more detail on neoplasia induction by hormonal derangement, the reader is referred to the reviews or monographs of Gardner *et al.* (1953), Russfield (1966), Furth and Clifton (1966), Kwa (1961), and Furth *et al.* (1973*d, e*).

2.1. Neurohypothalamic Areas and Neoplasia

The existence of hypothalamic substances regulating anterior pituitary function was postulated by Green and Harris (1947) and demonstrated by Harris (*cf.* 1955) by tapping the hypophyseal portal veins. Subsequent developments led to the isolation of several low molecular weight polypeptides in the hypothalamus and to the recognition of neural influences on the hypothalamus. Hypothalamic factors (hormones) are now known to control production and release of the pituitary hormones AtH, TtH, LH, FtH, StH, and MtH. Two adenohypophyseal hormones, MtH and StH, are also under the influence of hypothalamic inhibitory factors (hormones).

Figure 2 is the classic diagram of Lyons and Li (updated by Li, 1972) on the levels of hormonal communications, including the target organ hormones. Figure 3 is our cybernetic sketch indicating lines of communications (Furth *et al.*, 1973*d*). The fulcrum of the four levels of the regulatory system is the pituitary gland. It receives impulses from both the visceral cells and the hypothalamus. The impulses or responses of the cerebral system are transmitted to the hypothalamus by neural routes, at the long terminals of which these messages are expressed by neurohormones. The hypothalamus is the transmitter of impulses received from the cerebral or visceral areas and acts by discharging hormones of its own into the hypophysis by way of the portal system.

Neoplasia can be initiated not only by a change in the four integrated areas but also by a mere disruption of communication among them (Fig. 3), resulting in an excess of "target cell" stimulating influences or a deficiency of its inhibiting influences. The role of hypothalamic hormones in neoplasia seems to be limited to modulation of pituitary hormones. Tumors do occur in the hypothalamic area (*cf.* Turkington, 1972), but none has been actually identified as a direct secretor of hypothalamic hormones. The pituitary can give rise to monomorphous tumors of perhaps all of its tropic cellular components. The differentiated neurons do not multiply. Tumors of neurons are likely to be congenital. The same applies to the neural lobe of the pituitary, which is a storage organ of oxytocin and vasopressin.

The hypothalamic hormones have been extensively studied from the standpoint of their physiological effects, but with the exception of P.IF little is known of their influence in tumorigenesis. The following are some illustrative examples: GH.IH (StH.IH) was isolated from ovine hypothalami by Brazeau *et al.* (1973). It strongly lowers GH levels in patients with acromegaly without affecting prolactin levels (Hall *et al.*, 1973), but also impairs the normal TtH and FtH responses to T.RH. T.RH is one of the best studied hypothalamic polypeptides. Administration of T.RH causes a sharp and marked rise of TtH within 3 min, with a slow dropping thereafter. Grant *et al.* (1973) found two binding sites on Tt cells, differing in intensity of affinity for T.RH and its analogues. However, Clifton (1963) has presented some suggestive evidence for the essentiality of hypothalamic connections in induction of TtT in mice and has suggested that T.RH plays some role in development of TT.

As concerns mammary neoplasia, P.IF and P.RF are highly important. Their discovery was "inevitable" following the studies of Harris (*cf.* 1955) on their presence in the hypophyseal portal vessels. The enhanced pituitary MtH secretion occurring as a sequel to pituitary isografts is due to lack of hypothalamic P.IF. This discovery of Everett and Nikitovich-Winer (1963) followed the analysis of the phenomenon that pituitary isografts were conducive to the development of MT (Loeb and Kirtz, 1939).

A great impetus in this area came from the recognition of drugs which act on the central nervous system via P.IF or P.RF. Flückiger (1972) names nine tranquilizers, two psychomotor stimulants, two antihistamines, two antihypertensives, and other drugs that influence prolactin secretion. Ten of these, tested for their influence on prolactin secretion, exhibited diverse unwanted side-effects, but some ergot alkaloids (Shelesnyak, 1954) have proved to be of practical value.

In his pioneer studies, Meites (*cf.* 1973) indicated that administration of drugs that decrease prolactin release (such as L-dopa, iproniazid, pargyline, and certain ergot drugs) results in reduced MT growth; while other drugs that increase prolactin release (as reserpine, haloperiodol, or methyldopa) accelerate growth of MT in rats. Incidentally, these findings lent further support to earlier biological studies indicating that prolactin is a major, often the essential, hormone for induction and growth of many MT.

The rapid advancement in this area is indicated by the proceedings of three international conferences on prolactin (Wolstenholme and Knight, 1972; Boyns and Griffiths, 1972; Pasteels and Robyn, 1973) and one monograph (Horrobin, 1973) containing a wealth of information on the biochemistry and physiology of prolactin, including its role in carcinogenesis.

The pivotal role of these hypothalamic factors in the growth of established hormone-sensitive carcinomas is attested to by the flood of current experimental and clinical observations (e.g., Minton and Dickey, 1973). Suppression of serum prolactin by L-dopa alone can produce clinical remissions in carcinoma of the breast and relieve the bone pain, presumably as a result of suppression of tumor growth, with no consistent changes in FtH, GH, LH, estradiol, estrone, estriol, and progesterone levels (Dickey and Minton, 1972a,b).

All known drugs exerting their effects by way of the hypothalamus are short-acting. The synthetic ergot alkaloid CB-154 (2-bromo-α-ergocryptine; Flückiger, 1972) can be injected daily over long periods of time. The development of long-acting prolactin inhibitors is required to attain a lasting depression of prolactin discharge with inhibition of tumor growth. Welsch and Gribler (1973) found that CB-154 is an effective inhibitor of the developmental phases of murine MT, but not of MT in mature multiparous mice. Welsch *et al.* (1973) found that the combined administration of ergocornine and reserpine (but neither drug alone) produced as prolonged and as good a regression of DMBA-induced MT of mice as did hyperphysectomy. Buckman and Peake (1973) found that stimulation of prolactin by perphenazine is augmented by prior estrogen treatment.

The hypothalamic hormones do not seem as specific as would be required for homeostasis of a target organ function. For example, several investigators have demonstrated elevated serum MtH following administration of T.RH. Mt cells possess receptor sites for T.RH (*cf.* Grant *et al.*, 1973). Increase in the rate of synthesis of MtH produced by T.RH in cultures of rat pituitary cells was reported by Hinkle and Tashjiam (1973). However, no one, to our knowledge, has demonstrated biological MtH activity following administration of T.RH. To unravel the lack of specificity of these hormones is an intriguing problem. Mechanisms do exist to block biological activity by a circulating hormone. For example, in MtT F4-bearing rats, StH activity is blocked by adrenal corticoids. L-dopa has been reported to suppress T.RH-stimulated MtH release (Noel *et al.*, 1973). Dimethoxyphenylethylamine blocks the dopamine-inhibitory control of MtH secretion (Smythe and Lazarus, 1973). It is known that MtH and StH are related structurally and biologically, but Flückiger (*cf.* 1972) found that L-dopa and chlorpromazine have opposite actions on MtH and StH secretion. Competitive interaction can occur at hypothalamic, pituitary, or peripheral levels.

For more details on the rapidly evolving knowledge on neural and hypothalamic influences and other substances acting by way of the hypothalamus, the reader should see the respective mongraphs and reviews of Haymaker *et al.* (1969), Meites (1970), Knigge *et al.* (1972), Ganong and Martini (1973), Locke and Schally (1973) Vale *et al.* (1973), Schally *et al.* (1973), and Thomas and Mawhinney (1973).

Despite the problem of specificity, hypothalamic hormones hold considerable promise in cancer research, as either prophylactic or therapeutic agents, doing away with drastic surgical procedures in disease control (*cf.* Stoll, 1972).

2.2. Cell Types of the Adenohypophysis and Their Neoplasms

The adenohypophysis (pars distalis) is believed to be composed of five cell types secreting ten different hormones. On the basis of structural and biological effects, Li (1972) divides these hormones into three classes: I—AtH, melanocyte-stimulating hormones (α- and β-MSH), lipotropic hormones (β- and γ-LPH); II—StH (GH) and MtH (P); III—LH (luteinizing and interstitial cell stimulating hormone = ICSH), FSH, TtH. The principal functions of the ten hormones are as follows: (1) *AtH* stimulates the adrenal cortex to produce steroid hormones as cortisol and corticosterone; (2, 3) α- *and* β-*MSH* cause darkening of skin by melanogenesis in preexisting unpigmented melanocytes; (4, 5) β- *and* γ-*LPH* cause release of lipid from adipose tissue; (6) *StH (GH)* has an anabolic effect on various tissues of the body and affects fat, carbohydrate, and protein metabolism and general body growth; (7) *MtH(P)* is responsible for the growth, development, and lactation of the mammary gland; (8) *LH (ICSH)* in women, affects the development of interstitial cells in the ovaries and is related to reproduction and in men is responsible for development of interstitial cells in the testes and affects reproduction; (9) *FSH* in women induces the development of follicles in the ovaries and affects reproduction and in men stimulates seminiferous tubules and spermatogenesis; (10) *TtH* is responsible for the production and secretion of thyroid hormones. This schematic description, based mainly on Li's concepts, is given for general didactic purposes with the qualification that there are numerous "gray" areas concerning all unit systems of the adenohypophysis.

Structural relationships explain why one cell type can possess more than one hormonal potency. Although all hormones possess a high degree of specificity when used in physiological doses, they can exhibit several activities when their concentration is high, as is the case with various hormonal derangements. Classic examples of such structural relationships are those between StH and MtH and between TtH and GtH. The latter has been thoroughly analyzed (Canfield *et al.*, 1971; Pierce *et al.*, 1971; Rathnam and Saxena, 1971; Vaitukaitis and Ross, 1972; Furth *et al.*, 1973*b*).

A single macromolecular hormone such as TtH and LH can give rise to several antibodies. The cross-reactions can be analyzed by quantitative absorption or blocking tests. The type-specific antigenic groups are named "β," and the common subunit is "α." The overlapping biological activities were first discovered years ago during the course of transplantation of TtT. The "built-in" MSH activity of AtT was similarly discovered during the course of transplantation studies by Steelman *et al.* (1956) and Bahn *et al.* (1957). According to more recent investigations (Nakane, 1970; Phifer *et al.*, 1972, 1973), the two gonadotropic hormones (FSH and LH) are secreted by the same cell, but what controls their secretion is obscure.

The physical properties of human MtH and StH are so close that separation was unsuccessful until Pasteels (*cf.* 1972) indicated the existence of a separate human MtH [subsequently purified by Friesen *et al.*, 1970 (*cf.* Friesen, 1972; Friesen and Hwang, 1973) and Lewis *et al.*, 1971]. The structural similarities of these two hormones are indicated by the following findings of Li (1973): For each milligram of human MtH there are 25 IU of lactogenic and 0.4 USP U of StH activity, while each milligram of human StH possesses 2 IU of lactogenic and 2 USP U of StH activity.

The "chromophobe" is a poorly secreting cell, a degranulated, functional differentiated cell, or a reserve undifferentiated cell. The term is now obsolete. The terms "acidophil" and "basophil" have some qualifying value (see Table 1).

Speculating on the evolution of pituitary hormones, Li (1972) considers AtH-MSH the ancestral molecule (see his Fig. 11). It is noteworthy in relation to his classification of hormones that when a pituitary cell becomes neoplastic the common change is usually a shift in its hormonal spectrum. For example, some MtT often exhibit more StH than MtH activity, to such an extent that three investigators independently described the transformation of the same MtT into an StT (MacLeod *et al.*, 1966; Tashjian *et al.*, 1968; Hollander and Hollander, 1971). Rare transplantable MtT strains appear to be predominantly AtH secreting and cause hypertension attributed to heightened adrenal cortical activity (Molteni *et al.*, 1972). Bates *et al.* (1966) and Martin *et al.* (1968) analyzed the relation of MStT of rats to diabetes. Similarly, when a TtT becomes autonomous it can exhibit greater gonadotropic than thyrotropic activity (Messier and Furth, 1962). Acquisition by one cell type of the biological activity of cells of another class of Li has also been reported (for example, StH activity of autonomous TtT; Furth *et al.*, 1973*c*).

When hormonal derangement is lasting, as is the case with neoplasms, secondary (minor) components may be expressed biologically (clinically) to such an extent that the primary (main) hormonal stimulation is obscured by secondary and tertiary derangements (see Section 5). This explains why the human (unlike the experimental) pituitary tumors are usually not named by the type of cell causing the initial change. For example, AtT is called Cushing's disease, MtT is known as Forbes–Albright syndrome, and StT as acromegaly or gigantism. Turkington (1972) identified MtH secretion in patients having tumors associated with Forbes–Albright syndrome, Chiari–Frommel syndrome, and Nelson's syndrome and in those having hypothalamic tumors.

Inasmuch as various hormone-secreting pituitary tumors (MtT, StT, MStT, AtT, FtT, and GtT) have been reviewed elsewhere (Furth *et al.*, 1973*d*), I have cited here only a few recent related reports.

Immunohistochemical staining can visualize the hormone content of all accepted pituitary cell types of man and experimental animals. The latter has been extensively illustrated in reviews of Baker (1970) and Nakane (1970) and in our own review (Furth *et al.*, 1973*e*). The two acidophils (Mt and St) are spherical (Fig. 6a, b). The characteristic feature of Mt is the "caplike" localization of the hormone about the nucleus, well illustrated in Fig. 6e. The Gt are somewhat larger and tend to be polyhedral (Fig. 6c). The At are highly angular, often resembling macrophages (Fig. 6d). In a human prolactin-secreting pituitary tumor (Fig. 6f), almost all cells have an affinity for antiprolactin, and for no other antihormone.

The counterpart of immunohistochemical staining is radioimmunoassay, which quantitates the discharged hormone in circulation at a given time. These two techniques are extremely useful tools in diagnosis and analysis of complex situations. For example, the half-life of various pituitary hormones can be studied by injecting labeled hormones and following their disappearance from the circulation. Storage and discharge can be ascertained by the rebound phenomenon (Furth *et al.*, 1973*a*). The character of a hormone-secreting tumor can be determined by immunohistochemical staining of the tumor for various hormones. The pharmacological effects of drugs can be similarly tested. For example, utilizing immunohistochemical staining Baker *et al.* (1972) found that treatment of adult female rats with a progestational compound (medroxyprogesterone acetate) caused a marked reduction in size of Mt cells and enlargement and increase in relative number of St cells. Gt cells responded variably and At cells were not affected significantly.

2.3. Neoplasia in Peripheral Endocrine-Related Organs

Neoplasia induced in peripheral organs by pituitary tumors and tumors arising in hormone-secreting organs outside the cranial cavity (such as hormone-related neoplasms of the parathyroid and insulinomas, medullary adrenal tumors,

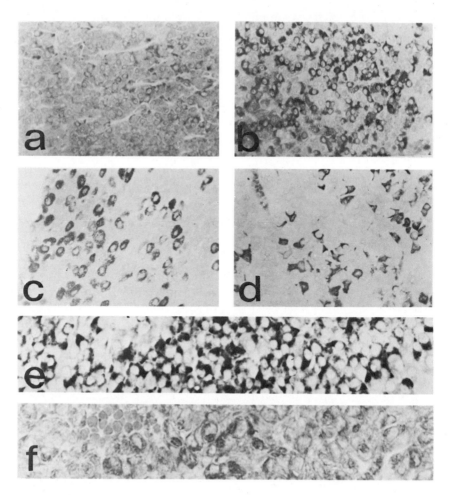

FIGURE 6. Normal and neoplastic cells of the adenohypophysis as visualized by immunohistochemical staining. (a) Normal female rat pituitary at 48 days of age, stained with anti-MtH. × 150. (b) Same, stained with anti-StH. × 150. (c) Same, stained with anti-LH. × 150. (d) Same, stained with anti-AtH. × 150. (e) Normal female rat pituitary at 124 days of age, stained with anti-MtH. × 350. (f) Human MtT stained with anti MtH. × 500. (Magnifications are approximate.)

melanomas, prostate tumors, and carcinoids) are omitted here. The following are brief general comments on tumors in peripheral areas illustrating the diversity of pathogenic mechanisms by which hormones can produce such tumors, notably those with which we have had personal experience. The character of hormone-related tumors varies with species, strain, tumor inducers, and the concentrations. For details on peripheral hormone-related tumors, the reader should see the comprehensive textbooks of Willis (1967) and Williams (1968) for general orientation, and subsequent volumes of this treatise.

Peripheral tumors are of two kinds: those affecting non-hormone-secreting organs, which do not feed back (as the mammary gland), and those affecting peripheral hormone-secreting organs, which do. The best example of the former is MT. Good examples of the second type are TT and OT. The latter are variously hormone secreting and can themselves induce tumors with different spectra. The male "analogy" of the mammary gland tumor is the prostate tumor. On clinical grounds, androgens are suspected of being the responsible hormone in the genesis of prostate tumors, but thus far attempts to develop a hormone-dependent prostatic carcinoma have been unsuccessful.

2.3.1. Ovarian Tumors

Experimental studies on induction of leukemias by X-rays led to the discovery of development of OT in most irradiated mice. Such tumors can arise from any cell of the ovary other than ova: from granulosa and lutein cells, which secrete characteristic steroid hormones, and from nonsecreting germinal, epithelial, stromal, and endothelial cells. By means of transplantation, monomorphous tumors can be obtained. The primary radiation-induced OT inevitably have a long latency; even if this inducer is applied very early in postnatal life, tumors will arise in the second half of the life span. Increasing the dose does not markedly hasten tumor induction. For references, see Bali and Furth (1949).

The identity of the GtH component in the mechanism of ovarian tumorigenesis was clarified following observations of Biskind and Biskind (1944) that mere transplantation of normal ovaries into the spleen of castrated rodents will also yield OT. This is attributed to (1) a break in the Gt–gonadal hormone feedback loop by diversion of the gonadal hormones to the liver, where they are inactivated as illustrated in Fig. 5 (Gardner *et al.*, 1959) (In cybernetics, this is said to "open the loop."), and (2) a consequential increase of GtH production. The primary tumors of ovarian grafts in the spleen are not autonomous—that is, transplantable into normal hosts—for about 9–12 months of the graft (Green, 1957). Numerous observations indicate the increase of GtH as one component of OT induction by radiation. The other is a direct injury to the ovary.

The transplanted granulosa cell tumors produce secondary changes indicative of estrogen secretion; those of luteomas point to progestin as the major steroid (Bali and Furth, 1949). Granulosa tumors produce a marked hypervolemia associated with anemia (Wish *et al.*, 1950), while the luteomas are associated with polycythemic hypervolemia and Cushing's syndrome (Gottschalk and Furth, 1951).

OT is one of the many tumors induced by the multipotent DMBA and other polycyclic aromatic hydrocarbons. The report of Howell *et al.* (1954) on the high incidence of granulosa cell OT in mice that had been repeatedly given oily solutions of DMBA was followed by numerous studies on the character and pathogenesis of those tumors. Jull and Phillips (1969) concluded that the carcinogenic effect of DMBA on mouse ovaries was direct but that it was modified by secretion of several pituitary hormones, notably gonadotropins. The tumors were autonomous, but gonadotropins accelerated tumorigenesis by DMBA (Orr, 1962). Some enzymatic and histochemical studies were made with such tumors by

Ueda *et al.* (1972), but the characterization of monomorphous OT from the standpoint of steroidogenesis and interrelationships and effects of serum and cell volumes remains to be fully explored. For further details on OT, the reader should consult Zuckerman (1962).

The most valuable technique for inducing OT is that of Biskind and Biskind (1944), because it is best suited for analysis of the sequential events from hyperplasia to dependent and this to autonomous OT.

2.3.2. Leydig Cell Tumors

Leydig cell tumors occur in small numbers of several strains of mice, rats, and dogs (*cf.* Gardner *et al.*, 1959; Russfield, 1966; Huseby, 1972). They are especially common in undescended testes and can be readily induced with estrogens. Experimental Leydig cell tumors were extensively studied by Huseby (1960) and Jacobs and Huseby (1972). The sequential changes from hyperplasia to neoplasia are similar to those of other estrogen-induced tumors (*cf.* Andervont *et al.*, 1957). The biological findings suggest that these tumors are usually androgen secreting, but the spectrum of steroids secreted by these tumors requires further study. Accumulation of ^{3}H-estradiol in mouse testes following prolonged treatment with estrogen was reported by Bollengier *et al.* (1972). Our observations (Clifton *et al.*, 1956) suggest that some tumors may secrete both estrogens and androgens. The very problem of the source of estrogens in male rodents, usually related to Sertoli cells (*cf.* Huggins and Moulder, 1945), also requires further study.

Hormone-independent Leydig cell tumors in the mouse have been well maintained in organ cultures, whereas those that were hormone dependent were poorly maintained (Elias and Rivera, 1959).

2.3.3. Thyroid tumors

There are two features common to the development of "spontaneous" and induced TT: (1) presence of thyroid cells that are capable of multiplication but are imparied in synthesis of thyroid hormones, and (2) elevated TtH levels. TH synthesis begins with "capture" of iodine, followed by sequential enzymatic processes and culminating in formation of L-triiodothyronine (T3) and L-thyroxine (T4). Nature provides ample opportunities for insult to this normal sequence, including iodine deficiency and goiterogenic agents in the diet. To these have been added man-made injuries to the thyroid epithelium, such as by "fallout" or accidental irradiation of the newborn. This subject has been thoroughly reviewed at two international conferences on thyroid cancer (see Hedinger, 1969; Young and Inman, 1968).

The sequential events in the goiterogen-induced adenomas and carcinomas have been well analyzed and reproduced in the laboratory. The initial hyperplasia is usually nodular and diffuse (unlike Grave's disease, in which the hyperplasia is diffuse but not nodular and seems to be unrelated to TtH). The malignant neoplasia appears late and varies in frequency in relation to intensity and maintenance of the thyroid damage. We studied the sequential changes from hyperplasia to highly malignant carcinoma by long-continued, uninterrupted exposure of normal thyroid grafts to very high levels of TtH produced by cografts of an autonomous TtH-secreting pituitary tumor. Several years of sequential transplantations yielded "sarcomatoid carcinomas" which were indistinguishable from human sarcomatoid carcinomas (often called sarcomas), leaving unresolved the question of whether a carcinoma cell can turn into a sarcoma cell (Ueda and Furth, 1967).

2.3.4. Other Tumors

a. Adrenal Tumors. Adrenal tumors (AT) are unique in that they can give rise to four or more types of tumors—estrogen, androgen, glucocorticoid, and mineralocorticoid secreting—and in that they have different types of inductive mechanisms, of which some have already been discussed. The type of AT extensively studied by my associates is glucocorticoid secreting. It proved suitable for assay of AtH (Cohen *et al.*, 1957) and was used to first establish the high AtH serum level in a patient with Cushing's syndrome in whom bilateral adrenalectomy was followed by manifestations of Cushing's disease AtT with MSH activity (Cohen and Furth, 1959). This condition was later named "Nelson's syndrome" after the investigator who thoroughly studied this event in numerous patients. The steroidogenesis by our AT was well investigated by Bloch *et al.* (1960). This tumor was used to first study the mechanism of adrenal stimulation by labeled AtH (Lefkowitz *et al.*, 1970a). It produces corticoid *in vitro* (Buonassisi *et al.*, 1962).

b. Renal Cortical Carcinomas. Renal cortical carcinomas induced by estrogens in male hamsters (Kirkman and Bacon, 1950; Horning, 1954) are among the most puzzling estrogen-dependent tumors. They are malignant yet hormone dependent and seem "specific" to hamsters.

c. Human Placental Lactogen. Human placental lactogen (HPL), a hormone with both MtH and StH activity, stimulates carcinogenesis by DMBA in young rats. It promotes mammary tumorigenesis during pregnancy, both directly and indirectly, through its promotion of progesterone secretion by the ovary (Nagasawa and Yanai, 1973).

d. Medullary Thyroid Carcinoma. Thyrocalcitonin is the hypocalcemic polypeptide hormone secreted by the medullary cells of the thyroid. These cells can give rise to tumors (Munson *et al.*, 1968; Taylor and Foster, 1970).

e. Ectopic Hormones. The ectopic hormones are discussed in Section 4.

3. Detection of Hormonal Activity

3.1. General Considerations

Hormonal stimulation or depression of an organ can be detected by clinical and anatomical changes. The criteria of malignancy are well defined in textbooks of pathological anatomy, but many hormone-dependent and responsive tumors do not possess such definitive identification marks as invasiveness and anaplasia, and masquerade as diffuse or nodular hyperplasia. Chromosomal abnormalities can be conspicuous in hyperplasia and, if marked, suggest cell transformation. However, the presence of transformed cells (commonly defined in tissue cultures by lack of contact inhibition) does not differentiate neoplastic from metabolic transformation. Both produce altered cells, either abnormally differentiated or mutated. Neoplastic cells possess a proliferative advantage over homeostatically controlled cells; metabolically altered cells usually do not. The latter are common in normal aging organs and may be a component of the aging process (*cf.* Furth, 1969). During sustained hyperplasia, as induced by hormonal derangement, an increasing number of cells undergo some transformation and exist intermingled with hyperplastic unaltered cells. Transformation of cells is hastened by chemical, viral, and radiation carcinogens. Depending on the dose of the carcinogen and other factors, the number of transformed cells may vary and some may be autonomous at the start. When neoplasia is rooted in a hormonal derangement, the initial phase is that of hyperplasia, which is usually followed by hormone-dependent and responsive neoplasia. Sustained hyperplasia may lead to neoplasia by means of spontaneous replication errors of the genetic apparatus (see Section 6).

It is likely that in their earlier (silent) phases, many tumors are hormone responsive or even hormone dependent—hence the importance of detecting such cells. For laboratory diagnosis of endocrine diseases, the reader should consult Sunderman and Sunderman (1971). For hormones in the blood, Gray and Bacharach (1967) should be consulted. Eckstein and Knowles (1963) have summarized the techniques in endocrine research. Some "footprints" of biochemical, histochemical, and immunological tests do exist; for evaluation of existing nodules of debatable character, transplantation assay is a useful tool.

Transplantation assays are suitable for both detection and characterization of neoplastic cells. They require the use of histocompatible strains of animals, and are therefore not feasible for assay of human tumors. As substitutes, techniques have been proposed which have one feature in common: the use of animals in which immunological antagonism is lacking or has been abolished. The older techniques are transplantation in the anterior chamber of the eye, or on the chorioallantoic membrane of the chick embryo, or in the cheek pouch of the hamster. These have been followed by the use of animals whose immunological capacity has been checked by administration of glucocorticoids, by neonatal thymectomy, or by cografts of transplantable AtT. Very recently, the congenital athymic nude mouse has become the host of choice. It is essential that the chosen method allow the expression of the hormonal effects of the grafts and of the added hormonal manipulations. No cell and organ culture method is known which faithfully imitates the homeostatic interplay of hormones *in vivo*.

In model animal systems using histocompatible hosts, the immunological antagonism of hosts, if at all expressed, is not much greater than that of the primary hosts. Histocompatible strains never have the 100% genetic identity of identical twins. Some genetic antagonism can be overcome by injection of large numbers of viable cells.*

3.2. Detection and Quantitation of Hormones

Three types of procedures for detection and quantitation of hormones are currently available: chemical assays and bioassays, radioimmunoassay, and immunohistochemical visualization of hormones by the use of fluorescent antibodies or immunohistochemical staining. None of these by itself is adequate for characterization of a given hormone-related neoplasm. The diverse techniques applied to hormone-related tumors have been reviewed by us (Furth *et al.*, 1973*d*). Listed below are other recent reviews and books. Utilization of these disciplines requires special expertise; the literature is replete with articles containing inconclusive reports and data due to lack of it. Problems requiring specialized techniques are best pursued by cooperative efforts of investigators majoring in the wanted areas.

Radioimmunoassay is now an indispensable tool in research in every area of endocrinology. The scope of its usefulness has rapidly expanded far beyond the quantitation of peptide hormones as introduced by Berson and Yalow (*cf.* 1973). Steroid hormones, enzymes, diverse antigens and antibodies, and many other substances of diagnostic and therapeutic value can now be measured in nanogram, some in picogram, quantities. Specific and group reactions can be estimated. As concerns hormone assays, it should be kept in mind that antigenic determinants, although related to biological activity are not identical with it. Conversely, biological activity can be expressed in the absence of detectable immunological reactivity. Consequently, purification by physicochemical procedures (such as gel filtration, electrophoresis, and ultracentrifugation) can yield immunologically active substances missed earlier, when purification was guided by bioassays. These substances may represent precursors or metabolic products of a biologically active hormone. Yalow (1974) reviewed the complex relationship of immunoreactive forms of five peptide hormones: parathormone, insulin, gastrin, AtH, and StH. Further, different antisera can detect different forms of the same peptide hormone, its precursor or metabolite, and relate them to its structure. Presently, the peptide hormones are named according to their molecular size: "big-big," "big," and "little." Goodman *et al.* (1972) demonstrated by Sephadex

---

* To make model systems available to qualified investigators, the National Cancer Institute has established a "bank" for hormone-related tumors. A word of warning: Because of the frequent changes occurring during the course of transplantations, one should not accept a studied tumor to be true to its name, but should verify its biological character.

G75 filtration that radioimmunoassayable StH in acromegalic and normal plasma contains a minor component (14–28%) of "big" StH, with molecular weight approximately 40,000, and a major component (67–86%) of "little" StH, with molecular weight approximately 21,000. Most original studies on heterogeneity were made on human hormone-related tumors; they have been extended recently to include experimental tumors. Studies along these lines will enhance our knowledge of the synthesis, storage, circulation time, and disposal of diverse hormones.

Immunohistochemical techniques (Nakane, 1970), by virtue of their great specificity, are increasingly replacing the chemical characterization of hormone-secreting cells. When coupled with electron microscopy, they visualize the organelles of cells and enable analysis of the synthesis, as well as disposal, of hormones in various physiological and pathological states. The techniques widely used have been reviewed and updated by Mazurkiewicz and Nakane (1972) and Moriarty (1973). Like radioimmunoassay, immunohistochemical staining is still subject to further refinements, but it is likewise sufficiently advanced for routine use. The appearance of the various types of pituitary hormone-secreting cells in rodents, as visualized by immunohistochemical staining, is characteristic for their identification (Fig. 6a–e).

The potentialities of electron microscopy in studies of the pathophysiology of the pituitary are well indicated by Farquhar (1971) and Hopkins and Farquhar (1973). These investigators also present excellent illustrations of the stages during the synthesis, intracellular transport, and excretion of synthesized hormones, and crinophagia. The various pituitary cell types have certain identifying features, of which the size and shape and location of the hormone are outstanding. The monograph of Benoit and DaLage (1963) and the abortive studies of Farquhar (personal communication) indicate the problems inherent in analysis of the neoplastic changes in the diverse pituitary tumors. Combining immunohistochemical staining with electron microscopy (Nakane, 1970) and other techniques (Hopkins and Farquhar, 1973) may be helpful in making some headway in this direction.

3.3. Steroid vs. Protein Hormones: Their Receptors and Translation of Their Messages

The disproportionate length of this section on steroid and protein hormones—with particular emphasis on estrogen and prolactin—is attributable to the temporal surge in establishing the pathogenesis of MT, the most common neoplasm in women, and the great promise of its control which followed the discovery of hypothalamic factors.

The discovery by Doisy et al. (1929) of the first neoplasia-related hormone (estrone) followed Beatson's intuitive studies (1896) on the relation of the ovary to human mammary cancers. This led to research on adrenal steroids and the disclosure that the adrenal is a reserve organ for production of gonadal steroids. Following their isolation, ovarian estrogens became the focal point in study of mammary carcinogenesis and the mouse the classic animal in MT research because of the high incidence of spontaneous MT in this species. Decades of thorough work led Bittner to formulate a triad in murine mammary carcinogenesis: genetics, estrogens, and his mammary tumor agent (MTA). He considered estrogen the basic carcinogen and his MTA a mere promoter (1946–1947, 1952). Subsequently, several investigators noted that natural and synthetic estrogens and certain nonsteroidal substances with estrogenic activity (as diethylstilbestrol) can induce pituitary tumors with high frequency in mice and rats. Furth and Clifton (*cf.* 1966) found that these tumors secreted prolactin and named them "mammotropic" (MtT). Transplanted MtT of rats and mice yield huge quantities of MtH. In our concept, prolactin is a major component in mammary tumorigenesis.

The recent discovery of hypothalamic P.IF and P.RF introduced a new set of factors which circumvent the gonads and operate via regulation of prolactin release. Thus there are three major types of hormones related to mammary tumorigenesis, but their relative roles and interrelationships remain to be fully clarified.

The discovery of Huggins *et al.* (1961) of the highly elevated sensitivity to DMBA of the mammary gland of female rats between the ages of 29 and 60 days (with a peak at about 55 days) has led many of us to investigate the hormonal status at this critical age. Beginning with immunohistochemical staining of the pituitaries, we found that at 5 and 10 days of age all pituitary hormones are present in the pituitary with the exception of prolactin, which begins to appear at about 15 days and becomes distinct at about 30 days (Furth *et al.*, 1974). Radioimmunoassays by Wuttke (1973) and Esber and Bogden (to be published) are in essential agreement with the results of immunohistochemical staining. (It should be noted that immunohistochemical staining represents storage of hormones, while radioimmunoassay detects their levels in the serum.)

Independent studies of Weisz and Gunsalus (1973) and Esber and Bogden (*cf.* Furth *et al.*, 1974) have shown that estrogens are present in the serum at birth and have a remarkable spurt at 19 days, that is, before ovarian follicular maturation. Their probable source is the adrenal. It is therefore reasonable to suppose that the primary factors in the differentiation of the mammary gland during the period of heightened susceptibility to carcinogens are estrogens, aided by other hormones, as will be discussed.

3.3.1. Steroid Hormones and Their Receptors

Jensen and his associates were among the first to investigate thoroughly the affinity of ovarian steroids for mammary and uterine tumors and the pathways of their actions (*cf.* Jensen and DeSombre, 1973). The gateways of hormone action are the receptors of their target organs. Jensen's team discovered that the estrogen receptor sites reside in the cytosol, where they combine with a specific 4S protein. The receptor–estrogen complex proceeds to the nucleus, where it interacts with DNA. How this interaction results in differentiation of primitive mammary tubules, proliferation of resting mammary gland during pregnancy, and the production of a functional lactating mammary gland or MT is the subject of much current research.

Advancing Jensen's findings, Bresciani *et al.* (1973) observed that the estrogen–receptor complex is modified by a proteolytic enzyme. The modified complex enters the nucleus and binds to a basic acceptor protein which is part of the chromatin; this is followed by "activation" of DNA synthesis and mitosis, especially when aided by oncogenic agents or viruses. However interesting, these findings have not yet lifted the veil surrounding the role of estrogens in cancer. The chain of events may be interrupted at some stage after fixation of the estrogen by its receptor. McCormick and Moon (1973) found that incremental doses of estradiol benzoate, either alone or in conjunction with progesterone, depressed tumor appearance in DMBA-treated female rats, but progesterone alone did not. Mešter *et al.* (1973) extracted an estrogen-binding protein from the nuclei of pituitary tumor cells (line GH₃) grown in culture. The nuclei contain an estradiol-binding system that functions independently of the presence or absence of cytosol in the incubation medium.

Most of the basic work of Jensen and associates was done with the uterus. Although estradiol is only mildly carcinogenic in the uterus, the sequence of events was found to be basically applicable to the mammary gland and its estrogen-responsive tumors. Estradiol reaches the nucleus unchanged. Agents such as nafoxidine, which inhibit its uptake *in vitro*, inhibit its growth effect *in vivo*. By means of dry-mount radioautography, Stumpf (1969) visualized in cells the intranuclear location of these steroids.

The estrogen-binding protein in rat MT is virtually indistinguishable from that in human MT. It has a high affinity for estradiol but does not bind nonestrogenic proteins such as hydrocortisone, progesterone, or testosterone (McGuire and DeLaGarza, 1973*a*).

The binding of steroid to a cell, or even its passage to nuclear DNA itself, is not adequate proof of carcinogenicity. The steroid–receptor–DNA complex may lead either to metabolic stimulation of a cell or to its growth. For example, cortisol uptake in the liver can lead to new formation of enzymes without neoplastic transformation, and estrogen uptake in the mammary gland to differentiation or milk secretion. Labeled estrogens are bound to several organs in varying grades of intensity. Corticoids are one of the factors known to stimulate milk production without being growth stimulating.

The estrogen receptors in human breast cancer are markedly labile under the conditions usually employed for assay. Significant increases in assay sensitivity can be achieved with the use of thiol reagents, such as dithiothreitol, at low temperatures. Such technical improvements may prevent misclassification of a tumor as being autonomous with regard to endocrine therapy (McGuire and DeLaGarza, 1973*b*).

The recent literature abounds in reports utilizing various methods to determine *in vitro* hormone responsiveness of experimental and human MT, correlating it with clinical progress. When tumors are cultured *in vitro* for hormone dependency, assays for DNA synthesis are the most useful parameter to explore; the site of

[3]H-thymidine uptake can be documented by radioautographs. Without the latter, the results may be paradoxical (Riley *et al.*, 1973). When model animal tumors are available, the results are best checked *in vivo* assays (*cf.* Takizawa *et al.*, 1970). Simultaneous receptor assays for steroids, MtH, and other agents which may affect the growth of MT are desirable (*cf.* Flaxman and Lasfargues, 1973). Flax (1973) maintained tumor cells *in vitro* cultures for 24 h in the presence of nearly physiological concentrations of 17 β-estradiol, testosterone, and prolactin. The results were determined by a histochemical reaction demonstrating total dehydrogenase activity of the pentose shunt, as well as by hematoxylin-eosin staining. The tumors were judged as hormone responsive by greater activity with a particular hormone. On this basis, 14% of 100 tumors were responsive to prolactin, 8% to estradiol, 10% to testosterone, 14% to both estradiol and prolactin, and 12% to prolactin and testosterone combined.

Much is yet to be learned about estrogen action. Even certain brain regions are known to stereospecifically bind estradiol, notably the hypothalamus-preoptic area–amygdala–midbrain. Nuclear uptake of estradiol rises in infancy through puberty (Plapinger and McEwen, 1973; Plapinger *et al.*, 1973). Kato (1970) demonstrated *in vitro* that estradiol is preferentially taken up by the anterior hypothalamus, as well as by the hypophysis, and is preferentially retained at these sites when the tissues are washed with estradiol-free medium. The precise location of the receptor sites in these organs is yet to be established. Eisenfeld (1970) studied the *in vitro* binding of ^{3}H-estradiol to sulfhydryl groups in macromolecules from the rat hypothalamus, pars distalis of the pituitary, and uterus. The macromolecular-bound radioactivity was separated by gel filtration. Higher concentrations of radioactive estradiol were found in the macromolecular fractions from the pituitary, uterus, and hypothalamus than from the cerebrum, cerebellum, heart, and plasma. By means of dry-mount radioautography, Keefer *et al.* (1973) demonstrated the topographical localization of estrogen-containing cells in the rat spinal cord following ^{3}H-estradiol administration.

Specific estradiol binding has been demonstrated in the mammary glands of the rat, the mouse, and man, and in experimental and spontaneous hormone-dependent MT of the rat. Tumors which do not regress after ovariectomy can be readily distinguished from the "hormone-dependent" tumors by both the magnitude of the estradiol uptake and the degree of sensitivity to inhibitors such as nafoxidine. The estradiol–receptor complex related to MT sediments at a well-defined 8S peak on sucrose density gradient ultracentrifugation. Tumors which do not regress after ovariectomy have only small 8S receptors (Jensen *et al.*, 1971). Of 84 primary human tumors investigated, 39 showed the presence of estrogen receptor. A Cooperative Breast Cancer Group (Engelsman *et al.*, 1973) studied 37 patients with progressive breast cancer. Two objective remissions were noted in 20 patients with estrogen receptor-negative tumors and 14 objective remissions in 17 patients with receptor-positive tumors. McGuire *et al.* (1973) found an estrogen receptor system in a mammotropic pituitary tumor corresponding to its biological activities. Neoplasia induction by estrogen seems to be maximum in the pituitary, next in the mammary gland, and greatly variable in different species. However, estrogen stimulates the synthesis and release of prolactin in the normal rat pituitary gland. Thus estrogen can act via the pituitary.

Watanabe *et al.* (1973) identified and partially characterized a receptor with specificity and high affinity for glucocorticoid hormones in the cytoplasmic fraction of a mouse adrenotropic pituitary tumor.

3.3.2. Protein Hormones and Their Receptors

The receptor sites and patterns of biochemical action of protein hormones were first demonstrated by the binding of AtH to cells of the adrenal cortex (Lefkowitz *et al.*, 1970a,b; Wolfsen *et al.*, 1972). Porcine ^{125}I-AtH bound to the plasma membrane of the cells of the adrenal cortex initiated the events discovered by Sutherland and Robison (1966). The generalization followed that all peptide hormones react with membrane-bound nucleotide cyclase systems to stimulate the conversion of a nucleotide triphosphate, such as adenosine triphosphate (ATP), to the corresponding 3′,5′-monophosphate, for example, cyclic adenosine monophosphate (cAMP). In line with these observations, the specific receptor site for MtH was found by Turkington (1971) and Birkinshaw and Falconer (1972) to reside in the plasma membrane.

There are many gray areas concerning the relative roles of estrogen and prolactin in mammary gland neoplasia (*cf.* Kim, 1965). Investigators are divided into two factions. The faction championed by Jensen explains most events by steroid actions; the other presents evidence indicating the primacy of prolactin in stimulation of the differentiated mammary epithelium and of transformed latent or overt mammary cancer cells (*cf.* Kim and Furth, 1960a,b). Another challenge has come with the discovery of hypothalamic P.RF and P.IF, which can also circumvent the ovaries and influence the growth of MT in the presence of the ovaries. My impression is that estrogens play a major role in bringing about differentiation of the mammary gland, while prolactin exerts a dominant action on the differentiated mammary gland. Estrogens are inducers of prolactin and have receptor sites in both the mammary gland and the pituitary. Since the adrenal is a "reserve" organ for secretion of estrogens, it can influence the mammary gland even after menopause, directly or indirectly. It seems that estrogens are ever present and may be the sole inducers of prolactin. The hypothalamic factors may merely regulate prolactin release and secretory rates, and perhaps also the number of prolactin-secreting cells. Until these circuits are clearly defined, several critical questions remain unanswered.

Cortisol appears to play some permissive role in hormonal stimulation of diverse cells. Its role in mammary tumorigenesis is debatable. An elevated rate of cortisol production was found in patients with advanced breast cancer. After hypophysectomy, it was found to fall to one-sixth of the original level. The high preoperative cortisol production was attributed to stress-induced elevation of AtH (Lewis and Deshpande, 1973) This is a common feature of most advanced tumors. It is noteworthy that milk secretion is usual in stimulated mammary gland and mammary tumors of the rat, but not in human tumors. Adrenal corticoids are one essential component of milk production. The physiological pathway of their secretion and their relation to prolactin and estrogen require further clarification.

Failure to consider the fact that estrogen is a (or the) physiological inducer of prolactin is a common shortcoming of many experiments attributing to estrogens an absolute role in mammary tumorigenesis. Isolated prolactin preparations stimulate the mammary gland in gonadectomized-adrenalectomized-hypophysectomized rats and can resuscitate mammary cancers which regressed following ovariectomy of hypophysectomy. Correspondingly, P.IF can also inhibit "hormone-responsive" mammary cancers of man and experimental animals, as described above.

It is known that some MT can regress following treatment with pharmacological doses of estrogen. Several explanations given for these events have been reviewed by Stoll (1973). He offers a hypothesis of his own: "the effect of high-dosage oestrogen therapy in breast cancer may depend critically on the absolute and relative concentrations of prolactin and oestrogen actively available at the tumor... Differences in site sensitivity in the same patient may depend on tumoral factors such as the level of oestradiol and prolactin binding receptors in the tissue." A similar explanation is that the binding of the estrogens to MT does not leave enough estrogen free to stimulate the secretion of MtH by Mt. Others suggest that MtH levels are elevated in the pituitary but are not released.

There are no satisfactory analytical studies in which the presence of receptors for both estrogen and prolactin and their role in regression of a "certified" hormone-responsive experimental MT were compared. Experiments aimed at clarifying the estrogen vs. prolactin controversy should consider the following: (1) MtH has a very short half-life (less than 30 min). Injecting MtH is not equivalent to grafting on the animal a highly prolactin-secreting tumor, in which the MtH levels are continuously high (thousands of nanograms per milliliter of serum). (2) Such high levels cannot be attained by isografts of pituitaries in hypophysectomized animals. (3) Estrogens do have a double action—a direct one on the mammary gland and an indirect one on pituitary Mt cells; thus, in the presence of the pituitary (Mt cell), it is uncertain as to which of the two stimulates the mammary gland. (4) High estrogen levels inhibit the mammary gland and MT (hence the use of pharmacological doses of estrogens in treatment of MT). (5) The "Huggins tumors" are variously deviated from normal to highly autonomous types, are probably multiclonal, and are subject to "progression." Stating that the tumor used was a "DMBA-induced tumor" is not satisfactory. Each experimental situation requires assays for analysis of the various factors that influence the growth of the mammary gland. (Takizawa *et al.*, 1970, used the sera of MtT-bearing rats, which contain such physiological costimulants as StH and insulin.) Whether injection of P.IF alone can inhibit and P.RF stimulate the mammary gland in the absence of the gonads and adrenals remains to be clarified.

Thus we face the apparent contradiction: Assays of Jensen for estrogen receptors suggest that they can predict almost all human hormone-responsive MT. In contrast, many others utilizing drugs which inhibit prolactin release claim the same results. Shall we conclude that hormone-responsive MT have receptors for both estrogens and prolactin?

Cell and organ cultures have been used extensively for the study of hormonal secretion and hormone responsiveness of neoplasms and for establishment of differentiated hormone-related cell lines (*cf.* Kruse and Patterson, 1973). An excellent compilation of articles written in this area from 1907 to 1971 is contained in *Readings in Mammalian Cell Culture* (Pollack and Sato, 1973).

4. Ectopic Hormones

The strongest argument in favor of the "dedifferentiation" theory of neoplasia is the finding that nonendocrine organs can give rise to tumors which secrete hormones (as AtH, insulin, TtH, GtH, and erythropoietin). Gellhorn (1966) gathered the evidence and stressed the association of ectopic hormone production with dedifferentiation. Certain tumors of infancy and childhood (such as neuro-blastomas) may be linked to disturbance in differentiation, but as for the majority of tumors the relationship may be incidental to mutation.

The immunological relationship of ectopic AtH with that secreted by adreno-tropes has been investigated by Yalow and associates. Gewirtz and Yalow (1973) found that ectopic AtH from all but one of 30 extracts of primary or metastatic carcinoma of the lung was immunoreactive with antinormal AtH. Its predomin-ant reactive form was big AtH. About 7% of laboratory controls and hospital patients had elevated afternoon plasma levels of AtH (in excess of 150 pg/ml), with big AtH as the predominant component, compared to about half of 59 patients with carcinoma of the lung. Nevertheless, for screening procedures for detection of carcinoma of the lung and for evaluation of response to therapeutic procedures, this test may be useful (*cf.* Yalow, 1974).

Braunstein *et al.* (1973) demonstrated ectopic production of human chorionic gonadotropin in 113 out of 918 cancer patients, with a high incidence in those with cancer of the stomach (25.5%), liver (17.3%), and pancreas (50%). Ectopic hormone production in diverse human neoplasms has been reviewed by Omenn (1973).

5. Sequential Events: Multiglandular Syndromes

Decades of experimental studies on diverse types of carcinogenesis have given me the impression that neoplasia is rarely a single-step process. Each class of carcinogens has its own *modus operandi* of transforming normal into neoplastic cells. Now that many evidently environmental and occupational cancers are under control, anatomical studies rarely disclose a carcinogen. Man cannot escape living in a world containing low levels of carcinogens (such as radiations), and it is my impression that subtle neoplastic changes evolve and progress silently through the cooperation of some carcinogen and some promoter.

Among the hormone-related experimental tumors, those induced by ionizing radiations demonstrate best the inducer–promoter cooperation. Theoretically, ionizing radiations properly applied should be able to produce a neoplasm in all cells, the numbers of which are homeostatically regulated. The following are relevant well-documented examples: (1) Irradiation of mice often induces leukemias which originate in the thymus, can be prevented by thymectomy, and are restored by thymic grafts. (2) Irradiated mice frequently develop OT, but not when only one ovary is exposed to radiation or when the animals receive grafts of normal ovaries following irradiation. (3) Radiothyroidectomy induces pituitary tumors in all strains of mice. Originally, this was attributed to "stress" or to incidental pituitary irradiation, but subsequent studies have shown that these tumors are all thyrotropic, while most pituitary tumors induced by radiations are mammosomatotropic. Further, induction of TtT can also be achieved by surgical thyroidectomy (Dent *et al.*, 1956). Radiation brings about homeostatic derangements by virtue of its mutagenic effect. The transformed cell can be either the cell irradiated or its regulator cell.

Examples in which the sequence of events in neoplasia occurs in "slow motion" have already been mentioned. The insult can occur early in life, progresses slowly, and terminates fatally in old age. The sequential events from normal to fully autonomous neoplasms can occur in one host, but the complete spectrum of sequential changes is best disclosed by serial subpassages in histocompatible animals.

Progression from normal cells to autonomous cancers has been extensively studied in the gonadotrope–ovary, thyrotrope–thyroid, estrogen–Leydig cell, and estrogen/prolactin–mammary gland systems. The inducibility of tumors and the timetable of transformation vary with the strain of animal used. None is strictly applicable to corresponding human tumors, but analysis of the dynamics of events yields valuable information on the pathogenesis of corresponding human tumors. The following examples will amplify the observations sketched in Sections 1 and 2.

5.1. Neonatal Ovariectomy

Neonatal ovariectomy is an example of how a single insult can induce a variety of tumors evolving in sequence during the life span of an animal. Studies on induction of tumors by gonadectomy were begun in 1945 and have been thoroughly worked out morphologically by Woolley *et al.* (*cf.* Woolley, 1958). The end result was a multiglandular "syndrome": AT, MT, and pituitary tumors. The character of the last is still uncertain: Were they estrogen-induced MtT or gonadectomy-induced GtT? The incidental observation that the adrenal compensates with estrogen production in the absence of the gonads paid rich dividends years later by the introduction of adrenalectomy to control breast cancer in women in whom the compensatory estrogens of the adrenal lead to recurrence of MT after ovariectomy.

Houssay *et al.* (1955) have undertaken an analysis of the genesis of the "Woolley tumors." With the aid of parabiosis, staining reactions ("basophilia" and periodic acid–Schiff positivity), and electron microscopy, they demonstrated that the pituitary tumors were gonadotropic. My associates have not been able to confirm this. The pituitary tumors found in old gonadectomized rats were the MtT type, as were the overwhelming majority of the spontaneous pituitary tumors of the rat (Kim *et al.*, 1960*b*; Ito *et al.*, 1972*a*). In our experience, hyperplasia of Gt occurs rapidly after gonadectomy in both sexes. The majority of cells in the pituitary 242 days after gonadectomy were Gt cells in various stages of hypertrophy. They can be well stained by labeled anti-LH. The hyperplasia of Gt appears to plateau and persists without formation of tumors.

The work of Griesbach and Purves (1960), confirming that of Houssay and associates, is open to doubt because inadequate techniques were used to identify the tumors. However, some tumors isolated by Iglesias *et al.* (1969, 1972) in the course of studies on gonadal tumorigenesis in AxC rats appear to be transplantable GtT of low hormonal potency.

These observations on hormonal interrelationships in the gonadal–gonadotrope axis may explain the extreme rarity of GtT in man and laboratory animals.

5.2. Thyroidal Carcinogenesis

The first thoroughly studied hormone-related tumors were those of the thyroid. They can be produced by several different methods in rats and mice, and develop through a series of gradual changes which include (1) hyperplasia, (2) focal areas of proliferation of altered cells, (3) formation of multicentric adenomas, and finally (4) carcinomas. The techniques used to induce them have been well summarized and illustrated by Morris (1955).

Two monographs on thyroid cancer (Young and Inman, 1968; Hedinger, 1969) present a wealth of facts and opinions on this subject by endocrinologists, oncologists, and immunogeneticists. Once a major worldwide problem, the importance of nodular enlargement of the thyroid gland (goiter) and its relation to cancer has been greatly minimized by the discovery of the various causative agents of goiters, ranging from iodine deficiency to substances in food and drugs which block TH synthesis. Figure 4 illustrates the simple feedback mechanism of the TH–TtH "axis" (see Section 1.4).

Goiters and TT (spontaneous and experimental) can be induced by the following procedures: (1) *without carcinogen*—(a) by blocking TH synthesis with antithyroidal chemicals thereby producing a sustained elevation of TtH; (b) by I_2-deficient diet; (c) by sustained administration of TtH; (2) *with carcinogen*—by low dose of ^{131}I (*cf.* Lindsay, 1969) or certain chemicals such as acetylaminofluorene; (3) *combination* of procedures (1) and (2). Procedure (1) promotes tumorigenesis by (2).

The experimentally induced TT begin as hormone-responsive lesions and slowly acquire autonomy, usually after several consecutive animal passages. To verify the role of TtH in thyroidal tumorigenesis, my associates studied the induction of TT by sustained administration of homologous TtH (Haran-Ghera *et al.*, 1960; Sinha *et al.*, 1965; Ueda and Furth, 1967). The greatly hyperplastic thyroids so induced consisted of a conglomeration of follicular and papillary nodules which failed to grow in euthyroid animals for about 2 yr, during which they were carried in consecutive passages in animals rendered hyperthyroid with highly elevated TtH levels. They gave rise to autonomous, but hormone-responsive, tumors. After being carried in normal hosts for about another 2 yr, the tumors gradually lost their "organoid" structure completely, took up less and less ^{131}I, and became less and less stimulated by TtH. Ultimately, they lost hormone responsiveness completely and became transformed into spindle- and giant-celled tumors as described by Russell (*cf.* Hedinger, 1969) in human TT. These sarcomatoid carcinomas were rapidly fatal. Why the nodularity of goiters in several species and the rarity of their giving rise to cancers is uncertain.

Thyroid cells in adults rarely multiply. Stimulation and inhibition are usually expressed by increased hormone production by the existing "resting" cells. Carcinogens, such as ionizing radiations, can readily induce tumors in immature, multiplying thyroid cells, but not in the adult thyroid. However, sustained elevation of TtH levels in adults can invariably induce the development of thyroid adenomas and the development of these into carcinomas, albeit very slowly, as our experiments indicate. We support the view that the first step in control of TT (benign or malignant) should be a trial of reduction of TtH levels (Astwood *et al.*, 1960).

Several ill-conceived notions, dogmatically held by many thyroidologists and not challenged by experimental observations, call for clarification:

1. Cold nodule formation (either adenomatoid or papillary) induced by goiterogens is not synonymous with cancer. We have failed to graft these in normal histocompatible hosts. Even such diagnostic points as presence of thyroid cells in venules do not unequivocally signify malignancy.
2. Chromosomal abnormalities may indicate mutations, but many mutants are not neoplastic. Thyroid remnants in mice given large does of ^{131}I (and irradiated tissues in general) often contain such cells, which persist until death of the host without giving rise to tumors.
3. Electron microscopy is a good adjunct in the characterization of cells, but profound cellular changes induced by differentiation or hormonal stimulation may resemble alterations now considered by some workers to be indicative of neoplasia.
4. A fatal neoplasm is not necessarily an autonomous cancer. Many fully hormone-dependent neoplasms are known which are fatal unless the hormonal derangement is controlled, and they often metastasize to regional lymph nodes.

Immunological changes with nonneoplastic thyroid diseases are common; they are "autoimmune," not related to TT. It is a sound practice to characterize localized thyroid neoplasms by the therapeutic approach: administration of cold TH to reduce TtH levels.

5.3. Multiglandular Diseases

There are several mechanisms by which a multiglandular disease can be induced by a single hormone deficiency: (1) That encountered in female mice bearing TtT is attained by virtue of the structural relationship between TtH and GtH (Furth *et al.*, 1973*b*). A direct mechanism is also possible by virtue of MtH stimulation by T.RH. Grant *et al.* (1973) found that Mt cells possess membrane receptors for T.RH *in vitro*. The biological mammotropic effect by T.RH *in vivo* has yet to be demonstrated. Another example in this category is the "transformation" of an MtT into and StT (Ito *et al.*, 1972*b*) related to the structural relationship between MtH and StH. Yet another example of this is the syndrome of hypersomatotropism consisting of pituitary and pancreatic changes due to the StH–insulin relationship (Garay *et al.*, 1971; Bates and Garrison, 1973). (2) TtT is also a good example of acquisition of new hormonal capabilities when it becomes fully autonomous (Furth *et al.*, 1973*c*). The TtT syndrome has been fully described elsewhere (Furth *et al.*, 1973*a,d*) and has been sketched in Section 2. (3) Evidence has been accumulated for the ability of a normal pituitary cell to produce more than one hormone when it becomes neoplastic. This has been summarized and illustrated by Ueda *et al.* (1973). The outstanding example is the acquisition by Mt of the ability to secrete three hormones, of which AtH is dominant (as in rat MtT strain F4). (For other examples, see Section 2.) The biological features of the AtH-secreting rat MtT/F4 are, in several respects, common with those of the purely AtH-secreting mouse AtT/20. Both are associated with marked hyperadrenolcorticoidism and thymic atrophy. While the mouse AtT also causes profound obesity similar to that of the genetically obese mouse (*cf.* Green, 1966), rats bearing MtT/F4 are not obese.

There are many human syndromes with multiple endocrine neoplasia (*cf.* Williams, 1968), the pathogenesis of which is subject to speculation. One of these, reported recently by Steiner *et al.* (1968), is a kindred with pheochromocytoma, medullary thyroid carcinoma, hyperparathyroidism, and Cushing's disease.

6. Problems and Prospects

6.1. The Basic Change in Neoplasia

Among the first attractive theories of neoplasia was that of somatic mutation (Boveri, 1929). Its first powerful opponent was Rous, who, following his excellent work with avian leukosis viruses, maintained that all tumors were caused by viruses (Rous, 1943). In the debates which followed, causation and basic nature were confused. The virus "theory" of cancer gained dominance until Rous himself, looking into the modes of chemical carcinogenesis, considered that viruses could not be the sole cause of cancer. A link between viruses and some genetic factor was demonstrated by the observations of the genetic inheritance of a leukemia factor in Ak mice (Cole and Furth, 1941), the isolation of a virus (Gross, 1953), and the association of viral RNA with the host cells' DNA by means of a reverse transcriptase (*cf.* Temin, 1972; Spiegelman and Schlom, 1972). The observation that thymectomy blocks the development of leukemia, but not the inheritance of leukemia virus, pointed to a thymus-related host factor essential for the expression of the somatic potentialities of this virus. Earlier, Bittner (1946–1947) discovered the presence of a similar causative agent in murine MT, calling it "milk factor" or "mammary tumor agent," now properly recognized as a virus.

Our present concept is based on the major discovery of Rous of the multifactorial concept of carcinogenesis (initiation, promotion, and the existence of latent cancers). The latter acquired solidity and popularity through subsequent studies of Berenblum (1947), Shubik, and others. The pathogenesis of neoplasia, the major roles of hormones, and other cybernetic forces (Wiener, 1948) became clarified, but the fundamental nature of neoplasia remained the subject of debates.

Mathematical analyses lent support to the hypothesis that sequential mutations were involved in the evolution of species (*cf.* Eigen, 1971) and probably also of neoplasia. As to the causative agents of mutations, three classes are generally accepted: radiations, certain chemicals, and viruses. All three are aided by some hormones. A fourth class of mutation, spontaneous DNA replication error, should, in my opinion, be included.

Promoters, by sustained enhancement of cell replication, increase the chances for spontaneous mutations. When the giant DNA molecule is replicating, it is indeed surprising that so few mistakes are made (or go unrepaired). Errors which do occur, spontaneous or induced, are now assumed to be more common than hitherto believed. Preferential replication of some mutants is conceived to be the basis of Darwinian evolution (Eigen, 1971). Mutants unable to recognize the homeostatic forces that limit the number of their normal ancestors, or defective in translating signals received by their receptors, gain a proliferative advantage over their normal ancestors. In his article "Cancer and the Evolution of Species: A Ransom," DeGrouchy (1973) states: "Evolution ... is a direct consequence of chromosomal instability. At meiosis chromosomal instability is responsible for the occurrence of individuals carrying new karyotypes and liable to be at the origin of a new species. At mitosis, chromosomal instability produces cells carrying new karyotypes. According to the chromosomal theory of carcinogenesis these cells are potential ancestors of novel clones liable to become malignant tumors. Carcinogenesis therefore appears as inexorable as the evolution of species." Genetic instability leads to further modifications, hence the progression from dependent to autonomous tumors. The precise characterization of a human tumor soon after its discovery, with the aim of checking its promoters, should be a major task of cancer research.

Related to the mutation theory are those of abnormal differentiation and dedifferentiation. These gained prominence by the discovery of ectopic hormones (see Section 4).

Differentiation yields the many organs with their specific cell types. It is commonly conceived as being nearly as irreversible as mutation, but differentiation is not accompanied by changes in the *basic* DNA code. The irreversibility of tissue differentiation is not without challenge. DeCosse *et al.* (1973) have reported on induction of differentiation in MT by embryonic tissue. A mouse MT was maintained *in vitro*, separated from embryonic mammary mesenchyme by a Millipore filter. Tubules developed in the tumor, DNA synthesis declined, and a presumptive acid mucopolysaccharide matrix, not evident in the controls, appeared.

It is assumed that differentiation is achieved by repression of certain genes and derepression of others (*cf.* Wolstenholme, 1966). Following failure to clearly associate basic proteins (notably histones) with repression of DNA, research has recently turned to DNA-associated acidophilic proteins which may accomplish this basic function (see review by Stein *et al.*, 1974).

There is one reservation to the mutation hypothesis. It is conceivable that some neoplasms—notably, those fully hormone dependent—are not due to modification of DNA but to that of an associated protein repressor. It has been shown that the λ-phage repressor can block RNA polymerase (Ptashne, 1973–1974), and it is conceivable that such repressors are the agents causing differentiation of diverse organs without modification of the associated DNA. The requirement of a neoplastic "derepressed" cell is the acquisition of a proliferative advantage. Obviously, this hypothesis cannot apply to neoplasms with marked chromosomal alterations indicative of some DNA change. In this sense, one is tempted to hypothesize the existence of two types of neoplastic transformation of cells—one based on DNA modification, another on that of a DNA-associated protein repressor. The latter allows reversal of some neoplasms (such as the hormone-dependent ones), the former does not. Solid evidence for this concept will come from developments identifying nucleotide sequences in DNA and identifying the DNA repressor proteins and the loci of genes involved in the neoplastic change. (It should be noted that the modification of the repressor could itself be a consequence of a change in the DNA.)

6.2. Carcinogenesis without Extrinsic Carcinogens

Five lines of evidence support the hypothesis of carcinogenesis without extrinsic carcinogens:

1. Numerous observations suggested that sustained specific growth stimulation of a cell, initiated either by removal of its homeostatic growth inhibitor or by sustained application of its physiological growth stimulant, can induce tumors without extrinsic carcinogenic agents. Tumors so induced are specific for the hyperstimulated cell type and their transplantability is, at first, usually dependent on their inducer. However, successive transplantations usually elicit autonomous variants. Such hormone-specific tumors can be induced in practically any member of any strain of any species and in any geographic region. Although carcinogens are everywhere in the environment, it seems unlikely that the induction of such tumors is dependent on a ubiquitous carcinogen or on the cell's DNA-integrated specific viruses. Examples are given in Sections 1 and 2.

2. A recent observation supporting this hypothesis resulted from the search for an explanation of Huggins' finding (Huggins *et al.*, 1961) of the hypersensitivity of female rats to induction of MT by chemical carcinogens between the ages of about 20 and 60 days (with a peak at 50–60 days), dropping sharply thereafter (Furth, 1973). The most conspicuous histological change in the mammary gland during this period is a burst of mitoses at the terminal buds of the rudimentary ducts, reaching a climax at 50–60 days (Fig. 7) and sharply declining thereafter. The mature breast of virgin female rats subsequently becomes rather stationary after 70 days of age. Differentiation of the mammary gland is directly initiated by gonadotropin-induced estrogens, aided by other hormones such as StH, insulin, somatomedins, and MtH, which the estrogens induce. It is well on its way at 20 days of age, when all major pituitary hormones are present at about normal levels, with the exception of MtH. The presumed factors contributing to the heightened sensitivity to tumor induction are (a) an early spurt of estrogens (which are nucleophilic); (b) rapid replication of DNA, enhancing susceptibility to carcinogens; (c) errors in DNA synthesis (spontaneous mutation); and (d) increase in MtH, the specific stimulator of the mammary gland, and in other nonspecific growth factors. The difficulty in excluding the role of a latent genetically integrated virus in seemingly spontaneous neoplastic transformation is an obstacle to acceptance of the spontaneous mutation hypothesis. The now accepted sequence of events is RNA virus → integration with the cell's DNA → release of RNA virus (with or without associated neoplastic transformation of cells). However remote it may appear to be, the sequence DNA → RNA virus, as conceived by Temin (personal communication), is a possible explanation for the genesis of some tumor viruses, but not for the genesis of all tumors. The finding of electron microscopic particles in man and other species (*cf.* Moore *et al.*, 1971; Dmochowski, 1973), as well as biochemical evidence for the presence of a presumably causative MTV in several species including man (Schlom and Spiegelman, 1973), raises the question of whether or not all members of a neoplasia-prone species carry a latent neoplasia-inducing virus.

3. A survey of several epidemiological studies (*cf.* MacMahon *et al.*, 1973) indicates an initial sharp rise in the incidence of breast cancers in women at about 25–45 yr of age. These tumors may have been initiated during the estrogen-triggered differentiation and growth of the mammary epithelium at puberty. This sharp initial rise occurs in all parts of the globe where such epidemiological studies have been made, suggesting that neoplastic transformation at puberty (yet to be solidly documented) is not likely to be due to an extrinsic carcinogen. (The many speculative interpretations proposed to explain the changes in breast cancer incidence at later ages have been well reviewed by MacMahon *et al.*, 1973.) A closer analysis of events during the pubertal period in mice (now in progress in our laboratory) may clarify this problem. Success hinges on the accuracy of the view that there are mouse strains free from MTV.

4. Choh Hao Li (1972) isolated ten hormones from the anterior pituitary, each possessing specific functions. On the basis of amino acid sequences, he divided them into three classes in their presumed phylogenetic order of evolution. The

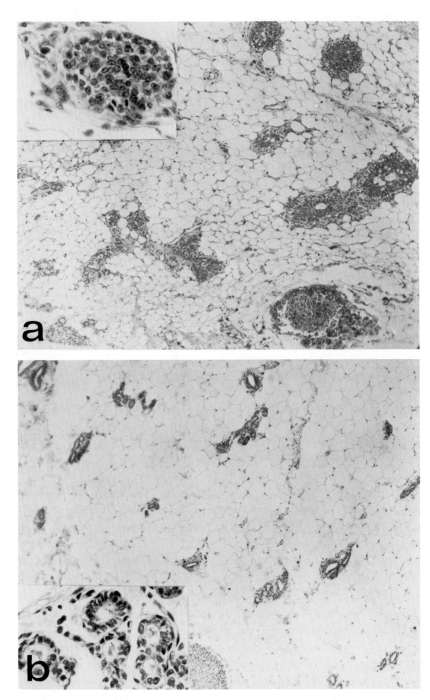

FIGURE 7. (a) The appearance of the female rat mammary gland at puberty. Note the bulbous growth of differentiating tubules containing numerous mitotic figures. Hematoxylin and eosin, × 75. Inset, × 400. (b) The fully differentiated ductal system of the virgin rat mammary gland at 87 days of age. Hematoxylin and eosin, × 75. Inset, × 400.

members of each class have strong common structural features and overlapping biological activities. During the past 20 yr, we have developed transplantable pituitary tumors of all three cell classes of Li, two of them by homeostatic derangement. The remarkable feature of the hormone-induced tumors is that they usually start as hyperplasia and only stepwise do they give rise to autonomous, fully hormone-independent tumors via fully hormone-dependent ones (see Section 5). A slight neoplastic code-change occurs within the class; marked derepression transgresses it. A single stable transplantable pituitary tumor cell can produce three separable hormones (Ueda *et al.*, 1973).

5. Indirect support to our hypothesis is given by the mathematical theories of Eigen (1971), solidified by DeGrouchy (1973). Recently, Macfarlane Burnet (1973) presented observations of his own supporting the spontaneous mutation hypothesis of neoplasia.

It is noteworthy that successive transplantation of normal cells *in vitro* often leads to transformation of the growth character of the cells, with acquisition of features known to characterize neoplastic cells. This occurs with or without acquisition of chromosomal abnormalities and with or without acquisition of transplantability. Because of the lack of homeostatic inhibitors *in vitro* and the oversupply of various nonspecific growth promoters, the opportunity for mutations is greatly enhanced. Possibly, the absence of a surveillance mechanism *in vitro* magnifies the chances for survival of many altered cells. It is surprising that despite decades of work on cell growth there has been no definitive study of the possibility of genetic and antigenetic modification of cells during the course of rapid replication without a carcinogen *in vitro* or *in vivo*.

6.3. Relation of Neoplasia to Aging

In Section 1.3, we postulated the existence of two types of mutations—metabolic and neoplastic—and related the former to aging. If one accepts the existence of mutations as an evolutionary force, one logically arrives at the conclusion that they can also be an involutionary force. If some transformed (mutated) cells have a proliferative advantage, they become cancer cells. Others, called metabolic mutants—that is, those disadvantaged in performing their physiological functions—may also slowly accumulate or may perish with age, depending on the existing homeostatic or immunological status. Cannon (1942), in his classical essay on homeostasis, writes: "The regulatory devices suffer a progressive impairment in most individuals as the decades pass after about the fortieth year." By "regulatory devices" he means homeostasis of temperature, salt, glucose, water, etc. To this we may add deterioration of immunosurveillance with age, which results in failure of the host to eliminate metabolically altered, as well as neoplastic, cells.

Chromosome analysis in relation to age sheds new light on the problem. Resting cells of the liver were studied at various ages and following exposure to mutagens. They were brought to division by subtotal resection of the organ (*cf.* Curtis, 1963,

1964). Curtis's findings indicate that the number of abnormal mitoses increases with age and that carcinogens administered early in life greatly enhance their number even late in life. Evidently, some of the transformed cells are compatible with life, some may even be functionally superior, but most of them seem inferior, hence senescence. Only a rare cell is a neoplastic mutant, and many of these may remain latent until some hormonal derangement or other homeostatic change induces them to multiply and form overt tumors (*cf.* Rous and Kidd, 1941; Kim and Furth, 1960*a,b*).

6.4. Prospects

Huggins (1967) lists seven hormone-responsive human cancers, three of which occur in both man and animals. None of the human tumors is surely curable by hormonal manipulation, although such treatment can produce lasting remissions. Many hormone-responsive tumors (including the three mentioned above) have been studied extensively in animals. Some were found to be curable because their pathogenesis was established, and they could be treated at the early phase of full hormone dependence.

Transformation of normal cells into cancer cells is, in our concept, no more preventable than evolution, senescence, and death. But with advancing knowledge in detecting liability to certain tumors, discovering latent tumors (from their "footprints"), and controlling the growth of frank neoplastic cells, an optimistic outlook of steady betterment of cancer control is well justified. As we have already learned, one can live with a highly carcinogenic, usually hidden, virus. The life span of the individual with cancer can be prolonged and made more comfortable. And the rare complete arrest of malignant growth (obtained by diverse therapeutic approaches) is, we believe, a portent of things to come.

ACKNOWLEDGMENTS

We gratefully acknowledge the assistance of our librarian, Ms. Betty Moore, in collecting the bibliography, and that of our photographer, Mr. Edward Hajjar. Special credit is due to numerous associates, whose dedicated work could not be adequately acknowledged in this review article.

7. References

ANDERVONT, H. B., SHIMKIN, M. B., AND CANTER, H. Y., 1957, Effect of discontinued estrogenic stimulation upon the development and growth of testicular tumors in mice, *J. Natl. Cancer Inst.* **18**:1.

ASTWOOD, E. B., CASSIDY, C. E., AND AURBACH, G. D., 1960, Treatment of goiter and thyroid nodules with thyroid, *J. Am. Med. Assoc.* **174**:459.

BAHN, R., FURTH, J., ANDERSON, E., AND GADSDEN, E., 1957, Morphologic and functional changes associated with transplantable ACTH-producing pituitary tumors of mice, *Am. J. Pathol.* **33**:1075.

BAKER, B. L., 1970, Studies on hormone localization with emphasis on the hypophysics, *J. Histochem. Cytochem.* **18**:1.

BAKER, B. L., ESKIN, T. A., AND CLAPP, H. W., 1972, The effect of medroxyprogesterone on cells of the pituitary pars distalis, *Proc. Soc. Exp. Biol. Med.* **140**:357.

BALI, T., AND FURTH, J., 1949, Morphological and biological characteristics of X-ray induced transplantable ovarian tumors, *Cancer Res.* **9**:449.

BATES, R. W., AND GARRISON, M. M., 1973, Synergism among growth hormone, ACTH, cortisol and dexamethasone in the hormonal induction of diabetes in rats and the diabetogenic effect of tolbutamide, *Endocrinology* **93**:1109.

BATES, R. W., SCOW, R. O., AND LACY, P. E., 1966, Induction of permanent diabetes in rats by pituitary hormones from a transplantable mammotropic tumor: Concomitant changes in organ weights and the effect of adrenalectomy, *Endocrinology* **78**:826.

BEATSON, G. T., 1896, On the treatment of inoperable cases of carcinoma of the mamma: Suggestions for a new method of treatment with illustrative cases, *Lancet* **2**:104.

BENOIT, J., AND DALAGE, C., eds., 1963, *Cytologie de l'Adénohypophyse*, Centre National de la Recherche Scientifique, No. 128, Paris.

BERENBLUM, I., 1947, Cocarcinogenesis, *Brit. Med. Bull.* **4**:343.

BERSON, S. A., AND YALOW, R. S., eds., 1973, *Methods in Investigative and Diagnostic Endocrinology*, Vol. 2: *Peptide Hormones*, American Elsevier, New York.

BIRKINSHAW, M., AND FALCONER, I. R., 1972, The localization of prolactin labelled with radioactive iodine in rabbit mammary tissue, *J. Endocrinol.* **55**:323.

BISKIND, M. S., AND BISKIND, G. R., 1944, Development of tumors in the rat ovary after transplantation into the spleen, *Proc. Soc. Exp. Biol. Med.* **55**:176.

BITTNER, J. J., 1946–1947, The causes and control of mammary cancer in mice, *Harvey Lect.* **42**:221.

BITTNER, J. J., 1952, The genesis of breast cancer in mice, *Texas Rep. Biol. Med.* **10**:160.

BLOCH, E., COHEN, A. I., AND FURTH, J., 1960, Steroid production *in vitro* by normal and adrenal tumor–bearing male mice, *J. Natl. Cancer Inst.* **24**:97.

BOLLENGIER, W. E., EISENFELD, A. J., AND GARDNER, W. U., 1972, Accumulation of ^{3}H-estradiol in testes and pituitary glands of mice of strains differing in susceptibility to testicular interstitial cell and pituitary tumors after prolonged estrogen treatment, *J. Natl. Cancer Inst.* **49**:847.

BOVERI, T., 1929, *The Origin of Malignant Tumors* (trans. Marcella Boveri), Williams and Wilkins, Baltimore.

BOYNS, A. R., AND GRIFFITHS, K., eds., 1972, *Prolactin and Carcinogenesis*, Alpha Omega Alpha, Cardiff.

BRAUNSTEIN, G. D., VAITUKAITIS, J. L., CARBONE, P. P., AND ROSS, G. T., 1973, Ectopic production of human chorionic gonadotropin by neoplasms, *Ann. Int. Med.* **78**:39.

BRAZEAU, P., VALE, W., BURGUS, R., LING, N., BUTCHER, M., RIVIER, J., AND GUILLEMIN, R., 1973, Hypothalamic polypeptide that inhibits the secretion of immunoreactive pituitary growth hormone, *Science* **179**:77.

BRESCIANI, F., NOLA, E., SICA, V., AND PUCA, G. A., 1973, Early stages in estrogen control of gene expression and its derangement in cancer, *Fed. Proc.* **32**:2126.

BUCKMAN, M. T., AND PEAKE, G. T., 1973, Estrogen potentiation of phenothiazine-induced prolactin secretion in man, *J. Clin. Endocrinol. Metab.* **37**:977.

BUONASSISI, V., SATO, G., AND COHEN, A. I., 1962, Hormone-producing cultures of adrenal and pituitary tumor origin, *Proc. Natl. Acad. Sci.* **48**:1184.

BURNET, F. M., 1970, *Immunological Surveillance*, Pergamon Press, Sydney.

BURNET, F. M., 1973, A genetic interpretation of ageing, *Lancet* **2**:480.

CANFIELD, R., MORGAN, F., KAMMERMAN, S., BELL, J., AND AGOSTO, G., 1971, Studies of human chorionic gonadotropin, *Rec. Prog. Hormone Res.* **27**:121.

CANNON, W. B., 1932, Homeostasis, *Cycloped. Med.* **6**:861.

CANNON, W. B., 1942, Ageing of homeostatic mechanisms, in: *Problems of Ageing* (E. V. Cowdry, ed.), pp. 567–582, Williams and Wilkins, Baltimore.

CLIFTON, K. H., 1963, Tumor induction in hypophyseal grafts in radiothyroidectomized mice; hypothalamico-hypophyseal relationships, *Proc. Soc. Exp. Biol. Med.* **114**:559.

CLIFTON, K. H., BLOCH, E., UPTON, A. C., AND FURTH, J., 1956, Transplantable Leydig-cell tumors in mice, *Arch. Pathol.* **62**:354.

COHEN, A. I., AND FURTH, J., 1959, Corticotropin assay with transplantable adrenocortical tumor slices: Application to the assay of adrenotropic pituitary tumors, *Cancer Res.* **19**:72.

COHEN, A. I., BLOCH, E., AND CELOZZI, 1957, *In vitro* response of functional experimental adrenal tumors to corticotropin (ACTH), *Proc. Soc. Exp. Biol. Med.* **95**:304.

COLE, R. K., AND FURTH, J., 1941, Experimental studies on the genetics of spontaneous leukemia in mice, *Cancer Res.* **1**:957.

CURTIS, H. J., 1963, Biological mechanisms underlying the aging process, *Science* **141**:686.

CURTIS, H. J., 1964, The biology of aging, in:*Brookhaven National Laboratory Lecture Series No. 34*, pp. 1–11, Associated Universities, Upton, N.Y.

DeCOSSE, J. J., GOSSENS, C. L., KUZMA, J. F., AND UNSWORTH, B. R., 1973, Breast cancer: Induction of differentiation by embryonic tissue, *Science* **181**:1057.

DeGROUCHY, J., 1973, Cancer and the evolution of species: A ransom, *Biomedicine* **18**:6.

DENT J. N., GADSDEN, E. L., AND FURTH, J., 1956, Further studies on induction and growth of thyrotropic pituitary tumors in mice, *Cancer Res.* **16**:171.

DICKEY, R. P., AND MINTON, J. P., 1972a, Levodopa relief of bone pain from breast cancer, *New Engl. J. Med.* **286**:843.

DICKEY, R. P., AND MINTON, J. P., 1972b, Levodopa effect on prolactin, follicle-stimulating hormone, and luteinizing hormone in women with advanced breast cancer, *Am. J. Obstet. Gynecol.* **114**:267.

DICKIE, M. M., AND LANE, P. W., 1956, Adrenal tumors, pituitary tumors and other pathological changes in F_1 hybrids of strain DE × DBA, *Cancer Res.* **16**:48.

DICKIE, M. M., AND WOOLLEY, G. W., 1949, Spontaneous basophilic tumors of the pituitary glands in gonadectomized mice, *Cancer Res.* **9**:372.

DMOCHOWSKI, L., 1973, The viral factor in the genesis of breast cancer: Present evidence, *Triangle* **12**:37.

ECKSTEIN, P., AND KNOWLES, F., eds., 1963 *Techniques in Endocrine Research*, Academic Press, London.

EIGEN, M., 1971, Self-organization of matter and evolution of biological macromolecules, *Naturwissenschaften* **58**:465.

EISENFELD, A. J., 1970, H^3-estradiol: *In vitro* binding to macromolecules from the rat hypothalamus, anterior pituitary and uterus, *Endocrinology* **86**:1313.

ELIAS, J. J., AND RIVERA, E. M., 1959, Comparison of the responses of normal, precancerous, and neoplastic mouse mammary tissues to hormones *in vitro*, *Cancer Res.* **19**:505.

ENGELSMAN, E., PERSIJN, J. P., KORSTEN, C. B., AND CLETON, F. J., 1973, Oestrogen receptor in human breast cancer tissue and response to endocrine therapy, *Brit. Med. J.* **2**:750.

EVERETT, J. W., AND NIKITOVITCH-WINER, M., 1963, Physiology of the pituitary gland as affected by transplantation or stalk transection, in: *Advances in Neuroendrocrinology* (A. V. Nalbanov, ed.), pp. 289–304, University of Illinois Press, Urbana.

FARQUHAR, M. G., 1971, Processing of secretory products by cells of the anterior pituitary gland, in: *Subcellular Structure and Function in Endocrine Organs* (H. Heller and K. Lederis, eds.), *Mem. Soc. Endocrinol.* **19**:79.

FLAX, H., 1973, A new method of determining the hormone dependence of human breast cancer, *Brit. J. Surg.* **60**:317.

FLAXMAN, B. A., AND LASFARGUES, E. Y., 1973, Hormone-independent DNA synthesis by epithelial cells of adult human mammary gland in organ culture, *Proc. Soc. Exp. Biol. Med.* **143**:371.

FLÜCKIGER, E., 1972, Drugs and the control of prolactin secretion, in: *Prolactin and Carcinogenesis* (A. R. Boyns and K. Griffiths, eds.), pp. 162–171, Alpha Omega Alpha, Cardiff.

FOULDS, L., 1969, *Neoplastic Development*, Academic Press, New York.

FRIESEN, H. G., 1972, Prolactin: Its physiologic role and therapeutic potential, *Hosp. Prac.* **7**:123.

FRIESEN, H., AND HWANG, P., 1973, Human prolactin, *Ann. Rev. Med.* **24**:251.

FRIESEN, H., GUYDA, H., AND HARDY, J., 1970, Biosynthesis of human growth hormone and prolactin, *J. Clin. Endocrinol. Metab.* **31**:611.

FURTH, J., 1969, Pituitary cybernetics and neoplasia, *Harvey Lect.* **63**:47.

FURTH, J., 1973, The role of prolactin in mammary carcinogenesis, in: *Human Prolactin* (J. L. Pasteels and C. Robyn, eds.), pp. 232–248, Excerpta Medica, Amsterdam.

FURTH, J., AND CLIFTON, K. H., 1966, Experimental pituitary tumors, in: *The Pituitary Gland* (G. W. Harris and B. T. Donovan, eds.), pp. 460–497, Butterworths, London.

FURTH, J., MOY, P., HERSHMAN, J. M., AND UEDA, G., 1973a, Thyrotropic tumor syndrome: A multiglandular disease induced by sustained deficiency of thyroid hormones, *Arch. Pathol.* **96**:217.

FURTH, J., MOY, P., SCHALCH, D. S., AND UEDA G., 1973b, Gonadotropic activities of thyrotropic tumors: Demonstration by immunohistochemical staining, *Proc. Soc. Exp. Biol. Med.* **142**:1180.

FURTH, J., MARTIN, J. M., MOY, P., AND UEDA, G., 1973c, Growth hormonal activity of thyotropic pituitary tumors, *Proc. Soc. Exp. Biol. Med.* **142**:511.

FURTH, J., UEDA, G., AND CLIFTON, K. H., 1973d, Pathophysiology of pituitaries and their tumors: Methodological advances, in: *Methods in Cancer Research*, Vol. X (H. Busch, ed.), pp. 201–277, Academic Press, New York.

FURTH, J., UEDA, G., AND CLIFTON, K. H., 1973d, Pathophysiology of pituitaries and their tumors: Methodological advances, in: *Methods in Cancer Research*, Vol. X (H. Busch, ed.), pp. 201–277, Academic Press, New York.

FURTH, J., NAKANE, P. K., AND PASTEELS, J. L., 1973e, Pathology and pathogenesis of spontaneous and experimental pituitary tumors, in: *Pathology of Tumors in Laboratory Animals*, Vol. 1, Part 2: *The Rat* (V. Turusov, ed.), IARC Scientific Publication No. 6, International Agency for Research on Cancer, Lyon, France, in press.

FURTH, J., ESBER, H. J., BOGDEN, A. E., AND MOY, P., 1974, Evolution of pituitary tropic cells and estrogens in relation to differentiation of the mammary gland and mammary tumorigenesis, *Proc. Endocrine Soc.*, Abst. No. 366, p. A-238.

GANONG, W. F., AND MARTINI, L., eds., 1973, *Frontiers in Neuroendocrinology, 1973*, Oxford University Press, New York.

GARAY, G. L., ÅKERBLOM, H. K., AND MARTIN, J. M., 1971, Experimental hypersomatotropism: Serum growth hormone and insulin, and pituitary and pancreatic changes in MtT-W15 tumor-bearing rats before and after tumor removal, *Horm. Metab. Res.* **3**:82.

GARDNER, W. U., PFEIFFER, C. A., TRENTIN, J. J., AND WOLSTENHOLME, J. T., 1953, Hormonal factors in experimental carcinogenesis, in: *The Physiopathology of Cancer*, 1st ed. (F. Homburger and W. H. Fishman, eds.), pp. 225–297, Hoeber-Harper, New York.

GARDNER, W. U., PFEIFFER, C. A., AND TRENTIN, J. J., 1959, Hormonal factors in experimental carcinogenesis, in: *The Physiopathology of Cancer*, 2nd ed. (F. Homburger, ed.), pp. 152–237, Harper, New York.

GELLHORN, A., 1966, Editorial on cancer: Facts and theories. Clinical physiology, chemotherapy, fundamental nature and mechanism of gene control, *Sem. Hematol.* **3**:99.

GEWIRTZ, G., AND YALOW, R. S., 1973, Ectopic ACTH production: Big and little forms, *Endocrinology (Suppl.)* **92**:A-53.

GOODMAN, A. D., TANENBAUM, R., AND RABINOWITZ, D., 1972, Existence of two forms of immunoreactive growth hormone in human plasma, *J. Clin. Endocrinol. Metab.* **35**:868.

GOTTSCHALK, R. G., AND FURTH, J., 1951, Polycythemia with features of Cushing's syndrome produced by luteomas, *Acta Haematol.* **5**:101.

GRANT, G., VALE, W., AND GUILLEMIN, R., 1973, Characteristics of the pituitary binding sites of thyrotropin-releasing factor, *Endocrinology* **92**:1629.

GRAY, C. H., AND BACHARACH, A. L., eds., 1967, *Hormones in Blood*, Vol. 1, Academic Press, London.

GREEN, E. L., ed., 1966, *Biology of the Laboratory Mouse*, McGraw-Hill, New York.

GREEN, J. A., 1957, Morphology, secretion and transplantability of ten mouse ovarian neoplasms induced by intrasplenic ovarian grafting, *Cancer Res.* **17**:86.

GREEN, J. D., AND HARRIS, G. W., 1947, The neurovascular link between the neurohypophysis and adenohypophysis, *J. Endocrinol.* **5**:136.

GRIESBACH, W. E., AND PURVES, H. D., 1960, Basophil adenoma in the rat hypophysis after gonadectomy, *Brit. J. Cancer* **14**:49.

GROSS, L., 1953, A filterable agent, recovered from Ak leukemic extracts, causing salivary gland carcinomas in C3H mice, *Proc. Soc. Exp. Biol. Med.* **83**:414.

HALL, R., SCHALLY, A. V., EVERED, D., KASTIN, A. J., MORTIMER, C. H., TUNBRIDGE, W. M. G., BESSER, G. M., COY, D. H. GOLDIE, D. J., MCNEILLY, A. S., PHENEKOS, C., AND WEIGHTMAN, D., 1973, Action of growth-hormone-release inhibitory hormone in healthy men and in acromegaly, *Lancet* **2**:581.

HARAN-GHERA, N., PULLAR, P., AND FURTH, J., 1960, Induction of thyrotropin-dependent thyroid tumors by thyrotropes, *Endocrinology* **66**:694.

HARRIS, G. W., 1955, *Neural Control of the Pituitary Gland*, Arnold, London.

HAYMAKER, W., ANDERSON, E., AND NAUTA, W. J. H., eds., 1969, *The Hypothalamus*, Thomas, Springfield, Ill.

HEDINGER, C., ed., 1969, *Thyroid Cancer*, UICC Monograph Series, Vol. 12, Springer, Berlin.

HINKLE, P. M., AND TASHJIAN, A. H., JR., 1973, Receptors for thyrotropin-releasing hormone in prolactin-producing rat pituitary cells in culture, *J. Biol. Chem.* **248**:6180.

HOLLANDER, N., AND HOLLANDER, V. P., 1971, Development of a somatotropic variant of the mammosomatotropic tumor MtT/W5, *Proc. Soc. Exp. Biol. Med.* **137**:1157.

HOPKINS, C. R., AND FARQUHAR, M. G., 1973, Hormone secretion by cells dissociated from rat anterior pituitaries, *J. Cell Biol.* **59**:276 (Part 1).

HORNING, E. S., 1954, The influence of unilateral nephrectomy on the development of stilbestrol-induced renal tumors in the male hamster, *Brit. J. Cancer* **8**:627.

HORROBIN, D. F., 1973, *Prolactin: Physiology and Clinical Significance*, MTP Medical and Technical Publishing Co., London.

HOUSSAY, A. B., HOUSSAY, B. A., CARDEZA, A. F., PINTO, R. M., AND FOGLIA, V. G., 1954, Estrogenic and adrenal tumors and gonadotropic pituitary tumors in gonadectomized rats, in: *Third Panamerican Congress of Endocrinology, Santiago de Chile*, p. 19.

HOUSSAY, B. A., HOUSSAY, A. B., CARDEZA, A. F., FOGLIA, V. G., AND PINTO, R. M., 1953, Adrenal tumors in gonadectomized rats, *Acta Physiol. Latinoam.* **3:**125.

HOUSSAY, B. A., HOUSSAY, A. B., CARDEZA, A. F., AND PINTO, R. M., 1955, Tumeurs surrénales oestrogéniques et tumeurs hypophysaires chez les animaux castrés, *Schweiz. Med. Wschr.* **85:**291.

HOWELL, J. S., MARCHANT, J., AND ORR, J. W., 1954, The induction of ovarian tumors in mice with 9:10-dimethyl-1:2-benzanthracene, *Brit. J. Cancer* **8:**635.

HUGGINS, C., 1967, Endocrine-induced regression of cancers, *Science* **156:**1050.

HUGGINS, C., AND MOULDER, P. V., 1945, Estrogen production by Sertoli cell tumors of the testis, *Cancer Res.* **5:**510.

HUGGINS, C., AND YANG, W. C., 1962, Induction and extinction of mammary cancer, *Science* **137:**257.

HUGGINS, C., BRIZIARELLI, G., AND SUTTON, H., 1959, Rapid induction of mammary carcinoma in the rat and the influence of hormones on the tumors, *J. Exp. Med.* **109:**25.

HUGGINS, C., GRAND, L. C., AND BRILLANTES, F. P., 1961, Mammary cancer induced by a single feeding of polynuclear hydrocarbon and its supression, *Nature* **189:**204.

HUSEBY, R. A., 1960, Studies of hormone dependency employing interstitial cell testicular tumors of mice, in: *Biological Activities of Steroids in Relation to Cancer* (G. Pincus, and E. P. Vollmer, eds.), pp. 211–223, Academic Press, New York.

HUSEBY, R. A., 1972, Hormonal factors in relation to cancer, in: *Environment and Cancer* (M. D. Anderson Hospital Symposium), pp. 372–393, Williams and Wilkins, Baltimore.

IGLESIAS, R., SALINAS, S., VUKUSIC, P., AND PANASEVICH, V., 1969, Transplantable gonadotrophic pituitary tumor of the AxC rat, *Proc. Am. Assoc. Cancer Res.* **10:**42.

IGLESIAS, R., SALINAS, S., VUKUSIC, P., GIRARDI, S., AND POLANCO, X., 1972, Functional transplantable ovarian tumors (OvT) developed in AxC rats grafted with the gonadotropic pituitary tumor (Gpic PT), *Proc. Am. Assoc. Cancer Res.* **13:**110.

ITO, A., MOY, P., KAUNITZ, H., KORTWRIGHT, K., CLARKE, S., FURTH, J., AND MEITES, J., 1972*a*, Incidence and character of the spontaneous pituitary tumors in strain CR and W/Fu male rats, *J. Natl. Cancer Inst.* **49:**701.

ITO, A., FURTH, J., AND MOY, P., 1972*b*, Growth hormone-secreting variants of a mammotropic tumor, *Cancer Res.* **32:**48.

IVERSEN, O. H., 1970, Some theoretical considerations on chalones and the treatment of cancer: A review, *Cancer Res.* **30:**1481.

JACOBS, B. B., AND HUSEBY, R. A., 1972, Brief communication: Hormone dependency of murine endocrine tumors *in vivo* and in organ culture: A correlative study, *J. Natl. Cancer Inst.* **49:**1205.

JENSEN, E. V., AND DeSOMBRE, E. R., 1973, Estrogen–receptor interaction, *Science* **182:**126.

JENSEN, E. V., BLOCK, G. E., SMITH, S., KYSER, K., AND DeSOMBRE, E. R., 1971, Estrogen receptors and breast cancer response to adrenalectomy, in: Prediction of Response in Cancer Therapy, *Natl. Cancer Inst. Monogr.* **34:**55.

JERNE, N. K., 1973, The immune system, *Sci. Am.* **229:**52.

JULL, J. W., AND PHILLIPS, A. J., 1969, The effects of 7,12-dimethylbenz(*a*)anthracene on the ovarian response of mice and rats to gonadotrophins, *Cancer Res.* **29:**1977.

KATO, J., 1970, *In vitro* uptake of tritiated oestradiol by the anterior hypothalamus and hypophysis of the rat, *Acta Endocrinol.* **64:**687.

KEEFER, D. A., STUMPF, W. E., AND SAR, M., 1973, Topographical localization of estrogen-concentrating cells in the rat spinal cord following ^{3}H-estradiol administration, *Proc. Soc. Exp. Biol. Med.* **143:**414.

KIM, U., 1965, Pituitary function and hormonal therapy of experimental breast cancer, *Cancer Res.* **25:**1146.

KIM, U., AND FURTH, J., 1960*a*, Relation of mammary tumors to mammotropes. II. Hormone responsiveness of 3-methyl-cholanthrene-induced mammary carcinomas, *Proc. Soc. Exp. Biol. Med.* **103:**643.

KIM, U., AND FURTH, J., 1960*b*, Relation of mammotropes to mammary tumors. IV. Development of highly hormone-dependent mammary tumors, *Proc. Soc. Exp. Biol. Med.* **105:**490.

KIM, U., AND FURTH, J., 1960c, Relation of mammary tumors to mammotropes. I. Induction of mammary tumors in rats, *Proc. Soc. Exp. Biol. Med.* **103**:640.

KIM, U., FURTH, J., AND CLIFTON, K. H., 1960a, Relation of mammary tumors to mammotropes. III. Hormone responsiveness of transplanted mammary tumors, *Proc. Soc. Exp. Biol. Med.* **103**:646.

KIM, U., CLIFTON, K. H., AND FURTH, J., 1960b, A highly inbred line of Wistar rats yielding spontaneous mammo-somatotropic pituitary and other tumors, *J. Natl. Cancer Inst.* **24**:1031.

KIRKMAN, H., AND BACON, R. L., 1950, Malignant renal tumors in male hamsters (*Cricetus auratus*) treated with estrogen, *Cancer Res.* **10**:122.

KLEIN, G., 1973–1974, Immunological surveillance against neoplasia, *Harvey Lect.*, in press.

KNIGGE, K. M., SCOTT, D. E., AND WEINDL, A., eds., 1972, *Brain–Endocrine Interaction. Medium Eminence: Structure and Function*, Karger, Basel.

KRUSE, P. F., JR., AND PATTERSON, M. K., JR., 1973, *Tissue Culture: Methods and Applications*, Academic Press, New York.

KWA, H. G., 1961, *An Experimental Study of Pituitary Tumors*, Springer, Berlin.

LEFKOWITZ, R. J., ROTH, J., AND PASTAN, I., 1970a, Effects of calcium on ACTH stimulation of the adrenal: Separation of hormone binding from adenyl cyclase activation, *Nature (Lond.)* **228**:864.

LEFKOWITZ, R. J., ROTH, J., PRICER, W., AND PASTAN, I., 1970b, ACTH receptors in the adrenal: Specific binding of ACTH-^{125}I and its relation to adenyl cyclase, *Proc. Natl. Acad. Sci.* **65**:745.

LEWIS, A. A. M., AND DESHPANDE, N., 1973, The effect of hypophysectomy on the cortisol secretion in 4 patients with advanced metastatic breast cancer, *Brit. J. Surg.* **60**:493.

LEWIS, U. J., SINGH, R. N. P., AND SEAVEY, B. K., 1971, Human prolactin: Isolation and some properties, *Biochem. Biophys. Res. Commun.* **44**:1169.

LI, C. H., 1972, Hormones of the adenohypophysis, *Proc. Am. Phil. Soc.* **116**:365.

LI, C. H., 1973, Prolactin, *Calif. Med.* **118**:55.

LINDSAY, S., 1969, Ionizing radiation and experimental thyroid neoplasms: A review, in: *Thyroid Cancer* (C. Hedinger, ed.), pp. 161–171, Springer, Berlin.

LOCKE, W., AND SCHALLY, A. V., 1973, *The Hypothalamus and Pituitary in Health and Disease*, Thomas, Springfield, Ill.

LOEB, L., AND KIRTZ, M. M., 1939, The effect of transplants of anterior lobes of the hypophysis on the growth of the mammary gland and on the development of mammary gland carcinoma in various strains of mice, *Am. J. Cancer* **36**:56.

LOWENSTEIN, W. R., 1968, Communication through cell junctions: Implications in growth and differentiation, *Develop. Biol.* **19**:151 (Suppl. 2).

MACLEOD, R. M., SMITH, C., AND DEWITT, G. W., 1966, Hormonal properties of transplanted pituitary tumors and their relation to the pituitary gland, *Endocrinology* **79**:1149.

MACMAHON, B., COLE, P., AND BROWN, J., 1973, Etiology of human breast cancer: A review, *J. Natl. Cancer Inst.* **50**:21.

MARTIN, J. M., ÅKERBLOM, H. K., AND GARAY, G., 1968, Insulin secretion in rats with elevated levels of circulating growth hormone due to MtT-W15 tumor, *Diabetes* **17**:661.

MAZURKIEWICZ, J. E., AND NAKANE, P. K., 1972, Light and electron microscopic localization of antigens in tissues embedded in polyethylene glycol with a peroxidase-labeled antibody method, *J. Histochem. Cytochem.* **20**:969.

MCCORMICK, G. M., AND MOON, R. C., 1973, Effect of increasing doses of estrogen and progesterone on mammary carcinogenesis in the rat, *Europ. J. Cancer* **9**:483.

MCGUIRE, W. L., AND DELAGARZA, M., 1973a, Similarity of the estrogen receptor in human and rat mammary carcinoma, *J. Clin. Endocrinol. Metab.* **36**:548.

MCGUIRE, W. L., AND DELAGARZA, M., 1973b, Improved sensitivity in the measurement of estrogen receptor in human breast cancer, *J. Clin. Endocrinol. Metab.* **37**:986.

MCGUIRE, W. L., DELAGARZA, M., AND CHAMNESS, G. C., 1973, Estrogen receptor in a prolactin-secreting pituitary tumor (MtTW5), *Endocrinology* **93**:810.

MEITES, J., ed., 1970, *Hypophysiotropic Hormones of the Hypothalamus: Assay and Chemistry*, Williams and Wilkins, Baltimore.

MEITES, J., 1973, Control of prolactin secretion in animals, in: *Human Prolactin* (J. L. Pasteels and C. Robyn, eds.), pp. 105–118, Excerpta Medica, Amsterdam.

MESSIER, B., AND FURTH, J., 1962, A reversely responsive variant of a thyrotropic tumor with gonadotropic activity, *Cancer Res.* **22**:804.

MEŠTER, B., BRUNELLE, R., JUNG, I., AND SONNENSCHEIN, C., 1973, Estrogen-sensitive cells: Hormone receptors in tumors and cells in culture, *Exp. Cell Res.* **81**:447.

MINTON, J. P., AND DICKEY, R. P., 1973, Levodopa test to predict response of carcinoma of the breast to surgical ablation of endocrine glands, *Surg. Gynecol. Obstet.* **136**:971.

MOLTENI, A., NICKERSON, P. A., LATTA, J., AND BROWNIE, A. C., 1972, Hypertension in rats bearing an adrenocorticotropic hormone-, growth hormone-, and prolactin-secreting tumor (MtTF4), *Cancer Res.* **32**:114.

MOON, H. D., SIMPSON, M. E., LI, C. H., AND EVANS, H. M., 1950a, Neoplasms in rats treated with pituitary growth hormone. I. Pulmonary and lymphatic tissues, *Cancer Res.* **10**:297.

MOON, H. D., SIMPSON, M. E., LI, C. H., AND EVANS, H. M., 1950b, Neoplasms in rats treated with pituitary growth hormone. II. Adrenal glands, *Cancer Res.* **10**:364.

MOON, H. D., SIMPSON, M. E., LI, C. H., AND EVANS, H. M., 1950c, Neoplasms in rats treated with pituitary growth hormone. III. Reproductive organs, *Cancer Res.* **10**:549.

MOON, H. D., SIMPSON, M. E., LI, C. H., AND EVANS, H. M., 1951, Neoplasms in rats treated with pituitary growth hormone. V. Absence of neoplasms in hypophysectomized rats, *Cancer Res.* **11**:535.

MOORE, D. H., CHARNEY, J., KRAMARSKY, B., LASFARGUES, E. Y., SARKAR, N. H., BRENNAN, M. J., BURROWS, J. H., SIRSAT, S. M., PAYMASTER, J. C., AND VAIDYA, A. B., 1971, Search for a human breast cancer virus, *Nature (Lond.)* **229**:611.

MORIARTY, G. C., 1973, Adenohypophysis: Ultrastructural cytochemistry. A review, *J. Histochem. Cytochem.* **21**:855.

MORRIS, H. P., 1955, Experimental thyroid tumors, in: *The Thyroid* (Brookhaven Symposia in Biology No. 7), pp. 192–219, Associated Universities, Upton, N.Y.

MUNSON, P. L., HIRSCH, P. F., BREWER, H. B., REISFELD, R. A., COOPER, C. W., WÄSTHED, A. B., ORIMO, H., AND POTTS, J. T., JR., 1968, Thyrocalcitonin, *Rec. Prog. Horm. Res.* **24**:589.

NAGASAWA, H., AND YANAI, R., 1973, Effect of human placental lactogen on growth of carcinogen-induced mammary tumors in rats, *Int. J. Cancer* **11**:131.

NAGASAWA, H., CHEN, C.-L., AND MEITES, J., 1973, Relation between growth of carcinogen-induced mammary cancers and serum prolactin values in rats, *Proc. Soc. Exp. Biol. Med.* **142**:625.

NAKANE, P. K., 1970, Classifications of anterior pituitary cell types with immunoenzyme histochemistry, *J. Histochem, Cytochem.* **18**:9.

NOEL, G. L., SUH, H. K., AND FRANTZ, A. G., 1973, L-Dopa suppression of TRH-stimulated prolactin release in man, *J. Clin. Endocrinol. Metab.* **36**:1255.

OMENN, G. S., 1973, Pathobiology of ectopic hormone production by neoplasms in man, in: *Pathobiology Annual*, Vol. 3 (H. L. Ioachim, ed.), pp. 177–216, Appleton-Century-Crofts, New York.

ORR, J. W., 1962, Tumors of the ovary and the role of the ovary and its hormones in neoplasia, in: *The Ovary*, Vol. 2 (S. Zuckerman, ed.), pp. 533–561, Academic Press, New York.

PASTEELS, J. L., 1972, Tissue culture of human hypophyses: Evidence of a specific prolactin in man, in: *Lactogenic Hormones* (G. E. W. Wolstenholme and J. Knight, eds.), pp. 269–286, Churchill-Livingstone, Edinburgh.

PASTEELS, J. L., AND ROBYN, C., eds., 1973, *Human Prolactin*, Excerpta Medica, Amsterdam.

PHIFER, R. F., MIDGLEY, A. R., AND SPICER, S. S., 1972, Histology of the human hypophyseal gonadotropin secreting cells, in: *Gonadotropins* (B. B. Saxena, C. G. Beling, and H. M. Gandy, eds.), pp. 9–25, Wiley, New York.

PHIFER, R. F., MIDGLEY, A. R. AND SPICER, S. S., 1973, Immunohistologic and histologic evidence that follicle-stimulating hormone and luteinizing hormone are present in the same cell type in the human pars distalis, *J. Clin. Endocrinol. Metab.* **36**:125.

PIERCE, J. G., LIAO, T., HOWARD, S., SHOME, B., AND CORNELL, J., 1971, Studies on the structure of thyrotropin: Its relationship to luteinizing hormone, *Rec. Prog. Hor. Res.* **27**:165.

PLAPINGER, L., AND MCEWEN, B. S., 1973, Ontogeny of estradiol-binding sites in rat brain. I. Appearance of presumptive adult receptors in cytosol and nuclei, *Endocrinology* **93**:1119.

PLAPINGER, L., MCEWEN, B. S., AND CLEMENS, L. E., 1973, Ontogeny of estradiol-binding sites in rat brain. II. Characteristics of a neonatal binding macromolecule, *Endocrinology* **93**:1129.

POLLACK, R., AND SATO, G., eds., 1973, *Readings in Mammalian Cell Culture*, Cold Spring Harbor Laboratory, Cold Spring Harbor, N.Y.

PTASHNE, M., 1973–1974, Repressor, operators and promotors in bacteriophage λ, *Harvey Lect.*, in press.

RATHNAM, P., AND SAXENA, B. B., 1971, Subunits of luteinizing hormone from human pituitary glands, *J. Biol. Chem.* **246**:7087.

RILEY, P. A., LATTER, T., AND SUTTON, P. M., 1973, Hormone assays on breast-tumour cultures, *Lancet* **2**:818.

ROUS, P., 1943, The nearer causes of cancer, *J. Am. Med. Assoc.* **122**:573.

ROUS, P., AND KIDD, J. G., 1941, Conditional neoplasms and subthreshold neoplastic states, *J. Exp. Med.* **73**:365.

RUSSFIELD, A. B., 1966, *Tumors of Endocrine Glands and Secondary Sex Organs*, Public Health Service Publication No. 1332, Government Printing Office, Washington, D.C.

SCHALLY, A. V., ARIMURA, A., AND KASTIN, A. J., 1973, Hypothalamic regulatory hormones, *Science* **179**:341.

SCHLOM, J., AND SPIEGELMAN, S., 1973, Evidence for viral involvement in murine and human mammary adenocarcinoma, *Am. J. Clin. Pathol.* **60**:44.

SHELESNYAK, M. C., 1954, Ergotoxine inhibition of deciduoma formation and its reversal by progesterone, *Am. J. Physiol.* **179**:301.

SINHA, D., PASCAL, R., AND FURTH, J., 1965, Transplantable thyroid carcinoma induced by thyrotropin, *Arch. Pathol.* **79**:192.

SMYTHE, G. A., AND LAZARUS, L., 1973, Blockade of the dopamine-inhibitory control of prolactin secretion in rats by 3,4-dimethoxyphenylethylamine (3,4-di-O-methyldopamine), *Endocrinology* **93**:147.

SPIEGELMAN, S., AND SCHLOM, J., 1972, Reverse transcriptase in oncogenic RNA viruses, in: *Virus–Cell Interactions and Viral Antimetabolites* (D. Sugar, ed.), pp. 115–133, Academic Press, London.

STEELMAN, S. W., KELLY, T. L., NORGELLO, H., AND WEBER, G. F., 1956, Occurrence of melanocyte stimulating hormone (MSH) in a transplantable pituitary tumor, *Proc. Soc. Exp. Biol. Med.* **92**:392.

STEIN, G. S., SPELSBERG, T. C., AND KLEINSMITH, L. J., 1974, Nonhistone chromosol proteins and gene regulation, *Science* **183**:817.

STEINER, A. L., GOODMAN, A. D., AND POWERS, S. R., 1968, Study of a kindred with pheochromocytoma, medullary thyroid carcinoma, hyperparathyroidism and Cushing's disease: Multiple endocrine neoplasia, type 2, *Medicine* **47**:371.

STERENTAL, A., DOMINGUEZ, J. M., WEISSMAN, C., AND PEARSON, O. H., 1963, Pituitary role in the estrogen dependency of experimental cancer, *Cancer Res.* **23**:481.

STOLL, B. A., 1972, Brain catecholamines and breast cancer: A hypothesis, *Lancet* **1**:431.

STOLL, B. A., 1973, Hypothesis: Breast cancer regression under oestrogen therapy, *Brit. Med. J.* **3**:446.

STUMPF, W. E., 1969, Nuclear concentration of ^{3}H-estradiol in tissues: Dry-mount autoradiography of vagina, oviduct, testis, mammary tumor, liver and adrenal, *Endocrinology* **85**:31.

SUNDERMAN, F. W., AND SUNDERMAN, F. W., JR., eds., 1971, *Laboratory Diagnosis of Endrocrine Diseases*, Green, St. Louis.

SUTHERLAND, E. W., AND ROBISON, G. A., 1966, The role of cyclic-3′,5′-AMP in responses to catecholamines and other hormones, *Pharmacol. Rev.* **18**:145.

TAKIZAWA, S., FURTH, J. J., AND FURTH, J., 1970, DNA synthesis in autonomous and hormone-responsive mammary tumors, *Cancer Res.* **30**:206.

TASHJIAN, A. H., YASUMURA, Y., LEVINE, L., SATO, G. H., AND PARKER, M. L., 1968, Establishment of clonal strains of rat pituitary tumor cells that secrete growth hormone, *Endocrinology* **82**:342.

TAYLOR, S., AND FOSTER, G., eds., 1970, *Calcitonin*, Springer, New York.

TEMIN, H. M., 1972, RNA-directed DNA synthesis, *Sci. Am.* **226**:24.

THOMAS, J. A., AND MAWHINNEY, M. G., 1973, *Synopsis of Endocrine Pharmacology*, University Park Press, Baltimore.

TURKINGTON, R. W., 1971, Measurement of prolactin activity in human plasma by new biological and radioreceptor assays, *J. Clin. Invest.* **50**:94a.

TURKINGTON, R. W., 1972, Secretion of prolactin by patients with pituitary and hypothalamic tumors. *J. Clin. Endocrinol. Metab.* **34**:159.

UEDA, G., AND FURTH, J., 1967, Sacromatoid transformation of transplanted thyroid carcinoma, *Arch. Pathol.* **83**:3.

UEDA, G., HAYAKAWA, K., HAMANAKA, N., YOSHINARE, S., SATO, Y., AND OKUDAIRA, Y., 1972, Enzyme histochemistry of experimental ovarian tumors in mice, *Acta Obstet. Gynecol. Jap.* **18**:16.

UEDA, G., MOY, P., AND FURTH, J., 1973, Multihormonal activities of normal and neoplastic pituitary cells as indicated by immunohistochemical staining, *Int. J. Cancer* **12**:100.

VAITUKAITIS, J. L., AND ROSS, G. T., 1972, Antigenic similarities among the human glycoprotein hormones and their subunits, in: *Gonadotropins* (B. B. Saxena, C. G. Beling, and H. M. Gandy, eds.), pp. 435–443, Wiley, New York.

VALE, W., GRANT, G., AND GUILLEMIN, R., 1973, Chemistry of the hypothalamic releasing factors—Studies on structure–function relationships, in: *Frontiers in Neuroendocrinology, 1973* (W. F. Ganong and L. Martini, eds.), pp. 375–413, Oxford University Press, New York.

WATANABE, H., ORTH, D. N., AND TOFT, D. O., 1973, Glucocorticoid receptors in pituitary tumor cells. I. Cytosol receptors, *J. Biol. Chem.* **248:**7625.

WEISZ, J., AND GUNSALUS, P., 1973, Estrogen levels in immature female rats: True or spurious—ovarian or adrenal? *Endocrinology* **93:**1057.

WELSCH, C. W., AND GRIBLER, C., 1973, Prophylaxis of spontaneously developing mammary carcinoma in C3H/HeJ female mice by suppression of prolactin, *Cancer Res.* **33:**2939.

WELSCH, C. W., ITURRI, G., AND MEITES, J., 1973, Comparative effects of hypophysectomy, ergocornine and ergocornine–reserpine treatments on rat mammary carcinoma, *Int. J. Cancer* **12:**206.

WIENER, N., 1948, *Cybernetics, or Control and Communication in the Animal and the Machine,* Technology Press, New York.

WILLIAMS, R. H., ed., 1968, *Textbook of Endocrinology,* Saunders, Philadelphia.

WILLIS, R. A., 1967, *Pathology of Tumours,* 4th ed., Butterworths, Washington, D.C.

WISH, L., FURTH, J., AND STOREY, R. H., 1950, Direct determinations of plasma, cell, and organ-blood volumes in normal and hypervolemic mice, *Proc. Soc. Exp. Biol. Med.* **74:**644.

WOLFSEN, A. R., McINTYRE, H. B., AND ODELL, W. D., 1972, Adrenocorticotropin measurement by competitive binding receptor assay, *J. Clin. Endocrinol. Metab.* **34:**684.

WOLSTENHOLME, G. E. W., ed., 1966, *Histones—Their Role in the Transfer of Genetic Information* (Ciba Foundation Study Group 24), Little Brown, Boston.

WOLSTENHOLME, G. E. W., AND KNIGHT, J., eds., 1972, *Lactogenic Hormones,* Churchill-Livingstone, Edinburgh.

WOOLLEY, G. W., 1958, Tumors of the adrenal cortex, in: *Ciba Foundation Colloquia on Endocrinology,* Vol. 12 (G. E. W. Wolstenholme and M. O'Connor, eds.), pp. 122–136, Churchill, London.

WUTTKE, W., 1973, Discussion, in: *Human Prolactin* (J. L. Pasteels and C. Robyn, eds.), p. 143, Excerpta Medica, Amsterdam.

YALOW, R. S., Heterogeneity of peptide hormones, *Rec. Prog. Horm. Res.,* **30:**597.

YOKORO, K., AND FURTH, J., 1962, Determining the role of "mammotropins" in induction of mammary tumors in mice by virus, *J. Natl. Cancer Inst.* **29:**887.

YOKORO, K., FURTH, J., AND HARAN-GHERA, N., 1961, Induction of mammotropic pituitary tumors by X-rays in rats and mice: The role of mammotropes in development of mammary tumors, *Cancer Res.* **21:**178.

YOUNG, S., AND INMAN, R., eds., 1968, *Thyroid Neoplasia,* Academic Press, London.

ZUCKERMAN, S., ed., 1962, *The Ovary,* Vol. II, Academic Press, New York.

5

Pathogenesis of Plasmacytomas in Mice

Michael Potter

1. Introduction

The malignant plasmacytoma is a rare tumor type that occurs naturally in several mammals—the dog (Osborne *et al.*, 1968), the cat (Farrow and Penny, 1971), the hamster (Cotran and Fortner, 1962), the rat (Bazin *et al.*, 1972), the mouse (Dunn, 1954, 1957), and man (Azar, 1973). Because plasmacytomas occur infrequently, it is difficult to study their pathogenesis. It is possible, however, to induce plasmacytomas in high frequency in a few uniquely susceptible inbred strains of mice by the intraperitoneal implantation of solid plastic materials (Merwin and Algire, 1959; Merwin and Redmon, 1963) or the intraperitoneal injection of mineral oils and related substances (Potter and Robertson, 1960; Potter and Boyce, 1962; Anderson and Potter, 1969). While this unusual method of induction is a laboratory method and has no apparent relationship to any known natural form of plasmacytoma development, it provides a means for studying the pathogenesis of plasmacytomas. In many forms of carcinogenesis, a specific differentiated cell type is the selective target. The reasons for cytotropism in the carcinogenic process are an intriguing problem. In plasma cell tumor formation in mice, the problem is even more complex because a segment of the plasma cell population appears particularly vulnerable. At present, immunology is an area of biology that has captured broad interest, and from many investigations have come a wealth of data on the differentiation, development, physiology, and proliferation of plasma cells. These data provide the background for understanding the normal plasma cell and the process of plasmacytoma formation. In this chapter, the pathogenesis of the induction of peritoneal plasmacytomas will

Michael Potter ● National Cancer Institute, Laboratory of Cell Biology, Bethesda, Maryland.

135

be the main topic. The underlying mechanisms of peritoneal plasmacytoma formation in the mouse are not yet established, but it is hoped that insight gained from this study will provide a basis for understanding how plasmacytomas may develop "spontaneously" in the mouse and in other species, including man.

2. "Spontaneous" Plasmacytomas

2.1. Ileocecal Plasmacytomas in Mice

Dunn (1954, 1957) described "spontaneous" plasmacytomas that appeared to develop in the ileocecum of old mice. The smallest lesions detected on routine autopsy were areas of inflammation in the wall of the ileocecum (approximately 5 mm in diameter). The mucosa overlying the area was ulcerated. Within the lesions in the ileocecum, inflammatory reactive tissues containing well-differentiated plasma cells as well as plasma cells with distorted morphology were seen infiltrating the wall of the intestine, the lymphatics, and the regional mesenteric lymph node. Dunn noted that these rare tumors were most commonly seen in C3H mice; however, one case occurred in a Carworth Farms No. 1 mouse, and subsequently Yancey (1964) described a case in a (BALB/c × A/He)F₁ hybrid mouse. Dunn had no difficulty in classifying the large ileocecal tumors as plasmacytomas.

Pilgrim established two C3H plasmacytomas (X5563, X5647) in transplant and sent them to Dunn, who in turn gave them to the author for serological study (Potter *et al.*, 1957). Both tumors were shown to produce immunoglobulin (Potter *et al.*, 1957; Fahey *et al.*, 1960): X5563 produced an IgG (γ2a type) M component and X5647 produced an IgA M component. Since the successful transplantation of these two tumors, only three more ileocecal tumors have been transplanted in the mouse (Potter and Fahey, 1960). Yancey (1964) described one of these, YPC-1, an ileocecal plasmacytoma associated with ascites formation that developed in a (BALB/c × A/He)F₁ mouse; this ileocecal tumor was also associated with a small adenocarcinoma of the cecum. Three of the transplanted plasmacytomas of ileocecal origin produced IgA myeloma proteins and one an IgG (γ2a) immunoglobulin.

Pilgrim (1965) made a detailed study of the ileocecal region in old C3H mice and found that over 90% of them had mucosal ulcers in the ileocecum. The small ulcerations in the ileocecum suggest an important pathogenetic sequence, mainly that the ulceration of the mucosa is the primary event that permits the development of infection and a chronically inflamed tissue. Among 125 ileocecums examined by Pilgrim, 28 plasmacytomas were found microscopically; however, none of these was successfully established in transplant.

2.2. Ileocecal Immunocytomas in Rats

Bazin *et al.* (1972) identified monoclonal immunoglobulin-secreting tumors in rats and named these tumors "immunocytomas." Immunocytomas are closely related, if not actually homologous, to the ileocecal plasmacytomas in mice. In contrast to the single mesenteric node in mice, the rat has a chain of mesenteric lymph nodes; the cecum is drained by one located near the ileocecal junction, the ileocecal lymph node, and this is where immunocytomas appear to develop.

A review of the literature by Bazin *et al.* (1972) indicated that ileocecal lymph node tumors in the rat have been known for many years, the first description dating back to 1911. The pathological classification of the tumors varied— "malignant lymphoma," "polymorphous cell sarcoma," "lymphoblastic lymphosarcoma," "reticulum cell sarcoma," "lymphosarcoma," and "lymphoblastic reticulosarcoma" having been employed by various authors. The first clue that these tumors were derived from immunoglobulin-secreting cell types was found by Deckers (1963), who demonstrated M components associated with four of these tumors. Immunocytomas in rats are readily transplantable. According to Bazin *et al.* (1972), histological and cytological studies show that cell types predominant in immunocytomas are poorly differentiated and cannot be readily classified as in plasmacytomas. However, the imprints and electron micrographs of the tumors are not unlike those of plasmacytomas in mice. Further detailed study is needed.

The histogenesis of these tumors has not been examined, chiefly because of the rarity of primary tumors. Bazin *et al.* (1973) have been able by selective breeding to obtain in strain LOU/Wsl rats a 23% incidence of immunocytomas. The mean age at appearance of immunocytomas is about 12–14 months. The possibility that these tumors originate in the wall of the cecum, as they all appear to do in the mouse, is not at all clear at present. In some earlier studies, ulceration of the ileocecum was described; however, the subsequent descriptions by Bazin's group suggest that the tumors involve the gut wall secondarily.

Roughly 73% of transplantable immunocytomas (Bazin *et al.*, 1973) have been shown to secrete immunoglobulin: of 184 examined, 23 or 3.3% produced IgM, 0.6% IgA, 35.9% IgG1, 6% IgG2a, 0.6% IgG2b, 6.0% IgG2c, and 32.4% IgE. The unusual and exciting finding of Bazin's group has been the existence of a large number of IgE myeloma proteins (this is the immunoglobulin class associated with reaginic antibody and with helminth infestations). IgE is a rare myeloma type in man and has not been seen in the mouse. The immunocytomas in rats offer an unusual new model system involving a very specialized component of the immune system.

2.3. Comment

The association of immunoglobulin-producing tumors in mice and rats with the gastrointestinal tract suggests that a regional disease in the gastrointestinal tract is a pathogenetic factor. The infestation of rats and mice with helminths and protozoans coupled with the normal flora could provide the specific agent that invades and damages the mucosa, thus beginning a chain of events from chronic inflammation to plasmacytoma development.

2.4. Plasma Cell Leukemias in Mice

Rask-Nielsen *et al.* (1968) and Ebbesen *et al.* (1968) have described the development of lymphomalike tumors in old BALB/c mice that produce monoclonal spikes or myeloma proteins. In these studies the mice had been inoculated as neonates with tumor extracts. Little is known about this system, and the long latent period presents a difficult experimental system.

3. Induced Plasmacytomas in Mice

3.1. Plasmacytomagenic Peritoneal Granuloma Inducing Agents

Merwin and Algire (1959) first found peritoneal plasmacytomas in BALB/c mice that had been implanted with Millipore diffusion chambers (MDC) containing allogeneic tissue. In later experiments, Merwin and Redmon (1963) placed MDC of different sizes, with and without tissue, as well as components of the chambers and related materials, intraperitoneally in BALB/c mice to determine the nature of the plasmacytomagenic material (Table 1). Fifty-four percent of mice implanted with large empty MDC, 21 mm in diameter, developed plasmacytomas. A much lower incidence was observed with empty 17.5-mm MDC, and no plas-

TABLE 1

Materials That Evoke a Chronic Peritoneal Granuloma and Plasmacytomas in BALB/c Mice

Material	Number of plasmacytomas/ total (%)	Reference
21.0-mm Millipore chamber, empty	14/26 (54)	Merwin and Redmon (1963)
17.5-mm Millipore chamber, empty	2/27 (7.3)	Merwin and Redmon (1963)
17.5-mm Millipore chamber + tumor tissue	21/96 (22)	Merwin and Redmon (1963)
14.0-mm Millipore chamber, empty	0/25 (0)	Merwin and Redmon (1963)
14.0-mm Millipore chamber + tumor tissue	7/177 (3.99)	Merwin and Redmon (1963)
14- or 17.5-mm Millipore discs	3/30 (10)	Merwin and Redmon (1963)
14- or 15.5-mm Lucite discs	2/11 (18.5)	Merwin and Redmon (1963)
Lucite borings	11/20 (56)	Merwin and Redmon (1963)
Freund's adjuvant, 0.5 ml × 1	37/64 (57.8)	Potter (1967)
Lieberman's staphylococcal adjuvant		Potter (1967)
Primol D, 0.5 ml × 1	27/56 (39.2)	Potter (1967)
Bayol F, 0.5 ml × 3, bimonthly intervals	78/128 (61.0)	Potter and Boyce (1962)
Bayol F, 0.5 ml × 1	14/119 (11.7)	Potter and Boyce (1962)
Drakeol 6VR, 0.5 ml × 3	15/32 (47.0)	Potter (1967)
Drakeol 6VR, 0.5 ml × 1	3/32 (9.4)	Potter (1967)
Pristane (2,6,10,14-tetramethylpentadecane), 0.5 ml × 3	73/120[a] (61)	Anderson and Potter (1969)
Pristane, 0.5 ml × 1	8/55[a] (14.3)	This chapter
Squalane	— (23)	Anderson (1970)
7n-Hexyloctadecane	— (60)	Anderson (1970)

[a] Based on incidence at 300 days; see Fig. 1.

macytomas were obtained with MDC of 14-mm diameter. Tissue-containing
17.5-mm MDC induced a greater incidence of plasmacytomas than empty chambers, suggesting an additive effect of the tissue. Discs of only Millipore membrane
or Lucite induced 10% and 18.5% plasmacytomas, respectively. Sharp-edged
borings from Lucite blocks 1 mm in diameter were placed intraperitoneally and
found to be highly effective materials: 50% of the mice developed plasmacytomas.
Discs and chambers caused the formation of both fibrosarcomas and plasmacytomas. The fibrosarcomas arose in the capsules surrounding the discs or
chambers, and the plasmacytomas were found elsewhere on the peritoneal
surfaces.

The induction in 1959 of plasmacytomas by MDC containing allogeneic tissue
suggested that some component of the chambers, in particular the allogeneic
tissue, was producing a sustained immune response. Other agents that stimulated
immune responses over extensive periods of time were tested for plasmacytomagenic activity in the BALB/c peritoneum. At that time, Lieberman *et
al.* (1960) had shown the effectiveness of a staphylococcal adjuvant mixture for
inducing ascites fluid containing antibody in mice. This mixture contained 1
part incomplete Freund's adjuvant (8.5 parts Bayol F, 1.5 parts mannide
monooleate) and 1 part heat-killed staphylococci. An intraperitoneal injection
of 0.5 ml of this mixture induced plasmacytomas in BALB/c mice (Potter and
Robertson, 1960), but multiple injections were more effective (Potter and Boyce,
1962). Since this adjuvant mixture contained several different materials, tests
were made on individual components to determine whether any alone was
plasmacytomagenic. It was found that the mineral oil component Bayol F actively
induced plasmacytomas (Potter and Boyce, 1962). A systematic dose study was
not made, but it was found that three 0.5 ml injections of the oil spaced 2 months
apart were more effective than a single injection (Potter and Boyce, 1962; Potter,
1967). A variety of light and heavy white mineral oils including oils of USP grade
that contain no fluorescent materials, e.g., Primol D, Drakeol 6VR, and Ervol,
have been shown to induce plasmacytomas in BALB/c mice (Potter, 1967;
Anderson, 1970). Mineral oils are chemically heterogeneous, and only a few
chemically defined light oily substances are available. The straight-chain alkane
n-hexadecane proved to be highly toxic (Potter, unpublished observations that
could not be evaluated); however, a branched-chain, low-viscosity oily substance,
pristane (2,6,10,14-tetramethylpentadecane), was very plasmacytomagenic
(Anderson and Potter, 1969). Pristane is well tolerated by mice, and when
intraperitoneally given to BALB/c mice in three 0.5-ml doses spaced 2 months
apart induced a high incidence (60–70%) of plasmacytomas (Fig. 1) (Anderson
and Potter, 1969). In subsequent studies, Anderson (1970) has shown
that squalane and the synthetically prepared 7*n*-hexyloctadecane are
plasmacytomagenic. These compounds, however, are available only in limited
quantities.

Crude petroleum from various geographic sources contains from 0.03 to 0.5%
pristane (Bendoraitis *et al.*, 1962). Commercially, pristane is obtained from the
livers of plankton-feeding vertebrates taken from the general vicinity of the Gulf

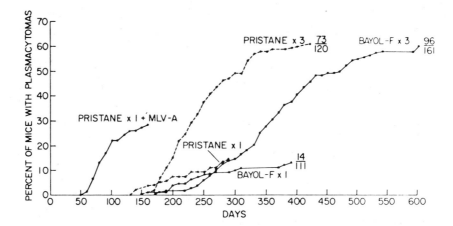

FIGURE 1. Induction of plasmacytomas. The percentage of plasmacytomas is the total number of plasmacytomas over the total number of mice at the start of the experiment and represents the total yield. Each curve represents the average of several experiments. "Pristane×1" and "Pristane×1+MLV-A" are the data from three experiments (Potter *et al.*, 1973) in Table 4. The "Pristane×1" group has been updated. "Pristane×3" represents two experiments run in 1969 and 1971. "Bayol-F×3" represents three experiments run in 1960, 1962, and 1970. "Bayol-F×1" represents three experiments run in 1960 and 1961 (Potter, 1967; Potter and Boyce, 1962).

of Maine (Blumer *et al.*, 1969). Blumer and his associates have outlined the migration of pristane in the food chain of marine animals (Fig. 2) (Blumer, 1965; Blumer and Thomas, 1965; Blumer *et al.*, 1969). Pristane is derived from phytol produced by phytoplankton. Phytol is converted to pristane and other intermediates by zooplankton and then consumed by plankton-feeding vertebrates such as the basking shark, sperm whale, alewife, and herring, where it is stored in the body fat and liver. The proportion of intermediates and other derivatives (Fig. 2) found in the body fat of zooplankton remains much the same in the vertebrate tissues, as these compounds are not further metabolized. From 1 to 3% of commercially pure pristane may contain mono- and diolefins described and identified by Blumer and colleagues (Blumer, 1965; Blumer and Thomas, 1965; Blumer *et al.*, 1969) as well as traces of squalane. The oxidation of olefins could give rise to epoxide derivatives. It is of interest, then, that Van Duuren *et al.* (1963, 1967) have shown that compounds such as 1,2-epoxyhexadecane and hexaepoxysqualane are weakly carcinogenic for the mouse epidermis.

Despite the evidence that pristane preparations can contain olefins, there is no evidence that active substances contained therein are indeed mutagenic or carcinogenic for B lymphocytes. No study has been made to determine if pristane (or other alkane or olefin) enters the plasma membranes of B lymphocytes, or further is ingested and converted to a proximal carcinogen inside the cell. The evidence is usually interpreted in the other way: mainly, that the metabolic inertness of pristane (and other alkanes) is the important property. This is a common characteristic of Lucite shavings, MDC, and mineral oils. The plasmacytomagenic effects of pristane appear to be indirect, and the consequence

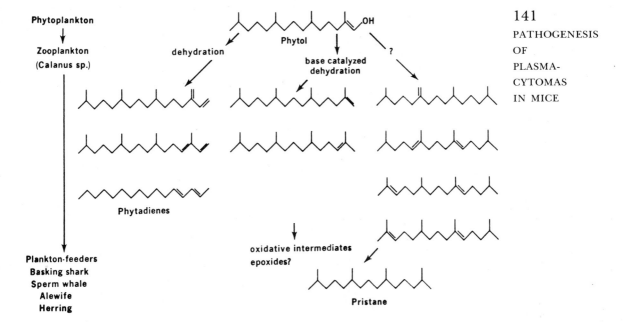

FIGURE 2. Isoprenoid hydrocarbons in the marine food chain. The data in this chart were derived from the publications of Dr. Max Blumer and associates of the Woods Hole Oceanographic Institute (Blumer, 1965; Blumer and Thomas, 1965; Blumer *et al.*, 1969).

of their ability to provoke a sustained, prolonged inflammatory process. This process not only stimulates inflammatory cells to liberate lymphokines and growth-stimulating factors, but in addition creates an abnormal tissue microenvironment.

3.1.1. Latent Period

The earliest plasmacytomas are detected between 138 and 180 days after the first injection of oil and continue thereafter to develop until the mice are 2 years old. The rate at which plasmacytomas develop varies with the type of oil used. With three injections of heterogeneous light oil such as Bayol F, plasmacytomas develop slowly over a prolonged period (Fig. 1) (180–600 days); by contrast, with three injections of pristane the tumors develop precipitously between 150 and 300 days after the first injection of oil.

The more rapid formation of tumors with pristane is as yet unexplained but suggests that pristane itself has a special property that accelerates plasmacytoma development or that it contains a cocarcinogenic substance as described above.

As may be seen from Fig. 1, three injections of oil given over a 4-month period are much more effective than a single injection. We are currently investigating the effects of two 0.5-ml intraperitoneal injections of pristane: given 48–120 days apart, they produce nearly as many plasmacytomas as three injections given at 0, 60, and 120 days. These results suggest that the presence of an excess of free oil in the peritoneum over an extended period of time is critical.

MICHAEL
POTTER

There have been a number of attempts to induce plasmacytomas in strains other than BALB/c (Merwin and Redmon, 1963; Potter, 1967; Yamada *et al.*, 1969; Warner, 1975; Morse *et al.*, 1978, 1980). A summary of the data is given in Table 2. As may be seen, only BALB/c and NZB are susceptible. The percentage of plasmacytomas is somewhat lower in NZB, and further the tumors produce predominantly IgG-class myeloma proteins (Morse *et al.*, 1978), suggesting a somewhat different pathogenesis.

A common genetic characteristic of these two strains has been the subject of discussion (see Morse *et al.*, 1980), but no clear picture has emerged. The two strains differ greatly in respect to integrated retrovirus loci. NZB is unusual in

TABLE 2

Effect of Intraperitoneal Implantation of Plastics or Injection of Mineral Oil in Strains of Mice Other Than BALB/c

	Number of plasmacytomas/total	
	Plastic	Mineral oil or pristane
Inbred strain		
C3H, C3Hf	4/224[a]	1/55[b]
DBA/2	0/63[a]	0/36[b]
C57BL/6	0/28[a]	
C57BL/Ka	—	0/52[b]
SWR	1/25[a]	0/30[b]
A/He	—	0/26[b]
AL/N	—	1/59[b]
BALB/cAn	11/20	73/120
NZB/Wehi		18/51[d]
NZB/BlWCri	—	340/2000[e]
NZC/Wehi	—	0/181[d]
NZW/Wehi	—	0/50[d]
C58/LwN	—	0/67[e]
Hybrids		
(NZB × BALB/c)F₁		7/31[c]
(BALB/c × A/He)F₁	3/40[a]	
(BALB/c × DBA/2)F₁	0/14[a]	0/82[b]
(BALB/c × AL/N)F₁		4/32[b]
(BALB/c × C57BL/Ka)F₁		5/25[b]
(BALB/c × NH)F₁		2/40[b]
(NZB/BLN × BALB/c)F₁	—	262/860[e]
(NZB × C57BL/Kn)F₁Wehi	—	1/38[d]
BALB/c × C57BL/6	—	16/227[f]
BALB/c × CBA	—	1/76[d]

[a] Adapted from Merwin and Redmon (1963).
[b] Potter (1967).
[c] Goldstein *et al.* (1966).
[d] Warner (1975).
[e] Morse *et al.* (1978, 1980).
[f] Potter *et al.* (1975).

that it produces a large amount of xenotropic type C retroviruses (Levy and
Pincus, 1970) throughout life (see Morse *et al.*, 1980). In contrast, in normal
BALB/c, loci coding for eco- and xenotropic type C viruses do not become active
until the mice are 6 months of age and then very little virus is produced as
compared with NZB (Aaronson and Stephenson, 1973; Aaronson *et al.*, 1969;
Peters *et al.*, 1972*a,b,c*). There seems to be no obvious retrovirus-related characteristic shared by the two strains. Further, high ecotropic virus-producing strains
such as C58 are not susceptible to pristane-induced plasmacytomagenesis (Morse
et al., 1980). F_1 hybrids of BALB/cAn and other strains of mice excepting
$(NZB \times BALB/c)F_1$ are not susceptible to the induction of plasmacytomas (Table
2). This suggests that resistance genes are dominant. However, penetrance of
susceptibility in F_1 hybrids differs. Some hybrids are absolutely resistant; others,
e.g., C57BL, develop a few tumors. This suggests several genes play a cooperative
role and some gene combinations permit a few plasmacytomas to develop. One
study has been made of BALB/c and C57BL/6 using the Bailey recombinant
inbred strains. These seven new inbred strains were derived from random pairs
of $(BALB/cAn \times C57BL/6)F_2$ mice. Four of the new strains were susceptible and
three were resistant. The Bailey RI strains have mixtures of many genes from
both parents. This study indicates that susceptibility can penetrate when on a
number of different backgrounds. Our laboratory is currently attempting to
identify resistance genes of DBA/2 origin, using BALB/c congenic strains carrying identifiable DBA/2 markers.

3.2.1. Karyological Changes

Early, cytogenetic studies of transplantable plasmacytomas in BALB/c mice
demonstrated a high frequency of polyploidy, aneuploidy, and marker chromosomes (Yosida *et al.*, 1968). Later Yosida *et al.* (1970) extended these studies to
14 primary plasmacytomas and found that 11 had modal numbers somewhere
between 60 (triploid) and 80 (tetraploid). All of the tumors changed to near
tetraploidy during transplantation. Moriwaki *et al.* (1971) followed one diploid
tumor MSPC-1 through 40 transfer generations and found that it repeatedly
gave rise to tetraploid variants. When individual chromosomes became
identifiable by specific chromosome-staining techniques, e.g., Giemsa banding
(see Nesbitt and Franke, 1973), the plasmacytomas have revealed several common
translocations (Shepard *et al.*, 1974*a*, 1976, 1978; Yosida and Moriwaki, 1975;
Yosida *et al.*, 1978). Shepard *et al.* (1974*a,b*, 1976, 1978) showed that five
long-term-transplanted plasmacytomas all carried deleted No. 15 chromosomes
with a common breakpoint at band D31E, as with all translocations of the distal
end of chromosome 15 to chromosome 12 or a reciprocal translocation of
chromosomes 6 and 15.

Ohno *et al.* (1979) have extended this analysis to seven primary and/or early
transfer generation tumors and found that all had either the deleted 15 (del
15)+T12;15 or less commonly rcp T(6/15). In diploid cells the del 15+T12;15
involved only one No. 15 chromosome, while in tetraploid cells two No. 15

chromosomes were involved. The association of chromosome 12 [which carries the structural genes for the Ig heavy (H) chains (Hengartner *et al.*, 1978; Meo *et al.*, 1980)] and chromosome 6 [which carries the structural genes for the Ig light (kappa) chains (Gibson *et al.*, 1978; Hengartner *et al.*, 1978; Swan *et al.*, 1979)] suggests that the translocations could be related to the differentiation of immunoglobulin structural gene complex loci. It is now established that the process of V-C joining involves the rearrangement of genomic DNA, and breaks in the DNA are essential to this process. The appearance of the chromosomal breaks in only one No. 6, 12, or 15 chromosome per haploid set is reminiscent of allelic exclusion. Immunoglobulin synthesis occurs for the most part on only one Ig-locus-bearing chromosome in a diploid cell, the other being excluded.

The consistent involvement of chromosome 15 in plasmacytomas is not explained. Little is known about the genes carried on this chromosome, but trisomy 15 has been repeatedly found in T-cell leukemias in the mouse (see Klein, 1979). It will be important in future studies to determine if genes on chromosome 15 play a role in plasmacytomagenesis.

3.3. The Peritoneal Site

Thus far, plasmacytomas have been induced only in the peritoneal cavity. Injection of oils or adjuvants subcutaneously results in the formation of large cysts. Fibrosarcomas develop in the cyst capsules surrounding adjuvants but have not been observed thus far around loculated subcutaneous mineral oils (Potter, unpublished observations). No subcutaneous plasmacytomas have been found in the mouse; however, Oppenheimer *et al.* (1955) reported one in a rat that had received a cellophane implant into the subcutaneous tissues. The peritoneal site as compared to other sites provides (1) a large area over which oil or plastic material may be distributed and (2) a potential space in which cells may enter. The peritoneum contains a population of free cells, the peritoneal exudate cells, that probably provide the precursors of plasmacytoma cells. The physiological function of these cells is to police the peritoneal space. The peritoneum of the mouse is very resistant to infection with most common bacteria, and this reflects in part the effectiveness of the local cellular defense system. Peritoneal exudate cells are macrophages, small and large lymphocytes, mast cells, and mesothelial cells (Carr, 1967). Peritoneal exudate cells originate from circulating cells (Volkman, 1966; Koster and McGregor, 1971) and from the small patches of lymphoreticular tissue in the omentum, the "taches laiteuses" of Ranvier or milk spots (Carr, 1967). The precursors of peritoneal macrophages are found chiefly in the bone marrow and blood (Volkman, 1966), while the precursors of the small and large lymphocytes are in the thoracic duct fluid (Koster and McGregor, 1971). In rats presensitized to *Listeria monocytogenes* antigen and then challenged intraperitoneally with *Listeria* organisms, the influx of short-lived, large and medium lymphocytes was particularly vigorous (Koster and McGregor, 1971). Evidence that long-lived small lymphocytes also enter the peritoneum could not be found in this study.

Inflammation is an important feature of plasmacytoma formation in the mouse. The only studies dealing directly with this problem (Takakura *et al.*, 1966; Hollander *et al.*, 1968) demonstrated that the subcutaneous administration of 0.1 or 0.5 mg cortisol five times per week to BALB/c mice continuously during and after the three intraperitoneal injections of mineral oil entirely prevented or vastly reduced the incidence of plasmacytomas. The total number of peritoneal exudate cells was $29.4 \times 10^4/\text{mm}^3$ in mineral-oil-treated mice and $1.4 \times 10^3/\text{mm}^3$ in those treated with cortisol plus mineral oil. Histologically the granulomatous tissue was reduced to only small pinpoint lesions on the omentum, and most of the mineral oil apparently remained in the peritoneal space.

Antigenic stimulation from the normal microbial flora is known to play an important role in plasmacytoma formation. McIntire and Princler (1969) found a greatly reduced incidence of plasmacytomas in germfree mice injected with mineral oil, and we (Asofsky and Potter, unpublished observations) have confirmed this. A relatively large number of myeloma proteins (about 5%) induced in BALB/c mice have been found to bind antigens of bacterial origin (Potter, 1970, 1971); many of these antigens are produced by microorganisms isolated from our BALB/c mouse colony. These observations suggest that cells sensitized by the normal microbial flora are potential precursors of some plasmacytomas. The migration of these cells into the peritoneum where plasmacytomas develop may require antigen to be present in the peritoneum, or possibly the sustained inflammation in the peritoneum may simply increase the entry of all circulating cells.

A characteristic of peritoneal plasmacytomas in the mouse is the relatively high frequency (66%) of tumors differentiated to make IgA-class myeloma proteins (see Potter, 1972). In multiple myeloma in man, the preponderant class is IgG (Zawadzki *et al.*, 1967). IgA-producing cells are found normally in great abundance in the lamina propria of the gastrointestinal tract, where they represent over 80% of all immunoglobulin-producing cells (Crabbé *et al.*, 1970). The bulk of IgA produced by lamina propria plasma cells is secreted across the mucosal epithelium into the lumen of the gut (Tomasi and Bienenstock, 1968). Comoglio and Guglielmone (1973) have demonstrated that IgA produced by subcutaneously transplanted plasmacytomas can be actively secreted across the gastrointestinal epithelium or into the saliva. This suggests that the proximity of plasma cells to the mucosal epithelium is not a necessary prerequisite for secretion. Secretory IgA is thought to interact with antigen in the lumen of the gastrointestinal tract and with other secretions and thereby form a first line of defense for the organism. The peritoneum has not yet been implicated in the formation of secretory immunoglobulin, and thus the location of IgA-producing plasmacytomas here may reflect an unnatural location. The preponderance of IgA-producing plasmacytomas in BALB/c may be explained in another way based on new insights in immunoglobulin molecular genetics. The chromosomal order of the IgC$_H$ genes has recently been established in the mouse to be $5'-\mu-\delta-\gamma3-\gamma1-\gamma2b-\gamma2a-\alpha-3'$ by Honjo and Kataoka (1978). Expression of heavy-chain classes in an IgA-producing clone is sequential and irreversible beginning with μ and switching to any other locus to the right. It has been proposed by Gearhart and Cebra (1979) and Gearhart *et al.* (1980) that switch in a B-lymphocyte clone is dependent upon mitotic activity and that cells that have undergone many divisions, as for example the rapidly dividing B lymphocytes in the lymphoid nodules of Peyers patches, progressively become end-stage IgA-producing cells. Thus, the IgA-secreting plasmacytomas may have arisen from B lymphocytes that have undergone prolonged mitotic divisions in the oil granuloma. This contrasts from the notion that the tumor cells are derived from B lymphocytes of the secretory (IgA) immune system.

3.4. Role of the Oil Granuloma

Because of the ease of injecting oily liquid substances intraperitoneally, the oil granuloma has been the most extensively studied peritoneal granulomatous tissue. This tissue begins to form almost immediately after the injection of oil. The oil first causes an inflammatory reaction characterized by the presence of lymphocytes, granulocytes, and plasma cells in the mesentery; furthermore, macrophages become very active and begin phagocytozing oil droplets. In the process the oil-laden macrophages adhere to the peritoneal surfaces and begin the buildup of oil granuloma tissue. This consists primarily of oil-laden macrophages or large drops of oil surrounded by many macrophages. Eventually these oil-containing cells become organized on the peritoneal surfaces and form a very extensive new tissue that is vascularized and covered with mesothelium (Potter and MacCardle, 1964).

3.4.1. Growth Dependence of Primary Plasmacytomas

Some insight into the mechanism of action of the oil granuloma in plasmacytoma development has been derived from studies on the transplantation of relatively low numbers of primary plasmacytoma cells (Potter *et al.*, 1972). It was found that when doses of 10^5 or fewer cells obtained from the peritoneal fluid of a mouse with a primary plasmacytoma were transplanted intraperitoneally in normal BALB/c mice, only 3 of 15 tumors grew progressively. By contrast, 10^5 or fewer cells from all of these same tumors grew in mice previously conditioned with a single intraperitoneal injection of pristane. The tumors developed within several weeks, and in all the cases studied the immunoglobulins produced by the tumors were the same as in the original primary tumor. In cases where the primary host lacked a demonstrable M component, the M components in all the recipients had the same electrophoretic mobility. In some of the cases investigated, as few as 10^5 primary plasmacytoma cells were successfully transplanted. In subsequent unpublished studies, it has been found that the conditioning injection of pristane can be given either simultaneously with the cells or within 7 days.

Cancro and Potter (1976) have studied the effects of the continuous injection of hydrocortisone on conditioning dependence of primary plasmacytomas. When

TABLE 3

Effect of Transplantation of 10^5 Plasmacytoma Cells from a Primary Case to Various Kinds of Conditioned Hosts[a]

Conditions		Number of primary tumors	Number of mice with progressively growing tumors[b]
Day 0	Day 3		
—	—	23	5/212 (3%)
Pristane[c]	—	23	227/228 (99%)
Pristane + hydrocortisone	—	11	32/150 (21%)
Pristane	Hydrocortisone[d]	11	150/150 (100%)
Thioglycollate[e]	—	6	0/60 (0%)

[a] Adapted from Cancro and Potter (1976).
[b] All mice were observed for at least 100 days.
[c] Pristane conditioning was begun at various intervals from 3 to 60 days before tumor inoculation.
[d] Hydrocortisone 0.5 mg/day 5×/week.
[e] Thioglycollate broth was given every 3 days for the duration of the experiment.

hydrocortisone was administered with or before the injection of pristane, only 21% of the mice developed progressively growing tumors after the injection of 10^5 viable tumor cells (Table 3). However, if hydrocortisone was begun 3 days after the injection of pristane, all of the mice developed progressively growing tumors. Histologically, pretreatment with hydrocortisone suppressed the development of the oil granuloma. This effect has been attributed to the ability of hydrocortisone to effectively suppress the entry of blood monocytes into the peritoneal cavity (Thompson and VanFurth, 1970). It is clear from this work that free pristane in the peritoneum is not responsible for the growth-promoting effect and further continuous treatment with hydrocortisone does not depress plasmacytoma growth.

Peritoneal inflammatory exudates are often elicited experimentally by the injection of thioglycollate broth. Cancro and Potter (1976) studied the effect of continuous thioglycollate injections on primary plasmacytoma growth and found that this treatment did not promote growth. Histologic studies showed that thioglycollate broth did not induce the formation of a granuloma. This evidence suggests that the growth-promoting effects of pristane or mineral oil are related to the adherent granulomatous tissue itself and the unusual microenvironment it creates.

3.4.2. Growth Factors for Established Tumors

There is evidence from *in vitro* studies of plasmacytoma growth that special factors may be required for the growth of plasmacytoma cells. Namba and Hanaoka (1972), in attempting to adapt the MOPC104E plasmacytoma to tissue culture, noted that their plasmacytoma cells grew initially in culture for a period of about 30 days and then began declining in numbers; simultaneously, the macrophages disappeared from the culture flask. Namba and Hanaoka (1972) were able to rescue cultures of MOPC104E cells by transfer of the declining cell cultures to dishes containing proliferating phagocytic cells, or by culturing the cells with conditioned medium from various types of cultures of phagocytic cells, including adherent cells obtained from the tumor itself, spleen, or peritoneum. Conditioned medium obtained from fibroblasts did not contain the factor. Normal mouse serum also contained a factor that stimulated growth. The potency of mouse serum could be increased over 18-fold that of normal serum if the mice were previously injected intraperitoneally with 0.2 ml complete Freund's adjuvant. The peak activity was observed on the 16th day after injection but remained high for over 30 days. These workers also found that mitotic activity of MOPC104E cells could be stimulated by the addition of 3′,5′-cyclic AMP (0.5 μg/ml) to the cultures.

In an independent study, Metcalf (1973) has been able to obtain microcolonies of plasmacytoma cells in agar. In this study, 25 different plasmacytomas were tested directly from *in vivo* transplant lines. Nineteen produced colonies in agar when a factor from whole mouse blood or from washed red blood cells of mouse or other mammals were added. Cloning efficiencies from 0.01 to 21.6% were obtained. The colony-enhancing factor was not present in normal serum but could be obtained from the serum of endotoxin-infected mice.

These *in vitro* studies of plasmacytoma growth indicate that special factors are required for growth and that they can be supplied from various sources. The Namba and Hanaoka (1972) serum factor appearing after intraperitoneal injection of Freund's adjuvant, which is also obtained from cultures of phagocytic cells, may possibly be produced by the large population of phagocytic cells in the oil granuloma. The serum factor described by Metcalf (1973) appearing after the injection of endotoxin may be similar to or even different from the factor described by Namba and Hanaoka. Other nutritional factors have been described by Park *et al.* (1971).

3.4.3. Local Immunosuppression

A second biological action of the oil granuloma on plasmacytoma formation may be in the form of a protective effect on tumor cell growth. It is known that transplantable plasmacytoma cells have several types of potential cell-surface antigens, e.g., PC1 and XVEA (Aoki and Takahashi, 1972; Herberman and Aoki, 1972), tumor-specific transplantation antigens (Lespinats, 1969; Röllinghoff *et al.*, 1973; Williams and Krueger, 1972), and immunoglobulin idiotypic determinants (Lynch *et al.*, 1972). Since these may also be found on developing primary tumor cells, the question of how the tumor escapes from some form of immune elimination arises. Possibly the oil granuloma has an immunosuppressive action. Kripke and Weiss (1970) postulated that the mineral oil might be immunosuppressive, but in their studies they looked for a general immunosuppressive effect and were able to obtain minimal evidence. We have observed that an established immunity to a transplantable plasmacytoma (Adj PC5) can be abrogated in mice that have been previously conditioned with an intraperitoneal injection of pristane (Potter and Walters, 1973). The effect is local, however, and occurs only when tumor cell challenges are introduced intraperitoneally into mice that have received a prior intraperitoneal injection of pristane. Similar challenge doses of tumor cells given subcutaneously to immune intraperitoneal pristane-treated mice were rejected as efficiently as in normal mice.

Several intriguing actions of macrophages on tumor immunity have been demonstrated in other systems that might be related to local abrogation of immunity in intraperitoneal pristane-conditioned mice. Hersey and MacLennan (1973) observed, for example, that macrophages can protect lymphoma tumor cells from cell-mediated and humoral immune cytolysis. In this system, they postulate that macrophages can actually phagocytose tumor cells, or provide protection by coming in close contact with them. They envisage that the macrophages in some way facilitate in clearing the antigenic materials from the fluid mosaic cell surface, thereby protecting against cytotoxic effects.

3.5. Role of Viruses in Plasmacytoma Development

Viruses have been strongly implicated in peritoneal plasmacytomagenesis in mice, but their precise mode of action has not yet been defined. Two general ways in which viruses may be involved in plasmacytoma formation are (1) by activation of endogenous viruses in cells that are precursors of plasmacytomas and (2) somatic infection of precursors with a plasmacytomagenic virus. There is substantial evidence that C-type RNA viruses of the murine leukemia virus (MuLV) complex are activated in plasmacytoma cells. Further, a defective C-type RNA virus (Abelson virus) has been shown to induce plasmacytomas rapidly in pristane-primed mice (Potter *et al.*, 1973).

3.5.1. Endogenous C-Type Viruses

In a number of studies, C-type RNA viral particles (Watson *et al.*, 1970; Volkman and Krueger, 1973) or viral-associated antigens (Stockert *et al.*, 1971; Hyman *et al.*, 1972; Takahashi *et al.*, 1970, 1971*a*,*b*; Aoki and Takahashi, 1972; Herberman and Aoki, 1972) have been demonstrated in transplantable plasmacytomas. The etiological significance of these findings is clouded by the fact that C-type RNA viruses of the MuLV system have been implicated in most neoplasms of the lymphoreticular tissues in mice and by the fact that the BALB/c strain of mouse in which these tumors developed is known to carry several different forms of C-type RNA viruses. Furthermore, many of these studies have been done with tissue culture lines of plasmacytomas, and *in vitro* cultivation alone is known to activate latent C-type RNA viruses (Aaronson *et al.*, 1969). Aoki *et al.* (1973) have more closely implicated the activation of C-type RNA viruses in plasmacytoma formation by demonstrating virus particles in primary plasmacytomas.

Xenotropic and ecotropic C-type RNA retroviruses have been isolated from lymphoid tissues and peritoneal exudate cells of BALB/c mice after the intraperitoneal injection of pristane (Armstrong *et al.*, 1978; Hartley and Potter, unpublished observations). In the study by Armstrong *et al.* (1978), xenotropic viruses first appeared about 9 weeks after the first injection of pristane, and N and B tropic viruses first appeared at about the time plasmacytomas emerged. Hartley and Potter (unpublished observations) found xenotropic virus expression in peritoneal exudate cells 2 weeks after the injection of pristane, and ecotropic viruses sporadically during the same period.

Primary and early transfer generation plasmacytomas readily yield both xeno- and ecotropic viruses (Morse *et al.*, 1980). Recombinant forms probably also exist, but at present only one dual tropic mink-cell-focus-forming virus (a recombinant of xeno- and ecotropic exogenous viruses) has been isolated from a plasmacytoma among 26 studied (Hartley and Potter, unpublished observations) (see Morse *et al.*, 1980).

Despite the obvious presence of endogenous retroviruses in plasmacytomas, a mechanistic effect of these viruses in plasmacytomagenesis has not been established. Continuous retrovirus production in B lymphocytes could lead to recombinatorial events between provirus DNA and integrated virus genomes or related sequences in chromosomes. Such recombinations might alter host gene expressions and disturb regulatory processes in the cells by turning "on" or "off" genes that are critical for the maturation of cells to a postmitotic state. Continuous virus production could lead to the integration of viral genes into new chromosomal sites.

C-Type retroviruses probably do not directly transform cells, but the process of virus replication, which creates proviral DNA, may have an important genetic impact on cells. First the viral DNA can recombine with host DNA, and second the viral DNA may integrate at new sites in the mouse genome. Somatic genetic changes such as these may increase the chances for a neoplastic variant to emerge.

3.5.2. Intracisternal A Particles

Intracisternal A particles (double-membrane particles that bud from the rough endoplasmic reticulum) have been found by electron microscopy in every plasmacytoma of BALB/c origin thus far examined (Dalton *et al.*, 1961; Dalton and Potter, 1968). In transplantable tumors, large numbers of particles are often seen. Relatively pure preparations of the particles have been isolated from plasmacytomas and found to contain a small amount of RNA (Kuff *et al.*, 1968, 1972), a DNA polymerase enzyme with somewhat unusual substrate requirements (Wilson and Kuff, 1972), and a structural protein that differs from gs antigen (Kuff *et al.*, 1972) of the MuLV system. Furthermore, intracisternal A particles do not have the MuLV-associated gs antigens.

Intracisternal A particles have not yet been shown to be infective for any other cell type as yet, and thus it has not been possible to demonstrate that they play a role in plasmacytoma formation. A number of other neoplastic and normal cell types have also been shown to have these particles (Wivel and Smith, 1971). In most studies of normal plasma cells, intracisternal A particles have not been found. If these particles represent a defective virus, it is possible that their activation may play a role in plasmacytoma development. Thus far, however, intracisternal A particles have been found to have an intracytoplasmic location, and they probably do not affect the cell membrane.

3.5.3 Rapid Induction of Plasmacytomas in Pristane-Primed Mice by Abelson Virus

A method for rapidly inducing plasmacytomas in BALB/c mice has been developed using pristane and Abelson virus (MLV-A) (Potter *et al.*, 1973). Adult mice are given a single 0.5-ml injection of pristane and 39–57 days later an injection of MLV-A. Plasmacytomas and lymphosarcomas begin to develop within 21 days after the injection of the virus, and 43–60% of the mice ultimately develop lymphosarcomas and 25–36% plasmacytomas (Table 4 and Fig. 1). The plasmacytomas develop long before the appearance of plasmacytomas in mice that receive only a single injection of pristane (Table 4 and Fig. 1). The rapidity with which these plasmacytomas develop indicates that they are derived from cells that have been transformed by MLV-A. The predominant form of immunoglobulin is IgA.

MLV-A was originally isolated by Abelson and Rabstein (1970*a,b*) from a BALB/c mouse that had received prednisolone continuously from birth and an intraperitoneal injection of Moloney leukemia virus (MolLV) (Pfizer Lot 3042-278) at 28 days of age. The purpose of the prednisolone was to maintain a steroid-induced atrophy of the thymus. It had been previously reported (Moloney, 1962; Dunn and Deringer, 1968) that MolLV produced different types of reticular neoplasms in surgically thymectomized mice than in intact hosts. In the intact host, the tropism of the virus was for thymic cells (Dunn *et al.*, 1961). In thymectomized hosts, myeloid leukemias and reticulum cell neoplasms developed. In the Abelson and Rabstein study (1970*a*), of 85 mice that were maintained on high doses of prednisolone and injected with MolLV, 50 developed lymphocytic leukemia, 7 granulocytic neoplasms, 1 a stem cell leukemia, and 6 lymphosarcomas. One mouse that developed a lymphosarcoma at 93 days of age was the source of MLV-A. The lymphosarcoma in the original mouse involved the peripheral lymph nodes as well as tumors extending from the right hip region and others from the thoracic, lumbar, and sacral vertebrae and from the parietal bones of the skull. There were large tumor follicles in the spleen, but the viscera were not infiltrated. The thymus was normal. Microscopically the tumor consisted of large immature lymphocytes, many of which had an indented nucleus. This same type of nonthymic lymphoma of bone marrow and lymph nodes was transmitted by cellular transfer or by inoculation of either newborn or adult noncortisonized mice with cell-free filtrates. Attempts to isolate a similar virus from the other five lymphosarcomas in the study were unsuccessful (Abelson and Rabstein, 1970*b*).

MLV-A is a defective C-type RNA virus that contains two viral elements. The first component is the Moloney leukemia virus, Mol-MuLV, which has a full complement of retrovirus genes and is self-replicating. The second component is defective and contains only a few Mol-MuLV genes (the p15 and p12 gag genes at the 5′ end and 730 base pairs derived from Mol-MuLV at the 3′ end)

TABLE 4

Induction of Plasmacytomas (PC) and Lymphosarcomas (LS) by MLV-A in Pristane-Treated BALB/c Mice

Experiment No.	Group	Pristane[a] (0.5 ml)	MLV-A on day[b]	Virus pool[c]	Total number of mice	Number of mice with		Average latent period (range)[d]	
						LS (%)	PC (%)	LS	PC
I	A	−	39	1	14	2 (14)	0 (0)	73 (58–89)	—
	B	+	—	—	16	0 (0)	1 (6)	—	(285)
	C	+	39	1	16	10 (62)	4 (24)	70 (40–129)	59 (46–73)
II	A1	−	57	2	16	10 (60)	0 (0)	44 (36–55)	—
	A2	−	57	2F	8	4 (50)	0 (0)	42 (32–47)	—
	B	+	—	—	24	0 (0)	6	—	217 (138–290)
	C1	+	57	2	32	20 (62)	8 (25)	55 (30–120)	49 (21–93)
	C2	+	57	2F	14	6 (43)	5 (36)	40 (30–48)	46 (20–82)
III	B	+	—	—	16	0 (0)	1 (6)	—	(189)
	C	+	39	3	30	18 (60)	9 (30)	37 (26–67)	47 (28–58)

[a] Pristane was injected intraperitoneally when the mice were approximately 2 months of age.

[b] Days after pristane.

[c] MLV-A pools 1 and 2 were 1.7 and 10% extracts of primary lymphosarcomas, respectively. Pool 2F was a 0.45-nm Millipore filtrate of pool 2. Pool 3 was a 10% extract of a transplanted lymphosarcoma. Infectivity titers (per 0.1 ml) were as follows: pool 1, $10^{4.9}$ plaque-forming units (pfu) and $10^{1.8}$ tumor (lymphosarcoma)-producing units 50 (TPD$_{50}$); pool 2, $10^{5.7}$ pfu and $10^{2.6}$ TPD$_{50}$; pool 2F, $10^{5.2}$ pfu; pool 3, 1.6×10^{5} pfu and 10^{2} TPD$_{50}$.

[d] Average latent period was determined as the number of days after the injection of MLV-A, except for mice in group B, for which it was determined as the number of days after pristane.

(Baltimore *et al.*, 1979). These are not enough to replicate the virus particles. The defective virus contains a new 3.6 kb element derived from the BALB/c mouse genome (Baltimore *et al.*, 1979) and is thought to have evolved by a recombination of a Moloney provirus element and genomic mouse DNA (Baltimore *et al.*, 1979).

When MLV-A is injected into adult BALB/c mice, it induces the formation of lymphosarcomas that develop chiefly in the bone marrow and peripheral lymph nodes. These tumors are clearly not of thymic origin and are probably derived from primitive B lymphocytes. MLV-A can also transform B lymphocytes *in vitro* to become lymphosarcomas (Rosenberg *et al.*, 1975; Rosenberg and Baltimore, 1976). A few of the *in vivo* or *in vitro* induced lymphosarcomas produce small amounts of sIgM and sIgD (Premkumar *et al.*, 1975; Potter *et al.*, 1978). Siden *et al.* (1979) have shown that 50–60% of lymphocytes transformed *in vitro* with MLV-A synthesize small amounts of cytoplasmic μ-heavy chains and occasionally *in vitro* cell lines will begin secreting Ig. The general picture that emerges from various studies is that MLV-A has a high predilection to transform a primitive lymphocyte in the B-lymphocyte series.

Most adult BALB/c mice injected intraperitoneally with pristane and subsequently infected with MLV-A also develop lymphosarcomas with short latent periods from 30 to 50 days. However, 5–25% of them develop plasmacytomas with very short latent periods—30 to 70 days after the injection of pristane (Potter *et al.*, 1973). In early experiments with this system (Table 4), the yield of plasmacytomas was quite high, but with passage of the virus, fewer developed plasmacytomas. This may have been due to a change in the virus, e.g., the ratio of Mol-MuLV to defective particles or a change in the 3.6 kb part of the defective viral component.

The role of MLV-A in the rapid formation of plasmacytomas in pristane-treated mice is not clearly defined. The MLV-A-induced plasmacytomas produce MLV-A, indicating the defective element has integrated into the plasmacytoma genome.

Several possible modes of action of MLV-A seem plausible. First, MLV-A can infect B lymphocytes at different stages of development. The intraperitoneal injection of pristane probably promotes both division and maturation of B lymphocytes to advance to immunoglobulin-secreting cell types. Intermediate cells such as the plasmacytic lymphosarcomas (Potter *et al.*, 1978) and plasma cells are transformed, simply because of their greater abundance. In the absence of such a stimulus, the hypersusceptible primitive lymphocyte is transformed and maturation is arrested.

A second role of MLV-A infection is related to the protein product of the 3.6 kb part of the defective fragment. There is a growing body of evidence that indicates that defective transforming C-type retroviruses (e.g., Rous sarcoma virus) and the viruses that induce acute leukemias in chickens (e.g., MC29) transform cells because of proteins, produced by the nonviral host genes that have been recombined into the retroviral genomes (Collett *et al.*, 1979; Graft *et al.*, 1980). Production of these proteins in abnormal amounts (because of the increased number of copies of viral genes, or because these recombined host genes are no longer subject to regulation) directly imbalances the cell, making growth regulation impossible. The MLV-A is no exception, as the 3.6 kb part of the defective element codes for a complete functional protein. This protein has been identified serologically by antisera prepared in strain C57BL mice by immunization with syngeneic MLV-A-transformed cells (Witte *et al.*, 1979). Immunization with MLV-A-transformed cells induces the formation of several types of antibodies including those to products of mouse genes in the MLV-A defective virus. These proteins made by the defective virus range from 90,000 to 160,000 daltons and are related to a normal 150,000-dalton cellular protein. This protein is called NCP150 by Baltimore *et al.* (1979) and not unexpectedly is found in normal cells. NCP150 is a phosphoprotein, and in cells is located within the plasma membrane as a transmembrane protein. In normal cells the content of this protein is quite low as compared with MLV-A-infected cells. Overproduction then could lead to severe changes in the capacity of the cells to regulate growth. Risser *et al.* (1978) have described another antigen associated with MLV-A-transformed cells; this antigen is probably not coded by the defective virus, but is considered by Baltimore and colleagues to possibly be a cell-surface antigen found on stem cells that is expressed on all MLV-A-transformed cells.

4. Summary

1. Rare spontaneous plasmacytomas in mice appear to arise in the lymphoid tissue associated with the gut, particularly the ileocecal region.

2. Plasmacytomas can be induced in high frequency in two susceptible inbred strains of mice, BALB/cAn and NZB, by the intraperitoneal implantation of plastics or the injection of mineral oils or specific alkanes such as pristane (2,6,10,14-tetramethylpentadecane).

3. These substances are neither metabolized nor effectively removed and cause the formation of a chronic granulomatous tissue. They probably also stimulate B-lymphocyte proliferation and maturation.

4. Plasmacytomas develop in the chronic granulomatous tissue, and depend upon this microenvironment or a product of the abnormal microenvironment for growth.

5. The role of C-type RNA viruses in plasmacytomagenesis remains obscure. These viruses are activated in the oil granuloma and virtually every BALB/c plasmacytoma actively produces xeno- and ecotropic viruses. These endogenous viruses are not plasmacytomagenic, but their production in cells may be a factor in deregulating the cells. The defective MLVA virus accelerates the induction process, but does not initiate plasmacytomas in the absence of an oil granuloma.

6. Karyological studies of BALB/c plasmacytomas have a very high incidence of translocations affecting chromosomes 6, 12, and 15.

5. References

AARONSON, S. A., AND STEPHENSON, J. R., 1973, Independent segregation of loci for activation of biologically distinguishable RNA C-type viruses in mouse cells, *Proc. Natl. Acad. Sci. USA* **70**:2055–2058.

AARONSON, S. A., HARTLEY, J. W., AND TODARO, G. J., 1969, Mouse leukemia virus "spontaneous" release by mouse embryo cells after long term *in vitro* cultivation, *Proc. Natl. Acad. Sci. USA* **64**:87.

ABELSON, H. T., AND RABSTEIN, L. S., 1970*a*, Influence of prednisolone on Moloney leukemogenic virus in BALB/c mice, *Cancer Res.* **30**:2208–2212.

ABELSON, H. T., AND RABSTEIN, L. S., 1970*b*, Lymphosarcoma: Virus-induced thymic-independent disease in mice, *Cancer Res.* **30**:2213–2222.

ANDERSON, P. N., 1970, Plasma cell tumor induction in BALB/c mice, *Proc. Am. Assoc. Cancer Res.* **11**:3 (abstract).

ANDERSON, P. N., AND POTTER, M., 1969, Induction of plasma cell tumors in BALB/c mice with 2,6,10,14-tetramethylpentadecane (pristane), *Nature (London)* **222**:994–995.

AOKI, T., AND TAKAHASHI, T. L., 1972, Viral and cellular surface antigens of murine leukemias and myelomas, *J. Exp. Med.* **135**:443–457.

AOKI, T., POTTER, M., AND STURM, M. M., 1973, Analysis by immunoelectron microscopy of type-C viruses associated with primary and short-term transplanted mouse plasma (H) tumors, *J. Natl. Cancer Inst.* **51**:1609–1617.

ARMSTRONG, M. Y. K., EBENSTEIN, P., KONIGSBERG, W. H., AND RICHARDS, F. F., 1978, Endogenous RNA tumor viruses are activated during chemical induction of murine plasmacytomas, *Proc. Natl. Acad. Sci. USA* **75**:4549–4552.

AZAR, H. A., 1973, Pathology of multiple myeloma and related growths, in: *Multiple Myeloma and Related Disorders* (H. A. Azar and M. Potter, eds.), pp. 1–85, Harper & Row, New York.

BALTIMORE, D., ROSENBERG, N., AND WITTE, O. N., 1979, Transformation of immature lymphoid cells by Abelson murine leukemia virus, *Immunol. Rev.* **48**:3–22.

BAZIN, H., DECKERS, C., BECKERS, A., AND HEREMANS, J. F., 1972, Transplantable immunoglobulin secreting tumours in rats. I. General features of Lou/Wsl strain rat immunocytomas and their monoclonal proteins, *Int. J. Cancer* **10**:568–580.

BAZIN, H., BECKERS, A., DECKERS, C., AND MORIAME, M., 1973, Transplantable immunoglobulin-secreting tumors in rats. V. Monoclonal immunoglobulins secreted by 250 ileocecal immunocytomas in Lou/Wsl rats, *J. Natl. Cancer Inst.* **51**:1359–1362.

BENDORAITIS, J. G., BROWN, B. L., AND HEPNER, L. S., 1962, Isoprenoid hydrocarbons in petroleum isolation of 2,6,10,14-tetramethylpentadecane by high temperature gas–liquid chromatography, *Anal. Chem.* **34**:49–53.

BLUMER, M., 1965, "Zamene," isomeric C_{19} mono-olefins from marine zooplankton, fishes, and mammals, *Science* **148**:370–371.

BLUMER, M., AND THOMAS, D., 1965, Phytadienes in zooplankton, *Science* **147**:1148–1149.

BLUMER, M., MULLIN, M. M., AND THOMAS, D. W., 1963, Pristane in zooplankton, *Science* **140**:974.

BLUMER, M., ROBERTSON, J. C., GORDON, J. E., AND SASS, J., 1969, Phytol derived C_{19} di- and triolefinic hydrocarbons in marine zooplankton and fishes, *Biochemistry* **8**:4067–4074.

CANCRO, M., AND POTTER, M., 1976, The requirement of an adherent substratum for the growth of developing plasmactyoma cells *in vivo*, *J. Exp. Med.* **144**:1554–1566.

CARR, I., 1967, The fine structure of cells of the mouse peritoneum, *Z. Zellforsch. Mikrosk. Anat.* **80**:534–555.

COLLETT, M. S., ERIKSON, E., PURCHIO, A. F., BRUGGE, J. S., AND ERIKSON, R. L., 1979, A normal cell protein similar in structure and function to the avian sarcoma virus transforming gene product, *Proc. Natl. Acad. Sci. USA* **76**:3159–3163.

COMOGLIO, P. M., AND GUGLIELMONE, R., 1973, Immunohistochemical study of IgA transepithelial transfer into digestive tract secretions in the mouse, *Immunology* **25**:71–80.

COTRAN, R. S., AND FORTNER, J. B., 1962, Serum protein abnormality in a transplantable plasmacytoma of the Syrian hamster, *J. Natl. Cancer Inst.* **28**:1193–1205.

CRABBÉ, P. A., NASH, D. R., BAXIN, H., EYSSEN, H., AND HEREMANS, J. F., 1970, Immunochemical observations on lymphoid tissues from conventional and germ free mice, *Lab. Invest.* **22**:448–457.

DALTON, A. J., AND POTTER, M., 1968, Electronmicroscope study of the mammary tumor agent in plasma cell tumors, *J. Natl. Cancer Inst.* **40**:1375–1385.

DALTON, A. J., POTTER, M., AND MERWIN, R. M., 1961, Some ultrastructural characteristics of a series of primary and transplanted plasma cell tumors of the mouse, *J. Natl. Cancer Inst.* **26:**1221–1267.

DECKERS, C., 1963, Etude electrophoretique et immunoelectrophoretique des proteines du rat atteint de leucosarcome, *Protides Biol. Fluids Proc. Colloq.* **11:**105–108.

DUNN, T. B., 1954, Normal and pathologic anatomy of the reticular tissue in laboratory mice with a classification and discussion of neoplasms, *J. Natl. Cancer Inst.* **14:**1281–1433.

DUNN, T. B., 1957, Plasma-cell neoplasms beginning in the ileocecal area in strain C3H mice, *J. Natl. Cancer Inst.* **19:**371–391.

DUNN, T. B., AND DERINGER, M. K., 1968, Reticulum cell neoplasm, type B or the "Hodgkin's-like lesion" of the mouse, *J. Natl. Cancer Inst.* **40:**771–821.

DUNN, T. B., MOLONEY, J. B., GREEN, A. W., AND ARNOLD, B., 1961, Pathogenesis of a virus induced leukemia in mice, *J. Natl. Cancer Inst.* **26:**189–221.

EBBESEN, P., RASK-NIELSEN, R., AND McINTIRE, K. R., 1968, Plasmacell leukemia in BALB/c mice inoculated with subcellular material. I. Incidence and morphology, *J. Natl. Cancer Inst.* **41:**473–493.

FAHEY, J. L., POTTER, M., GUTTER, F. J., AND DUNN, T. B., 1960, Distinctive myeloma globulins associated with a new plasma cell neoplasm of strain C3H mice, *Blood* **15:**103–113.

FARROW, B. R. H., AND PENNY, R., 1971, Multiple myeloma in a cat, *J. Am. Vet. Med. Assoc.* **158:**606–611.

GEARHART, P. J., AND CEBRA, J. J., 1979, Differentiated B-lymphocytes. Potential to express particular antibody variable and constant regions depends on site of lymphoid tissue and antigen load, *J. Exp. Med.* **149:**216–227.

GEARHART, P. J., HURWITZ, J. L., AND CEBRA, J. J., 1980, Successive switching of antibody isotypes expressed within the lines of a cell clone, *Proc. Natl. Acad. Sci. USA* **77:**5424–5428.

GIBSON, D. M., TAYLOR, B. A., AND CHERRY, M., 1978, Evidence for close linkage of a mouse light chain marker with the Ly 2.3 locus, *J. Immunol.* **121:**1585.

GOLDSTEIN, G. L., WARNER, N. L., AND HOLMES, M. C., 1966, Plasma cell tumor induction in (NZB × BALB/c)f1 hybrid mice, *J. Natl. Cancer Inst.* **37:**135–143.

GRAFT, T., BRUG, H., AND HAYMAN, M. J., 1980, Target cell specificity of defective avian leukemia viruses: Hematopoietic target cells for a given virus type can be infected but not transformed by strains of a different type, *Proc. Natl. Acad. Sci. USA* **77:**389–393.

HENGARTNER, H., MEO, T., AND MULLER, E., 1978, Assignment of genes for immunoglobulin K and heavy chains to chromosomes 6 and 12 in mouse, *Proc. Natl. Acad. Sci. USA* **75:**4494–4498.

HERBERMAN, R. B., AND AOKI, T., 1972, Immune and natural antibodies to syngeneic murine plasma cell tumors, *J. Exp. Med.* **136:**94–111.

HERSEY, P., AND MacLENNAN, I. C. M., 1973, Macrophage dependent protection of tumor cells, *Immunology* **24:**385–393.

HOLLANDER, W. P., TAKAKURA, K., AND YAMADA, H., 1968, Endocrine factors in the pathogenesis of plasma cell tumors, Recent Prog. Horm. Res. **24:**81–137.

HONJO, T., AND KATAOKA, T., 1978, Organization of immunoglobulin heavy chain genes and allelic deletion model, *Proc. Natl. Acad. Sci. USA* **75:**2140–2144.

HYMAN, R., RALPH, P., AND SARKAR, S., 1972, Cell-specific antigens and immunoglobulin synthesis of murine myeloma cells and their variants, *J. Natl. Cancer Inst.* **48:**173–184.

KLEIN, G., 1979, Lymphoma development in mice and men: Diversity of initiation is followed by a convergent cytogenetic evolution, *Proc. Natl. Acad. Sci. USA* **76:**2442–2446.

KOSTER, F. T., AND McGREGOR, D. C., 1971, The mediator of cellular immunity. III. Lymphocyte traffic from the blood into the inflamed peritoneal cavity, *J. Exp. Med.* **133:**864–876.

KRIPKE, M. L., AND WEISS, D. W., 1970, Studies on the immune responses of BALB/c mice during tumor induction by mineral oil, *Int. J. Cancer* **6:**422–430.

KUFF, E. L., WIVEL, N. A., AND LUEDERS, K. R., 1968, The extraction of intracisternal A particles from a mouse plasma cell tumor, *Cancer Res.* **28:**2137–2148.

KUFF, E. L., LUEDERS, K. K., OZER, H. L., AND WIVEL, N. A., 1972, Some structural and antigenic properties of intracisternal A particles occurring in mouse tumors, *Proc. Natl. Acad. Sci. USA* **69:**218.

LESPINATS, G., 1969, Induction d'une immunite vis-à-vis de la greffe de plasmacytosarcomes chez la souris BALB/c, *Eur. J. Cancer* **5:**421–426.

LEVY, J. A., AND PINCUS, T., 1970, Demonstration of biological activity of a murine leukemia virus of New Zealand black mice, *Science* **170:**326–327.

LIEBERMAN, R., DOUGLAS, J. O., AND MANTEL, N., 1960, Production in mice of ascitic fluid containing antibodies induced by *Staphylococcus–* or *Salmonella–*adjuvant mixtures, *J. Immunol.* **84:**514–529.

LYNCH, R. G., GRAFF, R. J., SIRISINHA, S., SIMMS, E. S., AND EISEN, H. N., 1972, Myeloma proteins as tumor-specific transplantation antigens, *Proc. Natl. Acad. Sci. USA* **69:**1540–1544.

MCINTIRE, K. R., AND PRINCLER, G. L., 1969, Prolonged adjuvant stimulation in germ-free BALB/c mice: Development of plasma cell neoplasia, *Immunology* **17:**481–487.

MEO, T., JOHNSON, J., BEECHEY, C. V., ANDREWS, S. J., PETERS, J., AND SEARLE, A. G., 1980, Linkage analysis of murine immunoglobulin heavy chain and serum prealbumin genes establish their location on chromosome 12 proximal to the T(5;12)3H breakpoint in band 12F$_1$, *Proc. Natl. Acad. Sci. USA* **77:**550–553.

MERWIN, R. M., AND ALGIRE, G. H., 1959, Induction of plasma cell neoplasms and fibrosarcomas in BALB/c mice carrying diffusion chambers, *Proc. Soc. Exp. Biol. Med.* **101:**437–439.

MERWIN, R. M., AND REDMON, L. W., 1963, Induction of plasma cell tumors and sarcomas in mice by diffusion chambers placed in the peritoneal cavity, *J. Natl. Cancer Inst.* **31:**998–1007.

METCALF, D., 1973, Colony formation in agar by murine plasmacytoma cells: Potentiation by hematopoietic cells and serum, *J. Cell. Physiol.* **81:**397–410.

MOLONEY, J. B., 1962, The murine leukemias, *Fed. Proc.* **21:**19–31.

MORIWAKI, K., IMAI, H. T., YAMASHITA, J., AND YOSIDA, T. H., 1971, Ploidy fluctuations of mouse plasma cell neoplasm MsPC-1 during serial transplantation, *J. Natl. Cancer Inst.* **46:**623–637.

MORSE, H. C., III, RIBLET, R., ASOFSKY, R., AND WEIGERT, M., 1978, Plasmacytomas of the NZB mouse, *J. Immunol.* **121:**1969–1972.

MORSE, H. C., III, HARTLEY, J. W., AND POTTER, M., 1980, Genetic considerations in plasmacytomas of BALB/c, NZB and (BALB/c × NZB)F$_1$ mice, in: *Progress in Myeloma, 1980* (M. Potter, ed.), Elsevier/North-Holland, New York.

NAMBA, Y., AND HANAOKA, M., 1972, Immunocytology of cultured IgM-forming cells of mouse. I. Requirement of phagocytic cell factor for the growth of IgM-forming tumor cells in tissue culture, *J. Immunol.* **109:**1193–1200.

NESBITT, M. N., AND FRANKE, U., 1973, A system of nomenclature for band patterns of mouse chromosomes, *Chromosoma* **41:**145–148.

OHNO, S., BABONITS, M., WIENER, F., SPIRA, J., KLEIN, G., AND POTTER, M., 1979, Nonrandom chromosome changes involving the Ig gene-carrying chromosomes 12 and 6 in Pristane-induced mouse plasmacytomas, *Cell* **18:**1001–1007.

OPPENHEIMER, B. S., OPPENHEIMER, E. T., DANISHETSKY, I., STOUT, A. P., AND ELRICH, F. R., 1955, Further studies of polymers as carcinogenic agents in animals, *Cancer Res.* **15:**333–340.

OSBORNE, C. A., PERMAN, V., SAUTTER, J. H., STEVENS, J. B., AND HANLON, G. F., 1968, Multiple myeloma in the dog, *J. Am. Vet. Med. Assoc.* **153:**1300–1319.

PARK, C. H., BERGSAGEL, D. E., AND MCCULLOCH, E. A., 1971, Mouse myeloma tumor stem cells: A primary culture assay, *J. Natl. Cancer Inst.* **46:**411–422.

PETERS, R. L., RABSTEIN, L. S., SPAHN, G. J., MADISON, R. M., AND HUEBNER, R. J., 1972a, Incidence of spontaneous neoplasms in breeding and retired breeder BALB/c Cr mice throughout the natural life span, *Int. J. Cancer* **10:**273–282.

PETERS, R. L., HARTLEY, J. W., SPAHN, G. J., RABSTEIN, L. S., WHITMORE, L. S., TURNER, H. C., AND HUEBNER, R. J., 1972b, Prevalence of the group-specific (gs) antigen and infectious virus expressions of the murine C-type RNA viruses during the life span of BALB/c Cr mice, *Int. J. Cancer* **10:**283–289.

PETERS, R. L., RABSTEIN, L. S., SPAHN, G. J., TURNER, H. C., AND HUEBNER, R. J., 1972c, Incidence of group-specific (gs) antigens of type C RNA tumor viruses in spontaneous neoplasms of BALB/c Cr mice, *Int. J. Cancer* **10:**290–295.

PILGRIM, H. I., 1965, The relationship of chronic ulceration of the ileocecal junction to the development of reticuloendothelial tumors in C3H mice, *Cancer Res.* **25:**53–65.

POTTER, M., 1967, The plasma cell tumors and myeloma proteins of mice, in: *Methods in Cancer Research*, Vol. II (H. Busch, ed.), pp. 105–157, Academic Press, New York.

POTTER, M., 1970, Mouse IgA myeloma proteins that bind polysaccharide antigens of enterobacterial origin, *Fed. Proc.* **29:**85–91.

POTTER, M., 1971, Antigen binding myeloma proteins in mice, *Ann. N.Y. Acad. Sci.* **190:**306–321.

POTTER, M., 1972, Immunoglobulin producing tumors and myeloma proteins in mice, *Physiol. Rev.* **52:**631–719.

POTTER, M., AND BOYCE, C., 1962, Induction of plasma cell neoplasms in strain BALB/c mice with mineral oil and mineral oil adjuvants, *Nature (London)* **193**:1086–1087.

POTTER, M., AND FAHEY, J. L., 1960, Studies on eight transplantable plasma cell neoplasms in mice, *J. Natl. Cancer Inst.* **24**:1153–1165.

POTTER, M., AND MACCARDLE, R. C., 1964, Histology of developing plasma cell neoplasia induced by mineral oil in BALB/c mice, *J. Natl. Cancer Inst.* **33**:497–515.

POTTER, M., AND ROBERTSON, C. L., 1960, Development of plasma cell neoplasms in BALB/c mice after intraperitoneal injection of paraffin oil adjuvant–heat killed staphylococcus mixtures, *J. Natl. Cancer Inst.* **25**:847–861.

POTTER, M., AND WALTERS, J. L., 1973, Effects of intraperitoneal pristane on established immunity to the Adj-PC-5 plasmacytoma, *J. Natl. Cancer Inst.* **51**:875–881.

POTTER, M., FAHEY, J. L., AND PILGRIM, H. I., 1957, Abnormal serum protein and bone destruction in transmissible mouse plasma cell neoplasm (multiple myeloma), *Proc. Soc. Exp. Biol. Med.* **94**:327–333.

POTTER, M., PUMPHREY, J. G., AND WALTERS, J. L., 1972, Growth of primary plasmacytomas in the mineral oil-conditioned peritoneal environment, *J. Natl. Cancer Inst.* **49**:305–308.

POTTER, M., SKLAR, M. D., AND ROWE, W. P., 1973, Rapid viral induction of plasmacytomas in pristane primed BALB/c mice, *Science* **182**:592–594.

POTTER, M., PUMPHREY, J. G., AND BAILEY, D. W., 1975, Genetics of susceptibility of plasmacytoma induction. I. BALB/cAnN(C), C57BL/6N(B6) C57BL/Ka(BK), (C×B6)F$_1$, (C×BK)F$_1$ and C×B recombinant inbred strains, *J. Natl. Cancer Inst.* **54**:1413–1417.

POTTER, M., PREMKUMAR-REDDY, E., AND WIVEL, N. A., 1978, Immunoglobulin production by lymphosarcomas induced by Abelson virus in mice, in: *Gene Expression and Regulation in Cultured Cells* (K. K. Sanford, ed.), pp. 311–320, NCI Monograph 48.

PREMKUMAR, E., POTTER, M., SINGER, P. A., AND SKLAR, M. D., 1975, Synthesis, surface deposition and secretion of immunoglobulins by Abelson virus-transformed lymphosarcoma cell lines, *Cell* **6**:149–159.

RASK-NIELSEN, R., MCINTIRE, K. R., AND EBBESEN, P., 1968, Plasma-cell leukemia in BALB/c mice inoculated with subcellular material. II. Serological changes, *J. Natl. Cancer Inst.* **41**:495–504.

RISSER, R., STOCKERT, E., AND OLD, L. J., 1978, Abelson antigen: A new viral tumor antigen that is also a differentiation antigen BALB/c, *Proc. Natl. Acad. Sci. U.S.A.* **75**:3918–3922.

RÖLLINGHOFF, M., ROUSE, B. T., AND WARNER, N. L., 1973, Tumor immunity to murine plasma cell tumors. I. Tumor-associated transplantation antigens of NZB and BALB/c plasma cell tumors, *J. Natl. Cancer Inst.* **50**:159–172.

ROSENBERG, N., AND BALTIMORE, D., 1976, A quantitative assay for transformation of bone marrow cells by Abelson murine leukemia virus, *J. Exp. Med.* **143**:1453–1463.

ROSENBERG, N., BALTIMORE, D., AND SCHER, C. D., 1975, *In vitro* transformation of lymphoid cell by Abelson murine leukemia virus, *Proc. Natl. Acad. Sci. USA* **72**:1932–1936.

SHEPARD, J. S., PETTENGILL, O. S., WURSTER-HILL, D. H., AND SORENSON, G. D., 1974a, Alterations of karyotype and oncogenicity in mouse myeloma MOPC315 and 5-bromodeoxyuridine-resistant cell line, *Cancer Res.* **34**:2852–2858.

SHEPARD, J. S., WURSTER-HILL, D. H., PETTENGILL, O. S., AND SORENSON, G. D., 1974b, Giemsa banded chromosomes of mouse myeloma in relationship to oncogenicity, *Cytogenet. Cell Genet.* **13**:279–304.

SHEPARD, J. S., PETTENGILL, O. S., WURSTER-HILL, D. H., AND SORENSON, G. D., 1976, Karyotype marker formation and oncogenicity in mouse plasmacytomas, *J. Natl. Cancer Inst.* **56**:1003–1011.

SHEPARD, J. S., PETTENGILL, O. S., WURSTER-HILL, D. H., AND SORENSON, G. D., 1978, A specific chromosome breakpoint associated with mouse plasmacytomas, *J. Natl. Cancer Inst.* **61**:225–258.

SIDEN, E. J., BALTIMORE, D., CLARK, D., AND ROSENBERG, N. E., 1979, Immunoglobulin synthesis by lymphoid cells transformed by *in vitro* Abelson murine leukemia virus, *Cell* **5**:389–396.

STOCKERT, E., OLD, L. J., AND BOYSE, E. A., 1971, The G$_{ix}$ system: A cell surface antigen associated with murine leukemia virus; implications regarding chromosomal integration of the viral genome, *J. Exp. Med.* **133**:1334–1355.

SWAN, D., E'EUSTACHIO, P., LEINWAND, L., SEIDMAN, J., KEITHLEY, D., AND RUDDLE, F. H., 1979, Chromosomal assignment for the mouse K light chain genes, *Proc. Natl. Acad. Sci. USA* **76**:2735–2739.

TAKAHASHI, T., OLD, L. J., AND BOYSE, E. A., 1970, Surface alloantigens of plasma cells, *J. Exp. Med.* **131**:1325–1341.

TAKAHASHI, T., OLD, L. J., HSU, C. J., AND BOYSE, E. A., 1971a, A new differentiation antigen of plasma cells, Eur. J. Immunol. 1:478.

TAKAHASHI, T., OLD, L. J., McINTIRE, K. R., AND BOYSE, E. A., 1971b, Immunoglobulin and other surface antigens of cells of the immune system, J. Exp. Med. 134:815–832.

TAKAKURA, K., MASON, W. B., AND HOLLANDER, W. P., 1966, Studies on the pathogenesis of plasma cell tumors. I. Effect of cortisone on development of plasma cell tumors, Cancer Res. 26:596–599.

THOMPSON, J., AND VANFURTH, R., 1970, The effect of glucocorticosteroids on the kinetics of mononuclear phagocytes, J. Exp. Med. 131:429–442.

TOMASI, T. B., JR., AND BIENENSTOCK, J., 1968, Secretory immunoglobulins, Adv. Immunol. 9:1–96.

VAN DUUREN, B. L., NELSON, N., ORRIS, L., PALMES, E. D., AND SCHMITT, F. L., 1963, Carcinogenicity of epoxides, lactones, and peroxy compounds, J. Natl. Cancer Inst. 31:41–55.

VAN DUUREN, B. L., LANGSETH, L., GOLDSCHMIDT, B. M., AND ORRIS, L., 1967, Carcinogenicity of epoxides, lactones and peroxy compounds. VI. Structure and carcinogenic activity, J. Natl. Cancer Inst. 39:1217–1228.

VOLKMAN, A., 1966, The origin and turnover of mononuclear cells in peritoneal exudates in rats, J. Exp. Med. 124:241–253.

VOLKMAN, L. E., AND KRUEGER, R. G., 1973, XC cell cytopathogenicity as an assay for murine myeloma C-type virus, J. Natl. Cancer Inst. 51:1205–1210.

WARNER, N. L., 1975, Review. Autoimmunity and the pathogenesis of plasma cell tumor induction in NZB and hybrid mice, Immunogenetics 2:1–20.

WATSON, J., RALPH, P., AND SARKAR, S., 1970, Leukemia viruses associated with mouse myeloma cells, Proc. Natl. Acad. Sci. USA 66:344–351.

WILLIAMS, W. H., AND KRUEGER, R. G., 1972, Tumor-associated transplantation antigens of myelomas induced in BALB/c mice, J. Natl. Cancer Inst. 49:1613–1620.

WILSON, S. H., AND KUFF, E. L., 1972, A novel DNA polymerase activity found in association with intracisternal-A particles, Proc. Natl. Acad. Sci. USA 69:1531–1536.

WITTE, O. N., ROSENBERG, N. E., AND BALTIMORE, D., 1979, Normal cell protein cross-reaction to the major Abelson murine leukemia virus gene product, Nature (London) 281:396–398.

WIVEL, N. A., AND SMITH, G. H., 1971, Distribution of intracisternal A particles in a variety of normal and neoplastic mouse tissues, Int. J. Cancer 7:167–175.

YAMADA, H., MASHBURN, L. T., TAKAKURA, K., AND HOLLANDER, W. P., 1969, The correlation between plasma cell tumor development and antibody response in inbred strains of mice, Proc. Soc. Exp. Biol. Med. 131:947–950.

YANCEY, S. T., 1964, Plasma cell neoplasm arising in a CAF$_1$ mouse: Characteristics and response to certain chemotherapeutic agents, J. Natl. Cancer Inst. 33:373–382.

YOSIDA, M. C., AND MORIWAKI, K., 1975, Specific marker chromosomes involving a translocation (12;15) in a mouse myeloma, Proc. Jpn. Acad. 51:588–592.

YOSIDA, M. C., MORIWAKI, K., AND MIGITA, S., 1978, Specificity of the deletion of chromosome No. 15 in mouse plasmacytoma, J. Natl. Cancer Inst. 60:235–238.

YOSIDA, T. H., IMAI, H. T., AND POTTER, M., 1968, Chromosomal alteration and development of tumors. XIX. Chromosome constitution of tumor cells in 16 plasma cell neoplasms of BALB/c mice, J. Natl. Cancer Inst. 41:1083–1087.

YOSIDA, T. H., IMAI, H. T., AND MORIWAKI, K., 1970, Chromosomal alteration and development of tumors. XXI. Cytogenetic studies of primary plasma cell neoplasms induced in BALB/c mice, J. Natl. Cancer Inst. 45:411–418.

ZAWADZKI, Z. A., EDWARDS, G. A., AND ADAMS, R. V., 1967, M-components in immunoproliferative disorders. Electrophoretic and immunological analysis of 200 cases, Am. J. Clin. Pathol. 48:418–430.

6

Immunocompetence and Malignancy

Cornelis J. M. Melief and Robert S. Schwartz

The essential feature of a strategy of discovery lies in determining the sequence of choice of problems to solve. Now it is in fact very much more difficult to see a problem than to find a solution for it. The former requires imagination, the latter only ingenuity.

—J. D. Bernal

1. Introduction*

In June of 1908, Paul Ehrlich, the founder of immunology, lectured at the University of Amsterdam on the subject of cancer. His remarks included the following: "the understanding of natural immunity really represents the key to carcinoma . . . . I have acquired the firm conviction that natural immunity does not depend on the presence of anti-microbial materials, but rather, it depends on purely cellular activities. I am certain that, in the enormously complicated course of fetal and post-fetal development, aberrant cells become unusually common. Fortunately, in the majority of people, they remain completely latent thanks to the organism's positive mechanisms. If such mechanisms did not exist, one might

* We assume that the reader has a working knowledge of the basic principles of immunology. Those who wish to brush up on recent advances may wish to consult either Roitt (1971) or Bach and Good (1972), both of which are excellent texts.

Cornelis J. M. Melief and Robert S. Schwartz ● Hematology Service, New England Medical Center Hospital, and the Department of Medicine, Tufts University School of Medicine, Boston, Massachusetts. Dr. Melief is the recipient of a fellowship from the Dutch Organization for the Advancement of Pure Research (ZWO). Supported by grants from USPHS (CA 10018) and the Damon Runyon Foundation.

expect carcinomas to have an enormous frequency. These cells may live in a latent state for 20, 30 or 40 years before changing to a significant tumor. This means, in light of my theory, that there has been a diminution of some vital cell activity [which] allows the rapid, parasitic growth of certain cells" (Ehrlich, 1957).*

Apparently, Ehrlich's amazing prescience was not appreciated, because, apart from a brief comment by Emery (1924), who expressed a similar notion, the idea that cellular immunity is important in the defense against neoplastic cells lay fallow for decades. However, the landmark experiments of Little (1941), Foley (1953), Prehn and Main (1957), and Klein (1966) revitalized immunological studies of cancer and set the stage for the development of one of the most powerful influences in the field. This is the theory of immunological surveillance.

There is general agreement that this concept in its modern form was formulated by Lewis Thomas, who, in 1959, proposed that "the phenomenon of homograft rejection will turn out to represent a primary mechanism for natural defense against neoplasia" (Thomas, 1959). This idea, which was offered extemporaneously in a discussion, fortunately recorded, of Medawar's experiments on transplantation immunity, was taken up by Burnet, who, besides expostulating on its profound biological and medical implications, first used the term *surveillance* as a coda for Thomas's concept (Burnet, 1963, 1970).

The theory that the immune system "represents a primary mechanism for natural defense against neoplasia" makes four predictions: (1) Neoplastic cells possess antigenic determinants that are absent from normal cells. (2) These antigens are immunogenic in the host of origin; i.e., they are autoantigens. (3) The immune response provoked by tumor-associated antigens protects the host by destroying neoplastic cells; i.e., the surveillance mechanism relies on an autoimmune reaction. (4) Tumor cells flourish in individuals with defective or suppressed immunity.

Abundant evidence supports the first three predictions, and we will not deal with them here because they have been thoroughly analyzed elsewhere (Hellström, 1969; Alexander, 1972; Klein, 1972). Instead, we will direct our attention to the theory's fourth prediction. This is its keystone. Moreover, the prediction that impaired immunity encourages the development and growth of cancer has important clinical implications. Investigations of the possibility of enhanced development of neoplasms during immunosuppressive therapy and renewed efforts toward the immunotherapy of cancer both originate from the notion that the immune system of the patient has failed to reject the neoplasm.

Before addressing ourselves to this problem, we should admit to the reader our skepticism. We feel that the theory of immunological surveillance has been overemphasized,† perhaps to the detriment of alternative views. We also believe that this theory has not been adequately challenged in the laboratory. Indeed, almost all experimental work stimulated by the theory seems to have been designed with the expressed or implied purpose of proving it. Yet a theory derives its strength from its ability to resist refutation (Popper, 1968). Left unchallenged,

---

* We are grateful to Dr. Barry Bloom for directing our attention to this article.
† Prehn (1970) has called it "overrated."

the theory of immunological surveillance is in danger of becoming a mere self-fulfilling prophecy. And when that stage in concept-making is reached, no further progress is possible. By writing this chapter, we hope to contribute toward breaking what we believe is a deadlock. By virtue of its extraordinary achievements, tumor immunology is becoming orthodox and predictable. Perhaps only the unorthodox and the unpredicted can advance it to the next major phase in its evolution.

2. Deliberate Immunosuppression and Malignancy in Experimental Animals

2.1. Immunosuppression and Infection with Oncogenic Viruses

2.1.1. DNA Viruses

The polyoma virus,* which commonly infects both wild and laboratory mice (Gross, 1970), does not produce tumors under natural conditions even though it is potentially very oncogenic. Solid evidence indicates that this is so because thymus-dependent (T) lymphocytes efficiently eliminate any cell transformed to a malignant state by the virus.

Cells infected by the polyoma virus elaborate a new antigen, which, because it provokes the specific rejection of transplanted syngeneic polyoma tumors, is called a tumor-specific transplantation antigen (TSTA) (Koldovsky, 1969) or transplantation-resistance antigen (Law, 1969). Even transformed cells free of intact polyoma virus elaborate the TSTA (Ting and Law, 1965; Ting, 1966), so the relevant immunogenic determinant is not part of the virus itself but is made by the cell as a result of infection by the virus. Moreover, even high levels of antiviral antibody cannot protect mice against transplanted syngeneic polyoma tumors (Law, 1966).

Abundant evidence supports the view that the immunological response to TSTA induced by polyoma virus is mediated via thymus-dependent lymphocytes. Thymectomy or antilymphocyte serum (ALS)† treatment permits the appearance of tumors in mice and rats deliberately or naturally infected with polyoma virus (Vandeputte and De Somer, 1965; Allison and Taylor, 1967; Allison and Law, 1968; Chesterman et al., 1969; Vandeputte, 1969). In such immunological cripples, reconstitution with thymus, spleen, or lymph node cells prevents development of the neoplasms (Law and Ting, 1965; Allison and Taylor, 1967; Sjögren and Borum, 1971). Immunotherapy with lymphoid cells from sensitized donors is more effective in eliminating the neoplasms than is treatment with cells from normal donors (Law, 1969). This supports the argument that the neoplasms are rejected by immunologically specific mechanisms.

---

* Because the general principles derived from experiments with polyma are applicable to SV40 and oncogenic adenoviruses (Kirschstein et al., 1964; Allison et al., 1967; Allison and Taylor, 1967; Hoosier et al., 1968; Law, 1970b), these viruses will not be dealt with separately.

† ALS selectively depletes rodents of circulating T cells (Lance et al., 1973).

Recent evidence indicates that neither neonatal thymectomy nor treatment with ALS completely abolishes cellular immunity. Although the tissues of mice treated in either of these ways are severely depleted of lymphocytes, those few that do remain can exert specific killing effects on tumor cells *in vitro* (Sjögren and Borum, 1971). Therefore, impaired cellular immunity may not be the only reason for the progressive growth of polyoma-induced neoplasms. Another possibility is "blocking factor," which probably consists of a complex of tumor antigen and its corresponding antibody (Sjögren *et al.*, 1971). This factor prevents the killing of tumor cells by sensitized lymphocytes, probably by masking antigenic sites on the neoplastic cell. "Blocking factor" has been found in the serum of mice dying of progressively growing polyoma tumors (Sjögren and Borum, 1971). The story is further complicated by an "unblocking factor," which nullifies the effect of the "blocking factor." Infusion of serum containing "unblocking factor" into animals has caused regression of spreading polyoma tumors (Bansal and Sjögren, 1971, 1973). Neither thymectomy nor ALS treatment affects the production of "blocking factor," so an animal treated with, say, ALS, would be in double jeopardy if inoculated with a polyoma tumor: grossly impaired cellular immunity compounded by the biological effects of unimpaired production of "blocking factor."

Although the polyoma system seems to fulfill the four predictions of the theory of immunological surveillance, it is noteworthy that polyoma tumors are strongly antigenic and give rise to durable, high-grade immunity (Law, 1970b). By contrast, most naturally occurring neoplasms are only weakly antigenic (Klein, 1969). Therefore, the principles derived from the polyoma system may not apply directly to spontaneous neoplasms. We have also seen that even in mice with rapidly growing polyoma tumors there is an immune response: the production of "blocking factor." However, unlike cellular immunity, this response protects, not the host, but the tumor.

2.1.2. RNA Viruses

By contrast with the findings in the polyoma system, neonatal thymectomy *reduces* the incidence of leukemia in mice deliberately or naturally infected with Gross or Moloney leukemia virus (Gross, 1959; Moloney, 1962; Furth *et al.*, 1966; Law, 1966). However, in this instance the effects of thymectomy are related, not to immunosuppression, but to the removal of a microenvironment required for the development of leukemia. Hence, any tumor-promoting effect provided by immunosuppression after thymectomy will be obscured (Law, 1966).

Alternative immunosuppressive procedures are thus required to establish the relationship between immunocompetence and leukemogenesis due to oncornaviruses. The consensus is that treatment with ALS (Allison and Law, 1968; Hirsch and Murphy, 1968; Law, 1970a; Law and Chang, 1971; Varet *et al.*, 1971; Stutman and Dupuy, 1972; Zisblatt and Lilly, 1972), irradiation (Stutman and Dupuy, 1972), or cortisone (Shachat *et al.*, 1968) can increase susceptibility to tumors induced by a variety of C-type RNA viruses in mice and rats. Moreover, in those cases where oncogenesis by C-type RNA viruses does not require the thymic microenvironment (Rous sarcoma virus or murine sarcoma virus), thymectomy enhances rather than inhibits the development of neoplasms (Radzichovskaja, 1967; Ting, 1967; East and Harvey, 1968).

The effects of immunosuppression on oncogenesis by oncornaviruses include a reduction of the latency period, a decreased threshold dose of virus, an increase in tumor incidence, and, sometimes, alteration in the pathology of the disease. For example, Allison and Law (1968) observed a high incidence of subcutaneous reticulum cell sarcomas in ALS-treated mice given Moloney leukemia virus (MLV), an agent that usually causes a generalized leukemic process. Law (1970a) and Law and Chang (1971) found much higher levels of infective virus in spleen extracts of mice treated with both ALS and MLV as compared to mice given either ALS or MLV alone. In addition, antiviral antibody titers were reduced in mice treated with ALS and MLV. These findings contrast with the case of oncogenic DNA viruses, where titers of infectious virus and antiviral antibody are not altered by immunosuppression (Law and Ting, 1965; Vandeputte and De Somer, 1965; Law, 1966). Thus it remains to be determined whether immunosuppression facilitates tumor formation by oncornaviruses by suppressing antiviral immunity or, as in oncogenesis by DNA viruses, by suppressing the immune response against virus-induced antigens on tumor cells. This problem is of paramount importance for the development of an anticancer vaccine: what is the protective immunogen?

Stutman and Dupuy (1972) recently discovered several interesting relationships between the effect of ALS treatment on leukemogenesis by the Friend virus and two genes of the mouse, *Fv-1* and *Fv-2*. Alleles at these loci determine resistance or susceptibility to the virus. ALS treatment could not overcome resistance to the virus in animals possessing "resistant" alleles at both *Fv-1* and *Fv-2*. However, the effect of the allele for resistance (*r*) at *Fv-1* was overcome by the ALS treatment provided that the animals had the allele for susceptibility (*s*) at *Fv-2*. In the reverse situation (*Fv-1ˢ, Fv-2ʳ*), ALS treatment also partially overcame the resistance. Thus ALS appears capable of modifying the effect of either *Fv-1ʳ* or *Fv-2ʳ*, but not the combined effect of the two alleles. The effect of *Fv-1* is especially noteworthy because it influences resistance to a wide range of murine leukemia viruses, including naturally occurring endogenous viruses (Pincus *et al.*, 1971). This study is of considerable importance to our understanding of the effects of immunosuppression on leukemogenesis because it demonstrates that unless a genetic factor permitting the action of an oncogenic agent is present, immunosuppression has no effect. The converse seems equally illuminating: in individuals "absolutely resistant" to an oncogenic virus, the immune mechanism is irrelevant.

2.2. Effects of Immunosuppression on Oncogenesis by Chemicals

Although the enhancing effect of immunosuppression, particularly by ALS, on oncogenesis following infection by oncogenic viruses is unquestionable, the evidence in the case of chemical carcinogens is less convincing.

In thymectomized animals, the incidence of lymphatic leukemia after carcinogen administration is as drastically reduced as it is in the case of oncornaviruses (Law and Miller, 1950; Cohen et al., 1973). Again, this observation is of no help in establishing the importance of cell-mediated immunity in the defense against neoplasia because thymectomy removes the microenvironment required for the generation of the neoplastic cells. More significant is the failure of thymectomy to influence the incidence of skin and mammary tumors induced in mice by methylcholanthrene (Law and Miller, 1950). There is no evidence that the thymus is required for the induction of these kinds of neoplasms. Cohen et al. (1973) observed a greatly increased incidence of papillomas of the forestomach in adult mice subjected to thymectomy and treated with the carcinogen N-[4-(5-nitro-2-furyl)-2-thiazolyl]acetamide. By contrast with neonatal thymectomy, it is doubtful that thymectomy of adult mice produces much immunosuppression (Miller, 1962). Nevertheless, it must be conceded that the effects of various immunosuppressants are greatly augmented by thymectomy (Schwartz, 1965); therefore, this result can be explained if the carcinogen is immunosuppressive. In the hands of several investigators, neonatal thymectomy followed by painting of the skin with a carcinogen shortened the latent period before the appearance of papillomas (Miller et al., 1963; Defendi and Roosa, 1964; Grant and Miller, 1965; Johnson, 1968). However, the final incidence of tumors in these studies was 100% in both the thymectomized and the control group, and no effects on the growth rate or conversion to carcinoma were noted. Several investigators not only failed to observe a shortening of the latent period before tumor appearance, but they also were unable to demonstrate any effect on the incidence, growth rate, and histological type of tumors in neonatally thymectomized mice treated with carcinogens (Balner and Dersjant, 1966; Law, 1966; Allison and Taylor, 1967).

Immunosuppression by ALS has resulted in either an increased incidence of tumors or a decreased latency period, or both, after treatment with chemical carcinogens (Balner and Dersjant, 1969; Cerelli and Treat, 1969; Friedrich-Freska and Hoffman, 1969; Woods, 1969; Rabbat and Jeejeebhoy, 1970). Others, however, have failed to uncover an enhancing effect of ALS treatment on chemical oncogenesis (Fisher et al., 1970; Wagner and Haughton, 1971). Grant and Roe (1969) found that ALS-treated germ-free mice did not develop tumors when given dimethylbenzanthracene, whereas about one-half of similarly treated, conventional mice did. The emergence of neoplasms in the latter group was perhaps due to the combined effects of immunosuppression and antigenic stimulation, a subject we shall return to later.

Denlinger et al. (1973) reported that the treatment of rats given N-methyl-N-nitrosourea (MNU), a potent neurological carcinogen, with ALS did not increase the incidence of tumors of the nervous system. The incidence of nonneural tumors was also unaffected, with the notable exception of bladder tumors, which developed in 25% of the rats given both MNU and ALS but in none of the animals given either one alone.

Results with ALS are often difficult to evaluate. For example, each batch of ALS must be calibrated in vivo for its immunosuppressive potency because in many cases "ALS" has little or no immunosuppressive action. Among the many reasons for this is the fact that, being a foreign protein, ALS elicits an antibody that sooner or later nullifies its effects. Rendering the experimental animal tolerant of the foreign protein (e.g., rabbit globulin) before treatment with ALS (e.g., rabbit anti–mouse lymphocyte globulin) can prevent this complication (Lance *et al.*, 1973). Such considerations were taken into account by Stutman (1969), who rendered mice immunologically tolerant of the foreign protein and found that prolonged treatment with ALS failed to influence the incidence and latency period of tumors appearing after exposure to methylcholanthrene. Interestingly, the same treatment in mice *not* tolerant to rabbit globulin did shorten the latency period. However, the same effect was also produced by treatment with normal rabbit globulin! Such results indicate that prolonged antigenic stimulation—and not immunosuppression—was the accelerating factor. In other experiments with mice of the I strain, which are relatively resistant to the carcinogenic effects of methylcholanthrene, Stutman (1969) showed that prolonged treatment with ALS (after induction of immunological tolerance to rabbit globulin) did increase the incidence of methylcholanthrene-induced tumors from 14% to 37%. He commented that the results can be interpreted by "supporters of the immune surveillance theory . . . that, in the protracted presence of effective immunosuppression, the relative resistance of I mice to MCA oncogenesis is overcome. On the other hand, it is also clear that 60% of the similarly immunosuppressed animals . . . remained tumor-free during their lifespan, which suggests that other factors of a nonimmunologic type are operative."

The evidence that immunosuppression consistently augments the development of neoplasms by chemical carcinogens therefore seems unconvincing. We base our conclusion on two considerations: technical inadequacy of experimental design, which vitiates many of the data dealing with this subject, and, in those experiments that are based on sound immunological technique, the contribution of important nonimmunological mechanisms to resistance to carcinogenesis.

2.3. Effects of Immunosuppression on Development of Spontaneous Tumors

2.3.1. Natural Infection with Mammary Tumor Virus

Martinez 1964) was the first to observe that thymectomy at an early age greatly reduces the incidence of mammary tumors in strains of mice positive for mammary tumor virus (MTV).* Moreover, the latent period before tumor appearance was significantly longer in the thymectomized animals. Law (1966) made similar observations in MTV⁺ female C3H/HeN mice. Extending these findings, Yunis *et al.* (1969) showed that reconstitution of thymectomized C3H MTV⁺ female mice with syngeneic thymus tissue from either MTV⁺ or MTV⁻ animals abolished the inhibitory effect of thymectomy on mammary

---

* Natural carriers of this virus are termed MTV⁺, whereas mice normally free of the agent are designated MTV

carcinogenesis. Estrogen deficiency as a consequence of thymectomy cannot explain these findings, since the reduced tumor incidence was still observed after stimulation with exogenous hormone (Heppner *et al.*, 1968). Prehn's (1971) provocative explanation of these findings is that an immune response to mammary tumor–associated antigens actually stimulates growth of the neoplasm (see below).

In contrast to these results, Burstein and Law (1971) found an increased incidence of mammary tumors in neonatally thymectomized F_1 hybrids of C57BL and C3H mice (BC3HF$_1$), which are MTV$^-$. At 23 months of age, 40% of thymectomized animals had developed mammary carcinomas *vs.* only 4% of control animals. However, the thymectomized animals did not show an altered incidence of the two other commonly occurring spontaneous neoplasms of BC3HF$_1$ mice, hepatomas and reticulum cell sarcomas. The divergent effects of thymectomy on MTV- and non-MTV-induced mammary tumors remain unexplained; they are possibly related to a difference in antigenicity of the two types of tumor (Burstein and Law, 1971).

C3H mice in which the H-2^k histocompatibility locus was replaced with H-2^b by repeated backcrossing were much less susceptible to the development of mammary tumors by MTV (Mühlbock and Dux, 1971). Conceivably, the chromosomal region determining H-2^b contains a gene coding for immunoresistance against either the MTV itself (Klein, 1973) or the tumor cell antigens it induces. However, this does not explain how thymectomy reduces the incidence of MTV-induced tumors, since most genes determining immunological responsiveness, such as the Ir gene, operate via the T-cell system (Katz and Benacerraf, 1972).

Like thymectomy, ALS was also shown to inhibit tumorigenesis by MTV (Lappé and Blair, 1970; Blair, 1971). Interestingly, a high proportion of animals had circulating antibodies against MTV after recovery from ALS-induced immunosuppression. This raises the possibility that thymectomy or ALS treatment in MTV$^+$ animals abrogates immunological tolerance to the virus or to virus-induced cellular antigens, as suggested by Yunis *et al.* (1969). Indeed, it is increasingly clear that thymus-derived lymphocytes consist of several subpopulations, which can either enhance or suppress immune responses (Katz and Benacerraf, 1972; Blair, 1972; Gershon *et al.*, 1972).

2.3.2. Murine Leukemia Viruses

Most, if not all, mice appear to carry the genetic information required for the assembly of murine leukemic viruses (MuLV) (Todaro and Huebner, 1972). Whether or not this information is actually expressed seems to depend on many other genes, an increasing number of which are being identified (Lilly, 1972; Lilly and Pincus, 1973). Some strains of mice, in which high levels of infectious virus are present very early in life, such as AKR, SJL, and NZB, have a high incidence of leukemia or lymphoma later in life. In the AKR mouse, the malignancy originates in the thymus or in the thymus-dependent lymphoid tissue (Siegler, 1968). It is thus not surprising that thymectomy early in life drastically reduces the incidence of leukemia in this animal (McEndy *et al.*, 1944; Allison, 1970).

In contrast to thymectomy, ALS treatment can shorten the latent period before tumor development in natural carriers of infectious MuLV (Allison, 1970; Burstein and Allison, 1970; Judd *et al.*, 1971; Hirsch *et al.*, 1973*a*). Vredevoe and Hays (1969), however, observed a tendency toward prolongation of the latent period of spontaneous leukemia in AKR mice treated with ALS; also, Nagaya and Sieker (1969) failed to affect the incidence of leukemia after treatment of AKR mice with ALS. Interpretation of these results is subject to the same pitfalls mentioned in the case of ALS-treated mice given carcinogenic chemicals: unless the immunosuppressive potency of the ALS employed by the investigator is proven by bioassay, no conclusion can be drawn.

As mentioned previously, ALS, apart from its immunosuppressive properties, also has certain actions not directly related to immunosuppression. One such effect relevant to the preceding is its ability to lyse neoplastic lymphoid cells (Judd *et al.*, 1971). Furthermore, it is not inconceivable that certain batches of anti-mouse lymphocyte serum contain neutralizing antibodies against MuLV. Considering the prevalence of MuLV virions or their antigens in mice (Todaro and Huebner, 1972), this possibility deserves serious consideration. The presence of such antibodies could, of course, offset any immunosuppressive effects of the preparation. Because of the diverse effects of ALS, it is difficult to ascribe solely to immunosuppression any influence of ALS on virus-induced lymphoid tumors. Once again we are faced with the problem of interpreting results of what are most likely inadequate experiments, experiments that have failed to take into account the very complex nature of the system under analysis.

More decisive results have been obtained in mice that do not harbor infectious virus early in life. Nehlsen (1971) studied the effect of long-term ALS treatment on the incidence of tumors in 250 CBA mice. The ALS injections were started on the day of birth and were continued every 4 days for 18 months. This treatment caused a severe deficiency in cell-mediated immune capabilities, including inability to cause graft vs. host reactions, anergy to a chemical sensitizer (oxazolon), impaired responses of lymphocytes to phytohemagglutinin, retention of skin allografts for 6–18 months, and survival of skin xenografts for as long as 20–60 days. Nevertheless, the mice survived normally for 18 months, and, with the exception of two lymphoblastic lymphomas in male mice 13 months of age, all tumors that developed could be attributed to the polyoma virus. Sanford *et al.* (1973) studied the incidence of spontaneous tumors in BALB/c mice The life spans of neonatally thymectomized and sham-thymectomized animals did not differ (758 days and 796 days, respectively), nor did the overall incidence of tumors (85% and 81%, respectively). However, the kinds of tumors as well as their behavior were different in the two groups. In comparison to the control mice, the incidence of lung and mammary tumors was lower in thymectomized animals, whereas the incidence of hemangioendothelioma was slightly higher. Also, 10% of the thymectomized mice developed tumors of a type not found in the control mice, including two myoepitheliomas, one squamous cell carcinoma, and one lipoma. Furthermore, multiple lung adenomas were seen in ten of 20 thymecto-mized mice, whereas only single adenomas occurred in control mice. Trainin and

Linker-Israeli (1971) similarly observed an increased incidence of presumably non-virus-induced lung adenomas in neonatally thymectomized SWR and Swiss mice. In addition to Nehlsen (1971) and Sanford *et al.* (1973), others have failed to note an increased incidence of neoplasms in virus-negative animals treated with ALS or thymectomy, or both (Law, 1970*a*; Denlinger *et al.*, 1973).

Thus present evidence concerning the development of spontaneous neoplasms in deliberately immunosuppressed mice is conflicting. On the one hand, some data indicate that treatment with ALS hastens the appearance of neoplasms in mice with a high spontaneous incidence of such tumors. On the other hand, there is evidence that documented, severe immunosuppression fails to influence the incidence of neoplasms in mice with a low rate of development of spontaneous tumors. On balance, the weight of the evidence favors the view that severe immunosuppression *by itself* does not influence the incidence of neoplasms in laboratory mice. Important evidence now emerging from studies of congenitally athymic mice, which are discussed next, supports this conclusion.

3. Spontaneous Immunosuppression and Malignancy in Experimental Animals

3.1. Congenitally Athymic (Nude) Mice

In "nude" mice, a single autosomal recessive mutant gene is responsible for both hairlessness and failure of thymic development (Flanagan, 1966; Pantelouris, 1968). The immunological deficiencies of nude mice are impressive and include inability to reject skin grafts from other mammals and even from birds, reptiles, or amphibians, as well as markedly impaired antibody production in response to thymus-dependent antigens* (Rygaard, 1969; Wortis, 1971; Reed and Jutila, 1972; Manning *et al.*, 1973). Wortis *et al.* (1971) showed that nude mice have a normal compartment of precursors for T cells and concluded that a defective thymic epithelium is responsible for their grossly impaired immunity. The B-cell system of these animals is intact, and immunological responses to so-called thymus-independent antigens,† such as lipopolysaccharide, are intact (Reed *et al.*, 1973).

There is every indication that these animals promise important information relevant to immunological surveillance. If cellular immunity is a principal defense against neoplastic cells, nude mice should have a very high incidence of spontaneous neoplasms. But as of this writing, there is no evidence from any group studying these mice that this prediction is upheld. In nude mice observed for as long as 7 months, no spontaneous tumors were found (in these studies the genetic background for the nude strain was BALB/c) (Reed and Jutila, unpublished observations).‡ One difficulty in evaluating these preliminary results is the

---

* Antigens requiring the presence of both T and B cells in order to stimulate the production of antibodies (Claman and Chaperon, 1969).
† Antigens requiring the presence only of B cells in order to stimulate the production of antibodies (Claman and Chaperon, 1969).
‡ A 6-month-old nude mouse that died of a reticulum cell sarcoma was recently reported (Custer *et al.*, 1973).

relatively early death of the nude mouse due to its extreme susceptibility to infection. Successful colonies require either specific pathogen-free or germ-free conditions. Conceivably, imposition of the germ-free environment could in itself lower the incidence of neoplasms, especially of the lymphoid type.

Nude mice were recently found to resist the carcinogenic effects of certain hydrocarbons such as 3,4-benzopyrene, methylcholanthrene, and dimethylbenzanthracene (DMBA) (Johnson *et al.*, 1974). In these experiments, 100% of the normal littermates of nudes developed tumors in response to skin painting with DMBA, but only one of 15 nude mice did so. The one nude animal developed a papilloma which spontaneously regressed after 1 month. Out of 12 nude mice grafted with thymic tissue (thus restoring their T-cell system) and treated with DMBA, all developed tumors. Hence skin abnormalities in nudes are unlikely to account for their unexpected resistance to chemical carcinogenesis. It should be mentioned here that mice carrying a hairless mutation not associated with congenital absence of the thymus (*hr/hr*) have also shown resistance to tumor formation after skin painting with chemical carcinogens (Giovanella *et al.*, 1970). The resistance in these mice has been ascribed to the skin abnormalities, although the evidence is circumstantial.

In addition to chemical oncogenesis, viral oncogenesis by Friend leukemia virus (FLV) was also found to be disturbed in nude mice. Kouttab *et al.* (1974) noted that although FLV administration shortened the life span of nude mice, they did not have evidence of leukemia at the time of death. Considerable evidence indicates that FLV suppresses B-lymphocyte function (Dent, 1972). More recently, T cells were also shown to be suppressed (see below), suggesting that both B and T cells or cooperative mechanisms between B and T cells are targets of FLV. Although it is not known to what extent interaction between B and T cells is required for the development of typical Friend disease, the evidence in nude mice indicates that T cells are involved.

It thus appears that nude mice fail to develop neoplasms spontaneously or when treated with either chemical carcinogens or oncogenic viruses, although the data are admittedly in a preliminary stage. The results are not inconsistent with the "immunostimulatory" theory—i.e., that immunity is *required* for the development of a neoplasm (Prehn, 1972). They are not consistent with the immunological surveillance theory, unless the notion that cellular immunity is a prime defense against neoplasms is abandoned.

3.2. Immunocompetence of Animals with a High Incidence of Tumors

Immunocompetence has been studied in three "high tumor" strains of mice, AKR, NZB, and SJL/J. Whereas most authors agree that leukemic AKR mice have decreased immunocompetence (Metcalf and Moulds, 1967), preleukemic AKR mice have been variously reported to have normal immune capabilities (Murphy and Syverton, 1961; Metcalf, 1963; Hechtel *et al.*, 1965; Metcalf and Moulds, 1967; Levine and Vas, 1970; Hargis and Malkiel, 1972) or decreased immunocompetence (Friedman, 1964; Doré *et al.*, 1969; Gottlieb *et al.*, 1972). These investigations were of both humoral and cell-mediated immunological functions, such as the capacity to produce antibody against sheep red blood cells, rejection of tumor transplants, capacity to mount graft vs. host reactions, production of IgG and reagin, and susceptibility to infection. Results of these studies lead us to conclude that if immunodeficiency exists in preleukemic AKR mice, its extent is certainly not impressive. The question of whether AKR mice are selectively hyporesponsive to the leukemia virus they harbor or to virus-induced cellular antigens remains largely unanswered (Hirsch et al., 1973a). In any case, AKR mice, like other MuLV-carrying mice, are not tolerant to their own virus, since both humoral and cell-mediated responses to viral antigens can be detected in vitro (Hirsch et al., 1969; Wahren and Metcalf, 1970; Oldstone et al., 1972; Profitt et al., 1973). Recently, evidence has been presented for the existence of two loci coding for virus expression in the genome of AKR mice (Rowe, 1972; Rowe and Hartley, 1972). Conceivably, the action of these genes can overcome the effects of antiviral immunity.

The immune status of SJL mice, which are genetically predisposed to the development of a "Hodgkin's-like" lymphoma, has been less extensively studied. In one experiment, antibody production to sheep red blood cells, rejection of skin allografts, delayed hypersensitivity, and capacity to cause graft vs. host reactions were determined (Haran-Ghera et al., 1973). No significant immune deficiencies were found in young SJL/J mice, but, as also noted in strains without a high incidence of spontaneous tumors (Makinodan and Peterson, 1964; Metcalf et al., 1966; Hanna et al., 1967; Legge and Austing, 1968), the immune reactions of SJL mice decreased with age. This occurred whether the animal was normal or had a tumor.

A third strain of mice in which tumors develop in an unusually high percentage and in which a diversity of immunological abnormalities occurs is the NZB line (East, 1970). Whereas young NZB mice produce unusually large amounts of antibodies (Playfair, 1968; Weir et al., 1968; Staples and Talal, 1969), old NZB mice have profoundly impaired cellular immunity (Stutman et al., 1968; Cantor et al., 1970; Leventhal and Talal, 1970; Teague et al., 1970; Gelfand and Steinberg, 1973). The deficiencies in cell-mediated immunity include retarded rejection of skin allografts, diminished capacity to mount graft vs. host reactions, and impaired in vitro responses of lymphocytes to phytohemagglutinin and allogeneic lymphocytes. A progressive loss of recirculating T cells was also demonstrated in NZB mice (Denman and Denman, 1970; Gelfand and Steinberg, 1973). It is not known to what extent the infection with oncornaviruses in NZB mice causes, results from, or is coincidental with the immunological abnormalities.

Recent developments in the genetics of leukemogenesis may shed new light on experiments of the type we have just described. There is clear evidence that viral oncogenesis in mice depends on multiple genes. For example, the combined action of several genes determines the ultimate balance between resistance and susceptibility to the induction of leukemia in mice by either endogenous or exogenous viruses (Lilly, 1972; Lilly and Pincus, 1973). Nonimmunological effects are exerted by some of these genes, the most notable being the Fv-1 and Fv-2 loci.

Another gene, *Rgv-1*, exerts its influences by immunological mechanisms.* *Rgv-1* is located within the *H-2* complex of linkage group IX and its position coincides with the *Ir* region. The latter contains several genes determining the ability to respond immunologically to a variety of antigens (McDevitt and Benacerraf, 1969). In view of its chromosomal location, it is not surprising that all current evidence indicates that *Rgv-1* regulates the capacity to respond immunologically to MuLV and the cellular antigens it induces. For example, the antigenic system X.1 occurs on the surface of both the virions and the cells of a murine radiation-induced leukemia. Immunological responsiveness to this antigen has been traced to *Rgv-1*; alleles at this locus determine the animal's ability to produce antibody against X.1 and to reject $X.1^+$ leukemia cells (Sato *et al.*, 1973). In addition, *Rgv-1* may influence the expression of virus-induced cellular antigens: the antigen usually induced by Friend virus is not expressed in animals having the *Rgv-1* allele governing susceptibility to this agent (Lilly and Pincus, 1973).

Thus, at least in viral leukemogenesis in the mouse, there is strong circumstantial evidence that the genetic capacity to react immunologically to tumor-associated antigens influences the development of neoplasms. This may be of considerable importance in protection against neoplasia since mice prone to tumors induced by endogenous oncornaviruses, such as AKR, C58, SJL/J, NZB, and C3H, possess the *Rgv-1* allele for susceptibility. However, not all strains of mice with this allele have a high incidence of tumors. Clearly, leukemogenesis by endogenous oncornaviruses is a complex, multifactorial process involving not only several genes but also variations of the infectivity and oncogenicity of the virus itself (Rowe, 1972; Lilly and Pincus, 1973; Peters *et al.*, 1973).

In view of this, it seems an oversimplification to connect diminished immunological reactions against antigens such as foreign erythrocytes, skin grafts, and bacteria with the pathogenesis of neoplasms. Failure to respond to the etiological agent (virus) or to tumor-associated antigens of a spontaneous neoplasm seems more to the point. Recent findings on the genetic control of immunological responsiveness to oncornaviruses and the cellular antigens they induce bring these doubts into sharp focus and strongly imply that the demonstration of poor immunological responsiveness to a limited number of antigens does not necessarily imply poor responsiveness to tumor-associated antigens.

3.3. Immunosuppression by Oncogenic Viruses

Immunosuppression by oncogenic viruses has been reviewed by several authorities (Salaman, 1969; Notkins *et al.*, 1970; Dent, 1972; Friedman and Ceglowski, 1973). Nevertheless, a brief discussion of the major findings seems appropriate.

---

* The *Rgv-1* gene (resistance to Gross virus) was first identified in experiments concerning susceptibility to the Gross virus (Lilly *et al.*, 1964); subsequently it was also found to influence susceptibility to other leukemia viruses (Lilly, 1968; Tennant and Snell, 1968) as well as the mammary tumor virus (Nandi, 1967).

Almost all laboratory strains of leukemia-inducing RNA viruses have been found to suppress antibody formation. FLV has been most extensively studied in this regard. In general, the longer FLV is administered before antigen injection, the more profound the degree of immunosuppression. However, immunosuppression by FLV clearly precedes the onset of malignancy. Both IgM and IgG antibody responses to sheep red blood cells are affected after FLV infection, although the latter more than the former (Dent, 1972). Production of antibodies to "thymus-dependent" antigens such as sheep erythrocytes requires cooperation between T and B cells (Claman and Chaperon, 1969). Initially, FLV appeared to suppress preferentially the function of B lymphocytes (Bennett and Steeves, 1970). More recently, however, FLV was also shown to suppress T-cell-mediated immune functions, such as immunity to mycobacteria and rejection of skin allografts (Friedman and Ceglowski, 1971). Nevertheless, B-cell function is suppressed more rapidly and more profoundly than is T-cell function (Friedman *et al.*, 1973). In an earlier report, Gross passage A virus was also shown to prolong survival of skin allografts, in this instance across a non-*H-2* barrier (Dent *et al.*, 1965). In addition, a lymphatic leukemia-inducing virus isolated from irradiated SJL/J mice was found to depress the function of both T and B cells (Shearer *et al.*, 1973).

The general picture emerging from the literature is that laboratory strains of leukemogenic RNA viruses suppress both B- and T-cell functions. The suppression of T-cell function is especially intriguing, since immunosurveillance against cancer is thought to function via the T-cell system. Consequently, the important issue is raised here of whether or not suppression of T-cell function is a necessary prerequisite for tumor induction by these viruses. Although much can be said in favor of the notion that a causal relationship exists between immunosuppression by tumor viruses and oncogenesis (Dent, 1972), the evidence is entirely circumstantial. It is noteworthy that immunosuppression by naturally occurring leukemogenic viruses in their endogenous hosts has not been demonstrated. Moreover, in contrast to the lymphotropic RNA leukemia viruses, RNA sarcoma viruses and oncogenic DNA viruses have not generally been found to suppress immunological functions (Dent, 1972), although immunosuppressive procedures clearly enhance oncogenesis by these viruses. In addition, many nononcogenic viruses are known to be immunosuppressive (Salaman, 1969; Notkins *et al.*, 1970). Therefore, it seems that the true biological significance, if any, of immunosuppression by oncogenic viruses remains to be elucidated.

3.4. Immunosuppression by Carcinogenic Chemicals

Carcinogenic chemicals suppress both antibody production (Malmgren *et al.*, 1952; Stjernsward, 1965, 1966, 1967, 1969; Stutman, 1969; Ball, 1970; Szakal and Hanna, 1972) and cell-mediated immunity (Prehn, 1963; Stjernsward, 1965; Doell *et al.*, 1967; Ball, 1970; Lappé and Prehn, 1970; Szakal and Hanna, 1972). A number of observations sustain the hypothesis that carcinogenesis by these compounds is at least facilitated by, if not dependent on, their immunosuppressive properties. Thus carcinogenic hydrocarbons were found to be immunosuppressive, whereas noncarcinogenic hydrocarbons were not (Stjernsward, 1966). And mice resistant to carcinogenesis by 3-methylcholanthrene were also resistant to immunosuppression by this compound (Stutman, 1969). The duration of suppression of antibody production after carcinogen administration generally corresponds to the latency period before tumor appearance (Stjernsward, 1969; Szakal and Hanna, 1972). In one study (Szakal and Hanna, 1972), the suppression of both regional and systemic humoral immunity after treatment of Syrian hamsters with 7,12-dimethylbenzanthracene was transient, and maximal suppression coincided with the appearance of papillomas. Cell-mediated immunity was found to be depressed permanently, as measured by the survival of skin allografts, and this was considered to be essential for further development of the papillomas.

The evidence from these studies seems circumstantial and should be compared with contrasting observations. For example, additional immunosuppression by thymectomy or ALS treatment does not greatly increase the incidence of tumor after treatment with chemical carcinogens. Decisive evidence on this point was obtained by Andrews (1971), who placed methylcholanthrene-treated skin allografts on severely immunodepressed (thymectomy plus 450 r plus ALS) mice. Although the allografts were never rejected, 80% of the papillomas on the grafts regressed. Clearly, then, important nonimmunological mechanisms are responsible for the rejection of at least this kind of carcinogen-induced tumor. In other work, of three carcinogenic hydrocarbons (DMBA, benz[a]pyrene, and 3-methylcholanthrene) injected subcutaneously into newborn CFW/D mice, only one (DMBA) was found to suppress antibody production to sheep red blood cells, although all compounds induced tumors (Ball, 1970).

4. Immunosuppression and Malignancy in Human Beings

4.1. Immunodeficiency Diseases

Although it is widely held that neoplasms are common in patients with deficient immunity (Fraumeni, 1969; Kaplan, 1971; Good, 1972), their frequency is difficult to determine. The literature dealing with this topic consists largely of case reports, which give a distorted impression of the actual incidence. Thus far, a prospective study of large groups of patients with these diseases has not been undertaken for the purpose of determining the incidence of neoplasms. Table 1 provides data from several series of apparently unselected cases. Of the 678 patients (some of these may be duplicates), 33 had a neoplasm, for an incidence of about 5%. However, this figure is only an approximation and the true value could be substantially higher or lower. Note, for example, that in one series of patients with ataxia-telangiectasia, only 3 of 101 had a neoplasm (Boder and Sedgwick, 1963), whereas in a series of patients with Wiskott–Aldrich syndrome, 4 of 16 had a malignancy (Waldmann et al., 1972). Moreover, inclusion of 70 cases of

TABLE 1
Tumors/Patients

Combined immunodeficiency	0/70	Hitzig (1968)
Wiskott–Aldrich syndrome	1/18	Cooper *et al.* (1968)
Wiskott–Aldrich syndrome	4/16	Waldmann *et al.* (1972)
Ataxia-telangiectasia	1/20	Waldmann *et al.* (1972)
Ataxia-telangiectasia	3/101	Boder and Sedgwick (1963)
Ataxia-telangiectasia	8/125	Peterson *et al.* (1964)
Hypogammaglobulinemia[a]	8/176	Editorial (1969)
Selective IgA deficiency	5/102	Ammann and Hong (1971)
Intestinal lymphangiectasia	3/50	Waldmann *et al.* (1972)

[a] Common variable type.

combined immunodeficiency in this table may bias the result toward a lower than actual frequency, since patients with this condition usually die in infancy. If we accept 5% as tentative, the incidence of malignancy in the various immunodeficiency disorders is about 200 times the expected rate.

4.1.1. Classification of Immunodeficiency Diseases

Immunodeficiency diseases are a heterogeneous group, in which defects in T cells, B cells, or both predominate. The major forms these conditions take are as follows:

a. Combined Immunodeficiency (Swiss-Type Agammaglobulinemia) (Hoyer et al., 1968). Both humoral and cellular responses are lacking in combined immunodeficiency, probably because of the failure of precursors of T and B cells to develop. Death during infancy because of overwhelming infection is the rule.

b. DiGeorge Syndrome (DiGeorge, 1968). The thymus fails to develop in DiGeorge syndrome, whereas the B-cell population is normal in this very rare disorder. Cellular immunity is lacking and immunoglobulin synthesis is normal, although antibody production against thymus-dependent antigens is impaired.

c. X-Linked Hypogammaglobulinemia (Bruton Type) (Gitlin and Janeway, 1956). The converse of the DiGeorge syndrome, X-linked hypogammaglobulinemia, is characterized by a failure to produce antibodies and intact cellular immunity. Plasma cells are lacking, and the structure of the thymus is normal. If untreated, the disease is associated with an extraordinary susceptibility to infections by pyogenic bacteria.

d. Common Variable Immunodeficiency (Douglas et al., 1970). The onset of common variable immunodeficiency occurs in adults, and both men and women can be affected. The syndrome is heterogeneous, with hypogammaglobulinemia as the hallmark. Autoimmunity and gastrointestinal disorders are common. Defective cellular immunity is frequent, and, despite hypogammaglobulinemia, B

cells can be detected in the blood in some cases (Cooper *et al.*, 1971). The
fundamental defect may be an inability to "switch on" B cells.

e. Dysgammaglobulinemia (Ammann and Hong, 1971). Dysgammaglobulinemia is
characterized by a selective deficiency of one or more classes of immunoglobulins.
IgA deficiency is by far the commonest form of this group of disorders; its
incidence may be as high as one in 600. Autoimmunity is common, but some
persons with IgA deficiency are ostensibly normal.

f. Ataxia-Telangiectasia (Waldmann, et al., 1972). Ataxia-telangiectasia consists of
a triad of cerebellar ataxia, telangiectasia of the skin and eyes, and immunodeficiency. The last is the basis of the frequent sinopulmonary infections in ataxia-
telangiectasia. The immunodeficiency is complex; the usual findings are normal
levels of IgG, deficiency of IgA and IgE, the presence of low molecular weight
IgM, and diminished cellular immunity. The thymus is often absent or atrophic,
and thymus-dependent areas of lymphoid tissue are depleted. The immunological disorder may result from the failure of thymus development.

g. Wiskott–Aldrich Syndrome (Waldmann et al., 1972). Wiskott–Aldrich syndrome
consists of the triad of thrombocytopenia, eczema, and repeated infections and is
inherited as an X-linked recessive. The immunodeficiency is severe and consists of
defects in both cellular and humoral immunity. Immunoglubulin levels are
normal or even increased (IgA and IgE). Both the synthetic and the catabolic rates
of immunoglobulins G, A, and M are greatly increased. Despite this, antibody
responses following immunization, especially with polysaccharide antigens, are
depressed. The defect in cellular immunity is also paradoxical, because, although
delayed hypersensitivity is absent, *in vitro* responses of lymphocytes to PHA are
normal. The disease may represent an abnormality of the afferent limb of the
immune response, perhaps in the recognition or processing of antigen.

4.1.2. Malignancy in Immunodeficiency Diseases

Table 2 lists 55 representative examples of patients with an immunodeficiency
disease who developed a malignancy. These examples were culled from case
reports and are not meant to provide epidemiological data, but rather to
demonstrate the major features of the literature.

Several problems arise in coming to an understanding of the phenomena
described in Table 2. First among these is whether the changes described in the
lymphoid organs of these patients are truly neoplastic. Although no doubt exists
in those examples where metastases revealed the malignant nature of the process
(e.g., cases 8 and 20), in others the picture is not clear. This is especially so in
combined immunodeficiency. The changes described in these cases are not, in our
opinion, diagnostic of a lymphoreticular malignancy. Although Reed–Sternberg
cells were noted in cases 3 and 4 (and therefore led to the diagnosis of Hodgkin's
disease), this is not proof of malignancy since such cells have been found in

TABLE 2

Fifty-Five Cases of Neoplasms in Patients with Immunodeficiency Diseases

Case	Immuno-deficiency	Age	Tumor	Comment	Reference
1	CID	5 months	Lymphoreticular neoplasm	—	Jung *et al.* (1969)
2	CID	3 months	"Histiocytosis"	GVHR?	Jung *et al.* (1969)
3	CID	4 months	Reticulum cell hyperplasia	Reed–Sternberg cell	McKusick and Cross (1966)
4	CID	5 months	Thymoma	Reed–Sternberg cell	Bermuth *et al.* (1970)
5	WAS	3 yr	Acute myelogenous leukemia	Brother of case 6	Ten Bensel *et al.* (1966)
6	WAS	6 yr	Reticulum cell sarcoma	Metastases	Ten Bensel *et al.* (1966)
7	WAS	13 yr	Reticulum cell sarcoma	Monoclonal gammopathy	Radl *et al.* (1967)
8	WAS	2½ yr	Reticulum cell sarcoma	Metastases	Kildeberg (1961)
9	WAS	2 yr	"Reticuloendotheliosis"	—	Coleman *et al.* (1961)
10	WAS	9 yr	Thymoma	Lymphoepithelioma	Chaptal *et al.* (1966)
11	WAS	3 yr	Reticulum cell sarcoma	Confined to brain	Brand and Marinkovich (1969)
12	WAS	8yr	Astrocytoma	Cerebellum	Amiet (1963)
13	WAS	4½ yr	Histiocytosis (Letterer–Siwe)	Widespread tumors	Huber (1968)
14	WAS	6½ yr	Malignant reticuloendotheliosis	Brother had WAS and acute leukemia	Taleb *et al.* (1969)
15	AT	21 yr	Malignant lymphoma	—	Peterson *et al.* (1966)
16	AT	10 yr	Reticulum cell sarcoma	—	Gotoff *et al.* (1967)
17	AT	9 yr	Acute lymphocytic leukemia	—	Taleb *et al.* (1969)
18	AT	18 yr	Glioma (frontal lobe)	—	Young *et al.* (1964)
19	AT	13 yr	Cerebellar medulloblastoma		Shuster *et al.* (1966)
20	AT	9 yr	Lymphosarcoma	Disseminated	Peterson *et al.* (1964)
21	AT	5 yr	"Reticuloendotheliosis"	Histiocytosis X?	Peterson *et al.* (1964)
22	AT	9 yr	Hodgkin's disease	Radiation reaction	Morgan *et al.* (1968)
23	AT	15 yr	Reticulum cell sarcoma	—	Miller (1967)
24	AT	14 yr	Acute lymphocytic leukemia	Brother of case 25	Lampert (1969)
25	AT	3 yr	Acute lymphocytic leukemia	—	Lampert (1969)
26	AT	5 yr	Acute lymphocytic leukemia	Sister of case 27	Hecht *et al.* (1966)

		Age			Reference
27	AT	6 yr	Acute lymphocytic leukemia	—	Hecht et al. (1966)
28	AT	21 yr	Adenocarcinoma of stomach	Sister of case 29	Haerer et al. (1969)
29	AT	19 yr	Adenocarcinoma of stomach		Haere et al. (1969)
30	AT	10 yr	Lymphosarcoma	Radiation reaction	Gotoff et al. (1967)
31	AT	30 months	Reticulum cell sarcoma	Thymus, mediastinum, lung	Feigin et al. (1970)
32	AT	17 yr	Ovarian dysgerminoma	—	Dunn et al. (1964)
33	AT	14 yr	Unspecified lymphoma	Stomach	Castaigne et al. (1969)
34	AT	—	Histiocytic lymphoma	Brother of case 13	Castaigne et al. (1969)
35	AT	—	Basal cell carcinoma		
36	CVI	12 yr	Lymphosarcoma	Localized to pharynx	Freeman et al. (1970)
37	CVI	3¾ yr	Generalized lymphosarcoma	Sister of case 36	Freeman et al. (1970)
38	CVI	67 yr	Chronic lymphocytic leukemia		Potolsky et al. (1971)
39	CVI	45 yr	Lymphocytic lymphoma		Potolsky et al. (1971)
40	CVI	70 yr	Lymphosarcoma	Sister of case 39	Potolsky et al. (1971)
41	CVI	54 yr	Chronic lymphocytic leukemia	Sister of case 39	Potolsky et al. (1971)
42	CVI	50 yr	Reticulum cell sarcoma	Sister of case 39	Potolsky et al. (1971)
43	CVI	47 yr	Reticulum cell sarcoma	Brother of case 39	Green et al. (1966)
44	CVI	50 yr	Lymphoblastic lymphoma	Hypo-γ 18 yr	Fudenberg and Solomon (1961)
45	CVI	54 yr	Lymphosarcoma	—	Douglas et al. (1970)
46	CVI	54 yr	Thymoma	No tumor 16 yr later	Douglas et al. (1970)
47	CVI	28 yr	Lymphosarcoma		Hermans and Huizenga (1972)
48	CVI	57 yr	Adenocarcinoma of stomach	Long history of infections	Hermans and Huizenga (1972)
49	CVI	56 yr	Adenocarcinoma of stomach	Long history of infections	Hermans and Huizenga (1972)
50	CVI	31 yr	Adenocarcinoma of stomach	Long history of infections	Forssman and Herner (1964)
51	CVI	27 yr	Carcinoma of stomach	Long history of infections	
52	BA	5 yr	Malignant lymphoma	Dermatomyositis	Page et al. (1963)
53	BA	—	Acute lymphocytic leukemia	Brother of case 52	Page et al. (1963)
54	BA	—	Hodgkin's disease	Identical twin	Pekonen et al. (1963)
55	BA	—	Monomyelocytic leukemia	—	Reisman et al. (1964)

[a] CID, combined immunodeficiency disease; WAS, Wiskott–Aldrich syndrome; AT, ataxia-telangiectasia; CVI, common variable immunodeficiency; BA, Bruton's agammaglobulinemia.

benign, reactive disorders of lymphoid tissue (Strum *et al.*, 1970). Many of the pathological changes in combined immunodeficiency are entirely consistent with a graft vs. host reaction (GVHR). For example, case 2 was diagnosed as "histiocytosis," a characteristic finding in the acute GVHR, and the authors speculated on the possibility that instead of a neoplasm they were dealing with the end result of a GVHR (Jung *et al.*, 1969). Some cases of combined immunodeficiency may represent the result of a GVHR induced in the fetus by maternal lymphocytes that traversed the placenta (Kadowaki *et al.*, 1965).

Case 47 is of interest because she was diagnosed as having a "lymphosarcoma," yet 16 yr later there was no trace of the tumor. This extraordinary behavior of a "malignancy" in a patient with an immunodeficiency disease raises doubts about the validity of the diagnosis. If the lesion in this case and others is not neoplastic, what could it be? Perhaps we are dealing with unusual forms of lymphoid reactivity in patients with frequent infections (i.e., repeated antigenic stimuli) who lack normal immunoregulatory mechanisms. Experimentally, deregulated immune responses can lead to prolonged hyperplasia of lymphoid tissue (Sahiar and Schwartz, 1966). Relevant to this is the marked hyperplasia of lymphoid tissue without changes diagnostic of malignancy that can occur in patients with ataxia-telangiectasia (Peterson *et al.*, 1966; Ammann *et al.*, 1965). Conceivably, such hyperplastic changes could be misdiagnosed as neoplastic. In this connection, it is worth noting that many of the "tumors" in these cases were diagnosed only at autopsy because there were no clinical manifestations.

A second, related problem is the very high proportion of lymphoid tumors in these patients. Of the 55 malignancies in Table 2, 42 (80%) involved lymphoid tissue. Why should this be? One possibility has already been mentioned; i.e., that at least some of the "tumors" were not malignant, but either GVH reactions or highly abnormal kinds of reactive hyperplasia. Another possibility, which we shall discuss later, is that under conditions of combined immunosuppression and immunostimulation, lymphoid tissue is particularly susceptible to neoplastic transformation. We believe that if impaired immunological surveillance were the sole explanation for these cases, a much more representative variety of cancers should have been found. It seems more than coincidental that the very tissue which is abnormal in patients with immunodeficiency is the seat of the malignant change. Moreover, we would expect multiple neoplasms in the same immunodeficient patient if the immunological surveillance theory had a bearing on these cases. We have found no examples of this phenomenon in any of the 55 cases we studied.

We now come to the nonlymphoid tumors in immunodeficiency diseases. The development of brain tumors (cases 18 and 19) and an ovarian tumor (case 32) in ataxia-telangiectasia is interesting because in this condition it is these organs that undergo severe degenerative changes (McFarlin *et al.*, 1972). Is it conceivable that this is the basis of the tumors of these organs rather than some immunological dysfunction? Similarly, in the category of common variable immunodeficiency we see several cases of cancer of the stomach (cases 48, 49, 50, and 51). Two of these (cases 49 and 51) also had pernicious anemia, a disease known to predispose to this kind of cancer. Moreover, patients with common variable immunodeficiency are prone to achlorhydria and atrophic gastritis (Twomey *et al.*, 1970; Hermans and Huizenga, 1972), which are also associated with a high incidence of cancer of the stomach.

The case for an increased incidence of malignancy in X-linked hypogammaglobulinemia seems unsubstantiated. In two patients reported by Page *et al.* (1963), one also had dermatomyositis, which by itself can be associated with a high incidence of neoplasms, although in children the association is not as striking as it is in adults. One case associated with acute lymphocytic leukemia (Reisman *et al.*, 1964) and one with Hodgkin's disease (Pekonen *et al.*, 1963) are also recorded, but in view of the relatively high frequency of X-linked hypogammaglobulinemia we would expect many more such examples than the literature reports.

Intestinal lymphangiectasia is of considerable relevance to the problem of immunodeficiency diseases and malignancy. This disorder is characterized by losses of immunoglobulins and circulating lymphocytes through abnormal lymphoid channels in the gut. The result is hypogammaglobulinemia and lymphocytopenia, the latter leading to a profound depression in cellular immunity (Weiden *et al.*, 1972). These patients are thus analogous to animals undergoing thoracic duct drainage. Thus far, three of 50 patients with intestinal lymphangiectasia have developed neoplasms; all three were lymphomas, two of which involved primarily the gastrointestinal tract (Waldmann *et al.*, 1972).

A long-term study of ataxia-telangiectasia has revealed a new element of importance. Girls with the disease who pass through adolescence normally seem to avoid the development of severe pulmonary disease and neoplasia, whereas those who fail to develop secondary sexual characteristics or who do not menstruate regularly because of ovarian failure are predisposed to the infectious and malignant complications of ataxia-telangiectasia (Boder, 1973).

Immunodeficiency as an *effect* of the malignancy rather than its precursor needs to be excluded. This is well known to occur in Hodgkin's disease (Brown *et al.*, 1967). Immunodeficiency secondary to acute leukemia has also been described (Hersh *et al.*, 1971). This may have been the situation in case 55 (but no details are given). It is probably not applicable to those patients (e.g., cases 44 and 45) in whom a long history of hypogammaglobulinemia preceded development of leukemia.

Finally, the strong familial incidence of cancer in some of these patients is worth noting. This occurs particularly in ataxia-telangiectasia, where numerous family members without stigmata of ataxia-telangiectasia have cancer (Reed *et al.*, 1966). Is there, then, a genetic basis (excluding genes determining the immunodeficiency) for malignancy in some of these patients? In other words, the relationship between immunodeficiency and malignancy may not necessarily be cause and effect. Hecht *et al.* (1973) have provided an important clue to our understanding of this problem by their extraordinary study of a patient with ataxia-telangiectasia. Initially, they found in the blood a single lymphocyte that had a chromosomal translocation. During the next 52 months they scored 2676 metaphases of blood lymphocyte cultures and observed a progressive increase in the number of cells with the translocation. By the end of the study, about three-fourths of the lymphocytes had the abnormality. The chromosomal alterations occurred in the D group, where abnormalities are found in other cases of ataxia-telangiectasia, suggesting to the authors that "accidents" of a D chromosome could occur preferentially in this disease. The relationship between chromosomal abnormalities and the emergence of new clones of lymphocytes—as in Hecht's case—may be important in the development of lymphoid neoplasms in ataxia-telangiectasia.

The lack of evidence of an increased incidence of neoplasms in diseases with a secondary immunodeficiency, such as sarcoidosis (Hirschhorn *et al.*, 1964) and leprosy (Waldorf *et al.*, 1966; Bullock, 1968), compounds the difficulties in interpreting the significance of neoplasms in patients with a primary immunodeficiency. Although a systematic analysis of this question has not been carried out in sarcoidosis, the literature fails to reveal that malignancy is a feature of this condition (L. Siltzbach, personal communication, 1973). The incidence of neoplasms has been determined in 848 lepers; 19.7 cancer deaths were expected and 21 were observed (Oleinick, 1969). The defect in cellular immunity in lepromatous leprosy can be as severe as in any primary immunodeficiency disease, although anergy in patients with tuberculoid leprosy is less common (Turk and Bryceson, 1971), so we are left with the paradox of severe immunodeficiency without an increased incidence of malignancy.

If impaired immunological surveillance against malignant cells were the sole explanation for the development of tumors in patients with primary immunodeficiency diseases, we would anticipate (1) an incidence of neoplasms much higher than 5%, (2) a representative variety of cancers, and (3) multiple neoplasms in individual patients. By contrast, impaired immunological surveillance against microorganisms in these patients results in (1) an almost universal susceptibility to infections (2) infectious disorders mediated by mechanisms representative of the immunodeficiency and (3) simultaneous or repeated infection by multiple organisms. Thus everything known about the role of the immune system in infection is upheld by clinical evidence. But a Scotch verdict must be handed down in the case for immunological surveillance against neoplasms.

4.2. Neoplasms in Recipients of Organ Allografts

The dramatic announcement in 1969 by Penn and his colleagues of five cases of malignant lymphoma in recipients of kidney allografts* was soon followed by a series of similar observations. Penn has continued his observations, and many of these cases are described in detail in his monograph (Penn, 1970). A registry of 5170 recipients (including 5000 kidney and 170 heart allografts) was compiled (Schneck and Penn, 1971). Fifty-two (1%) of the patients had developed a

---

* These tumors arose *de vovo* and are to be distinguished from (1) the inadvertent transplantation of malignant cells contained in the kidney of a donor with a neoplasm or (2) the growth of residual tumor in a recipient who had cancer before the transplant operation (Starzl *et al.*, 1971).

neoplasm; 28 of the tumors were of epithelial origin (usually involving the skin, cervix, and tongue), 22 were lymphomas, and two were leiomyosarcomas. These cases were collected on an informal basis from transplantation centers around the world, and therefore the incidence of 1% may not be accurate. Penn and Starzl (1972) analyzed 366 of their own patients who were alive 6 months to $9\frac{1}{2}$ years after receiving a kidney allograft. Tumors developed in 18 (4.9%). More recently, Penn (1974) reported 24 neoplasms in 347 (6.9%) recipients surviving at least 4 months after renal transplantation.

An analysis of 95 tumors arising in about 9000 transplant recipients revealed that the commonest type (30%) was a malignant lymphoma (Penn and Starzl, 1972). Other common neoplasms included skin cancer (21%), *in situ* carcinoma of the cervix (8%), and carcinoma of the lip (8%). Two patients had multiple neoplasms. Superficial epithelial cancers have been noted in other series of kidney allograft recipients; for example, 14% of 51 recipients developed malignant skin tumors (Walder *et al.*, 1971), and carcinoma of the cervix has been noted by others (Kay *et al.*, 1970). It is noteworthy that the high incidence of skin cancer in recipients of renal allografts has been reported from Australia, a sun-drenched continent known for the high incidence of skin cancer in its population.

Another analysis of recipients of renal allografts—this one involving 6297 persons—indicated that the risk of reticulum cell sarcoma in men was 350 times greater than expected. In women the figure was 700. But the incidence of the commonest neoplasm of women, breast cancer, was not increased. The excess risk appeared within a year of transplantation and remained at the same high level for at least 5 yr. Skin and lip cancers occurred up to 4 times more often than expected and other cancers were 2.5 times more common, in men only. The excess risk of other cancers appeared later than that for the lymphomas and became more pronounced as the interval since transplantation increased (Hoover and Fraumeni, 1973).

One puzzling feature of these patients is that the incidence of neoplasms at different institutions is highly variable. The development of tumors in 24 out of 347 of Penn's patients has already been mentioned. By contrast, neither Deodhar (1972) at the Cleveland Clinic nor R. Simmons (personal communication, 1973) at the University of Minneapolis has found such a high incidence. Only one of Deodhar's 330 patients had a tumor, and Simmons found as many neoplasms in transplant recipients as in patients maintained on hemodialysis. It seems important to determine the basis for this regional variation (Table 3).

In every case of the *de novo* appearance of a tumor, the transplant recipient was receiving immunosuppressive therapy. All of the 95 patients referred to previously (Penn and Starzl, 1972) were taking corticosteroids, and 92 of them were also taking azathioprine. Antilymphocyte globulin was given to 25 patients. The average time of appearance of the tumor was 30 months after initiation of the immunosuppressive therapy; 12% of the neoplasms appeared in less than 4 months after transplantation.

The overriding consideration in arriving at an explanation of how these neoplasms arose is the immunosuppressive therapy. Yet analysis of this obvious

TABLE 3

Incidence of Tumors in Kidney Transplant Recipients from Three Different Medical Centers

Series	Number of patients	Post-transplant tumors	Pretransplant tumors
Penn	347	24	—
Deodhar	330	1	—
Simmons	480	9	11[a]

[a] In two cases, nephrectomy was done because of renal tumor. In three other cases, the tumor was removed at least 10 yr before the transplantation procedure.

possibility raises some doubts. In the first place, the assumption that any patient taking an "immunosuppressive" drug is immunologically impaired is unwarranted. At least two studies have shown that patients treated either with azathioprine alone or with azathioprine plus prednisone can respond normally to conventional antigenic stimuli (Swanson and Schwartz, 1967; Lee *et al.*, 1971). Moreover, the observation that many of the transplant recipients who developed a tumor had suffered repeated rejection crises (McKhann, 1969) indicates a relatively intact immune system, at least with regard to the antigens of the graft. However, enhanced susceptibility to infection with organisms that are not pathogenic in nonimmunosuppressed individuals is common (Rifkind *et al.*, 1967). Studies of the immune status of these patients are clearly in order, and until an immunodeficient state is identified and related to those recipients who developed a neoplasm, the pathogenesis of the tumors remains an open question.

We deal next with the possibility that chronic uremia, which impairs cell-mediated immunity (Dammin *et al.*, 1957), is behind the development of the neoplasms. Virtually all the recipients were chronically uremic before the transplant operation, but no data state the duration of the pregrafting uremic state. We know of no demonstration that chronic uremia is associated with an increased incidence of cancer. Of 4600 patients treated with hemodialysis for chronic uremia, 1% died from malignancy (Burton *et al.*, 1971). But this figure cannot be evaluated because the ages of the patients are not given. Penn (1970), citing a personal communication from R. F. Barth, states that no case of antecedent chronic renal disease was found in a study of 500 patients with lymphoma. We therefore exclude uremia as a contributing factor in the transplant cases.*

The extraordinarily high incidence (at least 100 times the expected rate) of lymphomas (especially reticulum cell sarcomas) is as vexing in the transplant recipients as it is in the patients with immunodeficiency diseases. But a new element is added in the former instance: involvement primarily of the brain in the majority of cases. Involvement of the central nervous system is a remarkable and highly atypical feature of the lymphomas arising in recipients of organ allografts

* The immunological surveillance theory fails to explain why there is not an increased incidence of malignancy in chronic uremia in view of the profound suppression of cellular immunity associated with this condition.

(Schneck and Penn, 1970, 1971). Ordinarily, lymphomas involving primarily the brain are very rare (Rosenberg *et al.*, 1961). Yet of 22 tumors found in transplant recipients, the brain was the only site of neoplasm in eight cases. In three additional patients, the brain as well as other organs was involved (Schneck and Penn, 1971). Traditionally, the brain is thought of as immunologically "privileged" because it lacks a lymphatic system. In such a protected environment, antigenic neoplasms should flourish. But, if this were the case, why should lymphomas arise preferentially in the brain of an *already* immunosuppressed person? Why do the transplant recipients develop cerebral *lymphomas* and not gliomas? Why are central nervous system lymphomas rare in patients with immunodeficiency diseases?

If we assume that transplant recipients and patients with immunodeficiency diseases have comparable degrees of impaired immunosuppression (as mentioned above, this assumption may be false), then two outstanding differences between the two groups are apparent. The first is that the former group is treated with azathioprine and corticosteroids, which could alter the permeability of the blood–brain barrier to lymphoid cells. These agents might thus enhance the spread of neoplastic cells from microscopic extracerebral sites to the brain. The second difference between the two groups is, of course, the transplanted organ. It is known that a kidney graft contains large numbers of donor lymphocytes, presumably of the circulating type (Guttman and Lindquist, 1969). If only a few foreign lymphocytes gained entry into the brain, might this not provide a nidus for the development of a cerebral lymphoma?

This brings us to consider the more general relevance of the allograft in the development of neoplasms in transplant recipients. In order to analyze this question, the incidence of tumors in patients treated with immunosuppressive agents, but who are not allograft recipients, is required. Unfortunately, little is known about the incidence of cancer in these patients. Several case reports describe the development of tumors in patients receiving immunosuppressants for the treatment of systemic lupus erythematosus (Lipsmeyer, 1972; Manny *et al.*, 1972; Newman and Walter, 1973), nephrotic syndrome (Sharpstone *et al.*, 1969; Bashour *et al.*, 1973), and psoriasis (Rees *et al.*, 1964; Harris, 1971; Craig and Rosenbery, 1971). However, these are difficult to interpret because neoplasms may develop in some of these diseases even when no treatment is applied (Hoerni and Laporte, 1970). The most striking example of the complexities of this problem is the controlled trial of azathioprine in rheumatoid arthritis conducted by Harris *et al.* (1971). Of 54 patients, 27 received azathioprine and 27 a placebo. Three lymphomas developed, each in a patient treated with the placebo. The authors dryly noted, "it is interesting to speculate on the conclusions which might have been drawn had the (tumors) occurred in the azathioprine-treated group." McEwan and Petty (1972) state that they can find only three published cases of neoplasm in over 4000 cases of nontransplant patients treated with azathioprine. However, this figure cannot be accepted as the true incidence; only a prospective search for cancer in these patients (and appropriate controls) will provide the answer.

There is interesting new information concerning the occurrence of a *new* malignancy in patients treated for cancer with agents known to suppress immunity. Several cases of acute myelomonocytic leukemia have occurred in patients treated with melphalan for multiple myeloma (Kyle *et al.*, 1970). (It is our opinion that the leukemia is a natural evolution of multiple myeloma.) A greater than threefold risk of development of second neoplasms was found in 425 patients with Hodgkin's disease treated with intensive radiotherapy, with or without subsequent chemotherapy (Arseneau *et al.*, 1972). In light of the demonstration that the standard form of radiotherapy given following mastectomy depletes T cells from blood (Stjernsward *et al.*, 1972), it is of interest that irradiation to the mediastinum following removal of a seminoma may be associated with an increased risk of a second neoplasm (Ytredal and Bradfield, 1972).

5. Conclusions

According to Burnet (1970), "when aberrant cells with proliferative potential arise in the body, they will carry new antigenic determinants on their cell surface. When a significant amount of new antigen has developed, a thymus-dependent immunological response will be initiated which eventually eliminates the aberrant cells in essentially the same way as a homograft is destroyed." We fully agree that all the criteria of a surveillance mechanism have been met in certain instances, such as polyma virus-induced tumors. However, we remain doubtful of the *general* applicability of the theory to the pathogenesis of cancer. Some of our doubt springs from semantic and technical problems:

1. Proponents of the theory of immunological surveillance have stressed repeatedly that "adaptive immunity evolved to minimize the dangers of malignant disease." This kind of statement, we feel, puts the idea beyond the reach of orderly discussion. Such teleological reasoning fails to acknowledge the existence of a parallel system of adaptive immunity—blocking antibody—which, according to all present evidence, protects the tumor against the cell-mediated immunity of the host. We feel it is time to abandon this kind of argument, which is of no value in coming to grips with the substantive issues.

2. Let us admit that, apart from a few exceptions, the cause of spontaneous cancer is unknown. It seems highly unlikely, for example, that the virulent strains of Friend, Moloney, and Rauscher viruses that are used to demonstrate immunosuppression by oncogenic viruses have any relevance to malignancies as they develop naturally. The same comment applies to the administration of large doses of carcinogenic chemicals to newborn animals, to the study of immunity in strains of mice with a 100% incidence of neoplasms, to the use of viruses which are not oncogenic in the strain of origin, and to all other systems that skirt the fundamental problem of spontaneous malignancy in genetically heterogeneous populations.

3. Assuming that at least some human neoplasms are induced by viruses (and this to us seems reasonable), the issue of defense mechanisms against oncogenic

viruses *qua* infectious agents must be separated from that of the defense against the cells they have transformed to a malignant state.* Very important conceptual and practical implications flow from these different phenomena. Earlier, we pointed out that several genes determine susceptibility or resistance to certain oncogenic viruses; some of these genes operate via nonimmunological mechanisms and they can be of overriding importance in determining the development of malignancy, even in severely immunosuppressed individuals. We feel that, in most experiments designed to examine immunological surveillance against neoplasms, this fundamental problem has been neglected. The most glaring example is the deliberate superinfection of mice with highly virulent oncogenic viruses combined with profound immunosuppression. In our opinion, all experiments of this type are useless because they fail to mirror spontaneous neoplasia. Quite simply, they are artifacts.

4. Although "immunosuppression" is a key notion in the concept of immunological surveillance, it is nowhere defined satisfactorily. The result is that virtually all experimental models have relied on techniques that yield profound degrees of immunosuppression, such as neonatal thymectomy, ALS treatment, or thymectomy combined with ALS. Apart from those patients with certain immunodeficiency diseases, there is no evidence that individuals with early neoplasms or with premalignant lesions have comparable defects in immunity. Indeed, there is little evidence that they have *any* immunodeficiency. We therefore conclude that the relevance of all such data to spontaneous neoplasms is highly doubtful except in one respect: the *failure* of profoundly immunosuppressed experimental animals to develop neoplasms sharply diminishes the force of the surveillance theory.

Possibly, the search for immunodeficiency has been misguided. Instead of cataloging responses to antigens with no conceivable relationship to the neoplasm, investigators of this problem may be better advised to determine the subject's ability to respond to antigens of his own neoplasm. This has already begun, and the results thus far are startling: in virtually every case of cancer studied in human beings, evidence for cell-mediated immunity against antigens of the tumor (either from the patient or from a histologically similar allogeneic tumor) has been found. This has been reported in sarcoma (Cohen *et al.*, 1973), neuroblastoma (Hellström *et al.*, 1970*b*), melanoma (Hellström and Hellström, 1973), carcinoma of the colon (Hellström *et al.*, 1970*a*) and bladder (Bubenik *et al.*, 1970), Burkitt's lymphoma (Fass *et al.*, 1970), and several other malignancies (Chu *et al.*, 1967; Oren and Herberman, 1971; Herberman, 1973). In many instances, notably in patients with rapidly advancing tumors, a blocking factor that specifically inhibits the cytotoxic effect of sensitized cells is also present (Hellström *et al.*, 1969, 1971). Therefore, the immunological defect in these cases is not due to immunosuppression, but to an immune response that protects the tumor instead

---

* The role of antiviral immunity in protection against neoplasms is nicely illustrated by the case of herpes virus saimiri, which causes no disease in its natural host, the squirrel monkey. However, when it is injected into marmosets and owl monkeys, which are normally free of this virus, a malignant lymphoma develops. The squirrel monkey—the natural host of this agent—produces antibody to this virus more regularly than marmosets and owl monkeys do (Falk *et al.*, 1973).

of the patient. It could be argued that such data detract nothing from the central theme of the surveillance theory: after all, in the final analysis cellular immunity failed to eliminate the tumor. However, the practical implications of these results are vastly different from the proposal that immunodeficiency is a major element in the development of cancer. It is one thing to deal therapeutically with the problem of blocking factor and quite another to devise methods of augmenting the immune response.

Conceivably, the theory of immunological surveillance can surmount these difficulties—or its proponents may have immediate answers—but even so, there remains an issue which to us seems of great importance. This is the extraordinary susceptibility of immunologically impaired individuals to develop malignant lymphoproliferative diseases. The reader is reminded that over 80% of the neoplasms in patients with spontaneous immunodeficiency and about 60% of those in recipients of organ transplants are lymphomas. Put another way, in a woman who receives a kidney transplant the risk of developing a reticulum cell sarcoma is about 700 times the risk of her developing cancer of the breast (Hoover and Fraumeni, 1973). If these figures are sustained by further experience, the theory of immunological surveillance cannot have general validity.

Can we explain these events without invoking a surveillance mechanism? At least two alternatives occur to us. In the first place, impaired defense mechanisms against oncogenic viruses have not been excluded. The marked susceptibility of heavily immunosuppressed recipients of renal allografts to viral infections is well documented. The common kinds of malignancy that do occur in immunosuppressed persons—lymphomas and superficial epithelial cancers of the lip, skin, and cervix—are precisely those in which oncogenic viruses are suspected to be etiological. This is what we referred to earlier as immunity against an infectious agent—and not immunity against a neoplasm.

Another possibility is that the development of lymphoid tumors in immunodeficiency states results from impaired regulation of lymphoid tissue. In other words, defective negative feedback loops permit unchecked proliferative activity in lymphoid tissue (Schwartz, 1972).

Several important feedback loops control the activity of antibody-forming tissue (Schwartz, 1971). Apart from the amount of antigen available to lymphocytes, the most important among these is the control of antibody synthesis by antibody. The feedback control of the synthesis of IgM antibodies by IgG antibodies is a typical example. This mechanism is highly specific and presumably acts by neutralization of the antigen. When IgG antibodies are not made (as, for example, in a partially immunosuppressed individual), IgM synthesis and hyperplasia of lymphoid tissue continue for a long time. Infusion of antigen-specific IgG antibodies immediately stops the abnormalities (Sahiar and Schwartz, 1966). Recently, considerable interest has focused on cellular feedback mechanisms. Regulation of thymus-independent (B) lymphocytes by T lymphocytes has been clearly demonstrated in several systems (Katz and Benacerraf, 1972). Interestingly enough, certain schedules of ALS—and perhaps other immunosuppressants—eliminate "suppressor" T cells with a sharp *increase* in antibody formation (Baker *et al.*, 1970).

Two experimental models are consistent with the notion that unrestrained proliferative activity of lymphoid tissue can culminate in neoplasia: persistent antigenic stimulation combined with partial immunosuppression (Krueger, 1972), and chronic graft vs. host reactions (Armstrong *et al.*, 1970). We believe that the following clinical events are representative of similar phenomena: antigenic stimulation by organ allografts in partially immunosuppressed recipients; uncontrolled lymphoid hyperplasia in patients with spontaneous and partial immunodeficiency; development of Burkitt's lymphoma in individuals who are partially immunosuppressed as a result of infestation by malaria parasites (Greenwood *et al.*, 1972; O'Conor, 1970); appearance of malignant lymphoproliferative diseases in association with certain autoimmune disorders (Talal and Bunim, 1964; Hoerni and Laporte, 1970).

Recent work has added a new dimension to the implications of immunoregulation in the pathogenesis of certain malignancies. This is the finding that antigenic stimuli can activate latent endogenous oncornaviruses (Hirsch *et al.*, 1970). Indeed, a reaction as seemingly innocuous as the rejection of a skin allograft can lead to the appearance of infectious oncornaviruses in the spleens of mice (Hirsch *et al.*, 1973*b*). Such immunologically activated viruses can be oncogenic (Armstrong *et al.*, 1973). Evidence is now accumulating that C-type RNA viruses replicate preferentially in transformed lymphocytes; this means that a deregulated immune response—one in which recruitment of newly transformed lymphocytes is unimpeded—can provide the ideal environment favoring the activation and replication of oncornaviruses (Schwartz, 1971).

The theory of immunological surveillance has held centerstage for a dozen years. Its usefulness in provoking experiments and, more important, in bringing a sense of definition and purpose to tumor immunology cannot be overestimated. However, alternative ideas are now possible because of the incredibly rich body of data that has emerged since the theory was first advanced. Indeed, recent experimental results now permit a serious examination of the notion that the immune reaction *stimulates* the growth of tumors (Prehn, 1971).

We end this chapter as we began, with a quotation from Ehrlich's address to the University of Amsterdam: "The deeper one explores these mechanisms in the experimental animal, the greater are the chances of offering treatment in human disease. Indeed, this was the reason I have brought to your attention the purely theoretical interpretation of current advances in experimental cancer research—it is especially true for the art of medicine that *Natura artis magistra*" (Ehrlich, 1957).

6. References

ALEXANDER, P., 1972, Foetal "antigens" in cancer, *Nature (Lond.)* **235**:137.
ALLISON, A. C., 1970, Tumour development following immunosuppression, *Proc. Roy. Soc. Med.* **63**:1077.
ALLISON, A. C., AND LAW, L. W., 1968, Effects of antilymphocyte serum on virus oncogenesis, *Proc. Soc. Exp. Biol. Med.* **127**:207.

ALLISON, A. C., AND TAYLOR, R. B., 1967, Observations on thymectomy and carcinogenesis, *Cancer Res.* **27**:703.

ALLISON, A. C., BERMAN, L. D., AND LEVEY, R. H., 1967, Increased tumour induction by adenovirus type 12 in thymectomized mice and mice treated with antilymphocyte serum, *Nature (Lond.)* **215**:185.

AMIET, A., 1963, Aldrich's syndrome: A report of two cases, *Ann. Paediat.* **201**:515.

AMMANN, A. J., AND HONG, R., 1971, Selective IgA deficiency: Presentation of 30 cases and a review of the literature, *Medicine* **50**:223.

AMMANN, P., LOPEZ, R., AND BUTLER, R., 1965, Das Ataxia-telangiecktasie-syndrom (Louis-Bar syndrom) aus immunologischer Sicht, *Helv. Paediat. Acta* **20**:137.

ANDREWS, E. J., 1971, Evidence of the nonimmune regression of chemically induced papillomas in mouse skin, *J. Natl. Cancer Inst.* **47**:653.

ARMSTRONG, M. Y. K., GLEICHMANN, E., GLEICHMANN, H., BELDOTTI, L., AND ANDRE-SCHWARTZ, R. S., 1970, Chronic allogeneic disease. II. Development of lymphomas, *J. Exp. Med.* **132**:417.

ARMSTRONG, M. Y. K., RUDDLE, N. H., LIPMAN, M. B., AND RICHARDS, F. F., 1973, Tumor induction by immunologically activated murine leukemia virus, *J. Exp. Med.* **137**:1163.

ARSENEAU, J. C., SPONZO, R. W., LEVIN, D. L., SCHNIPPER, L. E., BONNER, H., YOUNG, R. C., CANELLOS, G. P., JOHNSON, R. E., AND DEVITA, V. T., 1972, Nonlymphomatous malignant tumors complicating Hodgkin's disease, *New Engl. J. Med.* **287**:1119.

BACH, F. H., AND GOOD, R. A., 1972, *Clinical Immunobiology*, Vol. 1, Academic Press, New York.

BAKER, P. J., BARTH, R. F., STASHOK, P. W., AND AMSBAUGH, D. F., 1970, Enhancement of the antibody response to type III pneumococcal polysaccharide in mice treated with antilymphocyte serum, *J. Immunol.* **104**:1313.

BALL, J. K., 1970, Immunosuppression and carcinogenesis: Contrasting effects with 7,12-dimethylbenz (a) anthracene benz (a) pyrene and 3-methylcholanthrene, *J. Natl. Cancer Inst.* **44**:1.

BALNER, H., AND DERSJANT, H., 1966, Neonatal thymectomy and tumor induction with methylcholanthrene in mice, *J. Natl. Cancer Inst.* **36**:513.

BALNER, H., AND DERSJANT, H., 1969, Increased oncogenic effect of methylcholanthrene after treatment with antilymphocyte serum, *Nature (Lond.)* **224**:376.

BANSAL, S. C., AND SJÖGREN, H. O., 1971, "Unblocking" serum activity *in vitro* in the polyoma system may correlate with antitumour effect of antiserum *in vivo*, *Nature New Biol.* **233**:76.

BANSAL, S. C., AND SJÖGREN, H. O., 1973, Regression of polyoma tumor metastasis by combined unblocking and BCG treatment: Correlation with induced alterations in tumor immunity status, *Int. J. Cancer* **12**:179.

BASHOUR, B. N., MANCER, K., AND RANCE, C. P., 1973, Malignant mixed mullerian tumor of the cervix following cyclophosphamide therapy for nephrotic syndrome, *J. Pediat.* **82**:292.

BENNETT, M., AND STEEVES, R. A., 1970, Immunocompetent cell functions in mice infected with Friend leukemia virus, *J. Natl. Cancer Inst.* **44**:1107.

BERMUTH, G. V., MINIELLY, J. A., LOGAN, G. B., AND GLEICH, G. J., 1970, Hodgkin's disease and thymic alymphoplasia in a 5 month old infant, *Pediatrics* **45**:792.

BLAIR, P. B., 1971, Immunological aspects of the relationship between host and oncogenic virus in the mouse mammary tumor system, *Israel J. Med. Sci.* **7**:161.

BLAIR, P. B., 1972, Effect of transient immunosuppression on host response to neonatally introduced oncogenic virus, *Cancer Res.* **32**:356.

BODER, E., 1973, Ataxia-telangiectasia: Recent clinical and pathological observations, in: *Proceedings of the Second International Workshop on Immunodeficiency Diseases in Man* (D. Bergsma and R. A. Good, eds.), The National Foundation, New York.

BODER, E., AND SEDGWICK, R. P., 1963, Ataxia telangiectasia: A review of 101 cases, in: *Cerebellum, Posture and Cerebral Palsy* Little Club Clinics in Developmental Medicine No. 8, (G. E. Walsh, ed.), pp. 110–118, J. B. Lippincott, Philadelphia.

BRAND, M. M., AND MARINKOVICH, V. A., 1969, Primary malignant reticulosis of the brain in Wiskott–Aldrich syndrome: Report of a case, *Arch. Dis. Child.* **44**:536.

BROWN, R. S., HAYNES, H. A., FOLEY, H. T., GODWIN, H. A., BERARD, C. W., AND CARBONE, P. P., 1967, Hodgkin's disease: Immunologic, clinical and histologic features of 50 untreated patients, *Ann. Int. Med.* **67**:291.

BUBENIK, J., PERLMANN, P., HELMSTEIN, K., AND MOBERGER, G., 1970, Cellular and humoral immune responses to human urinary bladder carcinomas, *Int. J. Cancer* **5**:310.

BULLOCK, W. E., 1968, Studies of immune mechanisms in leprosy. I. Depression of delayed allergic responses to skin test antigens, *New Engl. J. Med.* **278**:298.

BURNET, F. M., 1963, The evolution of bodily defense, *Med. J. Austral.* **2**:817.

BURNET, F. M., 1970, The concept of immunological surveillance, *Prog. Exp. Tumor Res.* **13**:1.

BURSTEIN, N. A., AND ALLISON, A. C., 1970, Effect of antilymphocyte serum on the appearance of reticular neoplasms in SJL/J mice, *Nature (Lond.)* **225**:1139.

BURSTEIN, N. A., AND LAW, L. W., 1971, Neonatal thymectomy and nonviral mammary tumors in mice, *Nature (Lond.)* **231**:450.

BURTON, B. T., KRUEGER, K. K., AND BRYAN, F. A., 1971, National Registry of Long-Term Dialysis Patients, *J. Am. Med. Assoc.* **218**:718.

CANTOR, H., ASOFSKY, R., AND TALAL, N., 1970, Synergy among lymphoid cells mediating the graft versus host response. I. Synergy in graft versus host reactions produced by cells from NZB/Bl mice, *J. Exp. Med.* **131**:223.

CASTAIGNE, P., CAMBIER, J., AND BRUNET, P., 1969, Ataxie-telangiectasies, desordres immunitaires, lymphosarcomatose terminale chez deux frères, *Presse Med.* **77**:347.

CERELLI, G. J., AND TREAT, R. C., 1969, The effect of antilymphocyte serum on the induction and growth of tumor in the adult mouse, *Transplantation* **8**:774.

CHAPTAL, J., ROYER, P., JEAN, R., ALAGILLE, D., BONNET, H., LAGARDE, E., ROBINET, M., AND RIEU, D., 1966, Syndrome de Wiskott–Aldrich avec survie prolongée (gans) évolution mortelle par thymosarcome, *Arch. Franc. Pediat* **23**:907.

CHESTERMAN, F. C., GAUGAS, J. M., HIRSCH, M. S., REES, R. J. W., HARVEY, J. F., AND GILCHRIST, C., 1969, Unexpected high incidence of tumours in thymectomized mice treated with anti-lymphocyte globulin and *Mycobacterium leprae*, *Nature (Lond.)* **221**:1033.

CHU, E. H. Y., STJERNSWARD, J., CLIFFORD, P., AND KLEIN, G., 1967, Reactivity of human lymphocytes against autochthonous and allogeneic normal and tumor cells *in vitro*, *J. Natl. Cancer Inst.* **39**:595.

CLAMAN, H. N., AND CHAPERON, E. A., 1969, Immunologic complementation between thymus and marrow cells—A model for the two-cell theory of immunocompetence, *Transpl. Rev.* **1**:92.

COHEN, A. M., KETCHAM, A. S., AND MORTON, D. L., 1973, Tumor-specific cellular cytotoxicity to human sarcomas: Evidence for a cell-mediated host immune response to a common sarcoma cell-surface antigen, *J. Natl. Cancer Inst.* **50**:585.

COHEN, S. M., HEADLEY, D. B., AND BRYAN, G. T., 1973, The effect of adult thymectomy and adult splenectomy on the production of leukemia and stomach neoplasms in mice by N-(4-(5-nitro-2-furyl)-2-thiazolyl) acetamide, *Cancer Res.* **33**:637.

COLEMAN, A., LEIKIN, S., AND GUIN, G. H., 1961, Aldrich's syndrome, *Clin. Proc. Child. Hosp. (Wash.)* **17**:22.

COOPER, M. D., CHASE, H. P., LOWMAN, J. T., KRURT, W., AND GOOD, R. A., 1968, Wiskott–Aldrich syndrome, *Am. J. Med.* **44**:499.

COOPER, M. D., LAWTON, A. R., AND BOCKMAN, D. E., 1971, Agammaglobulinemia with B lymphocytes: Specific defect of plasma-cell differentiation, *Lancet* **2**:791.

CRAIG, S. R., AND ROSENBERY, E. W., 1971, Methotrexate-induced carcinoma? *Arch. Dermatol.* **103**:505.

CUSTER, R. P., OUTZEN, H. C., EATON, G. J., AND PREHN, R. J., 1973, Does the absence of immunologic surveillance affect the tumor incidence in "nude" mice? First recorded spontaneous lymphoma in a "nude" mouse, *J. Natl. Cancer Inst.* **51**:707.

DAMMIN, G. J., COUCH, N. P., AND MURRAY, J. E., 1957, Prolonged survival of skin homografts in uremic patients, *Ann. N.Y. Acad. Sci.* **64**:967.

DEFENDI, V., AND ROOSA, R. A., 1964, The role of the thymus in carcinogenesis, in: *The Thymus* (V. Defendi and D. Metcalf, eds.), p. 121, Wistar Institute Press, Philadelphia.

DENLINGER, R. H., SWENBERG, J. A., KOESTNER, A., AND WECHSLER, W., 1973, Differential effect of immunosuppression on the induction of nervous system and bladder tumors by N-methyl N-nitrosurea, *J. Natl. Cancer Inst.* **50**:87.

DENMAN, A. M., AND DENMAN, E. J., 1970, Depletion of long-lived lymphocytes in old New Zealand Black mice, *Clin. Exp. Immunol.* **6**:457.

DENT, P., 1972, Immunosuppression by oncogenic viruses, *Prog. Med. Virol.* **14**:1.

DENT, P. B., PETERSON, R. D. A., AND GOOD, R. A., 1965, A defect in cellular immunity during the incubation period of passage A leukemia in C3H mice, *Proc. Soc. Exp. Biol. Med.* **119**:869.

DEODHAR, S., 1972, Discussion, in: *Conference on Immunology of Carcinogenesis*, p. 217, National Cancer Institute Monograph 35, National Cancer Institute, Bethesda, Md.

DIGEORGE, A. M., 1968, Congenital absence of the thymus and its immunologic consequences: Concurrence with congenital hypoparathyroidism, in: *Immunologic Deficiency Diseases of Man* (R. A. Good and D. Bergsma, eds.), pp. 116–123, The National Foundation, New York.

DOELL, R. G., DeVAUX ST. CYR, C., AND GRABAR, P., 1967, Immune reactivity prior to development of thymic lymphoma in C57Bl mice, *Int. J. Cancer* **2**:103.

DORÉ, J. F., SCHNEIDER, M., AND MATHÉ, G., 1969, Réactions immunitaires chez les souris AKR leucemiques ou preleucemiques, *Rev. Franc. Etudes Clin. Biol.* **14**:1003.

DOUGLAS, S. D., GOLDBERG, L. S., AND FUDENBERG, H. H., 1970, Clinical, serologic and leukocyte function studies on patients with idiopathic "acquired" agammaglobulinemia and their families, *Am. J. Med.* **48**:48.

DUNN, H. G., MEUWISSEN, H., LIVINGSTON, C. S., AND PUMP, K. K., 1964, Ataxia telangiectasia, *Canad. Med. Assoc. J.* **91**:1106.

EAST, J., 1970, Immunopathology and neoplasms in NZB and SJL/J mice, *Prog. Exp. Tumor Res.* **13**:88.

EAST, J., AND HARVEY, J. J., 1968, The differential action of neoatal thymectomy in mice infected with murine sarcoma virus-Harvey (MSV-H), *Int. J. Cancer* **3**:614.

EDITORIAL, 1969, Hypogammaglobulinemia in the United Kingdom, *Lancet* **1**:163.

EHRLICH, P., 1957, Uber den jetzigen Stand der Karzinomforschung, in: *The Collected Papers of Paul Ehrlich,* Vol. II, p. 550, Pergamon Press, London.

EMERY, C. W. A., 1924, Early pregnancy and epitheliomata, *Brit. Med. J.* **2**:1149.

FALK, L. A., WOLFE, L. G., AND DEINHARDT, F., 1973, Herpesvirus saimiri: Experimental infection of squirrel monkeys (*Saimiri sciureus*), *J. Natl. Cancer Inst.* **51**:165.

FASS, L., HERBERMAN, R. B., AND ZIEGLER, J. L., 1970, Cutaneous hypersensitivity reactions to autologous extracts of Burkitt's lymphoma cells, *New Engl. J. Med.* **282**:776.

FEIGIN, R. D., VIETTI, T. J., WYATT, R. G., KAUFMAN, D. G., AND SMITH, C. H., 1970, Ataxia telangiectasia with granulocytopenia, *J. Pediat.* **77**:431.

FISHER, J. C., DAVIS, R. C., AND MANNICK, J. A., 1970, The effects of immunosuppression on the induction and immunogenicity of chemically induced sarcomas, *Surgery* **68**:150.

FLANAGAN, S. P., 1966, "Nude," a new hairless gene with pleiotropic effects, *Genet. Res. (Camb.)* **8**:295.

FOLEY, E. J., 1953, Antigenic properties of methylcholanthrene-induced tumors in mice of the strain of origin, *Cancer Res.* **13**:835.

FORSSMAN, O., AND HERNER, B., 1964, Acquired agammaglobulinaemia and malabsorption, *Acta Med. Scand.* **176**:779.

FRAUMENI, J. F., 1969, *Constitutional disorders of Man Predisposing to Leukemia and Lymphoma,* p. 221, National Cancer Institute Monograph 32, National Cancer Institute, Bethesda, Md.

FREEMAN, A. I., SINKS, L. F., AND COHEN, M. M., 1970, Lymphosarcoma in siblings associated with cytogenetic abnormalities, immune deficiency and abnormal erythropoiesis, *J. Pediat.* **77**:996.

FRIEDMAN, H., 1964, Distribution of antibody plaque forming cells in various tissues of several strains of mice injected with sheep erythrocytes, *Proc. Soc. Exp. Biol. Med.* **117**:526.

FRIEDMAN, H., AND CEGLOWSKI, W. S., 1971, Defect in cellular immunity of leukemia virus–infected mice assessed by macrophage migration-inhibition assay, *Proc. Soc. Exp. Biol. Med.* **136**:154.

FRIEDMAN, H., AND CEGLOWSKI, W. S., 1973, Cellular immunity and leukemia virus infection, in: *Virus Tumorigenesis and Immunogenesis* (W. S. Ceglowski and H. Friedman, eds.), p. 299, Academic Press, New York and London.

FRIEDMAN, H., MELNICK, H., MILLS, L., AND CEGLOWSKI, W. S., 1973, Depressed allograft immunity in leukemia virus infected mice, *Transpl. Proc.* **5**:981.

FRIEDRICH-FRESKA, H., AND HOFFMAN, M., 1969, Immunological defense against preneoplastic stages of diethyl-nitrosamine-induced carcinomas in rat liver, *Nature (Lond.)* **223**:1162.

FUDENBERG, H., AND SOLOMON, A., 1961, "Acquired agammaglobulinemia" with auto-immune hemolytic disease: Graft versus host reaction? *Vox Sang.* **6**:68.

FURTH, J., KUNII, A., IOACHIM, H., SANEL, F. T., AND MOY, P., 1966, Parallel observations on the role of the thymus in leukaemogenesis, immunocompetence and lymphopoiesis, in: *The Thymus: Experimental and Clinical Studies* (G. E. W. Wolstenholme and R. Potter, eds.), p. 288, Little, Brown, Boston.

GELFAND, M. E., AND STEINBERG, A. D., 1973, Mechanism of allograft rejection in New Zealand mice. I. Cell synergy and its age-dependent loss, *J. Immunol.* **110**:1652.

GERSHON, R. K., COHEN, P., HENCIN, R., AND LIEBHABER, S. A., 1972, Suppressor T cells, *J. Immunol.* **108**:586.

GIOVANELLA, B. C., LIEGEL, J., AND HEIDELBERGER, C., 1970, The refractoriness of the skin of hairless mice to chemical carcinogenesis, *Cancer Res.* **30**:2590.

GITLIN, D., AND JANEWAY, C. A., 1956, Agammaglobulinemia, congenital, acquired and transient forms, *Prog. Hematol.* **1**:318.

GOOD, R. A., 1972, Relations between immunity and malignancy, *Proc. Natl. Acad. Sci.* **69**:1026.

GOTOFF, S. P., AMIRMOKRI, E., AND LIEBNER, E. J., 1967, Ataxia telangiectasia: Neoplasia, untoward response to x-irradiation and tuberous sclerosis, *Am. J. Dis. Child.* **114**:617.

GOTTLIEB, C. F., PERKINS, E. H., AND MAKINODAN, T., 1972, Genetic regulation of the thymus dependent humoral immune response in leukemia prone AKR ($H-2^k$) and nonleukemic C3H ($H-2^k$) mice, *J. Immunol.* **109**:974.

GRANT, G. A., AND MILLER, J. F. A. P., 1965, Effect of neonatal thymectomy on the induction of sarcomata in C57BL mice, *Nature (Lond.)* **205**:1124.

GRANT, G. A., AND ROE, F. J. C., 1969, Effect of germ free status and antilymphocyte serum on induction of various tumors in mice by a chemical carcinogen given at birth, *Nature (Lond.)* **223**:1060.

GREEN, T., LITURN, S., ADLERSBERG, R., AND RUBIN, I., 1966, Hypogammaglobulinemia with late development of a lymphosarcoma: A case report, *Arch. Int. Med.* **118**:592.

GREENWOOD, B. M., BRADLEY-MOORE, A. M., PALIT, A., AND BRIJCESON, A. D. M., 1972, Immunosuppression in children with malaria, *Lancet* **1**:1969.

GROSS, L., 1959, Effect of thymectomy on development of leukemia in C3H mice inoculated with leukemic "passage" virus, *Proc. Soc. Exp. Biol. Med.* **100**:325.

GROSS, L., 1970, *Oncogenic Viruses*, Pergamon Press, New York.

GUTTMAN, R. D., AND LINDQUIST, P. R., 1969, Renal transplantation in inbred rats: Reduction of allograft immunogenicity by cytotoxic drug pretreatment of donors, *Transplantation* **8**:490.

HAERER, A. F., JACKSON, J. F., AND EVERS, C. G., 1969, Ataxia telangiectasia with gastric carcinoma, *J. Am. Med. Assoc.* **210**:1884.

HANNA, M. G., NETTESHEIM, P., AND OGDEN, L., 1967, Reduced immune potential of aged mice: Significance of morphologic changes in lymphatic tissue, *Proc. Soc. Exp. Biol. Med.* **125**:882.

HARAN-GHERA, N., BEN YAAKOV, M., PELED, A., AND BENTWICH, Z., 1973, Immune status of SJL/J mice in relation to age and spontaneous tumor development, *J. Natl. Cancer Inst.* **50**:1227.

HARGIS, B. J., AND MALKIEL, S., 1972, The immunocapacity of the AKR mouse, *Cancer Res.* **32**:291.

HARRIS, C. C., 1971, Malignancy during methotrexate and steroid therapy for psoriasis, *Arch. Dermatol.* **103**:501.

HARRIS, J., JESSOP, J. D., AND DE SAINTONGE, D. M. C., 1971, Further experience with azathioprine in rheumatoid arthritis, *Brit. Med. J.* **4**:463.

HECHT, F., KOLER, R. D., RIGAS, D. A., DAHNKE, G. S., CASE, M. P., TISDALE, V., AND MILLER, R. W., 1966, Leukemia and lymphocytes in ataxia telangiectasia, *Lancet* **2**:1193.

HECHT, F., McCAW, B. K., AND KOLER, R. D., 1973, Ataxia-telangiectasia—Clonal growth of translocation lymphocytes, *New Engl. J. Med.* **289**:286.

HECHTEL, M., DISHON, T., AND BRAUN, W., 1965, Hemolysin formation in newborn mice of different strains, *Proc. Soc. Exp. Biol. Med.* **120**:728.

HELLSTRÖM, I., AND HELLSTRÖM, K. E., 1973, Some recent studies on cellular immunity to human melanomas, *Fed. Proc.* **32**:156.

HELLSTRÖM, I., HELLSTRÖM, K. E., EVANS, C. A., HEPPNER, G. H., PIERCE, G. E., AND YANG, J. P. S., 1969, Serum-mediated protection of neoplastic cells from inhibition by lymphocytes immune to their tumor-specific antigens, *Proc. Natl. Acad. Sci.* **62**:362.

HELLSTRÖM, I., HELLSTRÖM, K. E., AND SHEPARD, T. H., 1970a, Cell-mediated immunity against antigens common to human colonic carcinomas and fetal gut epithelium, *Int. J. Cancer* **6**:346.

HELLSTRÖM, I., HELLSTRÖM, K. E., BILL, A. H., PIERCE, G. E., AND YANG, J. P. S., 1970b, Studies on cellular immunity to human neuroblastoma cells, *Int. J. Cancer* **6**:172.

HELLSTRÖM, I., HELLSTRÖM, K. E., SJÖGREN, H. O., AND WARNER, G. A., 1971, Serum factors in tumor-free patients cancelling the blocking of cell-mediated immunity, *Int. J. Cancer* **8**:185.

HELLSTRÖM, K. E., AND HELLSTRÖM, I., 1969, Cellular immunity against tumor antigens, *Advan. Cancer Res.* **12**:167.

HEPPNER, G. H., WOOD, P. C., AND WEISS, D. W., 1968, Studies on the role of the thymus in viral tumorigenesis. I. Effect of thymectomy on induction of hyperplastic alveolar nodules and mammary tumors in BALB/c and C3H mice, *Israel J. Med. Sci.* **4**:1195.

HERBERMAN, R. B., 1973, *In vivo* and *in vitro* assays of cellular immunity to human tumor antigens, *Fed. Proc.* **32**:160.

HERMANS, P. C., AND HUIZENGA, K. A., 1972, Association of gastric carcinoma with idiopathic late-onset immunoglobulin deficiency, *Ann. Int. Med.* **76**:605.

HERSH, E. M., WHITECAR, J. P., McCREDIE, K. B., BODEY, G. P., AND FREIREICH, E. J., 1971, Chemotherapy, immunocompetence, immunosuppression and prognosis in acute leukemia, *New Engl. J. Med.* **285**:1211.

HIRSCH, M. S., AND MURPHY, F. A., 1968, Effects of antithymocyte serum on Rauscher virus infection of mice, *Nature (Lond.)* **218**:478.

HIRSCH, M. S., ALLISON, A. C., AND HARVEY, J. J., 1969, Immune complexes in mice infected neonatally with Moloney leukemogenic and murine sarcoma viruses, *Nature (Lond.)* **223**:739.

HIRSCH, M. S., BLACK, P. H., TRACY, G. S., LEIBOWITZ, S., AND SWARTZ, R. S., 1970, Leukemia virus activation in chronic allogeneic disease, *Proc. Natl. Acad. Sci.* **67**:1914.

HIRSCH, M. S., BLACK, P. H., WOOD, M. L., AND MONACO, A. P., 1973a, Effects of pyran copolymer on leukemogenesis in immunosuppressed AKR mice, *J. Immunol.* **111**:91.

HIRSCH, M. S., ELLIS, D. A., BLACK, P. H., MONACO, A. P., AND WOOD, M. L., 1973b, Leukemia virus activation during homograft rejection, *Science* **180**:500.

HIRSCHHORN, K., SCHREIBMAN, R. R., BACH, F. H., AND SILTZBACH, L. E., 1964, In vitro studies of lymphocytes from patients with sarcoidosis and lymphoproliferative diseases, *Lancet* **2**:842.

HITZIG, W. G., 1968, The Swiss type of agammaglobulinemia, in: *Immunologic Deficiency Diseases in Man* (R. A. Good and D. Bergsma, eds.), p. 53, The National Foundation, New York.

HOERNI, B., AND LAPORTE, G., 1970, Immunological disorders in the aetiology of lymphoreticular neoplasms, *Rev. Europ. Etud. Clin. Biol.* **15**:841.

HOOVER, R., AND FRAUMENI, J. F., JR., 1973, Risk of cancer in renal-transplant recipients, *Lancet* **2**:55.

HOYER, J. R., COOPER, M. C., GABRIELSON, A. E., AND R. A., 1968, Lymphopenic forms of congenital immunologic deficiency diseases, *Medicine* **47**:201.

HUBER, F., 1968, Experience with various immunologic deficiencies in Holland, in: *Immunologic Deficiency Diseases in Man* (R. A. Good and D. Bergsma, eds.) p. 53, The National Foundation, New York.

JOHNSON, E. A., REED, N. D., JUTILA, J. W., AND HILL, W. D., 1974, Submitted for publication.

JOHNSON, S., 1968, Effect of thymectomy on the induction of skin tumors by dibenzanthracene and of breast tumors by dimethylbenzanthracene in mice of the IF strain, *Brit. J. Cancer* **22**:755.

JUDD, K. P., STEPHENS, K., AND TRENTIN, J. J., 1971, Effects of heterologous antilymphocyte antibody on the development of spontaneous and transplanted lymphoma in AKR mice, *Cancer* **27**:1161.

JUNG, K. S. K., HOFFMAN, G. C., AND LONSDALE, D., 1969, Lymphoproliferative lesion in congenital thymic aplasia associated with agammaglobulinemia, *Am. J. Clin. Pathol.* **52**:726.

KADOWAKI, J. I., THOMPSON, R. I., ZUELZER, W. W., WOOLEY, P. V., BROUGH, A. J., AND GRUBER, D., 1965, XX/XY lymphoid chimaerism in congenital immunological deficiency syndrome with thymic alymphoplasia, *Lancet* **2**:1152.

KAPLAN, H. S., 1971, Role of immunologic disturbance in human oncogenesis: Some facts and fancies, *Brit. J. Cancer* **25**:620.

KATZ, D. H., AND BENACERRAF, B., 1972, The regulatory influence of activated T cells on B cell responses to antigen, *Advan. Immunol.* **15**:1.

KAY, S., FRABLE, W. J., AND HUME, D. M., 1970, Cervical dysplasia and cancer developing in women on immunosuppression therapy for renal homotransplantation, *Cancer* **26**:1048.

KILDEBERG, P., 1961, The Aldrich syndrome: Report of a case and discussion of pathogenesis, *Prediatrics* **27**:362.

KIRSCHSTEIN, R., RABSON, A. S., AND PETERS, E. A., 1964, Oncogenic activity of adenovirus 12 in thymectomized BALB/c and C3H/HeN mice, *Proc. Soc. Exp. Biol. Med.* **117**:198.

KLEIN, E., 1972, Tumor immunology, escape mechanisms, *Ann. Inst. Pasteur* **122**:593.

KLEIN, G., 1966, Tumor antigens. *Ann. Rev. Microbiol.* **20**:223.

KLEIN, G., 1969, Experimental studies in tumor immunology, *Fed. Proc.* **28**:1739.

KLEIN, G., 1973, Tumor immunology, *Transpl. Proc.* **5**:31.

KOLDOVSKY, P., 1969, *Tumor Specific Transplantation Antigen*, Springer, New York.

KOUTTAB, N. M., JUTILA, J. W., AND REED, N. D., Submitted for publication.

KRUEGER, G. R. F., 1972, Chronic immunosuppression and lymphomagenesis in man and mice, in: *Conference on Immunology of Carcinogenesis*, p. 138, National Cancer Institute Monograph 35, National Cancer Institute, Bethesda, Md.

KYLE, R. A., PIERRE, R. V., AND BAYRD, E. D., 1970, Multiple myeloma and acute myelomonocytic leukemia, *New Engl. J. Med.* **283**:1121.

LAMPERT, F., 1969, Akute lymphoblastische Leukämie bei Geschwistern mit progressiver Kleinhernataxie (Louis-Bar syndrom), *Deutsch. Med. Wschr.* **94**:217.

LANCE, E. M., MEDAWAR, P. B., AND TAUT, R. N., 1973, Antilymphocyte serum, *Advan. Immunol.* **17**:2.

LAPPE, M. A., AND BLAIR, P. B., 1970, Interference with mammary tumorigenesis by antilymphocyte serum, *Proc. Am. Assoc. Cancer Res.* **11**:47.

LAPPE, M. A., AND PREHN, R. J., 1970, The predictive value of skin allograft survival times during the development of urethan-induced lung adenomas in BALB/c mice, Cancer Res. 30:1357.

LAW, L. W., 1966, Studies of thymic function with emphasis on the role of the thymus in oncogenesis, Cancer Res. 26:551.

LAW, L., 1969, Studies of the significance of tumor antigens in induction and repression of neoplastic disease, Cancer Res. 29:1.

LAW, L. W., 1970a, Effects of antilymphocyte serum on the induction of neoplasms of lymphoreticular tissues, Fed. Proc. 29:171.

LAW, L. W., 1970b, Studies of tumor antigens and tumor specific immune mechanisms in experimental systems, Transpl. Proc. 2:117.

LAW, L. W., AND CHANG, S. S., 1971, Effects of antilymphocyte serum (ALS) on the induction of lymphocytic leukemia in mice, Proc. Soc. Exp. Biol. Med. 136:420.

LAW, L. W., AND MILLER, J. H., 1950, The influence of thymectomy on the incidence of carcinogen-induced leukemia in strain DBA mice, J. Natl. Cancer Inst. 11:425.

LAW, L. W., AND TING, R. C., 1965, Immunologic competence and induction of neoplasms by polyoma virus, Proc. Soc. Exp. Biol. Med. 119:823.

LEE, A. K. Y., MACKAY, I. R., ROWLEY, M. J., AND YAP, C. Y., 1971, Measurement of antibody-producing capacity to flagellin in man. IV. Studies in autoimmune disease, allergy and after azathioprine treatment, Clin. Exp. Immunol. 9:507.

LEGGE, J. S., AND AUSTING, C. M., 1968, Antigen localization and the immune response as a function of age, Austral. J. Exp. Biol. Med. Sci. 46:361.

LEVENTHAL, B. G., AND TALAL, N., 1970, Response of NZB and NZB/NZW spleen cells to mitogenic agents, J. Immunol. 104:918.

LEVINE, B. B., AND VAS, N. M., 1970, Effect of combinations of inbred strain, antigen, and antigen dose on immune responsiveness and reagin production in the mouse, Int. Arch. Allergy Appl. 39:156.

LILLY, F., 1968, The effect of histocompatibility-2 type on response to Friend leukemia virus in mice, J. Exp. Med. 127:465.

LILLY, F., 1972, Mouse leukemia: A model of a multiple gene disease, J. Natl. Cancer Inst. 49:927.

LILLY, F., AND PINCUS, T., 1973, Genetic control of murine viral leukemogenesis, Advan. Cancer Res. 17:231.

LILLY, F., BOYSE, E. A., AND OLD, L. J., 1964, Genetic basis of susceptibility to viral leukemogenesis, Lancet 2:1207.

LIPSMEYER, E. A., 1972, Development of malignant cerebral lymphoma in a patient with systemic lupus erythematosus treated with immunosuppression, Arthritis. Rheum. 15:183.

LITTLE, C. C., 1941, The genetics of tumor transplantation, in: Biology of the Laboratory Mouse (G. D. Snell, ed.), pp. 279–309, Blakiston, Philadelphia.

MAKINODAN, T., AND PETERSON, W. J., 1964, Growth and senescence of the primary antibody-forming potential of the spleen, J. Immunol. 93:886.

MALMGREN, R. A., BENNISON, B. E., AND McKINLEY, T. W., 1952, Reduced antibody titers in mice treated with carcinogenic and cancer chemotherapeutic agents, Proc. Soc. Exp. Biol. Med. 79:484.

MANNING, D. D., REED, N. D., AND SHAFFER, C. F., 1973, Maintenance of skin xenografts of widely divergent phylogenetic origin on congenitally athymic (nude) mice, J. Exp. Med. 138:488.

MANNY, N., ROSENMAN, E., AND BENBASSAT, J., 1972, Hazard of immunosuppressive therapy, Brit. Med. J. 2:291.

MARTINEZ, C., 1964, Effect of early thymectomy on development of mammary tumours in mice, Nature (Lond.) 203:1188.

McDEVITT, H. O., AND BENACERRAF, B., 1969, Genetic control of specific immune responses, Advan. Immunol. 11:31.

McENDY, D. P., BOON, M. C., AND FURTH, J., 1944, On the role of thymus, spleen and gonads in the development of leukemia in a high leukemia stock of mice, Cancer Res. 4:377.

McEWAN, A., AND PETTY, L. G., 1972, Oncogenicity of immunosuppressive drugs, Lancet 1:326.

McFARLIN, D. E., STROBER, W., AND WALDMANN, T. A., 1972, Ataxia telangiectasia, Medicine 51:281.

McKHANN, C. F., 1969, Primary malignancy in patients undergoing immunosuppression for renal transplantation, Transplantation 8:209.

McKUSICK, V. A., AND CROSS, H. E., 1966, Ataxia telangiectasia and Swiss-type agammaglobulinemia, J. Am. Med. Assoc. 195:119.

METCALF, D., 1963, The fate of parental preleukemic cells in leukemia susceptible and leukemia resistant F_1 hybrid mice, Cancer Res. 23:1774.

METCALF, D., AND MOULDS, R., 1967, Immune responses in preleukemic and leukemic AKR mice, *Int. J. Cancer* **2:**53.

METCALF, D., MOULDS, R., AND PIKE, B., 1966, Influence of the spleen and thymus on immune responses in aging mice, *Clin. Exp. Immunol.* **2:**109.

MILLER, D. G., 1967, The association of immune disease and malignant lymphoma, *Ann. Int. Med.* **66:**511.

MILLER, J. F. A. P., 1962, Role of the thymus in transplantation, *Ann. N.Y. Acad. Sci.* **99:**340.

MILLER, J. F. A. P., GRANT, G. A., AND ROE, F. J. C., 1963, Effect of thymectomy on the induction of skin tumors by 3,4-benzopyrene, *Nature (Lond.)* **199:**920.

MOLONEY, J. B., 1962, The murine leukemias, *Fed. Proc.* **21:**19.

MORGAN, J. L., HOLCOMB, T. M., AND MORRISSEY, R. W., 1968, Radiation reaction in ataxia telangiectasia, *Am. J. Dis. Child.* **116:**557.

MÜHLBOCK, O., AND DUX, A., 1971, Histocompatibility genes and susceptibility to mammary tumor virus in mice, *Transpl. Proc.* **3:**1247.

MURPHY, W. H., AND SYVERTON, J. T., 1961, Relative immunologic capacity of leukemic and low-leukemic strains of mice to resist infection, *Cancer Res.* **21:**921.

NAGAYA, H., AND SIEKER, H. O., 1969, Effects of antithymus serum and antilymphocyte serum on the incidence of lymphoid leukemia, *Proc. Soc. Exp. Biol. Med.* **131:**891.

NANDI, S., 1967, The histocompatibility-2 locus and susceptibility to Bittner virus borne by red blood cells in mice, *Proc. Natl. Acad. Sci.* **58:**485.

NEHLSEN, S. L., 1971, Immunosuppression, virus and oncogenesis in mice, *Transpl. Proc.* **3:**811.

NEWMAN, D. M., AND WALTER, J. B., 1973, Multiple dermatofibromas in patients with systemic lupus erythematosus on immunosuppressive therapy, *New Engl. J. Med.* **289:**842.

NOTKINS, A. L., MERGENHAGEN, S. E., AND HOWARD, R. J., 1970, Effect of virus infections on the function of the immune system, *Ann. Rev. Microbiol.* **24:**525.

O'CONOR, G. T., 1970, Persistent immunologic stimulation as a factor in oncogenesis, with special reference to Burkitt's tumor, *Am. J. Med.* **48:**279.

OLDSTONE, M. B. A., AOKI, T., AND DIXON, F. J., 1972, The antibody response to murine leukemia virus: Absence of classical immunologic tolerance, *Proc. Natl. Acad. Sci.* **69:**134.

OLEINICK, A., 1969, Altered immunity and cancer risk: A review of the problem and analysis of the cancer mortality experience in leprosy patients, *J. Natl. Cancer Inst.* **43:**775.

OREN, M. E., AND HERBERMAN, R. B., 1971, Delayed cutaneous hypersensitivity reactions to membrane extracts of human tumor cells, *Clin. Exp. Immunol.* **9:**45.

PAGE, A. R., HANSEN, A. E., AND GOOD, R. A., 1963, Occurrence of leukemia and lymphoma in patients with agammaglobulinemia, *Blood* **21:**197.

PANTELOURIS, F. M., 1968, Absence of thymus in a mouse mutant, *Nature (Lond.)* **217:**370.

PEKONEN, R., SIURALA, M., AND VUOPIO, P., 1963, Inherited agammaglobulinemia with malabsorption and marked alterations in the gastrointestinal mucosa, *Acta Med. Scand.* **173:**549.

PENN, I., 1970, *Malignant Tumors in Organ Transplant Recipients,* Springer, New York.

PENN, I., 1974, Malignancies in renal transplant recipients, in: *Seventh Miles International Symposium,* in press.

PENN, I., AND STARZL, T. E., 1972, Malignant tumors arising *de novo* in immunosuppressed organ transplant recipients, *Transplantation* **14:**407.

PENN, I., HAMMOND, W., BRETTSCHNEIDER, L., AND STARZL, T. E., 1969, Malignant lymphomas in transplantation patients, *Transpl. Proc.* **1:**106.

PETERS, R. L., SPAHN, G. J., RABSTEIN, L. S., KELLOFF, G. J., AND HUEBNER, R. J., 1973, Neoplasm induction by murine type-C viruses passaged directly from spontaneous non-lymphorecticular tumours, *Nature New Biol.* **244:**103.

PETERSON, R. D. A., KELLY, W. D., AND GOOD, R. A., 1964, Ataxia telangiectasia: Its association with a defective thymus, immunological deficiency disease, and malignancy, *Lancet* **1:**1189.

PETERSON, R. D. A., COOPER, M. D., AND GOOD, R. A., 1966, Lymphoid tissue abnormalities associated with ataxia-telangiectasia, *Am. J. Med.* **41:**342.

PINCUS, T., ROWE, W. P., AND LILLY, F., 1971, A major genetic locus affecting resistance to infection with murine leukemia viruses. II. Apparent identity to a major locus described for resistance to Friend murine leukemia virus, *J. Exp. Med.* **133:**1234.

PLAYFAIR, J. H. L., 1968, Strain differences in the murine response of mice. I. The neonatal response to sheep red cells, *Immunology* **15:**35.

POPPER, K., 1968, *The Logic of Scientific Discovery,* Harper and Row, New York.

POTOLSKY, A. I., HEATH, C. W., BUCKLEY, C. E., AND ROWLANDS, D. T., 1971, Lymphoreticular malignancies and immunologic abnormalities in a sibship, *Am. J. Med.* **50**:42.

PREHN, R. T., 1963, Function of depressed immunological reactivity during carcinogenesis, *J. Natl. Cancer Inst.* **31**:791.

PREHN, R. T., 1970, Critique of surveillance hypothesis, in: *Immune Surveillance* (R. T. Smith and M. Landy, eds.), p. 460, Academic Press, New York.

PREHN, R. T., 1971, Perspectives in oncogenesis: Does immunity stimulate or inhibit neoplasia? *J. Reticuloendothel. Soc.* **10**:1.

PREHN, R. T., 1972, The immune reaction as a stimulator of tumor growth, *Science* **176**:170.

PREHN, R. T., AND MAIN, J. M., 1957, Immunity to methylcholanthrene-induced sarcomas, *J. Natl. Cancer Inst.* **18**:769.

PROFITT, M. R., HIRSCH, M. S., AND BLACK, P. H., 1973, Absence of cell-mediated immunologic tolerance to leukemia virus in carrier mice, *J. Immunol.* **110**:1183.

RABBAT, A. G., AND JEEJEEBHOY, H. F., 1970, Heterologous antilymphocyte serum (ALS) hastens the appearance of methylcholanthrene-induced tumours in mice, *Transplantation* **9**:164.

RADL, MASOPUST, J., HOUSTEK, J., AND HRODEK, O., 1967, Paraproteinaemia and unusual dysgamma-globulinemia in a case of Wiskott–Aldrich syndrome: An immunochemical study, *Arch. Dis. Child.* **42**:608.

RADZICHOVSKAJA, R., 1967, Effect of thymectomy on Rous virus tumor growth induced in chickens, *Proc. Soc. Exp. Biol. Med.* **126**:13.

REED, N. D., AND JUTILA, J. W., 1972, Immune response of congenitally thymusless mice to heterologous erythrocytes, *Proc. Soc. Exp. Biol. Med.* **139**:1234.

REED, N. D., MANNING, J. K., AND RUDBACH, J. A., 1973, Immunological responsiveness of mice to LPS from *Escherichia coli, J. Infect. Diseases* (Endotoxin Suppl.).

REED, W. B., EPSTEIN, W. L., BODER, E., AND SEDGWICK, R., 1966, Cutaneous manifestations of ataxia telangiectasia, *J. Am. Med. Assoc.* **195**:746.

REES, R. B., BENNETT, J. H., HAMLIN, E. M., AND MAIBACH, H. I., 1964, Aminopterin for psoriasis, *Arch. Dermatol.* **90**:544.

REISMAN, L. E., MITANI, M., AND ZUELZER, W. W., 1964, Chromosome studies in leukemia. I. Evidence for the origin of leukemic stem lines from aneuploid mutants, *New Engl. J. Med.* **270**:591.

RIFKIND, D., MARCHIORO, T. L., AND SCHNECK, S. A., 1967, Systemic fungal infections complicating renal transplantation, *Am. J. Med.* **43**:28.

ROITT, I., 1971, *Essential Immunology,* Davis, London.

ROSENBERG, S. A., DIAMOND, H. D., JASLOWITZ, B., AND CRAVER, L. F., 1961, *Medicine* **40**:31.

ROWE, W. P., 1972, Studies of genetic transmission of murine leukemia virus by AKR mice. I. Crosses with $Fv\text{-}1^n$ strains of mice, *J. Exp. Med.* **136**:1272.

ROWE, W. P., AND HARTLEY, J. W., 1972, Studies of genetic transmission of murine leukemia virus by AKR mice. II. Crosses with $Fv\text{-}1^b$ strains of mice, *J. Exp. Med.* **136**:1286.

RYGAARD, J., 1969, Immunobiology of the mouse mutant "nude": Preliminary investigations, *Acta Pathol. Microbiol. Scand.* **77**:761.

SAHIAR, K., AND SCHWARTZ, R. S., 1966, The immunoglobulin sequence. II. Histological effects of the suppression of γM and γG antibody synthesis, *Int. Arch. Allergy* **29**:52.

SAINT GEME, J. W., JR., PRINCE, J. T., BURKE, B. A., GOOD, R. A., AND KRIVITT, W., 1966, Impaired cellular resistance to herpes-simplex virus in Wiskott–Aldrich syndrome, *New Engl. J. Med.* **273**:229.

SALAMAN, M. H., 1969, Immunosuppression by oncogenic viruses, *Antibiot. Chemother.* **15**:393.

SANFORD, B. H., KOHN, H. J., DALY, J. J., AND SOO, S. F., 1973, Longterm spontaneous tumor incidence in neonatally thymectomized mice, *J. Immunol.* **110**:1437.

SATO, H., BOYSE, E. A., AOKI, T., IRITANI, C., AND OLD, L. J., 1973, Leukemia associated transplantation antigens related to murine leukemia virus. The X.1 system: immune response controlled by a locus linked to *H-2, J. Exp. Med.* **138**:593.

SCHNECK, S. A., AND PENN, I., 1970, Cerebral neoplasms associated with renal transplantation, *Arch. Neurol.* **22**:226.

SCHNECK, S. A., AND PENN, I., 1971, *De-novo* brain tumors in renal-transplant recipients, *Lancet* **1**:983.

SCHWARTZ, R. S., 1965, Immunosuppressive drugs, *Prog. Allergy* **9**:246.

SCHWARTZ, R. S., 1971, Immunoregulation by antibody, *Prog. Immunol.* **1**:1081.

SCHWARTZ, R. S., 1972, Immunoregulation, oncogenic viruses and malignant lymphomas, *Lancet* **1**:1266.

SHACHAT, D. A., FEFER, A., AND MOLONEY, J. B., 1968, Effect of cortisone on oncogenesis by murine sarcoma virus (Moloney), *Cancer Res.* **28**:517.

SHARPSTONE, P., OGG, C. S., AND CAMERON, J. S., 1969, Nephrotic syndrome due to primary renal disease in adults. II. A controlled trial of prednisone and azathioprine, *Brit. Med. J.* **2**:535.

SHEARER, G, M., MOZES, E., HARAN-GHERA, N., AND BENTWICH, Z., 1973, Cellular analysis of immunosuppression to synthetic polypeptide immunogens induced by a murine leukemia virus, *J. Immunol.* **110**:736.

SHUSTER, J., HART, Z., STIMSON, C. W., BROUGH, A. J., AND POULIK, M. D., 1966, Ataxia telangiectasia with cerebellar tumor, *Pediatrics* **37**:776.

SIEGLER, R., 1968, Pathology of murine leukemias, in: *Experimental Leukemia* (M. A. Rich, ed.), p. 51, Appleton-Century-Crofts, New York.

SJÖGREN, H. O., AND BORUM, K., 1971, Tumor-specific immunity in the course of primary polyoma and Rous tumor development in intact and immunosuppressed rats, *Cancer Res.* **31**:890.

SJÖGREN, H. O., HELLSTRÖM, I., BANSAL, S. C., AND HELLSTRÖM, K. E., 1971, Suggestive evidence that the "blocking antibodies" of tumor-bearing individuals may be antigen–antibody complexes, *Proc. Natl. Acad. Sci.* **68**:1372.

STAPLES, P. J., AND TALAL, N., 1969, Relative inability to induce tolerance in adult NZB and NZB/NZW F_1 mice, *J. Exp. Med.* **129**:123.

STARZL, T. E., PENN, I., PUTNUM, C. W., GROTH, C. G., AND HALGRIMSON, C. G., 1971, Iatrogenic alterations of immunologic surveillance in man and their influence on malignancy, *Transpl. Rev.* **7**:112.

STJERNSWARD, J., 1965, Immunodepressive effect of 3-methylcholanthrene: Antibody formation at cellular level and reaction against weakly antigenic homografts, *J. Natl. Cancer Inst.* **35**:885.

STJERNSWARD, J., 1966, Effect of non-carcinogenic and carcinogenic hydrocarbons on antibody forming cells measured at cellular level *in vitro*, *J. Natl. Cancer Inst.* **36**:1189.

STJERNSWARD, J., 1967, Further immunological studies of chemical carcinogenesis, *J. Natl. Cancer Inst.* **38**:515.

STJERNSWARD, J., 1969, Immunosuppression by carcinogens, *Antibiot. Chemother.* **15**:213.

STJERNSWARD, J., JONDAL, M., VANKY, F., WIGZELL, H., AND SEALY, R., 1972, Lymphopenia and change in distribution of human B and T lymphocytes in peripheral blood induced by irradiation for mammary carcinoma, *Lancet* **1**:1352.

STRUM, S. B., PARK, J. K., AND RAPPAPORT, H., 1970, Observation of cells resembling Sternberg–Reed cells in conditions other than Hodgkin's disease, *Cancer* **26**:176.

STUTMAN, O., 1969, Carcinogen-induced immune depression: Absence in mice resistant to chemical oncogenesis, *Science* **166**:620.

STUTMAN, O., AND DUPUY, J. M., 1972, Resistance to Friend leukemia virus in mice: Effect of immunosuppression, *J. Natl. Cancer Inst.* **49**:1283.

STUTMAN, O., YUNIS, E. J., AND GOOD, R. A., 1968, Deficient immunologic functions of NZB mice, *Proc. Soc. Exp. Biol. Med.* **127**:1204.

SWANSON, M., AND SCHWARTZ, R. S., 1967, Immunosuppressive therapy: The relation between clinical response and immunologic competence, *New Engl. J. Med.* **277**:163.

SZAKAL, A. K., AND HANNA, M. G., 1972, Immune suppression and carcinogenesis in hamsters during topical application of 7,12-dimethylbenz(a)anthracene, in: *Conference on Immunology of Carcinogenesis*, p. 173, National Cancer Institute Monograph 35, National Cancer Instute, Bethesda, Md.

TALAL, N., AND BUNIM, J. J., 1964, The development of malignant lymphoma in the course of Sjögren's syndrome, *Am. J. Med.* **36**:529.

TALEB, N., TOHME, S., GHOSTINE, S., BARMADA, B., AND NAHAS, S., 1969, Association d'une ataxie telangiectasie avec une leucemie aigue lymphoblastique, *Presse Med.* **77**:345.

TEAGUE, P. O., YUNIS, E. J., RODEY, G., FISH, A. J., STUTMAN, O., AND GOOD, R. A., 1970, Autoimmune phenomena and renal disease in mice: Role of thymectomy, aging and involution of immunologic capacity, *Lab. Invest.* **22**:121.

TEN BENSEL, R. W., STADLAN, E. M., AND KRIVIT, W., 1966, The development of malignancy in the course of the Aldrich syndrome, *J. Pediat.* **68**:761.

TENNANT, J. R., AND SNELL, G. D., 1968, The *H-2* locus and viral leukemogenesis as studied in congenic strains of mice, *J. Natl. Cancer Inst.* **41**:597.

THOMAS, L., 1959, Discussion, in: *Cellular and Humoral Aspects of the Hypersensitive States* (H. S. Lawrence, ed.), pp. 529–532, Hoeber-Harper, New York.

TING, R. C., 1966, Effect of thymectomy on transplantation resistance induced by polyoma tumor homografts, *Nature (Lond.)* **211**:1000.

TING, R. C., 1967, Tumor induction in thymectomized rats by murine sarcoma virus (Moloney) and properties of the induced virus-free tumor cells, *Proc. Soc. Exp. Biol. Med.* **126**:778.

TING, R. C., AND LAW, L. W., 1965, The role of thymus in transplantation resistance induced by polyoma virus, *J. Natl. Cancer Inst.* **34**:521.

TODARO, G. J., AND HUEBNER, R. J., 1972, The viral oncogene hypothesis: New evidence, *Proc. Natl. Acad. Sci.* **69**:1009.

TRAININ, N., AND LINKER-ISRAELI, M., 1971, Increased incidence of spontaneous lung adenomas in mice following neonatal thymectomy, *Israel J. Med. Sci.* **7**:36.

TURK, J. L., AND BRYCESON, D. M., 1971, Immunological phenomena in leprosy and related diseases, *Advan. Immunol.* **13**:209.

TWOMEY, J. J., JORDAN, P. H., LAUGHTER, A. H., MEUWISSEN, H. J., AND GOOD, R. A., 1970, The gastric disorder in immunoglobulin-deficient patients, *Ann. Int. Med.* **72**:499.

VANDEPUTTE, M., 1969, Antilymphocyte serum and polyoma oncogenesis in rats, *Transpl. Proc.* **1**:100.

VANDEPUTTE, M., AND DE SOMER, P., 1965, Influence of thymectomy on viral oncogenesis in rats, *Nature (Lond.)* **206**:520.

VAN HOOSIER, G. L., GIST, C., AND TRENTIN, J. J., 1968, Enhancement by thymectomy of tumor formation by oncogenic adenoviruses, *Proc. Soc. Exp. Biol. Med.* **128**:467.

VARET, B., LEVY, J. P., LECLERC, J. C., AND KOURILSKY, F. M., 1971, Effect of antithymocytic serum on viral leukemia, erythroblastosis, and sarcoma in mice, *Int. J. Cancer* **7**:313.

VREDEVOE, D. L., AND HAYS, E. F., 1969, Effect of antilymphocytic and antithymocytic sera on the development of mouse lymphoma, *Cancer Res.* **29**:1685.

WAGNER, J. L., AND HAUGHTON, G., 1971, Immunosuppression by antilymphocyte serum and its effects on tumors induced by 2-methylcholanthrene in mice, *J. Natl. Cancer Inst.* **46**:1.

WAHREN, B., AND METCALF, D., 1970, Cytotoxicity *in vitro* of preleukaemic lymphoid cells on syngeneic monolayers of embryo or thymus cells, *Clin. Exp. Immunol.* **7**:373.

WALDER, B. K., ROBERTSON, M. R., AND JEREMY, D., 1971, Skin cancer and immunosuppression, *Lancet* **2**:1282.

WALDMANN, T. A., STROBER, W., AND BLAESE, R. M., 1972, Immunodeficiency disease and malignancy, *Ann. Int. Med.* **77**:605.

WALDORF, D. S., SHEAGREN, J. N., TRAUTMAN, J. R., AND BLOCK, J. B., 1966, Impaired delayed hypersensitivity in patients with lepromatous leprosy, *Lancet* **2**:773.

WEIDEN, P. L., BLAESE, R. M., STROBER, W., BLOCK, J. B., AND WALDMANN, T. A., 1972, Impaired lymphocyte transformation in intestinal lymphangiectasia: Evidence for at least two functionally distinct lymphocyte populations in man, *J. Clin. Invest.* **51**:1319.

WEIR, D. M., McBRIDE, W., AND NAYSMITH, J. D., 1968, Immune response to a soluble protein antigen in NZB mice, *Nature (Lond.)* **219**:1276.

WOODS, D. A., 1969, Influence of antilymphocyte serum on DMBA induction of oral carcinomas, *Nature (Lond.)* **224**:276.

WORTIS, H. H., 1971, Immunological responses of "nude" mice, *Clin. Exo. Immunol.* **8**:305.

WORTIS, H. H., NEHLSEN, S., AND OWEN, J. J., 1971, Abnormal development of the thymus in "nude" mice, *J. Exp. Med.* **134**:681.

YOUNG, R. R., AUSTEN, K. F., AND MOSER, H. W., 1964, Abnormalities of serum gamma-1-A globulin and ataxia telangiectasia, *Medicine* **43**:423.

YTREDAL, D. O., AND BRADFIELD, J. S., 1972, Seminoma of the testicle: Prophylactic mediastinal irradiation versus periaortic and pelvic irradiation alone, *Cancer* **30**:628.

YUNIS, E. J., MARTINEZ, C., SMITH, J., STUTMAN, O., AND GOOD, R. A., 1969, Spontaneous mammary adenocarcinoma in mice:Influence of thymectomy and reconstitution with thymus grafts or spleen cells, *Cancer Res.* **29**:174.

ZATZ, M. M., MELLORS, R. C., AND LANCE, E. M., 1971, Changes in lymphoid populations of aging CBA and NZB mice, *Clin. Exp. Immunol.* **8**:491.

ZISBLATT, M., AND LILLY, F., 1972, The effect of immunosuppression on oncogenesis by murine sarcoma virus, *Proc. Soc. Exp. Biol. Med.* **141**:1036.

7

Epidemiologic Approach to Cancer

Vincent F. Guinee

1. Introduction

An agent (or agents) acts on a host to cause disease. All three of the elements of this interaction are only partially understood. Descriptions of these elements are limited by our science and indeed by our vocabulary. In the ideal model one agent acting on one host would cause one disease. In an attempt to approximate this model, we instead say this host will more often develop this disease if exposed to this agent than if not exposed. The agent or environment (i.e., many agents) may then be considered to be causally associated with this disease.

The epidemiologist seeks the population from which the cases of disease emerge, and then attempts to distill from it the segment or subpopulation that most closely approximates the pure exposed population of the ideal model. Delineation of the exposed population by definition must lead toward identification of the agent. To the extent that this process identifies situations that are associated with disease occurrence, it can be the basis of avoiding these situations while the specific disease-causing agents are still being sought.

Epidemiology is thus based on knowledge of people as individuals and populations, knowledge of disease and its causes.

Vincent F. Guinee • Department of Epidemiology, The University of Texas System Cancer Center, M. D. Anderson Hospital and Tumor Institute, Houston, Texas.

2. The Definition of Disease

VINCENT F. GUINEE

2.1. Classification of a Disease

At present cancer is classified by descriptive terms of site and histology. Additional laboratory procedures are being proposed (Cox *et al.*, 1979) as part of more specific classification systems, but these remain descriptive (rather than etiologic).

As we learn more about cancer it may be reclassified into several new diseases or combined with another known disease entity. Yellow jaundice, a solely descriptive term, has been replaced by a group of diseases classified on etiologic grounds: hepatitis A and B, bile duct obstruction, cirrhosis, and so on. Certain maladies of the neck, lung, and kidney have been combined into the etiologic diagnosis of tuberculosis.

If cancer follows the pattern of previously unknown diseases (Fig. 1), we may see a shift in the disease spectrum from apparently high case fatality to recognition of mild symptoms and eventually identification of widespread subclinical cases. We have seen numerous examples of this process in recent years: poliomyelitis, Lassa fever, Legionnaires disease, childhood lead poisoning, and phenylketonuria, to name a few.

2.2. Definition of a "Case": The Diagnosis of a Disease

Because we are studying an unknown and evolving entity, numerous and disparate criteria will be proposed to denote the diseased population—the cases. Whether a single factor or multiple factors are used to make the diagnosis, this "test," which if "positive" designates the patient as having a particular disease or cancer, will have the inherent qualities of sensitivity, specificity, accuracy, and validity.

Criteria (the test) for a disease that are so strict as to include only true cases of the disease will omit other equally valid but less flagrant cases from study or treatment (Fig. 2). On the other hand, criteria so broad as to include every true case will include other disease entities with similar histories, signs, and laboratory

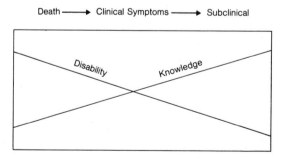

FIGURE 1. Evolution of our knowledge of disease. As knowledge of disease increases, disability associated with the disease decreases.

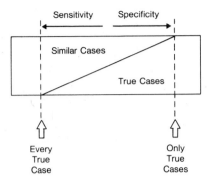

FIGURE 2. Qualities of a test. Selection of cases is affected by the degree of strictness of criteria and sensitivity of tests.

results. Thus, the highly specific test will create false negative cases, the highly sensitive test will create false positives. The shape of the interface curve will change from one test to another.

The balance and compromise between these two test qualities is constantly in evidence in the field of cancer screening, therapy, and research. Cases without histology are included in state and national statistics. False positives would not often be expected in reported cases of breast cancer, would be more likely to appear in lung cancer, and might be quite likely to appear in cases designated as liver cancer. The practical decision of not requiring histology has been made with the realization that a site-specific pattern of false positives and to a lesser degree false negatives will occur.

There is a wealth of literature concerning how best to deal with thyroid nodules. It starts with the consideration of screening high-risk groups and extends right to the physician's office where a decision to operate or not must be made. Criteria to designate who is at high risk will incorporate the test qualities of sensitivity and specificity. So too will the criteria for prompt surgical intervention.

The "test" or criteria to establish a series of cases to be studied at a medical center can and should be as specific as possible. However, these same criteria might be counterproductive in a community screening program. The latter situation is guided by two factors: how great is the risk to the undetected individual with the disease and what number of false positive cases can the screening system and the referral system process.

2.3. Accuracy and Validity

Two other inherent qualities of a test are accuracy and validity (Fig. 3). For a test to be useful it must be accurate, i.e., reproducible. Given the same test situations, the test should have the same results. The test should not be both positive and negative for the same patient on the same day, the clinical situation being constant. Two specimens obtained simultaneously should yield the same results. An observer who reads the test should interpret the results in the same

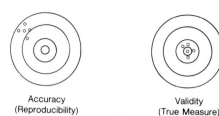

FIGURE 3. Qualities of a test. Two inherent qualities of a test are accuracy and validity.

way on different occasions. And finally, different observers should interpret the results in the same way.

Again, returning to the concept of sensitivity we can see how it enters into differing findings among observers. If a patient's cytology specimens or roentgenograms are examined by three observers for 5, 10, and 20 min, respectively, one can readily see a source of variation in reproducibility.

In the application of quality control to tests and observers, one rediscovers the art in the science of medicine. Written criteria and experienced eyes need to be aided by periodic blind readings, i.e., without knowledge of the patient's history or past test results, as well as duplicate readings by different observers. In one quality-control study the investigator concluded "examination of a section, on one occasion by one pathologist, was not a reliable way to answer the particular questions in which we were interested" (Sissons, 1975) (also see Penner, 1973).

A valid test is a true indicator of the presence of a condition or a disease. The concept of validity of a test is actually abstract. We approach it through circuitous reasoning since we only know a disease exists through a test. We do our best by stating the disease is present according to Test A and ask does Test B agree? If so, it is "valid." As can be seen in Fig. 3, validity implies accuracy. Accuracy on the other hand does not imply validity. Reproducibility does not guarantee you are measuring the appropriate aspect of the disease under study.

When inactivated measles vaccine was first administered to children, it produced antibody apparently similar to that produced by a measles illness. Subsequently, some of these children contracted measles—the first time a child with previously proven antibody had developed the disease. Further study showed that the appearance of this vaccine-produced antibody was not a sign of permanent immunity. Testing for the vaccine antibody was reproducible, but the validity of the test had changed in its prediction of permanent immunity.

3. The Distribution of Disease—Descriptive Epidemiology

3.1. Incidence and Prevalence

The terms "incidence" and "prevalence" have specific and different meanings in epidemiology than in everyday use in casual conversation.

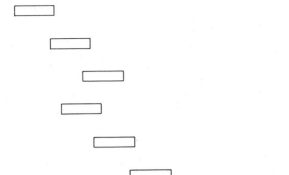

FIGURE 4. Incidence of a disease. The incidence of a disease is the number of cases that have their onset during a given period of time in a given population.

The incidence of a disease is the number of cases that have their onset during a given period of time in a given population (Fig. 4). It reflects the probability of *becoming* ill. Incidence represents *new* cases during a specified time.

The prevalence of a disease is the number of cases that exist at a given point of time in a given population (Fig. 5). It reflects the probability of *being* ill. Prevalence represents all *existing* cases at the time of observation.

The concept of prevalence is influenced by the duration of the disease as well as its incidence. A chronic disease of long duration such as diabetes is represented

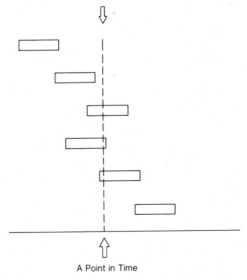

FIGURE 5. Prevalence of a disease. The prevalence of a disease is the number of cases that exist at a given point of time in a given population.

by numerous cases existing in the population. A prevalence rate of diabetes would include all of these existing cases whether their onset was 1 or 30 years before this observation.

Factors that modify the duration of a disease will modify its prevalence. If therapy is capable of curing a patient, he or she will no longer be counted in the prevalence rate. If therapy prevents death, the patient will live with the disease and thereby increase the prevalence.

If two types of cancer have exactly the same incidence but cancer "A" has a survival of 9 months and cancer "B" a survival of 18 months, the prevalence rates of cancer B will exceed those of cancer A (prevalence = incidence rate × average duration).

Incidence and prevalence are expressed as rates. It is to be noted that both the numerator and the denominator should refer to the same population under study.

Incidence rates are more useful in attempting to discuss the causes of a disease since all cases irrespective of their duration would be of interest for study. Prevalence on the other hand will be weighted to some degree with long-term survivors and will not include a portion of short-term survivors. However, if one were assessing the impact of a disease on the provision of health care in a community, the disease prevalence would be particularly important in projecting such items as bed utilization, clinic visits, and supportive care.

The best of circumstances, pure incidence or prevalence, can only be approximated. But these two measures are important for categorizing data measurements so that we are more aware of their advantages or disadvantages. For example, in the interpretation of mortality statistics, the mortality statistics of lung cancer (short survival) can be used to estimate its incidence, whereas mortality statistics of breast cancer (long survival) are much less a reflection of incidence either current or past.

3.2. Age, Sex, Race

A population is described first of all by age, sex, and race. A disease as it affects the population may be described using these same categories. Some diseases may affect a population quite uniformly. A new strain of influenza virus, for instance, will infect the entire age spectrum as it passes through a population. In contrast, prior to the introduction of measles vaccine, measles infected 95% of the population, but because it was so infectious almost all persons contracted measles during the first 10 years of life. Because of the ubiquitous presence of these viruses, both sexes and all racial segments of the community were infected.

Each cancer site has a characteristic pattern of age, sex, and race within the same population. The population tree of deaths due to thyroid cancer in Texas (1972–1976) demonstrates the well-known predilection of thyroid cancer for females (Fig. 6). A similar presentation of cancer of the kidney or larynx would essentially be a mirror image reflecting the male predominance of those cancer sites. It is seen that most of these deaths occur in persons 60 years or older.

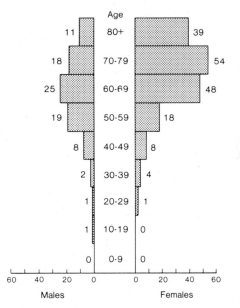

FIGURE 6. Deaths due to thyroid cancer by age and sex in Texas (1972–1976). This population tree demonstrates the well-known predilection of thyroid cancer for females.

The distribution of thyroid cancer deaths by race in Texas is compared with the racial distribution of the population (1970 census) in Table 1. Compared with the population as a whole, the percentage of thyroid cancer deaths is lower for Blacks (8% vs. 13%) and higher for those of Spanish surname (19% vs. 15%).

Among males, the ratio of thyroid cancer deaths for Black and Spanish surnames is about the same in relation to Whites (1:10). However, among females, the Spanish surname category has a 1:3 ratio to Whites, whereas the Black females have a 1:10 ratio.

A population tree of deaths due to acute leukemia in Texas (1972–1976) (Fig. 7) shows a pattern completely different from that of deaths due to thyroid cancer. Here, males and females are more equally affected, overall and in each decade. The striking difference is the appearance of deaths in the lower portion of the tree representing patients under 40 years of age.

TABLE 1

Deaths Due to Thyroid Cancer by Race and Sex in Texas (1972–1976)[a]

Race	Male	Female	Total	Percentage of thyroid cancer deaths	Percentage of 1970 population
White	68	120	188	73	72
Black	7	13	20	8	13
Spanish surname	10	39	49	19	15
Other	0	0	0	0	0
Total	85	172	257	100	100

[a] The distribution of thyroid cancer deaths by race in Texas is compared with the racial distribution of the population in the most recent census.

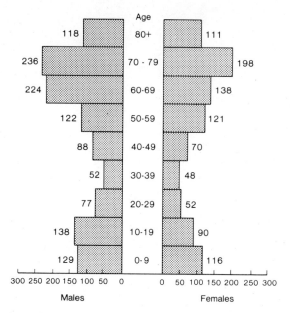

FIGURE 7. Deaths due to acute leukemia by age and sex in Texas (1972–1976). The population tree shows a completely different pattern from the thyroid death distribution shown in Fig. 6.

Examining the racial distribution of deaths (Table 2), the percentage of deaths is slightly higher for Whites and lower for Blacks when compared with the 1970 population.

These mortality data are presented in terms of the actual numbers of deaths; in practice, this is the manner in which data are initially presented to us. However, data tabulations as simple as these can be misleading if taken strictly on face value.

First, Blacks and those of Spanish surname are usually underenumerated in the census, thereby affecting their estimated percentage of the population. This then makes apparent death deficits more significant and apparent excess deaths less significant.

Second, the definition of a cancer death is that taken from a death certificate, the latter being dependent on a series of events. The individual must seek medical care, the diagnosis of cancer must be made, and later must be reported as the cause of death.

TABLE 2

Deaths Due to Acute Leukemia by Race and Sex in Texas (1972–1976)[a]

Race	Male	Female	Total	Percentage of acute leukemia deaths	Percentage of 1970 population
White	932	738	1670	78	72
Black	111	70	181	9	13
Spanish surname	134	134	268	13	15
Other	7	2	9	0	0
Total	1184	944	2128	100	100

[a] Examination of the racial distribution of deaths due to acute leukemia reveals a slight excess in whites and a deficit among blacks.

The third and most important factor is the age distribution of the Black and Spanish surname populations. Both are considerably younger than the White population. From the age distributions of the overall populations of the three groups, the percentages of those under 40 years of age are: Whites, 63.1%; Blacks, 70.7%; and Spanish surname, 77.1%. Thus, the latter two groups have a greater percentage of their population at risk for cancers that affect the young and a smaller percentage of their population at risk for cancers that affect the older age groups. Looking back at the deaths due to thyroid cancer (Table 1), the excess (19% vs. 15%) is of more interest considering the fact that we are studying a cancer known to affect older age groups in a much younger population. (Because the actual numbers are small, this apparent increase is barely at the level of statistical significance.)

In a heterogenous population, the concept of race and ethnic origin as a major element in the description of a disease on the national level is readily accepted. To the extent a nation has experienced significant immigration, or has come into being as a coalescence of ethnic populations, these concepts are appropriate for national statistics. Racial and ethnic variations of disease rates have been very useful in hypothesis formation. Though disease of genetic origin might become more apparent in these groups, ethnic differences are usually first attributed to the characteristic environment of the particular culture, especially diet.

The use of the term "Spanish surname" in vital statistics is an example of the ethnic classification difficulties that may be encountered. The alternative rubrics would be "Spanish origin" or "Spanish speaking," each with a somewhat different connotation. The administrative decision to classify a child with only one Spanish parent must be made. Then, too, in Texas, "Spanish" refers primarily to persons with a link to Mexico, whereas in New York, it usually refers to those linked to Puerto Rico.

3.3. Time

National time trend statistics for cancer mostly concern mortality rates. Incidence data produced by population-based registries usually representing smaller political units are also useful in following time trends. Dramatic differences in the behavior of cancer mortality can be observed over time. In the United States, since 1930, mortality due to cancer of the stomach in males has fallen markedly (Fig. 8). Mortality due to cancer of the lung in males has risen sharply, while that due to cancer of the colon has remained relatively unchanged. For both cancer of the lung and cancer of the stomach, the short survival after diagnosis allows us to equate mortality with incidence. As best as we can determine, these two curves therefore represent real increases and decreases of cancer cases during this time period, respectively. The increase in lung cancer mortality strengthens the hypothesis that it has been caused at least in part by cigarette smoking. The decrease in stomach cancer is still unexplained, and yet, a success in prevention. If that reason can be found, it would be available for other countries where this decrease has not yet occurred.

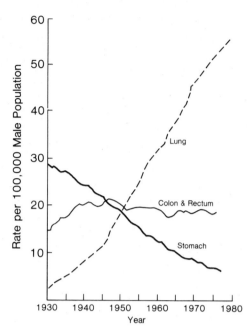

FIGURE 8. Age-adjusted cancer death rates of United States males for selected sites (1930–1977), standardized on the age distribution of the 1940 United States census population. Dramatic differences in the behavior of cancer mortality can be observed over time. From *Ca-A Cancer J. Clin.* **30**(1): 29 (1980).

The death rates shown are age-adjusted. This is necessary since there are often major shifts in the makeup of a population over several decades. All other factors remaining equal, an aging population will have a greater incidence of cancer on the basis of age alone. This would be reflected in the numbers of cancer deaths reported over time. Thus, time and age are interdependent.

A study of the incidence or mortality during a short period of time will likely utilize the same or hopefully similar definitions of cases that are represented in the numerator of the rates. In evaluating trends of disease over long periods of time, changes in definitions are likely to occur. These may be due to such factors as new diagnostic procedures or changes in procedures for registering deaths or disease occurrence. Not infrequently, changes in the classification of a disease are prompted by new pathological interpretations, which are then incorporated into different statistical rubrics.

In interpreting time trends of cancer incidence and mortality in a population, we must also be aware of the possible influence of confounding variables that may arise. The effect of hysterectomy on the mortality rates for uterine cancer is a case in point. Hysterectomy has become one of the most common operative procedures in the United States. Estimates of the number of hysterectomies performed in 1973 range from 689,000 to 778,000 (Walker and Jick, 1979). Calculations by Lyon and Gardner (1977) indicate that an adjustment for hysterectomy in the United States significantly increases the mortality rates of White females since 1960 for both cancer of the cervix and cancer of the corpus for those who are still at risk. They believe that failure to find an increasing incidence of endometrial cancer in the face of increasing use of a possible carcinogen is explained by the rising hysterectomy rates in the United States. Alderson and Donnan (1978) reported proportionally fewer hysterectomies in England and

Wales, and time trends in mortality from cervical cancer have not been similarly distorted.

3.4. Geography

The incidence and mortality rates of cancer have a surprisingly wide geographic variation. Considering the age-adjusted mortality rate for lung cancer, Scotland is close to 80 per 100,000 while Norway and Sweden are less than 20 per 100,000 (Fig. 9).

Geography, per se, may affect the incidence of disease. Climate and raw material will support a constellation of industries that in turn will support a socioeconomic milieu that will nourish the culture that chooses its own characteristic diseases.

Geography may also provide a selection of time frames for the study of disease. Medications, foods, and manufacturing processes are some of the obvious examples of potentially significant etiologic factors that are constantly appearing and fading from our cultures. In studying such etiologic factors in different countries, it is possible at a single point in time to observe populations at variable times—before, during, or after their exposures.

When a population shifts from one geographic area to another, it provides an opportunity to study the possible etiologic factors of the cancers of their

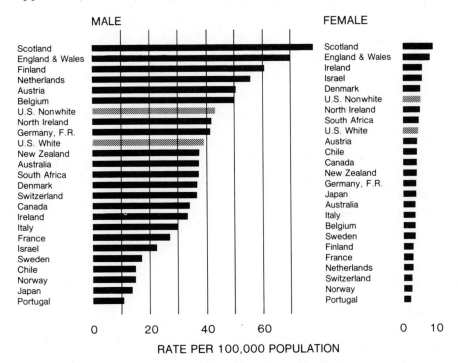

FIGURE 9. Age-adjusted mortality rates for malignant neoplasms of the lung, bronchus, and trachea in various countries, 1966–1967. The incidence and mortality rates of cancer have a surprisingly wide geographic variation. From *Cancer Rates and Risks* (2nd ed.), p. 41, 1974.

homeland, as well as the latent period of these cancers. One of the best known examples of this phenomenon is the mortality of stomach cancer among Japanese who immigrated to the United States. While the stomach cancer mortality rate has not dropped among the immigrants, it has declined for their offspring living in the United States (Haenszel and Kurihara, 1968; Haenszel *et al.*, 1972; Stemmermann, 1977). At the same time colon cancer rates increased about equally in both generations of Japanese living in the United States and are approaching those of American Whites (Dunn, 1975).

3.5. Occupation

It is usually possible to estimate the number of persons working in a particular industry in a geographic area during a particular time. It is often quite difficult to characterize the occupation of an individual or group of individuals. Indeed, in the same manufacturing plant both management and an outside governmental agency may have a different set of job descriptions for the same group of men.

If one is attempting to describe the employment history of a patient, occupation in terms of both the industry and the particular job is necessary, i.e., oil industry: secretary. Unfortunately, an occupational history is too often so involved as to seem impractical to obtain on a routine medical history. But to overlook this area of the patient's background would be to ignore many of the definitive carcinogens uncovered to date. A link between exposure to vinyl chloride monomer and angiosarcoma of the liver was recognized by Creech and Johnson (1974) in a medical care setting. Three patients, each treated by different physicians, had the same occupational background. The rarity of the tumor prompted their investigation. Only 25–30 cases a year would have been expected in the entire United States population (Heath *et al.*, 1975).

In studying occupational groups exposed to a potential disease-causing agent, comparison groups must be chosen with the "healthy work effect" in mind. As a group, those engaged in work are a self-selected cohort—healthy enough to be employed and therefore members of a group with a mortality rate lower than the population in general. When follow-up is achieved of a total worker cohort, including those that drop out for any reason, the healthy worker effect associated with active employment declines with time because of the absence of any continued selection process (McMichael, 1976).

4. Identification of Persons with Disease

4.1. Patient Populations

A study by White *et al.* (1961) concluded that in a population of 1000 adults in the United States or Great Britain, in an average month, 750 would experience an episode of illness, 250 would see a physician, but only 1 would be referred to a university medical center. This process of selection and self-selection has been further delineated by Feinstein and Spitz (1969) as it influences the manner

in which a patient comes to be included in a study of a particular disease. Some patients experience a symptom, others are detected through routine screening. Decisions to treat, not treat, or refer to a more specialized physician are made. The patient decides to accept or reject treatment at the community hospital or travel to the medical center. There, depending on associated conditions such as heart disease, age, or financial status, the patient may be included in a study.

There is real concern among physicians in community practice that the literature from specialized centers does not speak to their situation. Of course it can, but to do so it must put the reported cases in perspective, first by attempting to describe referral patterns and case selection, and second, by incorporating a healthy hesitation to generalize. As seen in Fig. 10, even if all patients with a rare disease are referred to a single specialty hospital, it is still difficult to put them into the perspective of their original community patient population.

A comparison of cancer diagnoses as seen by three categories of hospitals in Texas is shown in Table 3. The column labeled "MDAH" refers to M. D. Anderson Hospital, a comprehensive cancer center. Proportionally, there are fewer cancers such as lung and pancreas at M. D. Anderson Hospital, probably reflecting the unavailability of satisfactory treatment even at the most specialized center. The higher proportions of prostate and oral cavity cancer in the 200- and 500-bed hospitals suggest treatment is available in the community. The preponderance of melanoma and Hodgkin's disease at the specialized center suggests a definite referral pattern when specialized treatment holds greater promise of patient survival.

The comparison can be taken a step further into the community. Figure 11 compares the specialized cancer center patient population with a community-wide incidence survey, the Third National Cancer Survey. Again, the comprehensive center proportionally sees fewer cancers of the lung, colon and rectum, and prostate, and a higher proportion of head and neck cancer, lymphoma, and melanoma.

Among specialized cancer centers, there can also be considerable variation in patient population reflecting their referral system and service area.

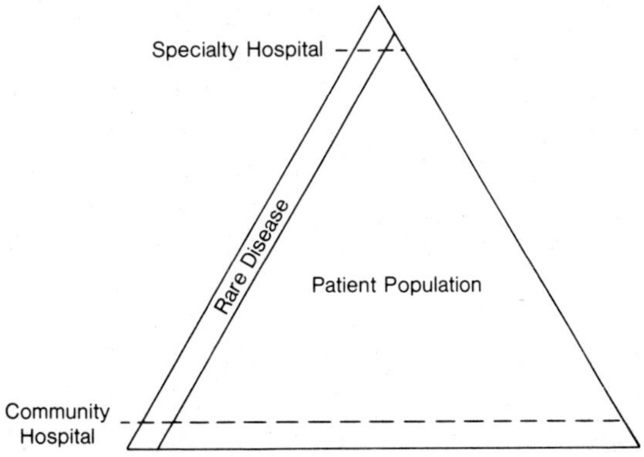

FIGURE 10. Referral effect on perspective of rare disease. Even if all patients with a rare disease are referred to a single specialty hospital, it is still difficult to put them into the perspective of their original community patient population.

TABLE 3

Percentage of Cancer Patients by Site for Hospitals in the
Cancer Information Service and a Comprehensive Cancer Center

Site	200 beds	500 beds	MDAH[a]
Lung	19.0	14.2	8.2
Breast	15.3	14.0	12.8
Prostate	7.6	8.3	2.4
Stomach	2.5	1.6	1.3
Bladder	4.9	3.6	2.4
Rectum	1.7	2.0	1.7
Cervix	5.5	6.6	8.5
Oral cavity	2.0	2.2	0.1
Non-Hodgkin's	1.7	2.8	4.5
Hodgkin's	0.0	0.9	2.3
Colon	8.4	8.0	3.6
Acute leukemia	0.1	1.0	2.9
Larynx	1.6	1.1	1.2
Melanoma	1.9	4.5	6.2
Pancreas	2.0	1.9	0.7
Ovary	2.2	1.7	3.5
Kidney	1.0	2.2	1.2
Uterus	2.8	3.2	2.7
Thyroid	1.3	1.1	1.2
Total	81.5	80.9	68.7

[a] M. D. Anderson Hospital and Tumor Institute.

4.2. Case Identification

4.2.1. Hospital Records

The hospital record is the primary source of information on an individual patient with cancer. It is the responsibility of the physician to see that it represents the patient's condition and experience, including both pertinent positive and negative findings. One cannot expect in retrospect uniform detailed accounts of social habits or exposures to agents newly suspected of causing cancer. A reasonably detailed description of the patient's status, the extent of cancer, the primary course of therapy, and the duration of survival will usually be found. Therefore, for studying these latter topics, it can be the best way to accumulate the experience of a large number of patients in a short time (Feinstein, 1968). The hospital cancer registry can characterize the hospital's experience with a particular type of cancer, describe the patient population seen in that hospital, and retrieve a set of hospital records for review.

4.2.2. Autopsy

If patients seen at a particular hospital represent a biased segment of the population, autopsy data are even less likely to represent the experience of a cross section of the community. In spite of the selection process that brings a

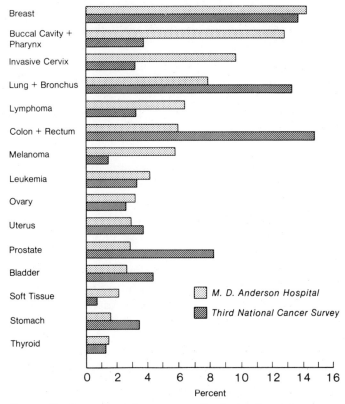

FIGURE 11. Comparison of percentage distribution for major cancer sites seen at M. D. Anderson Hospital, March 1944–August 1975, and the Third National Cancer Survey, 1969–1971. Cancer sites, as seen in a specialized cancer, do not occur in the same proportion as in the community. From V. F. Guinee and J. B. Arthaud, 1976, Epidemiology, in: *Cancer Patient Care at M. D. Anderson Hospital and Tumor Institute* (R. L. Clark and C. D. Howe, eds.), pp. 715–743, Year Book, Chicago.

group of individuals from their homes to autopsy, valuable information to support or reject hypotheses explaining clinical events can be obtained. The presence at autopsy of apparently quiescent cancer in the prostate (Liavag *et al.*, 1972) suggests that the malignant process in these instances may be held in check naturally. The paucity of undiagnosed endometrial cancer foci at pathologic examination has been used to counter claims that estrogen use affects these foci causing bleeding, thus prompting early detection of lesions that might otherwise have remained undetected. The end of the spectrum of cancer represented by those undetected until autopsy may be just as important as the obvious portion of the cancer spectrum represented by severe clinical disease in guiding us to new therapy or toward etiologic clues.

In its classic role autopsy data offer us insight into our diagnostic acumen. In a series of 10,977 autopsies from 1955 to 1965 at the Boston City Hospital, 2734 patients were found to have 3008 malignancies. Of these cancers, 797 (26.5%) were clinically undiagnosed. Of these, nearly two-thirds had extended beyond the primary site of origin. Bauer and Robbins (1972) concluded that undiagnosed cancer resulted chiefly from malignancies arising in the deep organ systems, which usually are inaccessible to adequate evaluation during routine physical examination.

4.2.3. Death Certificates

Death certificate data are the source of the mortality statistics published by governments. If the Director of the Bureau of Records and Statistics of the New York City Health Department writes an article entitled "What Is 'the Cause of Death'?," we too should be aware of the limitation of the present death certification systems. Erhardt (1958) alludes to factors that influence certification, among them being the habits of physicians, the concept of a single cause of death, the management of nosology problems, and the classification system used. He concludes "no more should be expected of them than they are capable of producing."

In an international comparison of the coding of death certificates, Percy and Dolman (1978) found that most of the differences among coders were due to a lack of specific instructions on how to select the underlying cause of death. Their study highlights the necessity for clearly written definitions of terms as a starting point for all types of research efforts extending from the realm of single-investigator studies to comparisons among nations.

In the Percy and Dolman study, an identical group of 1246 United States death certificates each with a cancer-related diagnosis was sent to the vital statistics departments of seven countries. The participants were asked to code the underlying cause of death according to the rules used in their office.

The difference between the percentage of malignant neoplasms coded in the United States and that coded in the other countries was statistically significant ($p < 0.01$). By the United States criteria, circulatory diseases were chosen over malignant neoplasms as the underlying cause of death more often than the other countries. In the United States, cancer was designated as the cause of death for 87.3% of the patients vs. 89.6–93.4% in the other countries.

A common problem encountered was the ambiguous use of the term "metastatic" when it was written without the qualification of "to" or "from," i.e., a designation "lung cancer—metastatic." Complications of treatment were also sources of confusion, as for example the coding of a myocardial infarct that occurred immediately after a pneumonectomy for lung cancer. Similarly confusing were conditions arising in cancer-debilitated patients such as mycotic infections. New coding rule classifications assigned both these latter diagnoses to the cancer as the underlying cause of death.

In Israel, the causes of death determined in 500 consecutive autopsies on patients aged 15 years or more were compared to diagnoses appearing on death certificates (Abramson *et al.*, 1971). In contrast to other disease entities, the death certificates gave a "fairly accurate indication of the presence of malignant neoplasms." Of those patients with a death certificate naming cancer as the cause of death, there was anatomical evidence in 95%. Of those who had cancer at autopsy, it was mentioned on the certificate in 80% of the cases. The false positive rate was very low (2.6%). However, there was considerably less agreement between death certificate data and autopsy data for specific categories of neoplasms than for neoplasms as a group. In only 74% of the cases in which a specific cancer was stated as the underlying cause of death was this specific site confirmed at autopsy.

4.3. Cancer Incidence Surveys

At present, to obtain cancer incidence data we must rely on survey techniques either periodic or continuous. The Introduction of the *Third National Cancer Survey: Incidence Data* details the massive effort involved (Cutler and Young, 1975). For the three-year period 1969–1971, 181,027 cancers were diagnosed in 177,504 persons in a population of 21 million. Over 900,000 documents were processed. Field staff abstracted information from hospital charts, pathology reports, radiotherapy records, outpatient clinics, and cancer registries. Copies of all death certificates that mentioned cancer were obtained. Computer programs compared data items on each individual for consistency. Duplicate cases were identified. It is interesting that although death certificates were the sole source of information for only 2.1% of the newly diagnosed cancers, they were the initial document that served to identify a cancer for more than 10% of the cases.

Microscopic confirmation was available for 90.1% of the cancers reported. This compared favorably with the 73.5% microscopic confirmation in a similar study in 1947–1948, a measure of the improved quality of medical practice in the United States. Microscopic confirmation did vary widely according to the primary site. Hodgkin's disease and cancers of the thyroid and testis were each confirmed microscopically in 98% of the cases. However, microscopic confirmation was available for only 81.5% of the reported stomach cancers and for 69.5% of the reported cancers of the pancreas. Considering these statistics, Cutler and Young noted that if a cancer survey or incidence reporting system relied solely on pathology laboratories for case ascertainment, 9.9% of the cases would not be identified, a serious understatement of cancer incidence.

An outgrowth of the National Cancer Surveys was the SEER program— Surveillance, Epidemiology and End Results. The purpose of this ongoing program, started in 1973, is the provision of incidence and survival data on cancer. Each of the participating areas, which collectively represent slightly more than 10% of the total United States population, attempts to identify all cases of cancer in a defined population. The different perspective of the cancer problem seen by incidence data, rather than mortality data, is illustrated by a recent SEER report (Young *et al.*, 1978). The three most frequent cancer sites are colorectal (incidence of 47.2 per 100,000), breast (46.3), and lung and bronchus (45.2), the incidence of each being essentially the same. In contrast, the death rates for these sites are markedly different: lung and bronchus, 36.9; colorectal, 22.3; and breast, 15.0.

Reports from population-based cancer registries from around the world are published in *Cancer Incidence in Five Continents* (Waterhouse *et al.*, 1976). The editors note that the main consideration for inclusion of data from a particular registry has been the reliability of data of both the numerator and the denominator. Adequacy of the data is judged by internal consistency, stability, the proportion of histological and death certificate diagnoses, and correlation with available mortality data. A recent and reliable census was considered necessary for documentation of the population at risk.

4.3.1. Census

Throughout the discussion of rates of cancer incidence and mortality, the denominator of 100,000 appears with the connotation of an unassailable standard. Its basis is the most recent census of that particular country.

The oldest continuous periodic census is that of the United States, which has been conducted every 10 years since 1790 (Taeuber, 1978). Commenting on recent United States censuses, Zelnik (1964) noted that females had relatively greater coverage than males. In the 1960 census it was estimated that 2.2% of White males were missed but only 0.8% of White females, the undercounting of males being especially prominent for the young adult and presumed to be due to "higher geographical mobility." The United States Census Bureau estimated the undercount of the Black population in the 1970 census at 8%.

The day-to-day problems of performing a national census are probably best followed in the press (Why the Census May Turn in a Miscount, *Business Week* June 16, 1980, p. 72). Typical of the reported factors that might contribute to a miscount of the 20th United States decennial census were that new subdivisions in Los Angeles and some centrally located apartments in Manhattan had not been included. Also, the Census Bureau relied on mailing lists bought from commerical vendors, lists less likely to include the lower socioeconomic population.

A major drawback of the current census system is the long period of time between counts. Over the space of a decade major population shifts may occur. In the past decade, the United States has experienced the "flight to the suburbs" of city populations and nationally the much-publicized migration to the "sun belt." These migrants then appear directly in the numerator data of state cancer morbidity and mortality but only through projected estimates are they represented in the denominator.

5. Analytic Epidemiology: Research Approach

The purpose of epidemiologic research is to formulate a statement that is true for the community as a whole. For this to be possible, the persons studied must be representative of that community. This is not to say that the conclusions apply to all persons in the community, but rather those individuals who might find themselves exposed to the disease-causing factor. Thus, one would not expect to generalize the findings of an occupational study to a pediatric age group.

The two basic approaches to epidemiologic research are the cohort study (prospective) and the case-control study (retrospective). As Sartwell (1974) points out, neither approach is experimental in character. These studies are best termed observational in contrast to the experimental method in which the investigator is able to manipulate the degree of exposure to the suspected disease-causing agent.

5.1. Cohort Studies

In a prospective study a cohort is formed of individuals who do not have the disease in question. At the outset of the study, these subjects are classified according to their exposure to the suspected disease-causing agent. The cohort is followed over a period of time in anticipation that in a number of cases the disease will occur. This study format produces actual incidence rates. Comparison of the disease incidence rates of subjects, with and without the suspected disease-causing agent, yields a relative risk.

This type of study approaches the planned experiment but is clearly different. In a comparable planned experiment, the study population would be defined and then half would be exposed by the investigator to the disease factor. In the prospective observational study, the population chosen arrives with its disease factor baggage already in tow, only the consequences have not been determined. As Dorn (1959) mentions, such studies need be prospective only in the sense that it is possible to define and identify the exposed population before observations are made. If the necessary records are available, a population could be defined as of some past date and study made of its disease occurrence subsequently.

5.2. Case-Control Studies

In the case-control study a group of patients with the disease is compared with a group that does not have the disease. An odds ratio is often used to express the results of a case-control study. It is a ratio of two ratios, namely the ratio of exposure in cases divided by the ratio of exposure in controls. The degree of association may also be expressed by comparing the resulting ratios and calculating the estimated relative risk. Estimation of the relative risk is discussed in detail by Mantel and Haenszel (1959). Writing on relative risks, Walter (1977) urges that specification of the magnitude of the relative risk, which it is meaningful to detect, should be decided first and then a study of a size adequate to demonstrate this risk designed. He also reminds us, "There is no equivalence between substantive significance and statistical significance." This caution is echoed through the literature. Mantel and Haenszel (1959) comment that a single retrospective (case-control) study does not yield conclusions, only leads (see also Copeland et al., 1977).

At first glance, a case-control study seems simple. In actual fact the choice of a control group is more complicated than the diagnosis of the patients with the disease to be studied. Janerich *et al.* (1979) state that although the cases have the condition of concern, it is the controls that constitute the key methodological part of the case-control method. Theoretically, the controls should be essentially identical to the disease group except for the disease-causing factor being investigated. Cases and controls are most often matched for such factors as age and sex. Other factors, such as previous symptoms, diagnostic tests, and treatments, have been used as well. It should be kept in mind, however, that if cases and controls are matched for a factor, it cannot be assessed as a study variable. In the analysis of studies (Ziel and Finkle, 1975; Smith *et al.*, 1975; Mack *et al.*, 1976) on the association of endometrial cancer and estrogen use, Horwitz and Feinstein (1978) postulated that estrogen therapy promoted bleeding and therefore detection. They called attention to the fact that bias will arise whenever a target disease that can occur in asymptomatic forms is likely to be preferentially diagnosed in persons exposed to the suspected etiologic agent. It was proposed that a more suitable matched control group for these studies would consist of patients undergoing dilatation and curettage for abnormal bleeding. However, this would probably have the effect of including more women taking estrogen in the control group. This would be matching in a partial fashion the cases and controls for estrogen use.

Commenting on this approach Vessey (1979) stated, "I am quite certain it is wrong." Shapiro (1979) added, "When one goes this route, it's almost guaranteeing that the estimate of association, or lack thereof will be biased." The reader is left with a question: Can you cure a bias with a bias?

Aside from that issue is another point—a bias once recognized does not necessarily vitiate a hypothesis. First, it may be a possible bias that in actual fact does not occur or occurs rarely. Second, there may be a preponderance of other information that supports the hypothesis and is unaffected by the bias. In the case of the link between endometrial cancer and estrogen use, Antunes *et al.* (1979) demonstrated that increasing duration of estrogen use and increasing dosage were associated with higher risks of endometrial cancer. They were unable to demonstrate a detection bias in their case series. A study by Weiss *et al.* (1979) also supported the link to duration of estrogen use.

A report on the very interesting Symposium on the Case-Control Study held in Bermuda in 1978 has been published (Ibrahim, 1979). In particular, Sackett's article (1979) includes an appendix listing 35 biases of case-control studies. He concludes that failure to develop improved standards for case-control studies may lead to the publication of seriously flawed studies with subsequent rejection of the entire approach by an inflamed scientific community.

With such strong feelings about the case-control study format, why is it used? In the same symposium, Inman (1979) stated that whereas a case-control study he performed in 1966 on "pill-mortality" involved 500 women and 2 years at a cost of about $20,000, a prospective cohort study by the University Group Diabetic Project cost many millions and took 8 years to complete. This then is the situation; prospective studies are expensive because of the large number of subjects included and the long period of time necessary for observation, waiting for the disease event to occur. This is more relevant in the study of cancer, a rare disease with a long latent period. Because of these latter factors, some prospective studies on cancer that ideally should be done are just not feasible.

There is probably no more interesting way to learn the thought process and approach of epidemiology than to review the literature on a particular subject through time. The review is not to ascertain facts per se, but rather to see in retrospect how facts have been produced and how their interpretation has evolved. The studies of Doll and Hill (1950, 1952, 1956) and Doll and Peto (1976) on the relation of smoking to lung cancer are a good example.

The initial studies used the case-control approach (1950, 1952), comparing lung cancer patients to control groups of other patients matched by sex and 5-year age groups. One is struck by the number of smokers in the population studied. Only 4.5% of the control patients were nonsmokers. This, however, differed from the rate of 0.5% among lung cancer patients. The findings that stood out were those concerning heavy smokers. Of male lung cancer patients, 25% reported smoking an average of 25 or more cigarettes daily versus only 13.4% for male control patients. Alternative hypotheses were extensively discussed including the possible role of the influenza pandemic of 1918–1919 (Iceland was visited by the pandemic but did not show an increase in lung cancer).

Serious consideration was given to interviewer bias affecting the results, since they did know which patients had cancer. To test this, a comparison was made of the smoking histories obtained from patients who were thought to have cancer of the lung but in whom the diagnosis was subsequently disproved. Their histories did not differ significantly from other control patients.

On the basis of these case-control studies, a large-scale prospective/cohort study was mounted (1956, 1976). Questionnaires on tobacco use were sent to 59,600 men and women on the Medical Register, of which 40,701 were sufficiently completed to be used. The fact of death was reported to the investigators by the Registrars-General and the British Medical Association. After a follow-up of 4 years and 5 months, among males over 35 years of age, a marked increase in lung cancer death rates was noted as the amount of cigarettes smoked increased. Doll and Hill estimated that the mortality of the doctors answering the questionnaires accounted for 92% of the mortality of all doctors whether they answered the questionnaire or not. Thus, they believed their results were not biased by those who chose not to respond to the survey.

Twenty years later the vital status of 99.7% of the cohort was known and 10,072 deaths were reported. Three repeat questionnaires had been answered by over 96% of the participants. By this time, the study population as a whole reduced its cigarette consumption substantially. At each successive survey fewer cigarettes were smoked. Mortality from lung cancer grew less common among these physicians and surgeons as a result of their participation in an epidemiologic study.

The author gratefully acknowledges the assistance of Miss Virgie McGuffee, Assistant Epidemiologist, for researching, collecting, and preparing the bibliography; and Mrs. Paula Stewart for her secretarial support in the preparation of the manuscript.

6. References

ABRAMSON, J. H., SACKS, M. I., AND CAHANA, E., 1971, Death certificate data as an indication of the presence of certain common diseases at death, *J. Chronic Dis.* **24**:417–431.

ALDERSON, M., AND DONNAN, S., 1978, Hysterectomy rates and their influence upon mortality from carcinoma of the cervix, *J. Epidemiol. Community Health* **32**:175–177.

ANTUNES, C. M. F., STOLLEY, P. D., ROSENSHEIN, N. B., DAVIES, J. L., TONASCIA, J. A., BROWN, C., BURNETT, L., RUTLEDGE, A., POKEMPNER, M., AND GARCIA, R., 1979, Endometrial cancer and estrogen use: Report of a large case-control study, *N. Engl. J. Med.* **300**:9–13.

BAUER, F. W., AND ROBBINS, S. L., 1972, An autopsy study of cancer patients. I. Accuracy of the clinical diagnoses (1955 to 1965) Boston City Hospital, *J. Am. Med. Assoc.* **221**:1471–1474.

COPELAND, K. T., CHECKOWAY, H., MCMICHAEL, A. J., AND HOLBROOK, R. H., 1977, Bias due to misclassification in the estimation of relative risk, *Am. J. Epidemiol.* **105**:488–495.

COX, E. B., LASZLO, J., AND FREIMAN, A., 1979, Classification of cancer patients beyond TNM, *J. Am. Med. Assoc.* **242**:2691–2695.

CREECH, J. L., JR., AND JOHNSON, M. N., 1974, Angiosarcoma of liver in the manufacture of polyvinyl chloride, *J. Occup. Med.* **16**:150–151.

CUTLER, S. J., AND YOUNG, J. L., JR. (eds.), 1975, *Third National Cancer Survey: Incidence Data*, Natl. *Cancer Inst. Monogr.* **41**.

DOLL, R., AND HILL, A. B., 1950, Smoking and carcinoma of the lung: Preliminary report, *Br. Med. J.* **2**:739–748.

DOLL, R., AND HILL, A. B., 1952, A study of the aetiology of carcinoma of the lung, *Br. Med. J.* **2**:1271–1286.

DOLL, R., AND HILL, A. B., 1956, Lung cancer and other causes of death in relation to smoking: A second report on the mortality of British doctors, *Br. Med. J.* **2**:1071–1081.

DOLL, R., AND PETO, R., 1976, Mortality in relation to smoking: 20 years' observations on male British doctors, *Br. Med. J.* **2**:1525–1536.

DORN, H. F., 1959, Some problems arising in prospective and retrospective studies of the etiology of disease, *N. Engl. J. Med.* **261**:571–579.

DUNN, J. E., JR., 1975, Cancer epidemiology in populations of the United States—with emphasis on Hawaii and California—and Japan, *Cancer Res.* **35**:3240–3245.

ERHARDT, C. L., 1958, What is "the cause of death"?, *J. Am. Med. Assoc.* **168**:161–168.

FEINSTEIN, A. R., 1968, Clinical epidemiology. III. The clinical design of statistics in therapy, *Ann. Intern. Med.* **69**:1287–1312.

FEINSTEIN, A. R., AND SPITZ, H., 1969, The epidemiology of cancer therapy. I. Clinical problems of statistical surveys, *Arch. Intern. Med.* **123**:171–186.

HAENSZEL, W., AND KURIHARA, M., 1968, Studies of Japanese migrants. I. Mortality from cancer and other diseases among Japanese in the United States, *J. Natl. Cancer Inst.* **40**:43–68.

HAENSZEL, W., KURIHARA, M., SEGI, M., AND LEE, R. K. C., 1972, Stomach cancer among Japanese in Hawaii, *J. Natl. Cancer Inst.* **49**:969–988.

HEATH, C. W., JR., FALK, H., AND CREECH, J. L., JR., 1975, Characteristics of cases of angiosarcoma of the liver among vinyl chloride workers in the United States, *Ann. N.Y. Acad. Sci.* **246**:231–236.

HORWITZ, R. I., AND FEINSTEIN, A. R., 1978, Alternative analytic methods for case-control studies of estrogens and endometrial cancer, *N. Engl. J. Med.* **299**:1089–1094.

IBRAHIM, M. A. (ed.), 1979, The case-control study: Consensus and controversy, *J. Chronic Dis.* **32**:1–144.

INMAN, W. H. W., 1979, Comment, *J. Chronic Dis.* **32**:89–90.

JANERICH, D. T., GLEBATIS, D., FLINK, E., AND HOFF, M. B., 1979, Case-control studies on the effect of sex steroids on women and their offspring, *J. Chronic Dis.* **32**:83–88.

LIAVAG, I., HARBITZ, T. B., AND HAUGEN, O. A., 1972, Latent carcinoma of the prostate, *Recent Results Cancer Res.* **39**:131–137.

LYON, J. L., AND GARDNER, J. W., 1977, The rising frequency of hysterectomy: Its effect on uterine cancer rates, *Am. J. Epidemiol.* **105**:439–443.

MACK, T. M., PIKE, M. C., HENDERSON, B. E., PFEFFER, R. I., GERKINS, V. R., ARTHUR, M., AND BROWN, S. E., 1976, Estrogens and endometrial cancer in a retirement community, *N. Engl. J. Med.* **294**:1262–1267.

MCMICHAEL, A. J., 1976, Standardized mortality ratios and the "healthy worker effect": Scratching beneath the surface, *J. Occup. Med.* **18**:165–168.

MANTEL, N., AND HAENSZEL, W., 1959, Statistical aspects of the analysis of data from retrospective studies of disease, *J. Natl. Cancer Inst.* **22**:719–748.

PENNER, D. W., 1973, Quality control and quality evaluation in histopathology and cytology, *Pathol. Annu.* **8**:1–19.

PERCY, C., AND DOLMAN, A., 1978, Comparison of the coding of death certificates related to cancer in seven countries, *Public Health Rep.* **93**:335–350.

SACKETT, D. L., 1979, Bias in analytic research, *J. Chronic Dis.* **32**:51–63.

SARTWELL, P. E., 1974, Retrospective studies: A review for the clinician, *Ann. Intern. Med.* **81**:381–386.

SHAPIRO, S., 1979, Discussion, *J. Chronic Dis.* **32**:47.

SISSONS, H. A., 1975, Agreement and disagreement between pathologists in histological diagnosis, *Postgrad. Med. J.* **51**:685–689.

SMITH, D. C., PRENTICE, R., THOMPSON, D. J., AND HERRMANN, W. L., 1975, Association of exogenous estrogen and endometrial carcinoma, *N. Engl. J. Med.* **293**:1164–1167.

STEMMERMANN, G. N., 1977, Gastric cancer in the Hawaii Japanese, *Gann* **68**:525–535.

TAEUBER, C., 1978, Census, in: *International Encyclopedia of Statistics* (W. H. Kruskal and J. M. Tanur, eds.), pp. 41–46, The Free Press, New York.

VESSEY, M. P., 1979, Discussion, *J. Chronic Dis.* **32**:46.

WALKER, A. M., AND JICK, H., 1979, Temporal and regional variation in hysterectomy rates in the United States, 1970–1975, *Am. J. Epidemiol.* **110**:41–46.

WALTER, S. D., 1977, Determination of significant relative risks and optimal sampling procedures in prospective and retrospective comparative studies of various sizes, *Am. J. Epidemiol.* **105**:387–397.

WATERHOUSE, J., MUIR, C., CORREA, P., AND POWELL, J., (eds.), 1976, *Cancer Incidence in Five Continents*, IARC Scientific Publication 15, Lyon, France.

WEISS, N. S., SZEKELY, D. R., ENGLISH, D. R., AND SCHWEID, A. I., 1979, Endometrial cancer in relation to patterns of menopausal estrogen use, *J. Am. Med. Assoc.* **242**:261–264.

WHITE, K. L., WILLIAMS, T. F., AND GREENBERG, B. G., 1961, The ecology of medical care, *N. Engl. J. Med.* **265**:885–892.

YOUNG, J. L., JR., ASIRE, A. J., AND POLLACK, E. S. (eds.), 1978, *SEER Program: Cancer Incidence and Mortality in the United States 1973-1976*, DHEW Publication No. (NIH) 78-1837, Washington, D.C.

ZELNIK, M., 1964, Errors in the 1960 census enumeration of native whites, *J. Am. Stat. Assoc.* **59**:437–459.

ZIEL, H. K., AND FINKLE, W. D., 1975, Increased risk of endometrial carcinoma among users of conjugated estrogens, *N. Engl. J. Med.* **293**:1167–1170.

7. Selected General References

Cervical Cancer Screening Programs

CLARKE, E. A., AND ANDERSON, T. W., 1979, Does screening by "Pap" smears help prevent cervical cancer? A case-control study, *Lancet* **2**:1–4.

GUZICK, D. S., 1978, Efficacy of screening for cervical cancer: A review, *Am. J. Public Health* **68**:125–134.

JOHANNESSON, G., GEIRSSON, G., AND DAY, N., 1978, The effect of mass screening in Iceland, 1965–74, on the incidence and mortality of cervical carcinoma, *Int. J. Cancer* **21**:418–425.

MILLER, A. B., LINDSAY, J., AND HILL, G. B., 1976, Mortality from cancer of the uterus in Canada and its relationship to screening for cancer of the cervix, *Int. J. Cancer* **17:**602–612.

TASK FORCE APPOINTED BY THE CONFERENCE OF DEPUTY MINISTERS OF HEALTH, 1976, Cervical cancer screening programs, *Can. Med. Assoc. J.* **114:**1003–1033.

Breast Cancer Screening Programs

BAILAR, J. C., III, 1976, Mammography: A contrary view, *Ann. Intern. Med.* **84:**77–84.

SHAPIRO, S., 1977, Evidence on screening for breast cancer from a randomized trial, *Cancer* **39:**2772–2782.

SNYDER, R. E., 1980, Mammography in 1980: An historical perspective and present state of the art, *Clin. Bull.* **10:**3–12.

Smoking and Cancer

FRIEDMAN, G. D., DALES, L. G., AND URY, H. K., 1979, Mortality in middle-aged smokers and nonsmokers, *N. Engl. J. Med.* **300:**213–217.

HAMMOND, E. C., AND HORN, D., 1958, Smoking and death rates—Report on forty-four months of follow-up of 187,783 men. II. Death rates by cause, *J. Am. Med. Assoc.* **166:**1294–1308.

ROGOT, E., AND MURRAY, J. L., 1980, Smoking and causes of death among U.S. veterans: 16 years of observation, *Public Health Rep.* **95:**213–222.

WYNDER, E. L., AND GRAHAM, E. A., 1950, Tobacco smoking as a possible etiologic factor in bronchiogenic carcinoma: A study of six hundred and eighty-four proved cases, *J. Am. Med. Assoc.* **143:**329–336.

Radiation and Cancer

COURT BROWN, W. M., AND DOLL, R., 1965, Mortality from cancer and other causes after radiotherapy for ankylosing spondylitis, *Br. Med. J.* **2:**1327–1332.

MARTLAND, H. S., 1929, Occupational poisoning in manufacture of luminous watch dials: General review of hazard caused by ingestion of luminous paint, with especial reference to the New Jersey cases, *J. Am. Med. Assoc.* **92:**466–473.

MARTLAND, H. S., 1931, The occurrence of malignancy in radioactive persons: A general review of data gathered in the study of the radium dial painters, with special reference to the occurrence of osteogenic sarcoma and the inter-relationship of certain blood diseases, *Am. J. Cancer* **15:**2435–2516.

REFETOFF, S., HARRISON, J., KARANFILSKI, B. T., KAPLAN, E. L., DE GROOT, L. J., AND BEKERMAN, C., 1975, Continuing occurrence of thyroid carcinoma after irradiation to the neck in infancy and childhood, *N. Engl. J. Med.* **292:**171–175.

SHARPE, W. D., 1978, The New Jersey radium dial painters: An occupational carcinogenesis, *Bull. Hist. Med.* **52:**560–570.

SOCOLOW, E. L., HASHIZUME, A., NERIISHI, S., AND NIITANI, R., 1963, Thyroid carcinoma in man after exposure to ionizing radiation: A summary of the findings in Hiroshima and Nagasaki, *N. Engl. J. Med.* **268:**406–410.

WRIGHT, E. S., AND COUVES, C. M., 1977, Radiation-induced carcinoma of the lung—The St. Lawrence tragedy, *J. Thorac. Cardiovasc. Surg.* **74:**495–498.

Occupational Mortality Studies

BAUMGARTEN, M., AND OSEASOHN, R., 1980, Studies on occupational health: A critique, *J. Occup. Med.* **22:**171–176.

ENTERLINE, P. E., 1964, The estimation of expected rates in occupational disease epidemiology, *Public Health Rep.* **79**:973–978.

MARSH, G. M., AND ENTERLINE, P. E., 1979, A method for verifying the completeness of cohorts used in occupational mortality studies, *J. Occup. Med.* **21**:665–670.

OLSEN, J., AND SABROE, S., 1979, Researching occupational mortality: The problem of comparison, *Scand. J. Soc. Med.* **7**:1–6.

Textbooks

FRAUMENI, J. F., JR. (ed.), 1975, *Persons at High Risk of Cancer: An Approach to Cancer Etiology and Control*, Academic Press, New York.

LILIENFELD, A. M., PEDERSEN, E., AND DOWD, J. E., 1967, *Cancer Epidemiology: Methods of Study*, The Johns Hopkins Press, Baltimore.

LILIENFELD, A. M., LEVIN, M. L., AND KESSLER, I. I., 1972, *Cancer in the United States*, Harvard University Press, Cambridge, Mass.

MacLENNAN, R., MUIR, C., STEINITZ, R., AND WINKLER, A., 1978, *Cancer Registration and Its Techniques*, IARC Scientific Publication 21, Lyon, France.

MacMAHON, B., PUGH, T. F. AND IPSEN, J., 1960, *Epidemiologic Methods*, Little, Brown, Boston.

MASON, T. J., McKAY, F. W., HOOVER, R., BLOT, W. J., AND FRAUMENI, J. F., JR., 1976, *Atlas of Cancer Mortality for U.S. Counties: 1950–1969*, DHEW Publication No. (NIH) 75-780, Washington, D.C.

Chemical Carcinogenesis

Chemical Agents, the Environment, and the History of Carcinogenesis

FREDERICK F. BECKER

1. Introduction

It is evident from the studies reported in other chapters that the examination of the interactions of chemical carcinogens (as modified by numerous factors) with target macromolecules of target cells has achieved a remarkable degree of sophistication and has resulted in an enormous increase in knowledge. Despite this, there is no aspect of this process, from the early macromolecular alterations within the exposed cells to the demise of the host, that is fully understood. Further, knowledge of these promising advances and the gaps that still exist, as well as the threat of the process of chemical carcinogenesis, has intruded into the awareness of the public and with it fear, misinformation, political intervention, and often conflicts between scientists in the public arena. The key to the impact of this area on scientists and the public has been the revelation of the intimate relationship between man and the world milieu that we term generically the *environment*. However, examination of the use of this term reveals a diversity of definition among differing interests, and the failure to hold a common meaning has led to further confusion. In the field of carcinogenesis, the term "environment" has often been equated with "pollution" (an equally ill-defined term); from there the extrapolation to "chemical agents" is but a word away, and the concept "occupation" is just around the semantic corner.

FREDERICK F. BECKER • Department of Anatomic and Research Pathology, M. D. Anderson Hospital and Tumor Institute, University of Texas System Cancer Center, Houston, Texas.

Indeed, the misconception that these terms are synonymous has caused a number of students of the impact of the environment to devote considerable effort to its clarification. The major exponent of clarification has been Higginson, who in his briefest exposition said, "... environment is what surrounds people and impinges on them. The air you breathe, the culture you live in, the agricultural habits of your community, the social cultural habits, the social pressures and the physical chemicals with which you come in contact, the diet and so on..." (Higginson, 1976, 1979). The enrichment of this term by increasing detail has been the contribution of many workers, as delineated by Wynder and Gori (1977). They categorized environmental carcinogens as follows:

> ... Environmental carcinogens, either established or suspected, may be categorized as being related either to personal lifestyle (tobacco, alcohol, sunlight, occupational exposure, and nutritional imbalances) or to general environmental factors (air and water pollution, drugs, and food additives as contaminants). Some are derived through individual choices; others are imposed by society....

In view of the vast implications of this redefined concept to the area of carcinogenesis and the potential role of physical and viral agents, this introductory chapter will focus only on the chemical aspects of the process. Further, it will focus mainly on the historical contributions of observation and epidemiologic and clinical studies, and only briefly on the early phases of laboratory investigation. Indeed, I will devote much of its content to the delineation of unanswered questions and areas of controversy.

Therefore, the first question to ask is, when did it all begin? Has chemical carcinogenesis (subsequently to be termed carcinogenesis) always been with us? Zimmerman (1977) summarized a vast number of studies of paleopathology and concluded that the relative absence of tumors in ancient times must be considered a reflection of a markedly lower incidence than that in recent populations. Indeed, tumors in thousands of preserved human species are not of the type(s) now considered to be related to exposure to chemicals.

Since "awareness" is an important operative term in the area of carcinogenesis, we might next ask what the sequence of "awareness" has been. In 1761, John Hill of London published his "Cautions Against Immoderate Use of Snuff," in which he reported six cases of "polypusses" related to indulgence in tobacco in the form of snuff.

> ... Whether or not polypusses, which attend snuff-takers, are absolutely caused by that custom; or whether the principals of the disorder were there before, and snuff only irritated the parts, and hastened the mischief, I shall not pretend to determine; but even supposing the latter only to be the case, the damage is certainly more than the indulgence is worth.... No man should venture upon snuff, who is not sure that he is not so far liable to cancer; and no man can be sure of that.... [See Shimkin, 1977, for this and many other valuable historical references.]

Hill's report preceded by over a decade the description of scrotal cancer in chimney sweeps by Percival Pott (Redmond, 1970). It is intriguing to note that some 200 years ago, Hill seemed to be cognizant of the multifaceted nature of the problem of carcinogenesis, i.e., a life-style that includes tobacco use and even the possible intervention of genetics. That this problem is current is indicated by the studies of Blot and Fraumeni (1977), who demonstrated a connection between snuff (and similar products) and oral cancer. The current advertising campaigns for "smokeless tobacco" suggest that the problem may eventually enter log phase and that at the very least, famous athletes are high-risk candidates.

If Hill's report can be considered to be the first to emphasize the involvement of life-style, Pott must be known as the instigator of awareness of the potential contribution of occupation. His description in 1775 of "Cancer of the scrotum in chimney sweeps" leaves no doubt that this was recognized as an occupational disease. From his "Chirurgical observations relative to the cataract, the polypus of the nose, the cancer of the scrotum, the different kinds of ruptures and mortification of the toes and feet" (Pott, 1775):

> . . . There is a disease as peculiar to a certain set of people which has not, at least to my knowledge been publicly noticed; I mean the chimney-sweepers' cancer. It is a disease which always makes its first appearance in the inferior part of the scrotum; where it produces a superficial, painful, ragged, ill-looking sore with hard and rising edges. The trade call it the soot-wart. I never saw it under the age of puberty, which is, I suppose, one reason, why it is generally taken, both by patient and surgeon, for venereal, and being treated with mercurials, is thereby soon, and much exasperated: in no great length of time, it pervades the skin, dartos, and membranes of the scrotum, and seizes the testicle, which it enlarges, hardens, and renders truly and thoroughly distempered; from whence it makes its way up the speramatic process into the abdomen, most frequently indurating, and spoiling the inguinal glands: when arrived within the abdomen it affects some of the viscera, and then very soon becomes painfully destructive.
>
> . . . the fate of these people seems singularly hard; in their early infancy, they are most frequently treated with great brutality, and almost starved with cold and hunger; they are thrust up narrow, and sometimes hot chimnies, where they are bruised, burned, and almost suffocated; and when they get to puberty, become peculiarly liable to a most noisome, painful, and fatal disease.
>
> Of this last circumstance there is not the least doubt, though perhaps it may not have been sufficiently attended to, to make it generally known. Other people have cancers of the same parts; and so have others, beside lead-workers, the Poictou colic and the consequent paralysis; but it it nevertheless a disease to which they are peculiarly liable; and so are chimney-sweepers to the cancer of the scrotum and testicles. The disease in these people seems to derive its origin from the lodgement of soot in the rugae of the scrotum, and at first not to be a disease of the habit.

Thus, with great clarity was delineated the differences between a selected occupational group that was at high risk for a specific cancer and the general population.

The factors preventing acceptance and public health intervention of this seminal finding of a relationship between occupation and cancer mirror strikingly the factors in the smoking controversy of more recent history. Populations of chimney sweeps in other countries, due to personal habits of cleanliness, did not demonstrate the disease, and the importance of the variation of life-style was not realized. Further, it would be many years before carcinogenic agents from soot would be isolated, purified, and demonstrated to be active. Lastly, any genetic variability that might affect incidence was unknown.

I have summarized my interpretation of the principles that Pott's findings have engendered as follows.

1. *Unusual population:* The clinical observation of tumor excess in a selected population must give rise to concern for an etiologic agent in the environment. Thus, whether in chimney sweeps (an occupational group) or pubescent females whose mothers were exposed to diethylstilbestrol (treatment-related group), it is the nature of the population that attracts attention. Thus, even a nation or a "people" could be construed to exemplify this "law," as in the case of hepatocellular carcinoma described below.

2. *Unusual tumors:* It is apparent that the likelihood of detecting the effect of a chemical agent is much greater if the tumor that results is rare. Thus, it was adenocarcinoma of the vagina, rare in any age group, occurring in pubescent females that suggested to an astute clinician that an etiologic agent might be involved. Of even greater rarity, angiosarcoma of the liver was the marker for the effect of vinyl chloride. Perhaps this then is a corollary; the rarer the tumor, the more we should question any increase in incidence. Perhaps, we should question the occurrence of a single tumor. As the tumor induced is more like the type that might be expected in the general population or age group, e.g., oropharyngeal tumors in smelter workers, mesotheliomas in asbestos workers, or bladder and lung tumors in chemical workers, the less likely a chemical etiology will be recognized. This leads to the third law, which applies to the greatest number of people.

3. *Endemic tumors:* Recognition that a specific tumor may be endemic to a given area has occurred with increasing frequency. That these tumors (foci in this instance being equated with areas as broad as segments of a continent) may be associated with an environmental agent has gained wide acceptance. Geographically determined entities such as hepatocellular carcinoma of Africa, Southeast Asia, and China or the esophageal malignancies of Iran, Yugoslavia, and China are now under intensive investigation.

Occupational foci, such as the lung cancers of those exposed to asbestos and uranium products and the bladder cancers of the chemical industry, have signaled the introduction of a carcinogen into the environment. Case numbers may range in the hundreds, potentially thousands, or be as few as one or two (such as the vinyl chloride-associated angiosarcoma of liver) and yet suggest an endemic quality. Indeed, these contrasts may even be evident in populations as close as adjacent hospitals. Thus, for more than 75 years, the rate of hepatocellular carcinoma per admission at Bellevue, the prototypic municipal hospital of New York City, exceeded that of its neighbor University Hospital, a private hospital, by 20-fold. So, too, has the rate of alcoholism and cirrhosis in the hospital for the indigent patient exceeded that of the fee-for-service hospital (Becker, 1975).

2. Laboratory Studies

Despite the clear evidence for the presence of environmental carcinogens that can be derived from the presence of endemic foci, an enormous effort may be required before the etiologic agent is identified, and the process is highly dependent on the state of the art. Although the presence of endemic foci of hepatocellular carcinoma in man has been known for many years, the etiologic factors suggested as the basis for this phenomenon depended upon the concepts of the pathogenesis of disease commonly accepted to be valid at the time. Thus, in sequence, it was suggested that these foci resulted from parasitic infestation, malnutrition, and iron excess (Becker, 1974). The next thrust forward was the recognition of the presence of the powerful, fungal hepatocarcinogen aflatoxin in these areas. First recognized as a potent hepatotoxin in animals, then as a hepatocarcinogen, and finally in a series of brilliant chemical–epidemiologic studies as a major contaminant of foodstuffs in the endemic areas, the incrimination of aflatoxin as the environmental carcinogen seemed one of the most successful searches of its type and lasted for a decade (Wogan, 1973, 1976). However, within the last few years we have been made aware that there exists a hepatitic virus carrier-state in these same endemic foci and in the same populations that demonstrate hepatocellular carcinomas (Ohta, 1976). Since the final answer is not yet available in this instance and although the possibility exists that immunization against the virus will eventually settle the question, it remains a classic example of environmental detection.

One other aspect of the hepatocellular "story" warrants mention. Both of the incriminated agents, aflatoxin and viruses, have been associated with endemic foci of animal tumors that were either recognized as an early signal of the effect of the agent or are now under study as a model for transmission and pathogenesis. Thus, for aflatoxin, an endemic focus in swine predated recognition of the carcinogen by approximately 20 years, and tumors of hatchery-raised trout were the final "signal" (Ninard and Hinterman, 1945). For the hepatitis virus, an almost identical viral carrier–hepatocellular carcinoma sequence has been identified in the eastern American woodchuck (Snyder, 1968). Our awareness, therefore, should be sharpened to include such animal foci as markers of the intrusion of a carcinogenic agent into our environment.

Another complication of unraveling the nature of carcinogenesis is the finding that the etiology of a given type of tumor in different endemic foci may differ. Thus, at present, the poasible bases suggested for widespread foci of esophageal malignancy have ranged from heavy metals through activation of nitrosamines by fungus-associated infections (Hutt and Burkitt, 1977).

The history of the 150 years following Pott's observation contains a series of observations that further implicated environmental and, in particular, occupational agents in the evocation of malignancy. Although occasionally contended, it is generally accepted that the work of Yamagiwa and Ichikawa in 1918 marked the transition from the stage of observatin to that of laboratory experimentation. By chronic painting of rabbit ears with coal tars, they were able to induce tumors, the first major link to modern carcinogenic research. Thus began a series of superb studies in which laboratory experiments would confirm impressions derived from clinical observation. In rapid order the relationship of lung cancer in workers in coal and gas manufacture with exposure to mustard gas was established, as was 4-aminodiphenyl with bladder tumors and many others (e.g., Table 1 of Davies, 1976, p. 256).

In more recent work, the end of that chain of association has been achieved, with laboratory studies suggesting the potential for carcinogenicity of substances in man prior to clinical observation. Thus, the laboratory work of Maltoni and Lefemine in 1974 first indicated the unusual carcinogenic capability of vinyl chloride in liver.

Today, an ever-lengthening list of tumors associated with occupational exposure is available, and many of these have been confirmed by exposure of laboratory animals. Many more remain controversial. Even more controversial, however, are estimates of the occupational contribution to the total cancer burden. Many reasons exist for this problem. The first may be the method of extrapolation, from the highest risk group (asbestos) and from maximum exposures. Perhaps the most important, however, is the difficulty of determining the levels and total time of exposure(s). Further complications include mobile populations, socioeconomic factors, race, and sex. Regardless of these problems, the message after 200 years should be clear: our suspicion must be high. Conditions associated with prolonged exposure to chemical agents should be subjected to maximum experimental expertise as quickly as possible.

Elsewhere in this volume, the approaches available for the evaluation of a potential carcinogenic exposure are discussed in detail. However, since a common sense evaluation of these new approaches is rarely evident in discussion of these topics, let us for a moment attempt an unusual approach. All other components being equal, the ultimate environmental protection would be based upon a rapid and accurate test of carcinogenicity (Ames *et al.*, 1973; McCann and Ames, 1976). Whether a worker has a prolonged or a short exposure to a carcinogenic substance, its immediate removal from his environment is of obvious benefit. The problems that exist in this approach are delineated by DeSerres, and they consist mainly of the need to develop a group of rapid assays with as few false-positive and false-negative results as possible. Although a positive assay would still leave the question of acceptable level (if such exists; see below) unanswered, it seems certain that eventually such assays will have a sufficient level of correlation with animal tumor studies to offer reasonable extrapolation.

One could fill the pages of several books with the steady, progressive steps by which we trace progress in the field of chemical carcinogenesis as related to the environment, from the papers of Yamagiwa and Ishikawa (1918) until today. For reference I recommend especially the work of Doll (1975), Davies (1976), Wynder and Gori (1977), Hiatt *et al.* (1977), Griffin and Shaw (1979), Fraumeni (1979), and Doll (1980).

3. Current Problems

It appears to me, however, that recent history can be best characterized by two major foci of interest. *The first is the realization that our life-style may be a major*

component of the total carcinogenic problem. The most potent finding of the current
scientific age in this regard was the association of smoking with cancer, and later
with a vast panorama of human ills (Doll and Hill, 1964). No other finding has
so influenced the attempt to alter the life-style of millions. The problem of tobacco
use has begotten a vast search for safer cigarettes, for filters, and for means of
reversing or making dormant the sequence of tissue alteration. This awareness
of the perpetual truth in Shakespeare's prose is nowhere better exemplified than
in "The fault is not in our stars, but in ourselves." Thus, the current major
studies of the effects of diet, alcohol, and a myriad of other factors, although
controversial and uncertain, seem to me to offer a prospect as bright as the
eventual removal of carcinogens (see Nagao and Sugimura, 1978; Hutt and
Burkitt, 1977; and the reviews discussed above).

The second major area of advance has resulted from *an increasing awareness
of the importance of cocarcinogens and, in particular, of the so-called promoting agents*
(Berenblum, 1979). Now classic as an example of the former is asbestos.
The story of its synergism with carcinogens is well reported (see Selikoff *et al.*,
1968). It is the prototype for a synergism that may require the regulation of
"noncarcinogenic" but highly active cocarcinogens. It has made us aware of
"incidental" contamination of the air and of the lag between exposure and
onset.

However, even this example is relatively uncomplicated compared to that
which may result from the regulation of promoters (see Farber, this volume).
These noncarcinogenic substances are highly active in inducing a full carcinogenic sequence after subcarcinogenic exposure to an active carcinogen. They
may range from esoteric derivatives of plants to common drugs. With increasing
speed, laboratory tests, which use animals, cells, or bacteria, are emerging and
have the potential for identifying these substances or this function. What then
will be the socioeconomic hazards and pressures to regulate these agents despite
their lack of carcinogenicity? Interestingly, almost 20 years ago, Roe, Salaman,
and Cohen (1959) presented evidence that cigarette smoke was a powerful
promoter as well as a carcinogen, a concept already proposed by Wynder (see
Roe *et al.*, 1959).

Perhaps the greatest problem of the next decade will be one of sorting the
important from the trivial. Of what importance is the finding (Commoner *et al.*,
1978) of small quantities of mutagens in a grilled hamburger? Is this experiment
as trivial as it would appear? If so, why would an important journal publish it
at all? Why would the media make it a major event? Perhaps it has significance
in terms of our total exposure to "mutagens" (Blum and Ames, 1977). However,
the significance of mutagens themselves remains to be demonstrated and represents a gap in our understanding of the process of carcinogenesis.

How will the political–scientific controversies be settled unless scientists answer
the basic and fundamental questions by focusing their efforts and funds and
avoiding trivia. For the response to a series of such announcements may lead
to what I have termed the saccharin backlash, which will be far from sweet
(Smith, 1980).

As I described at the beginning of this chapter, the socioeconomic implications of this field have assumed the status of media events; in the coliseum of the media, scientists are pitted in adversarial conflict, while political figures (to carry the image a bit further), like Roman senators, offer thumbs up or down on scientific–medical decisions. Diabetologists and obesiologists fight vigorously for saccharin; jokes are offered about "Canadian" rats. These conflicts stem from a plethora of questions that remain to be answered by appropriate experimentation and from the failure to explain the findings to the public appropriately. Some of these questions are discussed below.

1. *Why are such huge doses of carcinogens used?* In brief, the total dose of a chemical agent accumulated during exposure of man can only be simulated during the short life span of a rodent by these high doses. Further, to achieve a statistically significant result, limited as we are to relatively small numbers of animals (in comparison to man), we must accentuate the maximum opportunity for tumor development. This is especially true in the instance of weak carcinogens. Further, the long exposure, and often the subsequent long lag characteristic of human situations, must be reduced for a life span of 2 years.

2. *If all of these problems exist, why use the mouse or rat, and, further, are these results valid as extrapolated to man?*

Time, money, and statistics dictate the use of these animals. Only small animals can be maintained in sufficient numbers at "reasonable" cost to obtain statistically valid results in a relatively short period of time. The question of a valid extrapolation to man has been the keystone of arguments for and against this approach. Therefore, some comments on this topic are warranted.

A. Almost every agent that has been demonstrated to be carcinogenic in man has been carcinogenic in such animals. Further, several agents first demonstrated to be carcinogenic in animals were later shown to be so in man.

B. The metabolic activation and deactivation of carcinogenic agents and, when testable, the macromolecular interactions in these animals are similar or identical to those in man.

C. Perhaps the most controversial problem has been the interpretation of the significance of the tumors that result in rodents. Most of the malignancies induced in rodents by such agents simulate those seen in man. However, controversy occurs when the tumors are benign (or possibly premalignant) or demonstrate only very low-grade malignant behavior. These are lesions that morphologically do not possess the stigmata of malignancy and either fail to grow on transplantation or do so poorly. This is even more problematic when the test animal, such as the B6C3 mouse, has a basal level of spontaneous tumors. The assumption, legal or otherwise, has been offered that agents that evoke premalignant lesions should also be considered as carcinogens. However, as more data that characterize the malignancy of these tumors by objective biologic or biochemical means are accumulated, these problems should be reduced. For example, it is becoming evident that chemical agents induce a group of hepatocellular tumors that differ strikingly from those that arise spontaneously. Thus, it may be that in such mice the chemical agent acts as a promoter for spontaneous tumors and as a carcinogen for others.

D. What is the significance of the induction of a few tumors in a small number of animals? No definitive answer to this question now exists. However, a typical extrapolation to exposed human populations might suggest that several thousand tumors might result. Not an impressive number when the exposed population numbers in the millions, but very impressive to that person who is part of the positive population. And if there is validity to the argument that the number calculated might be excessive, the converse may also be true.

E. The no-dose or low-dose controversy has raged continuously for several decades. The infamous *Delaney clause* has been the keystone of much of this controversy:

> . . . no additive shall be deemed to be safe if it is found to induce cancer when ingested by man or animal, or if it is found, after tests which are appropriate for the evaluation of the safety of food additives, to induce cancer in man or animal. . . . [21 United States Code Service 348(c)(3)(a), 1972]

Such additives are therefore proscribed without regard to the magnitude of the risk at levels found in human exposure and without regard to possible benefits.

Even if we recognize the postulates upon which this law rests as reasonable and attempt to solve the problems of whether a given agent is carcinogenic, other major problems exist. Since this law was promulgated, analytic techniques have developed degrees of sensitivity not previously conceived of. It has been said, half in jest, that no safe level is possible on the face of this planet. These findings have led to the controversy of whether any level of exposure to such agents is noncarcinogenic. Such discussions cannot "factor" for the capacity of the cell to repair or for exposure to multiple agents, but are based mainly on statistical or mathematical arguments that are best examined directly by the reader (Kotin, 1976; Maugh, 1978; Wahrendorf, 1979). Currently, there is no single answer to this problem. However, all of these factors have added to the growing concept of a "sensible" Delaney clause. This approach would take into consideration whether an agent was weakly or strongly carcinogenic and, even more so, the risk/benefit ratio (Cornfield, 1977).

F. Risk/benefit ratio: It is recognized that several chemotherapeutic agents used in the treatment of malignancy may be carcinogenic. This is particularly true of the alkylating agents. Yet, faced with certain death from the primary tumor without treatment by the agent, the patient is offered little choice. This is risk/benefit at its most obvious level. However, when that ratio is controversial (Smith, 1980) and reputable scientist-physicians plead for an agent's retention, e.g., saccharin for diabetics, the decision is far from clear. Indeed, these problems await better scientific and perhaps philosophical definition before their solution.

Scientific data (or its lack), socioeconomic factors, and semantics are the components of the current controversies in environmental chemical carcinogenesis. Therefore, it is fitting to end this chapter by a brief discussion of the single phrase that best exemplifies to me all of these problems, i.e., "food additives" (Jukes, 1977; Lehmann, 1979). To the population at large this term has become a red flag, or a red dye, that connotes the evils of modern civilization and science. Conceived of as universally bad, often carcinogenic, they are better out, not in! In some cases this conception is obviously true, and several of these dyes and preservatives are now well-recognized, indeed laboratory models of, chemical carcinogens.

To further state the obvious, several of these are vital to the quality of food and some may even have anticarcinogenic properties. One of the factors that has been suggested to play a role in the decrease in stomach cancer during the last three decades has been the inclusion of antioxidants in our foods. Thus, lack of accepted methods for quickly testing these agents for carcinogenicity, of accepted extrapolation from animal to man, of acceptable no-threshold or low-threshold studies, and of methods for evaluating risk/benefit guarantee continuing controversy.

However, that some food additives may be beneficial offers one possible answer to the single most-puzzling question in the area of nonoccupational, environmental carcinogenesis: *Where are the tumors?* Despite some four decades of intense and increasing exposure to a variety of "carcinogens" in the environment, a very limited increase in human tumors is now evident (the quotation marks indicate that this designation was often based solely on a variety of animal test systems). Considering the length of exposure to this environment of at least three to four decades for millions of people, the fact that they were exposed through sensitive periods *in utero* and through childhood, and that a significant lag has been completed, it is reasonable to expect that a strikingly steep, rising slope should now be evident. At the very least, this should be evident for hepatocellular carcinoma, since a large number of the incriminated agents that were eventually proscribed from the environment are liver carcinogens. Further, it has been clearly documented that such agents can act synergistically, whether given together or sequentially (Becker, 1975).

Thus, where are the hepatocellular malignancies? I do not mean to end this chapter by suggesting that the problem of environmental chemical carcinogenesis is not a real one or that it is not threatening. Rather, I wish to end with the observation that this complex process is far from fully understood and remains one of the vital medical–scientific problems of our time.

References

AMES, B. N., MCCANN, J., LEE, F. D., AND DURSTON, W. E., 1973, An improved bacterial test system for the detection and classification of mutagens and carcinogens, *Proc. Natl. Acad. Sci. USA* **70:**782.

BECKER, F. F., 1974, Hepatoma: Nature's model tumor, *Am. J. Pathol.* **74:**179.

BECKER, F. F., 1975, Alteration of hepatocytes by subcarcinogenic exposure to *N*-2-fluorenylacetamide, *Cancer Res.* **35:**1734.

BERENBLUM, I., 1979, Theoretical and practical aspects of the two-stage mechanism of carcinogenesis, in: *Carcinogens: Identification and Mechanisms of Action* (A. C. Griffin and C. R. Shaw, eds.), pp. 25–36, Raven Press, New York.

BLOT, W. J., AND FRAUMENI, J. F., JR, 1977, Geographic patterns of oral cancer in the United States: Etiologic implications, *J. Chronic Dis.* **30**:745.

BLUM, A., AND AMES, B. N., 1977, Flame-retardant additives as possible cancer hazards, *Science* **195**:17.

COMMONER, J., VITHAYATHIL, A. J., DOLLARA, P., NAIR, S., MABYASTHA, P., AND CUCA, G. C., 1978, Formation of mutagens in beef and beef extract during cooking, *Science* **201**:913.

CORNFIELD, J., 1977, Carcinogenic risk assessment, *Science* **198**:693.

DAVIES, J. M., 1976, Occupational cancer, in: *Scientific Foundations in Oncology* (T. Symington and R. L. Carter, eds.), p. 256, Heinemann, London.

DOLL, R., 1975, Pott and prospects for prevention, *Br. J. Cancer* **32**:263.

DOLL, R., 1980, The epidemiology of cancer, *Cancer* **45**:2475.

DOLL, R., AND HILL, A. B., 1964, Mortality in relation to smoking: Ten years' observations of British doctors, *Br. J. Med.* **1**:1460.

FRAUMENI, J. F., JR., 1979, Epidemiological studies of cancer, in: *Carcinogens: Identification and Mechanisms of Action* (A. C. Griffin and C. R. Shaw, eds.), pp. 51–63, Raven Press, New York.

GRIFFIN, A. C., AND SHAW, C. R. (eds.), 1979, *Carcinogens: Identification and Mechanisms of Action*, Raven Press, New York.

HIATT, H. H., WATSON, J. D., AND WINSTEN, J. A. (eds.), 1977, *Origins of Human Cancer*, Books A–C, Cold Spring Harbor Laboratories, Cold Spring Harbor, N.Y.

HIGGINSON, J., 1976, A hazardous society? Individual vs. community responsibility in cancer prevention, *Am. J. Public Health* **66**: 359.

HIGGINSON, J., 1979, Cancer and environment, *Science* **205**:1363.

HIGGINSON, J., AND MUIR, C. S., 1979, Environmental carcinogenesis: Misconceptions and limitations to cancer control, *J. Natl. Cancer Inst.* **63**:191.

HUTT, M. S. R., AND BURKITT, D. P., 1977, Epidemiology of cancer, in: *Recent Advances in Medicine* (D. N. Baron, N. Compston, and A. M. Dawson, eds.), p. 1, Churchill Livingstone, London.

JUKES, T. H., 1977, Food additives, *N. Engl. J. Med.* **297**:427.

KOTIN, P., 1976, Dose–response relationship and threshold concepts, *Ann. N.Y. Acad. Sci.* **271**:22.

LEHMANN, T., 1979, *FDA Consumer* (June) **13**(5): 13–15.

MALTONI, G., AND LEFEMINE, G., 1974, Carcinogenicity bioassays of vinyl-chloride. I. Research plan and early results, *Environ. Res.* **7**:387.

MAUGH, T. H., 1978, Chemical carcinogens: How dangerous are low doses? *Science* **202**:37.

MCCANN, J., AND AMES, B. N., 1976, Detection of carcinogens as mutagens in the *Salmonella*/microsome test: Assay of 300 chemicals: Discussion, *Proc. Natl. Acad. Sci. U.S.A.* **73**:950.

NAGAO, M., AND SUGIMURA, T., 1978, Environmental mutagens and carcinogens, *Annu. Rev. Genet.* **12**:117.

NINARD, B., AND HINTERMAN, J., 1945, Les tumeurs de la tiaree hepatique chez le porc au maroc de 1944–1946, *Bull. Inst. Hyg. Maroc* **5**:59.

OHTA, Y., 1976, Viral hepatitis and hepatocellular carcinoma, in: *Hepatocellular Carcinoma* (K. Okada and R. L. Peters, eds.), p. 76, Wiley, New York.

POTT, P., 1775, *Chirurgical Observations Relative to the Cataract, the Polypus of the Nose, the Cancer of the Scrotum, the Different Kinds of Ruptures, and the Mortification of the Toes and Feet*, Hawkes, Clarke and Collins, London.

REDMOND, D. E., 1970, Tobacco and cancer: The first clinical report, 1776, *N. Engl. J. Med.* **282**:18.

ROE, F. J., SALAMAN, M. H., AND COHEN, J., 1959, Incomplete carcinogens in cigarette smoke condensate: Tumor promotion by a phenolic fraction, *Br. J. Cancer* **13**:623.

SELIKOFF, I. J., HAMMOND, C., AND CHURG, J., 1968, Asbestos exposure, smoking, and neoplasia, *J. Am. Med. Assoc.* **204**:106.

SHIMKIN, M. B., 1977, *Contrary to Nature*, U.S. Department of Health, Education and Welfare, U.S. Government Printing Offices, Washington, D.C.

SMITH, R. J., 1980, Latest saccharin tests kill FDA proposal, *Science* **208**:154.

SNYDER, R. L., 1968, Hepatomas of captive woodchucks, *Am. J. Pathol.* **52**:32a.

21 UNITED STATES CODE SERVICE 348(c)(3)(a), 1972, Lawyers Cooperative Publishing Co., Rochester, N.Y., p. 227.

WAHRENDORF, J., 1979, The problem of estimating safe dose levels in chemical carcinogenesis, *J. Cancer Res. Clin. Oncol.* **95**:101.

WOGAN, G. N., 1973, Aflatoxin carcinogenesis, *Methods Cancer Res.* **7**:309.

WOGAN, G. N., 1976, Aflatoxins and their relationship to hepatocellular carcinoma, in: *Hepatocellular Carcinoma* (K. Okada and R. L. Peters, eds.), p. 25, Wiley, New York.

240

FREDERICK F.
BECKER

WYNDER, E. K., AND GORI, G. B., 1977, Contribution of the environmental cancer incidence: An epidemiologic exercise, *J. Natl. Cancer Inst.* **58:**825.

YAMAGIWA, K., AND ISHIKAWA, K., 1918, Experimental study of the pathogenesis of carcinoma, *J. Cancer Res.* **3:**1.

ZIMMERMAN, M. R., 1977, An experimental study of mummification pertinent to the antiquity of cancer, *Cancer* **40:**1358.

9

Metabolism of Chemical Carcinogens

J. H. WEISBURGER AND G. M. WILLIAMS

1. Cancer, A Class of Diseases Due Mainly to Environmental Factors: Synthetic or Naturally Occurring

The concept that some types of cancer might be caused by environmental factors traces back to the observation of the English physician Pott in the late 18th century that human scrotal cancer in Great Britain was associated with the occupation of his affected patients as chimney sweeps. Since that time, people in other occupations have been demonstrated to have certain risks of developing cancer at some sites. Overall, however, occupational cancers are relatively rare events that affect only limited numbers of individuals (Saffiotti and Wagoner, 1976; Wynder and Gori, 1977; Higginson in Emmelot and Kriek, 1979; Higginson and Muir, 1981; Sontag, 1981). The bulk of human cancers were until recently considered to stem from unknown elements. It was primarily the examination of international incidence rates of various types of cancer, and the fact that the incidence depends in part on the site of residence, that led to the concept that many types of human cancer are caused, mediated, or modified by environmental factors (Higginson and Muir, 1981; Haenszel in Fraumeni, 1975;

J. H. WEISBURGER • American Health Foundation, Naylor Dana Institute for Disease Prevention, Valhalla, New York. Supported in part by Grants CA-17613, CA-15400, CA-21393, and CA-24217 and Contracts CP-75948 and CP-75940 from the National Cancer Institute, NIH, U. S. Public Health Service, and Grant OH00611 from the National Institute of Occupational Safety and Health.
G. M. WILLIAMS • American Health Foundation, Naylor Dana Institute for Disease Prevention, Valhalla, New York. Supported in part by Grants CA-17613, CA-12376, and CA-15400 and Contracts CP-55705, CP-85659, and CP-75952 from the National Cancer Institute, NIH, U. S. Public Health Service.

242

J. H.
WEISBURGER
AND
G. M.
WILLIAMS

Wynder and Hirayama, 1977; Doll in Emmelot and Kriek, 1979; Hirayama, 1979). Thus, examination of the incidence of two types of cancer of the digestive tract, namely stomach cancer and large-bowel cancer, in populations in Europe, Latin America, Japan, and the North American continent indicated clearly that they have quite different causative and modifying elements, but both are associated mainly with dietary factors. Lung cancer, on the other hand, has been definitely traced in most cases to the personal habit of cigarette smoking (Hammond in Hiatt *et al.*, 1977; Doll in Emmelot and Kriek, 1979; Wynder and Hoffmann, 1979). In all of these instances, it is quite certain that specific types of chemicals or mixtures of chemicals are the determining factors. Thus, overall, the majority of human cancer may be due to chemicals, either as naturally occurring chemicals or as chemical mixtures in diet, the nature of which remains to be defined in many instances, or as specific types of synthetic chemicals, for which exposure occurs mainly in the occupational setting.

The best way of controlling cancer is through primary prevention. This can be achieved most effectively by identification of the responsible carcinogens and their elimination. In addition, as will be developed in this chapter, many carcinogens are of a type that undergo biotransformation in the host. Such metabolism usually leads to detoxification and elimination but, unfortunately, also results in activation reactions leading to initiation of neoplastic development. This sometimes complex process proceeds to different extents as a function of many modulating, but not usually essential variables such as genetic background, age, sex, diet, and other environmental conditions. Thus, understanding of the factors involved in the ultimate disposition of carcinogens permits appreciation of environmental conditions that determine the risk for ultimate cancer development. Modification of these factors provides a means for the prevention or "chemoprevention" of neoplastic disease.

2. Types of Chemical Carcinogens

Chemical carcinogens are defined operationally by their ability to induce tumors. Four types of response have generally been accepted as evidence of tumorigenicity: (1) an increased incidence of the tumor types occurring in controls; (2) the occurrence of tumors earlier than in controls; (3) the development of types of tumors not seen in controls; and (4) an increased multiplicity of tumors in individual animals. Chemicals capable of eliciting one of these tumorigenic responses, and which are thereby classified as carcinogens, comprise a highly diverse collection, including organic and inorganic chemicals, solid-state materials, hormones, and immunosuppressants. For some of these chemicals, such as tumor enhancers or promoters, the designation "carcinogen" is perhaps unfortunate, but inescapable, since these chemicals in specific situations do increase the yield of spontaneously occurring cancers. In order to draw attention to the differences in properties of the diverse agents that can be considered as

TABLE 1
Classification of Carcinogenic Chemicals

Carcinogen class	Example
Genotoxic	
Activation-independent	Alkylating agent
Activation-dependent	Aromatic amine, polycyclic aromatic hydrocarbon
Inorganic[a]	Metal
Epigenetic	
Solid-state	Plastics, asbestos
Hormone	Estrogen, androgen
Immunosuppressor	Purine analog, antibody,
Cocarcinogen	Phorbol ester, catechol
Promoter	Phorbol ester, phenobarbital

[a] Tentatively categorized as genotoxic because of some evidence for direct interaction of some members with DNA.

carcinogens, Weisburger and Williams (1980) have developed a classification based on the mechanistic mode of action of carcinogens, which separates them into eight classes. These in turn can be divided into two general categories based on their ability to damage DNA. Carcinogens that undergo covalent reactions with DNA are categorized as genotoxic, and those lacking this property are designated as epigenetic. Based on the available data in the literature, the eight classes have been divided between these two categories (Table 1).

The genotoxic category contains those agents that function as electrophilic reactants, a property of carcinogens originally postulated by Miller and Miller in the early 1970s (in Searle, 1976; Hiatt *et al.*, 1977; Emmelot and Kriek, 1979; Griffin and Shaw, 1979; Miller and Miller, 1981). In addition, carcinogenic chemicals that give rise to DNA damage through formation of free radicals, derived either from their own molecular structure or from altered cellular macromolecules (e.g., lipid peroxides), would be considered genotoxic. Carcinogens that function as electrophilic reactants may have the necessary structure for reactivity and thus be direct acting (Section 4.1), or they may require biotransformation in order to give rise to a reactive species, in which case they are referred to as procarcinogens (Section 4.2). Also, because some inorganic chemicals have displayed DNA-damaging effects, they have tentatively been placed in this category (Section 4.3). However, the studies of Loeb and colleagues (*in* Kharasch, 1979) on effects of inorganic chemicals on the fidelity of DNA polymerases suggest that these might yield abnormal DNA by a mechanism distinct from the electrophilic genotoxic compounds.

The second broad category, designated as epigenetic carcinogens, comprises those carcinogens for which no evidence of direct interaction with genetic

244

J. H.
WEISBURGER
AND
G. M.
WILLIAMS

material exists. This category contains solid-state carcinogens, hormones, immunosuppressants, cocarcinogens, and promoters. The category of epigenetic carcinogens is currently the most controversial. Some investigators would object to calling agents of this type carcinogens at all, preferring terms such as tumor enhancers. While this view is understandable, it is perhaps unrealistic since many of the chemicals assigned to this category are widely accepted as carcinogens by authorities involved in the interpretation of bioassay results. Other reservations with this category have centered around the term "epigenetic" as being too definitive when "nongenotoxic" would suffice. The latter conveys the essential distinction in the proposed classification, but, as will be developed, the evidence for actual epigenetic mechanisms of action for carcinogens in this category is becoming increasingly evident. It is entirely possible that genotoxic carcinogens may also display epigenetic effects, perhaps through nongenotoxic metabolites (Williams in Borek and Williams, 1980).

Similar approaches to classifying carcinogens have been proposed (Kroes in Williams *et al.*, 1980a). Classifications of this type, if ultimately validated, have major implications for risk extrapolation to humans of data on experimental carcinogenesis. Genotoxic carcinogens, because of their effects on genetic material, pose a clear qualitative hazard to humans. These carcinogens are occasionally effective after a single exposure, act in a cumulative manner, and act together with other genotoxic carcinogens having the same organotropism. Thus, the level of human exposure acceptable for "no risk" to ensue needs to be evaluated most stringently in the light of existing data and relevant mechanisms.

On the other hand, with some classes of epigenetic carcinogens, it is known that their carcinogenic effects occur only with high and sustained levels of exposure that lead to prolonged functional abnormalities, hormonal imbalances, or tissue injury. Consequently, the risk from exposure may be of a quantitative nature. This is almost certainly the case with estrogens, which are carcinogenic only at unphysiologic, chronic exposure levels in animal studies; if it were otherwise, every individual would develop cancer. Thus, with epigenetic carcinogens, it may be possible to establish a "safe" threshold of exposure, once their specific mechanism of action is elucidated.

Within this broad definition of carcinogens, many structural types of chemicals are included. Some, such as those in the class of the direct-acting carcinogens, may have a chemical structure such that they do not require the participation of enzymes from the host organism to generate the key reactive intermediate— the ultimate carcinogen. This may also be true of inorganic carcinogens. Most direct-acting carcinogens are synthetic chemicals developed as laboratory tools for research; others are used in industry or as antitumor drugs. Some of these represent important occupational hazards and potential risks to exposed individuals. However, because of their high reactivity, they do not generally persist in the environment.

The second class of genotoxic carcinogens, termed procarcinogens, is comprised of organic chemicals that are active only after metabolic conversion by the host. This class includes most of the known chemical carcinogens, and in contrast to direct-acting carcinogens, procarcinogens can exist in the environment in a relatively stable condition until taken in by an exposed individual and activated through biotransformation. Thus, these chemicals appear to represent the greatest potential cancer threat to humans. A hazard of a similar nature is also posed by chemicals that, although not carcinogens themselves, are precursors from which carcinogens can be synthesized in the body.

Among the other classes of chemical carcinogens that are considered to operate by nongenotoxic (epigenetic) mechanisms are solid-state materials such as plastics and fiber materials. The carcinogenicity of these agents appears not to involve chemical reactivity (Weisburger and Williams, 1980) as host biotransformation has not been shown to have a role in their carcinogenicity. Nevertheless, the possibility that some polymers could release genotoxic monomers or other chemicals used in polymerization must not be overlooked.

The class of immunosuppressant chemical carcinogens (Section 5.1) is comprised primarily of drugs that are carcinogenic only under conditions in which suppression of the immune system is achieved (Weisburger, 1977; Weisburger and Williams, 1980). Mainly leukemias, lymphomas, or reticulum cell sarcomas are induced in mice, rats, and humans (Penn, 1978; Weisburger and Williams, 1980). The role of oncogenic viruses in causing these neoplasms deserves consideration. Immunosuppressant drugs such as azathioprine and 6-mercaptopurine are active as a result of their participation in host metabolic processes through which they lead to the death of immunocytes.

Hormones, especially those of the estrogen type, were shown over 40 years ago to cause cancer (Jull in Searle, 1976). Current work has established that estrogens, such as the naturally occurring hormone estradiol or the synthetic estrogen diethylstilbestrol, can cause cancer when administered chronically at high levels or when through disturbances of normal endocrine balances they are present in unphysiologic amounts for long periods of time. This may well be true even in the case of the female offspring of women treated with large amounts of diethylstilbestrol during pregnancy, for there exists an increased incidence of vaginal adenocarcinoma at about puberty (Herbst *et al.*, 1979). An important mechanism for neoplasia of this type at this stage of development may involve faulty differentiation of the complex endocrine apparatus in the fetus, exposed to abnormally high levels of natural or synthetic estrogens, which becomes apparent in the offspring at the time of sexual maturation. In animals and in humans, hormonally determined cancer development is most likely due to a promoting action and not to a direct modification of the genetic apparatus. Thus, hormones and hormonal balances act through epigenetic mechanisms (Section 5.2). The initiating agent leading to an altered DNA in humans, and in certain instances of animal neoplasms "induced" by excess estrogen, is not known. In certain animal models, for example, breast cancer in mice, a viral element is associated with carcinogenesis (this series, Volume 2; Hiatt *et al.*, 1977; Highman *et al.*, 1977; Moore *et al.*, 1979). For postmenopausal women maintained on estrogen, a high risk of endometrial cancer exists, the actual genotoxic agent

246

J. H.
WEISBURGER
AND
G. M.
WILLIAMS

being unknown. Likewise, in some relatively rare instances, among the millions of users of oral contraceptives, liver tumors have occurred (Pike *et al.* in Hiatt *et al.*, 1977). In all of these cases, the hormones can be considered to have promoted the lesions, actually caused by unknown initiating agents, which in the case of liver tumors may in fact be exposure to occult hepatocarcinogens or an agent akin to the hepatitis B virus (Weisburger and Williams, 1980).

The actual mechanism of promotion by estrogen is no doubt complex and may involve systemic general hormonal imbalances, including abnormalities in pituitary hormones such as prolactin and possibly also adrenal and thyroid hormones. Androgens have rarely caused cancer. There are a few case reports of liver cancer in males taking large amounts of androgens as anabolic agents or as muscle builders. As a rule, hormones need to be considered as powerful physiologic effectors, which when present in abnormally high amounts for a long time are likely to lead to neoplasia.

Naturally occurring hormones are, of course, metabolized by the enzyme systems that have evolved for the synthesis and degradation of these biologically active agents. Only in the case of diethylstilbestrol has it been suggested that biotransformation might give rise to a chemically reactive species (Gottschlich and Metzler, 1980), but this remains to be fully documented. Thus, for the remainder of the hormone class of carcinogens, metabolic processes that lead to formation of more hormonally active derivatives would enhance carcinogenic activity, whereas catabolism leading to the degradation, or conjugation, and excretion of hormones would diminish their carcinogenicity.

Cocarcinogens (Section 5.3) are agents that increase the overall carcinogenic process when administered together with a carcinogen. Present knowledge indicates that the action of cocarcinogens occurs only in conjunction with genotoxic carcinogens. The relevant mechanisms can be one or more of several possibilities: (1) The cocarcinogen may intervene in the metabolism of a genotoxic carcinogen by increasing the level of the active ultimate carcinogenic metabolite or by decreasing the detoxification process; (2) the cocarcinogen may sensitize the target tissue of the genotoxic carcinogen by stimulating proliferation; (3) the cocarcinogen may interfere with the repair of DNA damage produced by the genotoxic carcinogen; or (4) the cocarcinogen may increase nonspecifically or specifically the growth of cells with an altered genotype reflecting neoplastic change. The last mechanism is identical to that applying to promoters to be discussed below. As yet, however, none of these mechanisms have been specifically established for any cocarcinogen.

The demonstration of cocarcinogenesis was made over 40 years ago in the laboratories of Shear and especially of Berenblum and Shubik (see Berenblum, 1974; Slaga *et al.*, 1978; Diamond *et al.*, 1980). Berenblum's group noted that application of a carcinogenic polycyclic aromatic hydrocarbon to mouse skin together with croton oil, the oil of the euphorbia *Croton tiglium* L. seed, gave a much higher incidence of skin cancer than in controls given the carcinogen alone. The cocarcinogenic action of croton oil on skin was found to be species specific, not being demonstrable in the rabbit, rat, or guinea pig.

The active principles in croton oil, eventually isolated and identified by Hecker
(in Slaga *et al.*, 1978), were in the form of phorbol esters. These materials act
also as promoters. As cocarcinogens, it is not known whether they affect the
metabolism of the carcinogen.

Tobacco smoke, in addition to its relatively small content of genotoxic carcinogens such as polycyclic aromatic hydrocarbons, certain nitrosamines, and possibly certain pyrolysis products of proteins in the form of α- or β-carbolines and related materials (Hiatt *et al.*, 1977; Wynder and Hoffmann, 1979), also includes cocarcinogens typified by catechol and other phenolic compounds that are isolated mainly in the acidic fraction (Van Duuren in Searle, 1976). With these compounds also, the mechanism of cocarcinogenicity is not known. The cocarcinogenic factors in tobacco smoke are thought to play an important role in the overall effect of the smoke in leading to cancer in humans (Hammond *et al.* in Hiatt *et al.*, 1977; Wynder *et al.* in Slaga *et al.*, 1978). Thus, cocarcinogenicity represents not only a theoretical concept, valuable to dissect the complex sequence of events concerning cancer causation, but also has practical importance for human disease risk.

Promoters (Section 5.4) are agents that increase the tumorigenic response to a carcinogen when applied after the carcinogen. The demonstration of this phenomenon in the laboratories of Rous and of Berenblum and Shubik (see Berenblum, 1974) gave rise to the "two-stage" concept of carcinogenesis: initiation and promotion. Although promoters are typically thought of as being noncarcinogenic because they produce few or no tumors under the conditions in which they are active as promoters, virtually all produce a clear tumor response when applied under more strenuous test conditions (Weisburger and Williams, 1980). This includes even the phorbol esters (Iverson and Iverson, 1979).

Croton oil, studied by Berenblum and Shubik, has a highly specific and exquisite promoting activity on mouse skin, as with its cocarcinogenic action. In an impressive series of experiments, it has been shown that the exposure to a polycyclic aromatic hydrocarbon can be followed up to 1 year later by a promoting stimulus, such as an application of the phorbol esters from croton oil, and still result in production of skin tumors (Van Duuren *et al.*, 1978).

Promoters such as phorbol esters are cocarcinogenic, but not all promoters are cocarcinogens, nor are all cocarcinogens promoters. Thus, for example, phenol in tobacco tar is a promoter, but not cocarcinogenic.

Although phorbol esters remain a popular experimental model, a number of other promoters for different organ systems have been discovered. Bile acids have been shown to be promoters in colon carcinogenesis (Reddy *et al.*, 1980). Hormones increase tumor development through a mechanism of promotion when present in abnormal amounts. Certain inducers of liver metabolic enzyme systems, such as phenobarbital, DDT, and butylated hydroxytoluene, when administered after minimal doses of primary hepatocarcinogens, exert a substantial promoting effect (Peraino in Slaga *et al.*, 1978; Kaneko *et al.*, 1980; Peraino *et al.*, 1980). Most liver tumor promoters are not cocarcinogens, since when administered together with hepatocarcinogens they usually decrease

248

J. H.
WEISBURGER
AND
G. M.
WILLIAMS

carcinogenicity, most likely by increasing detoxification reactions, especially those concerned with conjugation (Weisburger and Weisburger, 1973; Irving, 1979). As indicated, all these agents are carcinogenic under some condition of exposure, and our current presumption is that this is as a result of their promoting effects.

The mechanism of the promoting effect of chemicals when administered after a primary carcinogen is not yet known. Recent findings with phorbol esters have revealed an ability to produce gene derepression and repression (see Slaga *et al.*, 1978), and this has been suggested to be indicative of the potential of promoters to enhance expression of the neoplastic phenotype in initiated cells. In a number of instances, vitamin A or retinoids have inhibited promotion (see Sporn and Newton, 1979). Since vitamin A is necessary for differentiation in some tissues, this has suggested further that promoters may operate at the level of gene expression. Alternatively, a substantial portion of the effects of phorbol esters on various cell types can be accounted for by their activity on cellular membranes (Sivak in Slaga *et al.*, 1978; Weinstein in Emmelot and Kriek, 1979). Such effects represent a particularly appealing basis for promoting action. As described above, initiated cells can remain persistent for up to 1 year before promotion is commenced. During this time, the initiated cells are presumably subject to the regulatory processes that govern normal cell turnover in tissues. This regulation could involve cell to cell communication mediated by chemical messages such as chalones. Alterations of cell membranes by promoters can thus be visualized to interrupt intercellular communication and release initiated cells for uncontrolled growth. Inhibition of cell to cell communication by promoters has been reported in several *in vitro* systems (Murray and Fitzgerald, 1979; Yotti *et al.*, 1979; Williams in Borek and Williams, 1980). The inhibiting effect of vitamin A in some situations could relate to its stimulation of gap junction formation (Elias *et al.*, 1980), the structures involved in cell to cell communication.

Many, if not all, liver tumor promoters, such as DDT, other chlorinated hydrocarbons, and phenobarbital, increase the incidence of mouse liver tumors and very rarely cause cancer in the rat liver. Enhancement of the development of preneoplastic liver lesions occurs with exposure to phenobarbital (Pitot *et al.* and Williams in Slaga *et al.*, 1978; Kaneko *et al.*, 1980), and thus it can be postulated that the tumorigency of these chemicals occurs by a mechanism of promotion of the preexisting abnormal liver cells that eventually give rise to the "spontaneously" occurring liver lesions and neoplasms in old mice and rats. The nature of the "inducing" agent yielding the abnormal cells is obscure. It could be genetic in these inbred strains, but variations in incidence between different colonies raise the possibility of an exogenous factor. In the mouse, this may be an agent akin to the hepatitis virus prevalent in mice. The few liver cancers occasionally seen in rats given phenobarbital or DDT may result from an intake of diets contaminated with mycotoxins or some nitrosamines.

There have been few studies on the metabolic fate of cocarcinogens or promoting agents in comparison to those on procarcinogens. Hecker and his associates (see Hecker in Miller *et al.*, 1979), Van Duuren (in Searle, 1976), and Boutwell

(1974) have developed information on the interaction of the classic agents of this type—croton oil and the active phorbol esters—with tissues, but more information is required as to the key metabolites derived from phorbol esters that exert the specific promoting effects. At this time, the evidence for several of these agents suggests that the molecule as a whole exerts the effect (Hecker in Miller *et al.*, 1979; Weinstein in Emmelot and Kriek, 1979); thus, metabolism may be primarily an inactivating reaction.

While it has been known for some time that phenols also have a promoting effect under certain conditions, the nature of the metabolites responsible for this reaction are likewise obscure. Yet it seems important to understand these processes in detail, for not only does this class of chemicals possess intrinsic theoretical interest, but it also appears that they are involved in potentiating lung cancer induction in animals, and possibly in humans, through their presence in sizable amounts in the smoke of tobacco products (Van Duuren in Searle, 1976; Hoffman *et al.*, 1978). Phenol is the main metabolite of benzene, and the question arises whether it is involved in the leukemogenic effect associated with certain sustained exposures of workers to benzene. There is no good animal model for this effect, perhaps because of the absence of a suitable initiating agent in the animals.

Data are beginning to appear that cancer of the large bowel may similarly stem from the cocarcinogenic or promoting effect of certain bile acid metabolites. These chemicals undergo metabolism by the microflora in the gut, the composition and enzyme activities of which appear to be modulated by diet (Reddy *et al.*, 1980). Diet also controls the conversion of cholesterol in the liver to bile acids through several mechanisms, including the activity of the cytochrome P-450 system, itself influenced in as yet unknown ways by ascorbic acid (Ginter, 1973; Zannoni and Sato, 1975).

Thus, most carcinogens of the promoting class undergo biotransformation, but since their active entities are not known the effect of metabolism is not always clear.

2.1. Chemical Carcinogens and Mutagens

For many years there was much controversy about whether mutagens were carcinogenic or whether carcinogens were mutagenic (Hollaender, 1971–1980). With the insight provided by the understanding of metabolic activation of chemical carcinogens to highly reactive products, it is now quite apparent that such ultimate carcinogens are also mutagenic (McCann and Ames, Sugimura *et al.* in Hiatt *et al.*, 1977; Matsushima *et al.* in Norpoth and Garner, 1980; Newbold *et al.*, 1980). Nevertheless, if the concept of genotoxic and epigenetic carcinogens is correct, there would still be a whole category of carcinogens, the epigenetic type, that would not be mutagenic. In addition, it would appear that not all mutagens are carcinogenic; examples are hydroxylamine, 8-hydroxyquinoline, and possibly sodium azide. The reason for this may be that such agents introduced

250

J. H.
WEISBURGER
AND
G. M.
WILLIAMS

into the microbiological system are not readily detoxified, whereas in a mammalian system they are (Williams in Butterworth, 1979). Evidence is now available that the metabolism performed by subcellular fractions used for activation in bacterial mutagenicity tests differs markedly from that in intact cells (Section 3.1.1), and this must always be kept in mind in the interpretation of results.

From a practical point of view, various methods including the Ames *Salmonella*/microsome test can now be applied to assess, in a preliminary way, the potential carcinogenic risk of chemicals or mixtures by determining their mutagenic potential (see Hiatt *et al.*, 1977; Jollow *et al.*, 1977; Emmelot and Kriek, 1979; Griffin and Shaw, 1979; Poirier and Weisburger, 1979; Sabadie *et al*, 1980; Coon *et al.*, 1980). In addition to bacterial mutagenicity, other test systems that have attained sufficient reliability to be used as prescreens are mammalian cell mutagenicity, mammalian cell DNA repair, mammalian cell chromosome damage (sister chromatid exchange), and mammalian cell transformation (Butterworth, 1979; Hollstein *et al.*, 1979; Stich *et al.*, 1979; International Agency for Research on Cancer, 1980; Williams *et al.*, 1980*a*). Other useful tests are also available, but the five test systems described represent a battery that appears to be sufficient for the *in vitro* screening of chemicals for genotoxicity and potential carcinogenicity (Williams *et al.*, 1980*a*; Williams and Weisburger, 1981). Needless to say, the results obtained warrant careful interpretation in the light of current knowledge.

Another method whereby metabolites of carcinogens in body fluids or in excreta may give an indication of exposure has been developed by Durston and Ames (1974) and by Bruce and co-workers (in Hiatt *et al.*, 1977), who detected materials possibly capable of inducing mutation in sensitive microorganisms. In addition, Albertini (in Hsie *et al.*, 1979) has described a technique for detecting mutations in peripheral lymphocytes of whole animals. These approaches, when further developed, could serve to monitor exposure of individuals to certain carcinogens, both voluntary exposure as in cigarette smoking and involuntary exposure as in diet and occupation.

Inasmuch as the ultimate genotoxic carcinogens derived from procarcinogens are most likely mutagenic in various sensitive and specific systems, the technique of mutagenicity testing can be used to rapidly find the relevant metabolites from the large numbers of metabolites produced *in vitro* and *in vivo*. Thus, mutagenicity testing has been employed to isolate mutagenic natural products in fried food, *in vitro* metabolites from various procarcinogens, and metabolites *in vivo* in laboratory animals and in humans. The presence of a mutagenic metabolite is thus one of the parameters that can be used to pinpoint potentially hazardous environmental chemicals whether they be naturally occurring or synthetic.

3. Metabolism of Chemical Carcinogens

Chemical carcinogens, both genotoxic and epigenetic (Section 2) of various classes, whether primary direct-acting carcinogens, secondary procarcinogens, hormones, immunosuppressants, cocarcinogens, or promoters, undergo a variety of chemical or biochemical reactions when introduced into a living system. These reactions can be mediated simply by body water, by selective tissue or cell chemicals, or by enzymes from mammalian and microbial cell systems. Many reactions can lead to detoxification, that is, to less carcinogenic or less active products. Indeed, this is the predominant result of biotransformation of most structural types of carcinogens, with a notable exception in the case of nitrosamines.

Importantly, metabolic conversion can also lead to more active metabolites and in the case of genotoxic carcinogens, to the key ultimate carcinogenic reactants, essentially as accidental reactions incidental to the process of detoxification. The balance of detoxification and activation reactions depends on the chemical structure of the agent, and is subject to many variables that are a function of this structure, or genetic background, sex, endocrine status, age, diet, and microbial environment, and of the presence of other chemicals (Sections 6 and 7). The possibilities for disposition and actions of a genotoxic procarcinogen are shown in Fig. 1. It is important to realize that the enzymes involved in carcinogen metabolism are also involved in the metabolism of a variety of

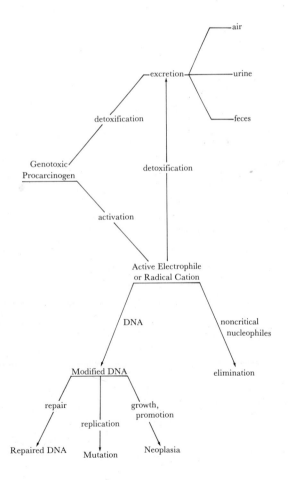

FIGURE 1. Schematic presentation of the diverse biochemical reactions involved in the metabolism of genotoxic procarcinogens. For many procarcinogens there are reactions leading to detoxified metabolites, facilitating excretion. Usually only a small fraction of a dose of a procarcinogen is converted, on one or more steps (Fig. 3), to more toxic and carcinogenic metabolites, which are reactive electrophiles or radical cations. These metabolites can undergo enzymatic detoxification reactions yielding excretable products, or they can react with nucleophiles noncritical to the carcinogenic or mutagenic process, in competition with the critical nucleophiles, especially DNA. *In vitro* systems have different ratios of activation/detoxification enzymes, and distinct levels of noncritical nucleophiles, thus accounting for differences found between *in vivo* and *in vitro* assays. The key reaction is with DNA, providing a parallel between mutagenesis and carcinogenesis. This lesion can be repaired, an effect that plays a role in quantitative carcinogenesis, and in the specific organ primarily affected by a given carcinogen. An essential element in the overall process toward mutation or neoplasia is production of altered DNA and cell duplication, growth, and promotion.

252

J. H.
WEISBURGER
AND
G. M.
WILLIAMS

substrates, and thus the introduction of specific xenobiotics may change the operating level and potential of these very enzymes, not only for the chemical under study but also for a diversity of other chemicals such as hormones. Since a number of carcinogen-metabolizing enzymes are in turn affected by such endogenous components as hormones, unexpected secondary metabolic, physiological, and, indeed, pathological reactions may occur (Conney et al., 1977, 1981). Also, in many cases repeated or chronic administration, without immediate overt cellular damage, leads to appreciable changes in enzymatic operating potential, in some cases through enzyme induction. Thus, the metabolism after chronic dosing may lead to qualitative and quantitative alteration in the products. Even diet as such, through normal constituents, or diets containing traces of contaminants, such as pesticides, can affect the bias toward certain products under the control of metabolic enzyme systems. Metabolism studies in humans are complicated by many such uncontrollable variables, which include, in addition, alcohol consumption and cigarette smoking (Conney et al., 1981).

Specific metabolic activation processes will be discussed in relation to each of the main types of chemical carcinogens. A few agents undergo activation by soluble enzyme systems in the cytoplasm of the cell. Thus, 4-nitroquinoline-N-oxide is reduced to the active hydroxylamino derivative by a reductase in the cytoplasm (Sugimura et al., 1979). Likewise, specific aromatic amines and substituted hydrazines appear to be activated by cytosolic N-acetyltransferases (Nelson et al., 1976; Lower et al., 1979; Tannen and Webber, 1979). Nevertheless, most carcinogens requiring metabolic activation are transformed by enzyme systems located on the membrane of the smooth endoplasmic reticulum. Ultracentrifugation of a cell homogenate sediments these activities with the microsome fraction.

The metabolism of most carcinogens involves cytoplasmic membrane-associated monooxygenases that belong to a family of cytochromes (White and Coon, 1980). Initially, these monooxygenases were labeled "cytochrome P-450" because a reduced form treated with carbon monoxide exhibits an absorption peak at 450 nm. Multiple forms of cytochrome P-450 exist (Levin et al. in Coon et al., 1980), as well as other cytochromes with spectral maxima at different wavelengths, i.e., 448 nm (P-448 or P_1-450). Just as isozyme variants are known for certain soluble enzymes such as aldolase and lactic dehydrogenase, it may be that the family of cytochromes mediating the metabolism of carcinogens and drugs, and exogenous or endogenous chemicals generally, are isozymes bound to membranes. All of these enzyme systems require NADPH as a cofactor and utilize molecular oxygen for their oxidative activity, but substrate specificities differ markedly (Gillette, 1979b; Kato, 1979; Nebert and Jensen, 1979a; Parke, 1979; Coon et al., 1980; Gelboin et al., 1980; Kawajiri et al., 1980). Because of the variety of substrates metabolized by the cytochrome oxygenases, the system is often referred to as mixed-function oxidases.

A scheme for the cytochrome P-450 monooxygenase-catalyzed reactions is shown in Fig. 2. In this scheme two electrons are transferred, probably sequentially, to the substrate–cytochrome P-450 complex. The reduced (Fe^{2+}) substrate–

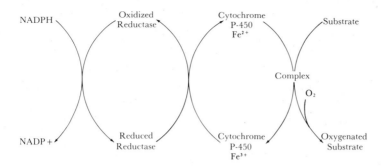

FIGURE 2. A set of membrane-bound enzymes, the cytochrome P-450 enzyme complex (or mixed-function oxidases), is present in many tissues. These enzymes catalyze a series of coupled reactions that activate molecular oxygen and convert a substrate to oxidized or hydroxylated products. Required cofactors are NADPH, magnesium, and flavins. The enzyme system can also perform reductions in the presence of a donor of hydrogen or of electrons. The enzyme system has been purified and its components studied. Cytochrome P-450 is so-named since it absorbs light at 450 nm in its reduced form in the presence of CO. An inducible cytochrome P-448, or cytochrome P_1-450 under the same conditions, absorbs at 448 nm and has distinct biochemical properties with regard to substrate affinity, specificity, and reaction rates.

cytochrome P-450 complex combines with oxygen (O_2), and one oxygen atom is introduced into the substrate while the other is reduced to water. The substrate–cytochrome P-450 complex then dissociates, releasing the oxygenated substrate and regenerated oxidized cytochrome P-450. This system is inducible by more than 200 chemicals and complex mixtures (Conney *et al.*, 1977; Alvares *et al.*, 1979*b*; Lee *et al.*, 1980). Although the monoxygenases have been best characterized on cytoplasmic membranes, the nucleus also possesses some of these enzyme systems (Sakai *et al.*, 1978; Stout and Becker, 1979; Bresnick, 1980) probably because the nuclear membrane is continuous with the cytoplasmic endoplasmic reticulum.

For aromatic or olefinic compounds that are metabolized to epoxides, a further hydrolytic reaction involves conversion to dihydrodiols by epoxide hydrolases (Oesch *et al.*, 1977; Coon *et al.*, 1980; Lu and Miwa, 1980; Ota and Hammock, 1980). This reaction is often a detoxification step, but with some substrates like 7,8-epoxy-7,8-dihydrobenzo[*a*]pyrene, it yields an active proximate carcinogen.

Following oxidation, which has been called Phase I metabolism, or formation of diols, the liver and to a lesser extent certain other tissues such as intestine are capable of carrying out a variety of conjugative or group transfer reactions as part of Phase II metabolism (Fishman, 1970; Aitio, 1978). This results in formation of glucuronic acid, sulfuric acid, mercapturic acid, amino acid conjugates, or acyl derivatives, which render the metabolite more water soluble for excretion. The formation of glucuronides is catalyzed by UDP-glucuronyltransferase, a membrane-associated, inducible enzyme. However, certain group

254

J. H.
WEISBURGER
AND
G. M.
WILLIAMS

transfer reactions, such as the effect of liver sulfotransferase on acylarylhydroxyl-amines, can also be activation steps (Section 4.2.4).

A family of multifunctional binding and catalytic proteins, the glutathione *S*-transferases, is widely distributed in the cytosol of tissues of many species (Chasseaud, 1979; Ketterer *et al.*, 1979; Lotlikar *et al.*, 1979). A number of distinct glutathione *S*-transferases have been identified in both human and rat livers. "Ligandin" was identified as one such enzyme (Litwack *et al.*, 1972; see Chasseaud, 1979). These enzymes catalyze transfer of the sulfhydryl group of glutathione. This process is important in the detoxification of reactive intermediates, which are eventually excreted as mercapturic acids. Depletion of the level of glutathione by this process increases the susceptibility of cells to toxicity (Jollow, 1980; Wells *et al.*, 1980). In contrast to the foregoing, conjugation with glutathione of certain haloalkanes is the first step leading to reactive intermediates, perhaps as a result of dehydrohalogenation (Van Bladeren *et al.*, 1979).

A variety of sequential or simultaneous reactions are carried out by other enzyme reactions including the "NIH shift," sulfoxidation and oxidative deamination, desulfuration, and dechlorination. Under some conditions, important reductive reactions such as those involving azo links or nitro groups are performed by mammalian and microbial enzymes (Huang *et al.*, 1979; Boxenbaum *et al.*, 1979; Koch and Goldman, 1979; Scheline, 1973; Hwang and Kelsey, 1978; Coon *et al.*, 1980; Goldman *et al.*, 1980). In addition, mammalian tissues contain a large number of nonspecific esterases and amidases that can hydrolyze ester and amide linkages in carcinogens. Thus, a variety of chemical and enzyme-catalyzed reactions take place on chemical carcinogens.

3.1. Metabolism by Mammalian Enzyme Systems

The metabolism of most structural types of procarcinogens takes place in ways leading to inactivation or to a lesser degree to activation, i.e., the ultimate production of a reactive moiety (Fig. 3). The capacity to metabolize foreign chemicals is probably a consequence of the presence of enzyme systems for metabolizing similar endogenous molecules. In view of the fact that the liver is involved in catabolism of many varied kinds of endogenous substances, it is not surprising that it has the greatest capacity to metabolize foreign carcinogens. Indeed, as pointed out in the first edition of this chapter, the liver possesses most of the specific activation systems to be discussed, and to our knowledge, apart from chemicals requiring biotransformation by microbial systems (Section 3.2), there is no carcinogen that cannot be metabolized by liver. This makes liver the logical source of enzyme or cell preparations for studying metabolism or providing metabolism for *in vitro* short-term tests.

In the past, many studies have dealt with drug- and carcinogen-metabolizing enzymes in liver. More recently, a beginning has been made to develop such information for other target organs in a variety of species, including humans (Hiatt *et al.*, 1977; Bartsch *et al.*, 1979*b*; Wolf *et al.*, 1979; Mattison and

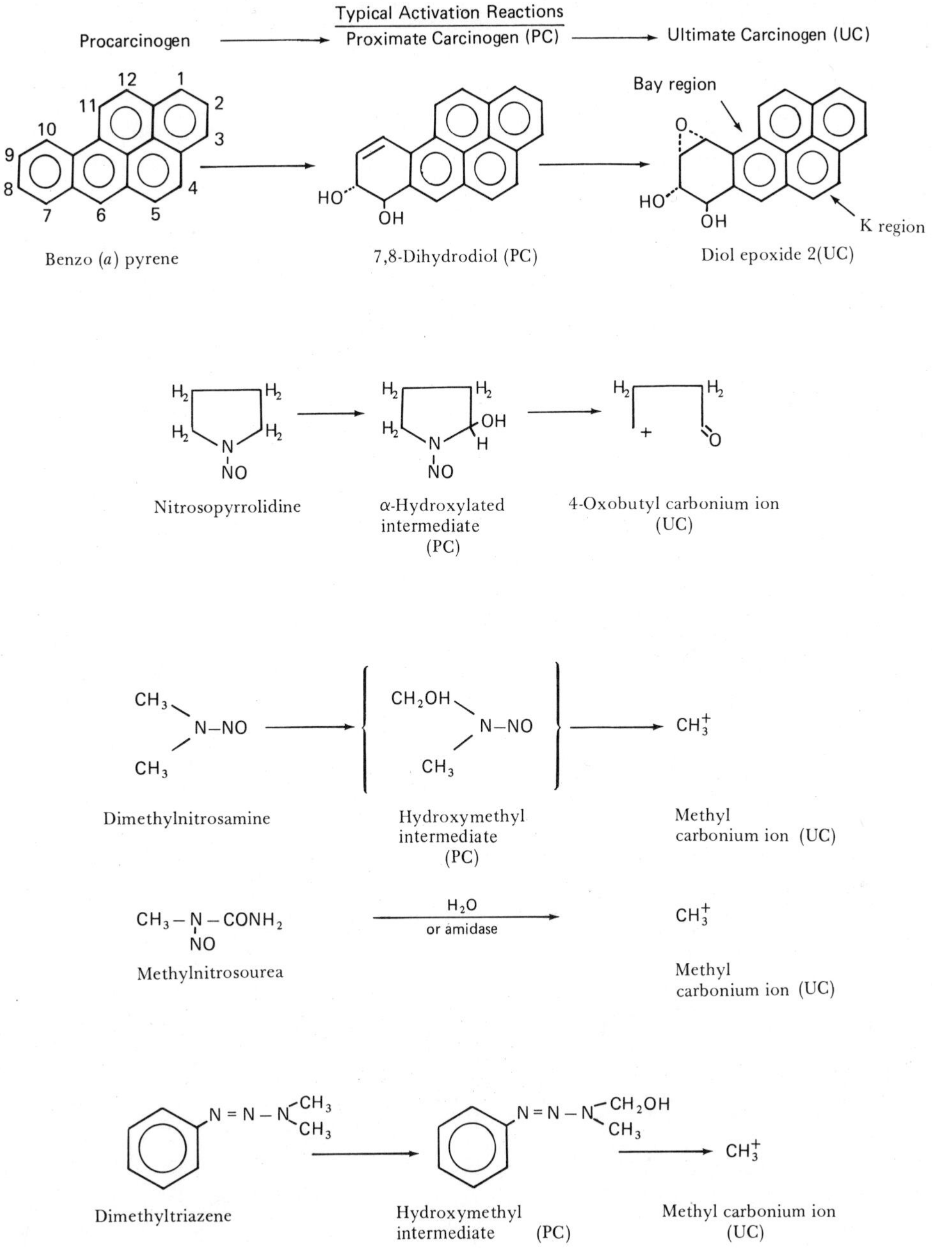

FIGURE 3. Schematic biochemical activation of typical procarcinogens. In some instances several reactions are involved in the conversion of a procarcinogen to a proximate carcinogen—an intermediate, more active molecule that does not have a structure such that it can interact directly with crucial macromolecular nucleophilic receptors in the cell. Nonetheless, in some instances, such as with arylamines, this step is a controlling event, highly dependent on the structure of the chemical and on the species, the strain, and certain environmental factors such as enzyme inducers or inhibitors. Formation of the ultimate carcinogen is also under enzymatic control. The exact nature of the ultimate carcinogen has not been fully documented in all cases. Because of the high reactivity of these chemicals, they often cannot be isolated. Their nature is usually elucidated on the basis of their precursors, or the products of interaction with macromolecules.

256

J. H.
WEISBURGER
AND
G. M.
WILLIAMS

Thorgeirsson, 1979; Autrup, 1980). Much more work along these lines is needed. Not only can various tissues carry out reactions that lead to formation of ultimate carcinogens, but they also have the enzymatic potential to split the active entities from their transport conjugates formed in the liver. For example, cancer in the urinary bladder most likely is due to the release of active carcinogens (such as arylhydroxylamine derivatives in the case of aromatic amine carcinogenesis) from glucuronides produced by hepatic metabolism (Kadlubar *et al.*, 1977; Poupko *et al.*, 1979).

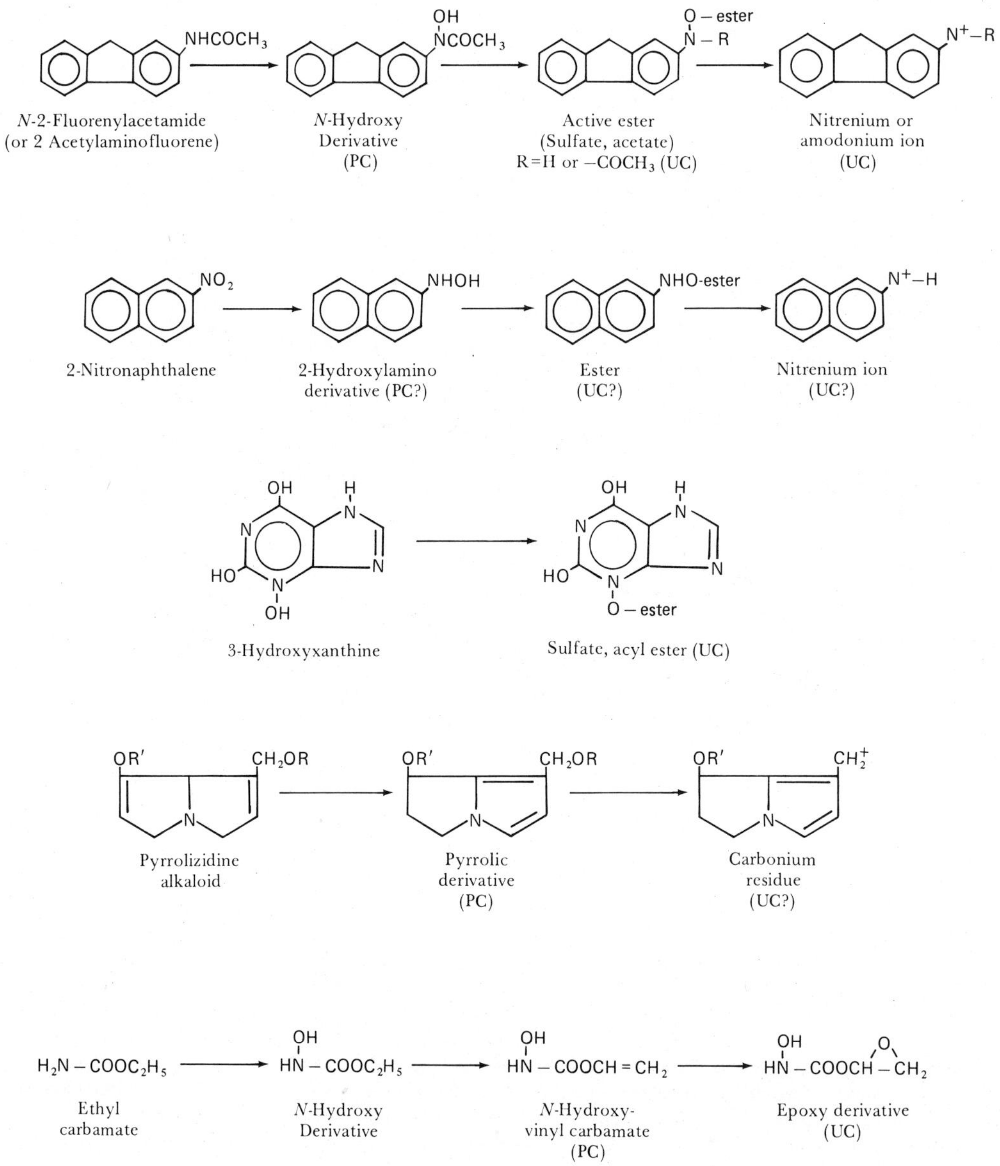

FIGURE 3 (*Continued*)

The target organ affected may depend on a combination of complex interactions (Magee in Margison, 1979). For example, 2',3-dimethyl-4-aminobiopenyl causes intestinal cancer in rats but urinary bladder cancer in hamsters. Probably, a transport form of the agent is excreted in the bile and thus reaches the intestine in the rat, but this occurs to a much lesser extent in the hamster (Fiala *et al.*, unpublished data). Biliary excretion of carcinogen metabolites in particular or drug metabolites in general is a function of molecular size, species, and other variables (Parke and Smith, 1977). This, in turn, determines whether metabolites are excreted into the gut via the bile or reach the kidneys via the blood for filtration and excretion in the urine. As a general rule, metabolites of a molecular weight less than 300 are excreted in the urine, while those greater are excreted in the bile. These processes, however, vary between species, a fact that needs consideration when extrapolating data obtained in rodents to humans. Metabolites reaching the intestine from bile may undergo further reactions mediated by microbial flora (see Section 3.2). The products so formed can be excreted in the feces or be resorbed (enterohepatic pathway) and are thus capable of further metabolism and interaction (Chhabra, 1979). These pathways may be important for the occurrence of certain types of cancer, such as that of the gallbladder, pancreas, and intestinal tract.

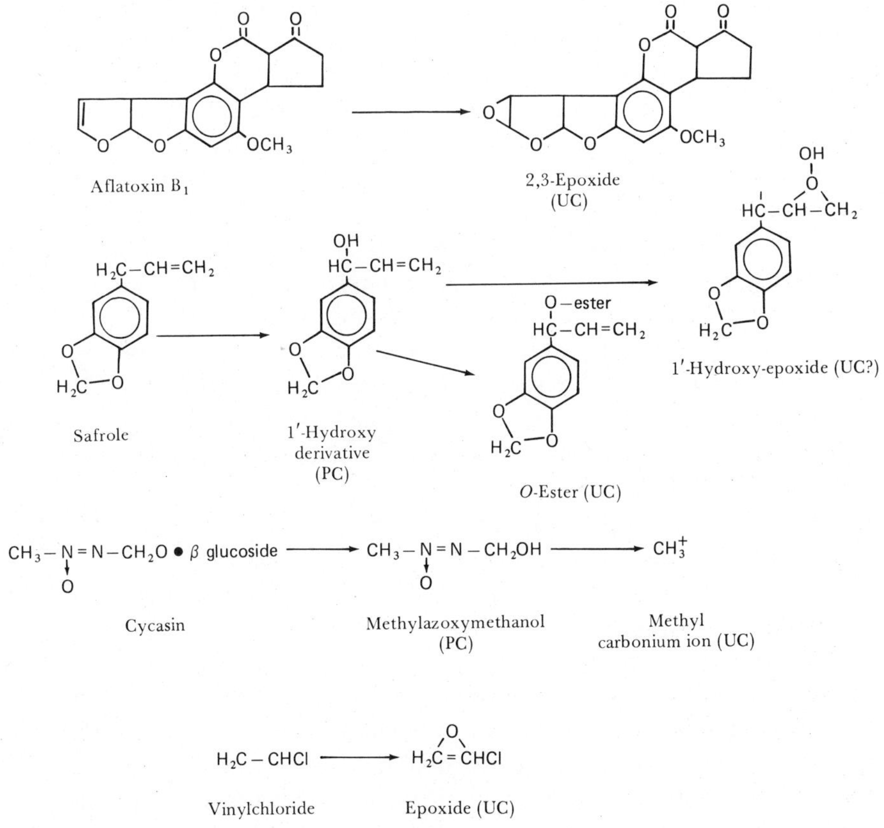

FIGURE 3 (*Continued*)

258

J. H.
WEISBURGER
AND
G. M.
WILLIAMS

The organs, apart from the liver, that have significant capabilities for biotransformation of carcinogens include kidney, lung, and gastrointestinal tract, although most organs possess metabolic enzymes to some degree. The placenta contains a variety of enzyme systems capable of modifying drugs and thereby affecting transplacental passage of chemicals (Juchau *et al.*, 1974; Lucier *et al.*, 1979; Rice, 1979; Rollins *et al.*, 1979). Enzymes metabolizing carcinogens are among those found in the placenta. On the other hand, tissues from aged animals contain such enzymes, but in quantitatively different ratios (Baird and Birnbaum, 1979*a*; Gilette, 1979*a*; Schmucker, 1979).

An organ such as mouse skin or subcutaneous tissue that contains enzyme systems for the activation of carcinogens like polycyclic aromatic hydrocarbons to yield epoxides, but that is poor in enzymes giving deactivated products or water-soluble conjugates, is extraordinarily sensitive to small amounts of such agents. On the other hand, an organ such as liver that is amply provided with such deactivating and conjugating enzymes is much less sensitive, even though it may also be capable of synthesizing sizable amounts of the active epoxide intermediates.

Many carcinogens under certain experimental conditions and in the human situation possess specific affinities for certain target organs. For example, some aromatic amine carcinogens give rise to cancer of the urinary bladder in man, dog, and hamster, but liver cancer in the mouse (Weisburger and Fiala in Thorgeirsson and Weisburger, 1981). Among the carcinogenic nitrosamines, there appears to be organ specificity related to structure (Schmähl, 1970; Preussmann, 1975; Druckrey, 1975; Magee *et al.* in Searle, 1976; Margison *et al.*, 1977; Magee *et al.* in Coon *et al.*, 1980). The exact reason for this specificity has not been fully documented in all cases, but in many cases the main effect appears to depend on specific metabolic activation. It must be emphasized, however, that metabolism is not the sole determinant of organotropism of carcinogens (Fig. 1). Rates of repair of the DNA damage produced by activated metabolites clearly play a major role in some situations (see Kleihues *et al.*, 1979; Singer, 1979; Montesano *et al.*, 1980*a*; Rajewsky, 1980; Setlow, 1980; Swann *et al.*, 1980). Furthermore, cell replication, growth, and development, in turn controlled by promotion (Section 5.4), need consideration as regards each specific target organ.

Through alteration of metabolic activity, the main target organ of a carcinogen can be protected, in which case a secondary organ may be involved. For example, it has been known for almost 30 years that administration of 3-methylcholanthrene together with 2-acetylaminofluorene protects rats against liver cancer induced by the latter (see Conney in Miller *et al.*, 1979). More recently, it has been noted that this combination produces an increased carcinogenic effect on the liver in hamsters. The difference in response is due to a specific alteration of the ratio of activated versus detoxified metabolites. Again, with 2-acetylaminofluorene, addition of tryptophan to the diet in part protects the liver, and urinary bladder cancer ensues (see Weisburger and Weisburger, 1973). In humans, similar relationships may obtain through as yet unclear mechanisms.

Heavy smokers may not necessarily develop lung cancer or heart disease, and it is suspected that there is a genetically controlled metabolic difference in susceptibility (Oesch *et al.*, 1977; Thorgeirsson and Nebert, 1977; Nebert and Jensen, 1979; Vesell, 1979, 1980). Such individuals, however, may develop cancer in the kidneys or the urinary bladder after a longer latent period (Hiatt *et al.*, 1977; Wynder and Gori, 1977; Wynder and Hoffmann, 1979).

3.1.1. Subcellular Fractions

The use of subcellular fractions to study carcinogen has received wide application. For the reasons indicated, liver is the usual source of these enzymes, although more effort is desirable to evaluate other tissues, especially target organs for selective carcinogens. The typical subcellular fraction consists of a postmitochondrial supernatant or microsomal suspension supplemented with an NADPH-regenerating system. The assay is usually for the production of a specific metabolite, of covalently bound carcinogen, or of a biologic endpoint such as mutagenicity. Grover and Sims (1968) and Gelboin (1969) demonstrated that such a system could be used to measure the generation of reactive metabolites that covalently bind to macromolecules. *In vitro* enzyme preparations are now routinely used to identify the ultimate reactive carcinogen metabolite, to study factors affecting metabolism, and to measure the metabolic activation of carcinogens to mutagens (Hiatt *et al.*, 1977; Emmelot and Kriek, 1979; Griffin and Shaw, 1979; Kawachi *et al.* in Miller *et al.*, 1979; Coon *et al.*, 1980; Matsushima *et al.* in Norpoth and Garner, 1980). In the latter situation, it has been pointed out that a paradox exists between the *in vitro* results and the *in vivo* effects (Williams in Butterworth, 1979). Whereas enzyme induction *in vivo* usually reduces the carcinogenicity of chemicals requiring biotransformation (Section 7.3), enzyme preparations from induced livers generate more mutagens. This discrepancy is due to the fact that conjugative–detoxification systems are poorly operative in subcellular enzyme preparations (Jollow *et al.*, 1977; Schmeltz *et al.*, 1978; Aitio, 1978; Dent in Hsie *et al.*, 1979), leaving a net enhancement of activation systems (Williams in Thorgeirsson and Weisburger, 1981). Subcellular fractions have many useful applications, but the imbalance in their metabolic systems must always be kept in mind.

3.1.2. Cell and Organ Culture

Cell culture offers many advantages in studying the metabolism of carcinogens. Most of the available cell cultures, however, are derived from fibroblasts. Few studies on metabolic capability have been performed with compounds other than the polycyclic hydrocarbon carcinogens, in which case important genetic controls were discovered. Epithelial liver cell cultures that retain the capability of the organ have been sought (Wigley, 1975). Rat liver epithelial cells have been shown to possess arylhydrocarbon hydroxylase and to be sensitive to a variety of carcinogens requiring metabolism (see Williams, 1976; Burke *et al.*, 1977; Schmeltz *et al.*, 1978). At present there is no reported culture known to possess

260
J. H.
WEISBURGER
AND
G. M.
WILLIAMS

all the *in vivo* carcinogen-metabolizing activities of liver, although primary cultures better maintain their metabolic capability compared to continuous lines or subcellular fractions such as the microsomal or $9000g$ supernatant fraction. In particular, cell cultures still have the conjugating capability of intact cells, in contrast to most subcellular preparations (Section 3.1.1). Recently it has also been shown that the DNA adducts produced by whole-cell metabolism of polynuclear aromatic hydrocarbons better reflect those formed *in vivo* than do adducts generated by subcellular metabolism (Bigger *et al.*, 1980*a,b*).

The metabolism of polycyclic hydrocarbon compounds in cell culture has been extensively studied by a number of groups (see Heidelberger, 1975). Both constitutive and inducible arylhydroxylase systems have been described. Metabolism by epoxidation, discussed in detail below, and by alternate pathways, such as formation of one-electron oxidation, free radical, or radical cation intermediates, have been reviewed (Coon *et al.*, 1980).

Culture of fragments of whole organs provides an important system in which to study the metabolism of organoselective carcinogens in isolated, but architecturally intact tissue. Recent studies have described metabolism by trachea (Mass and Kaufman, 1978), ovary (Mattison and Thorgeirsson, 1979), colon (Autrup *et al.*, 1978), bladder (Telang *et al.*, 1979), and esophagus (Harris *et al.*, 1979). This approach also permits study of metabolism by human tissues (Harris *et al.*, 1979; P. Okano *et al.*, 1970; Kuroki *et al.*, 1980).

Cell and organ culture systems also offer the possibility to examine the effect of modifiers such as enzyme inducers or inhibitors. However, it is hazardous to postulate that modifiers will have the same total effect in the whole organism as they do in culture. This is because blockage of metabolism in the intact animal at one site may result in an increase at another, such as has been described for dimethylnitrosamine in protein-deprived animals (Swann *et al.*, 1980).

3.2. Metabolism by Microorganisms

The intestines of all mammals are inhabited by a variety of bacteria. With respect to some carcinogens, the participation of microorganisms has been felt to be decisive in the development of certain neoplasms, particularly those of the colon and rectum. However, the contribution of these organisms to metabolism of carcinogens has not been extensively studied. It is clear, especially in mutagenesis studies, that certain bacteria cannot activate procarcinogens, but they do possess the enzymes to hydrolyze conjugates such as glucuronides (Aitio, 1978) and glucosides (Laqueur and Spatz, 1975; Miller *et al.*, 1979). These activities are critical to the fate of some carcinogens. For example, cycasin, a constituent of the cycad nut, is a β-glucoside that is not carcinogenic or mutagenic until methylazoxymethanol, an aglycone, is generated (Section 4.2.12). This is done by intestinal flora that possess glucosidase. Thus, in germfree animals, the glucoside is noncarcinogenic. Upon bacterial enzymatic splitting, the resulting methylazoxymethanol is absorbed and further distributed in a manner similar to that of some nitrosamines, yielding liver, colon, and sometimes kidney tumors.

Bacterial β-glucuronidase can split the glucuronides of carcinogen metabolites

excreted into the intestine via the bile and thereby liberate an active moiety
(Aitio, 1978). The flora also has N-dehydroxylase, which inactivates N-
hydroxy-N-2-fluorenylacetamide (see Weisburger and Weisburger, 1973), and
reductases, which split azo dyes or reduce nitroaryl compounds (Zacharia and
Juchau, 1974). To be thus affected by intestinal bacterial enzymes, the chemicals
must reach the large bowel. This is the case with poorly resorbed orally
administered chemicals or with metabolites excreted in the bile (Scheline, 1973;
Parke and Smith, 1977). Metabolites excreted as conjugates in urine may be
liberated in the urinary bladder, and thus be available for further metabolism
to an active bladder carcinogen (Kadlubar *et al.*, 1977; Poupko *et al.*, 1979).
Whereas phenols are not usually considered carcinogens, it was recorded recently
that 2-nitro-4-aminophenol fed at a high dietary level can induce bladder cancers,
presumably by such a mechanism.

3.3. Chemical Alteration; Endogenous Formation of Carcinogens

In addition to enzymatically mediated modification of carcinogens, there are
strictly chemical reactions leading either to activated or to detoxified products.

The broad class of direct-acting agents (Section 4.1), including dimethyl sulfate,
β-propiolactone, and alkylnitrosoureido compounds, undergoes hydrolytic reactions at neutral pH with release of the active electrophilic carcinogen
(Druckrey, 1975; Lawley in Searle, 1976; Lawley in Brookes, 1980). These
reactions can be accelerated by some compounds such as those with SH groups
or thiocyanate. The alkylnitrosoureido chemicals (Section 4.1) are often powerful
carcinogens because of their relative ease of hydrolysis. Chemical carcinogens
can also be formed in the host from suitable precursors. Sander *et al.* (1975)
noted that similar incidences of identical tumors were found when nitrite
and certain secondary amines were administered separately, as when the preformed nitrosamine was given. This discovery has led to a great deal of activity
in many laboratories and has extended the original findings. In addition to the
classical substrates, secondary amines, some tertiary amines can also react with
nitrite to produce a carcinogenic dialkylnitrosamine (Lijinsky and Taylor in Hiatt
et al., 1977). Inasmuch as many drugs and certain other environmental chemicals
possess such structures, these reactions need to be studied in detail in order to
delineate their importance in relation to the potential risk of carcinogenesis in
humans exposed to these agents and at the same time to nitrite. Most fresh foods
contain negligible amounts of nitrite, but some fruits and vegetables contain
sizable amounts of nitrate. Meats treated with the legal amount of nitrite,
80–160 ppm in the United States, contain low concentrations of about 5–20 ppm
residual nitrite by the time they reach the consumer. Ascorbic acid reacts with
nitrite, making it unavailable for nitrosation (Mirvish, 1977), and this finding
has been utilized to further decrease the potential risk of endogenous nitrite–
amide interaction leading to carcinogenic nitrosamides and nitrosamines. The
importance of past practices of extensively curing meats, fish, and other foods

262

J. H.
WEISBURGER
AND
G. M.
WILLIAMS

with large amounts of nitrate-containing salt has been noted as a source of nitrite. Of even more importance was the formation of nitrite in foodstuffs cooked with water of high nitrate content and then allowed to stand at room temperature (Weisburger *et al.*, 1980*a*) or the formation of nitrite in the oral cavity by bacterial enzymes (Tannenbaum *et al.*, 1976). Ingestion of large amounts of nitrite and subsequent reaction with specific substrates has led to substances of mutagenic activity with properties like those of alkylnitrosamides, which have induced gastric cancer (Weisburger *et al.*, 1980). The declining incidence of stomach cancer in the United States over the last 50 years may be ascribed to the decrease in pickling and curing of foods and the availability of mechanical refrigeration, leading to an overall reduction of nitrite intake. The effects ingested nitrites would be further reduced by more frequent coincident daily intake of the antidotes, namely foods with vitamin C and vitamin E (Mirvish, 1977; J. H. Weisburger *et al.*, 1980*a*).

In addition to the formation of carcinogens *in vivo*, they can also be produced during the processing or preparation of foods. Some human foods, in particular certain types of meats such as ham, have been shown to contain small amounts, on the order of parts per billion, of dimethylnitrosamine (see Walker *et al.*, 1978). Fried bacon may contain up to 80 ppb nitrosopyrrolidine, presumably derived from the nitrosation of proline followed by heat decarboxylation during frying. This level is now much lower owing to the addition of vitamin C during the processing of pork. Nitrosamines have also been identified in beers (Preussmann *et al.* in Emmelot and Kriek, 1979). The importance of these components in causing human cancer is not known.

A recent finding of considerable interest is formation of mutagens during the cooking of foods (Nagao *et al.*, 1978*a*). Some of these have been identified as pyrolysis products of amino acids, such as Trp-P1 and Trp-P2. Other heterocyclic amines have been isolated from cooked food (Kasai *et al.*, 1980). Their structural similarity to experimental breast and colon carcinogens such as 3′,2-dimethyl-4-aminobiphenyl is striking, and thus their role in human carcinogenesis is being actively evaluated (see Miller *et al.*, 1979; Ishii *et al.*, 1980).

4. Genotoxic Carcinogens

Genotoxic carcinogens are those capable of damaging DNA either in their parent form or following biotransformation. In addition to DNA interactions, genotoxic carcinogens react with other nucleophilic molecules such as RNA proteins, including those such as histones which are involved in neoplastic conversion, as well as others. These reactions are believed to underlie their mutagenic and carcinogenic properties, but as yet the specific reactions cannot be stated with certainty. Much available evidence points to the importance of DNA interactions. Regardless, this property can be used to distinguish these carcinogens from those lacking it. The most important pathways of metabolism for these carcinogens, therefore, are those leading to the formation of electrophilic reactants or free radicals capable of undergoing covalent interaction with DNA.

4.1. Direct-Acting Carcinogens

Direct-acting (activation-independent) carcinogens possess the proper reactivity inherent in their structure to take part in the key reactions with cellular and molecular receptors leading to cancer (Table 2). As the Millers have emphasized, this entails the generation of an electrophilic reagent or similar reactive entity (Miller and Miller in Searle, 1976; Miller and Miller in Hiatt *et al.*, 1977; Miller and Miller, 1980). While these chemicals do not, therefore, require metabolic activation, some, depending on structure, may be chemically or enzymatically

TABLE 2
Typical Direct-Acting Carcinogens

β-Propiolactone	$\overset{\displaystyle O \rule[0.5ex]{2em}{0.4pt} CO}{\underset{\displaystyle CH_2 \rule[0.5ex]{1em}{0.4pt} CH_2}{\vert \qquad \vert}}$
1,2,3,4-Diepoxybutane	$CH_2 \rule[0.5ex]{1em}{0.4pt} CH \quad CH \rule[0.5ex]{1em}{0.4pt} CH_2$ (epoxide)
Ethyleneimine	$CH_2 \rule[0.5ex]{1em}{0.4pt} CH_2$ (NH)
Propane sulfone	$\overset{\displaystyle O \rule[0.5ex]{4em}{0.4pt} SO_2}{\underset{\displaystyle CH_2 \rule[0.5ex]{1em}{0.4pt} CH_2 \rule[0.5ex]{1em}{0.4pt} CH_2}{\vert \qquad\qquad \vert}}$
Dimethyl sulfate	$CH_3OSO_2OCH_3$
Methylmethanesulfonate	$CH_3SO_2OCH_3$
Bis(2-chloroethyl)sulfide[a] (mustard gas or yperite)	$ClCH_2CH_2 \diagdown$ S $\diagup ClCH_2CH_2$
Nitrogen mustard (NH_2)[a]	$ClCH_2CH_2 \diagdown$ NCH$_3$ $\diagup ClCH_2CH_2$
Melphalan (sarcolysin)[a]	$ClCH_2CH_2 \diagdown$ N-p-L-C$_6$H$_4$CH$_2$CHCOOH $\diagup ClCH_2CH_2 \qquad$ NH$_2$
2-Naphthylamine mustard[a] (chlornaphazine)	$ClCH_2CH_2 \diagdown$ N $\diagup ClCH_2CH_2$ (naphthalene ring)
Bis(chloromethyl)ether	$ClCH_2OCH_2Cl$
Benzyl chloride	$C_6H_5CH_2Cl$
Dimethylcarbamyl chloride	$(CH_3)_2NCOCl$

[a] Such "mustards" may need biochemical activation.

264

J. H.
WEISBURGER
AND
G. M.
WILLIAMS

inactivated. For example, it has been shown that the mutagenicity of N-methyl-N'-nitro-N-nitrosoguanidine is reduced by the action of microsomal enzymes (Kawachi *et al.*, 1970; Popper *et al.*, 1973).

The direct-acting carcinogens include strained lactones such as β-propiolactone, propane sulfone, and α,β-unsaturated larger-ring lactones, epoxides, imines, some nitrogen mustard derivatives, alkylnitrosoureido compounds (see below), alkyl and other sulfate esters, and some active halogen derivatives, such as bis(chloromethyl)ether (Lawley in Searle, 1976; Van Duuren, 1979; Weisburger and Williams, 1980; Zajdela *et al.*, 1980).

Some quite reactive chemicals do not appear to be highly carcinogenic. The underlying reason may be not only enzymatic detoxification but also simple reaction with cell constituents such as water, proteins, and peptides, which neutralizes their reactivity so that the amount of active agent available at the target sites required for carcinogenicity is negligible. Even synthetically produced "ultimate" carcinogens, which serve as models for agents suspected of being derived metabolically from procarcinogens, have sometimes been found to be noncarcinogenic or of lower carcinogenicity than was initially expected. These highly reactive chemicals given exogenously may fail to reach key targets, but when produced intracellularly near the target they can lead to transformation and cancer. For example, some synthetic epoxides of carcinogenic polycyclic aromatic hydrocarbons, long suspected of being the reactive intermediates, are less carcinogenic than the parent compounds, unless administered under specialized conditions such as to newborn rodents (Buening *et al.*, 1978, 1979; Yang *et al.*, 1978). The sulfate ester of N-hydroxy-N-2-fluorenylacetamide fails to cause cancer in animals, yet there is strong evidence that agents such as this are metabolically produced active intermediates (Section 4.3.4).

Direct alkylating agents that do not require metabolic activation but do undergo biochemical detoxification can be detected under some conditions by their interaction with nitrobenzylpyridine, as developed by Preussmann (1975) and by Sawicki and Sawicki (1969). However, there does not appear to be a direct relationship between this reactivity and carcinogenic risk, probably because tissues and cells contain many competing nucleophilic reactants.

There have been relatively few studies on the metabolism of direct-acting alkylating agents, except insofar as attempts have been made to understand their action as drugs used in cancer chemotherapy. It would appear that most, if not all, of the alkylating agents used as anticancer drugs are also carcinogens (Weisburger, 1977). Apparently, in animal tests at least, their carcinogenic potential is greater than the anticancer potential.

Direct-acting carcinogens not only undergo oxidative enzymatic change but by virtue of their reactive centers also give rise to residues such as carbonium ions, often by a monomolecular SN_1 reaction or a bimolecular SN_2 reaction with a substrate (Jones and Edwards, 1973). Except for their interactions with genetic material, or macromolecules controlling the expression or repair of genetic information, metabolism of direct-acting mutagens and carcinogens usually yields inactive, or less active, detoxified metabolites.

Alkylnitrosoureido compounds do not seem to require enzymatic metabolic activation, although such a reaction is not ruled out and could possibly account for their high local reactivity and carcinogenicity. They are uniformly direct-acting mutagens (Anselme, 1978; Walker *et al.*, 1978; Lijinsky and Andrews, 1979). These chemicals do react at neutral pH with macromolecular and cellular receptors, and also with sulfhydryl compounds. They have limited half-life in aqueous media, especially above pH 6. Thus, it is not expected that such chemicals persist in the environment. However, they can be readily formed from precursors and nitrite (Section 3.3).

Kawachi *et al.* (1970) have described an enzyme system that removes the nitroso group and thus leads to an inactive compound. They ascribe the predominantly local action of this type of compound to such an inactivating reaction. However, large doses of compounds of this type may exhibit a remote effect, presumably because they exceed the capacity of the enzyme removing the nitroso group. Bralow and Weisburger (1976) have noted that *N*-methyl-*N'*-nitro-*N*-nitrosoguanidine, a highly active gastric carcinogen in the Wistar rat, is inactive in several inbred rat strains. It might be that these strains have high levels of the inactivating enzyme system.

Intrarectal administration of *N*-methyl-*N'*-nitro-*N*-nitrosoguanidine in rats readily induces colorectal cancer but no other lesions (Reddy *et al.*, 1980). However, the related nitrosomethylurea in mice leads not only to colorectal cancers but at high dose levels also to leukemias and lung tumors, indicating that this chemical can be absorbed from the large bowel and suggesting also that it is not denitrosated as readily as *N*-methyl-*N'*-nitro-*N*-nitrosoguanidine.

Methylureido derivatives, such as *N*-methylnitrosourea, even though administered intravenously, exhibit a selective carcinogenic effect on some organs, including rat mammary gland, brain, and nervous system. These compounds readily traverse the blood–brain barrier and the placenta. Shortly after injection of radioactive methylnitrosourea, radioactivity is found distributed in many organs. Thus, the distribution of carcinogen under these conditions does not seem to account for the significant organotropic effect. Other factors such as rates of DNA repair and the proliferative status of the tissue have been shown to significantly influence organ selectivity (Section 3.1).

Along these lines, orally administered methylnitrosourethan causes cancer in the stomach and to some extent in the exocrine pancreas in guinea pigs. Even so, liver nucleic acids are alkylated to a greater extent than pancreatic nucleic acids, perhaps a reflection of relative rates of metabolism and repair (Druckrey, 1975). These and similar data suggest that a much more detailed approach to the mode of action of these powerful carcinogenic and mutagenic agents is necessary in order to account for their selective effects.

The fact needs to be considered in all these models that alkylnitrosoureas and related chemicals are powerful carcinogens under virtually all conditions. With these compounds there have been proven chemical reactions in which the alkyl

266

J. H.
WEISBURGER
AND
G. M.
WILLIAMS

group is transferred to a macromolecular receptor (Morimoto *et al.*, 1979; Singer, 1979; Moschel *et al.*, 1980). Even here, however, it can be stated that specificity toward an organ under certain experimental conditions is not necessarily matched with a similar biochemical specificity. Nevertheless, except on intravenous injection, they are primarily local-acting carcinogens simply because the concentration of active electophile is usually greatest at the point of application, as for example in the stomach upon oral entry (Sugimura and Kawachi in Lipkin and Good, 1978).

The nitroso group is certainly essential for the carcinogenicity of this type of chemical. Interestingly, there is differential tissue labeling, depending on whether the material studied has carbon labeled in the methyl or alkyl, or in the guanidino portion (Sugimura and Kawachi in Lipkin and Good, 1978; Preussmann, 1975; Morimoto *et al.*, 1979; Pinsky *et al.*, 1980). The alkyl group appears to combine predominantly with nucleic acids, whereas the guanidino residue, and metabolites thereof, are found in proteins.

4.2. Procarcinogens

A great diversity of chemical structures have been demonstrated to possess the specific and unique property of leading to neoplasia under certain conditions in animals and in humans. Until recent years, it was not at all clear how chemicals as different as 4-dimethylaminoazobenzene, 2-acetylaminofluorene, dimethylnitrosamine, ethionine, pyrrolizidine alkaloids, and aflatoxin B_1 could all lead to liver cancer in rodents, or why 3-methylcholanthrene could inhibit this process with some of these agents under some conditions but enhance it with others, or why powerful sarcoma-inducing polycyclic aromatic hydrocarbons did not usually cause cancer in the liver, or why some carcinogens were excellent mutagens in microbial systems and other equally oncogenic agents were not.

Fortunately, considerable progress has been made in the last 30 years in the field of biochemical pharmacology. Advances have occurred in the area of metabolism of drugs and their mode of action, but it can be said that, in part, advances in this broader field have stemmed from pioneering investigations on the metabolism and mode of action of chemical carcinogens. Conney and colleagues in 1956 were the first to unravel the mechanism by which the carcinogenic effect of the azo dye 4-dimethylaminoazobenzene was inhibited in animals fed the carcinogen 3-methylcholanthrene at the same time. They discovered that the latter agent induced enzymes that converted the azo dye to inactive metabolites. This marked the beginning of detailed studies on enzyme induction, first in relation to the carcinogenic process, then in pharmacology as a whole (see Conney in Miller *et al.*, 1979).

The class of procarcinogens (activation-dependent carcinogens) was found to require metabolic activation, without which they are noncarcinogenic and nonmutagenic. Since most of the activation reactions are oxidative in nature and most microbiological systems used as indicators to detect mutagenic events are poorly endowed with such oxidative enzymes, these chemicals were not initially recognized as mutagens. A proper understanding of this area now permits the use of certain mammalian activation systems to detect potential carcinogenic risk via a mutagenic event in a bacterial indicator system (see Section 2). Such tests are much more rapid than the classical carcinogen bioassays, but must be interpreted with caution. Another important by-product of advances in genetic toxicology is that these short-term tests can serve as collateral supporting evidence in the delineation of possible carcinogenic risks where the results of the classical rodent bioassays are not clear-cut or are controversial (Weisburger and Williams, 1980).

Miller and Miller (see 1980) first generalized the concept that most procarcinogens are metabolized to electrophilic reagents, which appear to be the key intermediates for expression of carcinogenic activity. In some instances, the exact structure of the reagent derived from a chemical carcinogen is known (Fig. 3). For other carcinogens, the exact structure of the ultimate carcinogenic moiety is not yet known, e.g., thioacetamide (Section 4.2.16) or ethionine (Section 4.2.17). Also, it has been proposed that the intermediate may have free radical character, and this point for some kinds of chemicals deserves further experimental consideration. Some of the suggested intermediates, e.g., carbonium ions, have such an evanescent life that it is difficult to visualize how they could be produced at one place in the cell, for example, the endoplasmic reticulum, and then migrate to the receptor such as DNA within the nucleus. It could be that these and maybe all such intermediates are produced in close proximity to the target, and perhaps a concerted three-point interaction between procarcinogen, activating enzyme, and reactive site needs to be considered. This could occur at the membrane interface between endoplasmic reticulum and nucleus (Section 3). Isolated nuclei clearly have some of the metabolic systems to yield reactive electrophiles (Sakai *et al.*, 1978; Stout and Becker, 1979; Bresnick, 1980; Thorgeirsson and Weisburger, 1981).

4.2.1. Polycyclic and Heterocyclic Aromatic Hydrocarbons

Historically, polycyclic and heterocyclic aromatic hydrocarbons were the first pure chemical compounds that caused cancer in animal models. Consequently, investigations on their mode of action and metabolism have been a tradition. Even so, only quite recently has substantial progress toward the delineation of the activation process been made. These chemicals, typified by benz[*a*]anthracene, benzo[*a*]pyrene, dibenz[*a,h*]anthracene, 3-methylcholanthrene, and 7,12-dimethylbenz[*a*]anthracene, undergo numerous metabolic reactions (cf. Hathway, 1979 and previous volumes; Gelboin and Ts'o, 1978; Bjorseth and Dennis, 1980; Brookes, 1980; Coon *et al.*, 1980; Gelboin *et al.*, 1980) that have been delineated through new techniques such as high-performance liquid chromatography as developed by Selkirk and co-workers (Selkirk, 1980). The complicated metabolism of benzo[*a*]pyrene is illustrated in Fig. 4.

268

J. H.
WEISBURGER
AND
G. M.
WILLIAMS ·

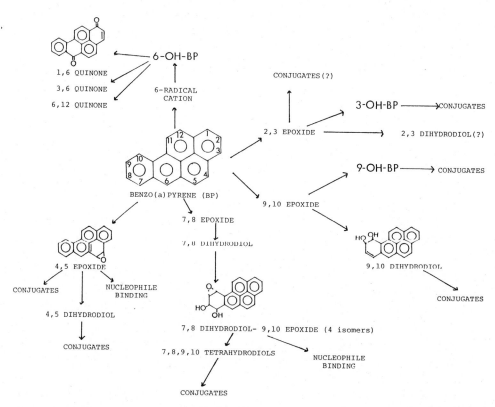

FIGURE 4. The complex metabolism of a typical polycyclic aromatic hydrocarbon, benzo[a]pyrene, a widely distributed environmental chemical in products such as tobacco and coal tar. The major reactions are mediated by the mixed-function oxidases and yield a number of epoxides at various positions on the ring. Also found are a radical cation and a phenol at the 6-position, in turn oxidized further to several quinones. The epoxides react with glutathione transferase to form water-soluble conjugates. The epoxides also rearrange to yield phenols, which are excreted as conjugates. Epoxide hydrases convert the phenols to the corresponding dihydrodiol, which can also be excreted as conjugates. A key activation step is epoxide formation and hydration at bonds 7,8. The resulting 7,8-dihydrodiol presents a reactive 9,10-double bond, subject to epoxidation. Thus, the 7,8-dihydrodiol is a proximate carcinogen. The 7,8-dihydrodiol-9,10-epoxide—specifically, one of the four stereo isomers, namely (+)-7β,8α-dihydroxy-9α,10α-epoxy-7,8,9,10-tetrahydrobenzo[a]pyrene—is the key reactive ultimate carcinogen. This area of the molecule has been termed the bay region in contrast to the 4,5 bond, historically named the K region. Reaction at 4,5 also forms an epoxide that is highly mutagenic, but much less carcinogenic than the active 7,8-dihydrodiol-9,10 epoxide. Possibly, all these activated products participate in the initiation of the overall carcinogenic process with benzo[a]pyrene.

Boyland proposed in 1952 that the key activation reaction might be the formation of an epoxide. However, for many years the polycyclic aromatic hydrocarbons were considered to be direct acting, mainly because very small amounts applied to the skin or injected subcutaneously produced tumors. The elegant theoretical studies of the Pullmans and Daudels pinpointed an electronically reactive area in these molecules that was proposed to be relevant to their carcinogenicity, the so-called K region (Bergmann and Pullman, 1969). The importance of metabolism to the activity of polycyclic aromatic hydrocarbons, however, was established when Gelboin, and Grover and Sims (see Bergmann and Pullman, 1969) showed that these carcinogens combined to a significant extent with DNA in the presence of a microsomal oxidative system. At the same time, Witkop, Daly, and Jerina noted that benzenic hydrocarbons could undergo epoxidation with formation of arene oxides (see Jerina *et al.* in Hiatt *et al.*, 1977). The epoxides are chemically reactive and are also substrates for further enzymatic reactions such as dihydrodiol formation (Lu and Miwa, 1980; Oesch in Coon *et al.*, 1980) and conjunction with sulfhydryl amino acids or peptides like glutathione (Benson *et al.*, 1978; Sarrif *et al.*, 1978; Chasseaud, 1979).

Epoxidation of aryl structures appears to be a common metabolic reaction undergone not only by the carcinogenic polycyclic aromatic hydrocarbons but even by simple noncarcinogenic mono- and dicyclic structures (Jerina *et al.* in Hiatt *et al.*, 1977). These are not usually carcinogenic, probably because the epoxides of the smaller hydrocarbons are good substrates for detoxifying enzymes.

Benzene itself has a leukemogenic effect in a few occupationally exposed individuals. Experimental production of tumors has only recently been reported (Maltoni and Scarnato, 1979). As would be expected, benzene is metabolized to phenolic compounds (Rickert *et al.*, 1979; Andrews *et al.*, 1979*b*), possibly via an intermediary arene oxide. The effect of benzene as a leukemogen may stem not only from an attack of a putative arene oxide on a macromolecular target (Nebert and Jensen, 1979*b*) but may also be accounted for indirectly by a possible immunosuppresive effect of phenolic compounds obtained through metabolism.

The higher homologs naphthalene and biphenyl are likewise metabolized through epoxidation followed by facile production of phenols and mercapturic acids. There are no data on any adverse aspects of these compounds. The capacity to induce enzymes for the specific hydroxylation of biphenyl to yield 2-hydroxy- vs. 4-hydroxybiphenyl, respectively, has been proposed by Parke (1979) as a possible indicator of a biochemical potential toward genotoxic activation.

Among the tricyclic compounds anthracene and phenanthrene, specific and sensitive techniques, combining synthetic approaches and an examination of *in vitro* and *in vitro* metabolic systems, have permitted the detection of small amounts of weakly mutagenic and carcinogenic metabolites as dihydrodiol epoxides (Buening *et al.*, 1979). For the first time, a metabolite of a tricyclic aromatic hydrocarbon has been found to be weakly and definitely mutagenic and carcinogenic. Under *in vivo* conditions, the major biochemical reactions are

270

J. H.
WEISBURGER
AND
G. M.
WILLIAMS

detoxification reactions, accounting for the fact that phenanthrene is not considered to be carcinogenic.

The higher homologs, namely systems with four or five rings exemplified by the weakly carcinogenic benz[a]anthracene and the powerful carcinogen benzo[a]pyrene, have been studied extensively to delineate the activation pathway. The larger molecules seem to have a strong affinity for large targets like DNA that facilitate intercalation and binding (Drinkwater et al., 1978). As noted above, historically the emphasis was on the demonstration that reactions on the so-called K region were related to this activation step. It was from the laboratory of Sims and his colleagues in London where the definite evidence first came that the activation might be more complex and involve an epoxidation, followed by hydration to a partially saturated dihydrodiol, exposing a highly reactive double bond that could further epoxidize. The postulated active ultimate carcinogen would thus be the dihydrodiol epoxide.

Active research in a number of centers, utilizing a great variety of techniques, has amply substantiated this concept with a number of polycyclic aromatic hydrocarbons. For further details the reader is referred to specific reviews in recent monographs (Gelboin and Ts'o, 1978; Bjorseth and Dennis, 1980; Miller et al., 1979; Emmelot and Kriek, 1979; Brookes, 1980; Coon et al., 1980).

The collaboration of the groups of Conney and of Jerina (in Hiatt et al., 1977) has developed the general and broadly applicable concept of bay-region activation, to denote the formation first of a dihydrodiol at a specific position of the ring system, followed by further expoxidation to yield the ultimate reactive species, a dihydrodiol epoxide (Fig. 3). Thus, the dihydrodiol is the proximate carcinogen, capable of detection as a mutagen for Salmonella typhimurium with, but not without, biochemical activation by the S-9 fraction rat liver. On the other hand, as the derived epoxide is active and thus does not require the S-9 fraction, it is the ultimate mutagenic metabolite.

More recently the stereochemistry has been elucidated. Among the several possible stereoisomers of a particular dihydrodiolepoxide, one specific isomer of the active form of benzo[a]pyrene is $(+)$-$7\beta,8\alpha$-dihydroxy-$9\alpha,10\alpha$-epoxy-7,8,9,10-tetrahydrobenzo[a]pyrene (Buening et al., 1978). The exact structure has been worked out by crystallographic analysis (Neidle et al., 1980), and the reactions with various cellular and molecular targets have established this particular metabolite as the key metabolite (Bartsch et al., 1979a; Huberman et al., 1977; Jeffrey et al., 1979; Marquardt et al., 1979; P. Okano et al., 1979; Pereira et al., 1979; Meehan and Straub, 1979; Backer and Weinstein, 1980; Slaga et al., 1980; Wood et al., 1980).

While this basic scheme has been demonstrated to occur for the known polynuclear aromatic hydrocarbons, it is possible that metabolites other than the bay-region epoxides may participate in the carcinogenic process (Perin-Roussel, et al., 1980). In fact, benzo[α]pyrene-4,5-epoxide is more mutagenic quantitatively than the bay-region epoxide, but it is less carcinogenic. Likewise, the bay-region dihydrodiols of the weak initiator dibenz[a,c]anthracene are less mutagenic than the non-bay-region dihydrodiol, but further research on initiation potential is needed to clarify those relationships (Malaveille *et al.*, 1980).

The explanation for the lack of quantitative correlation between mutagenicity
and carcinogenicity may stem from differences in the rates of detoxification in
bacterial vs. mammalian systems (Bartsch *et al.*, 1979a; Santella *et al.*, 1979;
Armstrong *et al.*, 1980; Bigger *et al.*, 1980a,b; Plummer *et al.*, 1980; Jerina *et al.*
in Coon *et al.*, 1980). Nonetheless, *in vivo*, particularly in diverse target organs,
all of the reactive electrophilic metabolites may play a role in the overall carcinogenic process (Okamoto *et al.*, 1978; Yang *et al.*, 1978; Thakker *et al.*, 1979;
Miller and Miller, 1980). There may be multiple reactive metabolites, and further
research, for example, on the nature of the macromolecular adducts, should
prove enlightening (Baird and Diamond, 1979; DiGiovanni *et al.*, 1979; Jeffrey
et al., 1979; Legraverend *et al.*, 1980).

Alkyl substitutition powerfully changes the carcinogenicity in this class of
compounds. For example, whereas benz[*a*]anthracene is a weak carcinogen,
7,12-dimethylbenz[*a*]anthracene is a powerful carcinogen (Chouroulinkov *et al.*,
1979). Chrysene is a weak carcinogen (Buening *et al.*, 1978; Levin *et al.*, 1978).
Of the six monomethyl chrysenes, the 5-methyl isomer is a highly active carcinogen, and the relevant activation process has been described in terms of a
bay-region dihydrodiol epoxide (Hecht *et al.*, 1979b,c, 1980). Less active alkyl-
substituted hydrocarbons have the alkyl group in a ring position such that
detoxification reactions are stimulated and activation reactions, by difference,
are less likely.

Whereas *C*-hydroxylation to phenols is often thought to be a detoxification
reaction, it seems that within the large molecules such as benzo[*α*]pyrene,
carcinogenicity and mutagenicity can be demonstrated, depending on the position of the hydroxy group, presumably because under these conditions the
bay-region dihydrodiol epoxide formation still occurs in target tissues (Chang
et al., 1979; Owens *et al.*, 1979; Cohen *et al.*, 1980; Kouri *et al.*, 1980).

One alternate way of oxidative metabolism in this class of compounds may
involve the formation of a radical cation, as for example at position 6 of
benzo[*a*]pyrene. This attack leads to certain of the known metabolites like
quinones, but it is not certain whether this particular reaction also relates to
carcinogenicity (Rogan *et al.*, 1979; Selkirk, 1980).

The sequence of the activation steps within the class of polycyclic aromatic
hydrocarbons and heterocyclic hydrocarbons draws attention also to the epoxide
hydrolases as playing a role both in the activation steps involving the production
of the dihydrodiol after the first oxidation reaction, and of a tetrahydrodiol or
tetrol from the addition of the elements of water to the second epoxide, or
indeed any other epoxides. The kinetics of the reaction of various epoxides
toward epoxide hydrolases are quite different. This accounts for the fact that
the 7,8-dihydrodiol of benzo[*a*]pyrene forms rather readily, whereas the 9,10-
epoxide is usually not a good substrate. This area has been summarized in
particular by Armstrong *et al.* (1980), Glatt *et al.* (1980), Lu and Miwa (1980),
and Oesch *et al.* (*in* Coon *et al.*, 1980). This enzyme is present not only
in mammalian systems but also in the intestinal microflora, which apparently

272

J. H.
WEISBURGER
AND
G. M.
WILLIAMS

convert, for example, cholesterol-5α,6α-epoxide to the corresponding cholestane-3β,5α,6β-triol, a fecal metabolite of cholesterol (Hwang and Kelsey, 1978).

A chemical system mimicking mammalian and microbiological reactions, namely oxidation with oxygen, catalyzed by ascorbic acid, iron, and a chelating agent, also has been shown to form dihydrodiols (Hewer *et al.*, 1979).

The biochemical reactions discussed account also for the subsequent formation of diols, and conjugates of such diols, the derived phenols, and also formation of glutathionine derivatives, and other metabolic products of polycyclic and heterocyclic hydrocarbons which have been known for many years. A combination of mutagenicity and carcinogenicity studies has provided an entirely new approach to the understanding of the essential pathways of activation of this class of chemical carcinogens. These reactions occur in varied organs and further studies may account for the organ specificity of certain of these chemicals (Okuda *et al.*, 1977; Benson *et al.*, 1978; Bartsch *et al.*, 1979*b*; Gehly *et al.*, 1979; Wolf *et al.*, 1979; Mattison and Thorgeirsson, 1979).

Polyheterocyclic aromatic hydrocarbons have the potential to undergo more complex metabolic reactions, since reaction on, or vicinal to the hetero-atom may lead to facile ring opening. Nonetheless, epoxides have been identified with such compounds (Kitahara *et al.*, 1978; P. Okano *et al.*, 1979; Okuda *et al.*, 1979).

Many polycyclic aromatic hydrocarbons can induce mixed-function oxidases (Section 7.3). However, there appears to be no relation between the property of inducting liver and intestinal tract metabolic enzymes and the facility of forming an electrophilic mutagen and carcinogen (Argus *et al.*, 1980).

Inasmuch as polycyclic hydrocarbons are a component of cigarette smoke and tobacco tar, the possibility is being explored that a differential sensitivity to these agents exists in humans. Development of more information might permit the assessment of the relative risk of cigarette smokers and thus provide an additional parameter in the worldwide efforts to reduce or prevent cancer (Hammond *et al.* in Hiatt *et al.*, 1977; Wynder and Gori, 1977; Wynder and Hoffmann, 1979).

4.2.2. Carcinogenic Nitrosamines and Related Compounds

Carcinogenic nitrosamines and related compounds have been the subject of study for only about 25 years. Dimethylnitrosamine, formerly an important industrial intermediate, was first found to cause cancer by Magee and Barnes in 1956 (see Magee *et al.* in Searle, 1976). Since that time, many different types of this broad class of chemicals have been synthesized and their carcinogenicity studied (see Schmähl, 1970; Druckrey, 1975; Preussmann, 1975; Magee *et al.* in Coon *et al.*, 1980; Walker *et al.*, 1978; Emmelot and Kriek, 1979). Virtually all of them exhibit some degree of carcinogenicity, except when there is no alkyl group, as in diphenylnitrosamine. At one high dose rate, but not a lower dose, this compound has induced bladder cancer in rats (Cardy *et al.*, 1979). The possibility of transnitrosation of secondary amines exists, but the mechanism may not involve genotoxicity at all.

As a function of structure, species, dose rate, and other variables, nitrosamines exhibit exquisite target specificity. A beginning has been made toward understanding this important tissue affinity on the basis of specific metabolic reactions (Druckrey, 1975; Magee *et al.* in Searle, 1976; Magee *et al.* in Coon *et al.*, 1980; LaVoie and Hecht in Saxena, 1980; Montesano *et al.*, 1980*a,b,c*).

Current concepts visualize the production of a reactive electrophilic intermediate. With the simplest of the nitrosamines, dimethylnitrosamine, this has been described as CH_3^+ (Fig. 3). In view of the very short half-life of such structures predicted by classical organic chemistry, it is possible that they are produced transitorily during a concerted reaction among substrate, enzyme system, and target, and the key active intermediate most likely is an alkyldiazonium hydroxide. Care must be taken to account for isotope effects in the metabolism of such small molecules (Singer and Lijinsky, 1979; Lijinsky and Reuber, 1980*a,b*). The complexity of the conversion of even simple prototypes in this class of compounds is attested to by the fact that dimethylnitrosamine is much more toxic than the diethyl higher homolog, but the latter appears to be more carcinogenic.

The first step in the metabolism of alkylnitrosamine appears to be a classical *C*-hydroxylation. The reaction sequence for dimethylnitrosamine is shown in Fig. 5. The eventual reactive product postulated is a methyl carbonium ion, although there could be a concerted effect between the methyl (or alkyl) diazonium hydroxide and the nucleophile attacked.

With a more complex alkyl group, the question is whether hydroxylation occurs proximate to the nitrogen on the α position, as proposed initially (Druckrey, 1975), or through a β-oxidation as in fatty acids, as visualized by Krüger (1973). With longer-chain alkylnitrosamines, ω-hydroxylation can also occur (Blattmann and Preussmann, 1973; Mochizuki *et al.*, 1980). There is evidence that all of these intermediates are metabolites, but α-hydroxylation is the key activation step with aliphatic and cyclic nitrosamines.

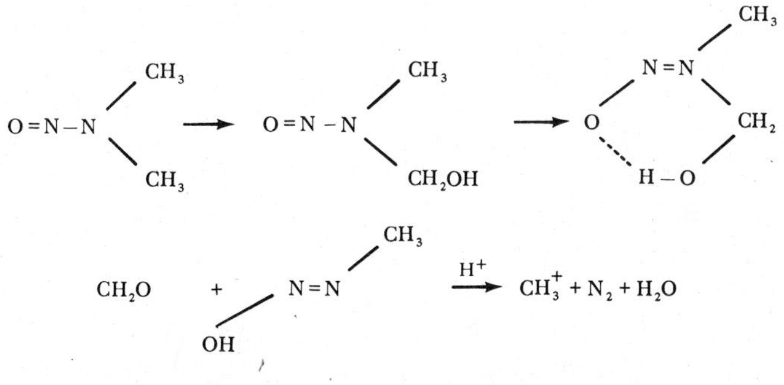

FIGURE 5. The metabolism of aliphatic nitrosamines involves a *C*-hydroxylation. Nominally, all carbons in a longer-chain alkane are subject to hydroxylation. With dimethylnitrosamine, the unstable intermediate hydroxymethyl compound releases formaldehyde (which can be measured), and via a methyl diazonium hydroxide yields a postulated highly reactive carbonium ion. In more complex aliphatic or cyclic nitrosamines, α-hydroxylation likewise is the key reaction (see the reactions for nitrosopyrrolidine in Fig. 3).

274

J. H.
WEISBURGER
AND
G. M.
WILLIAMS

Many species, including primates and humans, possess the necessary enzymes. Thus, these chemicals are reliably carcinogenic in rodents and in nonhuman primates (Adamson and Sieber, 1979), whereas in humans no case of cancer unambiguously related to exposure has been reported (Weisburger and Raineri, 1975).

In vitro studies, utilizing tissue slices or homogenates and subcellular fractions, have delineated a certain relationship between rate of metabolism and carcinogenicity. The metabolism was often measured by CO_2 or aldehyde evolution, recently made the subject of a new assay for nitrosamine metabolism (Farrelly, 1980), or a combination of radioactivity from the tagged carcinogens with cellular macromolecules such as RNA or DNA (Magee *et al.* in Searle, 1976; Pegg, 1980*a,b*).

Along these lines, a number of groups have demonstrated the conversion *in vitro* of dimethylnitrosamine by a microsome fraction of liver to a mutagen detected in the Ames system. The reaction is inhibited by carbon monoxide and appears to be cytochrome P-450 dependent. As the amount of enzyme preparation is crucial (Prival *et al.*, 1979), the liquid incubation introduced by Matsushima and by Bartsch is preferred (see Matsushima *et al.* in Norpoth and Garner, 1980; Bartsch *et al.*, 1979*a*).

Treatment of rats and mice with 3-methylcholanthrene decreases the carcinogenic effect of dimethylnitrosamine in the liver in rats but causes more extrahepatic tumors, especially in the lung. Decreased liver microsomal demethylation of dimethylnitrosamine was found on pretreatment with 3-methylcholanthrene or with phenobarbital. In mice, tumors at various sites were induced faster, especially in the lung and kidneys, by the mixture of dimethylnitrosamine and methylcholanthrene (Cardesa *et al.*, 1973; Uchida and Hirono, 1979). Thus, enzyme induction with this class of carcinogens often increases rather than decreases carcinogenicity, in contrast to polycyclic aromatic hydrocarbons or arylamine carcinogens, for which enzyme induction usually raises detoxification and excretion. Aminoacetonitrile inhibits both metabolism and carcinogenicity (see Magee *et al.* in Searle, 1976; Arcos *et al.*, 1980).

There is some controversy as to whether the mixed-function oxidases of the cytochrome P-450 system mediate the initial metabolic reaction concerned with the first step in the oxidation of the methyl group to the hydroxymethyl, which is thought to be the primary event. On the basis of inhibition experiments, there is evidence for several enzymes (Anselme, 1978; Appel *et al.*, 1979; Lotlikar *et al.*, 1978; Hutton *et al.*, 1979; Arcos *et al.*, 1980; Chin and Bosmann, 1980; Mostafa and Weisburger, 1980; Pegg, 1980*a*). Some data indicate that the Ziegler flavin-dependent oxidases oxidize the nitrogen followed by rearrangement (see Coon *et al.*, 1980). There are other data suggesting that hydroxylation on carbon involves several reaction sequences labeled demethylase I and II by Arcos *et al.* (1980), who base their views on selective inducibility and inhibition of the metabolic sequence. In any case, the reactions eventually lead to hydroxymethylmethylnitrosamine. This spontaneously decomposes to formaldehyde and the methyl diazonium hydroxide intermediate, which in turn leads to the methyl carbonium ion. As is true with the postulated ultimate carcinogens in the arylamine series where the active intermediate was stabilized through the chemical synthesis of an acyl derivative, a similar sequence was actually established with dimethylnitrosamine through the studies of the synthetic nitrosoacetoxymethylmethylamine (Roller *et al.*, 1975). This synthetic chemical exhibits many of the reactions of metabolically activated dimethylnitrosamine. It can be split by water or an esterase to yield the putative hydroxymethylmethylnitrosamine (Kleihues *et al.*, 1979; Frank *et al.*, 1980). Interestingly, intraperitoneal injection of this compound not only causes liver cancer but colon cancer, similar to the properties of methylazoxymethanol, the putative proximate carcinogen derived from 1,2-dimethylhydrazine (Section 4.2.12). Chronic intake affects the pattern of metabolism and repair (Stumpf *et al.*, 1979; Montesano *et al.*, 1980*b*).

With the more complex longer-chain aliphatic nitrosamines such as the dipropyl and dibutyl derivatives, and especially with the cyclic nitrosamines such as nitrosopyrrolidine and nitrosonornicotine, the activation reactions begin to be delineated (Magee *et al.* in Searle, 1976; Mirvish, 1977). While *C*-oxidation can and does occur at all possible carbon atoms, the significant *C*-oxidation forming a *C*-hydroxy derivative occurs on the α-carbon to the nitrosamine function. For example, with dibutylnitrosamine, a urinary bladder carcinogen in rats (Ito *et al.*, 1973; Druckrey, 1975; Irving *et al.*, 1979; Mochizuki *et al.*, 1980), there is also ω-hydroxylation, and interestingly, not only is the resulting alcohol still a urinary bladder carcinogen but also the further oxidized ω-carboxylic acid. Analyses of the residues bound to nucleic acids from the longer-chain aliphatic nitrosamines have given evidence not only of binding of the n-1 side chain but have also demonstrated methylation (see, for example, Leung *et al.*, 1980; LaVoie and Hecht in Saxena, 1980).

Just as the aliphatic and alkylaryl nitrosamines exhibit quite specific and selective organ affinity, in part a function of dose and other variables, probably owing to differences in metabolism related to them, the cyclic and heterocyclic nitrosamines do the same, but to an even more pronounced extent. The metabolism of cyclic nitrosamines has now been studied in some detail (Ross and Mirvish, 1977; Hecht *et al.*, 1978; Leung; *et al.*, 1978; Appel *et al.*, 1980; LaVoie and Hecht in Saxena, 1980). α-Hydroxylation is the primary event (Ross and Mirvish, 1977; Hecht *et al.*, 1978; Singer and Lijinsky, 1979; Chen *et al.*, 1980; Cottrell *et al.*, 1980; Gingell *et al.*, 1980). With unsymmetrical cyclic nitrosamines like nitrosonornicotine, both of the two possible α-hydroxylations have been shown to occur to form two distinct products (Chen *et al.*, 1980; Hoffmann *et al.*, 1980; LaVoie and Hecht in Saxena, 1980).

Dipropylnitrosamine causes cancer in rodents, including the hamster, at a number of different target organs. Importantly, in the hamster, bis(2-hydroxypropyl)nitrosamine is an excellent carcinogen for the pancreatic duct and thus a model for the disease that occurs in humans. The hydroxypropyl is readily metabolized to the hydroxypropyloxopropyl derivative and to the bisoxopropyl compound. These reactions are interconvertible: upon administration of one of these chemicals, the others are found as metabolites (Gingell *et*

276

J. H.
WEISBURGER
AND
G. M.
WILLIAMS

al., 1979, 1980; Whalley et al., 1980). Previously, Lijinsky's group (see Lijinsky and Reuber, 1980b) found that N-nitroso-2,6-dimethylmorpholine was a pancreatic carcinogen in the hamster. In this species, the overall metabolism of two possible isomers, cis and trans, is similar (see Gingell et al., 1979, 1980). In the rat, where this compound induces mainly tumors in the upper gastrointestinal tract and in the nasal cavity, the trans isomer seemed a more powerful carcinogen (Lijinsky and Reuber, 1980b). Thus, as is true for polycyclic aromatic hydrocarbons (Section 4.2.1), the carcinogenic effects are highly stereospecific. It was thought that this is due to the metabolic conversion of the cyclic nitrosamine to the hydroxypropylketopropylnitrosamine, which can exist in a cyclic form and in turn has a stereochemical conformation mimicking the cyclic form of carbohydrates. It has been proposed that this steric analogy might account for the preferential induction of pancreatic cancer in the hamster (Gingell et al., 1979, 1980). In rats the diketopropyl compound is a colon carcinogen, perhaps because of a reversible α-keto–α-alcohol conversion. As is true for the acetoxy analog derived from dimethylnitrosamine, which relates further to the organospecific action of methylazoxymethanol (Section 4.2.12), this kind of structure can induce colon cancer in rodents. Scarpelli et al. (1980) have established that a post-mitochondrial fraction from pancreas can metabolize 2,6-dimethyl-nitrosomorpholine and also nitrosobisoxopropylamine to mutagens.

Thus, virtually all biochemical metabolic reactions with aliphatic nitrosamines are concerned with activation eventually to the reactive carcinogenic and mutagenic electrophile. These reactions are complex and involve several enzymes, including the mixed-function oxidases, flavin dependent oxidases, and possibly even alcohol dehydrogenase, since the first oxidation of a CH_2 link leads to a CH_2OH alcoholic function. Nevertheless, there are now some data on deactivation reactions of nitrosamines and nitrosamides. Appel et al. (1980) reported that incubation of nitrosomorpholine with rat or mouse liver microsomes yielded nitrite. Nitrite removal was enhanced by phenobarbital treatment and was blocked by enhancers of the cytochrome P-450 system. A similar system but operating on alkylnitrosamides (see Section 4.1) was described by Kawachi et al. (1970).

4.2.3. Dialkyltriazines

The dialkyltriazines are related to the nitrosamines because, presumably, they form similar reactive intermediates during metabolism (Druckrey, 1975; Preussmann, 1975; Bartsch et al., 1979c). Except for the demonstration that labeled alkyltriazenes yield altered nucleic acids, with radioactivity attached to the guanylic acid in RNA, there have been no studies on the overall metabolism of these agents, some of which are related to dyestuff intermediates. It is obvious, however, that the key reaction is hydroxylation of the dialkyl groups attached to nitrogen, leading eventually to the production of a highly reactive intermediate.

4(5)-(3,3-Dimethyl-1-triazeno)imidazole-5(4)-carboxamide (DIC) was developed as a drug useful in the chemotherapy of certain neoplasms. As might be expected on the basis of its structure containing a dialkyltriazeno residue, this chemical is also a powerful carcinogen. Metabolism in animals and humans leads to microsomal dealkylation, with production of a residue described as a methylcarbonium ion similar to what is seen during the metabolism of dimethyl-nitrosamine or the 1-aryl-3,3-dialkyltriazenes, described earlier. The remainder of the DIC molecule, namely 4(5)-aminoimidazole-5(4)-carboxamide, is excreted in the urine of rodents and humans (Skibba *et al.*, 1970).

4.2.4. Aromatic Amines, Amides, and Aminoazo Dyes

The carcinogenic aromatic amines, azo dyes, and their derivatives and analogs do not usually cause cancer at the point of application. Thus, they have been the prototypes of agents that require metabolic activation. Exceptions are 2-anthramine, which Bielschowsky (see Clayson, 1962) found to cause skin tumors following cutaneous application to rats, and 6-aminochrysene, which failed to induce visceral tumors when fed to rats (see Franchi *et al.*, 1973; Grantham *et al.*, 1974a) but did cause tumors when applied to the skin of mice. It is probable and needs to be shown that these chemicals are thus active, not because of the aromatic amino group directly, but because of epoxide formation at a position activated by the amino group. Hence, these two and perhaps other aromatic amines are active through the aromatic carbon ring system of their molecule.

The concept of activation on the aromatic hydrocarbon portion of aromatic amines is further supported by the finding that *N*-2-fluorenylacetamide (or 2-acetylaminofluorene) appears to cause more skin tumors, on promotion with croton oil, than the *N*-hydroxy metabolite (Miller *et al.*, 1964). Indirect support for an epoxy metabolite with arylamines is based on the isolation of some mercapturic acids derived from acetanilide (Grantham *et al.*, 1974b), although Calder *et al.* (1974) have provided data indicating that such intermediates could result from hydroxylamine derivatives. It is not known whether such epoxy intermediates are involved in extrahepatic carcinogenesis by certain arylamines such as 6-aminochrysene or benzidine in the mammary gland, although with other arylamines a more conventional mechanism, the formation of electrophilic *N*-acetoxyarylamines (see below), has been observed (Bartsch *et al.*, 1973; Malejka-Giganti *et al.*, 1973).

The initial step in the activation of aromatic amines and their *N*-acetyl derivatives is well established to be hydroxylation on the nitrogen to form the corresponding hydroxylamino derivatives (Fig. 3). Evidence for this was first obtained in the laboratory of the Millers and has now been extended to other aromatic amines and amides (Miller *et al.*, 1964; Uehleke, 1973; Weisburger and Weisburger, 1973; Emmelot and Kriek, 1979; Griffin and Shaw, 1979; Miller *et al.*, 1979; Miller and Miller, 1980; Thorgeirsson and Weisburger, 1981). This reaction is stereospecific and takes place only when the amino group is on certain positions of the aromatic ring. Thus, 2-naphthylamine, 2-fluorenamine, and 2-anthramine are powerful carcinogens, whereas the pure 1-isomers are not. The groups of Radomski, Troll, and Gutmann have demonstrated that the hydroxylamines corresponding to the inactive 1- or 3-substituted arylamines are

278

J. H.
WEISBURGER
AND
G. M.
WILLIAMS

powerful carcinogens and mutagens. Just as in the case of the oxidation and further metabolism of the carcinogenic polycyclic aromatic hydrocarbons, the N-hydroxylation of aromatic amines likewise is probably under genetic control. Development of a simple clinical test for this property might be useful for delineating the risk of individuals with potential exposure to carcinogenic aromatic amines. New analytical techniques such as liquid chromatography and mutagenicity assays might help in this regard (see Gutmann, 1974; Gorrod, 1978; Raineri et al., 1978; Scribner et al., 1979; Hinson et al., 1979a).

Many of the key concepts in arylamine carcinogenesis were derived from studies with the powerful classic carcinogens 2-naphthylamine, 2-fluorenamine and derivatives, and 4-aminobiphenyl and derivatives. In recent years, systematic chronic toxicity tests of environmental carcinogens, including aromatic amines, have delineated the carcinogenicity of a number of smaller and larger molecular weight arylamines, such as those with a single benzene ring, or other more complex tricyclic arylamines, or alkyl-substituted arylamines (Weisburger and Williams, 1980).

Among single-ring compounds, aniline and the derived N-acetyl derivative acetanilide had been tested a number of times and found to be noncarcinogenic. In a recent NCI bioassay, however, where aniline was designed to be a negative control, tests of aniline itself appeared to induce a small but definite number of splenic sarcomas and hemangioendotheliomas. The metabolism of aniline has been studied in detail especially by Kiese and Uehleke (see Gorrod, 1978). Aniline undergoes N-hydroxylation to the corresponding hydroxylamine, which is in turn in equilibrium with the nitroso derivative. There are also ring hydroxylation reactions, especially to form p-aminophenol and the N-acetyl derivative. The latter can bind to protein (Youndes and Siegers, 1980). In addition, there is some evidence for an epoxy metabolite based on the isolation of the corresponding mercapturic acid (Grantham et al., 1974b). It is not certain whether the splenic sarcomas are the result of a direct interaction of an unidentified electrophilic reactant derived from aniline or whether these lesions stem from the well-known effect of the metabolically formed phenylhydroxylamine on the hematopoietic system (see Kiese in Gorrod, 1978). Establishment of the relevant mechanisms is important since the implications of a genotoxic interaction are quite different compared to the second possibility, a reversible dose- and time-dependent stress on the hematopoietic system.

The alkyl anilines, namely toluidines and xylidines, show great differences in carcinogenicity. The ortho derivatives are slightly but definitely carcinogenic. Son et al. (1980) have isolated an N-oxidation product of o-toluidine. The aniline metabolite, p-hydroxyacetanilide, is highly hepatotoxic but apparently, unlike the corresponding acetaminophen, not carcinogenic. The mode of toxicity of alkyl anilines is not yet well established, although protein binding has been detected (Black, 1980; Younes and Siegers, 1980; Rollins et al., 1979; Hinson et al., 1979b).

Phenacetin abuse, but not low periodic intake, has led to cancer of the urinary bladder in humans (Bengtsson et al., 1978). Whereas animal experimentation utilizing moderate dose levels failed to disclose carcinogenicity in animal models, high-level feeding parallel to the abuse situation in humans has confirmed the carcinogenicity of phenacetin (Nakanishi *et al.*, 1978; Isaka *et al.*, 1979). These findings have stimulated research on the metabolism of phenacetin, and an *N*-hydroxy derivative has been identified (Hinson *et al.*, 1979*b*; Pang *et al.*, 1979).

2,4-Toluenediamine was found carcinogenic to rodent liver, as was 2,4-diaminoanisole. Metabolism studies have yielded evidence that there is differential *N*-acylation of the amino group in different species (Glinsukon *et al.*, 1975; Unger *et al.*, 1980; King *et al.* in Gorrod, 1978; King *et al.* in Thorgeirsson and Weisburger, 1981). These compounds also yield mutagenic activity that is thought to be related to *N*-oxidation products (Aune and Dybing, 1979). The acylation reaction is in part under genetic control (Lower *et al.*, 1979; Tannen and Webber, 1979), and this reaction may have a role in certain of the carcinogenic aromatic amines.

With a number of aromatic amines, the effect noted is similar whether the chemical administered is the amine or an acylamide, especially if the acyl group is acetyl. It was known for many years, for example, that 2-fluorenamine and *N*-2-fluorenylacetamide have almost equivalent effects (E. K. Weisburger in Sontag, 1981). However, the benzoyl derivative has low carcinogenicity and the tosyl derivative is inactive. At one time, it was felt that this difference rested on the ease of hydrolysis and liberation of the amine. Since the discovery of *N*-hydroxylation as a key activation reaction for aromatic amines, it appears more likely that the difference in activity rests on the relative ease of *N*-hydroxylation. Synthetic *N*-hydroxyacyl derivatives are carcinogenic or mutagenic, although with bulky or complex acyl substituents a lower effect is noted. An extensive set of data in this area were provided by Malejka-Giganti *et al.* (1973), Bartsch *et al.* (1977), and Kuroki and Bartsch (1979).

Nonetheless, with certain other carcinogenic amines, there is a difference in carcinogenicity, such as the distinct effect of 2-naphthylamine and 2-naphthylacetamide in the dog. The dog may be unusual insofar as this species does not have acetyl transferase, and hence the equilibrium present in other species between acyl (specifically acetyl) derivatives and free amines does not hold. *N*-Formylation in rats was described in relation to the metabolism of 2-aminoanthraquinone (Gothoskar *et al.*, 1979).

Arylamines, carcinogenic or not, undergo several types of biochemical transformation *in vivo* and *in vitro* (Fig. 6). These involve oxidation on the ring, which, as noted above, implies a possible epoxide as intermediate, and oxidation on the nitrogen. The *N*-oxidation may involve not only the cytochrome P-450 enzyme system but also a flavine-adenine-dependent enzyme complex (Hlavica and Hülsmann, 1979; see Hlavica and Hülsmann in Coon *et al.*, 1980). Where the nitrogen is substituted with *N*-methyl, the latter enzyme system seems to be more relevant. In any case, oxidation on the nitrogen by either pathway leading to an arylhydroxylamine derivative appears to be an activation pathway for mutagenicity and carcinogenicity. As will be noted later on, this kind of

280
J. H.
WEISBURGER
AND
G. M.
WILLIAMS

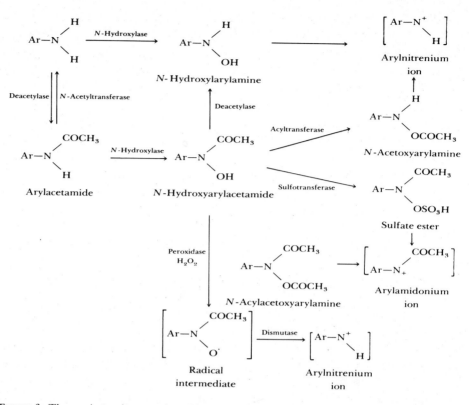

FIGURE 6. The carcinogenic aromatic amines or N-acyl derivatives can undergo ring hydroxylation to form phenolic products that are usually not carcinogenic since they can be excreted readily as conjugates. The major structure-, species-, and strain-specific controlling activation reaction is N-hydroxylation, yielding the corresponding N-hydroxy derivative. This metabolite can also form through reduction of the corresponding nitroaryl compounds, which are therefore also carcinogenic. Where the amino group is sterically unhindered through absence of large neighboring groups (e.g., methyl), there is a reversible deacetylation and acetylation, catalyzed by specific enzymes. With o-methyl substituents, these reactions, as well as N-hydroxylation, are sterically hindered. With the free hydroxylamine, a further oxidation step yields a reactive arylnitrenium ion, the ultimate carcinogen. With the N-acyl-N-hydroxy derivatives, a required second activation step is sulfate ester formation for liver carcinogenesis, or an O-acyl formation with an acyl transferase in specific other organs. These in turn can readily interact with nucleophiles, including DNA, as the arylnitrenium ion or the acyl amidonium ion. In addition, there is evidence of a peroxidation step which in the presence of hydrogen peroxide forms radical intermediates which in turn, through a dismutase, yield reactive products. Extrahepatic carcinogenesis appears to involve the acyl transferase or the peroxidation reactions. The overall process is a function of the structure of the chemical and many endogenous and exogenous controlling factors.

compound can be obtained also from the reduction of nitroaryl derivatives, thus accounting for their carcinogenicity.

Steric factors are important in the metabolism of aromatic amines and amides. Thus, extensive *ortho* substitution as, for example, in 2,4,6-trimethylacetanilide yields a noncarcinogenic compound whereas the corresponding amine, mesidine, is a weak carcinogen, as is also the case for 3,3',5,5'-tetramethylbenzidine versus benzidine. Likewise, the low extent of N-oxidation, relative to the more prevalent ring *C-oxidation of* α-amino-substituted arylamines, accounts for the low or negative mutagenicity and carcinogenicity of such compounds typified by 1-naphthylamine or 2-aminobiphenyl (McMahon and Turner, 1979).

The arylhydroxylamine and the corresponding *N*-acetyl derivatives can be conjugated with glucuronic acid or sulfuric acid (Irving in Fishman, 1970; Weisburger and Weisburger, 1973; Irving, 1979; Kriek, and Miller and Miller in Emmelot and Kriek, 1979). The former is a weak electrophile; the latter is a strong electrophile with good evidence that those arylamines that are liver carcinogens involve the sulfate ester as the ultimate carcinogenic form. Sakai *et al.* (1978) and Stout and Becker (1979) have provided evidence that enzymes in liver cell nuclei can activate this carcinogen to a mutagenic form. Recently a new metabolite of *N*-2-fluorenylacetamide in the form of a dimer was obtained; apparently this product arose secondarily from the sulfate ester (Andrews *et al.*, 1979*a*).

With the *N*-hydroxy acyl derivatives there is evidence of an *N-O* acyltransferase, which can thus lead to an active electrophilic reactant (Bartsch *et al.*, 1977; King *et al.* in Gorrod, 1978). It may be that cancer causation by this class of compounds in organs other than the liver involves this type of activation process (Irving, 1979).

In addition to the enzyme system mentioned, there is evidence that arylamines can also be metabolized through peroxidases such as was shown with the carcinogen *N*-2-fluorenylacetamide (see Walker and Floyd, 1979; Miller and Miller in Emmelot and Kriek, 1979). 4-Chloraniline and the 2-methyl derivative yielded the corresponding *N*-oxidation product, with mixed-function oxidases and with a peroxidase system (Hill *et al.*, 1979; Corbett *et al.*, 1980), and aminostilbenes, specific carcinogens for the rat Zymbal gland, appear metabolized also by such a system (Emmelot and Kriek, 1979; Osborne *et al.*, 1980).

In addition to *N-O* glucuronides, which may be considered to be mainly detoxification products, there are also hydroxylamine glucuronides, with the glucuronic acid group attached to the nitrogen. These conjugates have been demonstrated to be metabolites excreted in the bile, or in the urine via the kidney (Fig. 7). It is thought that cancer causation especially in the urinary bladder may involve this conjugate as a transport form from which an electrophilic nitrenium ion is released either enzymatically (colon) or at low pH prevailing in the urinary bladder (Kadlubar *et al.*, 1977; Poupko *et al.*, 1979; see Thorgeirsson and Weisburger, 1981). Biliary excretion followed by release in the intestine can lead to activation, by deconjugation and perhaps deacylation (Schut and Thorgeirsson, 1979).

Thus, with a great variety of arylamines and *N*-acyl arylamines, several kinds of activation reactions are important. The first step is *N*-oxidation mediated by at least three distinct enzyme systems: the cytochrome P-450 complex, the flavin-dependent enzymes, and a peroxidase system. The resulting hydroxylarylamines are often mutagenic, which could be interpreted to mean that they are the ultimate carcinogenic species. Yet, in mammalian systems there is good evidence for certain conjugates, eventually yielding a nitrenium ion as providing an essential additional activation step. Arylhydroxylamines are reactive

282

J. H.
WEISBURGER
AND
G. M.
WILLIAMS

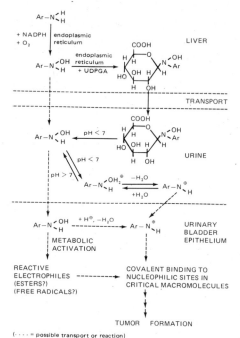

FIGURE 7. Formation and transport of possible proximate and ultimate carcinogenic metabolites of arylamines for the induction of bladder cancer (from Kadlubar *et al.*, 1977). This figure shows that production of an aryl hydroxylamine is followed by formation of the corresponding *N*-glucuronide, a stable transport form. At pH less than 7 in the urinary bladder, the hydroxylamine is released, which in turn yields the active nitrenium ion. The hydroxylamine *N*-glucuronide is also excreted in bile where the intestinal bacterial flora can release the hydroxylamine through enzymatic hydrolysis, thus accounting for the induction of intestinal cancer with specific arylamines. The intestinal microflora can also reduce the hydroxylamine to the arylamine, which can be reabsorbed and recycled or be excreted.

compounds chemically and biochemically. There are facile oxidation–reduction steps between the corresponding nitroso and hydroxylamine groups (Hecht *et al.*, 1979*a*; El-Bayoumy *et al.*, 1980). Isolation of the adducts with purines and pyrimidines has in part provided the background, not available by direct pharmacological techniques, that the key active intermediates are indeed nitrenium ions or in some instances the corresponding acyl derivatives (see Emmelot and Kriek, 1979; Miller *et al.*, 1979; Thorgeirsson and Weisburger, 1981). It is true that this concept stems mainly from studies involving liver, and more research is necessary to define the active intermediates for extrahepatic carcinogenesis.

There are considerable differences in the carcinogenicity of aromatic amines as a function of structure. The question of the location of the amino substituent has been discussed. In addition, the molecular size is important. Thus, *o*-toluidine is a very weak carcinogen compared to 3-methyl-2-naphthylamine or 3-methyl-4-aminobiphenyl. These differences may stem from the relative quantitative aspects of the essential *N*-oxidation reactions vs. the competitive ring metabolic reactions, which are usually detoxification steps. In some instances, additional parameters include the chain length of any acyl substituents, suggesting that the reactive centers around the nitrogen play a role as well (see Weisburger and Fiala in Thorgeirsson and Weisburger, 1981).

Variations in carcinogenicity of aromatic amines occur as a function of species and strain. In part these differences are accounted for by the ratio of *N*-oxidation to *C*-oxidation or of the further activation step of the corresponding hydroxylamine derivative to any competing detoxification reactions. The guinea pig has been found to be resistant to the carcinogenic action of *N*-2-fluorenylacetamide, and this has been ascribed to the low rate of *N*-oxidation in that species. However, recently it was found that microsomes from guinea pig liver were quite capable of converting 2-fluorenylacetamide to a mutagenic metabolic intermediate, which may be in the form of the hydroxylamine derivative (Takeishi *et al.*, 1979; see also Irving, 1979; Razzouk *et al.*, 1980). This finding points again to the need to carefully evaluate *in vitro* findings in relation to the *in vivo* situation where conjugative reactions, and in this case also more likely other *C*-hydroxylation reactions, may play an important role in leading to inactive detoxification products *in vivo*, but not *in vitro*.

The carcinogenic aromatic amines and acyl amides have distinct organotropic properties depending on their structure and on species, age, sex, and other variables. As noted, these properties are the result of the potential for stereo-specific activation to the corresponding arylhydroxylamines as a function of these variables. However, even the *N*-acetylarylhydroxylamines are not the ultimate carcinogenic entities in most cases. For rat liver, there is good evidence that a key activation step is conjugation to form the *O*-sulfate ester, mediated through a sulfotransferase (see Weisburger and Weisburger, 1973; Miller and Miller, 1980). In addition, for rat liver and possibly other organs such as breast, an acyl transferase, again yielding an active hydroxylamine ester, may be implicated (see Bartsch *et al.*, 1973; Emmelot and Kriek, 1979; Irving, 1979; Weeks *et al.*, 1980; Malejka-Giganti in Thorgeirsson and Weisburger, 1981).

Studies on the metabolism of several arylamines in humans have uniformly noted the heterogeneity of the metabolic capability of individuals (Alvares *et al.*, 1979*a*). This may account for the fact that drug metabolism in general, or cancer formation in abusers of drugs such as phenacetin, varies according to the individual. Furthermore, in contrast to animal data, which are usually obtained in a highly controlled laboratory environment as to diet, light cycle, and the like, humans are heterogeneous not only genetically but also as to customs such as the use of cigarettes, alcohol, or diet. All of these are known to have an impact on metabolic competence and, in particular, biochemical activation reactions (Conney *et al.*, 1977; Alvares *et al.*, 1979*a,b*; Dollery *et al.*, 1979).

Gorrod (see 1978) has proposed that *N*-hydroxylation of arylacetamides occurs by a cytochrome P-450-connected pathway, whereas free arylamines would be oxidized by a flavin-adenine nucleotide-dependent enzyme complex (see also Kato *et al.*, 1978; Irving, 1979; Ziegler and Prough *et al.* in Coon *et al.*, 1980). This interesting proposal deserves serious consideration and experimental documentation, for it does suggest clarification of certain currently obscure mechanisms.

Additional activation mechanisms operating on the hydroxylamino compounds may be required, for these chemicals are carcinogenic under conditions where neither of these types of ester formation is necessarily involved. Peroxidases or other means for generating one-electron intermediates have been implicated (Miller *et al.*, 1979; Walker and Floyd, 1979; Corbett *et al.*, 1980). Certain aromatic amines are carcinogenic to the urinary bladder through an intermediary hydroxylamine step by specific activation mechanisms. Transport to the bladder probably involves *N*-glucuronides (Kadlubar *et al.*, 1977; Poupko *et al.*, 1979;

284

J. H.
WEISBURGER
AND
G. M.
WILLIAMS

Thorgeirsson and Weisburger, 1981). In line with the concept that the higher-molecular-weight chemicals are more likely to be excreted in bile (Section 3.1), more dichlorobenzidine than benzidine was found in the bile of dogs, whereas more benzidine was excreted in urine (Kellner *et al.*, 1973). In rhesus monkeys, the urine contained some unmetabolized 3,3'-dichlorobenzidine, whereas with benzidine only metabolites were noted, including *N*-acetyl derivatives. Benzidine is activated, as arylamines are, via an *N*-oxidation step, followed by conjugation as the activation or transport mechanism (Morton *et al.*, 1979, 1980). In certain strains of female rats, some aromatic amines and derivatives such as benzidine, *N*-2-fluorenylacetamide, and its *N*-hydroxy derivative are highly active carcinogens for the mammary gland. When both amine and hydroxylamino derivatives were tested, the latter were usually more active, suggesting that a hydroxyl-amino metabolite is involved (see Malejka-Giganti in Thorgeirsson and Weisburger, 1981). However, a ring epoxy compound is also possible, as discussed above, especially since breast tissue is an excellent target for polycyclic aromatic hydrocarbons that are so activated.

Polyheterocyclic aromatic amines. In this class can be found a number of drugs as well as metabolites of aromatic amino acids like tryptophan. Recently, great interest has arisen in polyheterocyclic compounds since a series of these were identified as pyrolysis products of amino acids and proteins (Nagao *et al.*, 1978*a,b*, 1980). One of these compounds, namely 3-amino-1,4-dimethyl-5H-pyrido[4,3-*b*]-indole (Trp-P1), has induced liver cancer as well as subcutaneous sarcomas in rats. Weisburger *et al.* (1980*b*) have suggested that similar compounds obtained from fried meats may be relevant in relation to important human cancers such as those in the colon or breast. Kasai *et al.* (1980) have identified one of these compounds as being 2-amino-3-methylimidazo[4,5-*d*]quinoline. Kato (1979), Hashimoto *et al.* (1979, 1980), Nebert *et al.* (1979), and Ishii *et al.* (1980) have demonstrated that this class of compounds is metabolized by the mixed-function oxidase system. These chemicals are highly mutagenic with biochemical activation in strains of *S. typhimurium* sensitive to frameshift mutagens. The fact that cytochrome P-450 is involved suggests that the metabolic activation is similar to that prevailing for arylamines. In addition, as is true for any other heterocyclic compounds, *C*-hydroxylation proximate to a nitrogen can be conceived in two steps to lead to an imide, as was seen with metronidazole, and thus accounting for ring opening (Goldman *et al.*, 1980). A simple prototype, the liver carcinogen quinoline, undergoes epoxidation in position 2,3, vicinal to the nitrogen, or 3,4 and yields the appropriate DNA adducts (Tada *et al.*, 1980).

Aminoazodyes. The classic carcinogenic azo dyes, active mostly on rodent liver, and in some instances on hamster and dog urinary bladder, undergo activation via mechanisms similar to those described for the aromatic amines (Miller and Miller, 1980). The prototype, 4-dimethylaminoazobenzene, requires an *N*-methyl group. However, others, like *o*-aminoazotoluene, do not. The corresponding aminoazobenzene is very weakly carcinogenic.

With this class of compounds, *N*-oxidation is also an essential first activation step. This appears to be mediated by the flavin-dependent *N*-oxidation enzyme system (Ziegler and Prough *et al.* in Coon *et al.*, 1980). The participation by the cytochrome P-450 complex requires further definition. For liver cancer, the hydroxylamine requires further esterification as is true for other hepatocarcinogenic arylamines, and these form multiple key products upon reaction with DNA (Beland *et al.*, 1980; Tarpley *et al.*, 1980). The specific activation process relative to extrahepatic effects is not yet well established. Certain azo dyes such as *o*-aminoazotoluene are carcinogenic despite an absence of *N*-methyl substitution. They are most likely carcinogenic through mechanisms related to hydroxylamine formation, as described for the related *o*-methylarylamines.

In addition, carcinogenic azo dyes undergo detoxification reactions through reductive splitting of the azo link (purified enzymes; Huang *et al.*, 1979) and through hydroxylation on the ring system (Fig. 8). Reduction of the azo bond is also mediated to a considerable extent by the bacterial flora (Section 3.2). For this reason, feces usually do not contain azo dye, or metabolites with the azo bond intact, even though such chemicals are known to be excreted into the intestine via the bile. Conjugation with glutathione is important (Ketterer *et al.*, 1979).

Complex azo dyes containing carcinogenic components such as benzidine may be hazardous because of metabolic release and resorption of carcinogenic intermediates from the intestine (Rhinde and Troll, 1975; Robens *et al.*, 1980). They

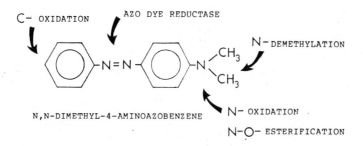

FIGURE 8. The carcinogenic azo dye typified by *N,N*-dimethyl-4-aminoazobenzene can undergo *N*-demethylation followed by *N*-oxidation, yielding the proximate *N*-hydroxy derivative. This is esterified with sulfate or acetate to reactive esters, the ultimate carcinogens, steps identical with those relevant to the carcinogenic arylamines. Detoxification steps involve *C*-oxidation yielding phenols, excreted as conjugates, and azo bond reduction yielding split products in the form of the respective amines. Azo dye reduction can take place through mammalian enzymes and even more readily through bacterial enzymes in the gut, the latter being more important with poorly absorbed polar azo dyes entering by the oral route. Polar substitution such as with carboxy or sulfonic acid in the aryl rings usually leads to inactive azo dyes because of ready azo bond splitting and excretion. However, for more complex tetraazo dyes, where the polar substituents such as sulfonate are present only in the terminal rings, and where the central part is not so substituted, azo dye reductase, particularly bacterial reductase in the gut, can lead to release of active carcinogenic diaryldiamines such as benzidine, tolidine, and the like, accounting for the carcinogenicity of such complex azo dyes.

286

J. H.
WEISBURGER
AND
G. M.
WILLIAMS

can be detected by mutagenicity assays (Lazear *et al.*, 1979; Matsushima *et al.* in Norpoth and Garner, 1980). On the other hand, amaranth, nonmutagenic and noncarcinogenic, is split to inactive products (Willes *et al.*, 1980).

4.2.5. *Nitroaryl Compounds*

The nitro analogs of the carcinogenic aromatic amines are usually also carcinogenic, mostly to the same target organs as the corresponding amines. In addition, however, most of them induce cancer in the forestomach of rodents on oral ingestion. It would seem that these nitroaryl derivatives are reduced in susceptible organs to the corresponding arylhydroxylamines (Fig. 3), which undergo further activation, as described above, as a function of structure, species, target organ, and the like (Gillette, 1979*b*; Weisburger and Weisburger, 1973; Johnson and Cornish, 1978). Inasmuch as the reduction of nitroaryl derivatives appears to be less stereospecific than the oxidation of the corresponding aromatic amines, it could be that such chemicals are more generally carcinogenic than the corresponding amines. Since most *Salmonella* systems used in mutagenicity testing have a nitroreductase, nitroaryl compounds often yield a positive response in such tests. However, such a response needs independent confirmation as to carcinogenicity since mammalian systems, especially *in vivo*, have great detoxification capacity not available in the bacterial system. For this reason false positives can occur in the bacterial mutagenicity assays. 1-Nitronaphthalene is such a mutagen (McCann *et al.*, 1975; El-Bayoumy *et al.*, 1980) that is not a carcinogen (E. K. Weisburger, 1981), and the reason may be rapid reduction to the inactive amine (Johnson and Cornish, 1978), without accumulation of the intermediate hydroxylamine. There is current interest in nitroaryl derivatives, since they are present in automobile and diesel exhausts (Wang *et al.*, 1978). Witness the results with 1-nitronaphthalene, and because of distinct metabolism, mammalian cell tests are required, in addition to bacterial mutagenicity, for the reliable screening of these compounds (Williams and Weisburger, 1981).

There have been few specific studies on the mechanism of reduction of carcinogenic nitroaryl compounds. It would appear that there are two distinct enzyme systems, one membrane bound and the other in the cytoplasm. In many instances, the membrane-bound system, requring NADPH and oxygen, is more active. It is presumed that the mechanism involved is an oxidation of NADPH by the nitroaryl compound.

The soluble enzyme also functions with NADH and may be similar to Ernster's enzyme, which in turn may be similar to xanthine oxidase (see Coon *et al.*, 1980). 4-Nitroquinoline-*N*-oxide and related carcinogens are reduced very effectively by a cytoplasmic enzyme similar to Ernster's enzyme (Sugimura, Endo, and Kondo in Sugimura *et al.*, 1979). In this instance, the nitro derivative is an excellent substrate, but the corresponding hydroxylamino derivative a poor one. Consequently, the active carcinogenic intermediate hydroxylamino derivative accumulates. A metal ion may facilitate binding to macromolecular receptors (Yamane and Ohtawa, 1979). Even the unstable 4-nitrosoquinoline-*N*-oxide can

be detected (Matsuyama and Nagata, 1973). This is not so with other carcinogenic
nitroaryl compounds, where the arylhydroxylamines seem to be a good substrate
for further reduction, and thus they are difficult to visualize by *in vitro* assays
since reduction to the arylamines occurs rapidly. In addition to mammalian
enzymes, bacterial enzymes from the intestinal flora may play an important role
in reducing aromatic nitro groups (Zachariah and Juchau, 1974; Goldman *et al.*,
1980) and also aromatic *N*-hydroxylamino derivatives (Weisburger and
Weisburger, 1973).

4.2.6. Nitrofurans

Bryan, Price, and associates discovered a series of nitrofuran thiazolyl derivatives
that were carcinogenic for a number of sites in rodents. While the exact mode
of action of these agents has not been delineated, it would appear that they can
be considered heterocyclic analogs of benzidine or more accurately of 4-nitro-4′-
aminobiphenyl (Bryan, 1978). Nitrofurans are mutagenic and damage DNA
(McCalla *et al.* in Margison, 1979). In rats and mice, the major portion of the
dose is excreted in the urine and much of the remainder in the feces in 4 days
after a single dose. A small portion of the urinary radioactivity is accounted for
by the drug administered. In accordance with the fate of other chemicals with
similar structures, reduction of the nitro group to the hydroxylamino constituent
should yield an active intermediate. However, such structures may be somewhat
unstable, and thus special techniques may be necessary to demonstrate their
transitory existence (Yahagi *et al.*, 1974). Metronidazole yields metabolites derived
from hydroxylation and reduction, often α to the heteroatoms (Koch and
Goldman, 1979).

4.2.7. 3-Hydroxyxanthine and Related Purine-N-Oxides

While studying the biological and biochemical properties of certain purine
derivatives, Brown discovered the carcinogenicity of certain purine-*N*-oxides.
These chemicals cause cancer at the point of application, but some of them are
also active at remote sites, mainly in the liver. It has been demonstrated that
certain of these hydroxylated derivatives are substrates for sulfotransferase, just
as are the hydroxy derivatives of certain carcinogenic aromatic amines. However,
there does not seem to be a relationship between the sulfoacceptor activity and
oncogenicity. It might be important to relate this biochemical parameter to the
ease of liver tumor formation, inasmuch as sulfate ester formation appears to
be involved mainly with carcinogenesis in the liver. Other reactions, to be
identified, relate to sarcoma formation and even mutagenicity. Stoehrer *et al.*
(1973) have identified the reaction product of the model-activated oncogen
3-acetoxyxanthine and tryptophan as a material attached to the 3-carbon of
tryptophan through position 8 of xanthine. A similar product appears to be
excreted in the urine of rats injected intraperitoneally with labeled 3-hydroxyxan-
thine.

288

J. H.
WEISBURGER
AND
G. M.
WILLIAMS

3-Hydroxyxanthine is produced metabolically through purine-3-oxide by the soluble xanthine oxidase (Teller *et al.*, 1978). As discussed above, this intermediate can be converted to an electrophilic reactant by conjugation with sulfate or by chemical conversion to an acetate ester. The result eventually is an electrophilic reactant (Parham and Templeton, 1980), through a pathway similar to that operating for the carcinogenic arylamines (Section 4.2.4). This feature also accounts for relative carcinogenic and mutagenic properties through reaction with critical cellular nucleophiles, in contrast to detoxification steps with competing nucleophiles such as glutathione, tryptophan, tyrosine, and the like (Matthews and Stoehrer, 1980).

4.2.8. Urethan

When administered as a single dose or repeatedly in smaller doses, urethan induces pulmonary tumors in mice (the effect depending in part on strain) and diverse tumors in other rodents after longer latent periods. It seems fairly well established that urethan is noncarcinogenic and requires biochemical activation (see Mirvish, 1968). *N*-Hydroxyurethan, a candidate metabolite, has never been detected reliably. This chemical, however, appears more reactive than the parent compound, but possibly not through the hydroxylamino group directly.

Inhibition of lung tumor induction was found when the metabolism of the *N*-hydroxy derivative was apparently blocked. However, it was demonstrated that vinyl carbamate, which could arise from the dehydrogenation of ethyl carbamate, was much more carcinogenic than urethan or ethyl carbamate. Also, vinyl carbamate is mutagenic, whereas the ethyl derivative is not. Even though the direct conversion of ethyl to vinyl carbamate has not yet been demonstrated, it seems likely that the activation process may involve dehydrogenation of the ethyl to the vinyl group, thereby accounting for the fact that methyl carbamate, unable to undergo this reaction, is noncarcinogenic. Thus, on the basis of the findings of Dahl *et al.* (1980), the dehydrogenation steps may be part of the activation pathway. Whether *N*-hydroxylation additionally plays a role is not yet clear. The final activation step can be visualized as epoxidation of the vinyl ester, although there is yet no evidence for this reaction. Urethan has been known to be carcinogenic for almost 40 years, but it is only recently that reasonable concepts accounting for the activation mechanism have been derived.

4.2.9. Naturally Occurring Carcinogens

A wide variety of carcinogens are formed as naturally occurring products of plants or microorganisms (Emmelot and Kriek, 1979; Hirono in Sugimura *et al.*, 1979; Miller and Miller, 1979; Miller *et al.*, 1979) (Table 3). The metabolism of some of these carcinogens is described in sections dealing with the specific structural type. Aflatoxin B_1, a major naturally occurring carcinogen, is described in Section 4.2.10, safrole in Section 4.2.11. For most of these agents, however, little is known of the biotransformation that they might undergo.

TABLE 3
Carcinogens Found in Microorganisms and Plants

Microorganisms	Plants
Aflatoxins	Tobacco, snuff
Sterigmatocystein	Betel nut
Luteoskyrin	Cycasin
Islanditoxin	Pyrrolizidine (*Senecio*)
Griseofulvin	alkaloids
Actinomycins	Coltsfoot
Mitomycin C	Bracken fern
Adriamycin	Mushroom toxins
Daunomycin	Safrole
Elaiomycin	β-Asarone (calamus oil)
Ethionine	Thiourea, goitrogens
Azaserine	Phorbol esters[a]
Nitrosonornicotine	Flavones
Streptozotocin	

[a] Cocarcinogen and promoter.

a. Pyrrolizidine Alkaloids. The pyrrolizidine or *Senecio* alkaloids are a family of naturally occurring hepatoxic and carcinogenic chemicals (Schoental in Searle, 1976). Their effect is highly modified by diet. The key activation process of this class of agents is enzymatic dehydrogenation to pyrrolic metabolites that exhibit high reactivity, accounted for as a redistribution of charges within the molecule (Mattocks and White, 1973; Miller and Miller, 1979; Styles *et al.*, 1980). The result is a leaving group and conversion to a carbonium ion or similar electrophilic reagent. Younger rats produce more pyrrolic metabolites than adults irrespective of sex, whereas in older animals, males form more pyrrolic metabolites. These metabolic conversions appear to account for the toxic effects of the alkaloids. Enzyme inducers and diet modify the effect. Isolated hepatocytes appear to retain a substantial capability for activation of pyrrolizidine alkaloids (Williams *et al.*, 1980*b*).

The tissue distribution of another hepatotoxin, luteoskyrin, has been reported by Uraguchi *et al.* (1972). In the mouse, this chemical is eliminated progressively, more in feces than in urine. A relationship has been found among toxicity, uptake by organs, and elimination.

b. Flavones. Flavones are polyhydroxylated cyclic compounds found widely distributed in the environment in plants and fruits, mostly as glycones or β-glucosides. Recently, two aglycones, quercetin and kaempferol, were found to be powerful mutagens (Nagao *et al.*, 1978*a*; Miller *et al.*, 1979). The mechanism of action is not clear. Characteristically the aglycones are unsaturated catechol derivatives, which may be the salient feature in the expression of mutagenicity. Ingestion of flavones would lead to bacterially mediated deconjugation in the intestine followed by absorption. In the liver, these compounds would be expected to be conjugated with glucuronic acid, sulfuric acid, and then excreted into bile

290

J. H.
WEISBURGER
AND
G. M.
WILLIAMS

or transferred to blood and filtered into urine. Upon reaching the intestinal flora, the biliary metabolites would be converted again to the deconjugated product (Section 3.2). A portion could be reabsorbed and thus recycled. Similarly, the portion excreted via the renal pathway can be deconjugated while in the urinary bladder. The mode of activation of this type of compound to a reactive electrophile is unknown.

4.2.10. Aflatoxins

Through the efforts of Büchi, Wogan, and their associates, the chemical structures of the aflatoxins, powerful carcinogenic mold products of environmental importance, were revealed (Wogan, 1973; Searle, 1976; Miller and Miller, 1979). Initially, four such chemicals were known. Aflatoxins B_1 and G_1 are characterized by a difuran ring system attached to a coumarin complex; the other two, aflatoxins B_2 and G_2, are similar but have a saturated double bond in the difuran ring. These latter chemicals are much less, if at all (aflatoxin G_2), carcinogenic. The low-level, but definite, carcinogenicity of aflatoxin B_2 may be accounted for by its metabolic conversion to aflatoxin B_1 through dehydrogenation (Swenson et al., 1977; Roebuck et al., 1978). Aflatoxins B_1 and G_1 and a compound with similar properties, sterigmatocystein, are potent liver carcinogens and also cause cancer at the point of application to mouse skin and subcutaneously in rats. Because of the latter, it was thought for many years that they might be direct acting, and attention was directed to the lactone portion of the molecule. This turned out to be a false lead, as also occurred in the case of polycyclic aromatic hydrocarbons. The key ultimate carcinogen is the epoxide at the 2,3-position in the furan ring (Fig. 3). The proof for the formation of an epoxide was elegantly provided by Swenson and co-workers (1974). They demonstrated the release of a dihydrodiol derivative of the epoxide upon hydrolysis of RNA-bound aflatoxin, thus showing that the attachment to nucleic acids is indeed through that part of the molecule. The ultimate carcinogen, namely the 2,3-epoxide of aflatoxin, is extraordinarily unstable. Attempts at chemical synthesis have uniformly failed. However, evidence that this is indeed the ultimate carcinogen from aflatoxin B_1 stems from the demonstration of the corresponding dihydrodiol in an in vitro reaction system (Lin et al., 1978). The isolation of glutathione conjugates (Degen and Neumann, 1978; Emerole, 1979; Lotlikar et al., 1979), and even more relevant the isolation of the reaction product with DNA with interaction at position 7 of guanine, all support the view that the 2,3-epoxide is the key intermediate (Lin et al., 1978; Autrup et al., 1979; Stark et al., 1979; Wogan et al. in Emmelot and Kriek, 1979; Miller and Miller, 1979; Miller et al., 1979).

In addition, aflatoxin is metabolized to a number of other hydroxylated products (Fig. 9), such as aflatoxins P_1, M_1, Q_1, and B_2a in which various ring positions undergo hydroxylation. The carbonyl group in the terminal five-membered ring is reversibly reduced to a hydroxy group to form aflatoxicol, thought to be a storage product (Wong et al., 1979). In addition, there is the O-demethylation and, in fact, permutations of several of these reactions. Most

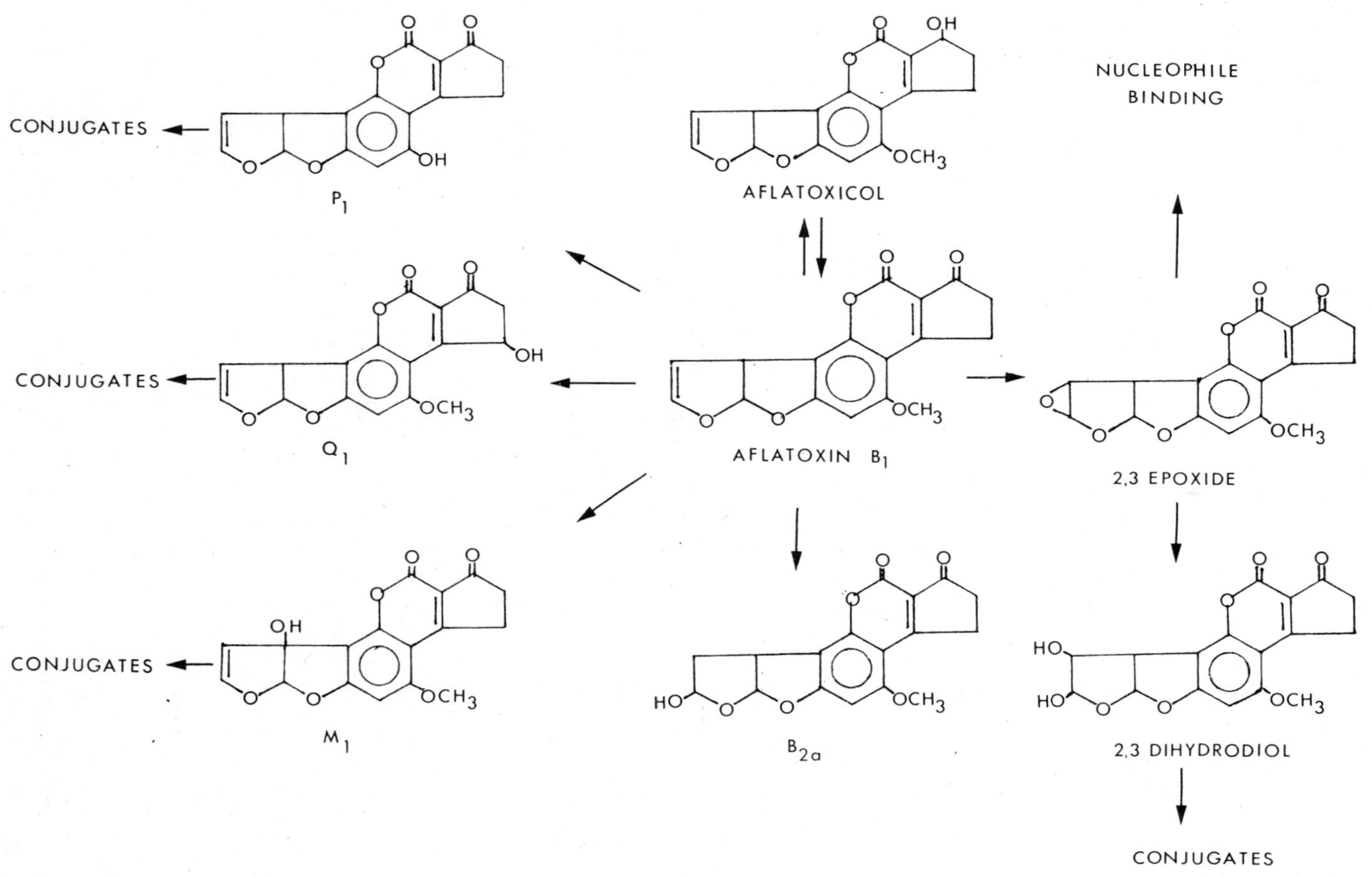

FIGURE 9. Aflatoxin B_1 is one of the most potent carcinogens known, inducing liver cancer with doses as low as 1 ppb in the diet. The metabolism involves hydroxylation, reversible oxidation–reduction of hydroxymethyl and keto groups, O-demethylation, and formation of conjugates of phenolic or alcoholic metabolites. The major activation reaction is formation of an epoxide on the double bond in the terminal furan ring.

292

J. H.
WEISBURGER
AND
G. M.
WILLIAMS

of these are less active mutagens or carcinogens. Colley and Neal (1979) developed analytical methods to separate many of these metabolites. The resistance of the mouse to carcinogenicity has not yet been fully explained through metabolic approaches. However, Ueno *et al.* (1980) have reported a considerably lower DNA binding with mouse liver, to which it is less carcinogenic (Vesselinovitch *et al.*, 1972; Patterson, 1973), than with rat liver. In addition to the classic cytochrome P-450 system or an S-9 fraction, Niranjan and Avadhani (1980) have noted a mitochondrial fraction that is able to metabolize aflatoxin B_1. Mainigi and Campbell (1980) have located radioactivity from labeled aflatoxin in various cell fractions, more so when the animals were on a high-protein diet compared to a low-protein diet.

4.2.11. Safrole

Safrole, a natural product and also a formerly used synthetic food additive, has caused cancer in rats when administered at high dose levels for extended periods of time. There are related compounds also found in nature, which may have similar properties. These include eugenol, anethole, estragole, myristicin, and asarone (Miller and Miller, 1979; Miller *et al.*, 1979). It was demonstrated that the carcinogenicity of safrole is not related to the presence of the methylenedioxy group, even though this structure provides the necessary bulk to constitute a bicyclic molecule.

The key metabolic reaction is a biochemical hydroxylation at the 1′-position in the allyl side chain (Miller and Miller, 1979). 1′-Hydroxysafrole is excreted in urine as a small fraction of the dose in rats, guinea pigs, and hamsters, and in larger amounts in mice. Pretreatment of rats with an enzyme inducer, phenobarbital or 3-methylcholanthrene, increases the excretion considerably. However, this is not seen in guinea pigs or hamsters. 1′-Hydroxysafrole appears to be a carcinogenic intermediate, for it causes tumors much faster at lower dose levels than safrole. Also, it causes tumors at the point of application or at the point of ingestion, the forestomach. However, 1′-hydroxysafrole appears to require additional activation, by esterification as with the corresponding aromatic amines and their N-hydroxy derivatives. Thus, 1′-acetoxysafrole is a potent local-acting oncogen. Also, 1′-hydroxysafrole fails to interact *in vitro* with model molecular receptors, whereas the 1′-acetoxy compound does. Other possible active metabolites are 1′-ketosafrole and the 1′-hydroxy-2′,3′-epoxy compound. Mutagenicity data support this view (Swanson *et al.*, 1979). Safrole and related compounds are relatively weak carcinogens *in vivo*, since metabolism yields relatively small ratios of activation/detoxification metabolites.

4.2.12. Cycasin, Dialkylhydrazines, Azoxyalkanes

Laqueur (see Laqueur and Spatz, 1975) discovered the carcinogenicity to small and large bowel, liver, and kidney of the plant product cycasin, the β-glucoside of methylazoxymethanol. He demonstrated that this product undergoes hydrolysis, mainly through enzymes provided by the intestinal microflora of rodents, with release of the aglycone. The tissues of infant animals apparently have a β-glucosidase capable of splitting cycasin, but this enzyme is repressed during development. Thus, cycasin exhibits toxic and carcinogenic effects in older animals only when administered by the oral route, leading to contact with and enzymatic activation by intestinal microflora. It is thus a unique carcinogen.

Cycasin is apparently not excreted appreciably in the bile, for parenteral injection has no pathological effect, indicating that the chemical does not reach the intestines in significant amounts. Rather, it is excreted unchanged in urine. Given orally, however, it is highly toxic, as is the aglycone methylazoxymethanol. Under these conditions, only about 50% cycasin is recovered from urine. Similar parenteral injections of methylazoxymethanol have induced cancer in the liver, kidney, gallbladder, and large bowel in hamsters, suggesting that this chemical can reach these sites. From the fact that cancer is seen in the gallbladder, the conclusion can be drawn that sufficient material is excreted in the bile under these conditions.

Attempts to synthesize methylazoxymethanol showed this was feasible but difficult (see Matsumoto in Miller *et al.*, 1979). Druckrey (see 1975) correctly reasoned that the readily available 1,2-dimethylhydrazine would be metabolized to methylazoxymethanol, an assumption that proved correct (Fig. 10).

In rats and less so in mice, 1,2-dimethylhydrazine induces mainly colon cancer, and to a smaller extent cancer in the duodenum, and depending on species and strain, cancer in the liver and the kidneys.

Druckrey (1975) proposed that 1,2-dimethylhydrazine is oxidized in a concerted manner by mixed-function oxidases via azoxymethane to methylazoxymethanol and then to an active methyldiazonium salt. Magee *et al.* and Fiala (see Fiala, 1980) observed that only small amounts of a dose of labeled 1,2-dimethylhydrazine are excreted in bile or feces. A small portion of the respiratory radioactivity is in the form of CO_2; the major part is azomethane. Administration of labeled dimethylhydrazine leads to concentration of radioactivity in liver, kidney, and intestinal tract, organs sensitive to cancer induction with this agent. On the other hand, with the diethyl analog, radioactivity is noted in the hematopoietic

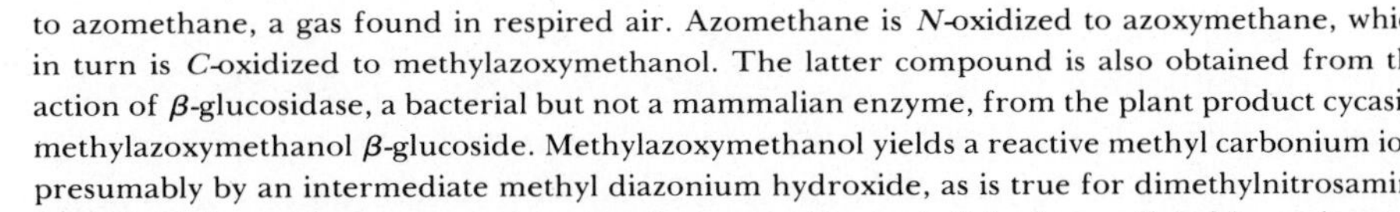

$$CH_3NHNHCH_3 \longrightarrow CH_3N=NCH_3 \longrightarrow CH_3N=NCH_3 \longrightarrow CH_3N=NCH_2OH \longrightarrow \left[CH_3^+\right]$$

1,2-DIMETHYLHYDRAZINE   AZOMETHANE   AZOXYMETHANE   METHYLAZOXYMETHANOL   METHYL-
(gas)   CARBONIUM
                                                                            ION

FIGURE 10. Symmetrical or 1,2-dimethylhydrazine is oxidized enzymatically or nonenzymatically to azomethane, a gas found in respired air. Azomethane is *N*-oxidized to azoxymethane, which in turn is *C*-oxidized to methylazoxymethanol. The latter compound is also obtained from the action of β-glucosidase, a bacterial but not a mammalian enzyme, from the plant product cycasin, methylazoxymethanol β-glucoside. Methylazoxymethanol yields a reactive methyl carbonium ion, presumably by an intermediate methyl diazonium hydroxide, as is true for dimethylnitrosamine (Fig. 5). This reaction occurs spontaneously to a small extent. It is also mediated by an isozyme of alcohol dehydrogenase, accounting in part for the pronounced specificity of this compound for the induction of colon cancer in rodents.

294

J. H.
WEISBURGER
AND
G. M.
WILLIAMS

system in the brain, again the target organ with these agents (Pozharisski *et al.*, 1979).

The key metabolic steps originally proposed by Druckrey, namely the conversion of 1,2-dimethylhydrazine to methylazoxymethanol via the easily volatilized azomethane found in expired air, and then to azoxymethane which is finally oxidized to methylazoxymethanol, has been fully validated by Fiala (1977). It would appear that these reactions occur primarily in the liver. Whereas 1,2-dimethylhydrazine rarely produces liver cancer in rats, it is an effective hepatocarcinogen in hamsters, perhaps because of more efficient DNA repair systems in rat liver.

By utilizing selective inhibitors such as disulfiram and other sulfur-containing compounds, Wattenberg (1978) and Fiala (1981) have selectively inhibited the metabolism of dimethylhydrazine at the N-oxidation and the C-oxidation steps, and thus inhibited the entire sequence to tumor formation. There is no evidence that methylazoxymethanol is conjugated with glucuronic acid. The chemical itself is fairly water soluble and readily transported by blood to the active sites. Zedeck (in Lipkin and Good, 1978) has shown that methylazoxymethanol may be specifically metabolized in the target organ, colon, by alcohol dehydrogenase, and Fiala *et al.* (1978) have further supported this concept by studies on the specific inhibition of alcohol dehydrogenase by pyrazole and other related chemicals.

More complex 1,2-dialkylhydrazines including 1,2-dimethylbenzylhydrazine and the related procarbazine are also carcinogenic. They are activated through mechanisms similar to those of the 1,2-dimethylhydrazine prototype (Lee and Dixon, 1978; Weinkam and Shiba, 1978; Dunn *et al.*, 1979; Solt and Neale, 1980).

Hydrazine itself, but more so 1-methylhydrazine and 1,1-dimethylhydrazine and analogous compounds are carcinogenic (Toth, 1980). The organotropism is quite different from that of the symmetrical 1,2-dimethylhydrazine, and the mode of action and metabolism have also been noted to be different. Such compounds appear to be activated by the mixed-function oxidases (Hines and Prough, 1980). In addition, a possible mechanism involved in the carcinogenic process may be like that described for other hydrazines and hydrazides extensively used in pharmacology, namely N-acylation followed by N-oxidation and the eventual release of an acylonium ion (Nelson *et al.* in Gorrod, 1978; Timbrell and Wright, 1979). More evidence that this pathway is involved in the carcinogenic process is necessary. Except for dimethylcarbamoyl chloride (Van Duuren *et al.*, 1979), there are few chemicals with the potential to form such acylonium ions, which have been described as carcinogens. It is of interest that low-level oral intake of 1,2-dimethylhydrazine yields similar kinds of tumors, namely endotheliomas, as does the unsymmetrical 1,1-dimethylhydrazine (Druckrey, 1975; Toth, 1980). Thus, it may be that under those conditions, the metabolism of 1,2-dimethylhydrazine is different compared to high-level intake, when intestinal cancer is the main lesion (Fiala, 1977). Perhaps a common intermediate is monomethylhydrazine.

4.2.13. 2-Nitropropane

Recent data show that inhalation of relatively low levels of 2-nitropropane rapidly induced liver cancer in rats (Lewis *et al.*, 1979). It will be of importance to study related compounds and acquire information on the relevant mechanisms. 1-Nitropropane is apparently not carcinogenic nor is nitromethane (Hadidian *et al.*, 1968). E. Fiala (personal communication) has suggested that the metabolism of 2-nitropropane yields an azoxy compound that may be a proximate carcinogen. He has shown the chemical reduction to operate via this pathway. Hite and Skeggs (1979) found 2-nitropropane but not nitroethane or 1-nitropropane to be mutagenic. The same mutagenic intermediates as azoxy compounds can be obtained by chemical and biochemical oxidation of precursor alkylamines (Fiala, 1980).

4.2.14. Halogenated Hydrocarbons

This class of compounds includes important industrial products, among them volatile liquids and gases. Thus, a considerable potential for occupational exposure exists. Recently, powerful analytical techniques have permitted the detection of such chemicals in raw and purified water to which the general public is exposed. Therefore, a delineation of the mechanisms of toxicity and possible carcinogenicity of these compounds is of great contemporary interest and purpose.

Carbon tetrachloride has been known for almost 40 years to induce liver tumors in mice. This chemical is highly hepatotoxic in many species, including humans. The mechanisms of toxicity or carcinogenicity have not led to an unambiguous explanation of its mode of action. Shah *et al.* (1979) have observed carbonyl chloride (or phosgene) during *in vitro* metabolism by rat liver. This metabolite was also found with chloroform, but the latter did not seem to be an intermediate metabolite. Carbon tetrachloride has many effects on cellular metabolism including interference with lipid metabolism, oxidation, and peroxidation reactions, and it is not yet clear whether one or more of these reactions are related to the effect of carbon tetrachloride (DiLuzio *et al.*, 1973). Zinc and other metals play a role in the hepatotoxicity of carbon tetrachloride, and metallothionine is thought to be involved in trapping toxic metabolites (Cagen and Klaassen, 1979).

Chloroform is also metabolized to phosgene (Uehleke *et al.*, 1973, 1977; Pohl *et al.*, 1979). Gomez and Castro (1980) observed covalent binding of chloroform metabolites to proteins but not to DNA or RNA, thus perhaps accounting for the severe renal and hepatic toxicity (Ilett *et al.*, 1973). This and related chemicals are not mutagenic (Uehleke *et al.*, 1977; Slacik-Erben *et al.*, 1980).

The higher homologs can be divided up into chlorinated and brominated compounds. Further classification needs to consider the number of halogenated atoms attached to the carbon chain. Thus, 1,2-dichloroethane appears to have reactivity with proteins and DNA *in vivo* and *in vitro*, and it is carcinogenic in mice but not in rats. It is also mutagenic (Livesky and Anders, 1979; Banerjee

296

J. H.
WEISBURGER
AND
G. M.
WILLIAMS

et al., 1980). While the overall mechanism of activation has not been totally delineated, Van Bladeren *et al.* (1979) postulated that glutathione transferase-mediated conjugates may constitute an active pathway. In agreement with this view, Banerjee *et al.* (1980) noted that the metabolic reactions leading to protein binding, however, may be different from those involved in DNA reactions. A microsomal dechlorination of chloroethane has been described, but it is not clear whether the mechanism rests on an oxidative or a conjugative step (Gandolfi and Van Dyke, 1973).

With unsaturated halogenated hydrocarbons derived from ethylene, including vinyl chloride, 1,1-dichloroethylene, and other dichloroalkenes, epoxidation of the double bond has been postulated for these and similarly unsaturated compounds (Henschler and Bonse, 1978; Bartsch *et al.*, 1979*a*; Van Duuren *et al.*, 1979). The prototype vinyl chloride, a carcinogen in humans and rodents, appears to be metabolized to such an active epoxide in the form of chloroethylene oxide (Fig. 3), which is mutagenic (see Zajdela *et al.*, 1980; Pessayre *et al.*, 1979; Filser and Bolt, 1979; Drevon and Kuroki, 1979; McCann *et al.*, 1975; Falk, 1977). Thus, the metabolic production of an epoxide from vinyl chloride and 1,1-dichloroethylene (or vinylidene chloride) appears well documented, even though the reaction, as measured by DNA repair and binding as the endpoint, is much less extensive than in a comparative study with dimethylnitrosamine (Reitz *et al.*, 1980). The main metabolic reaction of the epoxide from vinylidene chloride is conjugation with glutathione (Andersen *et al.*, 1980).

With higher chlorinated hydrocarbons based on saturated alkanes or unsaturated ethylenes, carcinogenicity seems to be restricted to mouse liver and there appears to be no evidence of reliable mutagenic activity in suitable tests. Metabolism may involve mainly conjugation with glutathione and similar sulfur amino acids with formation of an electrophilic intermediate, but only with compounds containing few halogen atoms, such as 1,2-dichloroethane (Van Bladeren *et al.*, 1979).

This may mean that the glutathione adduct has a structure simulating sterically vinyl chloride, with similar susceptibility to enzymatically mediated epoxidation. On the other hand, with more highly chlorinated compounds, conjugation with glutathione may occur, but the resulting product may have a hindered double bond, so that the rate of epoxidation is low and excretion of the glutathione conjugate leads to relatively rapid removal. The synthetic epoxides, like the epoxide derived from the more heavily substituted 1,1,2-trichloroethylene, have been found mutagenic, albeit weakly so. However, as just noted, it may be that epoxide formation in biochemical systems occurs to an insufficient extent with such extensive halogen substitution, possibly due to steric hindrance around the ethylene bond. The main metabolites are polychloroacetic acids in rodents, and chloral was detected in humans (Hathway, 1980). Thus, as was discussed by Weisburger and Williams (1980), chemicals such as trichloroethane, tetra-chloroethane, and the corresponding ethylene compounds, which behave alike *in vivo* (whether saturated ethanes or unsaturated ethylenes) in leading to liver tumors in mice of certain strains, probably do so via epigenetic mechanisms, rather than through production of an electrophilic reactant (see Section 5.4). Evidence is available that several halogenated polycyclic hydrocarbons (carcinogenic, again, only to mouse liver) are not genotoxic (Williams in Margison, 1979; see Nicholson and Moore, 1979).

In view of its importance as a commercial product, DDT has received extensive study with regard to tumorigenesis (Tomatis *et al.*, 1973) and metabolism. DDT induces mouse and rat liver tumors but, most interestingly, not hamster tumors. The suspected formation of an epoxide around the ethylene bond (Planche *et al.*, 1979) may occur to only a limited extent, again considering the steric hindrance at the active site. Other evidence suggests that DDT acts as an epigenetic agent (see Section 5.4).

Data on the carcinogenicity of acrylonitrile have not been published in detail, but mutagenicity data are available (DeMeester *et al.*, 1979). This chemical, however, can be conceived to undergo metabolic activation similar to vinyl chloride (Fig. 3), including epoxidation of the vinyl double bond, conjugation with glutathione, followed by further metabolism. Certain of these metabolites have been found (Langvardt *et al.*, 1980).

Brominated compounds have quite different carcinogenic effects than the comparable chlorinated compounds (see Banerjee *et al.*, 1979). For example, symmetrical ethylene dichloride is a relatively weak carcinogen and mutagen, affecting mostly mouse liver. In contrast, the corresponding dibromide is a much more powerful carcinogen, inducing cancer not only in the liver but in the stomach after oral intake in mice and rats. The bromo compounds are also mutagenic, with biochemical activation (Stolzenberg and Hine, 1979). The corresponding chloro and bromo halohydrins are mutagenic, with and without biochemical activation, suggesting that the activation pathway may involve dehalogenation without epoxidation or dehydrogenation (glutathione conjugation?), albeit a pathway requiring epoxidation has been described (Jones and Fakhouri, 1979).

4.2.15. Dioxane

Dioxane leads to liver tumors in rats and guinea pigs (Argus *et al.*, 1973). Tumors of the nasal cavity, as well as alterations in the kidney, are also noted. However, pretreatment of rats with 3-methylcholanthrene increases the toxicity of dioxane, suggesting that a metabolite is involved in the pathological effect of this agent. A metabolite resulting from α-oxidation, as with cyclic nitrosamines, is p-dioxane-2-one (Woo *et al.*, 1978; Young *et al.*, 1978), which may be involved in the biologic effects of dioxane.

4.2.16. Thioacetamide, Ethylenethiourea, and Acetamide

Thioacetamide, a powerful hepatotoxin and carcinogen to the liver of rodents in relatively small doses, has not been explored in detail with respect to metabolism or the specific metabolites that might be responsible for its effects. Other thioamides, such as thiouracil, act similarly, and this entire group deserves study.

298

J. H.
WEISBURGER
AND
G. M.
WILLIAMS

Recently, the complex metabolism of ethylenethiourea was described (Iverson *et al.*, 1980).

Acetamide is also hepatotoxic and carcinogenic, but this chemical is not a likely intermediate in the action of the thio analogs, mainly because much higher dose levels are required. The effect of acetamide is antagonized by arginine glutamate (Weisburger *et al.*, 1969), suggesting that the metabolism of ammonia is somehow involved. The alternative possibility of N-hydroxylation has been explored with inconclusive results (James Miller, personal communication). Considering the large, continuous dosing required and the unlikely production of an electrophilic metabolite, an epigenetic mechanism deserves serious consideration.

4.2.17. Ethionine

Ethionine, an antimetabolite to methionine, causes liver tumors in rats but not hamsters when relatively large amounts are fed chronically. Also, it is a tool for induction of experimental pancreatitis. Ethionine seems to undergo metabolism similar to that of methionine, including ATP-mediated incorporation into nucleic acids via S-adenosylethionine (Farber, 1973; Miller and Miller, 1979).

Similar to the dehydrogenation of aflatoxin B_2 to the highly carcinogenic aflatoxin B_1 (Section 4.2.10) and the postulated conversion of ethyl carbamate to the vinyl compound (Section 4.2.8), ethionine may be converted to vinyl homocysteine. Vinyl homocysteine is a mutagen for *S. typhimurium* (Leopold *et al.*, 1979*b*; Weisburger and Williams, 1980). However, it remains to be demonstrated that this particular intermediate arises from metabolism of ethionine.

4.3. Inorganic Carcinogens

Several heavy metals like chromium and nickel are carcinogenic in animal models and have been suspected of being involved in several cancer types in humans (Schrauzer, 1979; Sunderman in Emmelot and Kriek, 1979). In addition, the antitumor agent *cis*-dichlorodiamine platinum(II) has been shown to be carcinogenic (Leopold *et al.*, 1979*a*). A variety of carcinogenic metal ions have been reported to produce DNA damage, chromosomal aberrations, and mutagenesis (Hsie *et al.* and Flessel in Kharasch, 1979) in mammalian cells. However, Loeb and co-workers (in Kharasch, 1979; Kunkel and Loeb, 1979; Tkeshelashvilli *et al.*, 1980) have shown that these ions affect the fidelity of DNA polymerases and thus lead to the synthesis of abnormal DNA. If this proves to be the major mechanism of action of carcinogenic metals, then they would be better classified as epigenetic agents. The mutagenicity of carcinogenic metal ions is controversial.

Metals are transported in the blood bound to carrier proteins and associate with specific cellular ligands. Ions with more than one oxidation stage (e.g., chromium) undergo oxidation–reduction as metabolic steps, but this seems unrelated to carcinogenicity.

Selenium derivatives have been incriminated as carcinogens but current concepts disagree. In fact, selenium salts and organic selenium compounds inhibit the effect of genotoxic carcinogens (Griffin, 1979; Jacobs and Griffin, 1979; Schrauzer, 1979). In several instances, inhibition of the activation reaction leading to proximate or ultimate carcinogens has been documented, as for example with N-2-fluorenylacetamide (Marshall *et al.*, 1979) or azo dyes (Daoud and Griffin, 1980).

5. Epigenetic Carcinogens

As discussed in the introductory classification (Section 2), it has been proposed that chemical carcinogens can be considered under two major headings: genotoxic carcinogens and epigenetic agents. The preceding sections have dealt with the major classes of carcinogens that give rise to reactive electrophiles that in turn react with nucleophilic molecules such as DNA. These reactions are believed to underlie their mutagenic and carcinogenic activity, as well as certain other effects such as inhibition of enzymes, toxicity, and even in some instances effects on the immune system.

So far as is now known, epigenetic carcinogens are not converted to such reactive intermediates. The role of metabolism in the carcinogenicity of this group of carcinogens is thus more complicated and diverse than in the case of genotoxic carcinogens. The expression of epigenetic effects is not well known and may depend essentially on quite distinct, specific properties for each class and even for different chemicals within a class. For example, the effect of phenobarbital, DDT, or butylated hydroxytoluene in promoting liver carcinogenicity when administered after the appropriate genotoxic carcinogens is no doubt quite different from the effect of hormones in enhancing mammary or even pituitary gland carcinogenesis, or from the effect of immunosuppressants in increasing lymphomas, or from the effect of bile acids in increasing colon cancer, or from the effect of saccharin or of tryptophan metabolites in increasing bladder cancer. Thus, mechanistic studies must be conducted with specific reference to the agent and the target system.

Knowledge of epigenetic carcinogenesis bears on important kinds of human diseases such as cancer of the breast or colon. It also relates to the question of the significance of mouse liver tumors as sole pathological findings induced by certain chemicals such as some chlorinated hydrocarbons (DDT, trichloroethylene, tetrachloroethane, or perchloroethane) (see Section 4.2.14). Understanding of the mechanisms whereby mouse liver tumors are induced, as we postulate, through epigenetic rather than through genotoxic mechanisms would suggest a distinct kind of safety evaluation for "carcinogens" with this property.

5.1. Immunosuppressants

A number of genotoxic reactive carcinogens affect protein synthesis and thus the synthesis of the component of the immune system. In addition, genotoxic

300

J. H.
WEISBURGER
AND
G. M.
WILLIAMS

carcinogens are generally cytotoxic. Consequently, specific and general immunosuppressive effects have been noted with such chemicals. However, azathioprine, which is metabolized to 6-mercaptopurine as well as other select metabolites, has demonstrated an immunosuppressive effect through as yet unclear mechanisms, especially in relation to the actual metabolite of the drug involved. Long-term administration of these drugs has led to lymphoma in animals (Weisburger, 1977) and in humans (Penn, 1978). The underlying initiating event may well be a virus.

5.2. Hormones

There are numerous reports dealing with the metabolism and function of androgens and estrogens. The reader is referred to specialized treatises since the specific topic is outside the scope of this review of the metabolism of carcinogens. Hormones are conceived to affect and intervene in the carcinogenic process through indirect epigenetic mechanisms. Whereas under normal conditions the endocrine system maintains a balance between hormones from the gonads, adrenal, thyroid, and pituitary, the excessive production or exogenous intake of a specific hormone that leads to a long-lasting hormonal imbalance, disturbing the prevailing normal rhythmic cycles, might account for promoting effects in hormone-sensitive tissues. This is a complex area wherein the specific relevant mechanisms are not known. Hormonal balances are affected not only by administration of exogenous drugs or hormones but can be modified in more subtle ways via nutrition, including the state of obesity. Aging affects hormonal balances, accounting for the development of tumors in the endocrine organs late in life.

The role of specific receptors for hormones in relation to the mechanisms of action also requires further definition.

5.2.1. Diethylstilbestrol

Diethylstilbestrol (DES) acts as a promoter in enhancing breast cancer development in mice carrying the mammary tumor virus but not in mice lacking this virus (Highman *et al.*, 1977). It has led to a rare type of vaginal cancer in young girls about the time of puberty, consequent to the administration of large amounts of this drug to their mothers during pregnancy, but not when small amounts were given (see Hiatt *et al.*, 1977; Herbst *et al.*, 1979; Rice, 1979). The mechanism is unclear, but may be associated with the induction of a chronic hormonal imbalance in the offspring through the passage of the drug itself or unknown metabolites across the placenta. As a model, Fischer *et al.* (1973) have observed that labeled DES is absorbed more readily than the glucuronide from the intestine in weanling rats. However, in 5-day-old rats, the glucuronide may be absorbed intact, whereas in older animals bacterially mediated hydrolysis of the glucuronic acid conjugate precedes resorption. DES induces renal cancer in male but not female hamsters and not in male or female rats. Gabaldon and Lacomba (1972) noted much higher glucuronyl transferase activity for DES in hamsters than in rats but felt that this finding alone did not account for the carcinogenicity of DES in hamster kidney.

DES is a stilbene derivative with an ethylenic double bond, and the latter has attracted attention as a potential reactive point for the biochemical production of an epoxide, as occurs for other vinyl groups (Gottschlich and Metzler, 1980). A DES epoxide could be a potential genotoxic metabolite. Although a synthetic epoxide has been prepared, there is no evidence at this time for the occurrence of such a reactive metabolite *in vivo* or *in vitro*. It is possible that the highly hindered location, because of vicinal substituents, of the ethylene grouping does not permit the necessary steric conformation of the enzyme to the double bond, as has been postulated with tri- and tetrachloroethylene (Section 4.2.14). Thus, the competing facile detoxification reactions such as conjugation and excretion form the major metabolic pathway. A number of metabolites have been described, but the main metabolites in urine are glucuronic acid conjugates.

5.3. Cocarcinogens

By definition, an agent is a cocarcinogen if when administered together with a carcinogen it augments the tumor induction by the carcinogenic agent. As indicated in Section 2, the carcinogens whose activity has been enhanced by such agents have all been of the genotoxic type. Inasmuch as the activity of genotoxic carcinogens depends to a great extent on the ratio between the essential biochemical activation steps and the metabolic detoxification reactions, a cocarcinogen could either augment the activation steps, block the detoxification reactions, or do both. Another possibility is that cocarcinogens, through cell killing or other mechanisms, stimulate proliferation and thereby sensitize the organ to the carcinogenic effects of the genotoxic carcinogen. Thus, it appears possible for diverse types of chemicals to act as cocarcinogens through several possible mechanisms. The fact that cocarcinogens can occasionally produce tumors independent of additional carcinogen administration, as shown for 12-O-tetradecanoylphorbol-13-acetate (Iverson and Iverson, 1979), may relate to their effects in the presence of unidentified environmental carcinogens.

The classic cocarcinogen is the active ingredient in croton oil, namely phorbol esters. It would appear that this material itself is responsible for the cocarcinogenic effect inasmuch as metabolites are uniformly active or inactive (Hecker *et al.* and Van Duuren *et al.* in Slaga *et al.*, 1978; Hecker *et al.* in Miller *et al.*, 1979).

In the polycyclic aromatic hydrocarbons, a number of compounds have a cocarcinogenic effect, as for example dodecane (Bingham *et al.* in Slaga *et al.*, 1978), fluoranthrene, pyrene, and 9-methylcarbazole (Hoffmann *et al.*, 1978). Norharman and related products have been found to enhance the mutagenicity of a number of carcinogens (Nagao *et al.*, 1978*b*) and to affect their metabolism (Fugino *et al.*, 1978). It is not yet known whether such compounds can increase carcinogenicity. A test of norharman given together with aniline was negative

302

J. H.
WEISBURGER
AND
G. M.
WILLIAMS

(Hagiwara *et al.*, 1980), emphasizing the need to understand the mechanisms whereby norharman increases mutagenicity. Little is known of the metabolism of agents of this type.

Ethanol increases the risk of head and neck cancer in cigarette smokers. In a model situation, it was found that chronic ethanol intake by hamsters increased the metabolism of nitrosopyrrolidine and yielded more mutagenic products. Mixed-function oxidases, aniline hydroxylase, and especially the α-hydroxylation of nitrosopyrrolidine were more than doubled. Thus, ethanol is a cocarcinogen (McCoy *et al.*, 1979). Ethanol is itself metabolized by the mixed-function oxidases as well as by alcohol dehydrogenase to acetaldehyde. It seems likely that this metabolism leads to the induction of oxidase activities and thus cocarcinogenicity.

5.4. Promoters

Promoters are agents that increase the tumorigenic response to a carcinogen when applied after the carcinogen. They were usually conceived to be noncarcinogenic because by themselves under the conditions for obtaining promotion they did not produce tumors. However, as noted in Section 2, diverse kinds of promoters including phorbol esters, bile acids, hormones, and saccharin are now known to be carcinogenic under more strenuous test conditions. Thus, the enhancing effect of a second agent administered after a carcinogen cannot be taken as evidence of only a "promoting" or "tumor-enhancing" action. Indeed, even a genotoxic carcinogen can be administered at low enough doses in sequential exposure to augment the carcinogenicity of a previously administered carcinogen without itself being carcinogenic (Becker, 1975). For this reason, an important element in the definition of a promoter is that it is not genotoxic. The carcinogenic effects of promoters when administered singly are therefore considered to be due to the same epigenetic effects involved in their promoting activity in sequential studies.

Most promoters are quite specific as regards tissue or species affected. They exert a variety of effects (Sivak in Slaga *et al.*, 1978), but little is known of their actual mechanism of promoting action. Boutwell (1974) has noted the induction of ornithine decarboxylase, suggesting that the products, namely long-chain diamines, may be involved in the promoting process. Other promoters fail to induce this enzyme, and thus necessarily need to involve different effects as to mode of action. Recent findings with phorbol esters indicate an ability to produce gene derepression and repression (see Slaga *et al.*, 1978; Weinstein in Emmelot and Kriek, 1979; Diamond *et al.*, 1980), and this has been suggested to be indicative of the potential of promoters for enhancing expression of the neoplastic phenotype in initiated cells. Other evidence (Murray and Fitzgerald, 1979; Yotti *et al.*, 1979; Williams in Borek and Williams, 1980) supports an action of promoters in inhibiting intercellular communication.

Whereas most promoters undergo biotransformation, saccharin does not. Until such time as the relevant action for promotion is identified, the role of metabolic conversions will remain unclear. Nevertheless, for several agents, metabolism appears to reduce the promoting action. This seems to be the case for phorbol esters (Hecker in Miller *et al.*, 1979; Weinstein in Emmelot and Kriek, 1979) and DDT (Gingell and Wallcave, 1974). More detailed work on this subject is clearly needed.

6. Variation in Carcinogen Metabolism

As is apparent from the detailed description of the metabolic processes operating on chemical carcinogens, these are general systems akin to those that apply to exogenous chemicals and drugs in general and, indeed, also to certain endogenous products such as steroid hormones. There are rather specific activation reactions and also fairly broad detoxification processes mediated by cellular mammalian enzymes, as well as by microbiological systems. Whether or not a given carcinogen is active under certain conditions, the degree and extent of its activity, the site affected, and under some conditions the time required to elicit the effect depend more on the ratio of activation reactions vs. detoxification reactions than on virtually any other currently known parameter controlling the overall carcinogenic process (Weisburger and Williams, 1980). It is important, therefore, to understand fully the variables controlling this ratio, so that if a sensitive bioassay system is desired the ratio can be maximized, or if human cancer prevention is the goal it can be minimized.

These reactions depend on species, strain (and in humans, a truly heterogeneous population, on individuals), age, sex, endocrine status, diet, activities of intestinal flora, presence of other chemicals (synthetic or naturally occurring), mode and frequency of exposure, and numerous other parameters. Full discussion of these variables for each type of carcinogen is properly the subject of a separate monograph. Only a few essential and striking examples will be noted here.

6.1. Genetic Factors

In animal models, substantial species differences and, in fact, strain differences within the same species in the response to specific chemical carcinogens have been extensively documented. The underlying mechanisms require detailed study for each case, with special regard for the ratio of activation vs. detoxification metabolites.

Brodie first documented the concept that species differences in the pharmacological response to a drug correlate with its rate of metabolism (*see* Alvares *et al.*, 1979*a*, *b*). Species variations in the metabolism of xenobiotics have now been extensively documented (Kato, 1979; Thorgeirsson and Wirth, 1979; Vesell, 1979, 1980; Nebert, 1980). Likewise, the metabolism of carcinogens is genetically determined and varies greatly among species and individuals (Irving, 1979;

304

J. H.
WEISBURGER
AND
G. M.
WILLIAMS

Gelboin *et al.*, 1980). This has been useful in elucidating steps in activation reactions. For example, the guinea pig does not develop cancer after exposure to *N*-2-fluorenylacetamide, whereas the rat does (see Miller *et al.*, 1964). When it was suspected that *N*-hydroxylation was involved in the activation of *N*-2-fluorenylacetamide, the finding that the guinea pig could readily detoxify *N*-hydroxy compounds (thus accumulating little) confirmed the significance of this reaction (Section 4.2.4).

Some carcinogens, such as the nitrosamines, appear to be actively metabolized by most species, including humans (Magee *et al.* in Searle, 1976; Preussmann, 1975). Although there are no proven data for the carcinogenicity of nitrosamines in humans, they are active in all other species tested, including nonhuman primates, in agreement with metabolic parameters (Adamson and Sieber, 1979). On the other hand, hydrazine itself and asymmetrical hydrazines seem active predominantly in mice and hamsters (Toth, 1980). The induction of colon cancer by 1,2-dimethylhydrazine depends on mouse strain (Diwan and Blackman, 1980), as does the induction of gastric cancer by alkylnitrosoureas (Bralow *et al.*, 1973). It will be useful to relate these findings to information on metabolism as a function of species.

The responsiveness of various mouse strains to polycyclic aromatic hydrocarbons measured by inducibility of aryl hydrocarbon hydroxylase has been designated as the *Ah* locus (Nebert and Jensen, 1979*a*). Random-bred mice, about half of all inbred mouse strains, and about 20 inbred strains of rats are responsive, that is, possess the Ah^b dominant allele (the recessive allele is Ah^d). The methylcholanthrene-inducible *N*-hydroxylation of 2-acetylaminofluorene is also associated with the Ah^b allele in mice. Thus, heterozygous Ah^b/Ah^d mice are responsive, whereas Ah^d/Ah^d homozygous mice are not.

Other well-characterized genetic differences in carcinogen metabolism are known. For example, the *N*-acetyltransferase system, important in the metabolism of aromatic amines (Section 4.2.4), varies in activity between species (Weber in Fishman, 1973; Lower *et al.*, 1979; Tannen and Webber, 1979). Humans and rabbits show a polymorphic distribution of rapid and slow acetylation, with the slow-acetylation trait being recessive.

Species difference may be manifested primarily as a sex difference. For example, metabolism of certain drugs in the rat is less active in males, whereas there is no sex difference in other species. Such differences extend even to strains or to breeds within a species.

6.2. Sex and Endocrine Status

For most experimental species, males are more susceptible to some of the aromatic amine liver carcinogens than are females. On the other hand, female mice have been found to be more sensitive to carbon tetrachloride and *o*-aminoazotoluene and female rats more sensitive to diethylnitrosamine.

The basis for these various sex differences is not yet fully documented. In some special cases it could be that steroid hormones compete with carcinogens for metabolism or some other reaction such as binding. The cytosolic protein that binds corticosteroids also binds 4-dimethylaminoazobenzene and 3-methylcholanthrene. However, there is no significant competition between carcinogens and steroids for binding sites (Dao and Libby, 1972; Sarrif *et al.*, 1978; Tipping *et al.*, 1979; Smith *et al.*, 1980). These results may indicate that the covalent binding of activated carcinogens may be at a different site on the binding molecule than the noncovalent binding of steroids. On the other hand, steroids do compete with carcinogens for metabolism. Thus, steroids inhibit the metabolism of several carcinogens, including benzo[*a*]pyrene, aflatoxin, and 7,12-dimethylbenz[*a*]-anthracene (see Kato, 1974).

The other main possibility, that there are sex differences in the amount or activity of metabolizing enzymes, seems to be a more likely basis for sex differences. It is well known that metabolism of many drugs in rats is more active in males than in females (Alvares *et al.*, 1979*a*) and that after sexual maturation, mixed-function oxidase activity in liver is usually much greater in males (Kato, 1974). In addition, exogenous estrogens will reduce microsomal enzyme activities (Sweeney and Cole, 1980).

The fact that *N*-2-fluorenylacetamide is more hepatocarcinogenic in certain strains of rats to males than to females rests on the level of sulfotransferase (Miller and Miller, 1980). Diethylnitrosamine usually is slightly more active in female rats, but in mice, males respond better, a reflection of metabolism (Kato, 1979; Magee *et al.* in Searle, 1976).

Whenever experiments in chemical carcinogenesis reveal a difference in response between male and female animals, investigation of the underlying differences in enzymes concerned with activation and deactivation reactions contributes the key to the endocrine effect. However, in several instances in which a carcinogen has been administered to sexually immature animals, including developing fetuses and newborns, with no further exposure during the adult sexually differentiated stage, there still appears to be a sex-linked incidence of cancer, not only as might be expected in endocrine-responsive organs such as breast, but also in liver and other tissues (see Rice, 1979). This indicates that the hormonal status plays a role in neoplastic development at later stages beyond the metabolism of the agent and initial interaction with tissue constituents. One possible mechanism could be promotional effects (Section 5.2) even at physiological levels of endocrine activity. The question whether early exposure to reactive electrophilic carcinogens affects the differentiation and development of the endocrine system requires study.

6.3. Age

Newborn and young animals have been shown to be more susceptible to tumor induction at several sites than older animals (Toth, 1968). In some cases, this is probably because of the higher levels of cell proliferation in the affected organ, since susceptibility in older animals can be heightened by inducing cell replication. Drug-metabolizing enzymes are usually very low in newborn animals (Gillette,

306

J. H.
WEISBURGER
AND
G. M.
WILLIAMS

1979*a*, *b*), and this seems to be especially true of those involved with detoxification of chemical carcinogens, but perhaps is not so for activating enzymes (Lucier *et al.*, 1979). For example, the rate of total body clearance of 7,12-dimethyl-benz[*a*]anthracene is lower for newborn mice than for adults.

There is considerable concern about the possible effect of environmental carcinogens on unborn fetuses through placental transmission and possible fetal metabolism (see Rice, 1979). It is apparent that many of the ultimate carcinogens derived from procarcinogens through metabolic activation are highly reactive entities. Unless these are stabilized to a transport form that can subsequently be released in the fetus, it seems unlikely that activation to a final carcinogenic product in the mother would lead to the expression of carcinogenicity in the fetus. Thus, the question is whether placental transfer of a procarcinogen or a proximate but not ultimate carcinogen might lead to cancer in the offspring if the fetus possesses the necessary enzymatic potential to produce the ultimate carcinogenic metabolite. In recent years, a number of studies have documented the capability of fetuses to carry out such reactions (Rice, 1979; Hirakawa *et al.*, 1979; Schmucker, 1979).

From animal systems and from experiments with human fetuses in societies where this is considered permissible, useful comparative data have been obtained. Much more needs to be learned about the capability of fetuses of various species to effect biochemical alterations on substrates such as drugs and carcinogens as a function of fetal age. It would seem that in most cases the fetus has an enzymatic potential lower than that of the adult. However, fetuses do have many of the enzymes concerned with activation reactions, such as those that epoxidize polycyclic aromatic hydrocarbons (and perhaps aflatoxin) and nitroreductases, but seem to be deficient in the detoxification steps such as conjugation with glucuronic acid or epoxide hydrase. Thus, on balance, the fetus may be more sensitive for this reason, as is also documented by the demonstration that fetuses, or certainly newborn animals, are exquisitely sensitive to a variety of chemical carcinogens.

Metabolism of carcinogens in aged animals has not received much specific attention, although there have been recent studies on the metabolism of drugs (Baird and Birnbaum, 1979*a*; Gillette, 1979*a*; Schmucker, 1979). Such studies, incidentally, would be complicated by changes with age in the hormonal status, a component that also affects carcinogen metabolism (Section 6.2).

7. Modification of Carcinogen Metabolism

A number of factors have been found to alter the induction of cancer by certain carcinogens. Most of these factors function by altering the metabolism of the host. The host may be completely protected if the modifier inhibits activation while deactivation proceeds unimpaired in the same or another organ.

The enzymes concerned with the metabolism of carcinogens are in a dynamic equilibrium between the predominant detoxification activities and the activation reactions. The level of these enzymes depends on a number of endogenous and, more importantly, exogenous elements. These include the agent itself, other chemicals, carcinogenic or not, enzyme inducers or inhibitors, and also the dietary constituents. More subtle effects relate to variables such as light cycle and stresses such as temperature and crowding.

In the area of modification of carcinogen metabolism, liver enzymes have received extensive study for many reasons, including the central importance of this organ and also the ease of isolating cellular and molecular components. However, because of the need to understand carcinogen activation and detoxification at target sites other than the liver, such as the lung, the breast, the kidney, and the intestinal tract, a beginning has been made to understand enzymes in these organs in relation to environmental modifiers (Griffin and Shaw, 1979; Wattenberg in Emmelot and Kriek, 1979; Coon *et al.*, 1980). Much more remains to be done.

7.1. Diet

Many types of cancer in humans are mediated and controlled by diet. In recent years, much progress has been made by studying each type of cancer (e.g., colon, breast, stomach cancer) separately as to causes and modifiers (Reddy *et al.*, 1980). Such an approach has suggested the occurrence of specific carcinogens for each kind of target organ. Some of these have been partially elucidated; others have been postulated. It would appear that cancer causation in humans usually involves not one but a number of different factors, some of which are of the nature of genotoxic carcinogens and others are epigenetic agents, which can be conceived to enhance the process. Whether or not cancer occurs may depend on the efficiency and effectiveness of all the components involved.

Of course, diet can be the source of genotoxic carcinogens, such as nitrosamine- or aflatoxin-containing foods. The diet can also exert an important effect on metabolism, especially the absence of micronutrients (Wattenberg, 1978; Campbell, 1979; Conney *et al.*, 1977, 1981).

Nutrition thus affects the metabolism and specific activation of carcinogens. This includes not only macronutrients like fat but also micronutrients, including naturally occurring flavones and indole derivatives found in cabbage or brussels sprouts (Wattenberg, 1978). The effectiveness of many of these modifiers differs as a function of the carbohydrate/protein/fat ratio and, in fact, with the simple- vs. complex-carbohydrate distribution.

Inasmuch as the mixed-function oxidases and other enzymes have their own active life span and their own levels of continuing synthesis, the administration of a protein-deficient or protein-free diet has important considerations to nutrition and drug metabolism in general. For example, the metabolism of benzo[*a*]pyrene is reduced through a protein-deficient diet. In rats a protein-free diet results in greatly reduced metabolism of dimethylnitrosamine in the liver but not in the kidney. For this reason, animals on such a diet have virtually no

308

J. H.
WEISBURGER
AND
G. M.
WILLIAMS

liver tumors but eventually develop a high incidence of kidney tumors (Swann *et al.*, 1980). The mutagenicity of the direct-acting carcinogen N-methyl-N′-nitro-N-nitrosoguanidine is reduced by *in vitro* microsomal metabolism (Popper *et al.*, 1973) and a protein-deficient diet decreases the microsomal inactivation (Czygan *et al.*, 1974). These data illustrate the need for much more study on the influence of diet and any other modulators on the metabolic capability in specific organs (Lazear *et al.*, 1978; Newberne *et al.*, 1979). Specific components such as L-tryptophan can increase carcinogenesis in one organ, the urinary bladder (Cohen *et al.*, 1979), or protect an organ, such as the liver (Mostafa *et al.*, 1979).

Diet is also an important element in controlling the intestinal microflora, which intervene in the metabolism of certain carcinogens and promoters (Boxenbaum *et al.*, 1979; see Hill in Brookes, 1980; Reddy *et al.*, 1980). Indirectly, the intestinal microflora can affect mammalian enzymes in the liver perhaps through alteration of the feedback of metabolites in the enterohepatic circulation.

There have been numerous studies on the involvement of micronutrients such as vitamins and minerals in carcinogenesis. Vitamins A and E, as well as the synthetic retinoids, affect cancer causation in animal models and in humans (Genta *et al.*, 1974; Baird and Birnbaum, 1979b; Dashman and Kamm, 1979; Sporn and Newton, 1979; Daoud and Griffin, 1980). In part, their effect bears on the promoting process, but it is not yet known how these essential nutrients bear on cancer causation. Possibly, high levels of these substances may modify the metabolism of certain genotoxic carcinogens, but the precise mode of action requires further definition.

The involvement of riboflavin in the metabolism of carcinogenic dyes first called attention to the importance of nutrition in carcinogenesis. Animals on a high-flavin diet have a lower risk of liver cancer developing from carcinogenic azo dyes than animals with limited amounts of riboflavin. The classic explanation is that riboflavin and flavin are cofactors for azo dye reductase. Riboflavin plays additional roles reviewed by Rivlin (1973), and key older, classical literature reviewed by Clayson (1962).

Vitamin C is an essential contributor to the operation of mixed-function oxidases, although its precise role in complex reactions is not known (Zannoni and Sato, 1975; Coon *et al.*, 1980). Both vitamins C and E inhibit the endogenous formation of nitrosamines and nitrosamides (Section 3.3).

Schrauzer (1979) has reviewed the role of trace elements in carcinogenesis. This includes the inhibition of carcinogenesis by trace amounts of selenium, which appears to affect not only the production of active electrophiles from genotoxic carcinogens, but also involves the level of detoxification systems related to the sulfur-containing amino acids (Chasseaud, 1979; Griffin, 1979; Jacobs and Griffin, 1979; Sunderman in Emmelot and Kriek, 1979).

7.2. Effect of Mode and Frequency of Exposure

With a number of carcinogens distinct effects are noted as a function of mode of introduction. As already mentioned (Section 4.2.12), cycasin is active when given orally but not when injected parenterally, as this agent requires enzymatic hydrolysis mediated by intestinal flora. Dibutylnitrosamine induces mainly urinary bladder cancers on subcutaneous injection, but also liver and pulmonary tumors on oral intake. The reasons apparently are the distinct concentration effects in the liver and metabolism therein that result from administration by these two routes. It is well known that in many strains of mice small amounts of some polycyclic aromatic hydrocarbons are highly carcinogenic when applied cutaneously but not much so when given orally. The difference again rests on the balance of activating and detoxifying enzymes at these two sites. Thus, route of administration must always be carefully considered in carcinogenesis studies.

Some carcinogens such as polycyclic aromatic hydrocarbons are more active when the same total amount is administered subcutaneously in fractionated doses than when a single large dose is given. This is because the latter mode leads to extensive formation of detoxified metabolites, and hence reduces the total effective dose. Continuous low-dose intake may also be more effective than a few larger doses because of a chronic effect on repair and replication systems (Margison et al., 1977). With some nitrosamines, the target organ depends on dose schedule (Schmähl, 1970; Preussmann, 1975; Magee et al. in Searle, 1976; Magee in Coon et al., 1980). Some carcinogens, including most aromatic amines and azo dyes, must be administered for a minimal amount of time in order to allow accumulation of the necessary increasing amounts of active carcinogen in the form of N-hydroxy derivatives (see Weisburger and Weisburger, 1973), although in young rodents a single large dose can induce cancer after a long latent period. With other powerful carcinogens, including polycyclic hydrocarbons, nitrosamines and nitrosamides, azoxymethane, and aflatoxin B_1, a single large dose readily induces cancer. With weaker carcinogens like safrole and mesidine, this would be less likely, although there are no data.

In addition, it has been noted that multiple dosing of the same carcinogen, or of different carcinogens, sometimes affects to a considerable extent the level of DNA repair and cell replication, and therefore will eventually affect the overall carcinogenic process.

7.3. Effect of Other Agents

Due to the complexity of the environment, the induction of cancer in humans and in animal models requires careful analysis to dissect the manifold elements that eventually control whether a neoplasm does or does not occur. In animal models employing powerful carcinogens, such elements as quality and quantity of diet, including the possible presence of traces of pesticides and hormones as well as the amount of roughage, may not play a decisive role, whereas at lower dose levels or with weaker carcinogens, their role may be decisive. The effect can hinge on the relative activity of enzymes concerned with the metabolism of the carcinogen, but more data in this area are required.

310

J. H.
WEISBURGER
AND
G. M.
WILLIAMS

There are more than 200 chemicals known to stimulate the activity of microsomal enzymes (Coon *et al.*, 1980; Argus *et al.*, 1980). Many are compounds that are themselves metabolized by microsomal enzymes. Among the most studied are phenobarbital, polychlorinated hydrocarbons like DDT, 2,3,7,8-tetrachlorodibenzo-*p*-dioxin, and arachlor, polycyclic aromatic hydrocarbons such as 3-methylcholanthrene, benzo[*a*]pyrene, and benz[*a*]anthracene, and certain flavones. It is now established for several of these inducers that they promote synthesis of new enzymes including the cytochrome P-450 system (Section 3). The cytochrome induced by phenobarbital is P-450, whereas that induced by 3-methylcholanthrene and other polycyclic hydrocarbons is P_1-450 or P-448. These generate different ratios of metabolites from the same substrate (Parke, 1979; Kato, 1979; Nebert and Jensen, 1979*a*; Coon *et al.*, 1980). For example, the phenobarbital-induced P-450 catalyzes 4-hydroxylation of biphenyl, whereas the methylcholanthrene-induced P_1-450 mediates hydroxylation at the 2-position (Parke, 1979). Enzyme induction either enhances or decreases the tumorigenicity of a carcinogen according to whether activating or deactivating enzymes are predominantly induced. In most situations, however, enzyme induction inhibits carcinogenicity, often mainly because of increased levels of type II conjugation reactions (Section 3). Since simple nitrosamines do not undergo such type II conjugation, there is sometimes a related increased carcinogenicity (Section 4.2.2). There are also agents such as disulfiram (Antabuse) and related compounds, including carbon disulfide, that have a powerful inhibitory effect on mixed-function oxidases, and thus on carcinogen metabolism. Depending on the specific target organ affected, in turn a function of the metabolism of the carcinogen, partial or complete inhibition of carcinogenesis occurs (Wattenberg, 1978, 1980; Irving *et al.*, 1979; Fiala, 1981).

Many of the detoxification enzymes, such as UDP-glucuronyltransferase, glutathione *S*-transferase, and epoxide hydratase, are inducible. The outcome of a carcinogenicity experiment will depend on the relative increases of the activation steps compared to the detoxification steps.

An extensively studied example is that of the carcinogen *N*-2-fluorenylacetamide. Methylcholanthrene decreases carcinogenicity in the rat and increases it in the hamster. In both species, there is an increased formation of the proximate carcinogen, the *N*-hydroxy derivative. However, in the rat there is a more pronounced increase in glucuronyltransferase, leading to detoxified metabolites (Fishman, 1970; Aitio, 1978; Irving, 1979). Antioxidants such as butylated hydroxytoluene have similar effects (Grantham *et al.*, 1973; Talalay *et al.*, 1979). Phenobarbital given together with this carcinogen reduced the carcinogenic effect, again for a similar reason, namely increased detoxification through glucuronide formation (Weisburger and Weisburger, 1973). Interestingly, when phenobarbital is given after the carcinogen, it produces an enhancement as a result of different actions (Peraino *et al.*, 1980) (Section 5.4). Nevertheless, as a general rule, enzyme induction reduces the oncogenicity of procarcinogens due to predominant induction of detoxification pathways of metabolism. Such findings have more than theoretical importance, for Wattenberg (1978; in Emmelot and Kriek, 1979) has described the occurrence in foods consumed by humans of materials such as flavones, which are potent enzyme inducers and which can modify the response to carcinogens. Moreover, antioxidants such as butylated hydroxytoluene and 2(3)-*tert*-butyl-4-hydroxyanisole, which are also enzyme inducers (Grantham *et al.*, 1973; E. K. Weisburger *et al.*, 1977; Wattenberg, 1980; Talalay *et al.*, 1979), are used as food additives.

While the activation reactions for some types of carcinogens have been understood for some time now, as for example that of the aromatic amines and azo dyes, the background data for these processes with other agents are of recent date, and their modulation by enzyme inducers and inhibitors is not as well documented. This is especially true for carcinogens that affect extrahepatic sites. Thus, use of such enzyme inducers with carcinogens potentially affecting several tissues can yield a shift of the principal target organ.

In the case of carcinogens that are primarily inactivated by metabolism, inhibition of metabolism may actually increase the oncogenic effects. This appears to be the case with the effect of diet on the mutagenicity of N-methyl-N'-nitro-N-nitrosoguanidine (Section 7.1). The toxicity and probably also the carcinogenicity of direct-acting alkylating agents such as nitrogen mustards are decreased by enzyme induction.

In addition to effects on metabolism, other agents may affect the carcinogenicity of genotoxic carcinogens by providing competitive concentrations of nucleophilic trapping agents that interfere with the reaction of carcinogens with key cellular targets. A beginning success along these lines has been achieved, and more effort is warranted (Chasseaud, 1979; Jollow, 1980; Miller and Miller, 1980). Similar concepts are beginning to accumulate on the modification of DNA repair (O'Connor *et al.* in Emmelot and Kriek, 1979; Stumpf *et al.*, 1979; Montesano *et al.*, 1980*a*; Setlow, 1980), although noncarcinogenic modalities that affect such repair systems are needed.

8. Concluding Remarks and Prospects

Thirty years ago, the field of chemical carcinogenesis was concerned with the description of the effects of a few types of chemicals, mainly polycyclic aromatic hydrocarbons, aromatic amines and azo dyes, and several miscellaneous agents such as urethan. Their mechanism of action was obscure. In the intervening years, a number of additional structural types of chemical carcinogens have been discovered. Among these are the important nitrosamine derivatives, certain mycotoxins, other natural products such as safrole, and commercial chemicals such as vinyl chloride, asbestos, and chromates. Some of these chemicals are laboratory curiosities; others are tonnage industrial products that have caused cancer not only in animals but also in humans. Efforts have been and are being

312

J. H.
WEISBURGER
AND
G. M.
WILLIAMS

made to discover the carcinogenic principles responsible for certain important human cancers (Hiatt *et al.*, 1977; Higginson, Weisburger in Emmelot and Kriek, 1979).

An exciting development in the study of chemical carcinogens since the first edition of this series is the growing insight into their modes of action. It is now realized that the overall carcinogenic process is extremely complex. To conceptualize this process, carcinogens have been characterized as to mode of action. Those that are genotoxic have structures such that they interact with genetic material. Although a number of highly reactive compounds have this property inherent in their structure, most chemical carcinogens that can be classified as genotoxic first require metabolism.

The purpose of this chapter has been to summarize knowledge in this field which, for types of structures such as polycyclic aromatic hydrocarbons, has changed quite remarkably in the last 10 years, even though these were the first pure chemical carcinogens known. We have not reviewed in any detail the reactions of the active molecules, which are either electrophilic reactants or in some instances radical cations. The reactions include those with nucleophilic genetic material, those with other nucleophilic reactants in the cell, including proteins, peptides, and compounds with an SH bond (e.g., glutathione), and for highly reactive electrophilic molecules, even reactions with water.

The recognition of the genotoxic, electrophilic properties of ultimate carcinogens has also provided the basis for a link to mutagenicity in microbial and mammalian systems as well as the recognition that DNA damage, DNA repair, and cell transformation have a sound theoretical basis for the detection of chemicals that might be carcinogenic hazards to humans. Because of the known differences in biochemical activation, in contrast to biochemical detoxification steps, inherent in such short-term mutagenicity and related bioassay systems, it is also clear that a positive response in any one such system alone may not actually reflect *in vivo* carcinogenicity. Nonetheless, current thinking is that a uniformly positive reaction in a battery of such tests may approximate an expression of carcinogenic risk. As more such data accumulate, it may be possible to avoid long-term chronic bioassays. Also the information obtained in the short-term tests for genotoxicity or the production of electrophilic reactants aids in interpreting the results of long-term bioassays where these yield ambiguous results.

With the recognition that most genotoxic carcinogens require metabolic activation to produce neoplasms, it also became clear that this activation reaction, as opposed to detoxification metabolism, is subject to numerous modifying elements. These in turn can be divided into two subclasses. The first is endogenously controlled and involves genetics, age, and sex. Thus, whether or not a given individual of *Homo sapiens* or a given strain of rat or mouse responds to a specific carcinogenic stimulus depends on the individual's genetically controlled potential to produce electrophilic reactants from a given amount of carcinogen. The age and sex of such an individual would have similar roles. The second subclass is the complex area of environmental influences. Thus, there are enhancers of the activation reaction, termed cocarcinogens, and there are inhibitors. The latter might operate either by decreasing the activation process through the inhibition of a type I kind of reaction, or by increasing the detoxification through a type II reaction. A human, whether or not exposed to tobacco smoke, or depending on nutritional status, or whether environmentally exposed to certain industrial chemicals, would be at a greater or lesser risk for cancer development as a function of those variables.

Many experimental approaches have studied such interactions in animals. Owing to the complexity of the human environment, these approaches are sometimes not totally adequate since they involve highly controlled tests with two or at most three interacting chemicals. Nonetheless, such studies have provided much sound information on relevant mechanisms that can be used to begin to understand the more complex human situation. Much of the experimental knowledge of carcinogenesis is based on high-level exposure of animals during bioassay or even during metabolism studies. In some rare instances, it has been shown that high-dose experimental conditions represent metabolic overload, and cancer induction under such conditions would not be part of a normal metabolic sequence with lower dosage. This seems clearly to be the case with many epigenetic carcinogens, the other major category discussed. With genotoxic carcinogens, it would appear that there is a rather constant ratio of dosage to the production of electrophilic reactants and thus to potential risk, even in the presence of adequate repair. Considering the competition in any given tissue or cell between nongenetic nucleophiles and a key nucleophilic site on the genetic material, it may be that further research will demonstrate that even with genotoxic carcinogens there may be reliable no-effect levels. Such research is essential inasmuch as progress in analytical chemistry has permitted the detection of genotoxic carcinogens, as for example, alkylnitrosamines, at extremely low levels. The question is whether these levels are biologically significant.

That cancer causation can involve a promotion step has been known for over 40 years. Current research has shown that there are many kinds of chemicals that are not genotoxic and that are not metabolized to electrophilic reactants, but that nonetheless can powerfully influence the course of the carcinogenic process. Historically, there have been many studies with the active principle of croton oil. In recent years, however, many other kinds of chemicals have been found to promote cancer development; indeed, there are a number of situations where cancer induction in humans depends very heavily on promotion. This seems to be the case for the mechanisms through which nutrition impacts on carcinogenesis in breast, prostate, colon, and possibly several other organs that are major sites for cancer in the Western world. Even the powerful synergistic interaction of asbestos and cigarette smoking on the lung may represent a promoting action by asbestos. The mechanism of action of agents that operate through epigenetic routes is not clear and requires much more research. It may simply be a matter of permitting the growth of neoplastic cells. Or it may also involve an effect on differentiation and dedifferentiation or a combination of such actions. Not much is known about the metabolism or even the possible

314

J. H.
WEISBURGER
AND
G. M.
WILLIAMS

need of metabolic activation of agents that operate via epigenetic pathways. Phenobarbital, DDT, and butylated hydroxytoluene have been shown to promote liver carcinogenesis in mice and rats, but little is known about the mechanism of action or the actual metabolite of these diverse agents. This is true even though there are data on the metabolism of some of these agents such as phenobarbital and DDT.

Most studies on the mode of action of carcinogens have been conducted with a few select classes of chemicals such as N-2-fluorenylacetamide or phorbol esters—pure laboratory products representing a genotoxic carcinogen and an epigenetic agent, respectively. However, research during the last few decades has pinpointed natural products as major causes of cancer in humans in various parts of the world. This applies to mycotoxins as causes of primary liver cancer in Africa, the complex components of cigarette smoke in the Western world, and to an increasing extent in every part of the world, complex nutritional factors representing both genotoxic carcinogens and epigenetic agents. Curiously, and in the main, in many parts of the world, governmental regulatory activities are concerned mainly with synthetic chemicals simply because historically these were first used and demonstrated to be carcinogens under laboratory situations and because such chemicals were discovered to be causes of cancer in humans in an occupational, high-level-exposure setting. Also, through direct action, cancers due to occupational exposures can be controlled most readily through technology or elimination. The question is whether cancer causation brought about by lifestyle, namely smoking, nutrition, and alcohol use, can be controlled through chemopreventive measures, through understanding of the risk factors involved, both genotoxic and epigenetic in nature, for each kind of cancer, or whether product modification, such as the lower-tar cigarettes, will eventually be instrumental in reducing cancer risk. This chapter concerning the metabolism and mode of action of chemical carcinogens has described synthetic chemicals and some naturally occurring chemicals. It is hoped that much greater effort with the latter class of chemicals, associated with important kinds of cancer affecting large numbers of people, will become the emphasis in the future as part of broad approaches to generate a sound basis to cancer prevention.

ACKNOWLEDGMENTS

We are grateful to C. Horn and L. Stempel for excellent editorial and secretarial support and to S. Crescenzi for preparing the illustrations.

9. References

ADAMSON, R. H., AND SIEBER, S. M., 1979, The use of nonhuman primates for chemical carcinogenesis studies, in: *Regulatory Aspects of Carcinogenesis and Food Additives: The Delaney Clause* (F. Coulston, ed.), pp. 275–296, Academic Press, New York.

AITIO, A. (ed.), 1978, *Conjugation Reactions in Drug Biotransformations*, Elsevier/North Holland, Amsterdam.

ALVARES, A. P., KAPPAS, A., EISEMAN, J. L., ANDERSON, K. E., PANTUCK, E. J., HSIAO, K. C., GARLAND, W. A., AND CONNEY, A. H., 1979a, Intraindividual variation in drug disposition, *Clin. Pharmacol. Ther.* **26:**407–419.

ALVARES, A. P., PANTUCK, E. J., ANDERSON, K. E., KAPPAS, A., AND CONNEY, A. H., 1979b, Regulation of drug metabolism in man by environmental factors, *Drug Metab. Rev.* **9:**185–205.

ANDERSEN, M. E., THOMAS, O. E., GARGAS, M. L., JONES, R. A., AND JENKINS, L. J., JR., 1980, The significance of multiple detoxification pathways for reactive metabolites in the toxicity of 1,1-dichloroethylene, *Toxicol. Appl. Pharmacol.* **52:**422–432.

ANDREWS, L. S., POHL, L. R., HINSON, J. A., FISK, C. L., AND GILLETTE, J. R., 1979a, Production of a dimer of 2-acetylaminofluorene during the sulfation of *N*-hydroxy-2-acetylaminofluorene *in vitro*, *Drug Metab. Dispos.* **7:**296–300.

ANDREWS, L. S., SASAME, H. A., AND GILLETTE, J. R., 1979b, ^{3}H-Benzene metabolism in rabbit bone marrow, *Life Sci.* **25:**567–572.

ANSELME, J. (ed.), 1978, *N-Nitrosamines*, ACS Symposium Series 101, American Chemical Society, Washington, D.C.

APPEL, K. E., SCHWARZ, M., RICKARD, R., AND KUNZ, W., 1979, Influences of inducers and inhibitors of the microsomal monooxygenase system on the alkylating intensity of dimethylnitrosamine in mice, *J. Cancer Res. Clin. Oncol.* **94:**47–61.

APPEL, K. E., SCHRENK, D., SCHWARZ, M., MAHR, B., AND KUNZ, W., 1980, Denitrosation of *N*-nitrosomorpholine by liver microsomes: Possible role of cytochrome P-450, *Cancer Lett.* **9:**13–20.

ARCOS, J., MYERS, S. C., NEUBURGER, B. J., AND ARGUS, M., 1980, Comparative effects of indole and aminoacetonitrile derivatives on dimethylnitrosamine-demethylase and aryl hydrocarbon hydroxylase activities, *Cancer Lett.* **9:**161–167.

ARGUS, M. F., SOHAL, R. S., BRYANT, G. M., HOCK-LIGETI, C., AND ARCOS, J. C., 1973, Dose–response and ultrastructural alterations in dioxane carcinogenesis, *Eur. J. Cancer* **9:**237–243.

ARGUS, M. F., MYERS, S. C., AND ARCOS, J. C., 1980, Apparent absence of requirement of hydrocarbon metabolism for induction or repression of mixed-function oxidases, *Chem. Biol. Interact.* **29:**247–253.

ARMSTRONG, R. N., LEVIN, W., AND JERINA, D. M., 1980, Hepatic microsomal epoxide hydrolase: Mechanistic studies of the hydration of K-region oxides, *J. Biol. Chem.* **255:**4698–4705.

AUNE, T., AND DYBING, E., 1979, Mutagenic activation of 2,4-diaminoanisole and 2-aminofluorene *in vitro* by liver and kidney fractions form aromatic hydrocarbon responsive and nonresponsive mice, *Biochem. Pharmacol.* **28:**2791–2797.

AUTRUP, H., 1979, Separation of water-soluble metabolites of benzo(*a*)pyrene formed by cultured human colon, *Biochem. Pharmacol.* **28:**1727–1730.

AUTRUP, H., STONER, G. D., JACKSON, F., HARRIS, C. C., SHAMSUDDIN, A. K. M., BARRETT, L. A., AND TRUMP, B. F., 1978, Explant culture of rat colon: A model system for studying metabolism of chemical carcinogens, *In Vitro* **14:**868–872.

AUTRUP, H., ESSIGMANN, J. M., CROY, R. G., TRUMP, B. F., WOGAN, G. N., AND HARRIS, C. C., 1979, Metabolism of aflatoxin B$_1$ and identification of the major aflatoxin B$_1$–DNA adducts formed in cultured human bronchus and colon, *Cancer Res.* **39:**694–698.

BACKER, J. M., AND WEINSTEIN, I. B., 1980, Mitochondrial DNA is a major cellular target for a dihydrodiol-epoxide derivative of benzo(*a*)pyrene, *Science* **209:**297–299.

BAIRD, M. B., AND BIRNBAUM, L. S., 1979a, Increased production of mutagenic metabolites of carcinogens by tissues from senescent rodents, *Cancer Res.* **39:**4752–4755.

BAIRD, M. B., AND BIRNBAUM, L. S., 1979b, Inhibition of 2-fluorenamine-induced mutagenesis in *Salmonella typhimurium* by vitamin A, *J. Natl. Cancer Inst.* **63:**1093–1096.

BAIRD, W. M., AND DIAMOND, L., 1979, The nature of BaP–DNA adducts formed in hamster embryo cells depends on the length of time of exposure to BaP, *Biochem. Biophys. Res. Commun.* **77:**162–167.

BANERJEE, S., VAN DUUREN, B. L., AND KLINE, S. A., 1979, Interaction of potential metabolites of the carcinogen ethylene dibromide with protein and DNA *in vitro*, *Biochem. Biophys. Res. Commun.* **90:**1214–1220.

BANERJEE, S., VAN DUUREN, B. L., AND ORUAMBO, F. I., 1980, Microsome-mediated covalent binding of 1,2-dichloroethane to lung microsomal protein and salmon sperm DNA, *Cancer Res.* **40:**2170–2173.

316

J. H.
WEISBURGER
AND
G. M.
WILLIAMS

BARTSCH, H., DWORKIN, C., MILLER, E. C., AND MILLER, J. A., 1973, Formation of electrophilic N-acetoxyarylamines in cytosols from rat mammary gland and other tissues by transacetylation from the carcinogen N-hydroxy-4-acetylaminobiphenyl, *Biochim. Biophys. Acta* **304**:42–55.

BARTSCH, H., MALAVEILLE, C., STICH, H. F., MILLER, E. C., AND MILLER, J. A., 1977, Comparative electrophilicity, mutagenicity, DNA repair induction activity, and carcinogenicity of some N- and O-acyl derivatives of N-hydroxy-2-aminofluorene, *Cancer Res.* **37**:1461–1467.

BARTSCH, H., MALAVEILLE, C., BARBIN, A., AND PLANCHE, G., 1979a, Mutagenic and alkylating metabolites of halo-ethylenes, chlorobutadienes and dichlorobutenes produced by rodent or human liver tissues: Evidence for oxirane formation by P450-linked microsomal mono-oxygenases, *Arch. Toxicol.* **41**:249–277.

BARTSCH, H., MALAVEILLE, C., TIERNEY, B., GROVER, P. L., AND SIMS, P., 1979b, The association of bacterial mutagenicity of hydrocarbon-derived bay-region dihydrodiols with the Iball indices for carcinogenicity and with the extents of DNA-binding on mouse skin of the parent hydrocarbons, *Chem. Biol. Interact.* **26**:285–296.

BARTSCH, H., SABADIE, N., MALAVEILLE, C., CAMUS, A. M., AND BRUN, G., 1979c, Tissue specificity in metabolic activation, *Adv. Pharmacol. Ther.* **9**:93–102.

BECKER, F. F., 1975, Alteration of hepatocytes by subcarcinogenic exposure to N-2-fluorenyl-acetamide, *Cancer Res.* **35**:1734–1736.

BELAND, F. A., TULLIS, D. L., KADLUBAR, F. F., STRAUB, K. M., AND EVANS, F. E., 1980, Characterization of DNA adducts of the carcinogen N-methyl-4-aminoazobenzene *in vitro* and *in vivo*, *Chem. Biol. Interact.* **31**:1–17.

BENGTSSON, U., JOHANSSON, S., AND ANGERVALL, L., 1978, Malignancies of the urinary tract and their relation to analgesic abuse, *Kidney Int.* **13**:107–113.

BENSON, A. M., BATZINGER, R. P., OU, S. L., BUEDING, E., CHA, Y., AND TALALAY, P., 1978, Elevation of hepatic glutathione S-transferase activities and protection against mutagenic metabolites of benzo(a)pyrene by dietary antioxidants, *Cancer Res.* **38**:4486–4495.

BERENBLUM, I. (ed.), 1974, *Carcinogenesis as a Biological Problem, Frontiers of Biology*, Vol. 34, Elsevier/North Holland, Amsterdam.

BERGMANN, E. D., AND PULLMAN, B. (eds.), 1969, *Physico-chemical Mechanism of Carcinogenesis*, The Israel Academy of Science and Humanities, Jerusalem.

BIGGER, C. A. H., TOMASZEWSKI, J. E., ANDREWS, A. W., AND DIPPLE, A., 1980a, Evaluation of metabolic activation of 7,12-dimethylbenz(a)anthracene *in vitro* by aroclor 1254-induced rat liver S-9 fraction, *Cancer Res.* **40**:655–661.

BIGGER, C. A. H., TOMASZEWSKI, J. E., AND DIPPLE, A., 1980b, Limitations of metabolic activation systems used with *in vitro* test for carcinogens, *Science* **209**:503–504.

BJORSETH, A., AND DENNIS, A. (eds.), 1980, *Polynuclear Aromatic Hydrocarbons*, Batelle Press, Columbus, Ohio.

BLACK, M., 1980, Acetaminophen hepatotoxicity, *Gastroenterology* **78**:382–392.

BLATTMANN, L., AND PREUSSMANN, R., 1973, Struktur von metaboliten Carcinogener Dialkyl-nitrosamine im Rattenurin, *Z. Krebsforsch.* **79**:3–5.

BORCHERT, P., WISLOCKI, P. G., MILLER, J. A., AND MILLER, E. C., 1973a, The metabolism of the naturally occurring hepatocarcinogen safrole to 1'-hydroxysafrole and the electrophilic reactivity of 1'-acetoxysafrole, *Cancer Res.* **33**:575–589.

BORCHERT, P., MILLER, J. A., MILLER, E. C., AND LAIRD, T. K., 1973b, 1'-Hydroxysafrole: A proximate carcinogenic metabolite of safrole in the rat and mouse, *Cancer Res.* **33**:590–600.

BOREK, C., AND WILLIAMS, G. M., 1980, Differentiation and carcinogenesis in liver cell cultures, *Ann. N.Y. Acad. Sci.* **349**:1–419.

BOUTWELL, R. K., 1974, The function and mechanism of promoters of carcinogenesis, *CRC Crit. Rev. Toxicol.* **2**:419–443.

BOXENBAUM, H. G., BEKERSKY, I., JACK, M. L., AND KAPLAN, S. A., 1979, Influence of gut microflora on bioavailability, *Drug Metab. Rev.* **9**:259–279.

BOYLAND, E., 1952, Different types of carcinogens and their possible modes of action, *Cancer Res.* **12**:77–84.

BRALOW, S. P., AND WEISBURGER, J. H., 1976, Experimental carcinogenesis in the digestive organs, *Clinics in Gastroenterol.* **5**:527–542.

BRALOW, S. P., GRUENSTEIN, M., AND MERANZE, D. R., 1973, Host resistance to gastric adenocar-cinomatosis in three strains of rats ingesting N-methyl-N'-nitro-N-nitrosoguanidine, *Oncology* **27**:168.

BRESNICK, E., 1980, Nuclear activation of polycyclic hydrocarbons, *Drug. Metab. Rev.* **10**:209–224.

BROOKES, P., 1980, Chemical carcinogenesis, *Br. Med. Bull.* **36**:12–102.

BRYAN, G. T. (ed.), 1978, *Nitrofurans*, Raven Press, New York.

BUENING, M. K., WISLOCKI, P. G., LEVIN, W., YAGI, H., THAKKER, D. R., AKAGI, H., KOREEDA, M., JERINA, D. M., AND CONNEY, A. H., 1978, Tumorigenicity of the optical enantiomers of the diastereomeric benzo[a]pyrene 7,8-diol-9,10-epoxides in newborn mice: Exceptional activity of (+)-7-beta,8-alpha-dihydroxy-9-alpha,10-alpha-epoxy-7,8,9,10-tetrahydrobenzo[a]pyrene, *Proc. Natl. Acad. Sci. USA* **75**:5358–5361.

BUENING, M., LEVIN, W., KARLE, J. M., YAGI, H., JERINA, D. M., AND CONNEY, A. H., 1979, Tumorigenicity of bay region epoxides and other derivatives of chrysene and phenanthrene in newborn mice, *Cancer Res.* **39**:5063–5068.

BURKE, M. D., VADI, H., JERNSTROM, B., AND ORRENIUS, S., 1977, Metabolism of BaP with isolated hepatocytes and the formation and degradation of DNA-binding metabolites, *J. Biol. Chem.* **252**:6424–6431.

BUTTERWORTH, B. E., (ed.), 1979, *Strategies for Short-Term Testing for Mutagens/Carcinogens*, CRC Press, West Palm Beach, Fla.

CAGEN, S. Z., AND KLAASSEN, C. D., 1979, Protection of carbon tetrachloride-induced hepatotoxicity by zinc: Role of Metallothionine, *Toxicol. Appl. Pharmacol.* **51**:107–116.

CALDER, I. C., CREEK, M. J., AND WILLIAMS, P. J., 1974, *N*-Hydroxyphenacetin as a precursor of 3-substituted 4-hydroxyacetanilide metabolites of phenacetin, *Chem. Biol. Interact.* **8**:87–90.

CAMPBELL, T. C., 1979, Influence of nutrition on metabolism of carcinogens, *Adv. Nutr. Res.* **2**:29–255.

CARDESA, A., POUR, P., RUSTIA, M., ALTHOFF, J., AND MOHR, U., 1973, The syncarcinogenic effect of methylcholanthrene and dimethylnitrosamine in Swiss mice, *Z. Krebsforsch.* **79**:98–107.

CARDY, R. H., LIJINSKY, W., AND HILDEBRANDT, P. K., 1979, Neoplastic and nonneoplastic urinary bladder lesions induced in Fischer 344 rats and B6C3F hybrid mice by *N*-nitrosodiphenylamine, *Ecotoxicol. Environ. Safety* **3**:29–35.

CHANG, R. L., WISLOCKI, P. G., KAPITULNIK, J., WOOD, A. W., LEVIN, W., YAGI, H., MAH, H. D., JERINA, D. M., AND CONNEY, A. H., 1979, Carcinogenicity of 2-hydroxybenzo[a]pyrene and 6-hydroxybenzo[a]pyrene in newborn mice, *Cancer Res.* **39**:2660–2664.

CHASSEAUD, L. F., 1979, Role of glutathione and glutathione *S*-transferases in the metabolism of chemical carcinogens and other electrophilic agents, *Adv. Cancer Res.* **29**:176–275.

CHEN, C. B., HECHT, S. S., MCCOY, G. D., AND HOFFMANN, D., 1980, Assays for metabolic alpha-hydroxylation of *N′*-nitrosonornicotine and *N*-nitrosopyrrolidine and the influence of modifying factors, *IARC Sci. Publ.* **31**:349–357.

CHHABRA, R. S., 1979, Intestinal absorption and metabolism of xenobiotics, *Environ. Health Perspect.* **33**:61–69.

CHIN, A. E., AND BOSMANN, H. B., 1980, Hepatic microsomal metabolism of *N*-nitrosodimethylamine to its methylating agent, *Toxicol. Appl. Pharmacol.* **54**:76–89.

CHOUROULINKOV, I., GENTIL, A., TIERNEY, B., GROVER, P. L., AND SIMS, P., 1979, The initiation of tumours on mouse skin by dihydrodiols derived from 7,12-dimethylbenz(a)anthracene and 3-methylcholanthrene, *Int. J. Cancer* **24**:455–460.

CLAYSON, D. B., 1962, *Chemical Carcinogenesis*, Little, Brown, Boston.

COHEN, G. M., MACLEOD, M. C., MOORE, C. J., AND SILKIRK, J. K., 1980, Metabolism and macromolecular binding of carcinogenic and non-carcinogenic metabolites of benzo(a)pyrene by hamster embryo cells, *Cancer Res.* **40**:207–211.

COHEN, S., ARAI, M., JACOBS, J. B., AND FRIEDELL, G. H., 1979, Promoting effect of saccharin and DL-tryptophan in urinary bladder carcinogenesis, *Cancer Res.* **39**:1207–1215.

COLLEY, P. J., AND NEAL, G. E., 1979, The analysis of aflatoxins by high-performance liquid chromatography, *Anal. Biochem.* **93**:409–418.

CONNEY, A. H., PANTUCK, E. J., HSIAO, K. C., KUNTZMAN, R., ALVARES, A. P., AND KAPPAS, A., 1977, Regulation of drug metabolism in man by environmental chemicals and diet, *Fed. Proc.* **36**:1647–1652.

CONNEY, A. H., BUENING, M. K., PANTUCK, E. J., PANTUCK, C. B., FORTNER, J. G., ANDERSON, K. E., AND KAPPAS, A., 1980, Regulation of human drug metabolism by dietary factors, in: *Environmental Chemicals, Enzyme Function and Human Disease* (D. Evered and G. Lawrenson, eds.), Ciba Foundation Symposium 1976 (new series), pp. 147–167, Excerpta Medica, Amsterdam.

318

J. H.
WEISBURGER
AND
G. M.
WILLIAMS

COON, M. J., CONNEY, A. H., ESTABROOK, R. W., GELBOIN, H. V., GILLETTE, J. R., AND O'BRIEN, P. J. (eds.), 1980, *Microsomes, Drug Oxidations and Chemical Carcinogenesis*, 2 volumes, Academic Press, New York.

CORBETT, M., CHIPKO, B. R., AND BATCHELOR, A. O., 1980, The action of chloride peroxidase on 4-chloroaniline: *N*-oxidation and ring halogenation, *Biochem. J.* **187**:893–903.

COTTRELL, R. C., WALTERS, D. G., YOUNG, P. J., PHILLIPS, J. C., LAKE, B. G., AND GANGOLLI, S. D., 1980, Studies of the urinary metabolites of *N*-nitrosopyrrolidine in the rat, *Toxicol. Appl. Pharmacol.* **54**:368–376.

CZYGAN, P., GREIM, H., GARRO, A. J., SCHAFFNER, F., AND POPPER, H., 1974, The effect of dietary protein deficiency on the ability of isolated hepatic microsomes to alter the mutagenicity of a primary and secondary carcinogen, *Cancer Res.* **34**:119–123.

DAHL, G. A., MILLER, E. C., AND MILLER, J. A., 1980, Comparative carcinogenicities and mutagenicities of vinyl carbamate, ethyl carbamate, and ethyl *N*-hydroxycarbamate, *Cancer Res.* **40**:1194–1203.

DAO, T. L., AND LIBBY, P. R., 1972, Steroid sulphate formation in human breast tumors and hormone dependency, in: *Estrogen Target Tissues and Neoplasia* (T. L. Dao, ed.), pp. 181–200, Chicago University Press, Chicago.

DAOUD, A. H., AND GRIFFIN, A. C., 1980, Effect of retinoic acid, butylated hydroxytoluene, selenium and sorbic acid on azo-dye hepatocarcinogenesis, *Cancer Lett.* **9**:299–304.

DASHMAN, T., AND KAMM, J. J., 1979, Effects of high doses of vitamin E on dimethylnitrosamine hepatotoxicity and drug metabolism in the rat, *Biochem. Pharmacol.* **28**:1485–1490.

DEGEN, G. H., AND NEUMANN, H. G., 1978, The major metabolite of aflatoxin B_1 in the rat is a glutathione conjugate, *Chem. Biol. Interact.* **22**:239–255.

DEMEESTER, C., DUVERGER-VAN BOGAERT, M., LAMBOTTE-VANDEPAER, M., ROBERFROID, M., PONCELET, F., AND MERCIER, M., 1979, Liver extract mediated mutagenicity of acrylonitrile, *Toxicology* **13**:7–15.

DIAMOND, L., O'BRIEN, T. G., AND BAIRD, W. M., 1980, Tumor promoters and the mechanism of tumor promotion, *Adv. Cancer Res.* **32**:1–75.

DiGIOVANNI, J., ROMSON, J. R., LINVILLE, D., AND JUCHAU, M. R., 1979, Covalent binding of polycyclic aromatic hydrocarbons to adenine correlates with tumorigenesis in mouse skin, *Cancer Lett.* **7**:39–43.

DiLUZIO, N. R., STEGE, T. E., AND HOFFMAN, E. O., 1973, Protective influence of diphenyl-*p*-phenylenediamine on hydrazine induced lipid peroxidation and hepatic injury, *Exp. Mol. Pathol.* **19**:284–292.

DIWAN, B. A., AND BLACKMAN, K. E., 1980, Differential susceptibility of 3 sublines of C57BL/6 mice to the induction of colorectal tumors by 1,2-dimethylhydrazine, *Cancer Lett.* **9**:111–115.

DOLLERY, C. T., FRASER, H. S., MUCKLOW, J. C., AND BULPITT, C. J., 1979, Contribution of environmental factors to variability in human drug metabolism, *Drug Metab. Rev.* **9**:207–220.

DREVON, C., AND KUROKI, T., 1979, Mutagenicity of vinyl chloride, vinylidene chloride and chloroprene in V79 Chinese hamster cells, *Mutat. Res.* **67**:173–182.

DRINKWATER, N. R., MILLER, J. A., MILLER, E. C., AND YANG, N. C., 1978, Covalent intercalative binding to DNA in relation to the mutagenicity of hydrocarbon epoxides and *N*-acetoxy-2-acetylaminofluorene, *Cancer Res.* **38**:3247–3255.

DRUCKREY, H., 1975, Chemical carcinogenesis on *N*-nitroso derivatives, *Gann Monogr.* **17**:107–132.

DUNN, L. D., LUBET, R. A., AND PROUGH, R. A., 1979, Oxidative metabolism of *N*-isopropyl-alpha-(2-methylhydrazino)-*p*-toluamide hydrochloride (procarbazine) by rat liver microsomes, *Cancer Res.* **39**:4555–4563.

DURSTON, W. E., AND AMES, B. N., 1974, A simple method for the detection of mutagens in urine studies with the carcinogen 2-acetylaminofluorene, *Proc. Natl. Acad. Sci. USA* **71**:737–741.

EL-BAYOUMY, K., LaVOIE, E. J., HECHT, S. S., FOW, E. A., AND HOFFMANN, D., 1981, The influence of methyl substitution on the mutagenicity of nitronaphthalenes and nitrobiphenyls, *Mutat. Res.* **81**:143–153.

ELIAS, P. M., GRAYSON, S., CALDWELL, T. M., AND McNUTT, N. S., 1980, Gap junction proliferation in retinoic acid-treated human basal cell carcinoma, *Lab. Invest.* **42**:469–474.

EMEROLE, G. O., 1979, The detoxification of aflatoxin B_1 with glutathione in the rat, *Xenobiotica* **9**:737–743.

EMMELOT, P., AND KRIEK, E. (eds.), 1979, *Environmental Carcinogenesis*, Elsevier/North Holland, Amsterdam.

FALK, H. F. (Chairman), 1977, Conference on comparative metabolism and toxicity of vinyl chloride related compounds, *Environ. Health Perspect.* **21**:1–333.

FARBER, E., 1973, Hyperplastic liver nodules, *Methods Cancer Res.* **7**:345–375.

FARRELLY, J. G., 1980, A new assay for the microsomal metabolism of nitrosamines, *Cancer Res.* **40**:3241–3244.

FIALA, E. S., 1977, Investigations into the metabolism and mode of action of the colon carcinogens 1,2-dimethylhydrazine and azoxymethane, *Cancer* **40**:2436.

FIALA, E. S., 1980, The formation of azomethane, a colon carcinogen during the chemical oxidation of methylamine, *Carcinogenesis* **1**:57.

FIALA, E. S., 1981, Inhibition of carcinogen metabolism and action by disulfiram, pyrazole, and related compounds, in: *Inhibition of Tumor Induction and Development* (M. S. Zedeck and M. Lipkin, eds.), Plenum Press, New York.

FIALA, E. S., KULAKIS, C., CHRISTIANSEN, G., AND WEISBURGER, J. H., 1978, Inhibition of the metabolism of the colon carcinogen, azoxymethane, by pyrazole, *Cancer Res.* **38**:4515–4521.

FILSER, J. G., AND BOLT, H. M., 1979, Pharmacokinetics of halogenated ethylenes in rats, *Arch. Toxicol.* **42**:123–136.

FISCHER, I. J., KENT, J. H., AND WEISSINGER, J. L., 1973, Absorption of diethylstilbestrol and its glucuronide conjugate from the intestine of five- and twenty-five-day-old rats, *J. Pharmacol. Exp. Ther.* **185**:163–170.

FISHMAN, W. H. (ed.), 1970–1973, *Metabolic Conjugation and Metabolic Hydrolysis*, Vols. I, II, III, Academic Press, New York.

FRANCHI, G., FORGIONE, A., FILIPPESCHI, S., CSETENYI, J., AND GARATTINI, S., 1973, A spectrophotometric method for the estimation of the carcinostatic agent 6-chrysenamine (F.O.R.T.C. 116) in biological fluids and tissues, *Eur. J. Cancer* **9**:591–595.

FRANK, N., JANZOWSKI, C., AND WIESSLER, M., 1980, Stability of nitrosoacetoxymethylmethylamine in *in vitro* systems and *in vivo* and its excretion by the rat organism, *Biochem. Pharmacol.* **29**:383–387.

FRAUMENI, J. F., JR., 1975, *Persons at High Risk of Cancer: An Approach to Cancer Etiology and Control*, Academic Press, New York.

FUJINO, T., FUJIKI, H., NAGAO, M., YAHAGI, T., SEILNO, Y., AND SUGIMURA, T., 1978, The effect of norharman on the metabolism of benzo(*a*)pyrene by rat-liver microsomes *in vitro* in relation to its enhancement of the mutagenicity of benzo(*a*)pyrene, *Mutat. Res.* **58**:151–158.

GABALDON, M., AND LACOMBA, J., 1972, Glucuronyltransferase activity towards diethylstilbestrol in rat and hamster: Effect of activators, *Eur. J. Cancer* **8**:275–279.

GANDOLFI, A. J., AND VAN DYKE, R. A., 1973, Dechlorination of chloroethane with a reconstituted liver microsomal system, *Biochem. Biophys. Res. Commun.* **53**:687–692.

GEHLY, E. B., FAHL, W. E., JEFCOATE, C. R., AND HEIDELBERGER, C., 1979, The metabolism of benzo(*a*)pyrene by cytochrome P-450 in transformable and nontransformable C3H mouse fibroblasts, *J. Biol. Chem.* **254**:5041–5048.

GELBOIN, H. V., 1969, A microsome-dependent binding of benzo(*a*)pyrene to DNA, *Cancer Res.* **29**:1272–1276.

GELBOIN, H. V., AND TS'O, P. O. P. (eds.), 1978, *Polycyclic Hydrocarbons and Cancer*, Academic Press, New York.

GELBOIN, H. V., MacMAHON, B., MATSUSHIMA, T., SUGIMURA, T., TAKAYAMA, S., AND TAKEBE, H. (eds.), 1980, *Genetic and Environmental Factors in Experimental and Human Cancer*, University of Tokyo Press, Tokyo, and University Park Press, Baltimore.

GENTA, V. M., KAUFMAN, D. G., HARRIS, C. C., SMITH, J. M., SPORN, M. B., AND SAFFIOTTI, U., 1974, Vitamin A deficiency enhances binding of benzo(*a*)pyrene to tracheal epithelial DNA, *Nature (London)* **247**:48–49.

GILLETTE, J. R., 1979*a*, Biotransformation of drugs during aging, *Fed. Proc.* **38**:1900–1909.

GILLETTE, J. R., 1979*b*, Effects of induction of cytochrome P-450 enzymes on the concentration of foreign compounds and their metabolites and on the toxicological effects of the compounds, *Drug Metab. Rev.* **10**:59–87.

GINGELL, R., AND WALLCAVE, L., 1974, Species differences in the acute toxicity and tissue distribution of DDT in mice and hamsters, *Toxicol. Appl. Pharmacol.* **28**:385–394.

GINGELL, R., BRUNK, G., NAGEL, D., AND POUR, P., 1979, Metabolism of three radiolabeled pancreatic carcinogenic nitrosamines in hamsters and rats, *Cancer Res.* **39**:4579–4583.

GINGELL, R., BRUNK, G., NAGEL, D., WALLCAVE, L., WALKER, B., AND POUR, P., 1980, Metabolism and mutagenicity of *N*-nitroso-2-methoxy-2,6-dimethylmorpholine in hamsters, *J. Natl. Cancer Inst.* **64**:157–162.

GINTER, E., 1973, Cholesterol: Vitamin C controls its transformation to bile acids, *Science* **179**:702–704.

GLATT, H., KALTENBACH, E., AND OESCH, F., 1980, Epoxide hydrolase activity in native and in mitogen-stimulated lymphocytes of various human donors, *Cancer Res.* **40**:2552–2556.

320

J. H.
WEISBURGER
AND
G. M.
WILLIAMS

GLINSUKON, T., BENJAMIN, T., GRANTHAM, P. H., WEISBURGER, E. K., AND ROLLER, P. P., 1975, Enzymic N-acetylation of 2,4-toluenediamine by liver cytosols from various species, *Xenobiotica* **5**:475–483.

GOLDMAN, P., CARTER, J., AND WHEELER, L. A., 1980, Mutagenesis within the gastrointestinal tract determined by histidine autotrophs of *Salmonella typhimurium, Cancer* **45**:1068–1072.

GOMEZ, M. I., AND CASTRO, J. A., 1980, Covalent binding of chloroform metabolites to nuclear proteins—No evidence for binding to nucleic acids, *Cancer Lett.* **9**:213–218.

GORROD, J. W., (ed.), 1978, *Biological Oxidation of Nitrogen,* Elsevier/North-Holland, Amsterdam.

GOTHOSKAR, S. V., BENJAMIN, T., ROLLER, P. P., AND WEISBURGER, E. K., 1979, Metabolic fate of 2-aminoanthraquinone, a probable hepatocarcinogen and a nephrotoxic agent in the Fischer rat, *Cancer Detect. Prevent.* **2**:485–494.

GOTTSCHLICH, R., AND METZLER, M., 1980, Metabolic fate of diethylstilbestrol in the Syrian golden hamster, a susceptible species for diethylstilbestrol carcinogenicity, *Xenobiotica* **10**:317–328.

GRANTHAM, P. H., WEISBURGER, J. H., AND WEISBURGER, E. K., 1973, Effect of the antioxidant butylated hydroxytoluene (BHT) on the metabolism of the carcinogens N-2-fluorenylacetamide and N-hydroxy-N-2-fluorenylacetamide, *Food Cosmet. Toxicol.* **11**:209–217.

GRANTHAM, P. H., GIAO, NG. B., MOHAN, L. C., WEISBURGER, E. K., BUU-HOI, NG. P., AND RONCUCCI, R., 1974a, Metabolism of 6-aminochrysenes in the rat, *Toxicol. Appl. Pharmacol.,* **29**:95.

GRANTHAM, P. H., MOHAN, L. C., WEISBURGER, E. K., FALES, H. M., SOKOLOSKI, E. A., AND WEIS-BURGER, J. H., 1974b, Identification of new water soluble metabolites of acetanilide, *Xenobiotica* **4**:69–76.

GRIFFIN, A. C., 1979, Role of selenium in the chemoprevention of cancer, *Adv. Cancer Res.* **29**:419–442.

GRIFFIN, A. C., AND SHAW, C. R. (eds.), 1979, *Carcinogens: Identification and Mechanisms of Action,* Raven Press, New York.

GROVER, P. L., AND SIMS, P., 1968, Enzyme-catalysed reaction of polycyclic hydrocarbons with deoxyribonucleic acid and protein *in vitro, Biochem. J.* **110**:159–160.

GUTMANN, H. R., 1974, Isolation and identification of the carcinogen N-hydroxy-2-fluorenyl-acetamide and related compound by liquid chromatography, *Anal. Biochem.* **58**:469–478.

HADIDIAN, Z., FREDRICKSON, T. N., WEISBURGER, E. K., WEISBURGER, J. H., GLASS, R. M., AND MANTEL, N., 1968, Tests for chemical carcinogens. Report on the activity of derivatives of aromatic amines, nitrosamines, quinolines, nitroalkanes, amides, epoxides, aziridines, and purine antimetabolites, *J. Natl. Cancer Inst.* **41**:985–1036.

HAGIWARA, A., ARAI, M., HIROSE, M., NAKANOWATARI, J. I., TSUDA, H., AND ITO, N., 1980, Chronic effects of norharman in rats treated with aniline, *Toxicol. Lett.* **6**:71–75.

HARRIS, C. C., AUTRUP, H., STONER, G. D., TRUMP, B. F., HILLMAN, E., SCHAFER, P. W., AND JEFFREY, A. M., 1979, Metabolism of benzo(a)pyrene, N-nitrosodimethylamine, and N-nitrosopyrrolidine and identification of the major carcinogen–DNA adducts formed in cultured human esophagus, *Cancer Res.* **39**:4401–4406.

HASHIMOTO, Y., SHUDO, K., AND OKAMOTO, T., 1979, Structural identification of a modified base in DNA covalently bound with mutagenic 3-amino-1-methyl-5-H-pyrido[4,3-b]indole, *Chem. Pharm. Bull.* **27**:1058–1060.

HASHIMOTO, Y., SHUDO, K., AND OKAMOTO, T., 1980, Metabolic activation of a mutagen, 2-amino-6-methyldipyrido-[1,2-a:3′,2′-d]imidazole. Identification of 2-hydroxyamino-6-methyl-dipyrido[1,2-a:3′,2′-d]imidazole and its reaction with DNA, *Biochem. Biophys. Res. Commun.* **92**:971–976.

HATHWAY, D. E., 1979, *Foreign Compound Metabolism in Mammals,* Vol. 5, The Chemical Society, London.

HATHWAY, D. E., 1980, Consideration of the evidence for mechanisms of 1,1,2-trichloroethylene metabolism, including new identification of its dichloroacetic acid and trichloroacetic acid metabolites in mice, *Cancer Lett.* **8**:263–269.

HECHT, S. S., CHEN, C. B., AND HOFFMANN, D. H., 1978, Evidence for metabolic alpha-hydroxylation of N-nitrosopyrrolidine, *Cancer Res.* **38**:215–218.

HECHT, S. S., EL-BAYOUMY, K., TULLEY, L., AND LAVOIE, E., 1979a, Structure–mutagenicity relationships of N-oxidized derivatives of aniline, o-toluidine, 2′-methyl-4-aminobiphenyl, and 3,2′-dimethyl-4-aminobiphenyl, *J. Med. Chem.* **22**:981–987.

HECHT, S. S., LAVOIE, E., MAZZARESE, R., HIROTA, N., OHMORI, T., AND HOFFMANN, D. H., 1979b, Comparative mutagenicity, tumor-initiating activity, carcinogenicity, and *in vitro* metabolism of fluorinated 5-methylchrysenes, *J. Natl. Cancer Inst.* **63**:855–861.

HECHT, S. S., SHANTILAL, A., RIVENSON, A., AND HOFFMANN, D. H., 1979c, Tumor initiating activity of 5,11-dimethylchrysene and the structural requirements favoring carcinogenicity of methylated polynuclear aromatic hydrocarbons, *Cancer Lett.* **8:**65–70.

HECHT, S. S., RIVENSON, A., AND HOFFMANN, D. H., 1980, Tumor-initiating activity of dihydrodiols formed metabolically from 5-methylchrysene, *Cancer Res.* **40:**1396–1399.

HEIDELBERGER, C., 1975, Chemical carcinogenesis, *Annu. Rev. Biochem.* **44:**79–121.

HENSCHLER, D., AND BONSE, G., 1978, Metabolic activation of chlorinated ethylene derivatives, in: *Advances in Pharmacology and Therapeutics*, Vol. 9 (Y. Cohen, ed.), pp. 123–130, Pergamon Press, New York.

HERBST, A. L., COLE, P., NORUSIS, M. J., WELCH, W. R., AND SCULLY, R. E., 1979, Epidemiologic aspects and factors related to survival in 384 registry cases in clear cell adenocarcinoma of the vagina and cervix, *Am. J. Obstet. Gynecol.* **135:**876–883.

HEWER, A., RIBEIRO, O., WALSH, C., GROVER, P. L., AND SIMS, P., 1979, The formation of dihydrodiols from benz[a]pyrene by oxidation with an ascorbic acid/ferrous sulphate/EDTA system, *Chem. Biol. Interact.* **26:**147–154.

HIATT, H. H., WATSON, J. D., AND WINSTEN, J. A. (eds.), 1977, *Origins of Human Cancer*, Cold Spring Harbor Laboratory, Cold Spring Harbor, N.Y.

HIGGINSON, J., AND MUIR, C. S., 1981, Epidemiology, in: *Cancer Medicine* (J. F. Holland and E. Frei, III, eds.), 2nd ed., Lea & Febiger, Philadelphia.

HIGHMAN, B., NORVELL, M. J., AND SHELLENBERGER, T. E., 1977, Pathological changes in female C3H mice continuously fed diets containing diethylstilbestrol or 17-beta-estradiol, *J. Environ. Pathol. Toxicol.* **1:**1–30.

HILL, D., SHIH, T., AND STRUCK, R. F., 1979, Macromolecular binding and metabolism of the carcinogen 4-chloro-2-methylaniline, *Cancer Res.* **39:**2528–2531.

HINES, R. N., AND PROUGH, R. A., 1980, The characterization of an inhibitory complex formed with cytochrome P-450 and a metabolite of 1,1-disubstituted hydrazines, *J. Pharmacol. Exp. Ther.* **214:**80–86.

HINSON, J. A., POHL, L. R., AND GILLETTE, J. R., 1979a, A simple high pressure liquid chromatographic assay for the N-hydroxy derivatives of phenacetin, acetaminophen, 2-acetylaminofluorene, and other hydroxamic acids, *Anal. Biochem.* **101:**462–467.

HINSON, J. A., POHL, L. R., AND GILLETTE, J. R., 1979b, N-Hydroxyacetaminophen: A microsomal metabolite of N-hydroxyphenacetin but apparently not of acetaminophen, *Life Sci.* **24:**2133–2138.

HIRAKAWA, T., NEMOTO, N., YAMADA, M., AND TAKAYAMA, S., 1979, Metabolism of benzo[a]pyrene and the related enzyme activities in hamster embryo cells, *Chem. Biol. Interact.* **25:**189–195.

HIRAYAMA, T., 1979, Diet and cancer, *Nutr. Cancer* **1:**67–81.

HITE, M., AND SKEGGS, H., 1979, Mutagenic evaluation of nitroparaffins in the *Salmonella typhimurium*/mammalian microsome test and the micronucleus test, *Environ. Mutagenesis* **1:**383–389.

HLAVICA, P., AND HÜLSMANN, S., 1979, Studies on the mechanism of hepatic microsomal N-oxide formation: N-oxidation of N,N-dimethylaniline by a reconstituted rabbit liver microsomal cytochrome P-448 enzyme system, *Biochem. J.* **182:**109–116.

HOFFMANN, D., SCHMELTZ, I., HECHT, S. S., AND WYNDER, E. L., 1978, Polynuclear hydrocarbons in tobacco carcinogenesis, in: *Polycyclic Hydrocarbons and Cancer*, Vol. I (H. V. Gelboin and P. O. P. Ts'o, eds.), pp. 85–117, Academic Press, New York.

HOFFMANN, D., CHEN, C. B., AND HECHT, S. S., 1980, The role of volatile and nonvolatile N-nitrosamines in tobacco carcinogenesis, *Banbury Report 3: A Safe Cigarette?*, pp. 113–126, Cold Spring Harbor Laboratory, Cold Spring Harbor, N.Y.

HOLLAENDER, A. (ed.), 1971–1980, *Chemical Mutagens*, Vols. 1–7, Plenum Press, New York.

HOLLSTEIN, M., McCANN, J., ANGELSANTO, F. A., AND NICHOLS, W. W., 1979, Short-term tests for carcinogens and mutagens, *Mutat. Res.* **65:**133–226.

HSIE, A. W., O'NEILL, J. P., AND McELHENY, V. K. (eds.), 1979, *Banbury Report 2, Mammalian Cell Mutagenesis: The Maturation of Test Systems*, Cold Spring Harbor Laboratory, Cold Spring Harbor, N.Y.

HUANG, M., MIWA, G. T., AND LUE, A. Y. H., 1979, Rat liver cytosolic azoreductase, *J. Biol. Chem.* **254:**3930–3934.

HUBERMAN, E., YANG, S. K., McCAUST, D. W., AND GELBOIN, H. V., 1977, Mutagenicity to mammalian cells in culture by (+) and (−) *trans*-7,8-dihydrobenzo(a)pyrenes and the hydrolysis and reduction products of two stereoisomeric benzo(a)pyrene-7,8-diol-9,10-epoxides, *Cancer Lett.* **4:**35–43.

322

J. H.
WEISBURGER
AND
G. M.
WILLIAMS

HUTTON, J. J., HACKNEY, C., AND MEIER, J., 1979, Mutagenicity and metabolism of dimethyl-nitrosamine and benzo[a]pyrene in tissue homogenates from inbred Syrian hamsters treated with phenobarbital, 3-methylcholanthrene or polychlorinated biphenyls, *Mutat. Res.* **64**:363–377.

HWANG, K. K., AND KELSEY, M. I., 1978, Evidence of epoxide hydrase activity in human intestinal microflora, *Cancer Biochem. Biophys.* **3**:31–35.

ILETT, K. E., REID, W. D., SPIES, I. G., AND KRISHNA, G., 1973, Chloroform toxicity in mice: Correlation of renal and hepatic necrosis with covalent binding of metabolites to tissue macromolecules, *Exp. Mol. Pathol.* **19**:215–229.

INTERNATIONAL AGENCY FOR RESEARCH ON CANCER, 1980, *Long-Term and Short-Term Screening Assays for Carcinogens: A Critical Appraisal*, IARC Monographs, Suppl. 2, Lyon, France.

IRVING, C. C., 1979, Species and tissue variations in the metabolic activation of aromatic amines, in: *Carcinogens: Identification and Mechanisms of Action* (A. C. Griffin and C. R. Shaw, eds.), Raven Press, New York.

IRVING, C. C., TICE, A. J., AND MURPHY, W. M., 1979, Inhibition of N-n-butyl N-(4-hydroxy-butyl)nitrosamine-induced urinary bladder cancer in rats by administration of disulfiram in the diet, *Cancer Res.* **39**:3040–3043.

ISAKA, H., YOSHII, H., OTSUJI, A., KOIKE, M., NAGAI, Y., KOURA, M., SUGIYASU, K., AND KANABAYASHI, T., 1979, Tumors of Sprague–Dawley rats induced by long-term feeding of phenacetin, *Gann* **70**:29–36.

ISHII, K., ANDO, M., KAMATAKI, T., KATO, R., AND NAGAO, M., 1980, Metabolic activation of mutagenic tryptophan pyrolysis products (Trp-P-1 and Trp-P-2) by a purified cytochrome P-450-dependent monooxygenase system, *Cancer Lett.* **9**:271–276.

ITO, N., HIASA, Y., TOYOSHIMA, K., OKAJIMA, E., KAMAMOTO, Y., MAKIURA, S., YOKOTA, Y., SUGIHARA, S., AND MATAYOSHI, K., 1973, Rat bladder tumors induced by N-butyl-N-(4-hydroxy-butyl)nitrosamine, in: *Topics in Chemical Carcinogenesis* (W. Nakahara, S. Takayama, T. Sugimura, and S. Odashima, eds.), p. 175, University Park Press, Baltimore.

IVERSON, F., KHERA, K., AND HIERLIHY, S., 1980, In vivo and in vitro metabolism of ethylenethiourea in the rat and the cat, *Toxicol. Appl. Pharmacol.* **52**:16–21.

IVERSON, U. M., AND IVERSON, O. H., 1979, The carcinogenic effect of TPA (12-O-tetradecanoylphorbol-13-acetate) when applied to the skin of hairless mice, *Virchows Arch. B* **30**:33–42.

JACOBS, M. M., AND GRIFFIN, A. C., 1979, Effects of selenium on chemical carcinogenesis: Comparative effects of antioxidants, *Biol. Trace Element Res.* **1**:1–13.

JEFFREY, A. M., GRZESKOWIAK, K., WEINSTEIN, I. B., NAKANISHI, K., ROLLER, P., AND HARVEY, R. G., 1979, Benzo(a)pyrene-7,8-dihydrodiol 9,10-oxide adenosine and deoxyadenosine adducts: Structure and stereochemistry, *Science* **206**:1309–1311.

JOHNSON, D. E., AND CORNISH, H. H., 1978, Metabolic conversion of 1- and 2-nitronaphthalene to 1- and 2-naphthylamine in the rat, *Toxicol. Appl. Pharmacol.* **46**:549–553.

JOLLOW, J., 1980, Glutathione thresholds in reactive metabolite toxicity, *Arch. Toxicol. Suppl.* **3**:95–110.

JOLLOW, J., KOCSIS, J. J., SNYDER, R., AND VAINIO, H., 1977, *Biological Reactive Intermediates: Formation, Toxicity, and Inactivation*, Plenum Press, New York.

JONES, A. R., AND EDWARDS, K., 1973, Alkylating esters. VIII. The metabolism of iso-propyl methanesulphonate and iso-propyl iodide in the rat, *Experientia* **29**:538–539.

JONES, A. R., AND FAKHOURI, G., 1979, Epoxides as obligatory intermediates in the metabolism of alpha-halohydrins, *Xenobiotica* **9**:595–599.

JUCHAU, M. R., ZACHARIAH, P. K., COLSON, J., SYMMS, K. G., KRAMER, J., AND JAFFE, S. J., 1974, Studies on human placental carbon monoxide-binding cytochrome, *Drug Metab. Dispos.* **2**:79–86.

KADLUBAR, F. F., MILLER, J. A., AND MILLER, E. C., 1977, Hepatic microsomal N-glucuronidation and nucleic acid binding of N-hydroxy arylamines in relation to urinary bladder carcinogenesis, *Cancer Res.* **37**:805–814.

KANEKO, A., DEMPO, K., KAKU, T., YOKOYAMA, S., SATOH, M., MORI, M., AND ONOE, T., 1980, Effect of phenobarbital administration on hepatocytes constituting the hyperplastic nodules induced in rat liver by 3'-methyl-4-dimethylaminoazobenzene, *Cancer Res.* **40**:1658–1662.

KASAI, H., YAMAIZUMI, Z., WAKABAYASHI, K., NAGAO, M., SUGIMURA, T., YOKOYAMA, S., MIYAZAWA, T., SPINGARN, N. E., WEISBURGER, J. H., AND NISHIMURA, S., 1980, Potent novel mutagens produced by broiling fish under normal conditions, *Proc. Jpn. Acad.* **56**:278–283.

KATO, R., 1974, Sex-related differences in drug metabolism, *Drug. Metab. Rev.* **3**:1–32.

KATO, R., 1979, Characteristics and differences in the hepatic mixed function oxidases of different species, *Pharmacol. Ther.* **6:**41–98.

KATO, R., IWASAKI, K., AND NOGUCHI, H., 1978, Reduction of tertiary amine *N*-oxides by cytochrome P-450: Mechanism of the stimulatory effect of flavins and methyl viologen, *Mol. Pharmacol.* **14:**654–664.

KAWACHI, T., KOGURE, K., KAMIGO, Y., AND SUGIMURA, T., 1970, The metabolism of *N*-methyl-*N* -nitro-*N*-nitrosoguanidine in rats, *Biochim. Biophys. Acta* **222:**409–415.

KAWAJIRI, K., YONEKAWA, H., HARADA, N., NOSHIRO, M., OMURA, T., AND TAGASHIRA, Y., 1980, Immunochemical study on the role of different types of microsomal cytochrome P-450 in mutagenesis by chemical carcinogens, *Cancer Res.* **40:**1652–1657.

KELLNER, H. M., CARIST, O. E., AND LOTZSCH, K., 1973, Animal studies on the kinetics of benzidine and 3,3'-dichlorobenzidine, *Arch. Toxicol.* **31:**61–79.

KETTERER, B., KADLUBAR, F., FLAMMANG, T., CARNE, T., AND ENDERBY, G., 1979, Glutathione adducts of *N*-methyl-4-aminoazobenzene formed *in vivo* and by reaction of *N*-benzoyloxy-*N*-methyl-4-aminoazobenzene with glutathione, *Chem. Biol. Interact.* **25:**7–21.

KHARASCH, N., 1979, *Trace Metals in Health and Disease*, Raven Press, New York.

KITAHARA, Y., OKUDA, H., SHUDO, K., OKAMOTO, T., NAGAO, M., SEINO, Y., AND SUGIMURA, T., 1978, Synthesis and mutagenicity of 10-azabenzo[*a*]pyrene-4,5-oxide and other pentacyclic aza-arene oxides, *Chem. Pharm. Bull.* **26:**1950–1953.

KLEIHUES, P., DOERJER, G., KEEFER, L., RICE, J., ROLLER, P., AND HODGSON, R., 1979, Correlation of DNA methylation by methyl(acetoxymethyl)nitrosamine with organ-specific carcinogenicity in rats, *Cancer Res.* **39:**5136–5140.

KOCH, R., AND GOLDMAN, P., 1979, The anaerobic metabolism of metronidazole forms *N*-(2-hydroxyethyl)-oxamic acid, *J. Pharmacol. Exp. Ther.* **208:**406–410.

KOURI, R. E., WOOD, A. W., LEVIN, W., RUDE, T. H., YAGI, H., MAH, H. D., JERINA, D. M., AND CONNEY, A. H., 1980, Carcinogenicity of benzo(*a*)pyrene and thirteen of its derivatives in C3H/fCUM mice, *J. Natl. Cancer Inst.* **64:**617–623.

KRÜGER, F. W., 1971, Metabolism von Nitrosaminen *in vivo*, *Z. Krebsforsch.* **76:**145–154.

KRÜGER, F. W., 1973, New aspects in metabolism of carcinogenic nitrosamines, in: *Topics in Chemical Carcinogenesis* (W. Nakahara, S. Takayama, T. Sugimura, and S. Odashima, eds.), pp. 213–235, University Park Press, Baltimore.

KUNKEL, T. A., AND LOEB, L. A., 1979, On the fidelity of DNA replication: Effect of divalent metal ion activators and deoxyribonucleoside triphosphate pools on *in vitro* mutagenesis, *J. Biol. Chem.* **254:**5718–5725.

KUROKI, T., AND BARTSCH, H., 1979, Mutagenicity of some *N*- and *O*-acyl derivatives of *N*-hydroxy-2-aminofluorene in V79 Chinese hamster cells, *Cancer Lett.* **6:**67–72.

KUROKI, T., NEMOTO, N., AND KITANO, Y., 1980, Metabolism of benzo(*a*)pyrene in human epidermal keratinocytes in culture, *Carcinogenesis* **1:**559–565.

LANGVARDT, P. W., PUTZIG, C. L., BRAUN, W. H., AND YOUNG, J. D., 1980, Identification of the major urinary metabolites of acrylonitrile in the rat, *J. Toxicol. Environ. Health* **6:**273–282.

LAQUEUR, G. L., AND SPATZ, M., 1975, Oncogenicity of cycasin and methylazoxymethanol, in: *Recent Topics in Chemical Carcinogenesis* (S. Odashima, S. Takayama, and H. Sato), pp. 189–204, GANN Monograph 17, University Park Press, Baltimore.

LAZEAR, E. J., LOUIE, S. C., SHADDOCK, J. G., BARREN, P. R., AND NORVELL, M., 1978, The effects of dietary protein, fat and 2-acetylaminofluorene on the microsomal activity levels of liver from Balb/c mice, *Toxicol. Lett.* **2:**345–350.

LAZEAR, E. J., SHADDOCK, J. G., BARREN, P. R., AND LOUIE, S. C., 1979, The mutagenicity of some of the proposed metabolites of direct black 38 and pigment yellow 12 in the *Salmonella typhimurium* assay system, *Toxicol. Lett.* **4:**519–525.

LEE, I, P., AND DIXON, R. L., 1978, Mutagenicity, carcinogenicity and teratogenicity of procarbazine, *Mutat. Res.* **55:**1–14.

LEE, I. P., SUZUKI, K., LEE, S. D., AND DIXON, R. L., 1980, Aryl hydrocarbon hydroxylase induction in rat lung, liver, and male reproductive organs following inhalation exposure to diesel emission, *Toxicol. Appl. Pharmacol.* **52:**181–184.

LEGRAVEREND, C., NEBERT, D. W., BOOBIS, A. R., AND PELKONEN, O., 1980, DNA binding of benzo[*a*]pyrene metabolites: Effects of substrate and microsomal protein concentration *in vitro*, dietary contaminants, and tissue differences, *Pharmacology* **20:**137–148.

324

J. H.
WEISBURGER
AND
G. M.
WILLIAMS

LEOPOLD, W. R., MILLER, E. C., AND MILLER, J. A., 1979a, Carcinogenicity of antitumor cis-platinum(II) coordination complexes in the mouse and rat, *Cancer Res.* **39:**913–918.

LEOPOLD, W. R., MILLER, J. A., AND MILLER, E. C., 1979b, S-Vinyl homocysteine, an analog of ethionine that is highly mutagenic for *S. typhimurium* TA100, *Biochem. Biophys. Res. Commun.* **88:**395–401.

LEUNG, K. H., PARK, K. K., AND ARCHER, M. C., 1978, Alpha-hydroxylation in the metabolism of *N*-nitrosopiperidine by rat liver microsomes: Formation of 5-hydroxypentanal, *Res. Commun. Chem. Pathol. Pharmacol.* **19:**201–211.

LEUNG, K., PARK, K. K., AND ARCHER, M. C., 1980, Methylation of DNA by *N*-nitroso-2-oxopropylpropylamine; Formation of O^6 and 7-methylguanine and studies on the methylation mechanism, *Toxicol. Appl. Pharmacol.* **53:**29–34.

LEVIN, W., WOOD, A. W., CHANG, R. L., YAGI, H., MAH, H. D., JERINA, D. M., AND CONNEY, A. H., 1978, Evidence for bay region activation of chrysene 1,2-dihydrodiol to an ultimate carcinogen, *Cancer Res.* **38:**1831–1834.

LEWIS, T. R., ULRICH, C. E., AND BUSEY, W. M., 1979, Subchronic inhalation toxicity of nitromethane and 2-nitropropane, *J. Environ. Pathol. Toxicol.* **2:**233–249.

LIJINSKY, W., AND ANDREWS, A. W., 1979, The mutagenicity of nitrosamides in *Salmonella typhimurium,* *Mutat. Res.* **68:**1–8.

LIJINSKY, W., AND REUBER, M., 1980a, Carcinogenicity in rats of nitrosomethylethylamines labeled with deuterium in several positions, *Cancer Res.* **40:**19–21.

LIJINSKY, W., AND REUBER, M. D., 1980b, Comparison of carcinogenesis by two isomers of nitroso-2,6-dimethylmorpholine, *Carcinogenesis* **1:**501–503.

LIN, J. K., KENNAN, K. A., MILLER, E. C., AND MILLER, J. A., 1978, Reduced nicotinamide adenine dinucleotide phosphate-dependent formation of 2,3-dihydro-2,3-dihydroxyaflatoxin B_1 from aflatoxin B_1 by hepatic microsomes, *Cancer Res.* **38:**2424–2428.

LIPKIN, M., AND GOOD, R. A. (eds.), 1978, *Gastrointestinal Tract Cancer,* Plenum Press, New York.

LITWAK, G., MOREY, K. S., AND KETTERER, B., 1972, Corticosteroid binding proteins of liver cytosol and interactions with carcinogens, in: *Effects of Drugs on Cellular Control Mechanisms* (B. R. Rabin and R. B. Freedman, eds.), pp. 105–130, Macmillan, London.

LIVESKY, J. C., AND ANDERS, M. W., 1979, *In vitro* metabolism of 1,2-dihaloethanes to ethylene, *Drug Metab. Dispos.* **7:**199–203.

LOTLIKAR, P. D., HONG, Y. S., AND BALDY, W. J., JR., 1978, Effect of dimethylnitrosamine concentration on its demethylation by liver microsomes from control and 3-methylcholanthrene pretreated rats, hamsters and guinea pigs, *Cancer Lett.* **4:**355–361.

LOTLIKAR, P. D., INSETTA, S. M., LYONS, P. R., AND JHEE, E. C., 1979, Inhibition of microsome-mediated binding of aflatoxin B_1 to DNA by glutathione *S*-transferase, *Cancer Lett.* **9:**143–149.

LOWER, G. M., JR., NILSSON, T., NELSON, C. E., WOLF, H., GAMSKY, T. E., AND BRYAN, G. T., 1979, *N*-Acetyltransferase phenotype and risk in urinary bladder cancer: Approaches in molecular epidemiology. Preliminary results in Sweden and Denmark, *Environ. Health Perspect.* **29:**71–80.

LU, A. Y. H., AND MIWA, G. T., 1980, Molecular properties and biological functions of microsomal epoxide hydrase, *Annu. Rev. Pharmacol. Toxicol.* **20:**513–531.

LUCIER, G. W., LUI, E. M. K., AND LaMARTINIERE, C. A., 1979, Metabolic activation/deactivation reactions during perinatal development, *Environ. Health Perspect.* **29:**7–16.

MAINIGI, K. D., AND CAMPBELL, T. C., 1980, Subcellular distribution and covalent binding of aflatoxins as functions of dietary manipulation, *J. Toxicol. Environ. Health* **6:**659–671.

MALAVEILLE, C., HAUTEFEUILLE, A., BARTSCH, B., MacNICOLL, A. D., GROVER, P. L., AND SIMS, P., 1980, Liver microsome-mediated mutagenicity of dihydrodiols derived from dibenzo-(*a,c*)anthracene in *S. typhimurium* TA100, *Carcinogenesis* **1:**287–289.

MALEJKA-GIGANTI, D., GUTMANN, H. R., AND RYDELL, R. E., 1973, Mammary carcinogenesis in the rat by topical application of fluorenylhydroxamic acids, *Cancer Res.* **33:**2489–2497.

MALTONI, C., AND SCARNATO, C., 1979, First experimental demonstration of the carcinogenic effects of benzene, *Med. Lav.* **70:**352–357.

MARGISON, G. P. (ed.), 1979, *Carcinogenesis,* Vol. I, Pergamon, New York.

MARGISON, G. P., MARGISON, J. M., AND MONTESANO, R., 1977, Accumulation of O^6-methylguanine in non-target-tissue deoxyribonucleic acid during chronic administration of dimethylnitrosamine, *Biochem. J.* **165:**463–468.

MARQUARDT, H., BAKER, S., TIERNEY, B., GROVER, P. L., AND SIMS, P., 1979, Comparison of mutagenesis and malignant transformation by dihydrodiols from benz(*a*)anthracene and 7,12-dimethylbenz(*a*)anthracene, *Br. J. Cancer* **39:**540–547.

Marshall, M. V., Arnott, M. S., Jacobs, M. M., and Griffin, A. C., 1979, Selenium effects on the carcinogenicity and metabolism of 2-acetylaminofluorene, *Cancer Lett.* **7**:331–338.

Mass, M. J., and Kaufman, D. G., 1978, [^{3}H]Benzo(a)pyrene metabolism in tracheal epithelial microsomes and tracheal organ cultures, *Cancer Res.* **38**:3861–3866.

Matsuyama, A., and Nagata, C., 1973, Detection of the unstable intermediate 4-nitrosoquinolne 1-oxide, in: *Topics in Chemical Carcinogenesis* (W. Nakahara, S. Sakayama, T. Sugimura, and S. Odashima, eds.), pp. 35–51, University Park Press, Baltimore.

Matthews, R. A., and Stoehrer, G., 1980, Carcinogenic purine N-oxide ester modifies covalently all common bases in polynucleotides, *Chem. Biol. Interact.* **29**:57–66.

Mattison, D. R., and Thorgeirsson, S. S., 1979, Ovarian aryl hydrocarbon hydroxylase activity and primordial oocyte toxicity of polycyclic aromatic hydrocarbons in mice, *Cancer Res.* **39**:3471–3475.

Mattocks, A. R., and White, I. N. H., 1973, Toxic effects and pyrrolic metabolites in the liver of young rats given the pyrrolizidine alkaloid retrorsine, *Chem. Biol. Interact.* **6**:297–306.

McCann, J., Simmon, V., Stretiwieser, D., and Ames, B. N., 1975, Mutagenicity of chloroacetaldehyde, a possible metabolic product of 1,2-dichlorethane (ethylene dichloride), chloroethanol (ethylene chlorohydrin), vinyl chloride, and cyclophosphamide, *Proc. Natl. Acad. Sci. USA* **72**:3190–3193.

McCoy, G. D., Chen, C. B., Hecht, S. S., and McCoy, E., 1979, Enhanced metabolism and mutagenesis of nitrosopyrrolidine in liver fractions isolated from chronic ethanol-consuming hamsters, *Cancer Res.* **39**:793–796.

McMahon, R. E., and Turner, J. C., 1979, The microsomal metabolism of 2- and 4-aminobiphenyl. An example of the crucial role of metabolic activation in determining the mutagenic potential of a compound, *Environ. Mutagenesis* **1**:147.

Meehan, T., and Straub, K., 1979, Double-stranded DNA stereoselectively binds benzo(a)pyrene diol epoxides, *Nature* **277**:410–412.

Miller, E. C., and Miller, J. A., 1979, Naturally occurring chemical carcinogens that may be present in foods, in: *International Review of Biochemistry*, Vol. 27 (A. Neuberger and T. H. Jukes, eds.), pp. 123–165, University Park Press, Baltimore.

Miller, E. C., and Miller, J. A., 1981, Mechanisms of carcinogenesis, *Cancer* **47**:1055–1064.

Miller, E. C., Miller, J. A., and Enomoto, E., 1964, The comparative carcinogenicities of 2-acetylaminofluorene and its N-hydroxy metabolite in mice, hamsters, and guinea pigs, *Cancer Res.* **24**:2018–2026.

Miller, E. C., Miller, J. A., Hirono, I., Sugimura, T., and Takayama, S. (eds.), 1979, *Naturally Occurring Carcinogens—Mutagens and Modulators of Carcinogenesis*, Japan Sci. Societies Press, Tokyo, and University Park Press, Baltimore.

Mirvish, S. S., 1968, The carcinogenic action and metabolism of urethan and N-hydroxyurethan, *Adv. Cancer Res.* **11**:1–42.

Mirvish, S. S., 1977, N-Nitroso compounds: Their chemical and *in vivo* formation and possible importance as environmental carcinogens, *J. Toxicol. Environ. Health* **2**:1267–1277.

Mochizuki, M., Irving, C. C., Anjo, T., Wakabayashi, Y., Suzuki, E., and Okada, M., 1980, Synthesis and mutagenicity of 4-(N-butylnitrosamino)-4-hydroxybutyric acid lactone, a possible activated metabolite of the proximate bladder carcinogen N-butyl-N-(3-carboxypropyl)-nitrosamine, *Cancer Res.* **40**:162–165.

Montesano, R., Bartsch, H., and Tomatis, L. (eds.), 1980*a*, *Molecular and Cellular Aspects of Carcinogen Screening Tests*, IARC Scientific Publication 27, Lyon, France.

Montesano, R., Bresil, H., Planche-Martel, G., Margison, G. P., and Pegg, A. E., 1980*b*, Effect of chronic treatment of rats with dimethylnitrosamine on the removal of O^6-methyl guanine from DNA, *Cancer Res.* **40**:452–458.

Montesano, R., Pegg, A. E., and Margison, G. P., 1980*c*, Alkylation of DNA and carcinogenicity of N-nitroso compounds, *J. Toxicol. Environ. Health* **6**:1001–1008.

Moore, D. H., Long, C. A., Vaidya, A. B., Sheffield, J. B., Dion, A. S., and Lasfargues, E. Y., 1979, Mammary tumor viruses, *Adv. Cancer Res.* **29**:347–418.

Morimoto, K., Tanaka, A., and Yamaha, T., 1979, Comparative binding studies on 1,1'-ethylene bis(1-nitrosourea) and some 1-alkyl-1-nitrosoureas with nucleic acids and proteins *in vitro*, *Gann* **70**:693–698.

Morton, K. C., King, C. M., and Baetcke, K. P., 1979, Metabolism of benzidine to N-hydroxy-N,N'-diacetylbenzidine and subsequent nucleic acid binding and mutagenicity, *Cancer Res.* **39**:3107–3113.

326

J. H.
WEISBURGER
AND
G. M.
WILLIAMS

MORTON, K. C., BELAND, F. A., EVANS, F. E., FULLERTON, N. F., AND KADLUBAR, F. F., 1980, Metabolic activation of N-hydroxy-N,N'-diacetylbenzidine by hepatic sulfotransferase, *Cancer Res.* **40:**751–757.

MOSCHEL, R., HUDGINS, W. R., AND DIPPLE, A., 1980, Aralkylation of guanosine by the carcinogen N-nitroso-N-benzylurea, *J. Org. Chem.* **45:**533.

MOSTAFA, M. H., AND WEISBURGER, E. K., 1980, Effect of chlorpromazine-hydrochloride on carcinogen-metabolizing enzymess: Liver microsomal dimethylnitrosamine demethylase, 4-dimethylaminoazobenzene reductase, and aryl hydrocarbon hydroxylase, *J. Natl. Cancer Inst.* **64:**925–929.

MOSTAFA, M. H., EVARTS, R. P., AND WEISBURGER, E. K., 1979, *In vitro* effect of L-tryptophan and its metabolites on dimethylaminoazobenzene reductase of liver, *Biochem. Pharmacol.* **28:**815–829.

MURRAY, A. W., AND FITZGERALD, D. J., 1979, Tumor promoters inhibit metabolic cooperation in cocultures of epidermal and 3T3 cells, *Biochem. Biophys. Res. Commun.* **91:**395–401.

NAGAO, M., SUGIMURA, T., AND MATSUSHIMA, T., 1978a, Environmental mutagens and carcinogens *Annu. Rev. Genet.* **12:**17–59.

NAGAO, M., YAHAGI, T., AND SUGIMURA, T., 1978b, Differences in effects of norharman with various classes of chemical mutagens and amounts of S-9, *Biochem. Biophys. Res. Commun.* **83:**373–378.

NAGAO, M., TAKAHASHI, Y., YAHAGI, T., SUGIMURA, T., TAKEDA, K., SHUDO, K., AND OKAMOTO, T., 1980, Mutagenicities of gamma-carboline derivatives related to potent mutagens found in tryptophan pyrolysates, *Carcinogenesis* **1:**451–454.

NAKANISHI, K., FUKUSHIMA, S., SHIBATA, M., SHIRAI, T., OGISO, T., AND ITO, N., 1978, Effect of phenacetin and caffeine on the urinary bladder of rats treated with N-butyl-N-(4-hydroxybutyl)nitrosamine, *Gann* **69:**395–400.

NEBERT, D., 1980, Pharmacogenetics: An approach to understanding chemical and biologic aspects of cancer, *J. Natl. Cancer Inst.* **64:**1279–1290.

NEBERT, D. W., AND JENSEN, N. M., 1979a, The *Ah* locus: Genetic regulation of the metabolism of carcinogens, drugs, and other environmental chemicals by cytochrome P-450-mediated monooxygenases, *CRC Crit. Rev. Biochem.* **8:**401–438.

NEBERT, D. W., AND JENSEN, N. M., 1979b, Benzo[a]pyrene-initiated leukemia in mice, *Biochem. Pharmacol.* **27:**149–151.

NEBERT, D. W., BIGELOW, S. W., OKEY, A., YAHAGI, T., MORI, Y., NAGAO, M., AND SUGIMURA, T., 1979, Pyrolysis products from amino acids and protein: Highest mutagenicity requires cytochrome P_1-450, *Proc. Natl. Acad. Sci. USA* **76:**5929–5933.

NEIDLE, S., SUBBIAH, A., COOPER, C. S., AND RIBERIO, O., 1980, Molecular structure of (±)7-alpha, 8-beta-dihydroxy-9-beta, 10-beta-epoxy-7,8,9,10-tetrahydrobenzo[a]pyrene: An X-ray crystallographic study, *Carcinogenesis* **1:**249–255.

NELSON, S. D., SNODGRASS, W. R., AND MITCHELL, J. R., 1976, Chemical reaction mechanisms responsible for the tissue injury caused by monosubstituted hydrazines and their hydrazide drug precursors, in: *In Vitro Metabolic Activation in Mutagenesis Testing* (F. J. de Serres, J. R. Fouts, J. R. Bend, and R. M. Philpot, eds.), pp. 257–276, Elsevier/North Holland, Amsterdam.

NEWBERNE, P. M., WEIGERT, J., AND KULA, N., 1979, Effects of dietary fat on hepatic mixed-function oxidases and hepatocellular carcinoma induced by aflatoxin B in rats, *Cancer Res.* **39:**3986–3991.

NEWBOLD, R. F., WARREN, W., MEDCALF, A. S. C., AND AMOS, J., 1980, Mutagenicity of carcinogenic methylating agents is associated with a specific DNA modification, *Nature* **283:**596–599.

NICHOLSON, W. J., AND MOORE, J. A., (eds.), 1979, *Health Effects of Halogenated Aromatic Hydrocarbons*, The New York Academy of Sciences, New York.

NIRANJAN, B. G., AND AVADHANI, N. G., 1980, Activation of aflatoxin B_1 by a mono-oxygenase system localized in rat liver mitochondria, *J. Biol. Chem.* **255:**6575–6578.

NORPOTH, K. H., AND GARNER, R. C. (eds.), 1980, *Short-Term Test Systems for Detecting Carcinogens*, Springer-Verlag, Berlin.

OESCH, F., RAPHAEL, D., SCHWINDK, H., AND GLATT, H. R., 1977, Species differences in activating and inactivating enzymes related to the control of mutagenic metabolites, *Arch. Toxicol.* **39:**97–108.

OKAMOTO, T., SHUDO, K., MIYATA, N., KITAHARA, Y., AND NAGATA, S., 1978, Reactions of K-region oxides of carcinogenic and noncarcinogenic aromatic hydrocarbons: Comparative studies on reactions with nucleophiles and acid-catalyzed reactions, *Chem. Pharm. Bull.* **26:**2014–2026.

OKANO, P., MILLER, H. N., ROBINSON, R. C., AND GELBOIN, H. V., 1979, Comparison of benzo(a)pyrene and (-)-trans-7,8-dihydroxy-7,8-dihydrobenzo(a)pyrene metabolism in human blood monocytes and lymphocytes, *Cancer Res.* **39:**3184–3193.

OKANO, T., HORIE, T., KOKE, T., AND MOTOHASHI, N., 1979, Relationship of carcinogenicity, mutagenicity, and K-region reactivity in benz[o]acridines, *Gann* **70:**749–754.

OKUDA, H., KITAHARA, Y., SHUDO, K., AND OKAMOTO, T., 1979, Identification of an ultimate mutagen of 10-azabenzo[a]pyrene: Microsomal oxidation of 10-azabenzo[a]pyrene-4,5-oxide, *Chem. Pharm. Bull.* **27**:2547–2549.

OKUDA, T., VESELL, E. S., PLOTKIN, E., TARONE, R., BAST, R. C., AND GELBOIN, H. V., 1977, Interindividual and intraindividual variations in aryl hydroxylase in monocytes from monozygotic and dizygotic twins, *Cancer Res.* **37**:3904–3911.

OLSON, W. A., HABERMANN, R. T., WEISBURGER, E. K., WARD, J. M., AND WEISBURGER, J. H., 1973, Induction of stomach cancer in rats and mice by halogenated aliphatic fumigants, *J. Natl. Cancer Inst.* **51**:1993–1995.

OSBORNE, J. C., METZLER, M., AND NEUMANN, H. G., 1980, Peroxidase activity in the rat Zymbal gland and its possible role in the metabolic activation of aminostilbenes in the target tissue, *Cancer Lett.* **8**:221–226.

OTA, K., AND HAMMOCK, B. D., 1980, Cytosolic and microsomal epoxide hydrolases: Differential properties in mammalian liver, *Science* **207**:1479–1481.

OWENS, I. S., KOTEEN, G. M., AND LEGRAVEREND, C., 1979, Mutagenesis of certain benzo[a]pyrene phenols *in vitro* following further metabolism by mouse liver, *Biochem. Pharmacol.* **28**:1615–1622.

PANG, K. S., STROBL, K., AND GILLETTE, J. R., 1979, A method for the estimation of the fraction of a precursor that is converted to a metabolite in rat *in vivo* with phenacetin and acetaminophen, *Drug Metab. Dispos.* **7**:366–372.

PARHAM, J. C., AND TEMPLETON, M. A., 1980, Comparative reactivities of esters of oncogenic and nononcogenic purine *N*-oxides and evidence of the oxidation–reduction reactivity of aromatic nitrenium ions, *Cancer Res.* **40**:1475–1481.

PARKE, D. V., 1979, The role of the endoplasmic reticulum in carcinogenesis, in: *Regulatory Aspects of Carcinogenesis and Food Additives: The Delaney Clause* (F. Coulston, ed.), pp. 173–187, Academic Press, New York.

PARKE, D. V., AND SMITH, R. L., 1977, *Drug Metabolism—From Microbe to Man*, Taylor & Francis, London.

PATTERSON, D. S. P., 1973, Metabolism as a factor in determining the toxic action of the aflatoxins in different animal species, *Food. Cosmet. Toxicol.* **11**:287–294.

PEGG, A. E., 1980a, Metabolism of *N*-nitrosodimethylamine, in: *Molecular and Cellular Aspects of Carcinogen Screening Tests* (R. Montesano, H. Bartsch, and L. Tomatis, eds.), pp. 3–22, IARC Scientific Publication 27, Lyon, France.

PEGG, A. E., 1980b, Formation and subsequent repair of alkylation lesions in tissues of rodents treated with nitrosamines, *Arch. Toxicol. Suppl.* **3**:55–68.

PENN, I., 1978, Tumors arising in organ transplant recipients, *Adv. Cancer Res.* **28**:32–62.

PERAINO, C., STAFFELDT, E. F., HAUGEN, D. A., LOMBARD, L. S., STEVENS, F. J., AND FRY, R. J. M., 1980, Effects of varying the dietary concentration of phenobarbital on its enhancement of 2-acetylaminofluorene-induced hepatic tumorigenesis, *Cancer Res.* **40**:3268–3273.

PEREIRA, M. A., BURNS, F. J., AND ALBERT, R. E., 1979, Dose response for benzo(a)pyrene adducts in mouse epidermal DNA, *Cancer Res.* **39**:2556–2559.

PERIN-ROUSSEL, O., CROISY-DELCEY, M., MISPELTER, J., SAGUEM, S., CHALVET, O., EKERT, B., FOUQUET, J., JACQUIGNON, P., LHOSTE, J. M., MUEL, B., AND ZAJDELA, F., 1980, Metabolic activation of dibenzo(a,e)fluoranthene, a nonalternant carcinogenic polycyclic hydrocarbon, in liver homogenates, *Cancer Res.* **40**:1742–1749.

PESSAYRE, D., WANDSCHERR, J. C., DESCATOIRE, V., ARTIGOU, J. Y., AND BENHAMOU, J. P., 1979, Formation and inactivation of a chemically reactive metabolite of vinyl chloride, *Toxicol. Appl. Pharmacol.* **49**:505–515.

PINSKY, S. D., LEE, K. E., AND WOOLEY, P. V., 1980, Uptake and binding of 1-methyl-1-nitrosourea (MNU) and 1-methyl-3-nitro-1-nitrosoguanidine (MNNG) by the isolated guinea pig pancreas, *Carcinogenesis* **1**:567–575.

PLANCHE, G., CROISY, A., MALAVEILLE, C., TOMATIS, L., AND BARTSCH, H., 1979, Metabolic and mutagenicity studies on DDT and 15 derivatives. Detection of 1,1-bis(p-chlorophenyl)-2,2-dichloroethane and 1,1-bis(p-chlorophenyl)-2,2,2-trichloroethyl acetate (kelthane acetate) as mutagens in *Salmonella typhimurium* and of 1,1-bis(p-chlorophenyl)ethylene oxide, a likely metabolite, as an alkylating agent, *Chem. Biol. Interact.* **25**:157–175.

PLUMMER, J. L., SMITH, B. R., BALL, L. M., AND BEND, J. R., 1980, Metabolism and biliary excretion of benzo[a]pyrene 4,5-oxide in the rat, *Drug Metab. Dispos.* **8**:68–72.

POHL, L. R., GEORGE, J. W., MARTIN, J. L., AND KRISHMA, G., 1979, Deuterium isotope effect in *in vivo* bioactivation of chloroform to phosgene, *Biochem. Pharmacol.* **28**:561–563.

328

J. H.
WEISBURGER
AND
G. M.
WILLIAMS

POIRIER, L. A., AND WEISBURGER, E. K., 1979, Selection of carcinogens and related compounds tested for mutagenic activity, *J. Natl. Cancer Inst.* **62:**833–840.

POPPER, H., CZYGAN, P., GREIM, H., SCHAFFNER, F., AND GARRO, A. J., 1973, Mutagenicity of primary and secondary carcinogens altered by normal and induced hepatic microsomes, *Proc. Soc. Exp. Biol. Med.* **142:**727–729.

POUPKO, J. M., HEARN, W. L., AND RADOMSKI, J. L., 1979, N-Glucuronidation of N-hydroxyaromatic amines: A mechanism for their transport and bladder-specific carcinogenicity, *Toxicol. Appl. Pharmacol.* **50:**479–484.

POZHARISSKI, K. M., LIKHACHEV, A. J., KLIMASHEVSKI, V. F., AND SHAPOSHNIKOV, J. D., 1979, Experimental intestinal cancer research with special reference to human pathology, *Adv. Cancer Res.* **30:**166–238.

PREUSSMANN, R., 1975, Chemische Carcinogene in der Menschlichen Umwelt, in: *Handbuch der Allgemeinen Pathologie*, Vol. VI (II), pp. 421–594, Springer-Verlag, Berlin.

PRIVAL, M. J., KING, V. D., AND SHELDON, A. T., JR., 1979, The mutagenicity of dialkyl nitrosamines in the *Salmonella* plate assay, *Environ. Mutagenesis* **1:**95–104.

RAINERI, R., POILEY, J. A., ERNST, M. K., HILLESUND, T., AND PIENTA, J., 1978, A high pressure liquid chromatography procedure for the separation of metabolites of 2-acetylaminofluorene from cells in culture, *J. Liquid Chromatogr.* **1**(4):457–467.

RAJEWSKY, M. F., 1980, Specificity of DNA damage in chemical carcinogenesis, in: *Molecular and Cellular Aspects of Carcinogen Screening Tests* (R. Montesano, H. Bartsch, L. Tomatis, and W. Davis, eds.), pp. 41–54, IARC Scientific Publication 27, Lyon, France.

RAZZOUK, C., MERCIER, M., AND ROBERFROID, M., 1980, Characterization of the guinea pig liver microsomal 2-fluorenylamine and N-2-fluorenylacetamide N-hydroxylase, *Cancer Lett.* **9:**123–131.

REDDY, B. S., COHEN, L. A., MCCOY, G. D., HILL, P., WEISBURGER, J. H., AND WYNDER, E. L., 1980, Nutrition and its relationship to cancer, *Adv. Cancer Res.* **32:**237–345.

REITZ, R. H., WATANABE, P. G., MCKENNA, M. J., QUAST, J. F., AND GEHRING, P. J., 1980, Effects of vinylidene chloride on DNA synthesis and DNA repair in the rat and mouse: A comparative study with dimethylnitrosamine, *Toxicol. Appl. Pharmacol.* **52:**357–370.

RHINDE, E., AND TROLL, W., 1975, Metabolic reduction of azo dyes to benzidine in the rhesus monkey, *J. Natl. Cancer Inst.* **55:**181.

RICE, J. (ed.), 1979, Perinatal carcinogenesis, *Natl. Cancer Inst. Monogr.* **51:**1–282.

RICKERT, D. E., BAKER, T. S., BUS, J. S., BARROW, C. S., AND IRONS, R. D., 1979, Benzene disposition in the rat after exposure by inhalation, *Toxicol. Appl. Pharmacol.* **49:**417–423.

RIVLIN, R. S., 1973, Riboflavin and cancer, *Cancer Res.* **33:**1977–1986.

ROBENS, J. F., DILL, G. S., WARD, J. M., JOINER, J. R., GRIESEMER, R. A., AND DOUGLAS, J. F., 1980, Thirteen-week subchronic toxicity studies of direct blue 6, direct black 38, and direct brown 95 dyes, *Toxicol. Appl. Pharmacol.* **54:**431–442.

ROEBUCK, B. D., SIEGEL, W. G., AND WOGAN, G. N., 1978, *In vitro* metabolism of aflatoxin B_2 by animal and human liver, *Cancer Res.* **38:**999–1002.

ROGAN, E. G., KATOMSKI, P. A., ROTH, R. W., AND CAVALIERI, E. L., 1979, Horseradish peroxidase/hydrogen peroxide-catalyzed binding of aromatic hydrocarbons to DNA, *J. Biol. Chem.* **254:**7055–7059.

ROLLER, P. P., SHIMP, D. R., AND KEEFER, L. K., 1975, Synthesis and solvolysis of methyl(acetoxymethyl)nitrosamine: Solution chemistry of the presumed carcinogenic metabolite of dimethylnitrosamine, *Tetrahedron Lett.* **16:**2965–2968.

ROLLINS, D. E., VON BAHR, C., GLAUMANN, H., MODEUS, P., AND RANE, A., 1979, Acetaminophen: Potentially toxic metabolite formed by human fetal and adult liver microsomes and isolated fetal liver cells, *Science* **205:**1414–1416.

ROSS, A., AND MIRVISH, S. S., 1977, Metabolism of N-nitrosohexamethyleneimine to give 1,6-hexanediol bound to rat liver nucleic acids, *J. Natl. Cancer Inst.* **58:**651–655.

SABADIE, N., MALAVEILLE, C., CAMUS, A., AND BARTSCH, H., 1980, Comparison of the hydroxylation of benzo(*a*)pyrene with the metabolism of vinyl chloride, N-nitrosomorpholine, and N-nitroso-N'-methyl-piperazine to mutagens by human and rat liver microsomal fractions, *Cancer Res.* **40:**119–126.

SAFFIOTTI, U., AND WAGONER, J. K. (eds.), 1976, *Occupational Carcinogenesis*, *Ann. N.Y. Acad. Sci.* **271:**1–516.

SAKAI, S., REINHOLD, C. E., WIRTH, P. J., AND THORGEIRSSON, S. S., 1978, Mechanism of *in vitro* mutagenic activation and covalent binding of N-hydroxy-2-acetylaminofluorene in isolated liver cell nuclei from rat and mouse, *Cancer Res.* **38:**2058–2067.

SANDER, J., SCHWEINSBERG, F., LABAR, J., BUERKLE, G., AND SCHWEINSBERG, E., 1975, Nitrite and nitrosable amino compounds in carcinogenesis, *Gann Monogr.* **17**:145–164.

SANTELLA, R. M., GRUNBERGER, D., AND WEINSTEIN, I. B., 1979, DNA–benzo[a]pyrene adducts formed in a *Salmonella typhimurium* mutagenesis assay system, *Mutat. Res.* **61**:181–189.

SARRIF, A. M., MCCARTHY, K. L., NESNOW, S., AND HEIDELBERGER, C., 1978, Separation of glutathione *S*-transferase activities with epoxides from the mouse liver h-protein, a major polycyclic hydrocarbon-binding protein, *Cancer Res.* **38**:1438–1443.

SAWICKI, E., AND SAWICKI, C. R., 1969, Analysis of alkylating agents: Applications to air pollution, *Ann. N.Y. Acad. Sci.* **163**:895–920.

SAXENA, J. (ed.), 1980, *Hazard Assessment of Chemicals, Current Developments*, Vol. I, Academic Press, New York.

SCARPELLI, D. G., RAO, M. S., SUBBARAO, V., BEVERSLUIS, M., GURKA, D. P., AND HOLLENBERG, P. F., 1980, Activation of nitrosamines to mutagens by postmitochondrial fraction of hamster pancreas, *Cancer Res.* **40**:67–74.

SCHELINE, R. R., 1973, Metabolism of foreign compounds by gastrointestinal microorganisms, *Pharmacol. Rev.* **24**:451–523.

SCHMÄHL, D., 1970, *Entstehung, Wachstum und Chemotherapie maligner Tumoren*, Cantor, Aulendorf.

SCHMELTZ, I., TOSK, J., AND WILLIAMS, G. M., 1978, Comparison of the metabolic profiles of benzo(a)pyrene obtained from primary cell cultures and subcellular fractions derived from normal and methylcholanthrene-induced rat liver, *Cancer Lett.* **5**:81–89.

SCHMUCKER, D. L., 1979, Age-related changes in drug disposition, *Pharmacol. Rev.* **30**:455–456.

SCHRAUZER, G. N., 1979, Trace elements in carcinogenesis, *Adv. Nutr. Res.* **2**:219–244.

SCHUT, H. A., AND THORGEIRSSON, S. S., 1979, Mutagenic activation of *N*-hydroxy-2-acetylaminofluorene by developing epithelial cells of rat small intestine and effects of antioxidants, *J. Natl. Cancer Inst.* **63**:1405–1409.

SCRIBNER, J. D., FISK, S. R., AND SCRIBNER, N. K., 1979, Mechanisms of action of carcinogenic aromatic amines: An investigation using mutagenesis in bacteria, *Chem. Biol. Interact.* **26**:11–25.

SEARLE, C. E. (ed.), 1976, *Chemical Carcinogens*, ACS Monograph 173, American Chemical Society, Washington, D.C.

SELKIRK, J. K., 1980, Comparison of epoxide and free-radical mechanisms for activation of benzo[a]pyrene by Sprague–Dawley rat liver microsome, *J. Natl. Cancer Inst.* **64**:771–774.

SETLOW, R. B., 1980, Different basic mechanisms in DNA repair, *Arch. Toxicol. Suppl.* **3**:217–228.

SHAH, H., HARTMAN, S. P., AND WEINHOUSE, S., 1979, Formation of carbonyl chloride in carbon tetrachloride metabolism by rat liver *in vitro*, *Cancer Res.* **39**:3942–3947.

SINGER, B., 1979, *N*-Nitroso alkylating agents: Formation and persistence of alkyl derivatives in mammalian nucleic acids as contributing factors in carcinogenesis, *J. Natl. Cancer Inst.* **62**:1329–1338.

SINGER, G. M., AND LIJINSKY, W., 1979, Relative extents of hydrogen–deuterium exchange of nitrosamines: Relevance to biological isotope effect studies, *Cancer Lett.* **8**:29–34.

SKIBBA, J. L., BEAL, D. D., RAMIREZ, G., AND BRYAN, G. T., 1970, *N*-Demethylation of the antineoplastic agent 4(5)-(3,3-dimethyl-1-triazeno)imidazole-5(4)-carboxamide by rats and man, *Cancer Res.* **3**:147–150.

SLACIK-ERBEN, R., ROLL, R., FRANKE, G., AND UEHLEKE, H., 1980, Trichloroethylene vapours do not produce dominant lethal mutations in male mice, *Arch. Toxicol.* **45**:37–44.

SLAGA, T. J., SIVAK, A., AND BOUTWELL, R. K. (eds.), 1978, *Carcinogenesis: Mechanisms of Tumor Promotion and Cocarcinogenesis*, Raven Press, New York.

SLAGA, T. J., GLEASON, G. L., MILLS, G., EWALD, P. P., LEE, H. M., AND HARVEY, R. G., 1980, Comparison of the skin tumor-initiating activities of dihydrodiols and diol-epoxides of various polycyclic aromatic hydrocarbons, *Cancer Res.* **40**:1981–1984.

SMITH, G. J., OHL, V. S., AND LITWACK, G., 1980, Purification and properties of hamster liver ligandins, glutathione *S*-transferases, *Cancer Res.* **40**:1787–1790.

SOLT, A. K., AND NEALE, S., 1980, Natulan, a bacterial mutagen requiring complex mammalian metabolic activation, *Mutat. Res.* **70**:167–171.

SON, O. S., EVERETT, D. W., AND FIALA, E. S., 1980, Metabolism of *O*-[Methyl-^{14}C]toluidine in the F344 rat, *Xenobiotica* **10**:457–468.

SONTAG, J. (ed.), 1981, *Carcinogens in Industry and the Environment*, Dekker, New York.

SPORN, M., AND NEWTON, D., 1979, Chemoprevention of cancer with retinoids, *Fed. Proc.* **38**:2528–2534.

330

J. H.
WEISBURGER
AND
G. M.
WILLIAMS

STARK, A. A., ESSIGMANN, J. M., DEMAIN, A. L., SKOPEK, T. R., AND WOGAN, G. N., 1979, Aflatoxin B_1 mutagenesis, DNA binding, and adduct formation in *Salmonella typhimurium*, *Proc. Natl. Acad. Sci. USA* **76**:1343–1347.

STICH, H. F., WHITING, R. F., WEI, L., AND SAN, R. H. C., 1979, DNA fragmentation and DNA repair of mammalian cells as an indicator for the complex interactions between carcinogens and modulating factors, *Pharmacol. Rev.* **30**:493–499.

STOEHRER, G., SALEMNICK, G., AND BROWN, B. G., 1973, A chemical adduct of tryptophan and the oncogen 3-acetoxyxanthine, *Biochemistry* **12**:5084–5086.

STOLZENBERG, S. J., AND HINE, C. H., 1979, Mutagenicity of halogenated and oxygenated three-carbon compounds, *J. Toxicol. Environ. Health* **5**:1149–1158.

STOUT, D. L., AND BECKER, F. F., 1979, Metabolism of 2-aminofluorene and 2-acetylaminofluorene to mutagens by rat hepatocyte nuclei, *Cancer Res.* **39**:1158–1173.

STUMPF, R., MARGISON, G., MONTESANO, R., AND PEGG, A. E., 1979, Formation and loss of alkylated purines from DNA of hamster liver after administration of dimethylnitrosamine, *Cancer Res.* **39**:50–54.

STYLES, J., ASHBY, J., AND MATTOCKS, A. R., 1980, Evaluation *in vitro* of several pyrrolizidine alkaloid carcinogens: Observations on the essential pyrrolic nucleus, *Carcinogenesis* **1**:161–164.

SUGIMURA, T., ENDO, H., ONO, T., AND SUGANO, H., 1979, Progress in cancer biochemistry, *Gann Monogr.* **24**:1–281.

SWANN, P. F., KAUFMAN, D. G., MAGEE, P. N., AND MACE, R., 1980, Induction of kidney tumours by a single dose of dimethylnitrosamine: Dose response and influence of diet and benzo(a)pyrene pretreatment, *Br. J. Cancer* **41**:285.

SWANSON, A. B., CHAMBLISS, D. D., BLOMQUIST, J. C., MILLER, E. C., AND MILLER, J. A., 1979, The mutagenicities of safrole, estragole, eugenol, trans-anethole, and some of their known or possible metabolites for *Salmonella typhimurium* mutants, *Mutat. Res.* **60**:143–153.

SWEENEY, G. D., AND COLE, F. M., 1980, Effects of ethynyl estradiol on liver microsomal mixed function oxygenase activity in male rats, *Lab. Invest.* **42**:231–235.

SWENSON, D. H., MILLER, J. A., AND MILLER, E. C., 1974, Aflatoxin B_1-2,3-dichloride: A toxic and reactive derivative of aflatoxin B_1, *Proc. Am. Assoc. Cancer Res.* **15**:43.

SWENSON, D. H., LIN, J. K., MILLER, E. C., AND MILLER, J. A., 1977, Aflatoxin B_1-2,3-oxide as a probable intermediate in the covalent binding of aflatoxins B_1 and B_2 to rat liver DNA and ribosomal RNA *in vivo*, *Cancer Res.* **37**:172–181.

TADA, M., TAKAHASHI, K., KAWAZOE, Y., AND ITO, N., 1980, Binding of quinoline to nucleic acid in a subcellular microsomal system, *Chem. Biol. Interact.* **29**:257–266.

TAKEISHI, K., OKUNO-KANEDA, S., AND SENO, T., 1979, Mutagenic activation of 2-acetylaminofluorene by guinea-pig liver homogenates: Essential involvement of cytochrome P-450 mixed-function oxidases, *Mutat. Res.* **62**:425–437.

TALALAY, P., BATZINGER, R. P., BENSON, A. M., BUEDING, E., AND YOUNG-NAM CHA, 1979, Biochemical studies on the mechanisms by which dietary antioxidants suppress mutagenic activity, *Adv. Enzyme Regul.* **17**:23–36.

TANNEN, R. H., AND WEBBER, W. W., 1979, Rodent models of the human isoniazid acetylator polymorphism, *Drug Metab. Dispos.* **7**:274–279.

TANNENBAUM, S. R., WEISMAN, N., AND FETT, D., 1976, The effect of nitrate intake on nitrite formation in human saliva, *Food Cosmet. Toxicol.* **14**:459–552.

TARPLEY, W. G., MILLER, J. A., AND MILLER, E. C., 1980, Adducts from the reaction of *N*-benzoyloxy-*N*-methyl-4-aminoazobenzene with deoxyguanosine or DNA *in vitro* and from hepatic DNA of mice treated with *N*-methyl- or *N,N*-dimethyl-4-aminoazobenzene, *Cancer Res.* **40**:2493–2499.

TELANG, N., HECHT, S. S., AND WILLIAMS, G. M., 1979, Maintenance in organ culture of mouse bladder epithelium and response to a bladder carcinogen, *Fed. Proc.* **38**:1074.

TELLER, M. N., GINER-SORELLA, A., STOHRER, G., BUDINGER, J. M., AND BROWN, G. B., 1978, Oncogenicity of purine-3-oxide and unsubstituted purine in rats, *Cancer Res.* **38**:2229–2232.

THAKKER, D. R., LEVIN, W., YAGI, H., TADA, M., CONNEY, A. H., AND JERINA, D. M., 1980, Comparative metabolism of dihydrodiols of polycyclic aromatic hydrocarbons to bay region diol epoxides, in: *Polynuclear Aromatic Hydrocarbons: Chemistry and Biological Effects* (A. Bjorseth and A. J. Dennis, eds.), pp. 267–286, Batelle, Columbus, Ohio.

THORGEIRSSON, S. S., AND NEBERT, D. W., 1977, The *Ah* locus and the metabolism of chemical carcinogens and other foreign compounds, *Adv. Cancer Res.* **25**:119–194.

THORGEIRSSON, S. S., AND WEISBURGER, E. K. (eds.), 1981, *International Conference on Carcinogenic and Mutagenic N-Substituted Aryl Compounds*, Natl. Cancer Inst. Monograph 58, Bethesda, Maryland.

THORGEIRSSON, S. S., AND WIRTH, P. J., 1979, Genetic aspects of metabolic processing of chemical substances, *J. Toxicol. Environ. Health* 5:83–87.

TIMBRELL, J. A., AND WRIGHT, J. M., 1979, Studies on the effects of isoniazid on acetylhydrazine metabolism *in vivo* and *in vitro*, *Drug Metab. Dispos.* 7:237–240.

TIPPING, E., KETTERER, B., AND CHRISTODOULIDES, L., 1979, Interactions of small molecules with phospholipid bilayers. Binding to egg phosphosphatidylcholine of some organic anions (bromosulphophthalein, oestrone sulphate, haem and bilirubin) that bind to ligandin and aminoazo-dye-binding protein A, *Biochem. J.* 180:327–337.

TKESHELASHVILLI, L. K., SHEARMAN, C. W., ZAKOUR, R. A., KOPLITZ, R. M., AND LOEB, L. A., 1980, Effects of arsenic, selenium, and chromium on the fidelity of DNA synthesis, *Cancer Res.* 40:2455–2460.

TOMATIS, L., PARTENSKY, C., AND MONTESANO, R., 1973, The predictive value of mouse liver tumor induction in carcinogenicity testing—A literature survey, *Int. J. Cancer* 12:1–20.

TOTH, B., 1968, A critical review of experiments in chemical carcinogenesis using newborn animals, *Cancer Res.* 28:727–738.

TOTH, B., 1980, Actual new cancer causing hydrazines, hydrazides, and hydrazones, *J. Cancer Res. Clin. Oncol.* 97:97–108.

UCHIDA, E., AND HIRONO, I., 1979, Effect of phenobarbital on induction of liver and lung tumors by dimethylnitrosamine in newborn mice, *Gann* 70:639–644.

UEHLEKE, H., 1973, The role of cytochrome P-450 in the *N*-oxidation of individual amines, *Drug Metab. Dispos.* 1:299–313.

UEHLEKE, H., HELLMER, K. H., AND TABARELLI, S., 1973, Binding of ^{14}C-carbon tetrachloride to microsomal proteins *in vitro* and formation of $CHCl_3$ by reduced liver microsomes, *Xenobiotica* 3:1–11.

UEHLEKE, H., WERNER, T., GREIM, H., AND KRAMER, M., 1977, Metabolic activation of haloalkanes and tests *in vitro* for mutagenicity, *Xenobiotica* 7:393–400.

UENO, I., FRIEDMAN, L., AND STONE, C. L., 1980, Species difference in the binding of aflatoxin B_1 to hepatic macromolecules, *Toxicol. Appl. Pharmacol.* 52:177–180.

UNGER, P. D., SALERNO, A. J., NESS, W. C., AND FRIEDMAN, M. A., 1980, Tissue distribution and excretion of 2,4-^{14}C]toluenediamine in the mouse, *J. Toxicol. Environ. Health* 6:107–114.

URAGUCHI, K., UENO, I., UENO, Y., AND KOMAI, Y., 1972, Absorption, distribution and excretion of luteoskyrin with special reference to the selective action on the liver, *Toxicol. Appl. Pharmacol.* 21:335–347.

VAN BLADEREN, P. J., VAN GENDESEN, A., BREIMER, D. D., AND MOHN, G. R., 1979, Stereoselective activation of vicinal dihalogen compounds to mutagens by glutathione conjugation, *Biochem. Pharmacol.* 28:2521–2524.

VAN DUUREN, B. L., WITZ, G., AND SIVAK, A., 1974, Chemical carcinogenesis, in: *Pathophysiology of Cancer*, Vol. I (F. Homburger, ed.), pp. 1–63, S. Karger Verlag, Basel, Switzerland.

VAN DUUREN, B. L., SMITH, A. C., AND MELCHIONNE, S. M., 1978, Effect of aging in two-stage carcinogenesis on mouse skin with phorbol myristate acetate as promoting agent, *Cancer Res.* 38:865–866.

VAN DUUREN, B. L., GOLDSCHMIDT, B. M., LOEWENGART, G., SMITH, A. C., MELCHIONNE, S., SEIDMAN, I., AND ROTH, D., 1979, Carcinogenicity of halogenated olefinic and aliphatic hydrocarbons in mice, *J. Natl. Cancer Inst.* 63:1433–1439.

VESELL, E. S., 1979, Intraspecies differences in frequency of genes directly affecting drug disposition: The individual factor in drug response, *Pharmacol. Rev.* 30:555–563.

VESELL, E. S., 1980, Genetic and environmental factors affecting the metabolism of carcinogens, in: *Molecular and Cellular Aspects of Carcinogen Screening Tests* (R. Montesano, H. Bartsch, and L. Tomatis, eds.), pp. 23–40, IARC Scientific Publication 27, Lyon, France.

VESSELINOVITCH, S. D., MIHAILOVICH, N., WOGAN, G. N., LOMBARD, L. S., AND RAO, V. N., 1972, Aflatoxin B_1, a hepatocarcinogen in the infant mouse, *Cancer Res.* 32:2289–2291.

WALKER, E. A., CASTEGNARO, M., GRICIUTE, L., AND LYLE, R. E., 1978, *Environmental Aspects of N-Nitroso Compounds*, IARC Scientific Publication 19, Lyon, France.

WALKER, R. N., AND FLOYD, R. A., 1979, Free radical activation of *N*-hydroxy-2-acetylaminofluorene by methemoglobin and hydrogen peroxide, *Cancer Biochem. Biophys.* 4:87–93.

332

J. H.
WEISBURGER
AND
G. M.
WILLIAMS

WANG, Y. Y., RAPPAPORT, S. M., SAWYER, R. F., TALCOTT, R. E., AND WEI, E. T., 1978, Direct-acting mutagens in automobile exhaust, *Cancer Lett.* **5:**39–47.

WATTENBERG, L. W., 1978, Inhibitors of chemical carcinogenesis, *Adv. Cancer Res.* **26:**197–223.

WATTENBERG, L. W., 1980, Inhibition of polycyclic aromatic hydrocarbon induced neoplasia by sodium cyanate, *Cancer Res.* **40:**232–234.

WEEKS, C. E., ALLABEN, W. T., TRESP, N. M., LOUIE, S. C., LAZEAR, E. J., AND KING, C. M., 1980, Effects of structure of *N*-acyl-*N*-2-fluorenyl-hydroxylamines on arylhydroxamic acid acyltransferase, sulfotransferase, and deacylase activities, and on mutations in *Salmonella typhimurium* TA-1538, *Cancer Res.* **40:**1204–1211.

WEINKAM, R. M. J., AND SHIBA, D. A., 1978, Metabolic activation of procarbazine, *Life Sci.* **22:**937–946.

WEISBURGER, E. K., 1977, Bioassay program for carcinogenic hazards of cancer chemotherapeutic agents, *Cancer* **40:**1935–1949.

WEISBURGER, E. K., 1981, Species differences in response to aromatic amines, in: *Organ and Species Specificity in Chemical Carcinogenesis* (R. Langenbach, S. Nesnow, and J. Rice, eds.), Plenum Press, New York.

WEISBURGER, E. K., EVARTS, R. P., AND WENK, M. L., 1977, Inhibitory effect of butylated hydroxytoluene (BHT) on intestinal carcinogenesis in rats by azoxymethane, *Food Cosmet. Toxicol.* **15:**139–141.

WEISBURGER, E. K., MURTHY, A. S. K., FLEISCHMAN, R. W., AND HAGOPIAN, M., 1980, Carcinogenicity of 4-chloro-*O*-phenylenediamine, 4-chloro-*m*-phenylenediamine, and 2-chloro-*p*-phenylenediamine in Fischer 344 rats and B6C3F$_1$ mice, *Carcinogenesis* **1:**495–499.

WEISBURGER, J. H., AND RAINERI, R., 1975, Assessment of human exposure and response to *N*-nitroso compounds: A new view on the etiology of digestive tract cancers, *Toxicol. Appl. Pharmacol.* **31:**369–374.

WEISBURGER, J. H., AND WEISBURGER, E. K., 1973, Biochemical formation and pharmacological, toxicological, and pathological properties of hydroxylamines and hydroxamic acids, *Pharmacol. Rev.* **25:**1–66.

WEISBURGER, J. H., AND WILLIAMS, G. M., 1980, Chemical carcinogenesis, in: *Toxicology: The Basic Science of Poisons* (J. Doull, C. Klassen, and M. Amdur, eds.), 2nd ed., Macmillan, New York.

WEISBURGER, J. H., YAMAMOTO, R. S., GLASS, R. M., AND FRANKEL, H. H., 1969, Prevention by arginine glutamate of the carcinogenicity of acetamide in rats, *Toxicol. Appl. Pharmacol.* **14:**163–175.

WEISBURGER, J. H., MARQUARDT, H., MOWER, H. F., HIROTA, N., MORI, H., AND WILLIAMS, G., 1980*a*, Inhibition of carcinogenesis: Vitamin C and the prevention of gastric cancer, *Prev. Med.* **9:**352–361.

WEISBURGER, J. H., REDDY, B. S., SPINGARN, N. E., AND WYNDER, E. L., 1980*b*, Current views on the mechanisms involved in the etiology of colorectal cancer, in: *Colorectal Cancer: Prevention, Epidemiology, and Screening* (S. Winawer, D. Schottenfeld, and P. Sherlock, eds.), pp. 19–41, Raven Press, New York.

WELLS, P. G., BOERTH, R. C., OATES, J. A., AND HARBISON, R. D., 1980, Toxicologic enhancement by a combination of drugs which deplete hepatic glutathione: Acetaminophen and doxorubicin (adriamycin), *Toxicol. Appl. Pharmacol.* **54:**197–209.

WHALLEY, C. E., ZAFAR, M. I., AND EPSTEIN, S. S., 1980, The separation of *N*-nitroso-di-*n*-propylamine and its beta-oxidized carcinogenic metabolite by high pressure liquid chromatography, *J. Liquid Chromatogr.* **3:**693–703.

WHITE, R. E., AND COON, M. J., 1980, Oxygen activation by cytochrome P-450, *Annu. Rev. Biochem.* **4:**315–356.

WIGLEY, C. B., 1975, Differentiated cells *in vitro*, *Differentiation* **4:**25–55.

WILLES, R. F., STAVRIC, B., CRAIG, J. C., AND RUDDICK, J. A., 1980, Circulating naphthionic acid in nonpregnant and pregnant rats after feeding amaranth, *Toxicol. Appl. Pharmacol.* **54:**276–284.

WILLIAMS, G. M., 1976, The use of liver epithelial cultures for the study of chemical carcinogenesis, *Am. J. Pathol.* **85:**739–753.

WILLIAMS, G. M., AND WEISBURGER, J. H., 1981, Systematic carcinogen testing through the decision point approach, *Annu. Rev. Pharmacol. Toxicol.* **21:**393–416.

WILLIAMS, G. M., KROES, R., WAAIJERS, H. W., AND VAN DE POLL, K. W. (eds.), 1980*a*, *The Predictive Value of Short-term Screening Tests in Carcinogenicity Evaluation, Applied Methods in Oncology 3,* Elsevier/North-Holland, Amsterdam.

WILLIAMS, G. M., MORI, H., HIRONO, I., AND NAGAO, M., 1980*b*, Genotoxicity of pyrrolizidine alkaloids in the hepatocyte primary culture/DNA-repair test, *Mutat. Res.* **79:**1–5.

WOGAN, G. N., 1973, Aflatoxin carcinogenesis, *Methods Cancer Res.* **7:**309–344.

WOLF, C. R., SMITH, B. R., BALL, L. M., ŠERABJIT-SINGH, C., BEND, J. R., AND PHILPOT, R. M., 1979, The rabbit pulmonary monooxygenase system, *J. Biol. Chem.* **254:**3658–3663.

WONG, Z. A., DECAD, G. M., BYARD, J. L., AND HSIEH, D. P. H., 1979, Conversion of aflatoxicol to aflatoxin B_1 in rats *in vivo* and in primary hepatocyte culture, *Food Cosmet. Toxicol.* **17:**481–486.

WOO, Y.-T., ARGUS, M. F., AND ARCOS, J. C., 1978, Effect of mixed-function oxidase modifiers on metabolism and toxicity of the oncogen dioxane, *Cancer Res.* **38:**1621–1625.

WOOD, A. W., CHANG, R. L., HUANG, M. T., LEVIN, W., LEHR, R. E., KUMAR, S., THAKKER, D. R., YAGI, H., JERINA, D. M., AND CONNEY, A. H., 1980, Mutagenicity of benzo(*a*)pyrene and triphenylene tetrahydroepoxides and diol-epoxides in bacterial and mammalian cells, *Cancer Res.* **40:**1985–1989.

WYNDER, E. L., AND GORI, G. B., 1977, Contribution of the environment to cancer incidence: An epidemiological exercise, *J. Natl. Cancer Inst.* **58:**825–832.

WYNDER, E. L., AND HIRAYAMA, T., 1977, Comparative epidemiology of cancers in the United States and Japan, *Prev. Med.* **6:**567–594.

WYNDER, E. L., AND HOFFMANN, D. H., 1979, Tobacco and health: A societal challenge, *N. Engl. J. Med.* **300:**894–903.

YAHAGI, T., NAGAO, M., HARA, K., MATSUSHIMA, T., SUGIMURA, T., AND BRYAN, G. T., 1974, Relationship between the carcinogenic and mutagenic or DNA-modifying effects of nitrofuran derivatives, including AF-2, a food additive widely used in Japan, *Cancer Research* **34:**2266–2273.

YAMANE, Y., AND OHTAWA, M., 1979, Effect of aluminium chloride on binding of 4-hydroxyaminoquinoline 1-oxide to nucleotides, *Gann* **70:**316–364.

YANG, S. K., DEUTSCH, J., AND GELBOIN, H. V., 1978, Benzo(*a*)pyrene metabolism: Activation and detoxification, in: *Polycyclic Hydrocarbons and Cancer*, Vol. I (H. V. Gelboin and P. O. P. Ts'o, eds.), pp. 205–231, Academic Press, New York.

YOTTI, L. P., CHANG, C. C., AND TRASKO, J. E., 1979, Elimination of metabolic cooperation in Chinese hamster cells by a tumor promoter, *Science* **206:**1089–1091.

YOUNES, M., AND SIEGERS, C. P., 1980, Inhibition of the hepatotoxicity of paracetamol and its irreversible binding to rat liver microsomal protein, *Arch. Toxicol.* **45:**61–65.

YOUNG, J. D., BRAUN, W. H., AND GEHRING, P. J., 1978, Dose dependent fate of 1,4-dioxane in rats, *J. Toxicol. Environ. Health* **4:**709–726.

ZACHARIAH, P. K., AND JUCHAU, M. R., 1974, The role of gut flora in the reduction of aromatic nitro-groups, *Drug Metab. Dispos.* **2:**74–78.

ZAJDELA, F., CROISY, A., BARBIN, A., MALAVEILLE, C., TOMATIS, L., AND BARTSCH, H., 1980, Carcinogenicity of chloroethylene oxide, an ultimate reactive metabolite of vinyl chloride, and bis(chloromethyl)ether after subcutaneous administration and in initiation–promotion experiments in mice, *Cancer Res.* **40:**352–356.

ZANNONI, V. G., AND SATO, P. H., 1975, Effects of ascorbic acid on microsomal drug metabolism, *Ann. N.Y. Acad. Sci.* **258:**119–131.

10

Chemical Carcinogenesis: Interactions of Carcinogens with Nucleic Acids

S. RAJALAKSHMI, PREMA M. RAO, AND D. S. R. SARMA

1. Introduction

Some of the major conceptual advances in chemical carcinogenesis made during the past several years have been (1) the discovery of the enzymatic activation of procarcinogens to reactive ultimate carcinogens, (2) the characterization of interactions of the active metabolites of many carcinogens with a variety of tissue nucleophiles including DNA, RNA, and protein, and (3) the development of model systems for a sequential analysis of the initiation phase of carcinogenesis. This chapter primarily focuses on the interactions of chemical carcinogens and their activated metabolites with nucleic acids, both DNA and RNA.

Two important aspects of the interaction of carcinogens with nucleic acids are the nature and fate of the modified nucleic acids and their significance in carcinogenesis. Emphasis will naturally be given to the first, since this is our area of major knowledge. Although the second, viz. relevance to carcinogenesis, is the most important from the point of view of cancer, this must of necessity remain speculative today, for methods are not available for a scientific analysis of the process.

This chapter will summarize our current knowledge with regard to (1) the nature of the interactions between chemical carcinogens and nucleic acids, both DNA and RNA, with emphasis on interactions occurring *in vivo*, (2) the possible

S. RAJALAKSHMI, PREMA M. RAO, AND D. S. R. SARMA ● Department of Pathology, University of Toronto, Toronto, Ontario, Canada.

S. RAJALAKSHMI,
PREMA M. RAO,
AND
D. S. R. SARMA

importance of the DNA sequence and its conformation for such interactions, (3) the nature of the resultant structural and functional alterations of these macromolecules, and (4) the mechanisms by which the cell attempts to repair the altered macromolecules in order to restore normal structure and function. In addition, some general considerations regarding the possible relevance of alterations in nucleic acids to the initiation phase of carcinogenesis will be presented.

2. Interaction of Chemical Carcinogens with DNA

2.1. Covalent Interactions

2.1.1. General

Chemical carcinogens consist of organic and inorganic compounds differing widely in their structure and chemical reactivity. However, a common feature of the ultimate reactive form of the carcinogens is their electrophilic nature (Miller, 1970). With the exception of a few, the majority of carcinogens require metabolic activation to generate the electrophiles, which then interact with nucleophilic sites in nucleic acids and other cellular components. This sequence of events has been demonstrated for aromatic amines, azo dyes, polycyclic hydrocarbons, alkylating agents such as nitrosamines and nitrosamides, and several synthetic and naturally occurring carcinogens. In their reactive forms, most of the carcinogens interact with DNA covalently. It is becoming increasingly evident that covalent linkages can be formed with all of the four base residues in DNA as well as phosphodiester in some instances; but by far the most reactive groups are the purine nitrogens (Fig. 1A, B).

Except for those present at positions 3 and 7, the nitrogen atoms are engaged in either covalent or hydrogen bonding. The N-7 of guanine appears to be the most reactive site, followed by the N-3 and N-7 positions of adenine (Shapiro, 1969). This reactivity of N-7 of guanine has been attributed to its position peripherally in the wide groove of the Watson–Crick model of the DNA double helix in its B form (Reiner and Zamenhof, 1957). In the Z form of DNA recently postulated for the alternating pyrimidine–purine residues, the N-7 position of guanine is exposed outside the helical axis and is readily available to reactants (Wang et al., 1979; Arnott et al., 1980). Another possible basis for the high nucleophilicity of N-7 of guanine is the role of guanine as a hydrogen bond donor. It donates two bonds and accepts only one, thereby generating an increase in electron density over the guanine ring; this in turn may be reflected in the increased reactivity of the N-7 position. The increased nucleophilic activity of N-7 of guanine has also been suggested from wave-mechanical studies (Pullman and Pullman, 1959). It should be pointed out that chemical carcinogens interact at several other positions in the purines and pyrimidines of DNA, although to a considerably lesser degree. To date, interactions at the following sites have

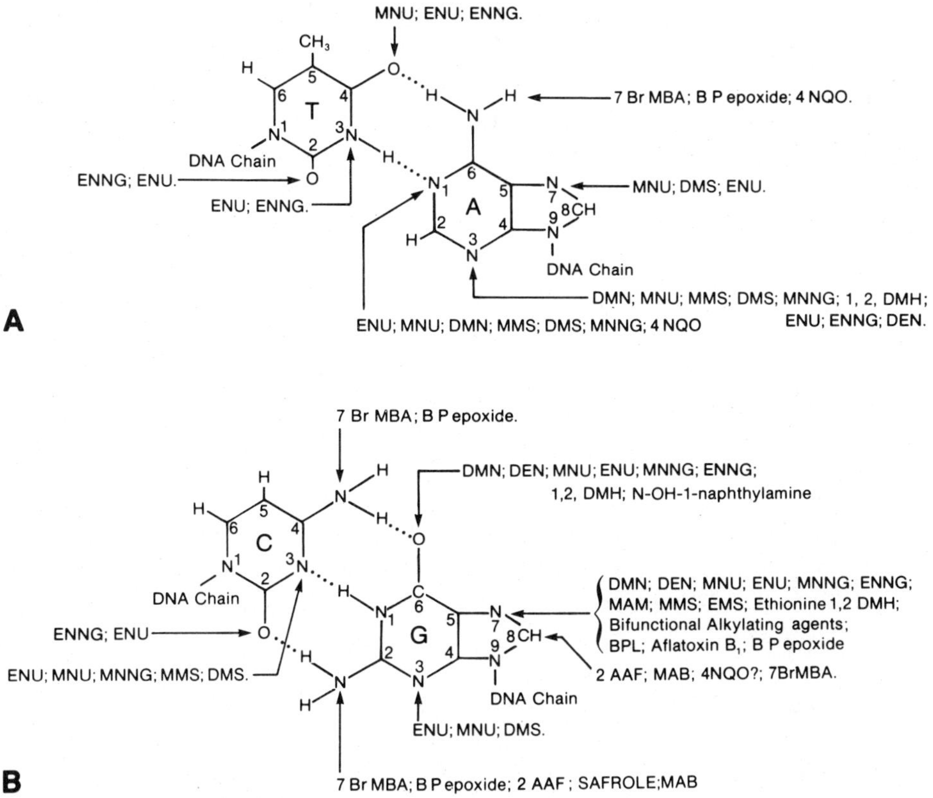

337

INTERAC-
TIONS OF
CARCINOGENS
WITH NUCLEIC
ACIDS

FIGURE 1. Sites of interaction of chemical carcinogens with DNA *in vivo* and *in vitro*.

been reported: N-7, O^6, N-3, 2-NH_2, and C-8 of guanine; 6-NH_2, N-1, N-3, and N-7 of adenine; N-3, 4-NH_2, O^2, and C-5 of cytosine; and O^2 and O^4 of thymine (Fig. 1A, B). Thus, there are very few positions in the four bases of DNA that have not been reported to be attacked by chemical carcinogens *in vivo* or *in vitro*. Much of this work has been reviewed recently (Lawley, 1976; E. C. Miller and Miller, 1971; Irving, 1973; Singer, 1975, 1979).

2.1.2. Alkylating Agents

The alkylating agents are a large and chemically diverse group of compounds that include ethyleneimines, methanesulfonates, epoxides, nitrogen and sulfur mustards, and certain lactones, nitrosamines, and nitrosamides.

There are two generally recognized mechanisms for alkylation, the SN_1 (unimolecular nucleophilic substitution) and SN_2 (bimolecular nucleophilic substitution) reactions (for details on these reactions, refer to Ingold, 1970; Pauling, 1970; Benfey, 1970). In the SN_1 mechanism, the reaction probably proceeds through the formation of a charged intermediate such as methyl or alkyl-diazonium ions (CH_3–N_2^+ or R–N_2^+), which are first attracted to the negatively charged phosphodiester backbone of the nucleic acid; subsequent interaction

S. RAJALAKSHMI,
PREMA M. RAO,
AND
D. S. R. SARMA

with other sites depends mainly on the stability of the diazonium intermediate, its Swain–Scott s value, the n value of the nucleophilic sites (Swain and Scott, 1953), and their steric accessibility to the reagent. In the SN_2 mechanism, the alkylation is governed principally by the nucleophilicity of the sites, the reaction occurring through the formation of a transition complex. In general, the reactivity of a selected methylating agent in the Ingold scheme (Ingold, 1970) increases as the s value decreases, and the relative ability to alkylate the oxygen atom of the bases in DNA (such as O^6 of guanine, O^4 of thymine) increases. Thus, N-nitroso-N-ethylurea (ENU), which has an s value of 0.26, has a higher ratio of O^6:N-7 alkylation of DNA guanine (0.7) than N-nitroso-N-methylurea (MNU), which has an s value of 0.42 and a ratio of O^6:N-7 alkylation of DNA guanine of 0.1. As predicted, methylmethanesulfonate (MMS), with an s value of 0.83, prefers the highly nucleophilic site N-7 compared to O^6 of DNA guanine and yields a ratio of O^6:N-7 alkylation of DNA guanine of 0.004 (Lawley, 1974; Lawley and Warren, 1975; Osterman-Golkar *et al.*, 1970; Veleminsky *et al.*, 1970). Similarly the nucleophilic reactivity of oxygen of the phosphodiester group in DNA was smallest for dimethylsulfate (DMS), which has a high s value (0.86) compared to ENU (Swenson and Lawley, 1978). For a more detailed discussion see Lawley (1976).

a. Nitrosamines and Nitrosamides. Among the potent alkylating carcinogens are nitroso compounds. In general, these compounds either are alkylating agents per se (nitrosamides and nitrosamidines) or are converted metabolically to such alkylating species (e.g., nitrosamines). The ultimate alkylating species are most probably carbonium ions (Magee and Schoental, 1964; Druckrey *et al.*, 1967), the nature of which has not been established for certain. It has been suggested that the formation of reactive alkylating species is via the formation of the

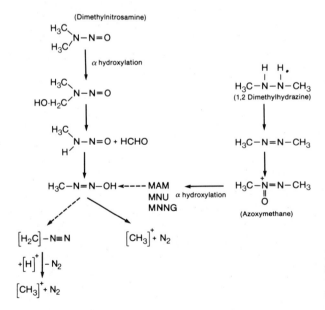

FIGURE 2. Probable mechanisms for the formation of reactive intermediates from some alkylating agents.

corresponding alkyldiazohydroxide, alkyldiazonium cation, and carbonium ion (Fig. 2) (Heath, 1961; Magee and Hultin, 1962). On the contrary, Lijinsky *et al.* (1968), using CD_3-labeled dimethylnitrosamine *in vivo*, have demonstrated that the methyl group enters 7-methylguanine (N-7-MeG) intact. Similar conclusions were reached using N-methyl-N'-nitro-N-nitrosoguanidine (MNNG) and *E. coli* DNA (Lingens *et al.*, 1971) and MNU and salmon sperm DNA (Lawley and Shah, 1973). These results suggest that diazomethane may not be the intermediate.

339

INTERAC-
TIONS OF
CARCINOGENS
WITH NUCLEIC
ACIDS

Unlike dialkylnitrosamines, the nitrosamides and nitrosamidines such as MNU, N-methylnitrosourethan (MNUT), and MNNG do not require enzymatic activation. The decomposition of MNNG to alkyl intermediates is stimulated by thiols (McCalla *et al.*, 1968; Schulz and McCalla, 1969; Lawley and Thatcher, 1970), while that of MNU is not (Lawley, 1972).

The lowest alkyl homologs, dimethylnitrosamine (DMN) and diethylnitrosamine (DEN), produce 7-methyl- and 7-ethylguanine, respectively, as one of the major products (Magee and Farber, 1962; Magee and Barnes, 1967; Swann and Magee, 1971). N-7-MeG has also been detected as the major product in nucleic acids after the administration of $[1-^{14}C]$-di-n-propyl- or $[1-^{14}C]$di-n-butylnitrosamine, but not when DEN or $[2-^{14}C]$di-n-propylnitrosamine is given. This suggests that higher di-n-alkylnitrosamines are metabolically converted to methylalkyl- or dimethylnitrosamine by a pathway analogous to fatty acid degradation. In support of this hypothesis is the *in vivo* formation of N-7-MeG in rat liver DNA and RNA after the administration of the probable intermediates of β-oxidation of di-n-propylnitrosamine such as $[1-^{14}C]$-β-hydroxypropyl propylnitrosamine, $[^3H]$-(2-oxopropyl)propylnitrosamine, and $[methyl-^3H]$ propylnitrosamine (Krüger, 1973; Krüger and Bertram, 1973).

N-7-MeG is not obtained with the cyclic $[2,5-^{14}C]$- and $[3,4-^{14}C]$-N-nitrosopyrrolidine, thus indicating that the hypothesis implicating β-oxidation may not apply to all complex nitroso compounds (Krüger, 1972). However, N-7-MeG was reported by Lee and Lijinsky (1966) to be produced from tritium-labeled nitrosopyrrolidine. Although a number of cyclic nitrosamines such as N-nitrosomorpholine, N-nitrosodihydrouracil, N-nitrosopiperidine, and N,N-nitrosopiperazine are carcinogens, very little is known about the mechanism of action of these agents or the nature of their interaction with nucleic acids. Circumstantial evidence indicates that with N-nitrosomorpholine (Stewart and Magee, 1972) and with N-nitrosopyrrolidine (Krüger, 1972), ring opening occurs and one or more derivatives are formed which interact with nucleic acids.

Alkylating agents in general, be they methylating or ethylating, produce 7-alkylguanine as the major alkylated base in DNA (Table 1). The quantitative and qualitative nature of the alkylation products vary with the agent, the type of DNA (single or double strand), and the source of DNA used. For example, very little guanine methylated at O^6 is found with MMS, while approximately 6% of the methylation with DMN or MNU is at this position.

Formation of phosphotriesters as a result of interaction between DNA and alkylating agents has been demonstrated (Elmore *et al.*, 1948; Stacey *et al.*,

TABLE 1

Patterns of Methylation of DNA in Intact Cells or in Isolated DNA by Methylating Agents[a]

Product	MMS in vitro	DMS In vitro	DMS In vivo	MNNG In vitro	MNNG In vivo	MNU in vitro	DMN in vivo	MAM acetate In vitro	MAM acetate In vivo
				Molar percentage of methylation of DNA by					
N-7-MeG	78–91[b]	76[c]	71–84[c]	67–76[c]	70–71[c]	Major product[c]	77–82[d]	Major product[e]	Major product[f] 61[g]
N-3-MeG	0.68[h]	1[i] (poly-G)		2[i] (poly-G)		1[i]	0.3–1.0[j]		
O-6-MeG	0.32[h]						6[j,k]		
N-1-MeA	ND[j]	0.2[c]	0.5–1[c]	6–7[c]	6[c]	7[i]	1.2–7[d,j]		
N-3-MeA	1–5[b]	3[c]	11–15[c]	1[c]	1[c]		2.6–9[d,j]		
N-1-MeC	8–20[b]	15–19[c]	1[b]	3–12[c]	7[c]		1–7		
O-4-MeT	1[b]	2[c]		2[c]	2[c]	Small concn[l]			
Phosphotriester	≦1[n]					18[m]			

[a] In vitro signifies reaction with isolated DNA (e.g., salmon sperm or calf thymus). In vivo signifies reaction with DNA in an intact cell. The cells used varied considerably—E. coli, T bacteriophages, rat liver (intact animal), hamster embryo cells, and mouse L cells.

[b] Lawley and Brookes (1963).
[c] Lawley et al. (1971–1972).
[d] Lawley et al. (1968).
[e] Matsumoto and Higa (1966).
[f] Shank and Magee (1967).
[g] Nagata and Matsumoto (1969).
[h] Lawley and Shah (1972).
[i] Lawley and Thatcher (1970).
[j] O'Connor et al. (1973).
[k] Craddock (1973).
[l] Lawley et al. (1973).
[m] Lawley (1973).
[n] Bannon and Verly (1972).

1957–1958; Rhaese and Freese, 1969; Walker and Ewart, 1973; Lawley, 1973; Shooter and Merrifield, 1976). Lett *et al.* (1962) have suggested that alkylating agents react primarily with phosphates in DNA and have presented spectrophotometric evidence for transalkylation from triester phosphates to bases in the DNA. It appears that the alkylation of phosphodiesters, like alkylation of O^6 of guanine, is associated mainly with the alkylating agents that are of the SN_1 type. For example, it has been shown that with MNU and ethylmethanesulfonate (EMS), 19 and 15% of DNA alkylation is on the phosphate, while with MMS only 1% is on the phosphate (Bannon and Verly, 1972; Lawley, 1973).

341

INTERAC-
TIONS OF
CARCINOGENS
WITH NUCLEIC
ACIDS

Ethylating agents differ markedly from methylating agents in their affinities for specific sites. When nucleic acids are interacted with ENU, approximately 80% of the ethyl groups are on the oxygens. Of these, 50–60% are ethyl substitutions on oxygens of either purines or pyrimidines irrespective of whether the alkylation was carried out *in vitro* with isolated nucleic acids, or with cells in culture, or *in vivo* with the intact animal (Singer, 1979). Interestingly, the pattern of alkylation also appears to be independent of both the extent of alkylation as well as the secondary structure of DNA (single or double stranded), except that N-1 of adenine and N-3 of cytosine are much less reactive in double-stranded DNA.

b. β-Propiolactone. β-Propiolactone is a highly strained four-member carcinogenic lactone that does not require metabolic activation (Walpole *et al.*, 1954). The hydrolysis product, β-hydroxypropionic acid, is not carcinogenic, thus indicating the need for an intact lactone ring for carcinogenesis (Dickens and Jones, 1963). Roberts and Warwick (1963) have shown that β-propiolactone interacts with RNA to yield 7-(2-carboxyethyl)guanine. Similar products have been obtained by interaction of β-propiolactone with mouse skin DNA (Boutwell *et al.*, 1969).

c. 1,2-Dimethylhydrazine. 1,2-Dimethylhydrazine (1,2-DMH) is carcinogenic to rat colon and rectum (Preussmann *et al.*, 1967; Druckrey *et al.*, 1967). This compound requires metabolic activation, and it is probably via the intermediates azomethane, azoxymethane, and methylazoxymethanol (MAM) (Fiala *et al.*, 1976, 1978) that it eventually yields carbonium ions (Fig. 2), which interact with DNA to give several methylated products including O^6-methylguanine (O^6-MeG) in DNA of both colon and liver of mice and rats (Hawks *et al.*, 1972; Swenberg *et al.*, 1979; Pegg, 1978a).

d. Methylazoxymethanol. Cycasin, a naturally occurring carcinogen, is the β-glucoside of MAM (Laqueur and Spatz, 1968). On oral administration, cycasin is hydrolyzed by bacterial β-glucosidase in the intestine to yield the ultimate carcinogen, MAM, which may be further metabolized (Schoental, 1973) to methylazoxyformaldehyde by alcohol dehydrogenase (Grab and Zedeck, 1977). Nonenzymatic methylation of DNA by MAM has been demonstrated, and the major reaction product is *N*-7-MeG (Matsumoto and Higa, 1966; Nagasawa *et* al., 1972). A similar pattern of alkylation of DNA by MAM and DMN was observed in the intact rat (Shank and Magee, 1967). It has been suggested that MAM may yield a methyldiazonium ion (Nagasawa et al., 1972), which on losing nitrogen yields a carbonium ion (Fig. 2).

e. *Azoxymethane.* Like 1,2-DMH, azoxymethane is a colon carcinogen (Druckrey, 1970). This agent may undergo enzymatic α-hydroxylation to yield MAM (Druckrey, 1972; Fiala et al., 1976, 1978) (Fig. 2).

f. *Urethan.* Urethan (ethylcarbamate), an aliphatic amide, is a multipotent carcinogen (Mirvish, 1968) and a "promoting" agent (Kawamoto et al., 1958; Berenblum and Trainin, 1960). Urethan requires metabolic activation, and the initial step may be N-hydroxylation to form N-hydroxyurethan, which may in turn be esterified. The ester may result in the formation of an ethoxycarboxylating agent and by subsequent loss of carbon dioxide may form the ethylating species (Nery, 1968, 1969; Williams and Nery, 1971). Administration of $[1\text{-}^{14}C]$ ethylcarbamate or $[carboxy\text{-}^{14}C]$ethylcarbamate results in the formation of a single radioactive compound in the RNA of mouse liver, which has been identified as the ethyl ester of cytosine-5-carboxylate (Boyland and Williams, 1969). It is not clear whether such a compound is formed in the DNA of urethan-treated animals. Several unidentified labeled components have been detected in the DNA of rats following the administration of $[1\text{-}^{14}C]$- or $[2\text{-}^{3}H]$urethan (Prodi et al., 1970a). Lawson and Pound (1973a) had suggested that the bound molecule does not contain the carbonyl carbon but probably only the ethyl group. Evidence in support of this was presented by Pound et al. (1976) by analyzing the ratio of $C^{12}\text{-}O^{18}O^{16}/C^{12}O^{16}O^{16}$ in CO_2 following decomposition of administered $C_2H_5\text{-}O^{18}\text{-}CONH_2$ and by identifying the DNA-bound radioactivity following administration of $^{14}C_2H_5 \cdot CONH_2$. The ethyl group was found neither on purine nor on pyrimidine residues of DNA but on phosphates.

g. *Ethionine.* Ethionine, the ethyl analog of methionine, is a hepatocarcinogen (Farber, 1963). Administration of large doses of ethionine results in the ethylation of rat liver DNA (Stekol, 1965), and the major product appears to be N-7-ethylguanine (Swann et al., 1971; Cox and Farber, 1972). *In vivo*, ethionine is metabolized in a manner similar to that of methionine yielding S-adenosyl-ethionine, which can substitute for S-adenosylmethionine in several reactions. Since N-7-MeG has not been found in normal DNA, Swann et al. (1971) suggested that ethylation of DNA by ethionine may not be mediated by a methyltransferase using S-adenosyl-L-ethionine as the ethyl-group donor.

h. *Nitrogen and Sulfur Mustards.* There are a great variety of mono- and bifunctional derivatives of nitrogen and sulfur mustards. Elmore et al. (1948) and later Alexander (1952) observed that mustard gas esterifies the primary phosphate groups of DNA. Bifunctional alkylating agents can interact with two nucleophilic centers, especially N-7 of two guanines, to form a bridge between them. The covalent cross-linking of DNA can be intra- or interstrand or between two separate duplex sturctures. Denatured DNA yields a lower proportion of diguaninyl product than does double-stranded DNA (Brookes and Lawley, 1961), thus suggesting that such a product arises preferentially from interstrand rather than intrastrand cross-linking. About 25% of the guanine alkylations in DNA by mustard gas is the diguaninyl product (Brookes and Lawley, 1961), the amount varying with the GC content of DNA (Lawley, 1966). For example, DNA from *Pseudomonas aeruginosa* (GC 67%) gave 26% diguaninyl product, that from *Escherichia coli* (GC 50%) gave 20%, and that from *Bacillis cereus* (GC 34%) 13%.

343

INTERAC-
TIONS OF
CARCINOGENS
WITH NUCLEIC
ACIDS

2.1.3. Aromatic Amines and Amides

a. 2-Acetylaminofluorene and Related Compounds. Aromatic amines and amides in general and 2-acetylaminofluorene (2-AAF) in particular require metabolic activation for their interaction with DNA; the initial step is a conversion to the *N*-hydroxy derivative followed by an esterification of the *N*-hydroxy derivative (Miller, 1970; Irving, 1970; Weisburger and Weisburger, 1973).

Glucuronide (Irving *et al.*, 1969; Irving and Russell, 1970) and sulfate (DeBaun *et al.*, 1970; Weisburger *et al.*, 1972) esters of *N*-hydroxy-2-AAF as well as nonenzymatic acylation of *N*-hydroxy-2-AAF by acetyl coenzyme A, carbamoylphosphate, or acetylphosphate have been demonstrated (Lotlikar and Luha, 1971*a, b*). It is not clear which of these esters is involved in the *in vivo* binding of *N*-hydroxy-2-AAF with DNA of the target tissue or in the induction of tumors. Thus, although the sulfate conjugate of *N*-hydroxy-2-AAF has been implicated in the induction of liver cancer by 2-AAF in rats (DeBaun *et al.*, 1970), *N*-hydroxy-2-AAF sulfotransferase activity is not detectable in two other tissues of rat susceptible to carcinogenesis by *N*-hydroxy-2-AAF: Zymbal's gland (the sebaceous gland of the external auditory canal) and the mammary gland (Irving *et al.*, 1971). It has been suggested that the glucuronide conjugate of *N*-hydroxy-2-AAF is involved in the binding of the carcinogen to rat liver DNA (Irving *et al.*, 1969; Irving, 1971; Irving and Russell, 1970), although this has by no means been established *in vivo*. Involvement of *O*-acetyl derivatives in the production of carcinogenic metabolites has also been suggested (King and Phillips, 1972; Bartsch *et al.*, 1972; King *et al.*, 1979). Furthermore, Weeks *et al.* (1978) reported that the metabolic events involved in the production of a mutagenic derivative of *N*-hydroxy-2-AAF in *Salmonella* may be different from those involved in the production of electrophilic chemical species that are believed to be involved in the carcinogenic process. The covalent interaction between the active derivative of *N*-hydroxy-2-AAF and DNA *in vivo* occurs at the C-8 position (Irving and Veazey, 1969) as well as the 2-NH_2 position of guanine; the major product (80%) is *N*-(deoxyguanosine-8-yl)-2-fluorenylacetamide (Kriek *et al.*, 1967), and the minor adduct has recently been identified as 3-(guanine-N^2-yl)-2-AAF (Kriek, 1974; Westra *et al.*, 1976).

Based on studies utilizing circular dichroism, proton magnetic resonance spectroscopy, and computer-generated molecular models of oligonucleotides

S. RAJALAKSHMI,
PREMA M. RAO,
AND
D. S. R. SARMA

containing bound 2-AAF, Nelson *et al.* (1971) suggested an interesting model for the interaction of 2-AAF with DNA. After interaction with 2-AAF, the guanine base rotates around the glycosidic bond at N-9, allowing an interaction of the fluorene compounds with the adjacent base in the nucleotide chain, thus producing a type of intercalation. One would anticipate localized regions of denaturation of the DNA at some sites of interaction with 2-AAF; the regions of denatured DNA observed in the electron microscopic studies of Epstein *et al.* (1969–1970) might well be gross manifestations of such an effect on DNA.

b. Naphthylamines. Several arylamines and arylamides are carcinogenic to the urinary bladder, liver, and other tissues of humans and experimental animals (see review by Clayson and Garner, 1976). The initial step in their activation is the formation of N-hydroxy derivatives, which are generally more carcinogenic than their corresponding parent compounds. One of the sites of interaction of N-hydroxy-1-naphthylamine is the O^6 position of guanine, and two products have been identified: a major adduct N-(deoxyguanosin-O^6-yl)- and a minor adduct 2-(deoxyguanosin-O^6-yl)-1-naphthylamine (Kadlubar *et al.*, 1978). In the urothelial and liver DNA of male beagle dogs administered 2-naphthylamine (2-NA), three DNA adducts have been characterized as 1-(deoxyguanosin-N^2-yl)-2-NA, 1-(deoxyadenosin-N^6-yl)-2-NA, and N-(deoxyguanosin-8-yl)-2-NA (Kadlubar *et al.*, 1980).

c. p-Dimethylaminoazobenzene and Derivatives. Relatively little is known about the mechanism involved in the binding of azo dyes to DNA *in vivo.* The Millers and co-workers have proposed that the activation of carcinogenic azo dyes may be similar to the activation of other aromatic amines (Poirier *et al.*, 1967; J. A. Miller and Miller, 1969). The activation of 4-dimethylaminoazobenzene (DAB) may involve the following steps: (1) mono$N$-demethylation, (2) N-hydroxylation, and (3) conjugation as a sulfate ester (Poirier *et al.*, 1967) or transacetylation (Bartsch *et al.*, 1972). In the case of ring-methylated azo dyes such as 3'-methyl-DAB, hydroxylation of the ring-methyl group followed by conjugation (e.g., as sulfate) may occur. This may lead to the formation of a carbonium ion by a route analogous to that hypothesized for methylated polycyclic aromatic hydrocarbons (Dipple, 1972). Roberts and Warwick (1961), using N,N'-dimethyl-4-aminoazobenzene labeled with tritium in the prime or aniline ring, have observed a low level of incorporation of tritium into rat liver DNA. More recently, Miller *et al.* (1970), using tritiated N-methyl-4-aminoazobenzene (radioactivity in the prime ring) and rat liver DNA, have isolated a product chromatographically identical to N-(deoxyguanosin-8-yl)-N-methyl-4-aminoazobenzene.

It is of interest to note that the binding of the weakly carcinogenic azo dye 2-methyl-DAB, following a single administration, is higher than can be obtained with the carcinogen DAB (Warwick, 1969). However, on continuous feeding, the level of binding of 2-methyl-DAB to liver DNA is somewhat lower than in the case of DAB (Roberts, 1969). 2-Methyl-DAB has been reported to induce liver cancer when fed to animals subjected to partial hepatectomy (Warwick, 1967).

345

INTERAC-
TIONS OF
CARCINOGENS
WITH NUCLEIC
ACIDS

*d. o-Aminoazotoluene. o-*Aminoazotoluene is the first azo dye shown to induce liver cancer in rats (Sasaki and Yoshida, 1935). Intragastric administration of tritiated *o*-aminoazotoluene to C57 mice results in liver DNA with covalently bound radioactivity (Lawson and Clayson, 1969). The nature of the interaction is not yet clearly established.

2.1.4. *Polycyclic Aromatic Hydrocarbons*

Since the first suggestion by Bergmann (1942) that in addition to aromaticity, geometry of the molecule is involved in hydrocarbon carcinogenicity, intercalation and other noncovalent interactions between DNA and certain planar polycyclic hydrocarbons such as benzo[*a*]pyrene (BP) and 3-methylcholanthrene (3-MC) have been suggested (Iball and MacDonald, 1960). This type of interaction may take place to a lesser extent with nonplanar compounds such as 7,12-dimethylbenz[*a*]anthracene (7,12-DMBA).

More recently, some polycyclic aromatic hydrocarbons have been shown to interact covalently with DNA following microsomal activation (Gelboin, 1969; Grover and Sims, 1968). Several suggestions have been advanced regarding the nature of the metabolically active intermediate(s) involved in the binding to DNA: (1) the formation of a radical cation, as a result of oxidation of the hydrocarbon (see Wilk and Girke, 1969), and (2) formation of K-region epoxides, e.g., 5,6-epoxydibenz[*a*]anthracene (Selkirk *et al.*, 1971) or 4,5-epoxide of 3,4-BP (Grover *et al.*, 1971*a*). Although the K-region epoxides interact with DNA to a greater extent than do the parent hydrocarbons (Grover and Sims, 1970; Grover *et al.*, 1971*b*; Kuroki *et al.*, 1971–1972), they have very little carcinogenic activity in mice or rats (see E. C. Miller and Miller, 1971). It may be pointed out, however, that they are mutagenic in several systems including mammalian cells in culture (Huberman *et al.*, 1971; Cookson *et al.*, 1971) and cause malignant transformation of cells in culture (Grover *et al.*, 1971*b*).

One of the advances in recent years is the finding that the critical or oncogenic metabolite of BP is not just a simple oxide (K-region) as it was thought to be, but a dihydrodiol epoxide ($\pm$)-7β, 8α-dihydroxy-9α,10α-epoxy-7,8,9,10-tetrahydrobenzo[*a*]pyrene (Kapitulnik *et al.*, 1977; Huberman *et al.*, 1976; Slaga *et al.*, 1977). The predominant RNA and DNA adduct present in human cells exposed to BP is formed by covalent linkage of the amino group at the 2 position of the guanine to the 10 position of a specific isomer, (+)-7β,8α-dihydroxy-9α,10α-epoxy-7,8,9,10-tetrahydrobenzo[*a*]pyrene (Jeffrey *et al.*, 1977). The adduct has also been detected in rodent cell cultures (Shinohara and Cerutti, 1977; Ivanovic *et al.*, 1978) and in mouse skin (Koreeda *et al.*, 1978), and its stereo chemistry has been elucidated (Nakanishi *et al.*, 1977). Lesser amounts of N^2-substituted deoxyguanosine adducts derived from ($\pm$)-7β,8α-dihydroxy-9β,10β-epoxy-7,8,9,10-tetrahydrobenzo[*a*]pyrene have also been detected *in vivo* (Cerutti *et*

S. RAJALAKSHMI,
PREMA M. RAO,
AND
D. S. R. SARMA

al., 1978), and there is indirect evidence for the reaction of BP diol epoxide at the N-7 position of guanine (Osborne *et al.*, 1978) and with phosphates of the DNA backbone (Koreeda *et al.*, 1978). *In vitro* studies with BP diol epoxide have revealed that under particular conditions there can be significant reactions with adenine and to a lesser extent with cytosine residues in synthetic homopolymers, RNA and DNA (Jennette *et al.*, 1977; Jeffrey *et al.*, 1979). The selective interaction of BP diol epoxide $7\beta,8\alpha$-dihydroxy-$9\alpha,10\alpha$-epoxy-7,8,9,10-tetrahydrobenzo[*a*]pyrene with the deoxyguanosine residues using SV40 DNA was demonstrated by Mengle *et al.* (1978).

Although these interactions are well demonstrated, the modification of nucleic acid by BP is considerably complicated since multiple isomers and enantiomers of BP diol epoxide exist and there can be both *cis* and *trans* attack during interaction with DNA. Future work may prove that interaction with DNA will depend on the cell type in which metabolism occurs (Ivanovic *et al.*, 1978) as well as the environment in which DNA exists and the conformation of DNA at the time of interaction. For example, Hsu *et al.* (1979) found that the diol derivative of BP interacts preferentially with single-stranded DNA, whereas the diol epoxide interacts with both single- and double-stranded DNA and RNA equally. Furthermore, these derivatives exhibit marked differences in their capacity to complex with specific deoxyhomopolymers, e.g., poly-dI. These observations suggest that the diol and diol epoxide derivatives and their isomers and enantiomers recognize different binding sites in nucleic acids. The results of Meehan and Straub (1979) demonstrate that the asymmetrical binding of the two enantiomeric *anti*-BP diol epoxides to the exocyclic amino group of guanine in double-stranded DNA is dependent on the secondary structure of the polymer. It is suggested that the ability of the secondary structure of DNA to distinguish two enantiomeric molecules is by stereoselective physical interaction, possibly intercalation, before covalent binding. In this study the interaction was studied with optically pure hydrocarbon after resolving the $(\pm)$-*anti*-BP diol epoxide using calf thymus and ϕX174 DNA.

Another mode of activation has been suggested for the methylated aromatic hydrocarbons such as 7,12-DMBA, some of which are potent carcinogens (Huggins *et al.*, 1964). The first probable step involved in such activation is oxidation to hydroxymethyl derivatives (Boyland and Sims, 1965; Sims and Grover, 1968) followed by esterification of the hydroxymethyl group. The model compounds 7-bromomethylbenz[*a*]anthracene [7-BrMeBA) and 7-bromomethyl-12-methylbenz[*a*]anthracene (7-BrMe-12-MeBA) react *in vitro* with DNA yielding several substitution products at the 2-amino group of guanine, the 6-amino group of adenine, and to a lesser extent the 4-amino group of cytosine (Dipple *et al.*, 1971). Substitution at the C-8 position of guanine has also been demonstrated (Pochon and Michelson, 1971). It may be noted that the model bromomethyl compounds are weak carcinogens (Dipple and Slade, 1970).

Ts'o *et al.* (1969), using *in vitro* conditions, studied the nature of the binding of benzopyrenes and other polycyclic hydrocarbons to DNA. They have reasoned that polycyclic hydrocarbon molecules bind to DNA by hydrophobic-stacking interaction in a face-to-face mode. If the system is properly activated either by supplying radiation energy or through free radical formation, the bases of DNA and polycyclic hydrocarbons may form covalent bonds.

347
INTERAC-
TIONS OF
CARCINOGENS
WITH NUCLEIC
ACIDS

Photoactivation of a mixture of thymine and 3,4-BP yields a photoproduct in which 3,4-BP is joined through a single covalent bond to C-6 of thymine (Blackburn *et al.*, 1972); whether a similar reaction occurs in DNA is not known. There is no a priori reason to believe that a single mechanism of activation operates in all tissues with all aromatic hydrocarbons. In general, one can visualize two types of interactions either separately or in combination: (1) complex formation with DNA, most probably by intercalation, particularly with planar compounds such as BP and 3-MC and to a lesser extent with nonplanar compounds such as 7,12-DMBA; and (2) covalent interaction with DNA after suitable activation *in vivo*. The latter pathway is probably the predominant one *in vivo*.

2.1.5. 4-Nitroquinoline-N-Oxide

4-Nitroquinoline-*N*-oxide (4NQO) and some of its derivatives are multipotent carcinogens (Nakahara *et al.*, 1957; Kawazoe *et al.*, 1969). Activated 4NQO or uncharacterized derivatives of 4NQO have been found to interact with DNA (Tada *et al.*, 1967; Matsushima *et al.*, 1967; Tada and Tada, 1971, 1976). Several probable mechanisms of interaction of 4NQ0 with DNA have been postulated. These are:

1. Reduction to the hydroxyamino derivatives (Kato and Takalashi, 1970) mediated by the diaphorase as shown in both bacterial and rat liver systems (Sugimura *et al.*, 1966; Fukuda and Yamamoto, 1972). 4-Hydroxyamino-quinoline-*N*-oxide (4OHAQO) by itself may not be the ultimate carcinogen, but free radicals produced from oxidation products (Nagata *et al.*, 1966; Ishizawa and Endo, 1967; Kosuge *et al.*, 1969) or from diesters (Araki *et al.*, 1969; Enomoto *et al.*, 1968) may be involved in the binding of DNA. Also, an ATP-requiring enzymatic acylation of 4OHAQO to yield the proximate carcinogen has been suggested (Tada and Tada, 1972).
2. Conversion to a nitroso intermediate, 4-nitrosoquinoline-1-oxide, as shown by Matsuyama and Nagata (1972) using a rapid-scan spectrophotometer. This may be an important reactive product in the interaction of 4NQO and 4OHAQO with DNA as well as in their carcinogenecity.
3. Formation of a carbonium ion through the intermediate formation of nitrous acid, which can react with primary amines *in vivo* to form diazonium ions (Kawazoe *et al.*, 1972). In bacteria as well as mammalian cells in culture, the covalent binding of 4NQO to purine residues in DNA and RNA yields 3-(N^6-adenyl)-4-aminoquinoline-1-oxide or 3(N-1-adenyl-4-aminoquino-line-1-oxide) (Kawazoe *et al.*, 1976).

Recently, a two-step binding mechanism for 4NQO has been postulated according to which intercalation of 4NQO or its metabolite precedes the covalent bond

348

S. RAJALAKSHMI,
PREMA M. RAO,
AND
D. S. R. SARMA

formation between the ultimate carcinogenic form and DNA. A complete empirical potential energy description of the base-sequence and metabolite specificities of the 4NQO interaction depicting the important force and structural interaction via decomposed energy functions (Ornstein and Rein, 1979) is presented.

2.1.6. Nitrofurans and Derivatives

Nitrofurans and their derivatives have been clinically used as antibacterial agents (Paul and Paul, 1964). They have been shown to be powerful carcinogens (Ertürk et al., 1971). In analogy to nitroaromatic carcinogens, such as 4NQO, reduction of the nitro group to a hydroxylamino derivative appears to be a necessary metabolic activation step for their interaction with macromolecules as well as for their carcinogenic property (Miura and Reckendorf, 1967; McCalla et al., 1971; Cohen et al., 1973). The nature of the interaction of these derivatives with nucleic acids has not been completely established.

2.1.7. Aflatoxin B_1

The aflatoxins are a group of naturally occurring compounds, some of which are highly carcinogenic for liver and other organs (Lancaster et al., 1961). These compounds apparently require metabolic activation prior to their reaction with DNA. Liver cells in culture convert aflatoxin B_1 (AFB_1) to a more potent cytotoxin (Scaife, 1970–1971). Garner et al. (1971) have reported that rat liver microsomes, in the presence of NADPH and oxygen, convert AFB_1 to a highly toxic product lethal to certain strains of S. typhimurium, and their data suggest that epoxidation at the 1,2-double bond might be involved in the in vivo activation of this compound. Microsomal-dependent binding of AFB_1 to DNA and RNA in vitro has been demonstrated (Garner, 1973; Swenson et al., 1973), and the aflatoxin B_1-2,3-oxide appears to be the reactive intermediate in the formation of the RNA–AFB_1 adduct (Swenson et al., 1973).

Recently, the DNA-bound aflatoxin adduct has been characterized using DNA interacted with AFB_1 in vivo and in vitro (Essigmann et al., 1977; Lin et al., 1977; Martin and Garner, 1977). The adduct was identified as 2,3-dihydro-2-(N-7-guanyl)-3-hydroxy-AFB_1. D'Andrea and Haseltine (1978) by modifying a DNA fragment of known sequence, containing the lactose promoter operator region, with activated AFB_1 and sequencing the modified DNA showed that AFB_1 induces alkali labile lesions primarily at guanine residues and to a minor extent with adenine residues. AFB_1 apparently reacts with the same guanines that were methylatable by DMS.

2.1.8. Safrole

Safrole, a component isolated from sassafras oil, is primarily a hepatocarcinogen. It has been shown that rat and mouse liver postmitochondrial supernatant, in the presence of NADPH, oxidizes safrole to 1'hydroxysafrole (Wislocki et al., 1973). Administration of $[2',3'-^3H]1'$-hydroxysafrole to rats yields tritium-labeled hepatic DNA (Wislocki *et al.*, 1973). One of the adducts of 1'-hydroxysafrole formed with mouse liver DNA *in vivo* has been characterized as N^2-(*trans*-isosafrol-3'-yl)deoxyguanasine (Phillips *et al.*, 1981).

349
INTERAC-
TIONS OF
CARCINOGENS
WITH NUCLEIC
ACIDS

2.1.9. Vinyl Chloride

The biological fate of vinyl chloride in relation to its carcinogenic and mutagenic effects has been elucidated (Green and Hathway, 1975; Bartsch and Montesano, 1975). Although epoxidation of vinyl chloride has been predicted (Salmon, 1976; Barbin *et al.*, 1975; Kappus *et al.*, 1976; Gothe *et al.*, 1976), convincing evidence has been reported only recently (Green and Hathway, 1977) for the *in vivo* participation of chloroethylene oxide and its chloroacetaldehyde rearrangement product. These two vinyl chloride metabolites are mutagens in the Ames test (Bartsch *et al.*, 1975; Malaveille *et al.*, 1975; McCann *et al.*, 1975) and in mammalian cells in culture (Huberman *et al.*, 1975). 9β-D-2'-Deoxyribofuranosyl-imidazo[2,1-*i*]purine ("etheno-deoxyadenosine") and 1β-D-2'-deoxyribofuranosyl-1,2-dihydro-2-oxoimidazo[1,2-*c*]pyrimidine ("etheno-deoxycytidine") have been identified in the enzyme hydrolysates of calf thymus DNA modified chemically with chloroacetaldehyde and from liver DNA of rats that had been administered vinyl chloride in drinking water for 2 years. Thus, vinyl chloride-derived metabolites (chloroethylene oxide and/or chloroacetaldehyde) behave as bifunctional alkylating agents toward deoxyadenosine and deoxycytidine residues of DNA (Green and Hathway, 1978).

2.2. Noncovalent Interactions

Noncovalent interactions can be broadly divided into two groups: (1) internal binding or intercalation, wherein the carcinogen is inserted between base pairs of the DNA duplex structure (Fig. 3), and (2) external binding, or adlineation,

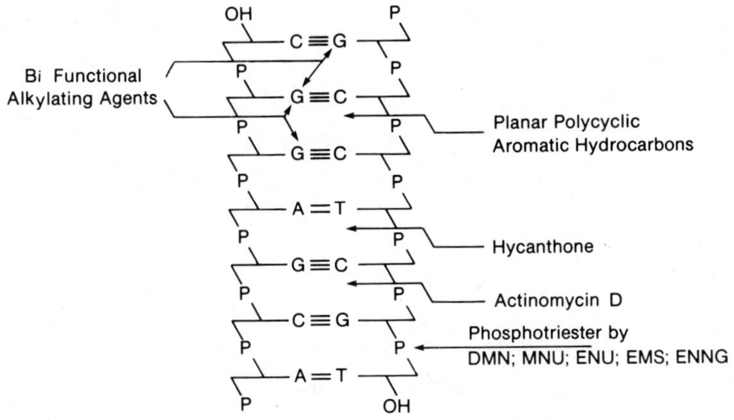

FIGURE 3. Schematic representation of chemical carcinogen–DNA interaction showing intercalation and inter- and intrastrand cross-linking.

wherein the agent interacts with bases at sites that are not involved in base pairing. In the latter event and in contrast to intercalation, the carcinogen binds perpendicular to the planes of the bases (Arcos and Argus, 1968).

2.2.1. Intercalation

Lerman (1964) postulated the intercalation model to explain the binding of acridine to DNA and the resultant frameshift mutations. Since then, this mechanism has been suggested to explain the binding of several drugs, antibiotics, alkaloids, and some carcinogens to DNA, a detailed discussion of which is presented by Hahn (1971). The primary requisite for intercalation is a suitable molecular geometry, planar compounds in general intercalating most easily. The ability of some carcinogens such as planar polycyclic aromatic hydrocarbons, hycanthone, and actinomycin D to intercalate into DNA has been studied *in vitro*. However, caution must be used in extrapolating these data to the intact animal or organism, since intercalation depends on many variables including the state of DNA.

The DNA in the nucleus is in a more compact or condensed form than it is in the purified state, and intercalation *in vivo* may therefore be less than in a more extended molecule. For example, within 10–70 min following the addition of phytohemagglutinin to lymphocytes, the binding of acridine orange is about four times that obtained before phytohemagglutinin treatment (Lerman, 1971), presumably due to an altered state of the DNA in the treated lymphocytes. Another interesting example is the binding to DNA of hycanthone, an intercalating agent that is used in the treatment of schistosomiasis. Hepatic DNA from rats treated with hycanthone methanesulfonate did not show any increase in T_m (Sarma *et al.*, 1977), in contrast to its effect on DNA *in vitro* where an obvious increase in T_m is observed (Weinstein and Hirschberg, 1971; Sarma *et al.*, 1977). This intercalating drug is a carcinogen in mice infected with schistosomiasis (Haese *et al.*, 1973) or subjected to partial hepatectomy (Tsuda *et al.*, 1979).

Intercalation has been suggested as a mechanism for the binding to DNA of planar carcinogenic polycyclic aromatic hydrocarbons such as 3,4-BP and 3-MC (Boyland, 1969; Liquori *et al.*, 1962; Ts'o *et al.*, 1969). However, this postulate is controversial (Giovanella *et al.*, 1964; Van Duuren *et al.*, 1968–1969).

Actinomycin D, a weak carcinogen (Kawamata *et al.*, 1958, 1959; DiPaolo, 1960; Svoboda and Reddy, 1970), also appears to intercalate into DNA *in vitro* (Müller and Crothers, 1968; Wells, 1971). Although a good correlation exists between frameshift mutagenicity and intercalation, a convincing correlation between carcinogenicity and extent of intercalation has yet to be established.

2.2.2. External Binding

External binding of several carcinogens, such as 4NQO (Malkin and Zahalsky, 1966; Paul *et al.*, 1971), aflatoxins (Sporn *et al.*, 1966; Clifford and Rees, 1967; Black and Jirgensons, 1967; Schabort, 1971), and polycyclic aromatic hydrocarbons (Arcos and Argus, 1968) with DNA has been suggested. This type of binding is relatively weak compared to that of intercalation, and it is not certain at present whether such binding occurs *in vivo*.

351

INTERAC-
TIONS OF
CARCINOGENS
WITH NUCLEIC
ACIDS

2.3. Purine-N-Oxides

The *N*-oxides of certain purines, such as adenine-1-oxide and 3-oxide derivatives of guanine and xanthine, are oncogenic and induce subcutaneous neoplasms at the site of injection and liver cancer in rats and mice (Sugiiura *et al.*, 1970; Brown *et al.*, 1973). Administration of ^{14}C-labeled 3-hydroxyxanthine does not result in any significant *in vivo* incorporation of radioactivity into adenine or guanine of RNA or DNA (Myles and Brown, 1969). However, 3-hydroxyxanthine induced alkali-sensitive lesions in rat liver DNA *in vivo* (Michael *et al.*, 1975).

2.4. Carcinogenic Metals

Many inorganic metal compounds are known to be carcinogenic. However, very little is known about mechanisms by which neoplasms are induced. By virtue of their being electrophilic cations, Be^{2+}, Cd^{2+}, Co^{2+}, and Ni^{2+} can interact with nucleophilic sites of macromolecules (Miller, 1970). Some of the metal ions are known to react with guanine (Shapiro, 1968) and to interact with phosphate groups of DNA (Eichhorn *et al.*, 1966); others interfere with the stability of the duplex structure by binding to the amino groups of the bases (Furst and Haro, 1969). Carcinogenic metal ions such as Ni^{2+} can depolymerize polynucleotides (Butzow and Eichhorn, 1965). The binding of some metals to the purine and pyrimidine bases can be through covalent bonds or π-electrons of the bases (Fuwa *et al.*, 1960). The nature of the *in vivo* interaction of the carcinogenic metals with nucleic acids remains to be elucidated.

3. Carcinogen–DNA Interactions at the Nucleoprotein Level

In eukaryotes, the DNA exists as a nucleoprotein complex, the chromatin, in which the DNA is associated with a stable complement of histones and a variable complement of nonhistone chromosomal proteins. The basic repeating unit of chromatin is the nucleosome, made up of a core particle of 140 base pairs of DNA associated with two molecules of each of the histones H2A, H2B, H3, and H4. These nucleosome cores are held together by a "spacer" or "linker" DNA strand and the histone H1 (Kornberg, 1977; Felsenfeld, 1978) (Fig. 4). The nonhistone proteins associated with the DNA are a very heterogeneous group and have been implicated in tissue specificity and regulation of gene expression (Wang *et al.*, 1976; Stein *et al.*, 1976).

Experimental evidence shows that although only about 10–15% of the eukaryotic genome is expressed, the nucleosomal structure is present in the transcriptionally active or euchromatin regions as well as in the transcriptionally inactive

S. RAJALAKSHMI,
PREMA M. RAO,
AND
D. S. R. SARMA

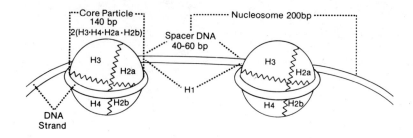

FIGURE 4. Schematic representation of DNA organization in chromatin at the nucleosomal level.

or heterochromatin regions. However, the conformation of the transcriptionally "active" chromatin is different from that of the "inactive" chromatin as judged by its susceptibility to nucleases (Weintraub and Groudine, 1976; Garel and Axel, 1976; Bonner *et al.*, 1975; Bloom and Anderson, 1978) and recognition by RNA polymerases (Silverman and Mirsky, 1973; Gilmour and Paul, 1973; Axel *et al.*, 1975). Furthermore, the euchromatin is characterized by the presence of unique sequences while the heterochromatin is enriched in repetitive sequences. In addition, certain regions such as promoter sequences are rich in AT base pairs. It was therefore not unreasonable to expect that the complexity of the organization of DNA and its conformational state in chromatin would influence the availability of the sites in DNA for interaction with carcinogens as well as repair enzymes. The studies of Segal *et al.* (1974) using β-propiolactone and Metzger and Daune (1975) using *N*-acetoxy-2-AAF had shown that the DNA in chromatin is less available for interaction compared to free DNA. The more important question, however, is whether there is any preferential interaction of carcinogens with different regions of chromatin DNA, e.g., transcribed as compared to nontranscribed. Of the several methods available for the fractionation of chromatin and DNA, only a few have been used to investigate the intragenomic distribution of carcinogens. Some of these are described below.

1. Fractionation of chromatin into core particles and linker regions:

Micrococcal nuclease
(preferentially digests the linker regions or gives limit digests of chromatin DNA)

Noll (1974), Axel (1975), Clark and Felsenfeld (1971)

2. Fractionation of chromatin into transcribable and nontranscribable regions:

DNase I
(under defined conditions digests the transcribable genes or gives limit digests of chromatin DNA)

Weintraub and Groudine (1976),
Garel and Axel (1976), Clark and Felsenfeld (1971)

353

INTERAC-
TIONS OF
CARCINOGENS
WITH NUCLEIC
ACIDS

DNase II   Bonner *et al.* (1975)
   (under defined conditions fractionates
   transcribable from nontranscribable
   genes)

3. Fractionation into eu- and heterochromatin:

Glycerol gradient centrifugation	Rodriguez and Becker (1976), Schwartz and Goodman (1979)
Linear sucrose gradients	Moyer *et al.* (1977)
Selective MgCl$_2$ aggregation	Arnold and Young (1974)
Fractionation on ECTHAM-cellulose	Tew *et al.* (1978)

4. Fractionation of DNA using reassociation kinetics

                     Britten and Kohne (1968)

5. Separation of satellite and main band DNA   Flamm *et al.* (1969)

6. Use of DNA-binding ligands: Rajalakshmi *et al.* (1978*a,b*, 1980)

Spermine (interacts with PO$_4^{2-}$)	Liquori *et al.* (1967)
Distamycin A and Netropsin (interacts with AT base pairs)	Zimmer (1975)
Actinomycin D (interacts preferentially with GC base pairs)	Krugh (1972), Wells and Larson (1970), Sobell *et al.* (1977)

Using the above-mentioned approaches it is observed that carcinogens exhibit a preferential interaction with some regions of DNA in chromatin. A brief discussion of these studies follows.

3.1. Alkylating Agents

3.1.1. Dimethylnitrosamine

Ramanathan *et al.* (1976*a*) fractionated rat liver chromatin DNA, methylated *in vivo* with [*methyl*-^{3}H]-DMN, into nuclease-accessible and -inaccessible regions using DNase I under conditions of limit digest (50% chromatin DNA) and found that 75% of the total methylated products were present in the DNase I-accessible regions of chromatin. The *in vivo* removal of alkylated products was also faster from this region. A further specificity apparently exists in the distribution of the individual alkylated bases; e.g., 72% of *N*-7-MeG was localized in the DNase I-accessible regions (Ramanathan *et al.*, 1976*a*) and O^6-MeG was preferentially released from the DMN-alkylated chromatin in the micrococcal nuclease-soluble fraction (Sarma *et al.*, 1978) suggesting its preferential location in the "spacer" regions. A similar heterogeneous distribution of N-7-MeG was reported by Cooper *et al.* (1975) and by Galbraith *et al.* (1979). Using DNA–DNA reassociation kinetics as a parameter for separating families of repetitive and unique sequences in DMN-methylated rat liver chromatin DNA, Galbraith *et al.* (1978), however, reported a random distribution of N-7-MeG between these classes of DNA. Since the technique only separated families of unique and repetitive sequences, non-random distribution within sequences of a given class was not ruled out. Pegg and Hui (1978) could not find a nonrandom alkylation of chromatin DNA using DMN and concluded that agents like DMN and MNU, which give rise to small, highly reactive, methylating species, are likely to interact randomly. However, this is not borne out by the nonrandom nature of MNU alkylation (see Section 3.1.2). On the other hand, these observed discrepancies could be due to the fact that the methods of fractionating chromatin are still not precise enough; only the location of the alkylated bases in a given nucleotide sequence can provide unequivocal proof for the nonrandomness or otherwise of the intragenomic distribution of alkylated bases.

3.1.2. Nitrosoureas

The interaction of two substituted nitrosoureas, chlorozotocin and 1-(2-chloroethyl)-3-cyclohexyl-1-nitrosourea, with HeLa cell chromatin and nucleosomal fractions was studied by Tew *et al.* (1978). Using ECTHAM-cellulose columns to fractionate HeLa cell chromatin into early- and late-eluting fractions, representing eu- and heterochromatins, the radioactivity from the two nitrosoureas was found to be preferentially located in the euchromatin fractions. Digestion of the alkylated chromatin with DNase I also showed that the interaction was greater in the transcriptionally active DNA in chromatin. Treatment of the cells with sodium butyrate (which increases the transcriptional activity of chromatin) prior to exposure to the nitrosoureas resulted in an increased alkylation of these fractions. Digestion of the labeled nuclei with micrococcal nuclease revealed that both compounds preferentially alkylated the nucleosomal core particle DNA. In contrast, MNU was found to interact more with the internucleosomal linker DNA than the core particle DNA (Sudhakar *et al.*, 1979). A similar nonrandom methylation by MNU in rat brain chromatin DNA was reported by Cox (1979). The specific activities of N-7-MeG and O^6-MeG were 4–5 times higher in the DNase I-sensitive fractions than in the DNase I-resistant fractions. The rate of loss of these products was also found to be faster from the nuclease-sensitive fractions.

3.2. Aromatic Amines

The most studied compound is 2-AAF and its derivatives N-hydroxy-2-AAF and N-acetoxy-2-AAF. The intragenomic distribution of 2-AAF (or its derivatives) binding in chromatin DNA has been studied both *in vivo* and *in vitro* using different procedures for fractionating chromatin.

355

INTERAC-
TIONS OF
CARCINOGENS
WITH NUCLEIC
ACIDS

Ramanathan *et al.* (1976*b*) showed that the radioactivity from the administered [^{3}H]-*N*-hydroxy-2-AAF bound to the DNase I-inaccessible regions of rat liver chromatin was 4 to 5 times higher than in the DNase I-accessible regions under conditions of limit digestion of chromatin DNA. The bound AAF-metabolite was also lost from these regions at different rates, being faster from the inaccessible regions. Nevertheless, at the end of 1 week, the carcinogen remaining bound to the nuclease-resistant region was 4 times greater than that in the accessible regions. Metzger *et al.* (1977) similarly found that 2-AAF interacted first with about 10% of the total chromatin DNA (the percentage easily digested by DNase I). However, the DNase I-resistant regions of chromatin DNA ultimately bound the maximum amount of the carcinogen. *In vitro* interaction of the direct-acting derivative, *N*-acetoxy-2-AAF, with duck erythrocyte chromatin was also found to be nonrandom, in that the DNA in the micrococcal nuclease-degradable regions of chromatin DNA was modified to a greater extent than the DNA in the nondigestible regions of chromatin. This preferential interaction with some regions of chromatin DNA was independent of the total amount of carcinogen bound to chromatin and was observed both *in vivo* and *in vitro* (Metzger *et al.*, 1976). Moyer *et al.* (1977) separated the 2-AAF-modified rat liver chromatin into eu- and heterochromatin by centrifugation on linear sucrose gradients and observed a fourfold greater binding in the euchromatin fractions. The loss of the bound carcinogen was also faster from the euchromatin. A similar preferential interaction of *N*-hydroxy-2-AAF metabolites with euchromatin was reported by Schwartz and Goodman (1979), who fractionated the chromatin into euchromatin, heterochromatin, and pelleted heterochromatin by two different methods: (1) glycerol density gradient centrifugation and (2) selective aggregation with MgCl$_2$. Irrespective of the method of fractionation, 2 h after administration of [^{3}H]-*N*-hydroxy-2-AAF, 40–60% of the total DNA-bound metabolites were found in the euchromatin and 20–30% in the pelleted heterochromatin. The rate of loss was also greater from the euchromatin, so that the pelleted heterochromatin had a higher percentage of bound metabolites a week after administration of the carcinogen. Furthermore, they found a differential distribution of the two AAF–DNA adducts in the chromatin fractions. Thus, although the C-8 adduct was the major component in all the fractions, the pelleted heterochromatin had a two- to threefold higher content of the minor N^2 adduct. Although it has been shown that the N^2 adduct has a longer half-life *in vivo* than the C-8 adduct, it is not known whether it represents the persistent form in the pelleted heterochromatin. The preferential loss of the carcinogen from some regions of chromatin could be due to a difference in the conformational states of DNA in the various regions of chromatin, as a result of interaction with proteins, rendering some regions more accessible to repair enzymes. Alternatively, depending on the nature of the distortions caused by the adducts in the DNA double helix, these are excised at different rates by the repair enzyme(s) (Levine *et al.*, 1974; Fuchs *et al.*, 1976). Kapuler and Michelson (1971) suggested that the formation of the C-8 adduct was possible only if the guanine was in a transient "open" state, which is more likely to occur in the extended regions of chromatin. On the other hand, Yamasaki *et al.* (1977*b*) found that the C-8 adducts of AAF in DNA were preferentially solubilized by S_1 nuclease and concluded that they caused conformational changes and localized regions of denaturation in the DNA, while the N^2 adducts did not. In the computer-generated models, the *N*-2 adduct has been shown to be located in the minor groove, causing little helical distortion (Beland, 1978), and therefore possibly escapes detection by repair enzymes, while the C-8 adducts (which cause base displacement and helix distortion) are recognized by the repair enzymes (Grunberger and Weinstein, 1976). In contrast to the above findings, Walker *et al.* (1979) did not find a preferential interaction of 2-AAF or *N*-hydroxy-2-AAF with euchromatin when the modified chromatin was fractionated using three different methods: glycerol gradient centrifugation, controlled digestion with DNase II, or treatment with micrococcal nuclease. However, the authors reported a twofold increase in *N*-hydroxy-2-AAF binding to the small fragments of DNA released by mild micrococcal nuclease digestion under conditions where the fragments are apparently enriched in transcriptionally active genes.

3.3. Polycyclic Aromatic Hydrocarbons

The binding of BP to different regions of DNA in calf thymus nuclei was studied by Jahn and Litman (1977) using a 3-MC-induced rat liver microsomal system to activate the BP and micrococcal nuclease to fractionate the modified chromatin. Most of the carcinogen was bound to the nuclease-digestible regions of chromatin. The digestion of the BP-modified nuclei by micrococcal nuclease and DNase I was followed as a function of time and the distribution of the bound carcinogen was determined in the isolated DNA as well as in the generated monomers, dimers, trimers, and tetramers (in the case of micrococcal nuclease) isolated by gradient centrifugation. While the specific activity of micrococcal nuclease-resistant fractions decreased as a function of loss of the spacer region, that from the DNase I-resistant fractions was found to increase. These results were interpreted to indicate that BP binding was clustered in the spacer region or at the very ends of the nucleosome core (Jahn and Litman, 1979). Similar preferential binding of BP epoxides to the internucleosomal spacer regions in duck reticulocyte chromatin was reported by Yamasaki *et al.* (1978) and in chicken erythrocyte nuclei and chromatin by Kootstra *et al.* (1979).

Moses *et al.* (1976) studied the binding of the polycyclic hydrocarbons, 3-MC, 5,6-dimethylbenzanthracene (5,6-DMBA), and its weakly carcinogenic analog 3,4-DMBA to nuclear subfractions from a clone of transformable AKR mouse embryo cells. They fractionated chromatin from cells exposed to the radioactively labeled compounds into template-active and -inactive fractions by sucrose density centrifugation and found that 3-MC and 5,6-DMBA exhibited a preferential binding to the template-active fractions. Zeiger *et al.* (1972) showed that 9,10-

DMBA quantitatively binds to the same extent to satellite and main band DNA in mouse skin.

357

INTERAC-
TIONS OF
CARCINOGENS
WITH NUCLEIC
ACIDS

The specificity of the interaction of 7-BrMeBA and 7-BrMe-12-MeBA in different chromatin fractions was studied by Ramanathan and Dipple (1976). They showed that the ratio of specific binding of 7-BrMeBA and 7-BrMe-12-MeBA to DNase I-sensitive and -resistant fractions was $1:3.5$ and $1:2$, respectively, and that this nonrandomness was independent of the extent of binding. In addition, Oleson et al. (1979) found that in confluent human fibroblasts exposed to 7-BrMeBA, 60–70% of the initial covalent binding was in the nucleosome core DNA and only 15–20% in the "linker" regions. The rate of loss from the two regions, however, was the same.

In all the foregoing studies, the carcinogen-interacted chromatin was fractionated on the basis of either accessibility to nucleases or transcriptionally active or inactive fractions. In a recent study, Rajalakshmi et al. (1978a, b, 1980) have developed a new approach to determine whether chemical carcinogens exhibit preferential interaction with certain regions of chromatin DNA. The method makes use of ligands that specifically interact with the minor groove of DNA and stabilize its structure; the ligands used are spermine (which interacts with the phosphate groups) and distamycin A (which binds to AT base pairs). Using this approach, it was found that both spermine and distamycin A inhibited the methylation of chromatin DNA by MNU at all three methylatable sites studied, viz. the N-7 and O^6 positions of guanine and the N-3 position of adenine (Rajalakshmi et al., 1978b, 1980). On the other hand, under identical conditions, the ligands had no effect on the alkylation of DNA by MMS and DMS. Based on the known mechanism of interaction of the ligands with DNA, it was concluded that MNU methylates regions of DNA that are readily denaturable, probably rich in AT base pairs located at or close to the binding sites of the ligands and/or the conformation DNA assumes in the presence of the ligands is unfavorable for methylation by MNU. Taken together, these results implicate DNA structure and/or its conformation in carcinogen–DNA interaction.

Another approach that has been used for determining the sites of modification of DNA by carcinogenic agents is the interaction DNA of fragments with carcinogen and determination of the site of interaction by sequencing. As pointed out in Section 2.1.7, using this technique, D'Andrea and Haseltine (1978) demonstrated that activated AFB_1 modifies the guanines and to a much lesser extent the adenines in a DNA fragment containing lactose promoter operator region, and that the guanines modified by AFB_1 and DMS were identical. The method should be useful in determining whether different carcinogens have identical or different site specificities for interactions with DNA.

4. Interaction of Chemical Carcinogens with Mitochondrial DNA

Almost all studies with DNA and chemical carcinogens have involved total tissue or organ DNA. Since nuclear DNA represents the overwhelming mass of cellular

DNA, it is usually assumed that what is being examined in these studies on cellular DNA pertains to nuclear DNA. However, the work by Wunderlich and associates and a few others calls for a reevaluation of this assumption.

Wunderlich et al. (1970, 1971–1972) have observed that mitochondrial DNA in liver has 3–7 times the specific activity of nuclear DNA in rats given single injections of methyl-labeled MNU or DMN. This has led them to suggest a cytoplasmic mutation hypothesis of carcinogenesis (Wunderlich et al., 1971–1972). In a recent study on the interaction of BP diol epoxide with mitochondrial DNA of three different cell lines, Backer and Weinstein (1980) observed that the extent of mitochondrial DNA modification was 40 to 90 times greater than that of nuclear DNA. They also observed that 30% of the cell-associated carcinogen was in the nuclear fraction wherein over 98% of the cellular DNA is present, whereas 15% of the carcinogen was localized in the mitochondrial fraction where less than 2% of the total DNA (Schneider and Kuff, 1965) is present. The suggestion was that lipophilic carcinogens can concentrate in the mitochondrial fraction and this may account for the increased extent of modification of mitochondrial DNA. In addition, since several factors influence carcinogen–DNA interaction (see Section 3), it is possible that the differential availability of regions in mitochondrial and nuclear DNA for carcinogen interaction is a reflection of the different organizational states of these two DNA species.

Wilkinson et al. (1975) also observed that DMN alkylated mitochondrial DNA to a greater extent than nuclear DNA (on a weight basis), whereas MMS alkylated both to relatively the same extent. The amount of mitochondrial DNA that could be isolated as closed circular forms decreased with increasing concentration of DMN and at high doses none were isolated, indicating introduction of strand breaks in a dose-dependent manner. No closed circular forms were detected even 24 h after treatment with DMN; on the other hand, with MMS at doses where it alkylated mitochondrial DNA to the same extent as DMN, no loss in closed circular forms was observed.

Morita et al. (1976) reported that short-term treatment of yeast with 4NQO induced a variety of mutants that had mitochondrial DNA of altered buoyant densities ranging from 1.682 to 1.675 g/cm^3. This was attributed to a decrease in the GC content from 24% to 15.3%. In a cytoplasmic respiration-deficient mutant of yeast induced by 4NQO, no mitochondrial DNA of normal density was detected. Miyaki et al. (1977) compared the effects of MNNG and 4NQO on mitochondrial DNA of rat ascites cells and HeLa cells. Both the carcinogens introduced strand breaks in mitochondrial DNA, but while the mitochondrial DNA from MNNG-treated cells was about 11 S, compared to 20 S for the control open circular form in alkaline sucrose gradients, that from the 4NQO-treated cells showed no difference in size, indicating that a single nick per strand was introduced by 4NQO. The closed circular forms were not restored even 20 h following treatment with MNNG while the damaged nuclear DNA became somewhat larger in size, indicating that mitochondrial DNA repair was slow compared to that of nuclear DNA. On the other hand, under these conditions the synthesis of mitochondrial DNA was restored to 70% of the control value, as was the synthesis of nuclear DNA. Whether this represents replication of mitochondrial DNA on damaged template with consequent alterations in base sequence or deletions in the daughter molecules is worth considering.

5. Interaction of Chemical Carcinogens with RNA

5.1. General

Cellular ribonucleic acids play a key role as mediators in the transfer of genetic information between DNA and protein. The ultraviolet absorption–temperature curve of RNA, reaction with formaldehyde, hyperchromicity in water and at high temperature, and several other parameters suggest that RNAs behave hydrodynamically as homologous single chains that are coiled in such a way to permit a substantial number of intramolecular hydrogen bonds (Kit, 1960). The three-dimensional structure of tRNAs (cloverleaf model) is maintained through intramolecular hydrogen bonds at specific locations (Holley *et al.*, 1965). The heterogeneous nuclear RNA (hnRNA) of HeLa cells and Ehrlich ascites carcinoma cells has been shown to contain double-stranded regions (Jelinek and Darnell, 1972; Ryskov *et al.*, 1972), while the mRNA of the same cells seems not to contain significant amounts of double-stranded regions. Thus, in RNA, unlike DNA, not all nucleotides are involved in the formation of hydrogen bonds, and theoretically one would expect more available sites in mRNA than in DNA for interaction of carcinogens. In general, however, the interaction of chemical carcinogens with RNA has not been as extensively investigated as that with DNA.

The importance of methylation in the processing of ribosomal precursor RNA (Darnell, 1968) and the structure and function of RNA has been documented (see Cohn and Volkin, 1976, for reviews). In addition, it has been shown that methylation of groups involved in base pair hydrogen bonding are either attenuators in the rate of transcription by AMV reverse transcriptase, e.g., N^2-MeG in the 16 S RNA of *E. coli* (Youvan and Hearst, 1979), or terminators, e.g., the N^6-dimethyladenine (Hagenbüchle *et al.*, 1978). In view of these, the interaction of carcinogens with hnRNA, mRNA, poly-A stretches in mRNA, and RNA species involved in DNA synthesis may prove to be important in our attempts to understand the role of altered RNA in carcinogenesis.

5.2. Alkylating Agents

5.2.1. Nitrosamines and Nitrosamides

Generally, the various sites capable of alkylation in RNA and their order of activity are N-7 of guanine >N-1 of adenine >N-3 of cytosine >N-7 of adenine >N-3 of adenine >N-3 of guanine (Shapiro, 1968, 1969). This general picture of activity is altered by (1) the type of alkylating agent, i.e., whether they act through an SN_1 or SN_2 mechanism, (2) the complex environment that exists when nucleic acids are bound to proteins, (3) the conformation of nucleic acids, and (4) the conditions under which the alkylation takes place.

The interaction of DMN with cellular RNA was first demonstrated by Magee and Farber (1962) and later by several other workers (Magee and Lee, 1963; Lee and Lijinsky, 1966; Lawley et al., 1968). DMN methylates the liver nucleic acids to a greater extent than those of other organs while MNU methylates nucleic acids of the various organs to the same extent (Swann and Magee, 1968). Both agents methylated RNA to a greater degree than DNA. MMS methylates the nucleic acids in several organs to the same extent as MNU, but methylation with DNA is more than with RNA. In all these cases, the alkylated base investigated was N-7-MeG. With respect to the formation of this major alkylated base, there seems to be no difference between DMN, MNU, MNNG, and MMS; however, the most striking difference was the formation of O^6-MeG by N-alkylnitroso compounds but not by either DMS or MMS (Lawley and Shah, 1972). The methylation of O^6 of guanine involves the anion form of guanine and presents an intriguing chemical problem. It is interesting to point out that the relative extent of methylation at the O^6 atom of guanine in RNA is about one-half of that in DNA. This finding is contrary to the expectation based on the concept that involvement of the O^6 atom in hydrogen bonding of the Watson–Crick type would decrease its reactivity as found with the N-1 of adenine. The possibility that the O^6 atom of guanine in RNA is hydrogen-bonded more strongly to water if not to cytosine is worth considering. The complex environment that exists in vivo may play a vital role in the alkylation reactions in addition to the other considerations mentioned above.

The nitroso compounds are relatively more reactive at N-7 of adenine and probably N-3 of guanine but less reactive at N-1 of adenine, N-3 of cytosine, and probably N-3 of uracil as compared to either DMS or MMS. Studies with TMV RNA or TMV virus indicate that the methylation reaction is conformation dependent (Singer and Fraenkel-Conrat, 1969). Methylation with DMS and MMS is affected mainly by hydrogen bonding, which therefore reduces the availability of N-1 of adenine and N-3 of cytosine. In contrast, with nitrosoguanidines, an effect in addition to that of hydrogen bonding is present, namely base stacking. The methylation of guanine and adenine is favored by base stacking, while with cytosine the opposite is found to be the case (Singer and Fraenkel-Conrat, 1969). A preferential methylation of cytosine has been noticed by these authors during the interaction of MNNG with TMV virus as compared to free TMV RNA. This is the only instance of an alkylation reaction of a base in RNA approaching in magnitude the alkylation of guanine.

Shooter et al. (1974a, b), using an RNA-containing bacteriophage R17, studied the inactivation of the phage with DMS, MMS, MNU, and MNNG. With DMS and MMS, the inactivation was mainly due to methylation at N-1 of adenine and N-3 of cytosine. However, with MNU and MNNG, only one-half of the inactivation observed could be accounted for by methylation at N-1 of adenine and N-3 of cytosine. The rest could be accounted for by methylation at O^6 of guanine and by breaks in RNA as a result of methylation of the phosphodiester group and the subsequent hydrolysis of the unstable triester formed (Shooter *et al.*, 1974*b*). In contrast to the instability of phosphotriester in RNA, the phosphotriester in DNA is relatively stable.

Recently, the extent of alkylation of various types of RNA such as mRNA, rRNA, nRNA, and tRNA was investigated by Pegg and Jackson (1976). It was found that mRNA and nRNA were alkylated to a lesser degree than rRNA by DMN *in vivo*. On the other hand, nRNA was alkylated to a greater extent than either mRNA or rRNA by MMS. The differences noticed were small; nevertheless, the influence of cellular environment on alkylation of nucleic acids cannot be ignored.

Pegg (1973) found no significant differences in the alkylation of tRNA^{fMet}, tRNA^{Phe}, tRNA^{Glu}, and tRNA^{Val} by MNU. The major product was N-7-MeG, accounting for 80% of the total, but 3-methylcytosine, O^6-MeG, and 1-methyl-, 3-methyl-, and 7-methyladenines were also identified as products of the reaction with tRNA^{fMet}. In addition, analysis of the methylated tRNA^{fMet} revealed that the distribution of 7-alkylguanine was in agreement with a random interaction with all guanosine residues in the tRNA molecule. The studies were carried out under conditions where the native configuration of tRNA was maintained and hence show that the tertiary structure of the tRNA does not impart any specificity to the reaction of MNU with guanine under the conditions of study. However, the possibility that such specificity may exist for the minor products of alkylation cannot be excluded. Also, whether the same random distribution would be found with the lower levels of methylation such as might be anticipated during carcinogenesis remains to be established. In this context, it is worth noting that the studies of Weinstein (1970) using 2-AAF, Fujimura *et al.* (1972) with N-acetoxy-2-AAF, and of Powers and Holley (1972) with DMS indicate that chemical interactions with tRNA can be highly specific for even single bases in complex macromolecules when the level of interaction is low.

5.2.2. Urethan

The binding of urethan to liver RNA has been studied by several workers. The level of binding of [^{3}H]urethan is higher in partially hepatectomized animals than in intact animals (Lawson and Pound, 1971–1972). However, the radioactivity declines very rapidly, a phenomenon that is apparently not due to the turnover of cellular RNAs. It is not known to which type of RNA urethan is bound or whether more than one type of RNA is involved. In mice, urethan labeled in the alkyl group and in the carbonyl carbon was found to react with nucleic acids of liver and lung. Only one radioactive spot, considered to be cytosine-5-carboxylic acid, was detected in the chromatogram (Boyland and Williams, 1969). In the rat, urethan labeled only in the alkyl group was found to bind to nucleic acids (Prodi *et al.*, 1970*a*). Lawson and Pound (1973*a*) have concluded that the bound molecule does not contain the carbonyl carbon but probably only the ethyl group.

S. RAJALAKSHMI,
PREMA M. RAO,
AND
D. S. R. SARMA

5.2.3. Ethionine

The hepatic carcinogen ethionine, which is an analog of methionine, reacts preferentially with liver tRNA *in vivo* (Farber and Magee, 1960; Stekol *et al.*, 1960; Natori, 1963; Farber *et al.*, 1967*a*, *b*; Rosen, 1968; Craddock, 1969). Ethionine has also been shown to produce specific modifications of isoaccepting tRNA^{Leu} species (Axel *et al.*, 1967). Rosen (1968) identified 7-ethyl- (10%), N^2-ethyl- (23%), and N^2-diethyl(2%)guanines among the ethylated purines and ribose (2-OH) ethylation of pyrimidine nucleotides. Pegg (1972) reported the presence of ethyluracil (5%), ethylcytosine (6%), N^2-ethyl- (25%), N^2-diethyl- (7%), 7-ethyl- (13%), and 1-ethyl(2%)guanines among the ethylated bases. Methyl substitutions at these positions are present in the normally methylated tRNA (Craddock *et al.*, 1968; Dunn, 1963; Smith and Dunn, 1959). Since large amounts of *S*-adenosylethionine accumulate in the liver of rats administered ethionine (Farber *et al.*, 1964; Smith and Salmon, 1965; Shull *et al.*, 1966), it has been suggested that the ethylation of RNA is catalyzed by the action of enzymes that normally utilize *S*-adenosyl-L-methionine as a donor of methyl groups (Stekol, 1965; Farber, 1967; Hancock, 1968). However, Ortwerth and Novelli (1969) have suggested that the ethylation of RNA by ethionine *in vivo* is not mediated through the RNA methyltransferases that can utilize *S*-adenosylethionine as a donor instead of *S*-adenosylmethionine but via a new, as yet unknown mechanism. It appears that there are some methyltransferases that cannot or do not use *S*-adenosylethionine. It is interesting to note that ethionine does not give rise to 5-ethylcytosine, although this is the major methylated base in eukaryotic DNA.

5.3. Aromatic Amines and Amides

5.3.1. 2-AAF and Derivatives

The binding of 2-AAF metabolites to liver tRNA and rRNA *in vivo* has been reported by several workers (Marroquin and Farber, 1965; E. C. Miller and Miller, 1969; Kriek *et al.*, 1967; Kriek, 1968; Irving *et al.*, 1967; Agarwal and Weinstein, 1970). The carcinogen *N*-acetoxy-2-AAF has been shown under certain conditions to interact preferentially with some nucleoside residues thought to be located in exposed regions of tRNA molecules (Weinstein *et al.*, 1971; Fujimura *et al.*, 1972). This carcinogen (or its derivatives) binds to the C-8 position of guanine in nucleic acids both *in vivo* and *in vitro* (Kriek *et al.*, 1967). It was observed that the *N*-acetyl group is retained in the binding to RNA (Irving *et al.*, 1967) but not to DNA (Kriek, 1968). The binding of *N*-acetoxy-2-AAF to tRNA in general (Fink *et al.*, 1970; Agarwal and Weinstein, 1970) and to tRNA^{fMet} in particular (Fujimura *et al.*, 1972) have been investigated in detail. The modified guanine is located in the single-stranded region at position 20 of the dihydrouridine loop. The cloverleaf model for tRNA^{fMet} (Dube *et al.*, 1968) predicts that 18 of the 25 guanine residues present in tRNA^{fMet} are in base-paired regions;

5 are presumably buried in the three-dimensional tertiary structure, leaving 2 of the remaining guanines present in the sequence G–G–Dh of the dihydrouridine loop free to react with N-acetoxy-2-AAF.

363

INTERAC-
TIONS OF
CARCINOGENS
WITH NUCLEIC
ACIDS

5.3.2. 2-Naphthylamine

Hughes and Pilczyk (1969–1970) showed the binding of 2-naphthylamine, a weak hepatocarcinogen for mice, to mouse liver RNA. The level of binding to liver RNA was higher in CBA mice, a strain susceptible to hepatocarcinogenesis, than in C57 mice.

5.3.3. DAB

The binding of DAB to ribosomal RNA has been demonstrated by Warwick and Roberts (1967).

5.3.4. o-Aminoazotoluene

The binding of o-aminoazotoluene to liver RNA as well as DNA has been shown by Lawson (1968). Binding to DNA reached a maximum 16 h after oral administration of the chemical, whereas the peak of RNA binding occurred at an earlier time.

5.4. Polycyclic Aromatic Hydrocarbons

The polycyclic hydrocarbons have been shown to bind to RNA of mouse skin *in vivo* (Brookes and Lawley, 1964; Prodi *et al.*, 1970*b*; Goshman and Heidelberger, 1967) and that of various cells in culture (Kuroki *et al.*, 1971–1972). In mouse embryo cells in culture, the RNA binding index is low for the noncarcinogen dibenz[a,c]anthracene and at least 10 times higher for the carcinogenic dibenz[a,l]anthracene (Duncan *et al.*, 1969; Kuroki and Heidelberger, 1971). In general, it has been found that there is a greater extent of binding to nucleic acids in normal and transformable cells in culture than in transformed tumor cells (Kuroki *et al.*, 1971–1972). The exact nature of the interactions is not clear. Considerable evidence has accumulated to show that the ultimate oncogenic metabolite of BP is a 7,8-dihydrodiol-9,10-epoxide. It was demonstrated that the predominant RNA adduct present in human cells exposed to BP is formed by covalent linkage of the amino group at the 2 position of guanine to the 10 position of the specific isomer. Under specific conditions there can be significant binding with adenine and to a lesser extent with cytosine residues in RNA and homopolymers (Straub *et al.*, 1977; Jennette *et al.*, 1977).

5.5. 4NQO

4NQO has been shown to bind to RNA (Andoh *et al.*, 1971; Tada and Tada, 1971), the binding sites apparently being limited in each of the nucleic acids studied, viz. tRNA, rRNA, and DNA. The binding ratios amounted to 2.6, 5.3, and 3.3 molecules of carcinogen per 10,000 nucleotide units for tRNA, rRNA, and DNA, respectively. One of the suggested sites of adduct formation is between the 4-amino nitrogen of 4NQO and the C-8 of purines.

5.6. AFB₁

An rRNA-bound AFB_1 adduct from rat liver was identified as 2,3-dihydro-2-(N-7-guanyl)-3-hydroxy-AFB_1 (Lin *et al.*, 1977).

6. Influence of Carcinogen–Nucleic Acid Interactions on the Structure, Synthesis, and Function of DNA and RNA

Interactions of carcinogens with nucleic acids exert a profound effect on the structure and synthesis of DNA and RNA, gene expression, and regulation of cellular development. Since the scope of this review does not permit a detailed account of these important aspects, only a brief discussion will be presented.

6.1. Alterations in DNA Structure

Because of their interaction with DNA, histones, and nonhistone chromosomal proteins, carcinogens cause structural alterations in DNA and chromatin. Such changes can be monitored by using physicochemical measurements such as viscosity, melting temperature, intercalation of ethidium bromide, binding of peptides containing aromatic amino acids, circular dichroism, and light scattering of DNA (Uhlenhopp and Krasna, 1971; Arcos *et al.*, 1971; Fuchs and Daune, 1974; Ramstein *et al.*, 1973; Nicolini *et al.*, 1976; Toulmé *et al.*, 1980); or by using enzymes such as S_1 nuclease (Fuchs, 1975; Yamasaki *et al.*, 1977*a*; Pulkrabek *et al.*, 1979; G. M. Ledda, A. Columbano, P. M. Rao, S. Rajalakshmi, and D. S. R. Sarma, unpublished observations, 1980). By their ability to interact with the phosphodiester backbone, carcinogens may decrease the net negative charge, which in turn may influence the binding of chromatin proteins to DNA. Aminoazo dyes have been shown to affect the binding of chromatin proteins to DNA *in vivo* (Dijkstra and Weide, 1972). In contrast, interaction of benzo[α]pyrene-7,8-dihydrodiol-9,10-oxide or N-acetoxy-2-AAF with DNA did not apparently influence the *in vitro* reconstitution of chromatin using such modified DNA and unmodified chromatin proteins (Yamasaki *et al.*, 1977*a*, 1978).

Intercalation of carcinogens in DNA alters the helical structure of DNA (Wagner, 1971). An interaction of this kind may induce conformational changes in the DNA, e.g., from the B form to some other form closely related to the A form (Yang and Samejima, 1969). Such a change in conformation would involve base tilting (Wagner, 1971). Bulky molecules such as 2-AAF and its derivatives interact at C-8 of guanine and cause local denaturation of the DNA (Nelson *et al.*, 1971).

365
INTERAC-
TIONS OF
CARCINOGENS
WITH NUCLEIC
ACIDS

S_1 nuclease, an enzyme that recognizes single-stranded as well as denatured regions in DNA, appears to preferentially release the C-8 adduct of guanine from DNA modified *in vitro* with *N*-acetoxy-2-AAF (Fuchs, 1975; Yamasaki *et al.*, 1977*b*). However, when rat liver DNA modified *in vivo* by administering *N*-hydroxy-2-AAF was subjected to S_1 nuclease digestion, neither a detectable preferential release of carcinogen–DNA adducts nor digestion of such modified DNA was noticed. These data suggest that the greater susceptibility of *in vitro* carcinogen-modified DNA towards S_1 nuclease may be because of the increased extent of modification of the DNA under these conditions, e.g., 0.65% (Yamasaki *et al.*, 1977*b*) as compared to 0.001% *in vivo* (Zahner, 1976). The presence of such local denatured regions in BP-modified DNA was also observed by Pulk-rabek *et al.* (1979) and Kakefuda and Yamamoto (1978) using S_1 nuclease.

Likewise, carcinogenic metal ions interact with the amino groups of the DNA bases (Furst and Haro, 1969) causing local denaturation, and metals such as Ni^{2+} in excess quantities can depolymerize polynucleotides (Butzow and Eich-horn, 1965). Some of the carcinogen–DNA adducts are unstable and result in depurination, and endonucleases that act at or near such apurinic sites can induce strand interruptions (see Section 7.4). A number of carcinogens appear to induce *in vivo* single- and/or double-strand breaks (see Table 2) (Cox *et al.*, 1973; Sarma, 1973; Sarma *et al.*, 1974; Saffhill *et al.*, 1974; Huang and Stewart, 1977; Parodi *et al.*, 1978) Carcinogens can cause local destabilization in DNA by binding to sites in the bases that are involved in hydrogen bonding, while others can cross-link the two strands of the DNA duplex, the same strand of DNA, or two DNA duplexes. These varied alterations in DNA structure induced by carcinogens may influence gene organization, DNA replication, transcription, and translation. Because of limitations of space, the influence of interactions of

TABLE 2
A Partial List of Chemicals That Induce Strand Breaks in Vivo in Liver DNA[a]

Hepatocarcinogens	Nonhepatocarcinogens
N-Nitrosodimethylamine	Methylmethanesulfonate
Methylazoxymethanol acetate	*N*-Methyl-*N'*-nitro-*N*-nitrosoguanidine
N-Nitrosodiethylamine	*N*-Nitrosomethylurea
2-Acetylaminofluorene	Ethylmethanesulfonate
N-Hydroxy-2-acetylaminofluorene	*N*-Nitrosoethylurea
N-Acetoxy-2-acetylaminofluorene	4-Nitroquinoline-*N*-oxide
3'-Methyl-4-dimethylaminoazobenzene	4-Hydroxyaminoquinoline-*N*-oxide
N-Nitrosomorpholine	
N-Nitrosopiperidine	Chemotherapeutic agents
N,N-Dinitrosopiperazine	Camptothecin
N-Nitrosodihydrouracil	Bleomycin
3-Hydroxyxanthine	
Aflatoxin B_1	
7,12-Dimethylbenz[*a*]anthracene	
Hycanthone methanseulfonate	
1,2-Dimethylhydrazine	

[a] For references see Sarma *et al.* (1974).

carcinogens with nucleic acids on translation and on cellular enzyme regulation is not discussed in this chapter.

6.2. Alterations in DNA Synthesis

6.2.1. In Vivo Studies

Carcinogens in general and liver carcinogens in particular inhibit DNA synthesis (see Sarma *et al.*, 1975, for references). In addition, they appear to inhibit DNA synthesis in a cell-cycle-dependent manner; the effect seems to depend on the nature of the carcinogen and the cell type used. For example, in HeLa cells damaged with MNU or with mustard gas, the replication of DNA occurs normally in the first cell cycle, while it is inhibited in the second cell cycle and the cells are killed subsequently. On the other hand, in Chinese hamster cells, addition of MNU during the G_1 phase of the cell cycle inhibits DNA synthesis in the second cell cycle, but addition of half mustard gas during the G_1 phase inhibits DNA synthesis in the first cell cycle itself (Roberts, 1972).

Attempts to understand the influence of chemical carcinogens on DNA synthesis revealed that in almost all systems studied, e.g., using the liver system in an intact rat (Rajalakshmi and Sarma, 1975; Zahner, 1976; Zahner *et al.*, 1977) or using mammalian cells in culture (Trosko *et al.*, 1973; D'Ambrosio and Setlow, 1976), replication of carcinogen-damaged DNA resulted initially in a newly made DNA of lower molecular weight. After a lag period, however, these chains are eventually elongated to normal size. Although other explanations are possible, one of the reasons for the generation of low-molecular-weight chains could be that certain lesions induced by the carcinogens in DNA can block the DNA polymerizing system. These gaps so created in the daughter strands are eventually filled in (see Section 7.5 for some of the possible pathways by which the gaps can be filled in).

Experiments for identifying the carcinogen-induced lesions that do or do not permit *in vivo* replication revealed that N-7-MeG, O^6-MeG, N-3-methyladenine, and possibly phosphotriesters induced by DMN (Abanobi *et al.*, 1980; Columbano *et al.*, 1980) and adducts of 8-(N-2-fluorenylamino)guanine induced by N-hydroxy-2-AAF permitted *in vivo* replication of rat liver DNA (Zahner, 1976; Zahner *et al.*, 1977).

6.2.2. In Vitro Studies

Experiments on the effect of carcinogen–DNA interaction on DNA synthesis using *in vitro* systems have shown that while some of the carcinogen-induced lesions act as blocks to DNA synthesis, others permit replication but with increased infidelity. For example, Moore and Strauss (1979) using ϕX174 DNA fragments of known sequence modified with N-acetoxy-2-AAF or irradiated with UV found that the lesions introduced by UV or the carcinogen were terminators for DNA synthesis. Similarly, Villani *et al.* (1978) found that UV-induced pyrimidine dimers inhibited chain elongation to a greater extent with *E. coli* Pol I than with

AMV DNA polymerase and mammalian DNA polymerase α; the inhibition with *E. coli* Pol I was attributed to the $3'$–$5'$ proofreading activity of the enzyme. Interaction of pBR 322 DNA with BP-7,8-dihydrodiol-9,10-epoxide was shown to result in a decrease in DNA synthesis, the decrease being proportional to the extent of modification. It was further concluded that while initiation was inhibited to some extent, the greater effect was on chain elongation (Mizusawa and Kakefuda, 1979). Similarly, Hsu *et al.* (1977) observed that modification of ϕX174 DNA with BP-7,8-dihydrodiol-9,10-epoxide not only resulted in a decreased DNA synthesis but also in a block in the propagation of complementary strands. Using BP-7,8-dihydrodiol-9,10-epoxide-modified poly-dC as template and AMV reverse transcriptase or *E. coli* Pol I, Yamaura *et al.* (1978) found that while modification with BP-4,5-oxide (K region) had no effect on the rate of synthesis, modification with the *cis-* or *trans*-7,8-dihydroxy-9,10-epoxy BP derivative decreased the initial rate of synthesis; the decrease was proportional to the extent of modification. However, the size of the product synthesized was found to be the same as that made on an unmodified template, and the result was interpreted to indicate that the enzyme had copied past the adduct. Furthermore, since no misincorporation was observed, the decrease in rate was ascribed to the higher affinity of the enzyme for the modified template.

In contrast to the above-mentioned studies, some carcinogen-induced lesions did permit copying *in vitro*, albeit with increased infidelity. For example, Shearman and Loeb (1979) studied the effect of the presence of apurinic sites in polynucleotide templates on the fidelity of DNA synthesis using *E. coli* Pol I, AMV DNA polymerase, and human placental polymerase β; they observed that DNA polymerases can copy past apurinic sites, generating molecules equal in size to those made on nondepurinated templates. However, misincorporation as single-base substitutions was observed; and misincorporation was abolished when the apurinic sites were removed by alkali treatment. Similarly, Abbott and Saffhill (1977) using poly-dA·dT methylated with DMS or MNU as templates found misincorporation of dGMP only with the MNU-alkylated template; furthermore, the extent was proportional to the O^4-methylthymine content. Likewise, using poly-dC·dG alkylated with DMS or MNU, miscoding was found only with the MNU-modified template (Abbott and Saffhill, 1979). Since both methylating agents gave *N*-3-MeC, *N*-3-MeG, and *N*-7-MeG, and only MNU gave O^6-MeG, the miscoding observed only with the MNU-alkylated template was attributed to the presence of O^6-MeG. Recently, Chan and Becker (1979) showed that the liver cytoplasmic and nuclear DNAα-polymerases from rats fed a carcinogenic regimen of 2-AAF were error prone, the former being more so; in contrast, the nuclear and cytoplasmic β-polymerases retained their fidelity through the feeding cycle.

6.3. Alterations in RNA Synthesis and Function

Although several carcinogens such as DMN, MNU, MAM, urethan, and AFB₁ have been shown to inhibit RNA synthesis, very few studies have correlated

367

INTERAC-
TIONS OF
CARCINOGENS
WITH NUCLEIC
ACIDS

S. RAJALAKSHMI,
PREMA M. RAO,
AND
D. S. R. SARMA

these changes with carcinogen–DNA interaction. Many of the effects are probably due to either a direct or an indirect effect of the carcinogen on the enzymes involved in the synthesis of macromolecules or due to some interference with the available pools of nucleotides.

Administration of ethionine results in the inhibition of *in vivo* hepatic RNA synthesis (Villa-Trevino *et al.*, 1966) and a decreased hepatic ATP level (Shull, 1962; Villa-Trevino *et al.*, 1963). Smuckler and Koplitz (1969) have shown that decreased RNA synthesis in ethionine-treated rats cannot be entirely due to the decreased substrate (ATP) concentration. More recently, it has been shown that the decreased RNA synthesis in whole nuclei of ethionine-treated rat liver can be related to the inhibition of the partially purified RNA polymerases solubilized from these nuclei (Farber *et al.*, 1975).

A single dose of MNU (100 mg/kg) reduces the labeling by [^{14}C]orotate of rat kidney and liver RNA by 40 and 15–20%, respectively, the maximum effect being reached by 1.5–3 h (Kleihues, 1972). The effect in kidney appears to be due to an inhibition of uptake of [^{14}C]orotate, while the decrease in labeling of liver RNA results from interference with the synthesis of pyrimidine nucleotides.

MAM acetate has been shown to inhibit hepatic RNA synthesis (Zedek *et al.*, 1970). Using isolated nuclei from MAM acetate-treated animals, Grab *et al.* (1973) reported that DNA template activity for RNA synthesis was unimpaired *in vitro* while template activity of chromatin was slightly decreased.

AFB$_1$ *in vivo* inhibits the synthesis of nuclear and nucleolar RNA, an effect attributed to its complexing with DNA (Edwards *et al.*, 1971; Floyd *et al.*, 1968; Gelboin *et al.*, 1966; Lafarge and Frayssinet, 1970; Pong and Wogan, 1970; Wagner and Drews, 1970).

Chronic feeding of 2-AAF to rats results in an inhibition of hepatic RNA synthesis (Troll *et al.*, 1968). The administration of a single dose of 2-AAF or *N*-hydroxy-2-AAF was found to produce a rapid inhibition of RNA synthesis in male mouse liver. The inhibition of the Mg^{2+}- and Mn^{2+}-activated RNA polymerase activities in nuclei isolated from *N*-hydroxy-2-AAF-treated rat liver was attributed to inactivation of polymerase (Zieve, 1972; Farber *et al.*, 1975). However, Grunberger *et al.* (1973) reported that the inhibition of RNA synthesis after the administration of an acute dose of *N*-hydroxy-2AAF to rats is due to an impairment of the nucleolar DNA template function rather than to an effect on RNA polymerase per se. Treatment of DNA with *N*-acetoxy-2-AAF *in vitro* also results in a drastic reduction in the ability of the DNA to function as a template for RNA synthesis (Zieve, 1973; Troll *et al.*, 1968).

The carcinogen nickel carbonyl has been demonstrated to inhibit both *in vivo* incorporation of radioactive orotate into rat liver RNA and DNA-dependent RNA polymerase activity (Sunderman and Estahani, 1968; Beach and Sunderman, 1970).

In contrast to the inhibition of RNA synthesis by several carcinogens, administration of azo dyes results in enhanced RNA synthesis. Nuclei from rats treated with aminoazo dyes exhibit enhanced RNA polymerase activity. However, when exogenous polymerase such as from *E. coli* is used for the enzyme assay, no such difference is observed. The increased activity is considered to be the result of enhanced binding of the enzyme to the template (Wu and Smuckler, 1971). *In vivo*, 3-MC causes an increase in the synthesis of all RNA species including hnRNA (Wiebel *et al.*, 1972). The nuclei exhibit an enhanced RNA polymerase activity *in vitro* also. This increase does not occur in adrenalectomized or hypophysectomized animals (Younger *et al.*, 1972). 3,4-BP and 7,12-DMBA cause a decrease in the rate of RNA synthesis initially, followed by an abrupt increase well above the normal rate. It is interesting to note that the early inhibitory effect is not observed with the noncarcinogen 1,2-BP (Alexandrov *et al.*, 1970). Leffler *et al.* (1977) observed that the presence of BP adducts in calf thymus DNA resulted in a reduced template activity for RNA polymerase and that the size of the transcript was small.

369
INTERAC-
TIONS OF
CARCINOGENS
WITH NUCLEIC
ACIDS

By virtue of their interaction with RNA and proteins, carcinogens may influence the composition of ribonucleoprotein particles (Patel and Holoubek, 1976; Yoshida and Holoubek, 1976) and further processing and transport of RNA from the nucleus to the cytoplasm. For example, intercalating agents appear to interfere with the processing of rRNA. rRNA formation in mammalian cells occurs through the formation of a high-molecular-weight 45 S precursor RNA that is synthesized in the nucleolus and then processed progressively in several steps, leading finally to 28 and 18 rRNA (reviewed by Darnell, 1968). Proflavin, ethidium bromide, and ellipticine, compounds known to bind to the nucleic acid helix by intercalation, were found to inhibit the processing of 45 S nucleolar ribosomal precursor RNA in L1210 lymphoma cells (Snyder *et al.*, 1971). The effect appears to be prompt and is not secondary to inhibition of RNA or protein synthesis. Similarly, carcinogens may also influence the processing of hnRNA, which not only contains the nuclear transcripts of mRNA sequences (Brawerman, 1974) but may also play an important regulatory role in transcription (Britten and Davidson, 1969). For example, Brinker *et al.* (1973) have reported that intercalating agents like proflavin, ethidium bromide, and daunomycin decrease the rate of degradation of hnRNA.

The interaction of carcinogens with mRNA is not known, although it has been suggested that such an interaction may prevent the translation of mRNA (Venitt *et al.*, 1968). Poly-A stretches in mRNA may play a role in its stability (Gorsky *et al.*, 1974) or protection from nucleases (Levy *et al.*, 1975). One wonders what influence the modification of poly-A stretches by carcinogens will have on mRNA metabolism. Poly-A-containing mRNA was found to increase in the cytoplasm following the administration of thioacetamide (Smuckler and Koplitz, 1976) and 3-MC (Lanclos and Bresnick, 1976).

Although several carcinogens have been shown to interact with tRNA, very little is known regarding the effects of such interactions, either qualitative or quantitative, on protein synthesis. The binding of an AAF derivative to a residue in the valine codon GUU, the lysine codon AAG, and poly-U·G completely inactivates the ability of the triplets to stimulate the binding of their respective aminoacyl tRNA (Grunberger and Weinstein, 1971; Grunberger *et al.*, 1970). In cases where the polymers with modified guanine residues are bound to ribosomes, polypeptide chain growth is blocked at the modified residue. Modification of poly-U·G by AAF also inhibits its template function in protein synthesis. However, no miscoding is observed.

Using an oocyte system, it has been demonstrated that ethylated tRNA obtained from the liver of ethionine-treated rats exhibited severe impairment in aminocylation capacity (Ginsburg *et al.*, 1979). This effect was not uniform for the various amino acid specific tRNAs. In addition, they also observed an impairment in the ability of these tRNAs to participate in protein synthesis. Since these tRNAs are both methyl deficient (Rajalakshmi, 1973) and ethylated, it is not clear whether undermethylation or ethylation is responsible for the impairment of their functions.

7. Carcinogen–DNA Interactions and Carcinogenesis

Although it is now a well-documented fact that carcinogens induce alterations in DNA, the relationship of any of these to carcinogenesis remains only speculative, largely because of the fact that interaction of carcinogen with cellular constituents is fast and is completed within minutes to hours, whereas the ultimate appearance of cancer may take months to years. Further, the latter is a multistep process and although some of the early steps have been characterized and can be experimentally modulated, the majority of them, particularly the rate-limiting ones, have not been identified.

Carcinogens in general interact with proteins, RNA, and DNA, and hypotheses have been formulated involving these major macromolecules as key components. In this short discussion on carcinogens and nucleic acid interactions, it should suffice to make a brief presentation of some of the quantitative and qualitative aspects of carcinogen–DNA interactions and the subsequent repair of the damage in relation to carcinogenesis.

7.1. Carcinogen–DNA Interactions: Quantitative Analysis

As can be seen from Table 3, the extent of interactions of the carcinogen or its derivative with nucleic acid is quite small. Several studies have tried to show a correlation between the extent of interaction and carcinogenesis.

In a comparative study using several hydrocarbons, Brookes (1966) pointed out that a binding of these agents to RNA or protein bore no correlation to the carcinogenic potency as expressed by the Iball index (1939), whereas such correlation did exist for DNA binding. In this context, it is noteworthy that the binding of metabolites of 2-naphthylamine to all types of macromolecules was found to be higher in CBA mouse liver (susceptible to the hepatocarcinogenic effect of 2-naphthylamine) than in C57 mouse liver (Hughes and Pilczyk, 1969–1970).

371

INTERAC-
TIONS OF
CARCINOGENS
WITH NUCLEIC
ACIDS

TABLE 3

Extent of Interaction of a Few Chemical Carcinogens with Nucleic Acids in Vivo

Carcinogen	Dose (μmol/kg) and route of administration	Duration of action (h)	Species and tissue	Extent of interaction (mol nucleotides/mol carcinogen)		Reference
				DNA	RNA	
MMS	1090, i.p.	4	Rat, liver	3.0×10^3		Mulivor et al. (1974)
DMN	67.5, i.p.	4	Rat, liver	0.2×10^3		Abanobi, Mulivor, and Sarma (unpublished data, 1974)
DEN	2700, i.p.	24	Rat, liver	—	3.8×10^2	Magee and Lee (1964)
DEN	2000, i.p.	24	Rat, kidney	—	2.4×10^3	Magee and Lee (1964)
Ethionine	26, i.p.	120	Rat, liver	2.7×10^7	5.6×10^{4a}	Farber et al. (1967b)
β-Propiolactone	97, skin	24	Mouse, skin	1.3×10^5	6.2×10^4	Brookes (1966)
Urethan	7500, i.p.	10	Mouse, liver	9.3×10^3	10.5×10^3	Lawson and Pound (1973b)
Mustard gas	13.3, i.p.	$\frac{1}{2}$	Mouse, tumor	2.0×10^4	2.5×10^4	Brookes and Lawley (1960)
DAB	675, i.p.	16	Rat, liver	2.3×10^5	2.7×10^4	Roberts and Warwick (1966)
2-AAF	2.8, i.p.	24	Rat, liver	4.0×10^5	1.2×10^{5a}	Farber (1968)
	14–15, i.p.	24	Rat, liver	1.1×10^5	1.0×10^5	Kriek (1969)
N-Hydroxy-2-AAF	14–15, i.p.	24	Rat, liver	1.3×10^5	1.0×10^5	Kriek (1969)
Benzo[a]pyrene	16, skin	42	Mouse, skin	2.9×10^5	6.2×10^4	Brookes and Lawley (1964)
7,12-DMBA	5.9, skin	22	Mouse, skin	2.4×10^5	4.8×10^5	Brookes and Lawley (1964)

[a] Largely soluble RNA.

In a study using β-propiolactone and several similar alkylating agents, it was also concluded that binding to DNA but not to RNA or protein correlated with tumor-initiating potency (Colburn and Boutwell, 1968). Dingman and Sporn (1967) and Brookes and Lawley (1964) also came to similar conclusions, on the basis of their studies with a series of aminoazo dyes and polycyclic aromatic hydrocarbons, respectively. On the other hand, using K-region epoxide and other derivatives of benz[a]anthracene and dibenz[a,b]anthracene and Chinese hamster celts, Kuroki et al. (1971–1972) concluded that a good correlation does not exist between the binding of the compounds to DNA and their ability to induce malignant transformations.

From the foregoing it appears that the quantitative binding of the carcinogen to DNA correlates well with carcinogenesis in the case of at least some chemical carcinogens. (For a detailed review see Lutz, 1979.)

7.2. Carcinogen–DNA Interactions: Qualitative Analysis

A qualitative analysis of carcinogen–DNA interaction will be of far greater importance than a quantitative analysis in relating carcinogen–DNA interaction to carcinogenesis. While considering this aspect it is important to focus not only on the site of modification on a particular purine or pyrimidine nucleotide, but also on the location of such modified nucleotide(s) in the DNA, the rationale being that perturbation in only certain regions of DNA may be relevant to the carcinogenic process. Data concerning the latter aspect are beginning to appear, and more information needs to be generated before any correlation between perturbation in a particular gene(s) and carcinogenesis can be established.

Nonetheless, several lines of evidence indicate that modification of groups involved in hydrogen bonding in the DNA duplex, such as the O^6 position of guanine, may be related to carcinogenesis. This implication was largely based on the following considerations: alkylating carcinogens like MNU accumulated O^6-MeG, a probable mutagenic lesion (Loveless, 1969), in the target tissue; the O^6-alkylguanines formed in brain DNA following the administration of the brain carcinogens ENU (Goth and Rajewsky, 1974a,b) and MNU (Kleihues and Buecheler, 1977) have a longer half-life, compared to that formed in the non-target organ liver; administration of large doses of DMN (doses that induce kidney tumors) increased the half-life of O^6-MeG in kidney DNA (Nicoll et al., 1977). A correlation between the formation and persistence of O^6-MeG and carcinogenesis has been demonstrated in other organs such as thymus (Frei et al., 1978), urinary bladder (Cox and Irving, 1977), and mammary gland (Cox and Irving, 1979). It should be pointed out that O^6-alkylguanine is formed in the DNA of nontarget organs but has a comparatively shorter half-life. The removal of O^6-MeG from DNA in vivo has presented several interesting problems; e.g., pretreatment with MNU or DMN was found to inhibit the removal of O^6-MeG formed by subsequent administration of the alkylating carcinogens and this was attributed to a saturation of the enzyme involved in O^6-MeG removal

(Kleihues and Margison, 1976; Stumpf *et al.*, 1979). However, recently Montesano *et al.* (1979) and Buckley *et al.* (1979) have found that chronic feeding of DMN or 2-AAF enhances the rate of removal of O^6-MeG formed by the administration of DMN. This phenomenon may be due to an adaptive response of the cell similar to the adaptive response reported in bacteria (Schendel and Robins, 1978; Robins and Cairns, 1979; Karran *et al.*, 1979).

373

INTERAC-
TIONS OF
CARCINOGENS
WITH NUCLEIC
ACIDS

The special significance of O^6-MeG as compared to other alkylated bases resides in the fact that substitution of the O^6 position of guanine facilitates the insertion of a wrong base during both replication and transcription by forcing the guanine into its enol form. Such a miscoding behavior of O^6-MeG was demonstrated *in vitro* using *E. coli* RNA and DNA polymerase and synthetic polyribo- or polydeoxyribonucleotides containing O^6-MeG (Gerchman and Ludlum, 1973; Abbott and Saffhill, 1979). It is not yet known whether in an *in vivo* system O^6-MeG will function as a miscoding lesion either during replication or during transcription. However, using different strains of mice with varying degrees of sensitivity toward MNU-induced carcinogenesis, it was found that the location of the tumors produced did not correlate well with the formation and persistence of O^6-alkylguanine in DNA (Buecheler and Kleihues, 1977). By measuring the number of precancerous lesions induced as a function of the time elapsed between DEN administration and partial hepatectomy, Scherer and Emmelot (1977) concluded that O^6-alkylation of guanine is not a relevant lesion for the first step in liver carcinogenesis. Similarly, Rabes *et al.* (1979) reported that in rats hepatocellular carcinomas were induced by a single administration of DMN only if given during the S phase, although the ratio of O^6-MeG:N-7-MeG was highest during G_1 and decreased rapidly during S and G_2-M phases.

Alkylation at the N-7 position of guanine is considerably greater compared to that at O^6, but alkylation at N-7 of guanine does not appear to be correlated with carcinogenecity. Surprisingly, the major interaction of the potent carcinogen AFB_1 with DNA is at N-7 of guanine (Lin *et al.*, 1977; Essigmann *et al.*, 1977).

Results from several laboratories indicate that the alkali-sensitive lesions induced by carcinogens in liver (Goodman and Potter, 1972; Sarma *et al.*, 1974, 1975; Den Engelse and Phillipus, 1977), intestine (Kanagalingam and Balis, 1975), and pancreas (Lilja *et al.*, 1978; Iqbal and Epstein, 1978) may be correlated to carcinogenesis. Similarly, in a few instances the formation of phosphotriesters has also been related to carcinogenesis (Shooter, 1978).

As pointed out earlier, all these correlations will remain speculative until each of the steps involved in the carcinogenic process are identified.

7.3. *Repair in Vivo of DNA Damage Induced by Chemical Carcinogens*

It is apparent from the above survey that the types of interactions between chemical carcinogens and nucleic acids (DNA and RNA) are varied, and that such interactions alter both the structure and the function of nucleic acids. In order to regain normal structure and function, the cell has devised several sophisticated processes to repair the altered nucleic acids. Virtually nothing is known about the repair of damaged RNA. However, several aspects of DNA repair have been investigated in bacteria and cells in culture following exposure to UV radiation (Hanawalt, 1972; Howard-Flanders, 1968), ionizing radiation (Lett *et al.*, 1970; Elkind and Redpath, 1977; Painter, 1970), and alkylating agents (Alexander, 1969; Coyle and Strauss, 1969–1970; Fox and Ayad, 1971; see also *Cold Spring Harbor Symp. Quant. Biol.* Vol. 33, 1968; Brash and Hart, 1978; Hanawalt and Setlow, 1975; Roberts, 1978). Very little is known about the repair of damage in DNA induced by chemical carcinogens in an intact animal (Goodman and Potter, 1972; Cox *et al.*, 1973; Damjanov *et al.*, 1973; Sarma *et al.*, 1974; Rajalakshmi and Sarma, 1973, 1975; Stewart and Farber, 1973).

Ideally, the repair of any nonphysiological alterations of the DNA molecule should result in the complete restoration of the original structure and function. The following is a brief survey of this presumably important area in chemical carcinogenesis.

7.3.1. Removal in Vivo of DNA-Bound Carcinogen or Carcinogen Metabolites

The dynamics and the mechanism by which the cell removes the bound carcinogen (or its metabolites) are not clearly understood. In the few investigations where this was studied, it was found that the removal of the DNA-bound carcinogen often followed multiphase kinetics and in many instances a certain percentage of bound carcinogen persisted for long periods of time.

Chemically, the simplest form of interaction between carcinogen and DNA is alkylation at one or more sites in the molecule. A few studies have been reported concerning the turnover of methyl or ethyl groups from various carcinogens. In many instances, elimination of such alkyl groups results in the loss of the alkylated bases from the DNA. Different methylated bases in DNA have different half-lives. For example, in *E. coli* O^6-MeG and N-3-methyladenine disappear more rapidly than does N-7-MeG (Lawley and Orr, 1970). In rat liver, the half-life of N-7-MeG is approximately 3 days (Margison *et al.*, 1973) while that of O^6-MeG is about 13 h (O'Connor *et al.*, 1973). It is noteworthy that the half-life *in vivo* of N-7-MeG is the same whether it is derived from MMS or from DMN (Margison *et al.*, 1973). However, the rate of removal of alkylated bases from different regions of the genome of the same organ or from different organs may not be the same. Mulivor *et al.* (1974) observed that significant amounts of depurinated sites were still present 7 days following the administration of DMN, even though the depurinatable sites were considerably decreased at this time compared to the number present at 4 h.

In general, it appears that the elimination of ethylated bases from DNA is slower than that of their methylated homologs (Lawley and Brookes, 1963). Further, interstrand cross-links in DNA of mouse L cells by sulfur mustard are unhooked faster ($t_{1/2} = 2$ h) than the rate of loss of mono adducts ($t_{1/2} = 18$ h) (Reid and Walker, 1969).

The removal of bulkier carcinogen adducts from DNA appears to have a more complex kinetics. Irving and Veazey (1969) reported that approximately 10%

of the radioactivity bound to rat liver DNA within 12–16 h persisted for at least 375

INTERAC-
TIONS OF
CARCINOGENS
WITH NUCLEIC
ACIDS
4–8 weeks following the administration of [9-^{14}C]2-AAF. The DNA-bound carcinogen decreased in two steps. Initially, the label was lost with a half-life of
10 h. Subsequently, the rate of loss was slower, with a half-life of 33 h (Szafarz
and Weisburger, 1969). As pointed out earlier, there appear to be at least two
types of reactions of N-acetoxy-2-AAF with guanine in DNA. The major component (80%), N-(deoxyguanosin-8-yl)-2-fluorenylacetamide, has a half-life of
days, while the other component (20%) remains on the DNA for periods of up
to 8 weeks. Warwick and Roberts (1967) have observed that after a single
administration of tritiated DAB the specific concentration of DNA-bound radioactivity decreased to approximately one-half its initial value in the first 7 days
and then remained nearly constant for 3 months. Similarly, 50% of the 7,12-
DMBA bound to DNA in parenchymal cells of mammary gland at 16 h was
present at 14 days and 31% at 42 days following the administration of tritiated
7,12-DMBA to rats (Janss et al., 1972).

7.3.2. Chromatin Structure and DNA Repair

The organization of the DNA in chromatin, which imposes restrictions on its
availability for interaction with carcinogens, also appears to affect the accessibility
of the carcinogen-induced damage to the repair enzymes. As pointed out earlier
(see Section 3), the rate of loss of the DNA-bound carcinogens or their metabolites
was not the same from different regions of chromatin DNA. This aspect of the
subsequent repair has been studied in systems where the DNA was damaged
either by chemicals or by physical agents such as UV irradiation and the repair
synthesis was monitored by measuring [^{3}H]-TdR incorporation in the presence
of hydroxyurea to inhibit replicative synthesis. The distribution of the incorporated label in chromatin DNA was determined by fractionating the chromatin
DNA on the basis of accessibility to endonucleases or by separating it into satellite
and main band DNA or eu- and heterochromatin. Harris et al. (1974) using
cytological techniques found that in human fibroblasts exposed to the chemical
carcinogens N-acetoxy-2-AAF, 7-Br-MeBA, or MNU or irradiated with UV, the
repair synthesis distribution was nonrandom, being greater in euchromatin than
in heterochromatin. Repair of damage induced by the monofunctional alkylating
agents, MMS and MNU, was reported by Bodell and Banerjee (1976) to be
reduced in mouse satellite DNA compared to main band DNA and it was
interepreted that the reduced repair activity in satellite DNA was due to its
location in a condensed chromatin fraction. Using micrococcal nuclease to fractionate the chromatin, Bodell (1977) showed that the "linker" region was the
primary site of DNA repair synthesis after MMS treatment of mouse mammary
gland fragments in culture. A similar preferential repair in linker regions of
nuclei was observed immediately after alkylation of mouse mammary tissue with
MNU or MMS (Bodell and Banerjee, 1979) but at later times, i.e., 6–12 h after
MNU or MMS treatment, the repair was more randomly distributed between
linker and core regions. They also showed that there was increased repair activity
in the transcriptionally active regions of chromatin alkylated by MMS or MNU

376

S. RAJALAKSHMI,
PREMA M. RAO,
AND
D. S. R. SARMA

as determined by the release of the incorporated thymidine in the DNase I-susceptible regions of chromatin.

Studies on the intragenomic distribution of repair synthesis in cultured mammalian cells exposed to N-acetoxy-2-AAF, 7-BrMeBA, or UV (Lieberman and Poirer, 1974a,b) indicate that DNA damage involving either pyrimidines or purines was repairable to about the same extent in both unique and repetitive sequences, although heterogeneity within any class was not ruled out. However, using microccocal nuclease to fractionate the repair-labeled chromatin from W1-38 fibroblasts exposed to N-acetoxy-2-AAF, Tlsty and Lieberman (1978) found that the initial repair synthesis occurs primarily in the nuclease-sensitive linker regions. However, continuous-labeling and pulse-chase experiments indicated that with time much of the repair-incorporated label was in the nuclease-insensitive regions, and nucleosome rearrangement in chromatin during repair was postulated. A similar preferential repair in the linker regions soon after treatment with 7-BrMeBA followed by a randomization at later time periods was reported by Oleson et al. (1979).

The most extensively studied repair system is that following UV irradiation. Wilkins and Hart (1974) determined the UV-endonuclease-accessible sites in UV-irradiated human fibroblasts treated with 0.15 and 2.0 M NaCl. Cells kept in high salt showed more endonuclease-susceptible sites than those kept in low salt, and this increase was attributed to sites being unmasked by the dissociation of bound proteins at the higher salt concentration. *In vivo* the nuclease-susceptible sites detectable under low-salt conditions were no longer present 44 h after irradiation whereas the sites detectable under high salt persisted, indicating a nonuniform repair process. Similarly, Buhl et al. (1974) found that in *P. tridactylus* irradiated with UV, 35% of the dimers are monomerized fast, and although 50% of the dimers are still present in the DNA 24 hr after UV treatment, these are not recognized by UV endonuclease. They postulated that the repair system that acts on a particular dimer is determined probably by the dimer's immediate environment, which changes with its position in the cell cycle and/or the extent of aggregation or coiling of the chromatin at the time after irradiation when the repair systems operate. The repair of UV-induced damage and the kinetics of rearrangement of nucleotides incorporated during repair were investigated by Smerdon and Lieberman (1978) and Smerdon et al. (1979) in normal human fibroblasts and fibroblasts from the C and D complementation groups of XP cells, which are partially deficient in excision repair. Initially (i.e., at the end of the pulse period) most of the repair was in microccocal nuclease-sensitive regions. The kinetics of rearrangement was found to be biphasic in that 85% of the repair synthesis sites undergo rapid rearrangement (4–5 h), while in the remaining sites rearrangement was minimal. It was speculated that nucleosome rearrangement may be induced by the repair process or the rate of repair synthesis may be regulated by the nucleosome rearrangement. Williams and Friedberg (1979) also found that although the distribution of thymine dimers, immediately after irradiation or at different times after irradiation, was similar in total DNA and core particle DNA, the repair synthesis was primarily in the microccocal

377

INTERAC-
TIONS OF
CARCINOGENS
WITH NUCLEIC
ACIDS

nuclease-sensitive regions. However, they detected only a limited (30%) rearrangement of these sites into nuclease-insensitive regions at later time periods. In contrast to the results obtained by these two groups, Cleaver (1977) found no evidence of nucleosome rearrangement during repair, although preferential repair in linker regions was observed. The reasons for these discrepancies are not clear at the present.

Although these studies point out several new aspects of carcinogen–DNA interaction—e.g., (1) that carcinogen-binding sites are distributed in a nonrandom fashion in the genome; (2) that DNA conformation and/or sequences play a significant role in such an interaction (see Section 3); (3) that the kinetics of repair from different regions are not the same; and (4) that carcinogens either per se or the resultant damage and/or repair appear to cause alterations in gene organization—they are not without discrepancies. Most of the discrepancies, however, may be due to the fact that different techniques are used to prepare and fractionate the chromatin DNA, some of which are not precise enough.

7.4. Probable Steps in the Removal of Bound Carcinogen and Subsequent Repair of the Damaged DNA

The enzymology of the steps involved in the *in vivo* removal of DNA-bound carcinogen or its metabolite in mammalian systems remains a challenging area for fruitful study. The probable steps in the removal of the DNA-bound carcinogen and subsequent repair of the damaged DNA are schematically presented in Fig. 5. Much of the work on DNA repair has been done in bacteria and deals

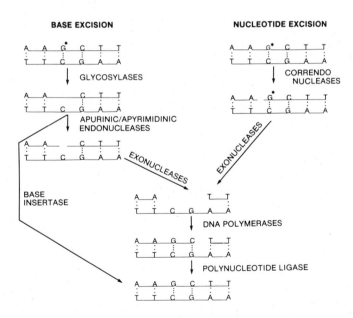

FIGURE 5. Probable steps in removal of bound carcinogen and repair of damaged DNA. Asterisk indicates the chemical modification.

378

S. RAJALAKSHMI,
PREMA M. RAO,
AND
D. S. R. SARMA

with the excision of pyrimidine dimers induced by UV irradiation and these offer a guide to the study in mammalian systems. Several aspects of DNA repair have been discussed in detail (for a review see Hanawalt et al., 1979). Basically there are two modes of removal of modified DNA bases, namely base excision and nucleotide excision (Fig. 5). In the base excision mode, only the modified base is removed, resulting in an apurinic or apyrimidinic DNA. Glycosylases in microorganisms that can remove N-3-methyladenine and N-3-ethyladenine from alkylated DNA have been reported (Laval, 1977; Riazuddin and Lindahl, 1978; Brent, 1979). Renard et al. (1978) reported an enzyme activity in rat liver nuclei that can remove O^6-ethylguanine from ethylated rat liver chromatin. Karran et al. (1979) have reported the presence of an enzyme activity in adapted E. coli that can remove O^6-MeG from methylated DNA. Although the detailed mechanism involved in this removal is not clear, it is apparently not mediated by a demethylase (Pegg, 1978b) or glycosylase or nuclease. Modification at certain sites of the DNA bases may create chemical instability and result in apurinic or apyrimidinic sites. For example, N-7-MeG is not actively excised enzymatically either in mammalian or in microbial systems but is slowly released from alkylated DNA nonenzymatically (Lawley and Orr, 1970; Prakash and Strauss, 1970; Margison et al., 1973). However, an enzyme activity in E. coli that can excise this modified base after the opening of the imidiazole ring has been reported recently (Chetsanga and Lindahl, 1979).

The first step involved in the restructuring of such apurinic or apyrimidinic DNA is the endonucleolytic attack by apurinic or apyrimidinic endonucleases. Apurinic endonucleases appear to be ubiquitous, and the activity has been demonstrated both in microbial as well as in mammalian systems including human tissues (Hadi et al., 1973; Verly et al., 1974; Teebor and Duker, 1975; Brent, 1976; Ljungquist and Lindahl, 1977; Linsley et al., 1977; Gossard and Verly, 1978; and also see reviews by Grossman et al., 1975; Roberts, 1978). The endonucleases nick the DNA on the 5' side of the apurinic sites giving 3'-OH and a 5'-phosphate. Since at least some of the apurinic endonucleases have no exonuclease activity, the DNA ligase can reseal the bond before the damage is corrected and thus may produce an abortive repair. However, it is possible that DNA-binding proteins could prevent this abortive repair (Grossman et al., 1975; Laval, 1977), and such binding proteins for UV-irradiated and apurinic DNA have been reported in human placenta (Feldberg and Grossman, 1976) and in cultured human fibroblasts (Deutsch and Linn, 1979), respectively. Alternatively, an exonuclease can excise the apurinic site, yielding a gap that in turn can be filled in by DNA polymerases, and the eventual restoration of the continuity of the phosphodiester chain can be achieved by a DNA ligase.

As pointed out in Fig. 5, the apurinic site may also be filled in by a base insertase. This enzyme preferentially incorporates purine bases and guanine in particular (Deutsch and Linn, 1979). A similar phenomenon was reported by Hennings and Michael (1976), who also observed the incorporation of radioactivity from deoxyguanosine rather than thymidine into the DNA of mouse skin cells following an exposure to low levels of MNNG. This enzymatic activity was not found to be deficient in the xeroderma pigmentosum D cell line, which lacks a major apurinic endonuclease species (Kuhnlein *et al.*, 1978).

379

INTERAC-
TIONS OF
CARCINOGENS
WITH NUCLEIC
ACIDS

As an alternative to the base excision mode, the damaged region may also be excised by nucleotide excision, a pathway that involves an endonucleolytic attack. Endonucleases that recognize and incise specifically at or near thymine dimers in the DNA have been reported. These are termed as correctional endonucleases or correndonucleases (Fig. 5) (see Grossman *et al.*, 1975, for a review). Although endonuclease preparations that attack carcinogen-modified DNA have been reported (Friedberg and Goldthwait, 1969; Van Lancker and Tomura, 1974; Maher *et al.*, 1974), their specificity toward any one particular carcinogen–DNA adduct has not been determined. The excision of the carcinogen–DNA adduct, however, is mediated by exonucleases. It is not yet clear whether the exonucleases that operate in nucleotide excision and base excision pathways are one and the same. The insertion of the nucleotides and the eventual resealing of the gap are mediated by DNA polymerases and polynucleotide ligase, respectively. The number of inserted nucleotides vary from 10 to a few thousand, depending on the type of cell, nature of DNA damage, and probably the intragenomic location of the DNA damage. For example, Regan and Setlow (1974) observed that *N*-acetoxy-2-AAF and UV induced a long patch repair, whereas X-rays and monofunctional alkylating agents such as MMS induced a short patch repair. Although the carcinogen-induced DNA damage may be repaired by either the base excision or the nucleotide excision mode, the relationship between the nature of the carcinogen-induced lesion and the mode of repair pathway is not yet thoroughly understood. Nonetheless, *N*-3-methyl- or ethyladenine (Riazuddin and Lindahl, 1978; Laval, 1977), N^6-(12)methylbenz[α]anthracenyl-7-methyl)adenine, and N^2-(12-methylbenz[α]anthracenyl-7-methyl-guanine (Kirtikar *et al.*, 1976) in DNA appear to be repaired via the base excision mode; others, e.g., 2–AAF adducts in DNA and pyridimidine dimers induced by UV are repaired by the nucleotide excision mode (Cleaver, 1978). Interestingly, O^6-MeG in DNA appears to be repaired by the nucleotide excision mode in mammalian systems and by the base excision mode in *E. coli* (Bodell *et al.*, 1979; Altamirano–Dimas *et al.*, 1979). Further, XP cell lines that have decreased capacity to repair pyrimidine dimers, a lesion that seems to be repaired by the nucleotide excision mode, also exhibit decreased ability to remove O^6-MeG, O^6-ethylguanine, and the lesions induced by *N*-acetoxy-2-AAF (Setlow and Regan, 1972; Goth-Goldstein, 1977; Bodell *et al.*, 1979; Altamirano-Dimas *et al.*, 1979).

7.5. Postreplicative Repair Processes

Despite the multiplicity of the excision repair processes, removal of some of the carcinogen–DNA adducts can be a relatively slow process; and especially in mammalian systems it may be incomplete before the cell traverses through the S phase. Replication of such carcinogen-modified DNA often results in newly made DNA of lower molecular weight compared to the corresponding control (see Section 6.2.1) probably because some of the lesions may not permit replication and thereby create gaps in the newly made strand. Since such an incomplete replication may result in chromosomal damage and eventual cell death, it would seem logical that the cell has developed mechanisms by which the gap is filled in. Some of the postreplicative repair processes by which the original damage is bypassed and the resulting gaps, if any, are filled in are schematically presented in Fig. 6, and are briefly discussed below.

If the gaps in the daughter strand occurred because certain carcinogen-induced lesions in DNA did not permit replication and these are eventually filled in by *de novo* synthesis (Fig. 6), then one wonders how the DNA polymerase system that was so stringent and did not copy the lesion initially becomes less stringent and copies the lesion later on. At least in bacteria, one of the mechanisms by which such a gap filling is achieved is by an inducible repair system termed "SOS" repair (SOS, the international distress signal) (see Witkin, 1976, for a detailed discussion).

The term "SOS repair" was coined by Radman (1974) to describe a group of inducible processes in *E. coli* that appear to be dependent on *lex A* and *rec A* genes. These processes, among many others, include induction of prophage in *E. coli* K-12, induced bacterial mutagenesis, and the so-called "Weigle reactivation" phenomenon, wherein UV-irradiated bacteriophages are able to survive better, albeit with an increased mutation rate, when plated on previously lightly irradiated *E. coli* as compared to plating on nonirradiated bacteria.

According to one hypothesis, under uninduced conditions, the lex A gene product binds to the SOS repressor and protects it from being attacked by a protease (a rec A gene product). During SOS induction, an activator (DNA degradation products) binds to the lex A gene product and removes it from the SOS repressor. The SOS repressor is now cleaved by the protease (a rec A gene product), thus permitting the induction of SOS functions (Witkin, 1976).

Since none of the constitutive DNA polymerases can copy UV-irradiated DNA past pyrimidine dimers and no new DNA polymerase has been identified during SOS repair, it was suggested that the product of SOS induction may be an

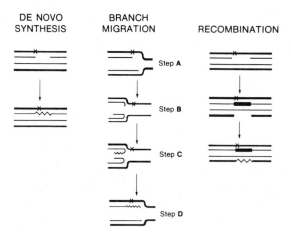

FIGURE 6. Probable mechanisms of postreplication repair of carcinogen-damaged DNA. **X** indicates carcinogen-induced lesion.

inhibitor to a proofreading $3'-5'$ exonuclease activity of the polymerase, thus permitting the filling up of gaps opposite to a noninstructive lesion (Villani *et al.*, 1978; Witkin, 1976). Accordingly, in the absence of this inhibitor, nucleotides inserted opposite pyrimidine dimers or other noninstructive lesions induced by carcinogens would be promptly removed. In its presence, the stable insertion of one or more wrong nucleotide would permit replication, albeit with a high probability of mutation. Indeed, induction of SOS functions increases cell survival, but is always accompanied by an increased mutation rate.

381
INTERAC-
TIONS OF
CARCINOGENS
WITH NUCLEIC
ACIDS

Exposure of Chinese hamster cells to *N*-acetoxy-2-AAF results initially in the synthesis of DNA of low molecular weight; after a lag period, the DNA becomes normal in size. However, exposure of cells to a lower concentration of this carcinogen prior to challenging them with a higher concentration decreased the lag period (D'Ambrosio and Setlow, 1976). The authors interpreted their results to indicate that prior treatment with low concentrations of *N*-acetoxy-2-AAF induced a repair system that was dependent on protein synthesis analogous to SOS repair in bacteria. Other explanations for this phenomenon were offered by Painter (1978) and Park and Cleaver (1979).

Chemical carcinogens have also been found to induce other types of SOS phenomena in bacteria. For example, several carcinogens induced prophage in *E. coli* K-12 (Moreau *et al.*, 1976), and AFB_1 enhanced reactivation of UV-damaged λ phage (Sarasin *et al.*, 1977). Similarly, enhanced survival of UV-irradiated SV40 (Sarasin and Hanawalt, 1978) and herpes virus (Lytle *et al.*, 1978) was demonstrated in host cells exposed to chemical carcinogens such as MMS, EMS, AFB_1, and 2-AAF metabolites prior to infection. This process is independent of the excision repair mechanism because reactivation of herpes virus occurs in XP cells also (Lytle *et al.*, 1976).

Alternate to this error-prone mechanism, the carcinogen-induced postreplicative gaps in the daughter strand may also be filled in by an error-free pathway that involves strand displacement and branch migration (see Fig. 6). According to this scheme, DNA synthesis stops at the lesion on one strand (step A); after the branch migration (step B), synthesis on the daughter DNA template occurs (step C). By another branch migration step, a completed double-stranded DNA results (step D) wherein the carcinogen-induced lesion is bypassed (Higgins *et al.*, 1976).

Carcinogen-induced postreplicative gaps in the daughter strand may also be filled in by another pathway involving a series of recombinational exchanges, which involves the insertion of an identical stretch of the parental strand of DNA into the daughter strand (Fig. 6), thus resulting in not only filling up the gap in the daughter strand but also bypassing the lesion in the parental strand (Rupp and Howard-Flanders, 1968). During such an exchange, some of the UV-induced pyrimidine dimers present in the parental strand are also exchanged into the daughter strand (Ganesan, 1974). Similarly, using a rat liver model some of the DMN-induced methylated bases present in the parental strand were also found in the daughter strand following DNA replication (Columbano *et al.*, 1980). These results raise the possibility that although the lesions in the parental

S. RAJALAKSHMI,
PREMA M. RAO,
AND
D. S. R. SARMA

strand are bypassed in the first cell cycle, it may take more than one cell cycle before this postreplicative gap-forming ability in the daughter strand is lost.

Crucial as it may be for cell survival, very little is known about the mechanism of recombination. However, in recent years, the biochemistry of the initiation of this process appears to be unraveling. A homogeneous rec A protein from *E. coli* has been shown to promote the exchange of a single-stranded DNA chain into homologous duplex DNA (strand assimilation). One of the products of such a reaction is a "D loop" structure, a locally triple-stranded region containing the paired exogenous strand and a displaced single-stranded loop from the duplex (McEntee *et al.*, 1979; Shibata *et al.*, 1979). A binding protein isolated from *E. coli* that specifically binds to single-stranded DNA appears to enhance strand assimilation (McEntee *et al.*, 1980).

7.6. DNA Repair and Carcinogenesis

Although the exact mechanism or mechanisms by which DNA damage and repair are involved in carcinogenesis cannot be understood with any accuracy at the present time, the overwhelming evidence, albeit circumstantial, indicating the causal relationship between these two processes warrants serious consideration. For example, carcinogens by and large interact with DNA, cause several types of DNA damage, and induce mutations in bacteriophages, microorganisms, and probably also in many eukaryotic cells (McCann *et al.*, 1976; Huberman and Sachs, 1974; Krahn and Heidelberger, 1977; Bridges, 1976). In at least a few human diseases like xeroderma pigmentosum (Cleaver, 1968, 1969), Fanconi's anemia (Sasaki and Tonomura, 1973), and ataxia telangiectasia (Paterson *et al.*, 1976), each associated with an unusually high incidence of various neoplasms, a deficiency of some kind in DNA repair is observed.

Cells from the thyroid and adjacent tissue of small fish (*Polcilia formosa*) irradiated with UV *in vitro* and then injected into an isogeneic recipient induced thyroid proliferation that was interpreted as a tumorous growth. However, if the UV irradiation was followed but not preceded by photoreactivating illumination (which is thought to monomerize the dimers), the yield of thyroid growths was decreased (Hart *et al.*, 1977). These results were interpreted to indicate that pyrimidine dimers are tumorigenic lesions. Similarly, treatment with caffeine, an inhibitor of postreplicative repair, suppressed the carcinogenic effects of UV (Zajdela and Latarjet, 1973) or cigarette smoke condensate (Rothwell, 1974) on mouse skin and of 4NQO (Nomura, 1976) or urethan (Theiss and Shimkin, 1978; Nomura, 1980) in the lung. As pointed out earlier (see Section 7.2), correlation also appears to exist between the extent and persistence of O^6-alkylguanine, a potential mutagenic lesion, and carcinogenicity.

One of the mechanisms by which DNA damage and repair may be implicated in carcinogenesis is the replication of DNA prior to the repair of a carcinogen-induced critical lesion. Evidence is being accumulated to indicate that cell proliferation in general and DNA replication in particular is an important step for the initiation of the carcinogenic process. For example, using the procedure described by Solt and Farber (1976) as modified by Cayama *et al.* (1978), wherein the carcinogen-initiated cells are selectively stimulated to grow into islands of presumptive preneoplastic hepatocytes, by a mitogenic stimulus in the presence of 0.02% 2-AAF, it was demonstrated that cell proliferation, prior to the repair of the carcinogen-induced critical lesion, is an essential step in the initiation of liver carcinogenesis by a single, nonnecrogenic dose of several carcinogens such as MNU (Cayama *et al.*, 1978), 1,2-DMH (Ying *et al.*, 1979), DMN, and DEN (Ying and Sarma, 1979). Similarly, cell transformation by radiation and viruses requires at least one round of cell proliferation prior to the repair of critical DNA damage (Borek and Sachs, 1967; Todaro and Green, 1966; Kakunaga, 1974).

383

INTERAC-
TIONS OF
CARCINOGENS
WITH NUCLEIC
ACIDS

Cell proliferation may exert its crucial effect in the initiation of chemical carcinogenesis at more than one step, e.g., (1) carcinogen–DNA interaction, (2) DNA repair, and (3) DNA replication. During replication the conformation and organization of DNA within the cell undergo changes, and it is perhaps logical to expect that these changes would affect carcinogen–DNA interaction and/or the subsequent repair, and such an altered interaction and/or repair may play a critical role in the initiation of carcinogenesis.

Studies on the quantitative aspects of the interaction of carcinogens like urethan and DMN with liver DNA revealed no differences between regenerating and nonregenerating liver. On the other hand, Marquardt *et al.* (1971) observed increased interaction of 7,12-DMBA with liver DNA during liver regeneration. Yuspa and Bates (1970) and Bowden and Boutwell (1973) observed that 7,12-DMBA interacted with both replicated and nonreplicated DNA. In all these studies no attempt was made to determine whether there were any differences in the qualitative nature of the interaction. During replication, the amount of transcribable genes increases. Recently, Tew *et al.* (1979) observed that the interaction of nitrosoureas with DNase II-solubilizable regions of DNA (probably representing transcribable genes) was preferentially increased in hydrocortisone-treated cells as compared with nontreated controls. One wonders, therefore, whether the interaction of carcinogens with the increased transcribable genes available during replication may have a role in the initiation of carcinogenesis. In addition, Rao *et al.* (1978) observed that [^{14}C]-DMN-induced N-3-methyl-adenine in rat liver chromatin that was initially completely susceptible to DNase I (under conditions of 50% digestion of chromatin DNA) was rendered partially nondigestible when the animal was treated with MNU after the [^{14}C]-DMN, suggesting an alteration in chromatin organization. If one extrapolates this interpretation to chromatin during replication, it is possible that alterations in chromatin organization during replication might affect the availability of carcinogen-induced lesions to repair enzymes. Indeed, during the S phase an inhibition of the removal of some of the methylated bases has been observed (Abanobi *et al.*, 1980; Smith *et al.*, 1980; Ying, 1980), thereby increasing (1) the persistence of carcinogen-induced critical lesions and (2) the chances of replication of DNA with such lesions.

384

S. RAJALAKSHMI,
PREMA M. RAO,
AND
D. S. R. SARMA

As pointed out earlier (see Section 6.2.1), replication of carcinogen- or mutagen-damaged DNA, in microbial and mammalian cell culture systems or *in vivo* using rat liver, often results in newly made DNA of low molecular weight; and after an initial lag period of hours to days, this low-molecular-weight DNA eventually becomes normal in size. It is not known whether these gaps are filled in by an error-prone inducible DNA polymerizing system, by a supposedly error-free branch migration pathway, by some recombinational events, or by a combination of the above-mentioned pathways. If they are filled in by the error-prone inducible DNA polymerizing system, the chances of inserting a wrong base are high and may thus result in altered DNA sequences and organization. In addition, replication of carcinogen-damaged DNA may also increase the recombinational events whereby the carcinogen-induced lesions are transferred to the daughter cell (Columbano *et al.*, 1980), and on further replication these lesions may again induce error-prone gap-filling mechanisms and the process may be continued for several cell cycles until the carcinogen-induced original damage is completely excised. Thus, replication of the carcinogen-damaged DNA and the recombinational events cause an amplification of the effects of the original DNA damage.

8. Perspectives and Conclusions

It is evident from this brief survey that any conclusions implicating altered nucleic acids in any proposed mechanism of chemical carcinogenesis must remain essentially speculative. Although there is an increasing body of information concerning various aspects of the interactions of carcinogens with nucleic acids, this factual base remains insufficient to permit anything but conjecture about how these interactions are related to carcinogenesis. Despite this inability to reach definitive conclusions, it has now become possible to begin to pinpoint areas of study that seem relevant to one or more aspects of the carcinogenic process.

In view of the short period of exposure to a chemical carcinogen that is often sufficient to trigger the carcinogenic process, it would seem that any relevant alterations in RNA or DNA would relate to initiation. Although variations in the control of gene action almost certainly play a major role in the new patterns of cell behavior seen during the cellular evolution to cancer, the primary effects of carcinogens can be most easily related to the initial events at this time. This is most easily viewed in terms of a permanent alteration in information content, either structural or regulatory or both.

What types of alterations in RNA or DNA induced by chemicals could lead to a permanent change, and how can such alterations be modified or nullified by repair processes? With respect to RNA, some of the possibilities are as follows. (1) The induction of a change in an RNA substrate for reverse transcriptase, resulting in a permanent transfer of misinformation to a DNA product. (2) The induction of a change in mRNA or tRNA leading to new proteins with different specificities. This could lead, in turn, to alterations either in the replication of those macromolecules (DNA, RNA) concerned with information storage or in the action of proteins involved in the control of DNA replication or transcription, e.g., "repressors." The repair of carcinogen-altered RNA has been essentially ignored, and yet it could be important in the study of the metabolic functions of RNA, especially as they relate to carcinogenesis.

385

INTERAC-
TIONS OF
CARCINOGENS
WITH NUCLEIC
ACIDS

With respect to DNA, there are many possibilities and uncertainties that relate to carcinogenesis. (1) Are interactions between carcinogens and DNA random or nonrandom? If it is nonrandom as is evident at least in some instances, what governs such regulated interaction? Is it the DNA sequence, conformation, and/or its organization within the nucleus that regulates the carcinogen–DNA interaction. This is especially important because DNA-binding ligands that alter the conformation appear to influence carcinogen–DNA interaction (Rajalakshmi *et al.*, 1978*a,b*, 1980). Similarly, the secondary structure of DNA seems to be one of the determinants in the interaction of BP derivatives with DNA (Hsu *et al.*, 1979; Meehan and Straub, 1979). Further, evidence is being accumulated that DNA can exist in more than one form. The recent structure, the Z form of DNA, proposed for an alternating purine-pyrimidine polymer (Wang *et al.*, 1979; Arnott *et al.*, 1980), exhibits certain interesting characteristics relevant to carcinogenesis. For example, in this conformation cytosine adopts the *anti* conformation relative to its deoxyribose as in B DNA, whereas guanine adopts the *syn* conformation and the N-7 and C-8 positions of guanine are thus exposed to the solvent and may facilitate the interaction at these sites. Since the conformation and organization of DNA seem to vary greatly as a function of the physiological state and needs of a cell, one wonders whether these changes influence the carcinogen–DNA interaction and the availability of the damaged regions to repair enzymes. If so, the role of physiological state in the initiation of carcinogenesis could be explained. (2) What are the ways by which *in vivo* (a) the DNA-bound carcinogen or its metabolite is removed and (b) the repair and subsequent restructuring of the DNA back to its normal state and function are achieved? Although a tremendous amount of information on these aspects has been generated using bacterial systems, unfortunately very little is known about this presumably important aspect using mammalian systems. The knowledge gained using bacterial systems can only be used as guidelines because the detailed mechanism by which a lesion is repaired in these two systems appears to be different. For example, O^6-MeG is removed in *E. coli* via the base excision mode, whereas in mammalian systems apparently it is removed via the nucleotide excision mode (see Section 7.4). (3) Can the role of cell proliferation in initiation be accounted for entirely as a means of converting transitory damage to DNA to permanent damage through DNA replication, or are there other considerations that are important, e.g., can such a replication induce legitimate recombinational events (homologous strand assimilation) and/or illegitimate recombinational events mediated by transposons that in turn may bring about an altered genetic organization within the cell, a step that may be very important for the initiation of carcinogenesis?

In spite of the extensive work that has been carried out in identifying various lesions induced by carcinogens in DNA, very little can be said with any accuracy concerning the critical lesion or lesions that are involved in the initiation of carcinogenesis. This is largely because carcinogenesis is a multistage process and several steps (especially the rate-limiting ones) have not yet been identified. However, in view of the recent advances in the development of model systems to study in a sequential manner liver carcinogenesis in general and the initiation process in particular (see Farber, this volume), it may now be possible to identify the critical lesion or lesions or at least identify the lesions that are not relevant for the initiation of liver carcinogenesis. Further, these model systems are also useful to define the role of DNA repair and replication of damaged DNA in the initiation of liver carcinogenesis.

The major problem, in the final analysis, is the potential usefulness of these studies to unravel the mechanisms of human carcinogenesis. Obviously, the information gained using experimental animals, mammalian cells in culture, or microbial systems and *in vitro* studies using nucleic acids as well as synthetic polynucleotides will serve as valuable guidelines. However, there is an urgency to develop model systems using human tissues to study carcinogen–nucleic acid interaction, DNA damage and repair, and other related aspects. Recent studies in this direction point out that *in vitro*, several human tissues do metabolize chemical carcinogens to active metabolites that can interact with DNA (e.g., see Harris *et al.*, 1978).

These considerations are only a few of the many that seem to have possible importance in understanding any relationship of carcinogen–nucleic acid interaction to carcinogenesis. It is hoped that the clarification of these and other problem areas will lead to progressively more insight into the processes by which chemicals trigger the evolution to malignant neoplasia.

Note added in proof: The removal of N-7-MeG from DNA was thought until recently to be nonenzymatic; however, an enzymatic activity for its removal has recently been reported (Cathcart and Goldthwait, 1981; Laval *et al.*, 1981; Singer and Brent, 1981; Margison and Pegg, 1981).

ACKNOWLEDGMENTS

The authors' research included in this review was supported in part by grants from the National Institutes of Health (CA 14689, CA 23958), the National Cancer Institute, and the Medical Research Council of Canada.

We wish to thank Mrs. Ayesha Alam, Miss Elizabeth Warner, and Ms. Helen Robitaille for their expert assistance and patience during the preparation of this manuscript.

9. References

ABANOBI, S. E., COLUMBANO, A., MULIVOR, R. A., RAJALAKSHMI, S., AND SARMA, D. S. R., 1980. *In vivo* replication of hepatic deoxyribonucleic acid of rats treated with dimethylnitrosamine: Presence of dimethylnitrosamine induced O^6-methylguanine, N-7-methylguanine and N-3-methyladenine in the replicated hybrid deoxyribonucleic acid, *Biochemistry* **19:**1382.

387
INTERAC-
TIONS OF
CARCINOGENS
WITH NUCLEIC
ACIDS

ABBOTT, P. J., AND SAFFHILL, R., 1977, DNA synthesis with methylated poly(dA-dT) template: Possible role of O^4-methylthymine as a promutagenic base, *Nucleic Acids Res.* **4**:761.

ABBOTT, P. J., AND SAFFHILL, R., 1979, DNA synthesis with methylated poly(dC-dG) templates: Evidence for competitive nature to miscoding by O^6-methylguanine, *Biochim. Biophys. Acta* **562**:51.

AGARWAL, M. K., AND WEINSTEIN, I. B., 1970, Modifications of ribonucleic acid by chemical carcinogens. II. *In vivo* reaction of N-2-acetylaminofluorene with rat liver ribonucleic acid, *Biochemistry* **9**:503.

ALEXANDER, P., 1952, Interference with the formation of a nucleoprotein complex by radiomimetic compounds, *Nature (London)* **169**:226.

ALEXANDER, P., 1969, Comparison of the mode of action by which some alkylating agents and ionizing radiations kill mammalian cells, *Ann. N.Y. Acad. Sci.* **163**:652.

ALEXANDROV, K., VENDRELY, C., AND VENDRELY, R., 1970, A comparative study of the action of carcinogenic substances on the RNA synthesis in mouse skin, *Cancer Res.* **30**:1192.

ALTAMIRANO-DIMAS, M., SKLAR, R., AND STRAUSS, B., 1979, Selectivity of the excision of alkylation products in a xeroderma-pigmentosum derived lymphoblastoid line, *Mutat. Res.* **60**:197.

ANDOH, T., KATO, K., TAKAOKA, T., AND KATSUTA, H., 1971, Carcinogenesis in tissue culture. XIII. Binding of 4-nitroquinoline-1-oxide-^{3}H to nucleic acids and proteins of L.P3 and JTC 25-P3 cells, *Int. J. Cancer* **7**:455.

ARAKI, M., KAWAZOE, Y., AND NAGATA, C., 1969, Chemical carcinogens. IX. Homolytic degradation of O,O'-diacetyl-4-hydroxyaminoquinoline-1-oxide (1-acetoxy-4-acetyloxyimino-1,4-dihydro-quinoline), *Chem. Pharm. Bull.* **17**:1344.

ARCOS, J. C., AND ARGUS, M. F., 1968, Molecular geometry and carcinogenic activity of aromatic compounds: New perspectives, *Adv. Cancer Res.* **11**:305.

ARCOS, J. C., VENKATESEN, N., AND ARGUS, M. F., 1971 Modification of the flow dichroism spectrum of rat liver nuclear DNA by *in vivo* alkylation with hepatocarcinogenic dialkylnitrosamines, *Gann* **62**:523.

ARNOLD, E. A., AND YOUNG, K. E., 1974, Heterogeneity of chromatin: Fractionation of sonicated rat liver chromatin by partial precipitation with Mg^{2+}, *Arch. Biochem. Biophys.* **164**:73.

ARNOTT, S., CHANDRASEKARAN, R., BIRDSALL, D. L., LESLIE, A. G. W., AND RETLIFF, R. L., 1980, Left handed DNA helices, *Nature (London)* **283**:743.

AXEL, R., 1975, Cleavage of DNA in nuclei and chromatin with staphylococcal nuclease, *Biochemistry* **14**:2921.

AXEL, R., WEINSTEIN, I. B., AND FARBER, E., 1967, Patterns of transfer RNA in normal rat liver during hepatic carcinogenesis, *Proc. Natl. Acad. Sci. USA* **58**:1255.

AXEL, R., CEDAR, H., AND FELSENFELD, G., 1975, The structure of the globin genes in chromatin, *Biochemistry* **14**:2489.

BACKER, J. M., AND WEINSTEIN, I. B., 1980, Modification of mitochondrial DNA by a dihydrodiolepoxide derivative of benzo(a)pyrene, *Proc. Am. Assoc. Cancer Res.* **21**:93.

BANNON, P., AND VERLY, W., 1972, Alkylation of phosphates and stability of phosphate triesters in DNA, *Eur. J. Biochem.* **31**:103.

BARBIN, A., BRESIL, H., CROSY, A., JACQUIGNON, P., MALAVEILLE, C., MONTESANO, R., AND BARTSCH, H., 1975, Liver microsome-mediated formation of alkylating agents from vinyl bromide and vinyl chloride, *Biochem. Biophys. Res. Commun.* **67**:596.

BARTSCH, H., AND MONTESANO, R., 1975, Mutagenic and carcinogenic effects of vinyl chloride, *Mutat. Res.* **32**:93.

BARTSCH, H., MILLER, J. A., AND MILLER, E. C., 1972, Activation of carcinogenic aromatic hydroxylamines by enzymatic O-acetylation, *Proc. Am. Assoc. Cancer Res.* **13**:12.

BARTSCH, H., MONTESANO, R., AND MALAVEILLE, C., 1975, Human, rat and mouse liver-mediated mutagenicity of the vinyl chloride in *S. typhimurium* strains, *Int. J. Cancer* **15**:429.

BEACH, D. J., AND SUNDERMAN, F. W., JR., 1970, Nickel carbonyl inhibition of RNA synthesis by a chromatin–RNA polymerase complex from hepatic nuclei, *Cancer Res.* **30**:48.

BELAND, F. A., 1978, Computer generated graphic models of the N^2-substituted deoxyguanosine adducts of 2-acetylaminofluorene and benzo(α)pyrene and the O^6-substituted deoxyguanosine adduct of 1-naphthylamine in the DNA double helix, *Chem. Biol. Interact.* **22**:329.

BENFEY, O. T., 1970, *Introduction to Organic Reaction Mechanisms*, McGraw-Hill, New York.

BERENBLUM, I., AND TRAININ, N., 1960, Possible two-stage mechanism in experimental leukemogenesis, *Science* **132**:40.

BERGMANN, F., 1942, On the mechanism of tumor production by chemical agents, *Cancer Res.* **2**:660.

BLACK, H. S., AND JIRGENSONS, B., 1967, Interactions of aflatoxin with histones and DNA, *Plant Physiol.* **42:**731.

BLACKBURN, G. M., FENWICK, R. G., AND THOMPSON, M. W., 1972, Structure of the thymine-3,4-benzopyrene photoproduct, *Tetrahedron Lett.* **7:**589.

BLOOM, K. S., AND ANDERSON, J. N., 1978, Fractionation of hen oviduct chromatin into transcriptionally active and inactive regions after selective micrococcal nuclease digestion, *Cell* **15:**141.

BODELL, W. J., 1977, Nonuniform distribution of DNA repair in chromatin after treatment with methylmethanesulfonate, *Nucleic Acids Res.* **4:**2619.

BODELL, W. J., AND BANERJEE, M. R., 1976, Reduced DNA repair in mouse satellite DNA after treatment with methylmethanesulfonate and N-methyl-N-nitrosourea, *Nucleic Acids Res.* **3:**1689.

BODELL, W. J., AND BANERJEE, M. R., 1979, The influence of chromatin structure on the distribution of DNA repair synthesis studied by nuclease digestion, *Nucleic Acids Res.* **6:**359.

BODELL, W. J., SINGER, B., THOMAS, G. H., AND CLEAVER, J. A., 1979, Evidence for removal at different rates of O-ethyl pyrimidines and ethyl phosphotriesters in two human fibroblast cell lines, *Nucleic Acids Res.* **6:**2819.

BONNER, J., GOTTESFELD, J., GERRARD, W., BELLING, R., AND UPHOUSE, L., 1975, Isolation of template active and inactive regions of chromatin, *Methods Enzymol.* **40E:**97.

BOREK, C., AND SACHS, L., 1967, The number of cell generations required to fix the transformed state in X-ray-induced transformation, *Proc. Natl. Acad. Sci. USA* **57:**1522.

BOUTWELL, R. K., COLBURN, N. H., AND MUCKERMAN, C. C., 1969, *In vivo* reactions of β-propiolactone, *Ann. N.Y. Acad. Sci.* **163:**751.

BOWDEN, G. T., AND BOUTWELL, R. K., 1973, The binding of 7,12-dimethylbenz(a)anthracene (DMBA) to replicating and non-replicating DNA *in vivo*, *Proc. Am. Assoc. Cancer Res.* **14:**28.

BOYLAND, E., 1969, The biochemistry of aromatic hydrocarbons, amines and urethane, in *Physicochemical Mechanisms of Carcinogenesis*, The Jerusalem Symposia on Quantum Chemistry and Biochemistry, Vol. 1 (E. D. Bergmann and B. Pullman, eds), p. 25, The Israel Academy of Science and Humanities, Jerusalem.

BOYLAND, E., AND SIMS, P., 1965, Metabolism of polycyclic compounds. The metabolism of 7,12-dimethylbenz(a) anthracene by rat liver homogenates, *Biochem. J.* **95:**780.

BOYLAND, E., AND WILLIAMS, K., 1969, Reaction of urethane with nucleic acids *in vivo*, *Biochem. J.* **111:**121.

BRASH, D. E., AND HART, R. W., 1978, DNA damage and repair *in vivo*, *J. Environ. Pathol. Toxicol.* **2:**79.

BRAWERMAN, G., 1974, Eukaryotic messenger RNA, *Annu. Rev. Biochem.* **43:**621.

BRENT, T. P., 1976, Purification and characterization of human endonucleases specific for damaged DNA, *Biochim. Biophys. Acta* **454:**172.

BRENT, T. P., 1979, Partial purification and characterization of a human 3-methyladenine-DNA glycosylase, *Biochemistry* **18:**911.

BRIDGES, B. A., 1976, Short term screening tests for carcinogens, *Nature (London)* **261:**195.

BRINKER, J. M., MADORE, A. P., AND BELLO, L. J., 1973, Stabilization of heterogeneous nuclear RNA by intercalating drugs, *Biochem. Biophys. Res. Commun.* **52:**928.

BRITTEN, R. J., AND DAVIDSON, E. H., 1969, Gene regulation for higher cells: A theory—New facts regarding the organization of genome provide clues to the nature of gene regulation, *Science* **165:**349.

BRITTEN, R. J., AND KOHNE, D. E., 1968, Repeated sequences in DNA. Hundreds and thousands of copies of DNA sequences have been incorporated into the genome of higher organisms, *Science* **161:**529.

BROOKES, P., 1966, Quantitative aspects of the reaction of some carcinogens with nucleic acids and the possible significance of such reactions in the process of carcinogenesis, *Cancer Res.* **26:**1994.

BROOKES, P., AND LAWLEY, P. D., 1960, The reaction of mustard gas with nucleic acids *in vitro* and *in vivo*, *Biochem. J.* **77:**478.

BROOKES, P., AND LAWLEY, P. D., 1961, The reaction of mono- and di-functional alkylating agents with nucleic acids, *Biochem. J.* **80:**496.

BROOKES, P., AND LAWLEY, P. D., 1964, Evidence for the binding of polynuclear aromatic hydrocarbons to the nucleic acids of mouse skin: Relation between carcinogenic power of hydrocarbons and their binding to deoxyribonucleic acid, *Nature (London)* **202:**781.

BROWN, G. B., TELLER, M. N., SMULLYAN, I., BIRDSALL, N. J. M., LEE, T.-C., PARHAM, J. C., AND STOHRER, G., 1973, Correlations between oncogenic and chemical properties of several derivatives of 3-hydroxyxanthine and 3-hydroxyguanine, *Cancer Res.* **33:**1113.

BUCKLEY, J. D., O'CONNOR, P. J., AND CRAIG, A. W., 1979, Pretreatment with acetylaminofluorene enhances the repair of O^6-methylguanine in DNA, *Nature (London)* **281:**403.

BUECHELER, J., AND KLEIHUES, P., 1977, Excision of O^6-methylguanine from DNA of various mouse tissues following a single injection of *N*-methyl-*N*-nitrosourea, *Chem. Biol. Interact.* **16:**325.

BUHL, S. N., SETLOW, R. B., AND REGAN, J. D., 1974, Recovery of the ability to synthesize DNA in segments of normal size at long times after UV irradiation of human cells, *Biophys. J.* **13:**1265.

BUTZOW, J. J., AND EICHHORN, G. L., 1965, IV. Degradation of polyribonucleotides by zinc and other divalent metal ions, *Biopolymers* **3:**95.

CATHCART, R., AND GOLDTHWAIT, D. A., 1981, Enzymatic excision of 3-methyladenine and 7-methylguanine by a rat liver nuclear fraction, *Biochemistry* **20:**273.

CAYAMA, E., TSUDA, H., SARMA, D. S. R., AND FARBER, E., 1978, Initiation of chemical carcinogenesis requires cell proliferation, *Nature (London)* **275:**60.

CERUTTI, P. A., SESSIONS, F., HARIHARAN, P. V., AND LUSBY, A., 1978, Repair of DNA damage induced by benzo(α)pyrene diol epoxides I and II in human alveolar tumor cells, *Cancer Res.* **38:**2118.

CHAN, J. Y. H., AND BECKER, F. F., 1979, Decreased fidelity of DNA polymerase activity during *N*-2-fluorenylacetamide hepatocarcinogenesis, *Proc. Natl. Acad. Sci. USA* **76:**814.

CHETSANGA, C., AND LINDAHL, T., 1979, Release of 7-methylguanine residues whose imidazole rings have been opened from damaged DNA by a DNA glycosylase from *Escherichia coli*, *Nucleic Acids Res.* **6:**3673.

CLARK, R. J., AND FELSENFELD, G., 1971, Structure of chromatin, *Nature (London)* **229:**101.

CLAYSON, D. B., AND GARNER, R. C., 1976, Carcinogenic aromatic amines and related compounds, in *Chemical Carcinogens* (C. E. Searle, ed.), p. 366, ACS Monograph 173, Washington, D.C.

CLEAVER, J. E., 1968, Defective repair replication of DNA in xeroderma pigmentosum, *Nature (London)* **218:**652.

CLEAVER, J. E., 1969, Xeroderma pigmentosum: A human disease in which an initial stage of DNA repair is defective, *Proc. Natl. Acad. Sci. USA* **63:**428.

CLEAVER, J. E., 1977, Nucleosome structure controls rates of excision repair in DNA of human cells, *Nature (London)* **270:**451.

CLEAVER, J. E., 1978, DNA repair and its coupling to DNA replication in eukaryotic cells, *Biochim. Biophys. Acta* **516:**489.

CLIFFORD, J. I. AND REES, K. R., 1967, The action of aflotoxin B_1 on the rat liver, *Biochem. J.* **102:**65.

COHEN, S. M., ALTER, A., AND BRYAN, G. T., 1973, Distribution of radioactivity and metabolism of formic acid 2-[4-(5-nitro-2-furyl)-2-^{14}C-2-thiazolyl]hydrazide following oral administration to rats and mice, *Cancer Res.* **33:**2802.

COHN, W. E., AND VOLKIN, E., (eds.), 1976, m-RNA: The relation of structure and function, *Prog. Nucleic Acid Res. Mol. Biol.* **19.**

COLBURN, N. H., AND BOUTWELL, R. K., 1968, The *in vivo* binding of β-propiolactone to mouse skin DNA, RNA and protein, *Cancer Res.* **28:**642.

COLUMBANO, A., RAO, P. M., RAJALAKSHMI, S., AND SARMA, D. S. R., 1980, Presence of dimethyl-nitrosamine (DMN) induced methylated products in the parental strand of the *in vivo* replicated, S_1 nuclease resistant, hybrid liver DNA, *Proc. Am. Assoc. Cancer Res.* **21:**86.

COOKSON, M. J., SIMS, P., AND GROVER, P. L., 1971, Mutagenicity of epoxides of polycyclic hydrocarbons correlates with carcinogenicity of parent hydrocarbons, *Nature (London)* **234:**186.

COOPER, H. K., MARGISON, G. P., O'CONNOR, P. J., AND ITZHAKI, R. F., 1975, Heterogenous distribution of DNA alkylation products in rat-liver chromatin after *in vivo* administration of *N,N*-di[^{14}C]methylnitrosamine, *Chem. Biol. Interact.* **11:**483.

COX, R., 1979, Differences in the removal of *N*-methyl-*N*-nitrosourea methylated products in DNase-I-sensitive and resistant regions of rat brain DNA, *Cancer Res.* **39:**2675.

COX, R., AND FARBER, E., 1972, Ethylation of DNA versus cancer induction with ethionine, *Proc. Am. Assoc. Cancer Res.* **13:**97.

COX, R., AND IRVING, C. C., 1977, Selective accumulation of O^6-methylguanine in DNA of rat bladder epithelium after intravesical administration of *N*-methyl-*N*-nitrosourea, *Cancer Lett.* **3:**265.

COX, R., AND IRVING, C. C., 1979, O^6-Methylguanine accumulates in DNA of mammary glands after administration of *N*-methyl-*N*-nitrosourea to rats, *Cancer Lett.* **6:**273.

COX, R., DAMJANOV, I., ABANOBI, S., AND SARMA, D. S. R., 1973, A method for measuring DNA damage and repair in the liver *in vivo*, *Cancer Res.* **33:**2114.

389

INTERAC-
TIONS OF
CARCINOGENS
WITH NUCLEIC
ACIDS

COYLE, M. B., AND STRAUSS, B. S., 1969–1970, Characteristics of DNA synthesized by methyl-methanesulfonate treated HEp-2 cells, *Chem. Biol. Interact.* **1**:89.

CRADDOCK, V. M., 1969, Methylation of t-RNA and ribosomal RNA in rat liver in the intact animal and the effect of carcinogens, *Biochim. Biophys. Acta* **195**:351.

CRADDOCK, V. M., 1973, Induction of liver tumours in rats by a single treatment with nitroso compounds given after partial hepatectomy, *Nature (London)* **245**:386.

CRADDOCK, V. M., VILLA-TREVINO, S., AND MAGEE, P. N., 1968, Occurrence of 7-methylguanine in nucleic acids of rat liver, *Biochem. J.* **107**:179.

D'AMBROSIO, S. M., AND SETLOW, R. B., 1976, Enhancement of post-replicative repair in Chinese hamster cells, *Proc. Natl. Acad. Sci. USA* **73**:2396.

DAMJANOV, I., COX, R., SARMA, D. S. R., AND FARBER, E., 1973, Patterns of damage and repair of liver DNA induced by carcinogenic methylating agents *in vivo*, *Cancer Res.* **33**:2122.

D'ANDREA, A. D., AND HASELTINE, W. A., 1978, Modification of DNA by aflatoxin B_1 creates alkali-labile lesions in DNA at positions of guanine and adenine, *Proc. Natl. Acad. Sci. USA* **75**:4120.

DARNELL, J. E., 1968, Ribonucleic acids from animal cells, *Bacteriol. Rev.* **32**:262.

DEBAUN, J. R., SMITH, J. Y. R., MILLER, E. C., AND MILLER, J. A., 1970, Reactivity *in vivo* of the carcinogen *N*-hydroxy-2-acetylaminofluorene: Increase by sulfate ion, *Science* **167**:184.

DEN ENGELSE, L., AND PHILLIPUS, E. J., 1977, *In vivo* repair of rat liver DNA damaged by dimethyl-nitrosamine or diethylnitrosamine, *Chem. Biol. Interact.* **19**:111.

DEUTSCH, W. A., AND LINN, S., 1979, DNA binding activity from cultured human fibroblasts that is specific for partially depurinated DNA and that inserts purines into apurinic sites, *Proc. Natl. Acad. Sci. USA* **76**:141.

DICKENS, F., AND JONES, H. E. H., 1963, Further studies on the carcinogenic and growth-inhibitory activity of lactones and related substances, *Br. J. Cancer* **17**:100.

DIJKSTRA, J., AND WEIDE, S. S., 1972, Changes in chromatin caused by aminoazo compounds, *Exp. Cell Res.* **72**:345.

DINGMAN, C. W., AND SPORN, M. B., 1967, The binding of metabolites of aminoazo-dyes to rat liver DNA *in vivo*, *Cancer Res.* **27**:938.

DIPAOLO, J., 1960, Experimental evaluation of actinomycin D, *Ann. N.Y. Acad. Sci.* **89**:408.

DIPPLE, A., 1972, Model studies for azo-dye carcinogenesis, *J. Chem. Soc. Perkin Trans.* **1**:447.

DIPPLE, A., AND SLADE, T. A., 1970, Structure and activity in chemical carcinogenesis: Reactivity and carcinogenicity of 7-bromomethylbenz(*a*)anthracene and 7-bromomethyl-12-methylbenz(*a*)-anthracene, *Eur. J. Cancer* **6**:417.

DIPPLE, A., BROOKES, P., MACKINTOSH, D. S., AND RAYMAN, M. P., 1971, Reaction of 7-bromomethyl-benz(*a*)anthracene with nucleic acids, polynucleotides and nucleosides, *Biochemistry* **10**:4323.

DRUCKREY, H., 1970, Production of colonic carcinomas by 1,2-dialkylhydrazines and azoxyalkanes, in *Carcinoma of the Colon and Antecedent Epithelium* (W. J. Burdette, ed.), p. 267, Thomas, Springfield, Ill.

DRUCKREY, H., 1972, Organospecific carcinogenesis in the digestive tract, in *Proceedings of the Second International Symposium of The Princess Takamatsu Cancer Research Fund* (W. Nakahara, S. Takayama, T. Sugimura, and S. Odashima, eds.), p. 73, University Park Press, Baltimore.

DRUCKREY, H., PREUSSMANN, R., MATZKUS, F., AND IVANKONIE, S., 1967, Selektive Erzeugung Von Darmkrebs bei Ratten durch 1,2-dimethylhydrazin, *Naturwissenschaften* **54**:285.

DUBE, S. K., MARCKER, K. A., CLARK, B. F. C., AND CORY, S., 1968, Nucleotide sequence of *N*-formyl-methionyl transfer RNA, *Nature (London)* **218**:232.

DUNCAN, M., BROOKES, P., AND DIPPLE, A., 1969, Metabolism and binding to cellular macromolecules of a series of hydrocarbons by mouse embryo cells in culture, *Int. J. Cancer* **4**:813.

DUNN, D. B., 1963, The isolation of 1-methyladenylic acid and 7-methylguanylic acid from ribonucleic acid, *Biochem. J.* **86**:14P.

EDWARDS, G. S., WOGAN, G. N., SPORN, M. B., AND PONG, R. S., 1971, Structure–activity relationships in DNA binding and nuclear effects of aflatoxin and analogs, *Cancer Res.* **31**:1943.

EICHHORN, G. L., CLARK, P., AND BECKER, E. D., 1966, Interactions of metal ions with polynucleotides and related compounds. VII. The binding of copper (II) to nucleosides, nucleotides and deoxyribonucleic acids, *Biochemistry* **5**:245.

ELKIND, M. M., AND REDPATH, J. L., 1977, Molecular and cellular biology of radiation lethality, in *Cancer: A Comprehensive Treatise*, Vol. 6 (F. F. Becker, ed.), p. 51, Plenum Press, New York.

ELMORE, D. J., GULLAND, J. M., JORDAN, D. O., AND TAYLOR, H. F. W., 1948, The reaction of nucleic acids with mustard gas, *Biochem. J.* **42**:308.

ENOMOTO, M., SATO, K., MILLER, E. C., AND MILLER, J. A., 1968, Reactivity of the diacetyl derivative of the carcinogen 4-hydroxyaminoquinoline-1-oxide with DNA, RNA and other nucleophiles, *Life Sci.* **7:**1025.

EPSTEIN, S. M., BENEDETTI, E. L., SHINOZUKA, H., BARTUS, B., AND FARBER, E., 1969–1970, Altered and distorted DNA from a premalignant liver lesion induced by 2-fluorenylacetamide, *Chem. Biol. Interact.* **1:**113.

ERTÜRK, E., MORRIS, J. E., COHEN, S. M., VON ESCH, A. M., CROVETTI, A. J., PRICE, J. M., AND BRYAN, G. T., 1971, Comparative carcinogenicity of formic acid 2-[4-(5-nitro-2-furyl)-2-thiazolyl]hydrazide and related chemicals in the rat, *J. Natl. Cancer Inst.* **47:**437.

ESSIGMANN, J. M., CROY, R. G., NAZDAN, A. M., BUSBY, W. F., JR., REINHOLD, V. N., BUCHI, G., AND WOGAN, G. N., 1977, Structural identification of the major DNA adduct formed by aflatoxin B$_1$ in vitro, *Proc. Natl. Acad. Sci. USA* **74:**1870.

FARBER, E., 1963, Ethionine carcinogenesis, *Adv. Cancer Res.* **7:**383.

FARBER, E., 1967, Ethionine fatty liver, *Adv. Lipid Res.* **5:**119.

FARBER, E., 1968, Biochemistry of carcinogenesis, *Cancer Res.* **28:**1859.

FARBER, E., AND MAGEE, P. N., 1960, The probable alkylation of liver ribonucleic acid by the hepatic carcinogens dimethylnitrosamine and ethionine, *Biochem. J.* **76:**58P.

FARBER, E., SHULL, K. H., VILLA-TREVINO, S., LOMBARDI, B., AND THOMAS, M., 1964, Biochemical pathology of acute hepatic adenosinetriphosphate deficiency, *Nature (London)* **203:**34.

FARBER, E., McCONOMY, J., FRANZEN, B., MARROQUIN, F., STEWART, G. A., AND MAGEE, P. N., 1967*a*, Interaction between ethionine and rat liver ribonucleic acid and protein *in vivo*, *Cancer Res.* **27:**1761.

FARBER, E., McCONOMY, J., AND FRUMANSKI, B., 1967*b*, Relative degrees of labeling of liver DNA and RNA with ethionine, *Proc. Am. Assoc. Cancer Res.* **8:**16.

FARBER, J. L., SHINOZUKA, H., SERRONI, A., AND FARMER, R., 1975, Reversal of the ethionine-induced inhibition of rat liver RNA polymerases *in vivo* by adenine, *Lab. Invest.* **31:**465.

FELDBERG, R. S., AND GROSSMAN, L., 1976, A DNA binding protein from human placenta specific for ultraviolet damaged DNA, *Biochemistry* **15:**2402.

FELSENFELD, G., 1978, Chromatin, *Nature (London)* **271:**115.

FIALA, E. S., KULAKIS, C., BOBOTAS, G., AND WEISBURGER, J. H., 1976, Separation of 1,2-dimethylhydrazine metabolites by high-pressure liquid chromatography, *J. Chromatogr.* **117:**181.

FIALA, E. S., KULAKIS, C., CHRISTIANSEN, G., AND WEISBURGER, J. H., 1978, Inhibition of the metabolism of the colon carcinogen, azoxymethane, by pyrazole, *Cancer Res.* **38:**4515.

FINK, L. M., NISHIMURA, S., AND WEINSTEIN, I. B., 1970, Modifications of ribonucleic acid by chemical carcinogens. I. *In vitro* modification of transfer ribonucleic acid by *N*-acetoxy-2-acetyl-aminofluorene, *Biochemistry* **9:**496.

FLAMM, W. G., WALKER, P. M., AND McCALLUM, M., 1969, Renaturation and isolation of single strands from the nuclear DNA of the guinea pig, *J. Mol. Biol.* **42:**441.

FLOYD, L. R., UNUMA, T., AND BUSCH, H., 1968, Effects of aflatoxin B$_1$ and other carcinogens upon nucleolar RNA of various tissues in the rat, *Exp. Cell Res.* **51:**423.

FOX, M., AND AYAD, S. R., 1971, Characteristics of repair synthesis in P388 cells treated with methyl methanesulphonate, *Chem. Biol. Interact.* **3:**193.

FREI, J. V., SWENSON, D. H., WARREN, W., AND LAWLEY, P. D., 1978, Alkylation of deoxyribonucleic acid *in vivo* in various organs of C57BL mice by the carcinogens *N*-methyl-*N*-nitrosourea, *N*-ethyl-*N*-nitrosourea and ethyl methanesulphonate in relaation to induction of thymic lymphoma. Some applications of high-pressure liquid chromatography, *Biochem. J.* **174:**1031.

FRIEDBERG, E. C., AND GOLDTHWAIT, D. A., 1969, Endonuclease II of *E. coli*. I. Isolation and purification, *Proc. Natl. Acad. Sci. USA* **62:**934.

FUCHS, R. P. P., 1975, *In vitro* recognition of carcinogen-induced local denaturation sites in native DNA by S$_1$ endonuclease from *Aspergillus oryzae*, *Nature (London)* **257:**151.

FUCHS, R. P. P., AND DAUNE, M. P., 1974, Dynamic structure of DNA modified with the carcinogen *N*-acetoxy-*N*-2-acetyl-aminofluorene, *Biochemistry* **13:**4435.

FUCHS, R. P. P., LEFEVRE, J. F., POUYET, J., AND DAUNE, M. P., 1976, Comparative orientation of the fluorene residue in native DNA, modified by *N*-acetoxy-*N*-2-acetylaminofluorene and two 7-halogeno-derivatives, *Biochemistry* **15:**3347.

FUJIMURA, S., GRUNBERGER, D., CARVAJAL, G., AND WEINSTEIN, I. B., 1972, Modification of RNA by chemical carcinogen. Modification of *E. coli* formylmethionine tRNA with *N*-acetoxy-2-acetyl-aminofluorene, *Biochemistry* **11:**3629.

391

INTERAC-
TIONS OF
CARCINOGENS
WITH NUCLEIC
ACIDS

FUKUDA, S., AND YAMAMOTO, N., 1972, Detection of activating enzymes for 4-nitroquinoline-1-oxide activation with a microbiology assay system, *Cancer Res.* **32**:435.

FURST, A., AND HARO, R. T., 1969, Possible mechanisms of metal ion carcinogenesis, in: *Physico-chemical Mechanisms in Carcinogenesis*, The Jerusalem Symposia on Quantum Chemistry and Biochemistry, Vol. 1 (E. D. Bergmann and B. Pullman, eds.), p. 310, The Israel Academy of Science and Humanities, Jerusalem.

FUWA, K., WARREN, W. E. C., DRUYAN, R., BARTHOLOMAY, A., AND VALLEE, B. L., 1960, Nucleic acids and metals. II. Transition metals as determinants of the conformation of ribonucleic acids, *Proc. Natl. Acad. Sci. USA* **46**:1298.

GALBRAITH, A. I., CHAPLEO, M. R., AND ITZHAKI, R. F., 1978, Distribution of 7-methylguanine and of replication sites in the different kinetic classes of DNA from rats treated with dimethyl-nitrosamine, *Nucleic Acids Res.* **5**:3357.

GALBRAITH, A. I., BARKER, M., AND ITZHAKI, R. F., 1979, Methylation of DNase digestible DNA and of RNA in chromatin from rats treated with dimethylnitrosamine, *Biochim. Biophys. Acta* **561**:334.

GANESAN, A. K., 1974, Persistence of pyrimidine dimers during post-replication repair in ultraviolet light irradiated *Escherichia coli* K12, *J. Mol. Biol.* **87**:103.

GAREL, A., AND AXEL, R., 1976, Selective digestion of transcriptionally active ovalbumin genes from oviduct nuclei, *Proc. Natl. Acad. Sci. USA* **73**:3966.

GARNER, R. C., 1973, Microsomal-dependent binding of aflatoxin-B_1 to DNA, RNA, polynucleotides and protein *in vitro*, *Chem. Biol. Interact.* **6**:125.

GARNER, R. C., MILLER, E. C., MILLER, J. A., GARNER, J. V., AND HANSON, R. S., 1971, Formation of a factor lethal for *S. typhimurium* TA 1530 and TA 1531 on incubation of aflatoxin B_1 with rat liver microsomes, *Biochem. Biophys. Res. Commun.* **45**:774.

GELBOIN, H. V., 1969, A microsome-dependent binding of benzo[*a*]-pyrene to DNA, *Cancer Res.* **29**:1272.

GELBOIN, H. V., WIRLHAM, J. S., WILSON, R. G., FRIEDMAN, M., AND WOGAN, G. N., 1966, Rapid and marked inhibition of rat liver RNA polymerase by aflatoxin B_1, *Science* **154**:1205.

GERCHMAN, L. L., AND LUDLUM, D. B., 1973, The properties of O^6-methylguanine in templates for RNA polymerase, *Biochim. Biophys. Acta* **308**:310.

GILMOUR, R. S., AND PAUL, J., 1973, Tissue specific transcription of the globin gene in isolated chromatin, *Proc. Natl. Acad. Sci. USA* **70**:3440.

GINZBURG, I., CORNELIS, P., GIVEON, D., AND LITTAUER, U. Z., 1979, Functionally impaired tRNA from ethionine treated rats as detected in injected *Xenopus* oocytes, *Nucleic Acids Res.* **6**:657.

GIOVANELLA, B. C., McKINNEY, L. E., AND HEIDELBERGER, C., 1964, On the reported solubilization of carcinogenic hydrocarbons in aqueous solutions of DNA, *J. Mol. Biol.* **8**:20.

GOODMAN, J. I., AND POTTER, V. R., 1972, Evidence for DNA repair synthesis and turnover in rat liver following ingestion of 3'-methyl-4-dimethylaminoazobenzene, *Cancer Res.* **32**:766.

GORSKI, J., MORRISON, M., MERKEL, C. G., AND LINGREL, J. B., 1974, Size heterogeneity of polyadeny-late sequences in mouse globin m-RNA, *J. Mol. Biol.* **86**:363.

GOSHMAN, L. M., AND HEIDELBERGER, C., 1967, Binding of tritium-labeled polycyclic hydrocarbons to DNA of mouse skin, *Cancer Res.* **27**:1678.

GOSSARD, F., AND VERLY, W. G., 1978, Properties of the main endonuclease specific for apurinic sites of *Escherichia coli* (endonuclease VI): Mechanism of apurinic site excision from DNA, *Eur. J. Biochem.* **82**:321.

GOTH, R., AND RAJEWSKY, M. F., 1974a, Persistence of O^6-ethylguanine in rat-brain DNA: Correlation with nervous system-specific carcinogenesis by ethyl nitrosourea, *Proc. Natl. Acad. Sci. USA* **71**:639.

GOTH, R., AND RAJEWSKY, M. F., 1974b, Molecular and cellular mechanisms associated with pulse-carcinogenesis in the rat nervous system by ENU ethylation of nucleic acid; elimination rates of ethylated bases from DNA of different tissues, *Z. Krebsforsch.* **82**:37.

GOTHE, R., CALLERMAN, C. J., EHRENBERG, L., AND WATCHMEISTER, C. A., 1976, Trapping with 3,4-dichlorobenzenethiol of reactive metabolites formed *in vitro* from the carcinogen, vinyl chloride, *Ambio* **3**:234.

GOTH-GOLDSTEIN, R., 1977, Repair of DNA damaged by alkylating carcinogens is defective in xeroderma pigmentosum-derived fibroblasts, *Nature (London)* **267**:81.

GRAB, D. J., AND ZEDECK, M. S., 1977, Organ specific effects of the carcinogen methylazoxymethanol related to metabolism by nicotinamide adenine dinucleotide-dependent dehydrogenases, *Cancer Res.* **37**:4182.

393

INTERAC-
TIONS OF
CARCINOGENS
WITH NUCLEIC
ACIDS

GRAB, D. J., ZEDECK, M. S., SURSTOCKI, N. I., AND SONENBERG, M., 1973, In vitro synthesis of RNA with "aggregate" enzyme, chromatin and DNA from liver of methylazoxymethanol acetate-treated rats, Chem. Biol. Interact. **6**:259.

GREEN, T., AND HATHWAY, D. E., 1975, The biological fate in rats of vinyl chloride in relation to its oncogenicity, Chem. Biol. Interact. **11**:545.

GREEN, T., AND HATHWAY, D. E., 1977, The chemistry and biogenesis of the S-containing metabolites of vinyl chloride in rats, Chem. Biol. Interact. **17**:137.

GREEN, T., AND HATHWAY, D. E., 1978, Interactions of vinyl chloride with rat-liver DNA in vivo, Chem. Biol. Interact. **22**:211.

GROSSMAN, L., BRAUN, A., FELDBERG, R., AND MAHLER, G., 1975, Enzymatic repair of DNA, Annu. Rev. Biochem. **44**:19.

GROVER, P. L., AND SIMS, P., 1968, Enzyme-catalysed reactions of polycyclic hydrocarbons with deoxyribonucleic acids and protein in vitro, Biochem. J. **110**:159.

GROVER, P. L., AND SIMS, P., 1970, Interactions of the K-region epoxides of phenanthrene and dibenz(a,h)anthracene with nucleic acids and histone, Biochem. Pharmacol. **19**:2251.

GROVER, P. L., FORRESTER, J. A., AND SIMS, P., 1971a, Reactivity of the K-region epoxides of some polycyclic hydrocarbons towards the nucleic acids and proteins of BHK 21 cells, Biochem. Pharmacol. **20**:1297.

GROVER, P. L., SIMS, P., HUBERMAN, E., MARQUARDT, H., KUROKI, T., AND HEIDELBERGER, C., 1971b, In vitro transformation of rodent cells by K-region derivatives of polycyclic hydrocarbons, Proc. Natl. Acad. Sci. USA **68**:1098.

GRUNBERGER, D., AND WEINSTEIN, I. B., 1971, Modifications of ribonucleic acid by chemical car- cinogens. III. Template activity of polynucleotides modified by N-acetoxy-2-acetylaminofluorene, J. Biol. Chem. **246**:1123.

GRUNBERGER, D., AND WEINSTEIN, I. B., 1976, The base displacement model: An explanation for the conformational and functional changes in nucleic acids modified by chemical carcinogens, in: Biology of Radiation Carcinogenesis (J. M. Yuhas, R. W. Tennat, and J. D. Regan, eds.), p. 175, Raven Press, New York.

GRUNBERGER, D., NELSON, J., CANTOR, R. C., AND WEINSTEIN, I. B., 1970, Coding and conformational properties of oligonucleotides modified with the carcinogen N-2-acetylaminofluorene, Proc. Natl. Acad. Sci. USA **66**:488.

GRUNBERGER, G., YU, F. L., GRUNBERGER, D., AND FEIGELSON, P., 1973, Mechanism of N-hydroxy-2- acetylaminofluorene inhibition of rat hepatic ribonucleic acid synthesis, J. Biol. Chem. **248**:6278.

HADI, I. S. M., KIRTIKAR, D., AND GOLDTHWAIT, D. A., 1973, Endonuclease II of Escherichia coli, degradation of double- and single-stranded deoxyribonucleic acid, Biochemistry **12**:2747.

HAESE, W. H., SMITH, D. L., AND BUEDING, E., 1973, Hycanthone induced hepatic changes in mice injected with Schistosoma mansoni, J. Pharmacol. Exp. Ther. **186**:430.

HAGENBÜCHLE, O., SANTER, M., STEITZ, J. A., AND MANS, R. J., 1978, Conservation of the primary structure at the 3' end of 18s rRNA from eukaryotic cells, Cell **13**:551.

HAHN, F. E., (ed.), 1971, Progress in Molecular and Subcellular Biology, Vol. 2, Springer-Verlag, New York.

HANAWALT, P. C., 1972, Repair of genetic material in living cells, Endeavour **31**:83.

HANAWALT, P. C., AND SETLOW, R. B., (eds.), 1975, Molecular Mechanism for Repair of DNA, Parts A and B, Plenum Press, New York.

HANAWALT, P. C., COOPER, P. K., GANESAN, A. K., AND SMITH, C. A., 1979, DNA repair in bacteria and mammalian cells, Annu. Rev. Biochem. **48**:783.

HANCOCK, R. L., 1968, Soluble RNA ethylase activity of normal and neoplastic mouse tissues, Cancer Res. **28**:1223.

HARRIS, C. C., CONNER, R. J., JACKSON, F. E., AND LIEBERMAN, M. W., 1974, Intranuclear distribution of DNA repair synthesis induced by chemical carcinogens or ultraviolet light in human diploid fibroblasts, Cancer Res. **34**:3461.

HARRIS, C. C., AUTRUP, H., STONER, G., AND TRUMP, B. F., 1978, Model systems using human lung for carcinogenesis studies, in: Pathogenesis and Therapy of Lung Cancer (C. C. Harris, ed.), p. 559, Marcel Dekker, New York.

HART, R. W., SETLOW, R. B., AND WOODHEAD, A. D., 1977, Evidence that pyrimidine dimers in DNA can give rise to tumors, Proc. Natl. Acad. Sci. USA **74**:5574.

HAWKS, A., SWANN, P. F., AND MAGEE, P. N., 1972, Probable methylation of nucleic acids of mouse colon by 1,2-dimethylhydrazine in vivo, Biochem. Pharmacol. **21**:432.

S. RAJALAKSHMI,
PREMA M. RAO,
AND
D. S. R. SARMA

HEATH, D. F., 1961, Mechanism of the hepatotoxic action of dialkylnitrosamine, *Nature (London)* **192**:170.

HENNINGS, H., AND MICHAEL, D., 1976, Guanine-specific DNA repair after treatment of mouse skin cells with N-methyl-N'-nitro-N-nitrosoguanidine, *Cancer Res.* **36**:2321.

HIGGINS, N. P., KATO, K., AND STRAUSS, B., 1976, A model for replication repair in mammalian cells, *J. Mol. Biol.* **101**:417.

HOLLEY, R. W., APGAR, J., EVERETT, G. A., MADISON, J. T., MARQUISEE, M., MERRILL, S. H., PENSWICK, J. R., AND ZAMIR, A., 1965, Structure of a ribonucleic acid, *Science* **147**:1462.

HOWARD-FLANDERS, P., 1968, DNA repair, *Annu. Rev. Biochem.* **37**:175.

HSU, W. T., LIN, E. J., HARVEY, R. G., AND WEISS, S. B., 1977, Mechanism of phage ϕX174 DNA inactivation by benzo[a]pyrene-7,8-dihydrodiol-9,10-epoxide, *Proc. Natl. Acad. Sci. USA* **74**:3335.

HSU, W. T., SAGHER, D., LIN, E. J., HARVEY, R. G., FU, P. P., AND WEISS, S. B., 1979, Benzo(a)pyrene-7,8-dihydrodiol: Selective binding to single stranded DNA and inactivation of ϕX174 DNA infectivity, *Biochem. Biophys. Res. Commun.* **87**:416.

HUANG, P. H. T., AND STEWART, B. W., 1977, Differences in patterns of structural change in rat liver DNA following administration of dimethylnitrosamine and methylmethanesulfonate, *Cancer Res.* **37**:3796.

HUBERMAN, E., AND SACHS, L., 1974, Cell-mediated mutagenesis of mammalian cells with chemical carcinogens, *Int. J. Cancer* **13**:326.

HUBERMAN, E., ASPIRAS, L., HEIDELBERGER, C., GROVER, P. L., AND SIMS, P., 1971, Mutagenicity to mammalian cells of epoxides and other derivatives of polycyclic hydrocarbons, *Proc. Natl. Acad. Sci. USA* **68**:3195.

HUBERMAN, E., BARSTCH, H., AND SACHS, L., 1975, Mutation induction in Chinese hamster V79 cells by two vinyl chloride metabolites, chloroethylene oxide and 2-chloroacetaldehyde, *Int. J. Cancer* **16**:539.

HUBERMAN, E., SACHS, L., YANG, S. K., AND GELBOIN, H., 1976, Identification of mutagenic metabolite of benzo(α)pyrene in mammalian cells, *Proc. Natl. Acad. Sci. USA* **73**:607.

HUGGINS, C., GRAND, L., AND FUKINISHI, R., 1964, Aromatic influences on the yields of mammary cancers following administration of 7,12-dimethylbenz(a)anthracene, *Proc. Natl. Acad. Sci. USA* **51**:737.

HUGHES, P. E., AND PILCZYK, R., 1969–1970, The *in vivo* binding of metabolites of 2-naphthylamine to mouse-liver DNA, RNA and protein, *Chem. Biol. Interact.* **1**:307.

IBALL, J., 1939, The relative potency of carcinogenic compounds, *Am. J. Cancer* **35**:188.

IBALL, J., AND MACDONALD, S. G. G., 1960, The crystal structure of 20-methylcholanthrene, *Z. Kristall. Mineral.* **114**:439.

INGOLD, C. K., 1970, *Structure and Mechanism in Organic Chemistry*, 2nd ed., pp. 421–555, Bell, London.

IQBAL, Z. M., AND EPSTEIN, S. S., 1978, Evidence of DNA repair in the guinea pig pancreas *in vivo* and *in vitro* following exposure to N-methyl-N-nitrosourethane, *Chem. Biol. Interact.* **20**:77.

IRVING, C. C., 1970, in *Metabolic Conjugation and Metabolic Hydrolysis*, Vol. 1 (W. H. Fishman, ed.), p. 53, Academic Press, New York.

IRVING, C. C., 1971, Metabolic activation of N-hydroxy compounds by conjugation, *Xenobiotica* **1**:387.

IRVING, C. C., 1973, Interaction of chemical carcinogens with DNA, in *Methods in Cancer Research*, Vol. VII (H. Busch, ed.), p. 189, Academic Press, New York.

IRVING, C. C., AND RUSSELL, L. T., 1970, Synthesis of the O-glucuronide of N-2-fluorenylhydroxylamine: Reaction with nucleic acids and with guanosine 5'-monophosphate, *Biochemistry* **9**:2471.

IRVING, C. C., AND VEAZEY, R. A., 1969, Persistent binding of 2-acetylaminofluorene to rat liver DNA *in vivo* and consideration of the mechanism of binding of N-hydroxy-2-acetylaminofluorene to rat liver nucleic acids, *Cancer Res.* **27**:1799.

IRVING, C. C., VEAZEY, R. A., AND WILLIARD, R. F., 1967, The significance and mechanism of the binding of 2-acetylaminofluorene and N-hydroxy-2-acetylaminofluorene to rat liver ribonucleic acid *in vivo*, *Cancer Res.* **27**:720.

IRVING, C. C., VEAZEY, R. A., AND HILL, J. T., 1969, Reaction of the glucuronide of the carcinogen N-hydroxy-2-acetylaminofluorene with nucleic acids, *Biochim. Biophys. Acta* **179**:189.

IRVING, C. C., JANSS, D. H., AND RUSSELL, L. T., 1971, Lack of N-hydroxy-2-acetylaminofluorene sulfotransferase activity in the mammary gland and Zymbal's gland of the rat, *Cancer Res.* **31**:387.

ISHIZAWA, M., AND ENDO, H., 1967, On the mode of action of a potent carcinogen, 4-hydroxylaminoquinoline 1-oxide, on bacteriophage T$_4$, *Biochem. Pharmacol.* **16**:637.

IVANOVIC, V., GEACINTOV, N. E., YAMASAKI, H., AND WEINSTEIN, I. B., 1978, DNA and RNA adducts formed in hamster embryo cell cultures exposed to benzo(α)pyrene, *Biochemistry* **17**:1597.

395

INTERAC-
TIONS OF
CARCINOGENS
WITH NUCLEIC
ACIDS

JAHN, C. L., AND LITMAN, G. W., 1977, Distribution of covalently bound benzo(α)pyrene in chromatin, *Biochem. Biophys. Res. Commun.* **76**:534.

JAHN, C. L., AND LITMAN, G. W., 1979, Accessibility of deoxyribonucleic acid in chromatin to the covalent binding of the chemical carcinogen benzo(α)pyrene, *Biochemistry* **18**:1442.

JANSS, D. H., MOON, R. C., AND IRVING, C. C., 1972, The binding of 7,12-dimethylbenz(a)anthracene to mammary parenchymal DNA and protein *in vivo, Cancer Res.* **32**:254.

JEFFREY, A. M., WEINSTEIN, I. B., JENNETTE, K. W., GRZESKOWIAK, K., NAKANISHI, K., HARVEY, R. G., AUTRUP, H., AND HARRIS, C., 1977, Structure of benzo(α)pyrene nucleic acid adducts formed in human and bovine bronchial explants, *Nature (London)* **269**:348.

JEFFREY, A. M., GRZESKOWIAK, K., WEINSTEIN, I. B., NAKANISHI, K., ROLLER, P., AND HARVEY, R. G., 1979, Benzo(α)pyrene-7,8-dihydrodiol-9-10-oxide adenosine and deoxyadenosine adducts: Structure and stereochemistry, *Science* **206**:1309.

JELINEK, W., AND DARNELL, J. E., 1972, Double-stranded regions in heterogeneous nuclear RNA from HeLa cells, *Proc. Natl. Acad. Sci. USA* **69**:2537.

JENNETTE, K. W., JEFFREY, A. M., BLOBSTEIN, S. H., BELAND, F. A., HARVEY, R. G., AND WEINSTEIN, I. B., 1977, Nucleoside adducts from the *in vitro* reaction of benzo(α)pyrene-7-8-dihydrodiol-9,10-oxide or benzo(α)pyrene-4,5-oxide with nucleic acids, *Biochemistry* **16**:932.

KADLUBAR, F. F., MILLER, J. A., AND MILLER, E. C., 1978, Guanyl O^6-arylamination and O^6-arylation of DNA by the carcinogen N-hydroxy-1-natphthylamine, *Cancer Res.* **38**:3628.

KADLUBAR, F. F., DOOLEY, K. L., AND BELAND, F. A., 1980, Urothelial and hepatic DNA adducts from the carcinogen 2-naphthylamine, *Proc. Am. Assoc. Cancer Res.* **21**:119.

KAKEFUDA, T., AND YAMAMOTO, H., 1978, Modification of DNA by the benzo(α)pyrene metabolite diol epoxide, r-7, t-8-dihydroxy-t-9,10-oxy-7,8,9,10-tetrahydrobenzo(α)pyrene, *Proc. Natl. Acad. Sci. USA* **75**:415.

KAKUNAGA, T., 1974, Requirement for cell proliferation in the fixation and expression of the transformed state in mouse cells treated with 4-nitroquinoline 1-oxide, *Int. J. Cancer* **14**:736.

KANAGALINGAM, K., AND BALIS, M. E., 1975, *In vivo* repair of rat intestinal DNA damage by alkylating agents, *Cancer* **36**:2364.

KAPITULNIK, J., LEVIN, W., CONNEY, A. J., YAGI, H., AND JERINA, D. M., 1977, Benzo(α)pyrene-7,8-dihydrodiol is more carcinogenic than benzo(α)pyrene in newborn mice, *Nature (London)* **266**:378.

KAPPUS, H., BOLT, H. M., BUCHTER, A., AND BOLT, W., 1976, Liver microsomal uptake of [^{14}C]-vinyl chloride and transformation of protein by alkylating metabolites *in vitro, Toxicol. Appl. Pharmacol.* **37**:461.

KAPULER, A. M., AND MICHELSON, A. M., 1971, The reaction of the carcinogen N-acetoxy-2-acetylaminofluorene with DNA and other polynucleotides and its stereochemical implications, *Biochim. Biophys. Acta* **232**:436.

KARRAN, P., LINDAHL, T., AND GRIFFIN, B., 1979, Adaptive response to alkylating agents involves alterations *in situ* of O^6-methylguanine residues in DNA, *Nature (London)* **280**:76.

KATO, M., AND TAKALASHI, A., 1970, Characteristics of nitro reduction of the carcinogenic agent, 4-nitroquinoline N-oxide, *Biochem. Pharmacol.* **19**:45.

KAWAMATA, J., NAKABAYASHI, N., KAWAI, A., AND USHIDA, T., 1958, Experimental production of sarcoma in mice with actinomycin, *Med. J. Osaka Univ.* **8**:753.

KAWAMATA, J., NAKABAYASHI, N., KAWAI, A., FUJITA, H., IMANISHI, M., AND IKEGAMI, R., 1959, Studies on the carcinogenic effect of actinomycin, *Biken J.* **2**:105.

KAWAMOTO, S., IDA, N., KIRSCHBAUM, A., AND TAYLOR, G., 1958, Urethan and leukemogenesis in mice, *Cancer Res.* **18**:725.

KAWAZOE, Y., ARAKI, M., AOKI, K., AND NAKAHARA, W., 1969, Structure–carcinogenicity relationship among derivatives of 4-nitro and 4-hydroxyaminoquinoline-1-oxides, *Biochem. Pharmacol.* **16**:631.

KAWAZOE, Y., ARAKI, M., AND HUANG, G. F., 1972, Chemical aspects of carcinogenesis by 4-nitroquinoline 1-oxide, in: *Proceedings of the Second International Symposium of the Princess Takamatsu Cancer Research Fund* (W. Nakahara, S. Takayama, T. Sugimura, and S. Odashima, eds.), p. 1, University Park Press, Baltimore.

KAWAZOE, Y., ARAKI, M., HUANG, G. F., OKAMOTO, T., TADA, M., AND TADA, M., 1976, Chemical structure of QAII, one of the covalently bound adducts of carcinogenic 4-nitroquinoline 1-oxide with nucleic acid bases of cellular nucleic acids, *Chem. Pharm. Bull.* **23**:3041.

KING, C. M., AND PHILLIPS, B., 1972, Mechanism of introduction of fluorenylamine (FA) substituents into nucleic acid by rat liver, *Proc. Am. Assoc. Cancer Res.* **13**:43.

KING, C. M., TRAUB, N. R., LORTZ, Z. M., AND THISSEN, M. R., 1979, Metabolic activation of arylhydroxamic acids by N-O-acetyltransferase of rat mammary gland, *Cancer Res.* **39**:3369.

S. RAJALAKSHMI,
PREMA M. RAO,
AND
D. S. R. SARMA

KIRTIKAR, D. M., CATHEART, G. R., AND GOLDTHWAIT, D. A., 1976, Endonuclease II. Apurinic acid endonuclease and exonuclease III, *Proc. Natl. Acad. Sci. USA* **73:**4324.

KIT, S., 1960, Studies on structure, composition, metabolism of tumour RNA in *Cell Physiology of New Phases*, 14th Annual Symposium on Fundamental Cancer Research, p. 337, M. D. Anderson Hospital and Tumor Institute, University of Texas Press, Austin.

KLEIHUES, P., 1972, *N*-Methyl-*N*-nitrosourea induced changes in the labeling by (^{14}C) orotate of RNA and acid-soluble fractions in rat kidney and liver, *Chem. Biol. Interact.* **5:**309.

KLEIHUES, P., AND BUECHELER, J., 1977, Long-term persistence of O^6-methylguanine in rat brain DNA, *Nature (London)* **269:**625.

KLEIHUES, P., AND MARGISON, G. P., 1976, Exhaustion and recovery of repair excision of O^6-methylguanine from rat liver DNA, *Nature (London)* **259:**153.

KOOTSTRA, A., SLAGA, T. J., AND OLINS, D. E., 1979, Interaction of benzo(α)pyrene diol-epoxide with nuclei and isolated chromatin, *Chem. Biol. Interact.* **28:**225.

KOREEDA, M., MOORE, P. D., WISLOCKI, P. G., LEVIN, W., CONNEY, A. H., YAGI, H., AND JERINA, D. M., 1978, Binding of benzo(α)pyrene 7,8-diol-9,10-epoxides to DNA, RNA, and protein of mouse skin occurs with high stereo selectivity, *Science* **199:**778.

KORNBERG, R. D., 1977, Structure of chromatin, *Annu. Rev. Biochem.* **46:**931.

KOSUGE, T., ZENDA, H., YOKOTA, M., SAWANISHI, H., AND SUZUKI, Y., 1969, Further evidence for formation of 4-nitrosoquinoline 1-oxide, *Chem. Pharm. Bull.* **17:**2181.

KRAHN, D. F., AND HEIDELBERGER, C., 1977, Liver homogenate-mediated mutagenesis in Chinese hamster V79 cells by polycyclic aromatic hydrocarbons and aflatoxins, *Mutat. Res.* **46:**27.

KRIEK, E., 1968, Difference in binding of 2-acetylaminofluorene to rat liver deoxyribonucleic acid and ribosomal ribonucleic acid *in vivo*, *Biochim. Biophys. Acta* **161:**273.

KRIEK, E., 1969, On the mechanism of action of aromatic amines *in vivo*. Differences in binding to ribosomal RNA and DNA in *Physico-chemical Mechanisms of Carcinogenesis*, The Jerusalem Symposia on Quantum Chemistry and Biochemistry, Vol. 1 (E. D. Bergmann and B. Pullman, eds.), p. 136, The Israel Academy of Science and Humanities, Jerusalem.

KRIEK, E., 1974, Carcinogenesis by aromatic amines, *Biochim., Biophys. Acta* **355:**177.

KRIEK, E., MILLER, J. A., JUHL, V., AND MILLER, E. C., 1967, 8-(*N*-2-fluorenylacetamide) guanosine, an arylamidation reaction product of guanosine and the carcinogen *N*-acetoxy-*N*-2-fluorenyl-acetamide in neutral solution, *Biochem. J.* **6:**177.

KRÜGER, F. W., 1972, New aspects in metabolism of carcinogenic nitrosamines, in: *Proceedings of the Second International Symposium of the Princess Takamatsu Cancer Research Fund* (W. Nakahara, S. Takayama, T. Sugimura, and S. Odashima, eds.), p. 213, University Park Press, Baltimore.

KRÜGER, F. W., 1973, Metabolism of nitrosamines *in vivo*. II. On the methylation of nucleic acids by aliphatic di-*n*-alkyl-nitrosamines *in vivo*, caused by β-oxidation: The increased formation of 7-methylguanine after application of β-hydroxypropyl-propyl-nitrosamine compared to that after application of di-*n*-propyl-nitrosamine, *Z. Krebsforsch.* **79:**90.

KRÜGER, F. W., AND BERTRAM, B., 1973, Metabolism of nitrosamines *in vivo*. III. On the methylation of nucleic acids by aliphatic di-*n*-alkyl-nitrosamines *in vivo* resulting from β-oxidation: The formation of 7-methylguanine after application of 2-oxo-propyl-propyl-nitrosamine and methyl-propyl-nitrosamine, *Z. Krebsforsch.* **80:**189.

KRUGH, T. R., 1972, Association of actinomycin-D and deoxyribonucleotides as a model for binding of the drug to DNA, *Proc. Natl. Acad. Sci. USA* **69:**1911.

KUHNLEIN, V., LEE, B., PINHOET, E. E., AND LINN, S., 1978, Xeroderma pigmentosum fibroblasts of the D-group lack an apurinic DNA endonuclease species with a low apparent K_m, *Nucleic Acids Res.* **5:**951.

KUROKI, T., AND HEIDELBERGER, C., 1971, The binding of polycyclic aromatic hydrocarbons to the DNA, RNA and proteins of transformable cells in culture, *Cancer Res.* **31:**2168.

KUROKI, T., HUBERMAN, E., MARQUARDT, H., SELKIRK, J. K., HEIDELBERGER, C., GROVER, P. L., AND SIMS, P., 1971–1972, Binding of K-region epoxides and other derivatives of benz(*a*)anthracene and dibenz(*a,h*)anthracene to DNA, RNA, and proteins of transformable cells, *Chem. Biol. Interact.* **4:**389.

LAFARGE, C., AND FRAYSSINET, C., 1970, The reversibility of inhibition of RNA and DNA synthesis induced by aflatoxin in rat liver, a tentative explanation for carcinogenic mechanism, *Int. J. Cancer* **6:**74.

LANCASTER, M. C., JENKINS, H. P., AND PHILIPS, J. M., 1961, Toxicity associated with certain samples of dry nuts, *Nature (London)* **192:**1095.

LANCLOS, K. D., AND BRESNICK, E., 1976, The formation of poly-A containing RNA in rat liver after administration of 3-methylcholanthrene, *Chem. Biol. Interact.* **12**:341.

LAQUEUR, G. L., AND SPATZ, M., 1968, Toxicology of cycasin, *Cancer Res.* **28**:2262.

LAVAL, J., 1977, Two enzymes are required for strand incision in repair of alkylated DNA, *Nature (London)* **269**:829.

LAVAL, J., PIERRE, J., AND LAVAL, F., 1981, Release of 7-methylguanine residues from alylated DNA by extracts of *Micrococcus luteus* and *Escherichia coli, Proc. Natl. Acad. Sci. USA* **78**:856.

LAWLEY, P. D., 1966, Effects of some chemical mutagens and carcinogens on nucleic acids, *Prog. Nucleic Acid Res. Mol. Biol.* **5**:89.

LAWLEY, P. D., 1972, The action of alkylating mutagens and carcinogens on nucleic acids: *N*-methyl-*N*-nitroso compounds as methylating agents, in *Proceedings of the Second International Symposium of the Princess Takamatsu Cancer Research Fund* (W. Nakahara, S. Takayama, T. Sugimura, and S. Odashima, eds.), p. 237, University Park Press, Baltimore.

LAWLEY, P. D., 1973, Reaction of *N*-methyl-*N*-nitrosourea (MNUA) with ^{32}P-labelled DNA: Evidence for formation of phosphotriesters, *Chem. Biol. Interact.* **7**:127.

LAWLEY, P. D., 1974, Some chemical aspects of dose–response relationships in alkylation mutagenesis, *Mutat. Res.* **23**:283.

LAWLEY, P. D., 1976, Carcinogenesis by alkylating agents, in *Chemical Carcinogens* (C. E. Searle, ed.), p. 83, ACS Monograph 173, Washington, D.C.

LAWLEY, P. D., AND BROOKES, P., 1963, Further studies on the alkylation of nucleic acids and their constituent nucleotides, *Biochem. J.* **89**:127.

LAWLEY, P. D., AND ORR, D. J., 1970, Specific excision of methylation products from DNA of *Escherichia coli* treated with *N*-methyl-*N'*-nitro-*N*-nitrosoguanidine, *Chem. Biol. Interact.* **2**:154.

LAWLEY, P. D., AND SHAH, S. A., 1972, Methylation of ribonucleic acid by the carcinogens dimethylsulfate, *N*-methyl-*N*-nitrosourea and *N*-methyl-*N'*-nitro-*N*-nitrosoguanidine: Comparisons of chemical analysis at the nucleoside and base levels, *Biochem. J.* **128**:117.

LAWLEY, P. D., AND SHAH, S. A., 1973, Methylation of DNA by ^{3}H-^{14}C-methyl-labelled *N*-methyl-*N*-nitrosourea—evidence for transfer of the intact methyl group, *Chem. Biol. Interact.* **7**:115.

LAWLEY, P. D., AND THATCHER, C. J., 1970, Methylation of deoxyribonucleic acid in cultured mammalian cells by *N*-methyl-*N'*-nitro-*N*-nitrosoguanidine. The influence of cellular thiol concentrations on the extent of methylation and the O^6-oxygen atom of guanine as a site of methylation, *Biochem. J.* **116**:693.

LAWLEY, P. D., AND WARREN, W., 1975, Specific excision of ethylated purines from DNA of *Escherichia coli* treated with *N*-ethyl-*N*-nitrosourea, *Chem. Biol. Interact.* **11**:55.

LAWLEY, P. D., BROOKES, P., MAGEE, P. N., CRADDOCK, V. M., AND SWANN, P. F., 1968, Methylated bases in liver nucleic acids from rats treated with dimethylnitrosamines, *Biochim. Biophys. Acta* **157**:646.

LAWLEY, P. D., ORR, D. J., AND SHAH, S. A., 1971–1972, Reaction of alkylating mutagens and carcinogens with nucleic acids: N-3 of guanine as a site of alkylation by *N*-methyl-*N*-nitrosourea and dimethylsulfate, *Chem. Biol. Interact.* **4**:431.

LAWLEY, P. D., ORR, D. J., SHAH, S. A., FARMER, P. B., AND JARMAN, M., 1973, Reaction products from *N*-methyl-*N*-nitrosourea and deoxyribonucleic acid containing thymidine residues: Synthesis and identification of a new methylation product, O^4-methylthymidine, *Biochem. J.*, **135**:193.

LAWSON, T. A., 1968, The binding of *O*-aminoazotoluene to deoxyribonucleic acid, ribonucleic acid and protein in the C57 mouse, *Biochem. J.* **109**:917.

LAWSON, T. A., AND CALYSON, D. B., 1969, Differences in binding of *ortho*aminoazotoluene to macromolecules in female and male C57 mouse liver, in *Physico-chemical Mechanisms of Carcinogenesis*, The Jerusalem Symposia on Quantum Chemistry and Biochemistry, Vol. 1 (E. D. Bergmann and B. Pullman, eds.), p. 226, The Isreal Academy of Science and Humanities, Jerusalem.

LAWSON, T. A., AND POUND, A. W., 1971–1972, The interaction of (^{3}H) ethyl carbamate with nucleic acids of regenerating mouse liver, *Chem. Biol. Interact.* **4**:329.

LAWSON, T. A., AND POUND, A. W., 1973*a*, The interaction of carbon-14-labeled alkyl carbamates, labeled in the alkyl- and carbonyl-positions, with DNA *in vivo, Chem. Biol. Interact.* **6**:99.

LAWSON, T. A., AND POUND, A. W., 1973*b*, The prolonged binding of ethyl carbamate-(^{14}C) to DNA in regenerating and intact mouse liver, *Eur. J. Cancer* **9**:491.

397

INTERAC-
TIONS OF
CARCINOGENS
WITH NUCLEIC
ACIDS

S. RAJALAKSHMI,
PREMA M. RAO,
AND
D. S. R. SARMA

LEE, K. Y., AND LIJINSKY, W., 1966, Alkylation of rat liver RNA by cyclic N-nitrosamines *in vivo*, *J. Natl. Cancer Inst.* **37**:401.

LEFFLER, S., PULKRABEK, P., GRUNBERGER, D., AND WEINSTEIN, I. B., 1977, Template activity of calf thymus DNA modified by a dihydrodiol epoxide derivative of benzo(a)pyrene, *Biochemistry* **16**:3133.

LERMAN, L. S., 1964, Acridine mutagens and DNA structure *J. Cell. Comp. Physiol.* **64**:1 (Suppl. 1).

LERMAN, L. S., 1971, Intercalability, the "y" transition, and the state of DNA in nature, in *Progress in Molecular and Subcellular Biology*, Vol. 2 (F. E. Hahn, ed.), p. 382, Springer-Verlag, New York.

LETT, J. T., PARKINS, G. M., AND ALEXANDER, P., 1962, Physiochemical changes produced in DNA after alkylation, *Arch Biochem. Biophys.* **97**:80.

LETT, J. T., KLUCIS, E. S., AND SUN, C., 1970, On the size of the DNA in the mammalian chromosome substructural subunits, *Biophys. J.* **10**:277.

LEVINE, A. F., FINK, L. M., WEINSTEIN, I. B., AND GRUNBERGER, D., 1974, Effect of N-2-acetyl-aminofluorene modification on the conformation of nucleic acids, *Cancer Res.* **34**:319.

LEVY, C. C., SCHMUKLER, M., FRANK, J. J., KARPETSKY, T. P., JEWETT, P. B., HIETER, P. A., LeGANDRE, S. M., AND DORRIS, G., 1975, Possible role of poly(A) as an inhibitor of endonuclease activity in eukaryotic cells, *Nature (London)* **256**:340.

LIEBERMAN, M. W., AND POIRER, M. C., 1974a, Distribution of deoxyribonucleic acid repair synthesis among repetitive and unique sequences in the human diploid genome, *Biochemistry* **13**:3018.

LIEBERMAN, M. W., AND POIRER, M. C., 1974b, Intragenomal distribution of DNA repair synthesis: Repair in satellite and main band DNA in cultured mouse cells, *Proc. Natl. Acad. Sci. USA* **71**:2461.

LIJINSKY, W., LOO, J., AND ROSS, A. E., 1968, Mechanism of alkylation of nucleic acids by nitrosodimethylamine, *Nature (London)* **218**:1174.

LILJA, H. S., CURPHEY, T. J., YAGER, J. D., JR., AND LONGNECKER, D. S., 1978, Persistence of DNA damage in rat pancreas following administration of three carcinogens and/or mutagens, *Chem. Biol. Interact.* **22**:287.

LIN, J. K., MILLER, J. A., AND MILLER, E. C., 1977, 2,3-Dihydro-2-(guan-7-yl)-3-hydroxy-aflatoxin B_1, a major acid hydrolysis product of aflatoxin-B_1-DNA or ribosomal-RNA adducts formed in hepatic microsome mediated reactions and in rat liver *in vivo*, *Cancer Res.* **37**:4430.

LINGENS, F., HAERLIN, F., AND SUSSMUTH, R., 1971, Mechanisms of mutagenesis by N-methyl-N'-nitro-N-nitrosoguanidine (MNNG). Methylation of nucleic acids by N-trideuteriomethyl-N'-nitro-N-nitrosoguanidine (D_3-MNNG) in the presence of cysteine and in cells of *Escherichia coli*, *FEBS Lett.* **13**:241.

LINSLEY, W. S., PENHOET, E. E., AND LINN, S., 1977, Human endonuclease specific for apurinic/apyrimidinic sites in DNA. Partial purification and characterization of multiple forms from placenta, *J. Biol. Chem.* **252**:1235.

LIQUORI, A. M., DeLERMA, B., ASCOLI, F., BOTRÉ, C., AND TRASCITTI, M., 1962, Interaction between DNA and polycyclic aromatic hydrocarbons, *J. Mol. Biol.* **5**:521.

LIQUORI, A. M., COSTANTINO, L., AND CRESCEZI, V., 1967, Complexes between DNA and polyamides: "A molecular model," *J. Mol. Biol.* **24**:113.

LJUNGQUIST, S., AND LINDAHL, T., 1977, Relation between *Escherichia coli* endonucleases specific for apurinic sites in DNA and exonuclease III, *Nucleic Acids Res.* **4**:2871.

LOTLIKAR, P. D., AND LUHA, L., 1971a, Enzymatic N-acetylation of N-hydroxy-2-aminofluorene of liver cytosol from various species, *Biochem. J.* **123**:287.

LOTLIKAR, P. D., AND LUHA, L., 1971b, Acylation of carcinogenic hydroxamic acids by carbamoylphosphate to form reactive esters, *Biochem. J.* **124**:69.

LOVELESS, A., 1969, Possible relevance of O^6 alkylation of deoxyguanosine to the mutagenicity and carcinogenicity of nitrosamines and nitrosamides, *Nature (London)* **223**:206.

LUTZ, W. K., 1979, *In vivo* covalent binding of organic chemicals to DNA as a quantitative indicator in the process of chemical carcinogenesis, *Mutat. Res.* **65**:289.

LYTLE, C. D., DAY, R. S., HELLMAN, K. B., AND BOCKSTAHLER, L. E., 1976, Infection of UV irradiated xeroderma pigmentosum fibroblasts by herpes-simplex-virus: Study of capacity and Weigle reactivation, *Mutat. Res.* **36**:257.

LYTLE, C. D., COPPEY, J., AND TAYLOR, W. D., 1978, Enhanced survival of ultraviolet-irradiated herpes-simplex virus in carcinogen pretreated cells, *Nature (London)* **272**:60.

MAGEE, P. N., AND BARNES, J. M., 1967, Carcinogenic nitroso compounds, *Adv. Cancer Res.* **10**:163.

MAGEE, P. N., AND FARBER, E., 1962, Methylation of rat-liver nucleic acids by dimethylnitrosamine *in vivo*, *Biochem. J.* **83**:114.

399

INTERAC-
TIONS OF
CARCINOGENS
WITH NUCLEIC
ACIDS

MAGEE, P. N., AND HULTIN, T., 1962, Toxic liver injury and carcinogenesis. Methylation of rat liver slices by dimethylnitrosamine *in vitro, Biochem. J.* **83**:106.

MAGEE, P. N., AND LEE, K. Y., 1963, Experimental toxic liver injury by some nitrosamines, *Ann. N.Y. Acad. Sci.* **104**:916.

MAGEE, P. N., AND LEE, K. Y., 1964, Cellular injury and carcinogenesis: Alkylation of ribonucleic acid of rat liver by diethylnitrosamine and *n*-butylmethylnitrosamine *in vivo, Biochem. J.* **91**:35.

MAGEE, P. N., AND SCHOENTAL, R., 1964, Carcinogenesis by nitroso compounds, *Br. Med. Bull.* **20**:102.

MAHER, V. M., DOUVILLE, D., TOMURA, T., AND VAN LANCKER, J. L., 1974, Mutagenicity of reactive derivatives of carcinogenic hydrocarbons: Evidence of DNA repair, *Mutat. Res.* **23**:113.

MALAVEILLE, C., BARTSCH, H., BARBINA CAMUS, A. M., MONTESANO, R., CROISY, A., AND JACQUIGNON, P., 1975, Mutagenicity of vinyl chloride, chloroethylene oxide, chloroacetaldehyde and chloroethanol, *Biochem. Biophys. Res. Commun.* **63**:363.

MALKIN, M. F., AND ZAHALSKY, A. C., 1966, Interaction of the water-soluble carcinogen 4-nitroquinoline *N*-oxide with DNA, *Science* **154**:1665.

MARGISON, G. P., AND PEGG, A. E., 1981, Enzymatic release of 7-methylguanine from methylated DNA by rodent liver extracts, *Proc. Natl. Acad. Sci. USA* **78**:861.

MARGISON, G. P., CAPPS, M. J., O'CONNOR, P. J., AND CRAIG, A. W., 1973, Loss of 7-methylguanine from rat liver DNA after methylation *in vivo* with methylmethanesulphonate or dimethyl-nitrosamine, *Chem. Biol. Interact.* **6**:119.

MARQUARTDT, H., BENDICH, A., PHILIPS, F. S., AND HOFFMANN, D., 1971, Binding of G-^{3}H-7,12-dimethylbenz(α)anthracene to DNA of normal and rapidly dividing hepatic cells of rats, *Chem. Biol. Interact.* **3**:1.

MARROQUIN, F., AND FARBER, E., 1965, The binding of 2-acetylaminofluorene to rat liver ribonucleic acid *in vivo, Cancer Res.* **25**:1262.

MARTIN, C. N., AND GARNER, R. C., 1977, Aflatoxin B$_1$ oxide generated by chemical or enzymic oxidation of aflatoxin B$_1$ causes guanine substitution in nucleic acids, *Nature (London)* **267**:863.

MATSUMOTO, H., AND HIGA, H. H., 1966, Studies on methylazoxymethanol, the aglycone of cycasin: Methylation of nucleic acids *in vitro, Biochem. J.* **98**:20C.

MATSUSHIMA, T., KOBUNA, I., AND SUGIMURA, T., 1967, *In vivo* interaction of 4-nitroquinoline-1-oxide and its derivatives with DNA, *Nature (London)* **216**:508.

MATSUYAMA, A., AND NAGATA, C., 1972, Detection of the unstable intermediate 4-nitrosoquinoline-1-oxide, in: *Proceedings of the Second International Symposium of the Princess Takamatsu Cancer Resarch Fund* (W. Nakahara, S. Takayama, T. Sugimura, and S. Odashima, eds.), p. 35, University Park Press, Baltimore.

MCCALLA, D. R., REUVERS, A., AND KITAI, R., 1968, Inactivation of biologically active *N*-methyl-*N*-nitroso compounds in aqueous solution: Effect of various conditions of pH and illumination, *Can. J. Biochem.* **46**:807.

MCCALLA, D. R., REUVERS, A., AND KAISER, C., 1971, Activation of nitrofurazone in animal tissues, *Biochem. Pharmacol.* **20**:3532.

MCCANN, J., SIMON, V., STREITWISER, D., AND AMES, B. N., 1975, Mutagenicity of chloroacetaldehyde, a possible metabolic product of 1,2-dichloroethane (ethylene-dichloride), chloroethanol (ethylene-chlorohydrin), vinyl chloride and cyclophosphamide, *Proc. Natl. Acad. Sci. USA* **72**:3190.

MCCANN, J., CHOI, E., YAMASAKI, E., AND AMES, B. N., 1976, Detection of carcinogens as mutagens in the *Salmonella*/microsome test: Assay of 300 chemicals, *Proc. Natl. Acad. Sci. USA* **72**:5135.

MCENTEE, K., WEINSTOCK, G. M., AND LEHMAN, I. R., 1979, Initiation of general recombination catalyzed *in vitro* by the Rec.A protein of *E. coli. Proc. Natl. Acad. Sci. USA* **76**:2615.

MCENTEE, K. WEINSTOCK, G. M., AND LEHMAN, I. R., 1980, Rec.A protein-catalyzed strand assimilation: Stimulation by *Escherichia coli* single stranded DNA-binding protein, *Proc. Natl. Acad. Sci. USA* **77**:857.

MEEHAN, T., AND STRAUB, K., 1979, Double-stranded DNA stereoselectively binds benzo(*a*)pyrene diol epoxides, *Nature (London)* **277**:410.

MENGLE, L., GAMPER, H., AND BARTHOLOMEW, J., 1978, Base specificity in the binding of benzo(α)pyrene diol epoxide to simian virus 40 DNA, *Cancer Lett.* **5**:131.

METZGER, G., AND DAUNE, M., 1975, *In vitro* binding of *N*-acetoxy-*N*-2-acetylaminofluorene to DNA in chromatin, *Cancer Res.* **35**:2738.

METZGER, G., WILHELM, F. X., AND WILHELM, M. L., 1976, Distribution along DNA of the bound carcinogen *N*-acetoxy-*N*-2-acetylaminofluorene in chromatin modified *in vitro, Chem. Biol. Interact.* **15**:257.

METZGER, G., WILHELM, F. X., AND WILHELM, M. L., 1977, Non-random binding of a chemical carcinogen to the DNA in chromatin, *Biochem. Biophys. Res. Commun.* **75**:703.

MICHAEL, R. O., PARODI, S., AND SARMA, D. S. R., 1975, *In vivo* repair of rat liver DNA damaged by 3-hydroxyxanthine, *Chem. Biol. Interact.* **10**:19.

MILLER, E. C., AND MILLER, J. A., 1969, Studies on the mechanism of activation of aromatic amine and amide carcinogens to ultimate carcinogenic electrophilic reactants, *Ann. N.Y. Acad. Sci.* **163**:731.

MILLER, E. C., AND MILLER, J. A., 1971, The mutagenicity of chemical carcinogens: Correlations, problems and interpretations, in: *Chemical Mutagens: Principles and Methods for Their Detection*, Vol. I (A. Hollaender, ed.) p. 83, Plenum Press, New York.

MILLER, J A., 1970, Carcinogenesis by chemicals: An overview—G. H. A. Clowes memorial lecture, *Cancer Res.* **30**:559.

MILLER, J. A., AND MILLER, E. C., 1969, Metabolic activation of carcinogenic aromatic amines and amides via *N*-hydroxylation and *N*-hydroxy-esterification and its relationship to ultimate carcinogens as electrophilic reactants, in: *Physico-chemical Mechanisms of Carcinogenesis*, The Jerusalem Symposia on Quantum Chemistry and Biochemistry, Vol. 1 (E. D. Bergmann and B. Pullman, eds.), p. 237, The Israel Academy of Science and Humanities, Jerusalem.

MILLER, J. A., LIN, J.-K., AND MILLER, E. C., 1970, *N*-(guanosin-8-yl) and *N*-(deoxyguanosin-8-yl)-*N*-methyl-4-aminoazobenzene: Degradation products of hepatic RNA and DNA in rats administered *N'*-methyl-4-aminoazobenzene, *Proc. Am. Assoc. Cancer Res.* **11**:56.

MIRVISH, S. S., 1968, The carcinogenic action and metabolism of urethan and *N*-hydroxyurethan, *Adv. Cancer Res.* **11**:1.

MIURA, K., AND RECKENDORF, H. K., 1967, The nitrofurans, *Prog. Med. Chem.* **5**:320.

MIYAKI, M., YATAGAI, K., AND ONO, T., 1977, Strand breaks of mammalian mitochondrial DNA induced by carcinogens, *Chem. Biol. Interact.* **17**:321.

MIZUSAWA, H., AND KAKEFUDA, T., 1979, Inhibition of DNA synthesis *in vitro* by binding of benzo(α)pyrene metabolites diol-epoxide I to DNA, *Nature (London)* **279**:75.

MONTESANO, R., BRÉSIL, H., AND MARGISON, G., 1979, Increased excision of O^6-methylguanine from rat liver DNA after chronic administration of dimethylnitrosamine, *Cancer Res.* **39**:1798.

MOORE, P., AND STRAUSS, B. S., 1979, Sites of inhibition of *in vitro* DNA synthesis in carcinogen and UV-treated ϕX174 DNA, *Nature (London)* **278**:664.

MOREAU, P., BAILONE, A., AND DEVORET, R., 1976, Prophage λ induction in *E. coli* K12 envA uvrB: A highly sensitive test for potential carcinogens, *Proc. Natl. Acad. Sci. USA* **73**:3700.

MORITA, T., FUKUNAGA, M., AND MIFUCHI, I., 1976, Loss of mitochondrial DNA in respiration deficient mutant of yeast induced by 4-nitroquinoline 1-oxide, *Gann* **66**:697.

MOSES, H. L., WEBSTER, R. A., MARTIN, G. D., AND SPELSBERG, T. C., 1976, Binding of polycyclic aromatic hydrocarbons to transcriptionally active nuclear subfractions of AKR mouse embryo cells, *Cancer Res.* **36**:2905.

MOYER, G. H., GUMBINER, B., AND AUSTIN, G. E., 1977, Binding of *N*-hydroxy-2-acetylaminofluorene to eu- and heterochromatin fractions of rat liver *in vivo, Cancer Lett.* **2**:259.

MULIVOR, R. A., ABANOBI, S. E., AND SARMA, D. S. R., 1974, Hepatic DNA damage induced by methylmethanesulfonate (MMS) and dimethylnitrosamine (DMN) *in vivo, Proc. Am. Assoc. Cancer Res.* **15**:85.

MÜLLER, W., AND CROTHERS, D. M., 1968, Studies on the binding of actinomycin and related compounds to DNA, *J. Mol. Biol.* **35**:251.

MYLES, A., AND BROWN, G. B., 1969, Purine *N*-oxides. XXX. Biochemical studies of the oncogen 3-hydroxyxanthine, *J. Biol. Chem.* **244**:4072.

NAGASAWA, H. T., SHIROTA, F. N., AND MATSUMOTO, H., 1972, Decomposition of methylazoxy-methanol, the aglycone of cycasin, in D_2O, *Nature (London)* **236**:234.

NAGATA, C., KATAOKA, N., IMAMURA, A., KAWAZOE, Y., AND CHIHARA, G., 1966, Electronic spin resonance study on the free radicals produced from 4-hydroxyaminoquinoline 1-oxide and its significance in carcinogenesis, *Gann* **57**:323.

NAGATA, Y., AND MATSUMOTO, H., 1969, Studies on methylazoxymethanol: Methylation of nucleic acids in the fetal rat brain, *Proc. Soc. Exp. Biol. Med.* **132**:383.

NAKAHARA, W., FUKUOKA, F., AND SUGIMURA, T., 1957, Carcinogenic action of 4-nitroquinoline 1-oxide, *Gann* **48**:129.

NAKANISHI, K., KASAI, H., CHO, H., HARVEY, R. G., JEFFREY, A. M., JENNETTE, K. W., AND WEINSTEIN, I. B., 1977, Absolute configuration of a ribonucleic acid adduct formed *in vivo* by metabolism of benzo(α)pyrene, *J. Am. Chem. Soc.* **99**:258.

401

INTERAC-
TIONS OF
CARCINOGENS
WITH NUCLEIC
ACIDS

NATORI, Y., 1963, VI. Sex-dependent behavior of methionine and ethionine in rats, *J. Biol. Chem.* **238**:2075.

NELSON, J. H., GRUNBERGER, D., CANTO, C. R., AND WEINSTEIN, I. B., 1971, Modification of ribonucleic acid by chemical carcinogens. IV. Circular dichroism and proton magnetic resonance studies of oligonucleotides modified with *N*-2-acetylaminofluorene, *J. Mol. Biol.* **62**:331.

NERY, R., 1968, Some aspects of the metabolism of urethane and *N*-hydroxyurethane in rodents, *Biochem. J.* **106**:1.

NERY, R., 1969, Acylation of cytosine by ethyl *N*-hydrocarbamate and its acyl derivatives and the binding of these agents to nucleic acids and proteins, *J. Chem. Soc. C* **1969**:1860.

NICOLINI, C., RAMANATHAN, R., KENDALL, F., MURPHY, J., PARODI, S., AND SARMA, D. S. R., 1976, Physicochemical alterations in the conformation of rat liver chromatin induced by carcinogens *in vivo*, *Cancer Res.* **36**:1725.

NICOLL, J. W., SWANN, P. F., AND PEGG, A. E., 1977, The accumulation of O^6-methylguanine in the liver and kidney DNA of rats treated with dimethylnitrosamine for a short or a long period, *Chem. Biol. Interact.* **16**:301.

NOLL, M., 1974, Subunit structure of chromatin, *Nature (London)* **251**:249.

NOMURA, T., 1976, Diminution of tumorigenesis initiated by 4-nitroquinoline 1-oxide by post-treatment with caffeine in mice, *Nature (London)* **260**:547.

NOMURA, T., 1980, Timing of chemically induced neoplasia in mice revealed by the antineoplastic action of caffeine, *Cancer Res.* **40**:1332.

O'CONNOR, P. J., CAPPS, M. J., AND CRAIG, A. W., 1973, Comparative studies of the hepatocarcinogen *N,N*-dimethylnitrosamine *in vivo*: Reaction sites in rat liver DNA and the significance of their relative stabilities, *Br. J. Cancer* **27**:153.

OLESON, F. B., MITCHELL, B. L., DIPPLE, A., AND LIEBERMAN, M. W., 1979, Distribution of DNA damage in chromatin and its relation to repair in human cells treated with 7-bromomethyl-benzo(*a*)anthracene, *Nucleic Acids Res.* **7**:1343.

ORNSTEIN, R. C., AND REIN, R., 1979, Nucleic acid base and carcinogen metabolites specificities during intercalative interactions between DNA and 4NQO, *Chem. Biol. Interact.* **27**:291.

ORTWERTH, B. J., AND NOVELLI, G. D., 1969, Studies on the incorporation of L-ethionine-ethyl-1-^{14}C into the transfer RNA of rat liver, *Cancer Res.* **29**:380.

OSBORNE, M. R., HARVEY, R. G., AND BROOKES, P., 1978, The reaction of *trans*-7,8-dihydroxy-*anti*-9,10-epoxy-7,8,9,10-tetrahydrobenzo(*a*)pyrene with DNA involves attack at the N-7 position of guanine moieties, *Chem. Biol. Interact.* **20**:123.

OSTERMAN GOLKAR, S., EHRENBERG, L., AND WACHTMEISTER, C. W., 1970, Reaction kinetics and biological action in barley of monofunctional methanesulfonic esters, *Radiat. Bot.* **10**:303.

PAINTER, R. B., 1970, Repair of DNA in mammalian cells, *Curr. Top. Radiat. Res.* **7**:45.

PAINTER, R. B., 1978, Does ultraviolet light enhance postreplication repair in mammalian cells?, *Nature (London)* **275**:243.

PARK, S. D., AND CLEAVER, J. E., 1979, Postreplication repair: Question of its definition and possible alteration in xeroderma pigmentosum cell strains, *Proc. Natl. Acad. Sci. USA* **76**:3927.

PARODI, S., TANINGHER, M., SANTI, L., CANANNA, M., SCIABA, L., MAURA, A., AND BRAMBILLA, G., 1978, A practical procedure for testing DNA damage *in vivo*, proposed for a prescreening of chemical carcinogens, *Mutat. Res.* **54**:39.

PATEL, N. T., AND HOLOUBEK, V., 1976, Protein composition of liver nuclear ribonuclear protein particles of rats fed carcinogenic amino azo-dyes, *Biochem. Biophys. Res. Commun.* **73**:112.

PATERSON, M. C., SMITH, B. P., LOHMAN, P. H. M., ANDERSON, A. K., AND FISHMAN, L., 1976, Defective excision repair of X-ray damaged DNA in human (ataxia telangiectasia) fibroblasts, *Nature (London)* **260**:444.

PAUL, H. E., AND PAUL, M. F., 1964, The nitrofurans—Chemotherapeutic properties, in: *Experimental Chemotherapy*, Vol. II (R. J. Schnitzer and F. Hawkins, eds.), p. 307, Academic Press, New York.

PAUL, J. S., MONTGOMERY, P. O'B., JR., AND LOUIS, J. B., 1971, A proposed model of the interaction of 4-nitroquinoline 1-oxide with DNA, *Cancer Res.* **31**:413.

PAULING, L., 1970, *General Chemistry*, Freeman, San Francisco.

PEGG, A. E., 1972, Ethylation of rat liver t-RNA after administration of L-ethionine, *Biochem. J.* **128**:59.

PEGG, A. E., 1973, Alkylation of transfer RNA by *N*-methyl-*N*-nitrosourea and *N*-ethyl-*N*-nitrosourea, *Chem. Biol. Interact.* **6**:393.

PEGG, A. E., 1978*a*, Inhibition of the alkylation of nucleic acids and of the metabolism of 1,2-dimethylhydrazine by amino acetonitrile, *Chem. Biol. Interact.* **23**:273.

S. RAJALAKSHMI,
PREMA M. RAO,
AND
D. S. R. SARMA

PEGG, A. E., 1978*b*, Enzymatic removal of O^6-methylguanine from DNA by mammalian cell extracts, *Biochem. Biophys. Res. Commun.* **84**:166.

PEGG, A. E., AND HUI, G., 1978, Removal of methylated purines from rat liver DNA after administration of dimethylnitrosamine, *Cancer Res.* **38**:2011.

PEGG, A. E., AND JACKSON, A., 1976, Alkylation of messenger RNA by dimethylnitrosamine, *Chem. Biol. Interact.* **12**:279.

PHILLIPS, D. H., MILLER, J. A., MILLER, E. C., AND ADAMS, B. 1981, N^2 atom of guanine and N^6 atom of adenine residues as sites for covalent binding of metabolically activated 1'-hydroxy safrole to mouse liver DNA in vivo, *Cancer Res.* **41**:2664.

POCHON, F., AND MICHELSON, A. M., 1971, Action of the carcinogen 7-bromomethyl-benz(a)anthracene on synthetic polynucleotides, *Eur. J. Biochem.* **21**:144.

POIRIER, L. A., MILLER, J. A., MILLER, E. C., AND SATO, K., 1967, *N*-Benzoyloxy-*N*-methyl-4-aminoazobenzene. Its carcinogenic activity in the rat and its reactions with proteins and nucleic acids and their constituents *in vitro*, *Cancer Res.* **27**:1600.

PONG, R. S., AND WOGAN, G. N., 1970, Time course and dose–response characteristics of aflatoxin B_1 effects on rat liver RNA polymerase and ultrastructure, *Cancer Res.* **30**:294.

POUND, A. W., FRANKE, F., AND LAWSON, T. A., 1976, Binding of ethyl carbamate to DNA of mouse liver *in vivo*. The nature and site of binding, *Chem. Biol. Interact.* **14**:149.

POWERS, D. M., AND HOLLEY, R. W., 1972, Selective chemical methylation of yeast alanine transfer RNA, *Biochim. Biophys. Acta* **287**:456.

PRAKASH, L., AND STRAUSS, B., 1970, Repair of alkylation damage: Stability of methyl groups in *Bacillus subtilis* treated with methylmethanesulfonate, *J. Bacteriol.* **102**:760.

PREUSSMANN, R., DRUCKREY, H., IVANKOVIC, S., AND HODENBERG, A. V., 1967, Chemical structure and carcinogenicity of aliphatic hydrazo, azo and azoxy compounds and of triazenes, potential *in vivo* alkylating agents, *Ann. N.Y. Acad. Sci.* **163**:697.

PRODI, G., ROCCHI, P., AND GRILLI, S., 1970*a*, *In vivo* interaction of urethan with nucleic acids and proteins, *Cancer Res.* **30**:2887.

PRODI, G., ROCCHI, P., AND GRILLI, S., 1970*b*, Binding of 7,12-dimethylbenz(a)anthracene and benzopyrene to nucleic acids and proteins of organs in rats, *Cancer Res.* **30**:1020.

PULKRABEK, P., LEFFLER, S., GRUNBERGER, D., AND WEINSTEIN, I. B., 1979, Modification of deoxyribonucleic acid by a diol epoxide of benzo(α)pyrene. Relation to DNA structure and conformation and effects on transfectional activity, *Biochemistry* **18**:5128.

PULLMAN, B., AND PULLMAN, A., 1959, The electronic structure of the purine–pyrimidine pairs of DNA, *Biochim. Biophys. Acta* **36**:343.

RABES, H. M., KERLER, R., WILHELM, R., RODE, G., AND RIESS, H., 1979, Alkylation of DNA and RNA by [^{14}C] dimethylnitrosamine in hydroxyurea synchronized regenerating rat liver, *Cancer Res.* **39**:4228.

RADMAN, M., 1974, in: *Molecular and Environmental Aspects of Mutagenesis* (L. Prakash, F. Sherman, M. W., MILLER, C. W. LAWRENCE, AND H. W. TEBER, eds.), p. 128, Thomas, Springfield, Ill.

RAJALAKSHMI, S., 1973, A liver tRNA for the assay of rat liver methylase *in vitro*, *Proc. Am. Assoc. Cancer Res.* **14**:39.

RAJALAKSHMI, S., AND SARMA, D. S. R., 1973, Rapid repair of hepatic DNA damage induced by camptothecin in the intact rat, *Biochem. Biophys. Res. Commun.* **53**:1268.

RAJALAKSHMI, S., AND SARMA, D. S. R., 1975, Replication of hepatic DNA in rats treated with dimethylnitrosamine, *Chem. Biol. Interact.* **11**:245.

RAJALAKSHMI, S., RAO, P. M., AND SARMA, D. S. R., 1978*a*, Modulation of carcinogen chromatin DNA interaction by polyamines, *Biochem. Biophys. Res. Commun.* **81**:936.

RAJALAKSHMI, S., RAO, P. M., AND SARMA, D. S. R., 1978*b*, Studies on carcinogen chromatin-DNA interaction: Inhibition of *N*-methyl-*N*-nitrosourea-induced methylation of chromatin-DNA by spermine and distamycin-A, *Biochemistry* **17**:4515.

RAJALAKSHMI, S., RAO, P. M., AND SARMA, D. S. R., 1980, Carcinogen–DNA interaction: Differential effects of distamycin-A and spermine on the formation of 7-methylguanine in DNA by *N*-methyl-*N*-nitrosourea, methylmethanesulfonate and dimethylsulfate, *Teratogenesis Carcinogenesis and Mutagenesis* **1**:97.

RAMANATHAN, R., AND DIPPLE, A., 1976, Specificity of interaction of directly acting carcinogens with DNA, *Proc. Am. Assoc. Cancer Res.* **17**:77.

403

INTERAC-
TIONS OF
CARCINOGENS
WITH NUCLEIC
ACIDS

RAMANATHAN, R., RAJALAKSHMI, S., SARMA, D. S. R., AND FARBER, E., 1976a, Non-random nature of *in vivo* methylation by dimethylnitrosamine and subsequent removal of methylated products from rat liver chormatin DNA, *Cancer Res.* **36**:2073.

RAMANATHAN, R., RAJALAKSHMI, S., AND SARMA, D. S. R., 1976b, Non-random nature of *in vivo* interaction of ^{3}H-*N*-hydroxy-2-acetylaminofluorene and its subsequent removal from rat liver chromatin DNA, *Chem. Biol. Interact.* **14**:375.

RAMSTEIN, J., HOUSSIER, C., AND LENG, M., 1973, Electro-optical properties of nucleic acids and nucleoproteins, IV. Influence of base composition and methylation on the properties of DNA and DNA–proflavin complexes, *Biochim. Biophys. Acta* **335**:54.

RAO, P. M., RAJALAKSHMI, S., AND SARMA, D. S. R., 1978, Carcinogen induced alterations in DNase I rlease of N^3-methyladenine from liver chromatin, *Chem. Biol. Interact.* **22**:347.

REGAN, J. D., AND SETLOW, R. B., 1974, Two forms of repair in the DNA of human cells damaged by chemical carcinogens and mutagens, *Cancer Res.* **34**:3318.

REID, B. D., AND WALKER, I. G., 1969, The response of mammalian cells to alkylating agents. II. On the mechanism of the removal of sulfur-mustard-induced crosslinks, *Biochim. Biophys. Acta* **179**:179.

REINER, B., AND ZAMENHOF, S., 1957, Studies on the chemically reactive groups of deoxyribonucleic acids, *J. Biol. Chem.* **228**:475.

RENARD, A., THIBODEAU, L., AND VERLY, W. G., 1978, O^6-Ethylguanine excision from DNA of liver nuclei treated with ethylnitrosourea, *Fed. Proc.* **37**:1412.

RHAESE, H. J., AND FREESE, E., 1969, Chemical analysis of DNA alteration. IV. Reactions of oligodeoxynucleotides with monofunctional alkylating agents leading to backbone breakage, *Biochim. Biophys. Acta* **190**:418.

RIAZUDDIN, S., AND LINDAHL, T., 1978, Properties of 3-methyl-adenine-DNA glycosylase from *Escherichia coli, Biochemistry* **17**:2110.

ROBERTS, J. J., 1969, The binding of metabolites of 4-dimethylaminoazobenzene and 2-methyl-4-dimethylaminoazobenzene to hooded rat macromolecules during chronic feeding, in: *Physicochemical Mechanisms of Carcinogenesis*, The Jerusalem Symposia on Quantum Chemistry and Biochemistry, Vol. 1 (E. D. Bergmann and B. Pullman, eds.), p. 229, The Israel Academy of Science and Humanities, Jerusalem.

ROBERTS, J. J., 1972, Repair of alkylated DNA in mammalian cells, in: *Molecular and Cellular Repair Processes* (R. F. Beers, R. M. Herriott, and R. C. Tilghman, eds.), p. 226, The Johns Hopkins Press, Baltimore.

ROBERTS, J. J., 1978, The repair of DNA modified by cytotoxic, mutagenic and carcinogenic chemicals, *Adv. Radiat. Biol.* **7**:211.

ROBERTS, J. J., AND WARWICK, G. P., 1961, Reactions of ^{3}H-labelled butter yellow *in vivo* and *N*-hydroxy-methylaminoazobenzene *in vitro, Biochem. J.* **93**:1897.

ROBERTS, J. J., AND WARWICK, G. P., 1963, The reaction of β-propiolactone with guanosine, deoxyguanylic acid and RNA, *Biochem. Pharmacol.* **12**:1441.

ROBERTS, J. J., AND WARWICK, G. P., 1966, The covalent binding of metabolites of dimethylaminoazobenzene, β-naphthylamine and aniline to nucleic acids *in vivo, Int. J. Cancer* **1**:179.

ROBINS, P., AND CAIRNS, J., 1979, Quantitation of the adaptive response to alkylating agents, *Nature (London)* **280**:74.

RODRIGUEZ, L. V., AND BECKER, F. F., 1976, Rat liver chromatin, fractionation into eu- and heterochromatin with localization of ribosomal genes, *Arch. Biochem. Biophys.* **173**:428.

ROSEN, L., 1968, Ethylation *in vivo* of purines in rat liver t-RNA by L-ethionine, *Biochem. Biophys. Res. Commun.* **33**:546.

ROTHWELL, K., 1974, Dose related inhibition of chemical carcinogenesis in mouse skin by caffeine, *Nature (London)* **252**:69.

RUPP, W. D., AND HOWARD-FLANDERS, P., 1968, Discontinuities in the DNA synthesized in an excision-defective strain of *Escherichia coli* following ultraviolet irradiation, *J. Mol. Biol.* **31**:291.

RYSKOV, A. P., FARASHYAN, V. R., AND GEORGIEV, G. P., 1972, Ribonuclease-stable base sequences specific exclusively for giant dRNA, *Biochim. Biophys. Acta* **262**:568.

SAFFHILL, R., COOPER, H. K., AND ITZHAKI, R. F., 1974, Detection by DNA polymerase I of breaks produced in rat liver chromatin *in vivo* by alkylating agents, *Nature (London)* **248**:153.

SALMON, A. G., 1976, Cytochrome P450 and the metabolism of vinyl chloride, *Cancer Lett.* **2**:109.

SARASIN, A. R., AND HANAWALT, P. C., 1978, Carcinogens enhance survival of UV-irradiated simian virus 40 in treated monkey kidney cells: Induction of a recovery pathway, *Proc. Natl. Acad. Sci. USA* **75**:346.

SARASIN, A. R., GOZE, A., DEVORET, R., AND MOULE, Y., 1977, Induced reactivation of UV-damaged phage λ in *E. coli* K12 host cells treated with aflatoxin B₁ metabolites, *Mutat. Res.* **42**:205.

SARMA, D. S. R., 1973, Chemical interaction measurements, in: *Carcinogenesis Testing of Chemicals* (L. Golberg, ed.), p. 95, CRC Press, Cleveland.

SARMA, D. S. R., ZUBROFF, J., MICHAEL, R. O., AND RAJALAKSHMI, S., 1974, DNA damage and repair *in vivo*—A measurement of *in vivo* carcinogen–DNA interaction and a possible bioassay for carcinogens, *Excerpta Med. Int. Congr. Ser.* **350**:82.

SARMA, D. S. R., RAJALAKSHMI, S., AND FARBER, E., 1975, Chemical carcinogenesis: Interactions of carcinogens with nucleic acids, in: *Cancer: A Comprehensive Treatise*, Vol. 1 (F. F. Becker, ed.), p. 235, Plenum Press, New York.

SARMA, D. S. R., ZUBROFF, J., AND RAJALAKSHMI, S., 1977, Repair *in vivo* of liver deoxyribonucleic acid damaged by hycanthone and related compounds, *Mol. Pharmacol.* **13**:719.

SARMA, D. S. R., RAJALAKSHMI, S., UDUPA, R., FARBER, E., AND RAO, P. M., 1978, Factors influencing DNA damage and its repair with cellular implications for toxicology, in: *Advances in Pharmacology and Therapeutics*, Vol. 9 (Y. Cohen, ed.), p. 71, Pergamon Press, Oxford.

SASAKI, M. S., AND TONOMURA, A., 1973, A high susceptibility of Fanconi's anemia to chromosome breakage by DNA crosslinking agents, *Cancer Res.* **33**:1829.

SASAKI, T., AND YOSHIDA, T., 1935, Production of carcinoma of the liver by feeding *o*-aminoazotoluene, *Arch. Pathol. Anat.* **295**:175.

SCAIFE, J. J., 1970–1971, Aflatoxin B₁: Cytotoxic mode of action evaluated by mammalian cell cultures, *FEBS Lett.* **12**:143.

SCHABORT, J. C., 1971, The differential interaction of aflatoxin B₂ with deoxyribonucleic acids from different sources and with purines and purine nucleosides, *Chem. Biol. Interact.* **3**:371.

SCHENDEL, P. F., AND ROBINS, P. E., 1978, Repair of O^6-methylguanine in adapted *Escherichia coli*, *Proc. Natl. Acad. Sci. USA* **75**:6017.

SCHERER, E., AND EMMELOT, P., 1977, Pre-cancerous transformation in rat liver by diethylnitrosamine in relation to the repair of alkylated site in DNA, *Mutat. Res.* **46**:153.

SCHNEIDER, W. C., AND KUFF, E. L., 1965, The isolation and some properties of rat liver mitochondrial deoxyribonucleic acid, *Proc. Natl. Acad. Sci USA* **54**:1650.

SCHOENTAL, R., 1973, The mechanisms of action of the carcinogenic nitroso and related compounds, *Br. J. Cancer* **28**:436.

SCHULZ, U., AND McCALLA, D. R., 1969, Reactions of cysteine with *N*-methyl-*N*-nitroso-*p*-toluenesulfonamide and *N*-methyl-*N*′-nitro-*N*-nitrosoguanidine, *Can. J. Biochem.* **47**:2021.

SCHWARTZ, E. L., AND GOODMAN, J. I., 1979, Quantitative and qualitative aspects of the binding of *N*-hydroxy-2-acetylaminofluorene to hepatic chromatin fractions, *Chem. Biol. Interact.* **26**:287.

SEGAL, A., SCHROEDER, M., BARNETTE, O., AND VAN DUUREN, B. L., 1974, Studies on the effects *in vitro* of β-propiolactone and β-propiolact[¹⁴C]one on whole mouse skin chromatin, *Biochem. Pharmacol.* **23**:937.

SELKIRK, J. K., HUBERMAN, E., AND HEIDELBERGER, C., 1971, An epoxide is an intermediate in the microsomal metabolism of the chemical carcinogen dibenz(*a, h*)anthracene, *Biochem. Biophys. Res. Commun.* **43**:1010.

SETLOW, R. B., AND REGAN, J. D., 1972, Defective repair of *N*-acetoxy-2-acetylaminofluorene-induced lesions in the DNA of xeroderma pigmentosum cells, *Biochem. Biophys. Res. Commun.* **46**:1019.

SHANK, R. C., AND MAGEE, P. N., 1967, Similarities between the biochemical actions of cycasin and dimethylnitrosamine, *Biochem. J.* **105**:521.

SHAPIRO, R., 1968, Chemistry of guanine and its biologically significant derivatives, *Prog. Nucleic Acid Res. Mol. Biol.* **8**:73.

SHAPIRO, R., 1969, Reactions with purines and pyrmidines, *Ann. N.Y. Acad. Sci.* **163**:624.

SHEARMAN, C. W., AND LOEB, L. A., 1979, Effects of depurination on the fidelity of DNA synthesis, *J. Mol. Biol.* **128**:197.

SHIBATA, T., DASGUPTA, C. CUNNINGHAM, R. P., AND RADDING, C. M., 1979, Purified *Escherichia coli* rec-A-protein catalyzed homologous pairing of superhelical DNA and single stranded fragments, *Proc. Natl. Acad. Sci. USA* **76**:1638.

SHINOHARA, K., AND CERUTTI, P. A., 1977, Excision repair of benzo(α)pyrene–deoxyguanosine adducts in baby hamster kidney 21/C13 cells and in secondary mouse embryo fibroblasts—C57BL/6J, *Proc. Natl. Acad. Sci. USA* **74**:979.

405

INTERAC-
TIONS OF
CARCINOGENS
WITH NUCLEIC
ACIDS

SHOOTER, K. V., 1978, DNA phosphotriesters as indicators of cumulative carcinogen-induced damage, *Nature (London)* **274**:612.

SHOOTER, K. V., AND MERRIFIELD, K., 1976, An assay for phosphotriester formation in the reaction of alkylating agents with deoxyribonucleic acid *in vitro* and *in vivo, Chem. Biol. Interact.* **13**:223.

SHOOTER, K. V., HOUSE, R., SHAH, S. A., AND LAWLEY., P. D., 1974*a*, The molecular basis for biological interaction of nucleic acid: The action of methylating agents on the RNA containing bacterophage R-17, *Biochem. J.* **137**:303.

SHOOTER, K. V., HOUSE, R., AND MERRIFIELD, K., 1974*b*, Biological effects of phosphotriester formation, *Biochem. J.* **137**:313.

SHULL, K. H., 1962, Hepatic phosphorylase and adenosine triphosphate levels in ethionine treated rats, *J. Biol. Chem.* **237**:p.c. 1734.

SHULL, K. H., McCONOMY, J., VOGT, M., CASTILLO, A., AND FARBER, E., 1966, On the mechanism of induction of hepatic adenosine triphosphate deficiency by ethionine, *J. Biol. Chem.* **241**:5060.

SILVERMAN, B., AND MIRSKY, A. E., 1973, Accessibility of DNA in chromatin to DNA polymerase and RNA polymerase, *Proc. Natl. Acad. Sci. USA* **70**:1326.

SIMS, P., AND GROVER, P. L., 1968, Quantitative aspects of the metabolism of 7,12-dimethyl-benz(*a*)anthracene by liver homogenates from animals of different age, sex and species, *Biochem. Pharmacol.* **17**:1751.

SINGER, B., 1975, Chemical effects of nucleic acid alkylation and their relation to mutagenesis and carcinogenesis, *Prog. Nucleic Acid Res. Mol. Biol.* **15**:219.

SINGER, B., 1979, *N*-Nitrosoalkylating agents: Formation and persistence of alkyl derivatives in mammalian nucleic acid as contributing factors in carcinogenesis, *J. Natl. Cancer Inst.* **62**:1329.

SINGER, B., AND BRENT, T. P., 1981, Human lymphoblasts contain DNA glycosylase activity excising N-3 and N-7 methyl and ethyl purines but not O^6-alkylguanines, *Proc. Natl. Acad. Sci. USA* **78**:856.

SINGER, B., AND FRAENKEL-CONRAT, H., 1969, Chemical modification of viral ribonucleic acid. VIII. The chemical and biological effects of methylating agents and nitrosoguanidine on tobacco mosaic virus, *Biochemistry* **8**:3266.

SLAGA, T. J., BRACKEN, W. M., VIAJE, A., LEVIN, W., YAGI, H., JERINA, D. M., AND CONNEY, A. H., 1977, Comparison of the tumor-initiating activities of benzo(α)pyrene-arene-oxides and diol-epoxides, *Cancer Res.* **37**:4130.

SMERDON, M. J., AND LIEBERMAN, M. W., 1978, Nucleosome re-arrangement in human chromatin during UV-induced DNA-repair synthesis, *Proc. Natl. Acad. Sci. USA* **75**:4238.

SMERDON, M. J., KASTAN, M. B., AND LIEBERMAN, M. W., 1979, Distribution of repair-incorporated nucleotides and nucleosome re-arrangement in the chromatin of normal and xeroderma pigmentosum human fibroblasts, *Biochemistry* **18**:3732.

SMITH, G. J., KAUFMAN, D. G., AND GRISHAM, J. W., 1980, Decreased excision of O^6-methylguanine and *N*-7-methylguanine during the S-phase in $10T\frac{1}{2}$ cells, *Biochem. Biophys. Res. Commun.* **92**:787.

SMITH, J. D., AND DUNN, D. B., 1959, The occurrence of methylated guanines in ribonucleic acids from several sources, *Biochem. J.* **72**:294.

SMITH, R. C., AND SALMON, W. D., 1965, Formation of *S*-adenosylethionine by ethionine-treated rats, *Arch. Biochem. Biophys.* **111**:191.

SMUCKLER, E. A., AND KOPLITZ, M., 1969, The effects of carbon tetrachloride and ethionine on RNA synthesis *in vivo* and in isolated rat liver nuclei, *Arch. Biochem. Biophys.* **132**:62.

SMUCKLER, E. A., AND KOPLITZ, M., 1976, Polyadenylic acid content and electrophoretic behavior of *in vitro* released RNA's in chemical carcinogenesis, *Cancer Res.* **36**:881.

SNYDER, A. L., KANN, H. E., JR., AND KOHN, K. W., 1971, Inhibition of the processing of ribosomal precursor RNA by intercalating agents, *J. Mol. Biol.* **5**:555.

SOBELL, H. M., TSAI, C. C., JAIN, S. C., AND GILBERT, S. G., 1977, Visualization of drug nucleic acid interactions at atomic resolution. III. Unifying structural concepts in understanding drug–DNA interactions and their broader implications in understanding protein–DNA interactions, *J. Mol. Biol.* **114**:333.

SOLT, D. B., AND FARBER, E., 1976, A new principle for the sequential analysis of chemical carcinogenesis, including a quantitative assay for initiation in liver, *Nature (London)* **263**:701.

SPORN, M. B., DINGMAN, C. W., PHELPS, H. L., AND WOGAN, G. N., 1966, Aflatoxin B_1: Binding to DNA *in vitro* and alteration of RNA metabolism *in vivo, Science* **151**:1539.

STACEY, K. A., COFF, M., COUSENS, S. F., AND ALEXANDER, P., 1957–1958, The reactions of the "radiomimetic" alkylating agents with macromolecules *in vitro, Ann. N.Y. Acad. Sci.* **68**:682.

STEIN, G., STEIN, J., KLEINSMITH, L., PARK, W., JANSING, R., AND THOMSON, J., 1976, Non-histone chromosomal proteins and histone gene-transcription, *Prog. Nucleic Acid Res. Mol. Biol.* **19**:421.

STEKOL, J. A., 1965, in: *Transmethylation and Methionine Biosynthesis* (S. K. Shapiro and F. Schiewk, eds.), p. 231, University of Chicago Press, Chicago.

STEKOL, J. A., MODY, U., AND PERRY, J., 1960, The incorporation of the carbon of the ethyl group of ethionine into liver nucleic acids and the effect of ethionine feeding on the content of nucleic acids in rat liver, *J. Biol. Chem.* **235**:p.c.54.

STEWART, B. W., AND FARBER, E., 1973, Strand breakage in rat liver DNA and its repair following administration of cyclic nitrosamines, *Cancer Res.* **33**:3209.

STEWART, B. W., AND MAGEE, P. N., 1972, Metabolism and some biochemical effects of *N*-nitrosomorpholine, *Biochem. J.* **126**:21P.

STRAUB, K. M., MEEHAN, T., BURLINGAME, A. L., AND CALVIN, M., 1977, Identification of major adducts formed by reaction of benzo(α)pyrene diol epoxide with DNA *in vitro*, *Proc. Natl. Acad. Sci. USA* **74**:5285.

STUMPF, R., MARGISON, G. P., MONTESANO, R., AND PEGG, A. E., 1979, Formation and loss of alkylated purines from DNA of hamster liver after administration of dimethylnitrosamine, *Cancer Res.* **39**:50.

SUDHAKAR, S., TEW, K. D., SCHEIN, P. S., WOOLLEY, P. V., AND SMULSON, M. E., 1979, Nitrosourea interaction with chomatin and effect on poly(adenosine diphosphate ribose) polymerase activity, *Cancer Res.* **39**:1411.

SUGIMURA, T., OKABE, K., AND NAGAO, M., 1966, The metabolism of 4-nitroquinoline-1-oxide, a carcinogen. III. An enzyme catalyzing the conversion of 4-nitroquinoline-1-oxide to 4-hydroxyaminoquinoline-1-oxide in rat liver and hepatomas, *Cancer Res.* **26**:1717.

SUGIURA, K., TELLER, M. N., PARHAM, J. C., AND BROWN, G. B., 1970, A comparison of the oncogenicities of 3-hydroxyxanthine, guanine-3-*N*-oxide and some related compounds, *Cancer Res.* **30**:184.

SUNDERMAN, F. W. JR., AND ESTAHANI, M., 1968, Nickel carbonyl inhibition of RNA polymerase activity in hepatic nuclei, *Cancer Res.* **28**:2565.

SVOBODA, D., AND REDDY, J., 1970, Invasive tumors induced in rats with actinomycin D., *Cancer Res.* **30**:2271.

SWAIN, C. G., AND SCOTT, C. B., 1953, Quantitative correlation of relative rates. Comparison of hydroxide ion with other nucleophilic reagents toward alkyl halides, esters, epoxides and acyl halides, *J. Am. Chem. Soc.* **75**:141.

SWANN, P. F., AND MAGEE, P. N., 1968, Nitrosamine induced carcinogenesis: The alkylation of nucleic acids of the rat by *N*-methyl-*N*-nitrosourea, dimethylnitrosamine, dimethylsulfate and methylmethanesulphonate, *Biochem. J.* **110**:39.

SWANN, P. F., AND MAGEE, P. N., 1971, The alkylation of N-7 of guanine of nucleic acids of the rat by dimethylnitrosamine, *N*-ethyl-nitrosourea and ethylmethanesulphonate, *Biochem. J.* **125**:841.

SWANN, P. F., PEGG, A. E., HAWKS, A., FARBER, E., AND MAGEE, P. N., 1971, Evidence for ethylation of rat liver deoxyribonucleic acid after administration of ethionine, *Biochem. J.* **123**:175.

SWENBERG, J. A., COOPER, H. K., BUECHLER, J., AND KLEIHUES, P., 1979, 1,2-Dimethylhydrazine induced methylation of DNA bases in various rat organs and the effect of pretreatment with disulfiram, *Cancer Res.* **39**:465.

SWENSON, D. H., AND LAWLEY, P. D., 1978, Alkylation of deoxyribonucleic acid by carcinogens dimethylsulphate, ethylmethanesulphonate, *N*-ethyl-*N*-nitrosourea and *N*-methyl-*N*-nitrosourea: Relative reactivity of the phosphodiester site thymidylyl (3′–5′) thymidine, *Biochem. J.* **171**:575.

SWENSON, D. H., MILLER, J. A., AND MILLER, E. C., 1973, 2,3-Dihydro-2,3-dihydroxy-aflatoxin B₁: An acid hydrolysis product of an RNA–aflatoxin B₁ adduct formed by hamster and rat liver microsomes *in vitro*, *Biochem. Biophys. Res. Commun.* **53**:1260.

SZAFARZ, D., AND WEISBURGER, J. H., 1969, Stability of binding of label from *N*-hydroxy-*N*-2-fluorenylacetamide to intraceullar targets, particularly deoxyribonucleic acid in rat, *Cancer Res.* **29**:962.

TADA, M., AND TADA, M., 1971, Interaction of a carcinogen, 4-nitroquinoline-1-oxide, with nucleic acids: Chemical degradation of the adducts, *Chem. Biol. Interact.* **3**:225.

TADA, M., AND TADA, M., 1972, Enzymatic activation of the carcinogen 4-hydroxyaminoquinoline-1-oxide and its interaction with cellular macromolecules, *Biochem. Biophys. Res. Commun.* **46**:1025.

TADA, M., AND TADA, M., 1976, Main binding sites of the carcinogen 4-nitroquinoline-1-oxide in nucleic acids, *Biochim. Biophys. Acta* **454**:558.

407

INTERAC-
TIONS OF
CARCINOGENS
WITH NUCLEIC
ACIDS

TADA, M., TADA, M., AND TAKAHASHI, T., 1967, Interaction of a carcinogen, 4-hydroxyaminoquino-line-1-oxide, with nucleic acids, Biochem. Biophys. Res. Commun. 29:469.

TEEBOR, G. W., AND DUKER, N. J., 1975, Different ultraviolet DNA endonuclease activity in human cells, Nature (London) 255:82.

TEW, K. D., SUDHAKAR, S., SCHEIN, P. S., AND SMULSON, M. E., 1978, Binding of chlorozotocin and 1-(2-chloroethyl)-3-cyclohexyl-1-nitrosourea to chromatin and nucleosomal fraction of HeLa-cells, Cancer Res. 38:3371.

TEW, K. D., SCHEIN, P., SASLAW, L. D., AND SMULSON, M. E., 1979, Steroid chromatin interactions modify nuclear alkylation by nitrosoureas, Proc. Am. Assoc. Cancer Res. 20:191.

THEISS, J. C., AND SHIMKIN, M. B., 1978, Inhibiting effect of caffeine on spontaneous and urethan-induced lung tumors in strain A mice, Cancer Res. 38:1757.

TLSTY, T. D., AND LIEBERMAN, M. W., 1978, The distribution of DNA repair synthesis in chromatin and its re-arrangement following damage with N-acetoxy-2-acetylaminofluorene, Nucleic Acids Res. 5:3261.

TODARO, G. J., AND GREEN, H., 1966, Cell growth and the initiation of transformation by SV40, Proc. Natl. Acad. Sci. USA 55:302.

TOULMÉ, F., HÉLÈNE, C., FUCHS, R. P. P., AND DAUNE, M., 1980, Binding of a tryptophan-containing peptide (lysyltryptophyllysine) to deoxy-ribonucleic acid modified by 2-(N-acetoxy acetyl-amino)fluorene, Biochemistry 19:870.

TROLL, W., BELMAN, S., BERKOWITZ, E., CHMIELEWICZ, Z. F., AMBRUS, J. L., AND BARDOS, T. J., 1968, Differential responses of DNA and RNA polymerase to modifications of the template rat liver DNA caused by action of the carcinogen acetylaminofluorene in vivo and in vitro, Biochim. Biophys. Acta 157:16.

TROSKO, J. E., FRANK, P., CHU, E. H. Y., AND BECKER, J. E., 1973, Caffeine inhibition of postreplication repair of N-acetoxy-2-acetylaminofluorene damaged DNA in Chinese hamster cells, Cancer Res. 33:2444.

TS'O P. O. P., LESKO, S. A., AND UMANS, R. S., 1969, The physical binding and the chemical linkage of benzopyrene to nucleotides, nucleic acids and nucleohistones, in: Physico-chemical Mechanisms of Carcinogenesis, The Jerusalem Symposia on Quantum Chemistry and Biochemistry, Vol. 1 (E. D. Bergmann and B. Pullman, eds.), p. 106, The Israel Academy of Science and Humanities, Jerusalem.

TSUDA, H., SARMA, D. S. R., RAJALAKSHMI. S., ZUBROFF, J., FARBER, E., BATZINGER, R. P., NAM CHA, Y., AND BUEDING, E., 1979, Induction of hepatic neoplastic lesions in mice with a single dose of hycanthone methanesulfonate after partial hepatectomy, Cancer Res. 39:4491.

UHLENHOPP, E. L., AND KRASNA, A. I., 1971, Alterations in the structure of deoxyribonucleic acid on chemical methylation, Biochemistry 10:3290.

VAN DUUREN, B. L., GOLDSCHMIDT, B. M., AND SELTZMAN, H. H., 1968–1969, The interaction of mutagenic and carcinogenic agents with nucleic acids, Ann. N.Y. Acad. Sci. 153:744.

VAN LANCKER, J. L., AND TOMURA, T., 1974, Purification and some properties of a mammalian repair endonuclease, Biochim. Biophys. Acta 353:99.

VELEMINSKY, J., OSTERMAN GOLKAR, S., AND EHRENBERG, L., 1970, Reaction rates and biological action of N-methyl and N-ethylnitrosourea, Mutat. Res. 10:169.

VENITT, S., BROOKES, P., AND LAWLEY, P. D., 1968, Effects of alkylating agents on the induced synthesis of β-galactosidase by Escherichia coli B$_{s-1}$, Biochim. Biophys. Acta 155:521.

VERLY, W. G., GOSSARD, F., AND CRINE, P., 1974, In vitro repair of apurinic sites in DNA, Proc. Natl. Acad. Sci. USA 71:2273.

VILLANI, G., BOITEUX, S., AND RADMAN, M., 1978, Mechanism of ultraviolet-induced mutagenesis: Extent and fidelity of in vitro DNA synthesis on irradiated templates, Proc. Natl. Acad. Sci. USA 75:3037.

VILLA-TREVINO, S., SHULL, K. H., AND FARBER, E., 1963, The role of adenosine triphosphate deficiency in ethionine-induced inhibition of protein synthesis, J. Biol. Chem. 238:1757.

VILLA-TREVINO, S., SHULL, K. H., AND FARBER, E., 1966, The inhibition of liver ribonucleic acid synthesis by ethionine, J. Biol. Chem. 241:4670.

WAGNER, L., AND DREWS, J., 1970, The effect of aflatoxin B$_1$ on RNA synthesis and breakdown in normal and regenerating rat liver, Eur. J. Cancer 6:465.

WAGNER, T. A., 1971, Physical studies on the interaction of lysergic acid diethylamide and trypano-cidal dyes with DNA and DNA-containing genetic material, in: Progress in Molecular and Subceulluar Biology, Vol. 2 (F. E. Hahn, ed.) p. 152, Springer-Verlag, New York.

WALKER, I. G., AND EWART, D. F., 1973, The nature of single-strand breaks in DNA following treatment of L-cells with methylating agents, *Mutat. Res.* **19**:331.

WALKER, M. S., BECKER, F. F., AND RODRIGUEZ, L. V., 1979, *In vivo* binding of N-2-acetyl-aminofluorene and its N-hydroxy-derivative to the DNA of fractionated rat liver chromatin, *Chem. Biol. Interact.* **27**:177.

WALPOLE, A. L., ROBERTS, D. C., ROSE, F. L., HENDRY, J. A., AND HOMES, R. F., 1954, Cytotoxic agents. IV. The carcinogenic actions of some monofunctional ethyleneimine derivatives, *Br. J. Pharmacol. Chemother.* **9**:306.

WANG, A. H. J., QUIGLEY, G. J., KOLPAK, F., CRAWFORD, J. L., VAN-BOOM, J. H., VANDER MARCEL, G. AND RICH, A., 1979, Molecular structure of a left handed double helical DNA fragment at atomic resolution, *Nature (London)* **282**:680.

WANG, T. Y., KOSTRABA, N. C., AND NEWMAN, R. S., 1976, Selective transcription of DNA mediated by non-histone proteins, *Prog. Nucleic Acid Res. Mol. Biol.* **19**:447.

WARWICK, G. P., 1967, The covalent binding of metabolites of tritiated 2-methyl-4-dimethyl-aminoazobenzene to rat liver nucleic acids and proteins and the carcinogenicity of the unlabelled compound in partially hepatectomised rats, *Eur. J. Cancer* **3**:227.

WARWICK, G. P., 1969, The covalent binding of metabolites of 4-dimethylaminoazobenzene to liver nucleic acids *in vivo*. The possible role of cell proliferation in cancer initiation, in: *Physico-chemical Mechanisms of Carcinogenesis*, The Jerusalem Symposia on Quantum Chemistry and Biochemistry, Vol. 1 (E. D. Bergmann and B. Pullman, eds.), p. 218, The Israel Academy of Science and Humanities, Jerusalem.

WARWICK, G. P., AND ROBERTS, J. J., 1967, Persistent binding of butter yellow metabolites to rat liver DNA, *Nature (London)* **213**:1206.

WEEKS, C. E., ALLABER, W. T., LOUIE, S. C., LAZEAR, E. J., AND KING, C. M., 1978, Role of aryl-hydroxamic acid acyltransferase in the mutagenicity of N-hydroxy-N-2-fluorenylacetamide in *Salmonella typhimurium*, *Cancer Res.* **38**:613.

WEINSTEIN, I. B., 1970, Modifications in transfer RNA during chemical carcinogenesis, in: *Genetic Concepts and Neoplasia*, p. 380, Williams & Wilkins, Baltimore.

WEINSTEIN, I. B., AND HIRSCHBERG, E., 1971, Mode of action of miracil D, in: *Progress in Molecular and Subcellular Biology*, Vol. 2 (F. E. Hahn, ed.), p. 232, Springer-Verlag, New York.

WEINSTEIN, I. B., GRUNBERGER, D., FUJIMURA, S., AND FINK, L. M., 1971, Chemical carcinogens and RNA, *Cancer Res.* **31**:651.

WEINTRAUB, H., AND GROUDINE, M., 1976, Transcriptionally active and inactive conformation of chromosomal subunits, *Science* **193**:848.

WEISBURGER, J. H., AND WEISBURGER, E. K., 1973, Biochemical formation and pharmacological, toxicological and pathological properties of hydroxylamines and hydroxamic acids, *Pharmacol. Rev.* **25**:1.

WEISBURGER, J. H., YAMAMOTO, R. S., WILLIAMS, G. M., GRANTHAM, P. H., MATSUSHIMA, T., AND WEISBURGER, E. K., 1972, On the sulphate ester of N-hydroxy-N-2-fluorenylacetamide as a key ultimate hepatocarcinogen in the rat, *Cancer Res.* **32**:491.

WELLS, R. D., 1971, The binding of actinomycin D to DNA, in: *Progress in Molecular and Subcellular Biology*, Vol. 2 (F. E. Hahn, ed.), p. 21, Springer-Verlag, New York.

WELLS, R. D., AND LARSON, J. E., 1970, Studies on the binding of actinomycin-D to DNA and DNA model polymers, *J. Mol. Biol.* **49**:319.

WESTRA, J. G., KRIEK, E., AND HITTEN HOUSEN, H., 1976, Identification of the persistently bound carcinogen N-acetyl-2-aminofluorene to rat liver DNA *in vivo*, *Chem. Biol. Interact.* **15**:149.

WIEBEL, F. J., MATTHEWS, E. G., AND GELBOIN, H. V., 1972, Ribonucleic acid synthesis-dependent induction of aryl hydrocarbon hydroxylase in the absence of ribosomal ribonucleic acid synthesis and transfer, *J. Biol. Chem.* **242**:4711.

WILK, W., AND GIRKE, W., 1969, Radical action of carcinogenesis alternant hydrocarbons, amines, and azo-dyes and their reactions with nucleobases, in: *Physico-Chemical Mechanisms of Carcinogenesis*, The Jerusalem Symposia on Quantum Chemistry and Biochemistry, Vol. 1 (E. D. Bergmann and B. Pullman, eds.), p. 91, The Israel Academy of Science and Humanities, Jerusalem.

WILKINS, R. J., AND HART, R. W., 1974, Preferential DNA repair in human cells, *Nature (London)* **247**:35.

WILKINSON, R., HAWKS, A., AND PEGG, A. E., 1975, Methylation of rat liver mitochondrial deoxyribonucleic acid by chemical carcinogens and associated alterations in physical properties, *Chem. Biol. Interact.* **10**:157.

Williams, J. I., and Friedberg, E. C., 1979, Deoxyribonucleic acid excision repair in chromatin after ultraviolet irradiation of human fibroblasts in culture, *Biochemistry* **18**:3965.

Williams, K., and Nery, R., 1971, Aspects of the mechanism of urethane carcinogenesis, *Xenobiotica* **1**:545.

Wislocki, P. G., Borchert, P., Miller, E. C., and Miller, J. A., 1973, Further studies on the metabolism and carcinogenicity of safrole, *Proc. Am. Assoc. Cancer Res.* **14**:19.

Witkin, E. M., 1976, Ultraviolet mutagenesis and inducible DNA repair in *Escherichia coli, Bacteriol. Rev.* **40**:869.

Wu, Y. S., and Smuckler, E. A., 1971, The acute effect of aminoazobenzene and some of its derivatives on RNA polymerase activity in isolated rat liver nuclei, *Cancer Res.* **31**:239.

Wunderlich, V., Schütt, M., Böttger, M., and Graffi, A., 1970, Preferential alkylation of mitochondrial deoxyribonucleic acid by *N*-methyl-*N*-nitrosourea, *Biochem. J.* **118**:99.

Wunderlich, V., Tezlaff, I., and Graffi, A., 1971–1972, Studies on nitrosodimethylanamine: Preferential methylation of mitochondrial DNA in rats and hamsters, *Chem. Biol. Interact.* **4**:81.

Yamasaki, H., Leffler, S., and Weinstein, I. B., 1977*a*, Effects of *N*-2-acetylaminofluorene modification on the structure and template activity of DNA and reconstituted chromatin, *Cancer Res.* **37**:684.

Yamasaki, H., Pulkrabek, P. G., Grunburger, D., and Weinstein, I. B., 1977*b*, Differential excision from DNA of the C-8 and N^2-guanosine adducts of *N*-acetyl-2-aminofluorene by single strand specific endonucleases, *Cancer Res.* **37**:3756.

Yamasaki, H., Roush, T. W., and Weinstein, I. B., 1978, Benzo(*a*)pyrene-7,8-dihydrodiol-9,10-oxide modification of DNA: Relation to chromatin structure and reconstitution, *Chem. Biol. Interact.* **23**:201.

Yamaura, I., Marquardt, H., and Cavalieri, L. F., 1978, Effects of benzo(α)pyrene adducts on DNA synthesis *in vitro, Chem. Biol. Interact.* **23**:399.

Yang, J. T., and Samejima, T., 1969, Optical rotatory dispersion and circular dichroism of nucleic acids, *Prog. Nucleic Acid Res. Mol. Biol.* **9**:224.

Ying, T. S., 1980, Studies on acute cell injury, cell replication and DNA repair during the initiation of liver carcinogenesis, Ph.D. thesis, University of Toronto.

Ying, T. S., and Sarma, D. S. R., 1979, Role of liver cell necrosis in the induction of preneoplastic lesions, *Proc. Am. Assoc. Cancer Res.* **20**:14.

Ying, T. S., Sarma, D. S. R., and Farber, E., 1979, Induction of presumptive preneoplastic lesions in rat liver by a single dose of 1,2-dimethylhydrazine, *Chem. Biol. Interact.* **28**:363.

Yoshida, M., and Holoubek, V., 1976, Early effects of carcinogenic amino dyes on the protein patterns and metabolism in rat liver, *Int. J. Biochem.* **7**:259.

Younger, L. R., Salomon, R., Wilson, R. W., Peacock, A. C., and Gelboin, H. V., 1972, Effects of polycyclic hydrocarbons on ribonucleic acid synthesis in rat liver nuclei and hamster embryo cells, *Mol. Pharmacol.* **8**:452.

Youvan, D. C., and Hearst, J. E., 1979, Reverse transcriptase pauses at N^2-methylguanine during *in vitro* transcription of *Escherichia coli* 16S ribosomal RNA, *Proc. Natl. Acad. Sci. USA* **76**:3751.

Yuspa, S. H., and Bates, R. R., 1970, The binding of benzo(*a*)anthracene to replicating and non-replicating DNA in cell culture, *Proc. Soc. Exp. Biol. Med.* **135**:732.

Zahner, A. J., 1976, Possible role of DNA replication in chemical carcinogenesis: An investigation of the *in vivo* replication of rat liver DNA arylated by the hepatocarcinogen *N*-hydroxy-2-acetylaminofluorene, Ph.D. thesis, Temple University.

Zahner, A. J., Rajalakshmi, S., and Sarma, D. S. R., 1977, Isolation of *in vivo* replicated rat liver DNA containing *N*-OH-2-AAF metabolites(s), *Proc. Am. Assoc. Cancer Res.* **18**:99.

Zajdela, F., and Latarjet, R., 1973, Effect inhibiteur de la cafeine sur l'induction de cancers cutanes par les rayons ultraviolets chez la souris, *C. R. Acad. Sci. Ser. D* **277**:1073.

Zedek, M. S., Steinberg, S. S., Poynter, R. N., and McGowan, J., 1970, Biochemical and pathological effects of methylazoxymethanolacetate, a potent carcinogen, *Cancer Res.* **30**:801.

Zeiger, R. S., Salomon, R., Kinoshita, N., and Peacock, A. C., 1972, The binding of 9,10-dimethyl-1,2-benzanthracene to mouse epidermal satellite DNA *in vivo, Cancer Res.* **32**;643.

Zieve, F. J., 1972, Inhibition of rat liver ribonucleic acid polymerase by the carcinogen *N*-hydroxy-2-fluorenylacetamide, *J. Biol. Chem.* **247**:5987.

Zieve, F. J., 1973, Effects of the carcinogen *N*-acetoxy-2-fluorenylacetamide on the template properties of deoxyribonucleic acid, *Mol. Pharmacol.* **9**:658.

Zimmer, C., 1975, Effect of antibiotics netropsin and distamycin A on the structure and function of nucleic acids, *Prog. Nucleic Acid Res. Mol. Biol.* **15**:285.

409

INTERAC-
TIONS OF
CARCINOGENS
WITH NUCLEIC
ACIDS

11

Some Effects of Carcinogens on Cell Organelles

DONALD J. SVOBODA AND JANARDAN K. REDDY

1. Introduction

In the first edition of this chapter, several acute and chronic effects of selected hepatocarcinogens on the histology and ultrastructure of rodent liver cells were reviewed briefly. That review covered the period from the emergence of the application of ultrastructural studies to the problem of carcinogenesis in the early 1960s through publications available in 1972. The purpose of this chapter is to present several observations regarding effects of carcinogens on cell ultrastructure that have been published from 1972 through 1979 and to update our present knowledge in this area by relating the more recent publications to those discussed previously.

Since most available reports deal with effects of commonly used chemical carcinogens on rodent liver cells *in vivo*, these effects comprise the major portion of this chapter. A brief section summarizing recent reports on the carcinogenicity of hypolipidemic drugs that also cause proliferation of hepatic peroxisomes has been added. A brief introduction to selected site-specific models of chemical carcinogenesis (other than liver) that have been developed in recent years has also been added.

DONALD J. SVOBODA ● Department of Pathology and Oncology, University of Kansas College of Health Sciences, Kansas City, Kansas.
JANARDAN K. REDDY ● Department of Pathology, Northwestern University Medical School, Chicago, Illinois.

While it is still generally true that no specific ultrastructural features are characteristic or consistent markers of neoplastic cells, observation of modulations, cytological adaptation, and abnormalities in the ultrastructure, number, or distribution of cell organelles may be useful in selecting other experimental approaches to study malignant transformation of cells. Also, study of the effects of chemical carcinogens on cell organelles permits a comparison of similarities and possible differences between effects of carcinogens and other forms of cell injury.

1.1. A Brief Review of Acute and Chronic Cytological Effects of Some Common Hepatocarcinogens

The carcinogens to be considered in this section include the aflatoxins, diethylnitrosamine (DEN), dimethylnitrosamine (DMN), ethionine, pyrrolizidine, alkaloids (notably lasiocarpine), 3'-methyl-4-dimethylaminoazobenzene (3'-Me-DAB), tannic acid, and thioacetamide.

The doses, routes, intervals of sacrifice, and resulting acute and chronic light and electron microscopic changes in rat liver induced by these carcinogens have been reviewed systematically in a previous publication, and the reader seeking greater detail regarding these changes and their interpretation is referred to that publication (Svoboda and Higginson, 1968). For convenience, the acute and chronic responses in rat liver cells due to these carcinogens are summarized briefly.

The acute histological changes included nuclear enlargement with DMN and thioacetamide and an increase in the number of nucleoli with thioacetamide. Decreased basophilia of centrilobular parenchymal cells and of the periportal zone followed administration of tannic acid and aflatoxin B_1, respectively, while thioacetamide and DEN induced increased acidophilia. Lysosomes were conspicuous after lasiocarpine, and 3'-Me-DAB caused cytoplasmic swelling. Most of the carcinogens, in the doses administered, caused slight to moderate necrosis and variable degrees of inflammatory infiltrate.

Regarding acute ultrastructural effects, all carcinogens caused an increase in the smooth endoplasmic reticulum (SER) and detachment of ribosomes from the rough endoplasmic reticulum (RER), resulting in an increased number of free ribosomes in the cytoplasm (Fig. 1). Similarly, all carcinogens caused a zonal or diffuse decrease in glycogen and a variable increase in cytoplasmic fat. Lysosomes were increased in number slightly with all carcinogens. Mitochondrial swelling was present to a variable degree with all carcinogens; with thioacetamide and aflatoxin B_1, there are dense matrix granules resembling calcium in some cells. The most uniform ultrastructural changes in the nucleus consisted of redistribution or rearrangement and/or quantitative differences in the fibrillar and granular components of the nucleus. The term "macrosegregation" (also called "nucleolar capping") indicates separation of granules and fibrils in large, distinct, and relatively pure zones. It was most characteristic with aflatoxin B_1, lasiocarpine, 3'-Me-DAB, and tannic acid (Fig. 2). In such instances, the nucleolar

413
SOME
EFFECTS OF
CARCINOGENS
ON CELL
ORGANELLES

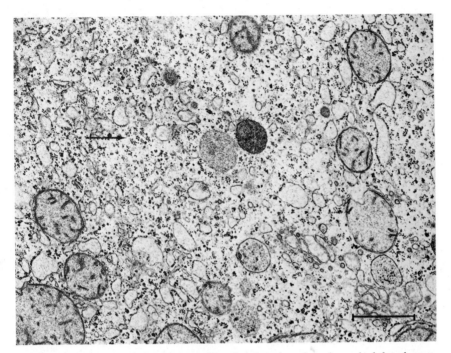

FIGURE 1. Two hours following lasiocarpine administration, there is marked detachment of ribosomes from membranes of the ER and numerous free ribosomes are present in the cytoplasm. ×15,000.

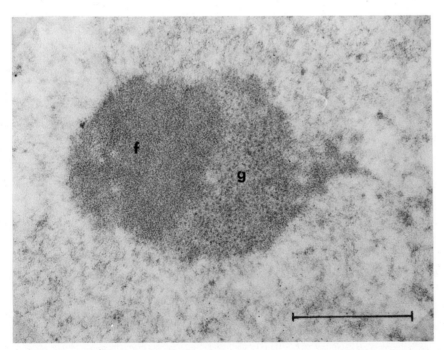

FIGURE 2. 3′-Methyldimethylaminoazobenzene, 24 h. There is distinct separation of the fibrillar (f) portion of the nucleolus from the granular (g) area, resulting in macro-segregation. ×33,000.

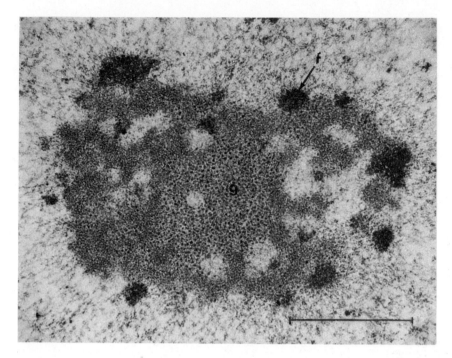

FIGURE 3. Dimethylnitrosamine, 36 h. The fibrillar (f) portion of the nucleolus is irregularly separated from the granular (g) portion and forms numerous condensations most prominent at the periphery of the nucleolus. This change is termed "microsegregation." ×33,000.

diameter was usually greater than normal. "Microsegregation," by comparison, is used to designate definite, compact condensations of the fibrillar component of the nucleolus. Condensations are multiple, irregular in size and shape, smaller and less pure than in macrosegregation and tend to occur as plaquelike configurations within or at the periphery of the dispersed nucleolus (Fig. 3). Microsegregation was conspicuous with DMN (6 days) and lasiocarpine at 1 h, after which macrosegregation was more evident. It was present in some cells 18 h after administration of tannic acid. It is evident that the terms "macrosegregation" and "microsegregation" do not necessarily imply functional differences nor need they be mutually exclusive after administration of a single carcinogen. To date, no noncarcinogenic agent has been shown to induce nucleolar segregation. Simple nucleolar enlargement, consisting principally of an increase in the granular component, was most evident after thioacetamide and, to a lesser extent, after ethionine.

In chronic studies, most of the carcinogens listed earlier caused alterations either in the proportion or configuration of nucleolar constituents. There was an increase in interchromatin and perichromatin granules with ethionine and enlargement of interchromatinic spaces with thioacetamide. The most consistent cytoplasmic changes were increased SER and detachment of ribosomes from ergastoplasmic membranes, changes that appeared to persist from the acute intervals. DMN caused a marked enlargement of mitochondria and bizarre-shaped profiles with a decrease in length and number of cristae. Golgi areas were often dilated but with empty vesicles and vacuoles. The number of lysosomes were increased slightly with all carcinogens.

415

SOME
EFFECTS OF
CARCINOGENS
ON CELL
ORGANELLES

None of these carcinogens caused specific changes in either acute or chronic stages that were sufficiently characteristic to identify the carcinogen by the alterations it caused.

2. The Carcinogens

In this section, some of the earlier literature dealing with specified carcinogens has been retained and more recent morphological observations have been incorporated. Much of the recent literature dealing with purely biochemical effects of these carcinogens has been omitted.

2.1. Aflatoxins

Among the first observations regarding abnormality of function of rat liver cells after treatment *in vivo* and *in vitro* with aflatoxin B_1 was early inhibition of RNA synthesis (Sporn *et al.*, 1966; Clifford and Rees, 1966). The early electron microscopic changes due to aflatoxin B_1 were macrosegregation of the nucleolus and an increase in interchromatin granules (Bernhard *et al.*, 1965; Butler, 1966; Svoboda and Higginson, 1968). In chronic experiments there was microsegregation of the nucleus. Detachment of ribosomes was conspicuous in both acute and chronic experiments.

By light microscopy, aflatoxin B_1 was associated, in chronic experiments, with the appearance of small foci of hyperbasophilic cells as well as aggregates of large pale cells lacking glycogen. Newberne and Wogan (1968) suggested that the basophilic cells progressed to poorly differentiated carcinomas while the large, pale, eosinophilic cells developed into well-differentiated carcinomas. The appearance of nontumor areas of rat liver bearing aflatoxin B_1-induced hepatomas is unusual in that it is not cirrhotic nor does it show cholangiofibrosis, or proliferation of bile ducts or oval cells.

In the rhesus monkey, Svoboda *et al.* (1966) noted macrosegregation of the nucleolus 48 h after a dose of 2.6 mg/kg body wt of pure aflatoxin B_1. The histological changes in livers of rhesus monkeys given 2.6 mg/kg of pure aflatoxin B_1 did not show periportal necrosis, in contrast to rats and ducklings. Instead, there was focal necrosis with sparse inflammatory infiltrate, individual cell necrosis, and eosinophilic Councilman bodies, the entire spectrum bearing some resemblance to acute viral hepatitis in humans.

In recent years, the aflatoxins as a group, and aflatoxin B_1 in particular, have assumed greater importance as potential, if not actual, injurious agents in humans. Their potential for acute and chronic injury to humans has been delineated from epidemiological, agricultural, and experimental observations. Shank (1976) and Linsell and Peers (1977) have recently reviewed the possible role of aflatoxins in liver cancer and other diseases in humans. Studies by Van Rensburg *et al.* (1974) showed that the highest rate of primary liver cancer in humans coincides geographically with the highest measured aflatoxin intake. Similarly, a study by Peers *et al.* (1976) showed a significant correlation between the calculated ingested daily dose of aflatoxins and the adult male incidence of primary liver cancer in different parts of Swaziland. Consumption of corn heavily contaminated with *Aspergillus flavus* was associated with hepatitis in western India (Krishnamachari *et al.*, 1975). Campbell *et al.* (1974) found that an extract of urine specimens (2-day collection period) from humans known to have consumed an average of 21 g of aflatoxin B_1 (via a diet of trout for a period of only 30 days) contained a potent hepatocarcinogen.

There have been several reports of aflatoxin contamination in a variety of foods in the United States (Fuller *et al.*, 1977; Scott and Kennedy, 1975; Wilson and Flowers, 1978). Although it was originally believed that growth of *A. flavus* and elaboration of aflatoxins were due primarily to poor storage of cereal grains, especially in developing countries, it is now known that in several parts of the United States, contamination of cereal grains occurred while still in the field prior to harvest or shortly after, indicating that aflatoxins may be a more serious hazard in the United States than suspected previously (Tuite and Caldwell, 1971; Anderson *et al.*, 1975), Lillehoj *et al.*, 1975*a,b*, 1976).

Aflatoxin M has been found in milk samples (Purchase and Vorster, 1968; Suzangar *et al.*, 1977) and has been reported to be approximately as toxic as aflatoxin B_1. Given subcutaneously, aflotoxin M caused subcutaneous tumors in two rats at 60 and 80 weeks, suggesting that it is carcinogenic (Purchase and Vorster, 1968). Although synthetic aflatoxin M_1 causes electron microscopic changes in rat liver similar to those due to aflatoxin B_1 and appears to be equal to B_1 in potency as measured by acute toxicity, M_1 is a much less potent hepatocarcinogen than B_1 (Wogan and Paglialunga, 1974).

In the jejunum and ileum of hamsters, a mixture of aflatoxins intraperitoneally caused reduction in mucosal thickness and villous atrophy as well as periportal megalocytosis in the liver and enlargement of renal proximal tubular epithelial cells (Herrold, 1969). Pong and Wogan (1970) showed that after administration of aflatoxin B_1 to rats, maximal inhibition of RNA polymerase activity (60%) occurred at 15 min but returned to normal by 36 h while the most extensive nucleolar structural changes did not occur until 1 h, indicating that macrosegregation is not a prerequisite for maximum enzyme inhibition.

Noyes (1975) reported that exposure of organ cultures of adult human liver cells (maintained for 5 weeks) to aflatoxin B_1, at a concentration of 0.01 g/liter, resulted in changes in morphology of parenchymal cells consisting of cells with enlarged, pale, eosinophilic cytoplasm similar to hepatic parenchymal cells of rats fed a diet containing aflatoxin as described by Newberne and Wogan (1968).

Liver tumors were induced in 2 of 22 male Fischer rats given 1 ppb of aflatoxin B_1, suggesting that, under experimental conditions, the sensitivity of the Fischer rat to hepatic carcinogenesis is approximately the same as that previously reported for rainbow trout (Wogan *et al.*, 1974). *Butler et al.* (1969) reported that of 26 rats that received a total of 6 mg of aflatoxin G_1, 21 developed liver tumors and 6 developed kidney tumors, the latter occurring only in males. The liver tumors were trabecular, adenomatous, or anaplastic. Cirrhosis was not present in nonmalignant areas of liver. Although aflatoxin B_2 did not induce carcinomas, atypical hyperplastic hepatic nodules were seen in rats that received this agent. Aflatoxin B_2 may be a less potent hepatocarcinogen than B_1; the data from these experiments are inconclusive.

417

SOME
EFFECTS OF
CARCINOGENS
ON CELL
ORGANELLES

In a study of acute toxicity of aflatoxin G_1 in the rat (Butler and Lijinsky, 1970), a common change in liver cells was diffuse cell necrosis, especially periportal, at 2–3 days. The most consistent hepatic change was early (2 days) proliferation of oval cells and bile duct epithelium in all portal tracts. This proliferation reached a maximum by 7 days when about one-fourth of the lobule was involved. In severely affected animals, hyperplastic nodules and areas of cholangiofibrosis were present. In the adrenal, there was extensive hemorrhagic necrosis of the zona reticularis and part of the zona fasciculata. By 3–4 weeks, the hemorrhagic zone was replaced by a narrow band of fibrous tissue and hemosiderin pigment. One of the most consistent lesions induced in the kidney by aflatoxin G_1 was massive necrosis of proximal tubules of the inner cortex. The epithelium regenerated so that by 3–4 weeks, the only evidence of damage was the presence of epithelial cells with large, bizarre nuclei. The authors concluded that aflatoxin B_1 is predominantly hepatotoxic while G_1 consistently affects kidney and adrenal and less consistently the liver. Whether this is a result of differing metabolism, solubility, or distribution of the toxins is not known. Examination of the interaction of aflatoxins B_1 and G_1 with nucleic acids and proteins of liver and kidney did not reveal differences to explain variations in acute toxicity.

Kim et al. (1972) showed that aflatoxin G_1, given at approximately threefold the dose of B_1, also caused nucleolar segregation in rat liver. The cytoplasmic changes were similar to those caused by B_1.

Using the Ames test to study the mutagenicity of several aflatoxins, Wong and Hsieh (1976) found the order of mutagenic potency to be aflatoxin B_1 > aflatoxicol > aflatoxins G_1 and M_1 > aflatoxicol H_1 and aflatoxins Q_1, B_2, P_1, G_2, B_{2a}, and G_{2a}. All required metabolic activation by addition of a preparation of rat liver.

In young marmosets (Saquinus oedipomidas) given 2 ppm of aflatoxin B_1 in the diet for 7–11 weeks, the most conspicuous change was giant cell transformation of hepatic parenchymal cells with many large, multinucleate cells extending from the portal tracts (Svoboda et al., 1971b). In another study, among 24 marmosets of both sexes, 2 males and 1 female developed trabecular hepatomas between 50 and 87 weeks after a cumulative dose of aflatoxin B_1 ranging from 3 to 5 g (Lin et al., 1974). The chronic ultrastructural changes in marmoset liver were similar to those reported in rat liver cells. The degree of hepatic injury was parallel to the cumulative dose of aflatoxin B_1, and males appeared to be more sensitive. A cholangiocarcinoma in a female rhesus monkey that had been given a mixture of aflatoxins B_1, G_1, and G_2 for 5 years was reported by Tilak (1975). Liver tumors have also been produced in a lower nonhuman primate, the tree shrew (Tupaia glis) (Reddy et al., 1976c). Of 12 animals that survived the experiment, all 6 females and 3 males developed hepatocellular carcinomas between 74 and 172 weeks after a total dose of aflatoxin ranging from 24 to 66 mg. Of these 9, the tumors of 2 animals were associated with severe post-necrotic scarring, while in the other 7 animals there was only mild to moderate portal fibrosis. Unlike the situation in rhesus monkeys in which liver damage appeared proportional to the dose of aflatoxin B_1, in shrews there was considerable variation in the degree of liver damage among the animals; in many instances, animals that received a relatively low dose showed considerably more hepatic injury than those that received a cumulatively higher dose and vice versa. Individual variation in hepatocellular responses to aflatoxin in this outbred species suggests caution in proposing permissible levels of aflatoxin contamination in human foodstuffs.

Though mice originally appeared to be relatively refractory to carcinogenic effects of aflatoxin B_1, Vesselinovitch *et al.* (1972) found that 89–100% of C57BL× C3H male mice given aflatoxin B_1 by intraperitoneal injection during infancy had hepatomas, often multiple. Females were free of tumors at 82 weeks. The study concluded that infancy and male sex renders mice susceptible to aflatoxin B_1 hepatocarcinogenicity. A variety of malignancies in Swiss mice given a mixture of aflatoxins B and G subcutaneously, by force feeding, or by aerosol was reported by Louria *et al.* (1974). Those given aflatoxins by the subcutaneous route developed local sarcomas, while those given the toxin by any route showed an incidence of lymphatic leukemia significantly greater than in age-matched controls.

Aflatoxin was given at a dose of 2 ppm to fish (*Brachydanio rero*) and to a freshwater snail (*Planorbarus carneus*) (Bauer *et al.*, 1972). In fish liver and in epithelium of snail tentacles, the principal changes were macrosegregation of nucleoli but with no loss of ribosomes from ER membranes. One peculiar and possibly specific change occurring in fish liver was the appearance of 360- to 400-Å granules in clusters within the fibrillar zone of the nucleolus. These have not been observed with other agents and their identity is uncertain. No neoplasms were found after 9 months, suggesting that in these species, nucleolar changes are not necessarily related to carcinogenesis.

While most attention to aflatoxin effects have been given to the liver, significant pancreatic changes have been reported in rats given aflatoxin B_1 (Rao *et al.*, 1974). Male rats given an i.p. dose of 250 g/kg body wt of aflatoxin B_1 showed markedly dilated ER by 24 h. Numerous aggregates of free ribosomes were present in the cytoplasm, and the number of mature zymogen granules was reduced. These changes progressed between 48 and 96 h when most acinar cells were devoid of zymogen granules. There was moderate enlargement of nucleoli but no other nucleolar alterations. At 48 and 72 h the pancreatic amylase concentration in rats given two doses of aflatoxin was appreciably lower than in controls. Taken together, these observations suggest that aflatoxin B_1 may inhibit protein synthesis in the pancreas and indicate that it is toxic to the pancreas.

The effect of lifetime exposure of rats to aflatoxin was reported by Ward *et al.* (1975). Aflatoxin B_1 was fed at 2 ppm in the diet to a group of pregnant F-344 rats from the time of conception and then to their offspring until death.

The diet was also given to another group of rats 6–7 weeks old for comparison. 419

SOME
EFFECTS OF
CARCINOGENS
ON CELL
ORGANELLES
Survival of male rats was significantly shorter than for female rats of both groups. The major causes of death were hepatic neoplasms with metastases. Most deaths resulted from a malignant hemorrhagic liver tumor histologically diagnosed as a hemangiosarcoma, which caused rupture and hemorrhage into the peritoneal cavity or metastases to the lungs. Ultrastructurally the tumors in the liver were composed of poorly differentiated cells resembling endothelium. The hemorrhagic tumors were characterized by vascular structures containing blood cells and resembling sinusoids. Anaplastic cells with vesicular or bizarre nuclei and scant or abundant eosinophilic cytoplasm formed small vessels or cords of cells lining large vascular spaces.

2.2. Azo Compounds

The sequence of light microscopic changes in livers of rats given carcinogenic azo compounds has been well documented (Opie, 1944; Firminger and Mulay, 1952).

In experiments in our laboratories dealing principally with 3′-Me-DAB the typical hyperplastic nodules with bile duct proliferation were apparent by 14 weeks. During the first 48 h, the most pronounced changes were swelling of the cytoplasm with a decrease in glycogen and the centrilobular infiltration of mononuclear cells. By electron microscopy, both micro- and macrosegregation of the nucleolus, detachment of ribosomes, increase in SER, focal mitochondrial swelling, and slight increase in lysosomes were apparent. "Coated" vesicles were also apparent. Ketterer *et al.* (1967) found a close relationship between biochemical and ultrastructural injury induced in rat liver by DAB. The earliest change after one dose was detachment of polyribosomes with disorganization and vesiculation of cisternae of granular ER followed by disaggregation of the polyribosomes and impaired microsomal amino acid incorporation that reached a maximum at 24 h. Reports from other laboratories dealing with ultrastructural effects of azo dyes may be consulted (Porter and Bruni, 1959; Timme and Fowle, 1963; Nigam, 1965).

In chronic experiments using 3′-Me-DAB, occasional nucleoli showed condensation of the fibrillar component; in the cytoplasm, detachment of ribosomes increased the amount of SER in close association with glycogen, and dilated empty Golgi vacuoles were prominent. Fat vacuoles were closely associated with mitochondria.

Hyperbasophilic areas appear with some regularity in the liver of rats given carcinogenic azo dyes. Such foci appear to be sites of accelerated DNA synthesis in preneoplastic liver (Simard and Daoust, 1966). Karasaki (1969) showed that the hyperbasophilic foci contained poorly differentiated proliferating cells that had several features of DAB-induced tumors (Svoboda, 1964) and suggested that hyperbasophilic foci represented sites of dedifferentiated liver cells having accelerated rates of proliferation leading to growth of liver tumors.

The feeding of 3'-Me-DAB for as short a period as 2 weeks has been found to be sufficient to cause cholangiofibrosis, which continued in severity up to 25 weeks (Terao and Nakano, 1974). The ultrastructure of the epithelial lining cells in the lesions of cholangiofibrosis showed typical intestinal cell metaplasia including goblet cells, enterochromaffin cells, and Paneth cells. Goblet cells showed various stages of mucus production.

LaFontaine and Allard (1964) demonstrated that ultrastructural changes produced in rat liver cells by a noncarcinogenic azo dye, 2-Me-DAB, duplicated most of the ultrastructural changes induced by the closely related potent carcinogen 3'-Me-DAB. Perhaps the most important interpretation to be drawn from this study is that noncarcinogenic chemicals closely related structurally to their carcinogenic analogs are capable of causing remarkably similar ultrastructural alterations in parenchymal liver cells of rats.

2.3. Ethionine

For a complete discussion of the role of ethionine in hepatocarcinogenesis, the reader should consult the review by Farber (1963). By light microscopy the most conspicuous changes 24 h after a single dose of DL-ethionine to male rats were an increase in the number of nucleoli and a slight, diffuse vacuolization of the cytoplasm. By 2 weeks, the liver of rats given 0.25% ethionine showed a slight fat accumulation and large, often multiple eosinophilic nucleoli. By electron microscopy, the most apparent changes were microsegregation of nucleoli and an increase in the number of interchromatin granules at 72 h. In chronic experiments, nucleoli were markedly enlarged because of an increase in both the granular and the fibrillar components, but no form of separation of these components was present. There was a marked increase in the amount of interchromatin granules, which commonly formed complex branching patterns. This change was more severe after 12 weeks and was accompanied by an increase in the number of perichromatin granules. The normal dense granules in the mitochondrial matrix were reduced or absent in various organelles. SER remained increased. Both nuclear and cytoplasmic changes persisted at 18 weeks. Similar changes in the ultrastructure of interphase nuclei of rat liver cells in ethionine intoxication were described by Miyai and Steiner (1965). They concluded that the nuclear changes were attributable to the toxic action of ethionine either through competition with methionine, alterations in energy balance, production of ethylated metabolites, incorporation of ethionine into protein, production of abnormal nucleic acids, or a combination of these processes.

In addition to other cytoplasmic changes that occur in chronic ethionine intoxication in rat liver cells, Steiner et al. (1964) described complex concentric circular arrays of membranes associated with glycogen granules. The authors indicated that liver cells of hyperplastic nodules had resumed glycogen storage and considered it likely that neoplasms arose from such cells. Similarly, Epstein et al. (1967) showed that nodules induced with ethionine retained glycogen despite a period of fasting or administration of glucagon. Also, the ethionine-induced nodules showed decreased activity of glucose-6-phosphatase and glycogen phosphorylase. It was Farber (1963) who initially suggested that the nuclear lesions were related to a fall in hepatic ATP concentration. Similarly, Meldolesi *et al.* (1967) felt that many of the ethionine-induced ultrastructural changes in the cytoplasm were correlated with the decrease of ATP.

421

SOME
EFFECTS OF
CARCINOGENS
ON CELL
ORGANELLES

Shinozuka *et al.* (1968) confirmed the earlier findings that 12 h after ethionine injection, there was almost complete fragmentation of nucleoli, and that prior administration of adenine prevented the nucleolar changes. If adenine was given 8 h after ethionine, it reversed the nucleolar lesions by 12 h. Methionine given at 8 h also caused earlier partial recovery of ethionine-induced nucleolar changes. In a later but related study, Shinozuka and Farber (1969) suggested that synthesis of new protein is not essential for recovery of nucleolar ultrastructure after ethionine and that such recovery probably results from reaggregation and restoration of preexistent nucleolar fragments. Later studies by Shinozuka *et al.* (1970) presented evidence that re-formation of the nucleoli takes place in the absence of significant protein synthesis but not in the absence of RNA synthesis. The observations suggest that ethionine-induced nucleolar lesions are probably related to ATP deficiency induced by ethionine. Following administration of ethionine, the decrease in nuclear ATP is considerably less than the decrease in cytoplasmic ATP (Okazaki *et al.*, 1968). The lesser degree of ATP inhibition in the nucleus may allow earlier recovery of nucleolar ultrastructure than of cytoplasmic changes. Natural recovery of nucleolar ultrastructure after ethionine was reported by Miyai and Ritchie (1970). They showed that after i.p. injection of 1 mg/g body wt of DL-ethionine to female rats, the ultrastructure of the nucleolus was normal and some ribosomes had reaggregated. Between 84 and 96 h, the ultrastructure of the cytoplasm was almost completely recovered.

Comparing the localization of acid phosphatase activity and of very-low-density lipoproteins in ethionine and control rats, Arstila and Trump (1972) suggested that ethionine induces a blockage in the transfer of materials from the ER to the Golgi apparatus.

2.4. Hypolipidemic Agents

In recent years, it has become apparent that a number of drugs that lower serum lipids in humans or in experimental animals are carcinogenic to rats and mice. These drugs characteristically cause a proliferation of hepatic peroxisomes (Fig. 4) and a simultaneous increase in hepatic catalase activity that is sustained as long as the respective drug is administered (Hess *et al.*, 1965; Svoboda and Azarnoff, 1966), but the peroxisome proliferation is not necessarily dependent on or proportional to catalase content (Reddy *et al.*, 1970). The function of peroxisomes in mammalian tissues has recently been reviewed briefly by Masters and Holmes (1979). Peroxisomes are ubiquitous cell organelles that contain not only catalase but several hydrogen peroxide-generating oxidases and carnitine

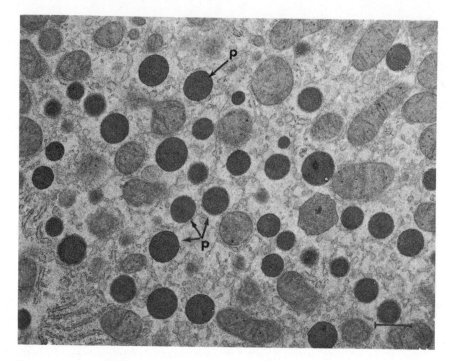

FIGURE 4. Male rat liver after 0.25% clofibrate in the diet *ad lib* for 7 days. There is a marked increase in the number of peroxisomes (p). ×9600.

acetyltransferase (Masters and Holmes, 1977). Recently Lazarow (1978) reported that rat liver peroxisomes may be specialized for β-oxidation of long-chain fatty acids. It is not known whether peroxisome proliferation following administration of hypolipidemic drugs is related to the carcinogenicity of these drugs.

The first report of malignant tumors caused by a hypolipidemic agent was that by Reddy *et al.* (1976*b*), who described hepatocellular carcinomas in mice given nafenopin (2-methyl-2-[*p*-(1,2,3,4-tetrahydro-1-naphthyl)phenoxyl]pro-pionic acid). Between 18 and 20 months, 9 male and 12 female mice developed hepatocellular carcinomas in which the number of peroxisomes varied. In lung metastases, peroxisomes were numerous. Later Reddy and Rao (1977*a*) found that nafenopin also caused hepatocellular carcinomas and acinar cell carcinomas of the pancreas in male Fischer rats. Reddy *et al.* (1977*b*) also found that Wy-14,643 [4-chloro-6-(2,3-xylidino)-2-pyrimidinylthio] acetic acid), a hypolipidemic drug with a chemical configuration unlike that of nafenopin but which also causes proliferation of hepatic peroxisomes, was capable of causing hepatocellular carcinomas containing numerous peroxisomes in male rats and mice. Wy-14,643 also accelerated the appearance of liver nodules induced with DEN in rats (Reddy and Rao, 1978). Clofibrate, another hypolipidemic drug, also enhanced DEN-induced liver tumors but to a lesser degree than Wy-14,643.

Reddy *et al.* (1979*a*) have also found that Br-931 [4-chloro-6-(2,3-xylidino)-2-pyrimidinylthio(N-β-hydroxyethyl)]-acetamide) and tibric acid (2-chloro-5-(3,5-dimethyl-piperidinosulfonyl)benzoic acid), two hypolipidemic chemicals that cause peroxisome proliferation, also induce hepatocellular carcinomas in mice and rats. The tumor cells contained numerous peroxisomes as noted in liver tumors induced with nafenopin or Wy-14,643.

423

SOME
EFFECTS OF
CARCINOGENS
ON CELL
ORGANELLES

Historically, the first hypolipidemic drug to be investigated extensively in terms of its effect on liver ultrastructure was clofibrate (ethylchlorophenoxyisobutyrate, atromid-S). Unlike the hypolipidemic chemicals previously discussed, clofibrate has been widely used in treating humans for several years and is the hypolipidemic drug most widely used in Europe and in the United States (Havel and Kane, 1973). It has been used for more than 15 years in the treatment of hyperlipoproteinemia, often in doses of 2000 mg/day. In view of the large number of people receiving clofibrate and the implications for public health and considering that it contains a chlorinated phenoxy moiety, Svoboda and Azarnoff (1979) tested it for carcinogenicity. The drug was administered at a concentration of 0.5% in the diet of 25 male F-344 rats from 72 to 97 weeks. The animals were followed to a maximum of 129 weeks. Between 72 and 129 weeks, 10 rats developed a total of 16 tumors. The tumors included four hepatocellular carcinomas, an adenocarcinoma of the glandular stomach, a papillary carcinoma of the urinary bladder, an acinar cell carcinoma of the pancreas, acinar cell adenomas of the pancreas, and others. The hepatocellular carcinomas were of the trabecular type (Fig. 5); ultrastructurally, the tumor cells contained abundant mitochondria lacking dense granules, several peroxisomes, and elongated cisternae of the ER. The pancreatic carcinoma was composed of acinar cells containing numerous eosinophilic granules. Most cells were elongated with basal nuclei and

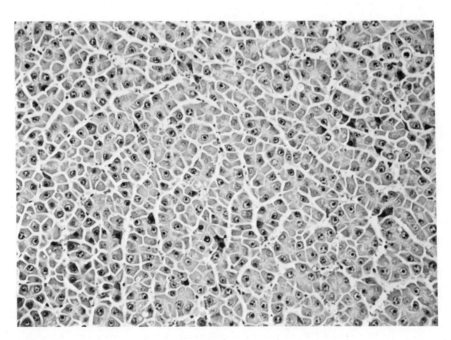

FIGURE 5. Trabecular pattern of hepatocellular carcinoma induced in male rat liver with long-term feeding of 0.5% clofibrate in the diet *ad lib.* ×520.

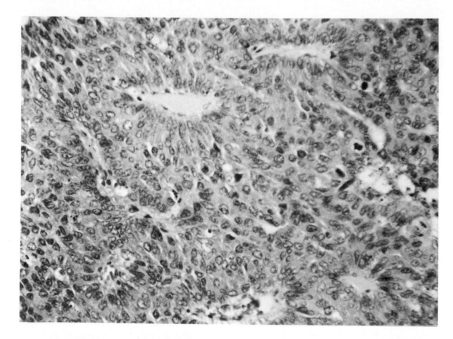

FIGURE 6. Acinar cell carcinoma of the pancreas in male rat after long-term feeding of 0.5% clofibrate in the diet *ad lib*. ×300.

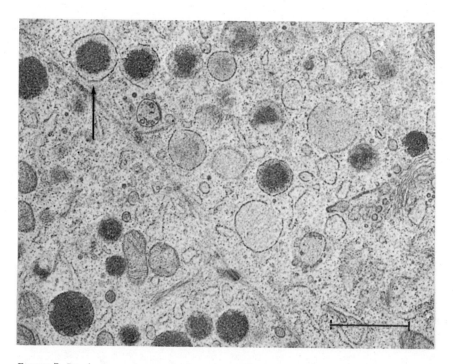

FIGURE 7. By electron microscopy, the acinar cell carcinoma of the pancreas contained several typical zymogen granules. In addition, other granules were only partially filled with electron-dense material (arrow) and empty vesicles were also present. ×19,500.

were arranged as pseudorosettes around a delicate fibrovascular stalk (Fig. 6). 425

SOME
EFFECTS OF
CARCINOGENS
ON CELL
ORGANELLES

By electron microscopy, in addition to numerous electron-dense zymogen granules, there were granules only partially filled or of reduced electron density, and in most cells, several empty cytoplasmic vesicles were present (Fig. 7). The carcinogenicity of clofibrate was confirmed by Reddy and Qureshi (1979), who reported hepatocellular carcinomas in 10 of 11 male F-344 rats and acinar cell carcinomas of the pancreas in 2 rats given clofibrate for 24–28 months.

The animal data indicating carcinogenicity of clofibrate are of special interest in view of a collaborative study in humans wherein it was shown that there were more deaths from malignant tumors in the clofibrate group than in a high-cholesterol control group (Report from the Committee of Principal Investigators, 1978). There are now five hypolipidemic drugs that are carcinogenic, clofibrate being the only one used in humans. The mechanism of carcinogenesis by these agents, of differing chemical structure, is not known at the present time. None of them caused mutagenic activity in the Ames *Salmonella*/microsome assay nor did they produce DNA damage in concanavalin A-stimulated lymphocytes *in vitro* (Warren *et al.*, 1980).

2.5. Nitrosamines

For detailed reports of the histological changes, the biochemical and carcinogenic effects, and the metabolism of *N*-nitroso compounds, the reader is referred to the reviews by Magee (1963) and Magee and Barnes (1967). In acute experiments (24–72 h), the light microscopic changes following administration of DEN or DMN were quite similar. Both caused centrilobular hemorrhagic necrosis and loss of glycogen. Moderate nuclear enlargement was apparent with DMN. In chronic experiments, DEN caused irregularity in the size of liver cells and subsequent nodular hyperplasia. DMN caused acidophilic degeneration of centrilobular cells and occasional large hyperchromatic nuclei. By electron microscopy, an early ultrastructural change induced by DMN was microsegregation; both DMN and DEN caused detachment of ribosomes and an increase in the amount of SER. Emmelot and Benedetti (1961) showed that a single dose of DMN caused a breakdown of the characteristic lamellar organization of the ER and a marked increase in the number of free ribosomes. Williams and Hultin (1973) found that administration of DMN to mice for 2 h resulted in 60% inhibition of hepatic protein synthesis accompanied by disaggregation of both free and membrane-bound polysomes.

Butler and Hard (1976) showed that after a single DMN treatment there was a wave of fibroblast proliferation in rat kidney after 6 days. After 12 weeks, there was rapid proliferation of mesenchymal cells leading to microscopic neoplasms after 20 weeks. The cell of origin was thought to be an interstitial cortical fibroblast or possibly an extramural pericyte.

A detailed study of the light and electron microscopic changes in rat liver following administration of nitrosomorpholine was reported by Bannasch (1968).

Observations were limited to the cytoplasm and included description of cells with prominent accumulations of glycogen associated with membranes resembling the complexes described by Steiner *et al.* (1964) after ethionine. Like Steiner *et al.*, Bannasch considered that hepatomas induced with nitrosomorpholine developed from those parenchymal cells that showed enhanced glycogen storage. From histochemical studies of liver of rhesus monkeys given DEN, Ruebner *et al.* (1976) suggested that foci of glycogen-containing cells might be the first step in the development of neoplasia in that species as well. Shinozuka and Estes (1977) found that administration of DEN to mice in drinking water greatly enhanced the appearance of intracisternal A particles. Such viruslike particles are occasionally present in normal liver cells of adult mice and in certain hepatomas. Their biological significance remains unknown.

DEN given to dogs in drinking water for several weeks was reported to cause a wide variety of neoplasms in the liver including fibromas, hemangioendotheliomas, fibrosarcomas, leiomyosarcomas, hepatocellular carcinoma, and cholangiocarcinoma (Hirao *et al.*, 1974).

In long-term cultures of liver cells from DEN-treated rats, persistent aggregates of 100-Å filaments resembling Mallory bodies developed (Borenfreund and Higgins, 1979). In organ cultures from humans, *N*-nitrosomethylurea caused hyperplasia of bronchial epithelium and connective tissue as well as hyperplasia of renal tubular epithelium (Shabad *et al.*, 1975).

2.6. Pyrrolizidine Alkaloids

The pyrrolizidine alkaloids constitute a large group of naturally occurring toxins derived from several families of plants distributed in various parts of the world (Kingsbury, 1964). Their chemistry and metabolism and the pathologic alterations resulting from both acute and chronic alkaloid poisoning in animals have been reviewed comprehensively by McLean (1970). In humans, these agents have been incriminated in veno-occlusive disease, cirrhosis, and Chiari's syndrome in those parts of the world where they are given as a medicinal tonic or consumed in flour contaminated with alkaloid-containing seeds.

The pyrrolizidine alkaloids, esters of a basic alcohol containing a pyrrolizidine group, differ from most hepatotoxic and carcinogenic substances in that they are capable of causing severe chronic and progressive liver disease after a single dose. In addition, some of these alkaloids induce formation of cellular aggregates in the lumens of central veins, often causing total occlusion of vessels. Some of the alkaloids, such as lasiocarpine, cause an atypical regenerative response, termed megalocytosis, in which liver cells three to four times the normal size, or greater, occur. Functionally, the RNA polymerase activity of megalocyte nuclei was comparable to that of normal nuclei. Further, the inducibility of tryptophan pyrrolase activity by hydrocortisone, in livers of rats exhibiting megalocytosis, indicates that translational mechanisms are intact. However, the increased uptake of [^{3}H]thymidine by megalocytes in the absence of observable mitotic activity suggests that the cells are in the process of hypertrophy. Megalocytes appear capable, therefore, of carrying on several normal functions except that they are in the process of hypertrophy and incapable of division due to the potent antimitotic action of the alkaloid (Svoboda et al., 1971a). It has been suggested that the alkaloids act as alkylating agents and are mutagenic.

427

SOME
EFFECTS OF
CARCINOGENS
ON CELL
ORGANELLES

The first study of the pyrrolizidine alkaloids lasiocarpine and monocrotaline on the fine structure of liver cells was reported by Svoboda and Soga (1966). In these studies, administration of lasiocarpine or an extract of *Crotalaria* caused microsegregation of the nucleolus by 30 min. Macrosegregation of the nucleolus and an increase in interchromatin granules were prominent between 2 and 8 h. The nucleolar changes returned to normal by 72 h. In a later study (Svoboda and Higginson, 1968) of the early (24 h) changes due to lasiocarpine in the liver of male rats, the nuclear alterations were essentially similar to those described above. In the cytoplasm, there was detachment of ribosomes with extensive dilatation of the RER and an increase in SER. An early report by Reddy and Svoboda (1968) pointed out that abnormalities in nucleolar ultrastructure and disaggregation of polyribosomes in liver cells were associated with the simultaneous inhibition of hepatic RNA and protein synthesis.

Monneron (1969) found that within 10 min after injection of lasiocarpine or aflatoxin to intact or partially hepatectomized rats, numerous helical polysomes occurred in hepatic parenchymal cells and in Kupffer cells. They appeared prior to the nucleolar changes produced by these agents, and their occurrence was not prevented by previous administration of actinomycin D. The sudden, early occurrence of helical polysomes may be related to the production of a special type of transient messenger RNA (Monneron et al., 1971).

Lasiocarpine given by i.p. injection to male rats for 52 weeks induced tumors between 60 and 76 weeks. Approximately 61% (11 of 18) developed hepatocellular carcinomas and 33% (6 of 18) developed well-differentiated squamous cell carcinomas. Tumors were transplanted through five generations. A long experimental interval (52 weeks) plus a period of observation after dosing is discontinued, may be necessary to allow cessation of the antimitotic effect of the alkaloid to permit expression of its carcinogenicity (Svoboda and Reddy, 1972). In contrast, dietary administration of lasiocarpine (50 ppm) led to development of angiosarcomas of the liver (Rao and Reddy, 1978). In another study, lasiocarpine was given in conjunction with aflatoxin B_1 to rats to determine whether lasiocarpine, because of its antimitotic effect, might inhibit initiation of liver tumors by aflatoxin B_1. Lasiocarpine did not inhibit liver tumors induced by aflatoxin B_1 but altered the appearance of the liver inasmuch as, in rats receiving both agents, the liver tumors were associated with postnecrotic cirrhosis, in contrast to rats that developed liver tumors with aflatoxin only (Reddy and Svoboda, 1972). Thioacetamide, which stimulates cell division in rat liver (Reddy et al., 1969), given in combination with lasiocarpine to rats for 15 weeks produced numerous grossly apparent hyperplastic nodules and postnecrotic cirrhosis. There were no hyperplastic nodules or cirrhosis in animals given either agent alone. These results, like others, suggest that cell proliferation, induced by thioacetamide, enhances the appearance of neoplasms (Reddy et al., 1976a).

2.7. Thioacetamide

The acute histological changes within 24–48 h after administration of thioacetamide were enlargement of nuclei and occasional acidophilic cells in the centrilobular zone. Glycogen was decreased and there was slight centrilobular necrosis. By electron microscopy, there was nucleolar enlargement due to an increase in the granular component. In addition, there was an increase in interchromatin granules. In the cytoplasm, as with other carcinogens, there was detachment of ribosomes and an increase in SER. Polysomes were conspicuous, as were dense deposits, possibly calcium, in occasional mitochondria. In chronic experiments, the most notable change was an increase in the size of the nucleolus, again principally due to an increase in the granular component. In the cytoplasm, the acute changes persisted. Two weeks after withdrawal of the carcinogen, only a few enlarged nucleoli remained. Some oval cells and small amounts of ceroid were present until 8 weeks when cytoplasmic basophilia was uniformly restored and most nucleoli recovered their normal structure.

Smith *et al.* (1968) reported that liver cell nuclei of mice fed thioacetamide contained lipid cysts by 3 days; similar cysts were found in the nuclei of mouse hepatomas transplanted subcutaneously. Date *et al.* (1976) demonstrated that partial hepatectomy accelerated thioacetamide-induced neoplasms in Swiss male mice.

Koshiba *et al.* (1971) found the nucleoli of thioacetamide-treated rat liver to exhibit two major differences from normal. First, there was a marked increase in the relative number of RNP particles, giving the nucleolus a far more granular appearance than normal, an observation confirmed in the authors' laboratories. Second, the size of the RNP particles was greater than normal. Extraction produced a 30-fold increase in the yield of nucleolar RNP particles per 100 g of liver.

In comparing effects of thioacetamide to those of acetamide in rat liver, Olason and Smuckler (1976) found that both agents caused nuclear enlargement but nuclei reverted to normal size within 16 h after acetamide while it persisted for at least 24 h after thioacetamide. Acetamide produced minimal cytoplasmic change, whereas thioacetamide caused centrilobular necrosis and lipid deposition. Despite these differences in nuclear and cytoplasmic responses with the two related agents, it is not possible to separate the components that merely represent reaction to injury from those related to carcinogenesis. In experiments with thioacetamide-induced liver tumors, Anghileri *et al.* (1977) found that tumor development was accompanied by a drastic modification in the permeability of the cell membrane, which led to an increase in the cellular concentration of calcium and sodium and a decrease in magnesium and potassium.

3. Summary of Response of Organelles to Several Carcinogens

In assessing the response of cell organelles to carcinogens, it is important to bear in mind the severe limitations in sampling imposed by electron microscopic methods. Similarly, variables such as nutrition, sex, age, and diurnal variations must be appreciated. For example, Nair *et al.* (1970) showed that there was a diurnal rhythm of enzyme activity in rat liver cells accompanied by proliferation of SER. At the time when enzyme activity was maximal, the amount of SER was also maximal and vice versa. When the rhythm of enzyme activity was abolished in blinded rats, the diurnal changes in ER were also abolished. Loud (1968) studied the fractional volumes in the cytoplasm of liver cells occupied by mitochondria, peroxisomes, lysosomes, lipid, and glycogen as well as the surface density of SER, RER, mitochondrial envelope, and cristae. The results provide a basis for ultrastructural quantitative comparisons between normal and pathologically altered cells. The study showed that parenchymal cells in normal rat liver are at least 80% homogeneous with respect to the structural features measured. The most pronounced lobular differences are in the two or three layers of cells surrounding the central vein. Weibel *et al.* (1969) showed that 1 ml of normal rat liver contains 1.7×10^8 nuclei of parenchymal cells and 9×10^7 nuclei of other cells as well as 2.8×10^{11} mitochondria. Hepatocyte cytoplasm accounts for 77% of liver volume and mitochondria for 18%. The surface area of ER membranes in 1 ml of liver was estimated at $11 \, \text{m}^2$, two-thirds of that being in the RER. The surface area of mitochondrial cristae in 1 ml of liver was estimated at $6 \, \text{m}^2$. One hepatocyte contains approximately 370 peroxisomes, which contribute only 1.5% of the cytoplasmic volume. Although somewhat laborious, this type of morphometric analysis allows one to compare normal with abnormal liver cells far more accurately than by mere visual inspection of electron micrographs and subjective impressions. The paper of Weibel *et al.* (1969) should be consulted for quantification of organelles in liver cells expressed in several different terms. The authors also point out problems that may arise in quantitative estimation of cell organelles and the artifacts that may originate from homogenization and preparation of cell fractions for biochemical analysis.

3.1. Endoplasmic Reticulum

For a recent general review of the structure and cytochemistry as well as morphological specializations and interactions of ER, the recent review by Novikoff (1976) should be consulted. A paper by Apffel (1978) updates the modulations in ER that result from the process of carcinogenesis. Since 1957, over 30 studies have been concerned with the ultrastructural changes in ER during carcinogenesis. Almost all of them indicated a decrease in the ratio of membrane-bound to free ribosomes. There is a decrease of ribosomes bound to ER while numerous unattached free ribosomes are scattered in the cytoplasm. This rather constant feature has been related to carcinogenesis, to progress of experimental tumors, and to spontaneous tumors in mice and in established tumors of mice, rats, hamsters, and in transformed monkey kidney cells. The decreased ratio of bound to free ribosomes characterizes tumors of all histologic categories so far investigated including mouse ascites tumors, hepatomas, breast carcinoma, Walker carcinosarcoma, lymphosarcoma, leukemia, plasmacytoma, melanoma, and rhabdomyoblastoma. This same characteristic has been found in human tumor cells of very diverse nature, such as endometrial carcinoma, urinary bladder carcinoma, glioblastoma, medulloblastoma, chronic lymphoid leukemia, Hodgkin's disease, and lymphosarcoma. In addition to increased detachment of ribosomes from ER membranes, a few less constant and more variable morphological aspects have been described in carcinogenesis. The alterations in RER may consist of either concentric, whorl, or fingerprint patterns, annulate lamellae, haphazard distribution of the cisternae along with aggregates of vesicles of SER, clustering of free ribosomes, decrease of ER, and hypertrophy of Golgi areas. Detachment of ribosomes has been described in embryonal liver cells and after administration of noncarcinogens as well (Herdson *et al.*, 1964; Fouts and Rogers, 1965; Hruban *et al.*, 1965; Orrenius and Ericsson, 1966; Rubin *et al.*, 1968). Liver cells of regenerating liver, however, may display an unchanged ratio of bound to free ribosomes. Detached polysomes and stripped RER both originating from normal cells will rebind *in vitro* under appropriate conditions of pH, ionic strength, and medium composition. Free polysomes of tumor cells may bind with membranes of stripped ER from normal cells, but free polysomes are irreversibly separated from ER membranes if both originate from neoplastic cells.

In view of interference in the membrane–ribosome association being such a common property in carcinogenesis, Williams and Rabin (1971) suggested that carcinogens occupy or destroy a site on the membrane for steroid hormones. They also speculated that interaction of the carcinogen and membrane *in vivo* would seriously disturb the pattern of template RNA lifetime because the messenger is probably more stable if attached to a membrane. Degranulation could thus bring about selective labilization of the same species of messenger RNA originally bound to the membrane. Such a hypothesis would be consistent with the hypothesis of malignancy proposed by Pitot (1964).

3.2. Plasma Membrane

Coated vesicles were prominent in acute experiments after administration of DEN, DMN, and 3′-Me-DAB. They were not present in chronic experiments. They appear to arise from the plasma membrane though they may be located deep in the cytoplasm. Coated vesicles have been noted in several cell types, and Novikoff and Shin (1964) suggested that these vesicles transport material from the ER. Friend and Farquhar (1967) suggested that coated vesicles could reflect accelerated transport of material through specialized portions of the plasma membrane. For additional references to coated vesicles, the reader is referred to the review by Svoboda and Higginson (1968). Additionally, the papers by Emmelot (1973), Sachs (1974), and Walborg *et al.* (1979) should be consulted for review of characteristic cell membrane changes in malignancy. Recently, the cell surface has been found to participate in growth control, and changes in the membrane have been related to the altered growth patterns of transformed cells. The demonstration that the plasma membrane is associated with cytoskeletal elements, particularly the interaction of membrane protein with microfilaments, has provided a structural and functional link between the cell environment and the cytoplasm (Nicolson, 1976).

431
SOME
EFFECTS OF
CARCINOGENS
ON CELL
ORGANELLES

In rats treated with 2-acetylaminofluorene (2-AAF) for 6–8 weeks, the number of microvilli of isolated hepatocytes was about half that of normal liver cells, but such cells had about four times as many protrusions and blebs as normal cells. The authors suggested that the reduced number of microvilli in 2-AAF-treated rats might be consistent with an inverse relationship between the level of cyclic AMP and the number of microvilli. By scanning electron microscopy, the presence of increased numbers of microvilli, blebs, and ruffles has been described in a variety of transformed cells including Chinese hamster ovary (Porter *et al.*, 1973) and mouse fibroblasts (Willingham and Pastan, 1975) compared to smooth surfaces in nontransformed cells. On the other hand, Collard and Temmink (1976) found that SV40-transformed fibroblasts throughout the life cycle have a smoother surface than normal fibroblasts.

Glioma cells induced in rats by ethylnitrosourea were shown by scanning electron microscopy to have large numbers of blebs, filopodia, and microvilli, whereas control lines had little surface activity (Winslow *et al.*, 1978).

Using freeze-fracture methods for demonstrating intrinsic membrane proteins, which are intramembranous particles of 70 Å, Scott and Furcht (1976) demonstrated that in contact-inhibited 3T3 cells, the particles were aggregated; in cells transformed by oncogenic viruses, chemical carcinogens, or spontaneous events, the intramembranous particles were randomly distributed. This difference in distribution of intramembranous particles in normal and transformed cells may reflect differences in intrinsic organization of plasma membrane protein. Cloyd and Bigner (1977) reported several parameters of cell shape, surface topography, and cellular interaction for a variety of neoplastic and nonneoplastic cultured rat cells. These cells showed a spectrum of features ranging from flat shape and smooth surfaces to rounded or pleomorphic shapes and abundant surface projections. Cells with any of these features were found in any line irrespective of tumorigenicity. Comparing several reports of surface morphology of nontransformed cells and cells transformed by various means, the results indicate that cell shape, topography, and interaction often do change upon neoplastic transformation but not always in consistent patterns nor in any pattern that can be specifically associated with the transforming agent. It can be concluded from the available studies that random sampling of external cell morphology may not necessarily predict neoplastic properties.

The presence and various types of cell junctions of normal and malignant tissues were compared and reviewed by Weinstein *et al.* (1976). These junctions not only serve as structural attachments between cells, but also provide a mechanism for cell to cell interactions and mediate communication between cells through transfer of ions, small molecules, and electrochemical impulses. The intermediate cells of normal cervical epithelium have as many as 225 gap junctions per cell, whereas invasive squamous cell carcinomas of the cervix are deficient in gap junctions. In well-differentiated areas of human tumors, up to four junctions per cell were present; in poorly differentiated tumors, none were found. In cultured cells in general, no correlation could be demonstrated between tumorigenicity and presence or absence of gap junctions. Desmosomes were also less frequent in invasive cervical squamous cell cancer than in normal cervix. From this review, the authors concluded that various types of cell junctions are present in many kinds of epithelial or mesenchymal tumors and their occurrence often is less frequent than in normal tissue.

3.3. Mitochondria, Lysosomes, Peroxisomes

In the authors' studies, the most conspicuous and consistent mitochondrial abnormalities occurred in rat liver cells in the immediate periportal area following DMN treatment. The changes consisted of marked enlargement, sometimes to a diameter equal to that of the nucleus, occasional rupture of limiting membranes and many bizarre profiles, with an abnormal number and distribution of cristae. These abnormal forms apparently occurred in too few cells to be reflected in alterations in P:O ratios. Mukherjee et al. (1963) showed that liver tissue does not react uniformly to DMN, and this could cause variation in electron microscopic and biochemical observations following administration of this carcinogen. Emmelot and Benedetti (1961) found that mitochondria isolated from rat liver 3 h after in vivo administration of 10 mg of DMN behaved normally but by 24 h after a dose of 20 mg there was some degree of respiratory inhibition and diminished oxidative phosphorylation. In these studies, although there was swelling of some mitochrondria, most retained normal ultrastructure.

As a general rule, in human tissues, it appears that mitochondrial pleomorphism is expressed only slightly in normal tissue, to a variable extent in nonmalignant tissue of tumorous organs, and to a much greater extent by all cancer lines (Springer et al., 1979). Stereological analysis of electron micrographs of hepatocytes of three hematoma cell lines, one slow-growing and two fast-growing, were compared. The relative mitochondrial volume in the cytoplasm appeared decreased with increased growth rate. It was concluded that hepatoma cells have fewer mitochondria than normal liver cells but the organelles had a normal content of inner membranes (Volman, 1978).

In experiments with carcinogens reported by Svoboda and Higginson (1968), there was a slight to moderate increase in the number of lysosomes in both acute and chronic experiments and in tumor cells. Because of the great variety of morphology and number of lysosomes in many pathological conditions, it is difficult to formulate conclusions regarding their reaction to carcinogens. Allison and Mallucci (1964) showed that the carcinogens dimethylbenzanthracene, methylcholanthrene, 1,2,5,6-dibenzanthracene, and 3,4-benzpyrene (studied in monkey kidney cells, HeLa cells, macrophages, and chick embryo cells as well as in vivo in mice given subcutaneous injections of dimethylbenzanthracene) concentrated in lysosomes and appeared to decrease the stability of their limiting membrane so that high concentrations of the carcinogens could cause release of lysosomal enzymes into the cytoplasm. The same phenomena were reported following X-irradiation (Brandes *et al.*, 1967). Studies of thioacetamide and DMN injury in rat liver gave no evidence of early lysosomal rupture during the prenecrotic period (Slater and Greenbaum, 1965), but aflatoxin induced an increase in the permeability of lysosomal membranes (Pokrovsky *et al.*, 1972), and feeding 2-AAF to rats caused a marked increase in the size of lysosomes in liver cells (Berg and Christoffersen, 1974). Increased lysosomal fragility of rat liver lysosomes after treatment with ethionine has also been reported (Zuretti and Baccino, 1975). In a review of lysosomes and cancer, Allison (1969) hypothesized that lysosomes accumulate carcinogens that promote release of lysosomal enzymes into the cytoplasm by increasing the permeability of their membranes. This in turn might allow the released lysosomal DNase to induce mutagenic changes in chromosomes.

At present, it is not known whether peroxisomes bear a relationship to neoplasia. They are present in a wide variety of tissues and cells of several species of animals and plants but have not been studied extensively in neoplasms originating from tissue other than liver where they vary in number and size depending on the specific tumor line. In liver tumors, the number of peroxisomes may be directly related to the degree of differentiation and inversely related to the rate of growth. As discussed previously, there is a significant increase in rat hepatic peroxisomes following administration of certain hypolipidemic drugs

433
SOME
EFFECTS OF
CARCINOGENS
ON CELL
ORGANELLES

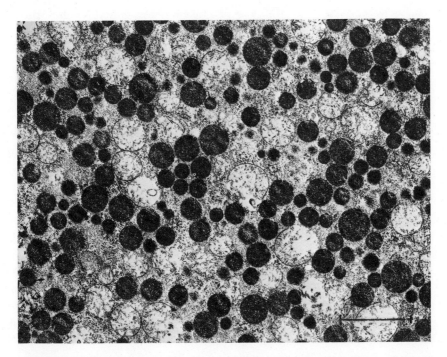

FIGURE 8. Pulmonary metastasis from a hepatocellular carcinoma induced with nafenopin. The tumor cell contains numerous electron-dense peroxisomes. ×18,000. Courtesy of Reddy *et al.* (1976*b*).

that cause malignant liver neoplasms. The increase is accompanied by an increase in hepatic catalase, one of their principal enzymes. The increase in peroxisomes and catalase occurs within as short a time as 3 days following initiation of the drug and typically reaches a plateau at approximately 2 weeks. The peroxisomes are increased significantly in number in nontumor cells of liver bearing tumors induced by clofibrate but are reduced in number in the tumor cells. Metastases from hepatocellular carcinoma induced by nafenopin may contain an exceedingly large number of peroxisomes (Fig. 8) (Reddy *et al.*, 1976*b*).

3.4. Nucleus, Nucleolus

A comparative study of the effects of various carcinogens and noncarcinogens on mitosis of rat hepatocytes was reported by Maini and Stich (1961).

Thioacetamide and 3'-Me-DAB were chosen as substances of strong carcinogenic activity, 4-monomethylaminoazobenzene was used as a substance of moderate activity, and *o*-aminoazotoluene, 4'-Me-DAB, ethionine, and thiourea were used as weak carcinogens. 2-Me-DAB and 4-aminoazobenzene were used as noncarcinogens. The ability of these chemicals to induce proliferation of hepatic tissue to cause formation of highly polyploid cells and to cause mitotic irregularities was compared. A correlation existed between carcinogenic activity of a chemical and its ability to produce proliferation and a large number of mitotic irregularities in the precancerous liver. Of the noncarcinogens, 4-aminoazobenzene lacked the ability to produce a heterogeneous cell population in the rat liver. The mitotic irregularities varied from chromosome fragmentation to incomplete spindle formation and were similar in all precancerous livers independent of the molecular structure of the carcinogens used. The chromosome injury persisted for several months. It was concluded that hepatomas are produced only when chromosome injury is combined with active cell proliferation.

The size of nuclei in HeLa cells exposed *in vitro* for 1–3 days to carcinogens was found to increase markedly at 48 h (Agrelo, 1978). Similarly, enlargement of liver cell nuclei containing numerous large nucleoli was reported following long-term ingestion of 2-AAF (Dobre *et al.*, 1976).

Purified nuclear membranes from normal rat liver and hepatomas were studied with emphasis on the nuclear pore complex using several methods for negative staining as well as freeze-cleavage. No significant differences in the dimensions of the pore complex were found (Harris *et al.*, 1974*b*). Dimensions of pore complexes may vary considerably, however, depending on the method for electron microscopic preparation.

The most comprehensive review of the biology of the nucleolus in tumor cells, especially liver nucleoli and the effects of drugs on nucleoli, is to be found in the monograph by Busch and Smetana (1970).

Yasuzumi *et al.* (1970) compared the nucleolar changes occurring after administration of 3'-Me-DAB, 2-AAF, and DL-ethionine; in all instances, there was nucleolar enlargement due principally to an increase in the granular component. The authors also described a decrease in the number of perichromatin granules. These granules may originate in the nucleolus (Derenzini and Moyne, 1978). Paul *et al.* (1971) showed that carcinogenic derivatives of 4-nitro-quinoline-*N*-oxide resulted in a preponderance of Chang cell nucleoli showing macrosegregation, while weakly carcinogenic ones resulted primarily in micro-segregation. Thus, there may be a relationship between type of nucleolar segrega-tion and carcinogenicity among the 4-nitroquinoline oxides; however, it may be valid only for this group of carcinogens. Reddy and Svoboda (1968) showed that 3'-Me-DAB, lasiocarpine, DMN, and tannic acid all inhibited nuclear and ribo-somal RNA synthesis at a time when nucleolar segregation was most pronounced. Further, the specific activity of nuclear and ribosomal RNA in rats treated with hepatocarcinogens was significantly lower than that of controls. In addition to inhibition of RNA synthesis, the RNA polymerase activity in segregated nucleoli was decreased. RNA synthesis returned to normal when nucleolar morphology recovered. Simard and Bernhard (1966) suggested that segregation and zoning of granular and fibrillar nucleolar components is a characteristic alteration produced by substances that bind with DNA and interfere with its template activity in DNA-directed RNA synthesis. It should not be construed, however, that structural or biochemical modifications in nuclear behavior represent necessary or specific events in the carcinogenic process; in fact, reports of nucleolar capping (macrosegregation) with noncarcinogenic agents in rat liver suggest the contrary. Many of the nucleolar changes recovered or did not occur when carcinogens were given in low chronic doses sufficient to induce tumors.

Although 2-AAF did not cause nuclear changes in rat hepatocytes in acute experiments (Flaks, 1970), infrequent nucleolar microsegregation was seen after 8–10 months (Flaks, 1971).

In general, it would appear that although some degree of redistribution of fibrillar and granular nucleolar constituents occurs with several carcinogens, the importance of such changes is questionable since, with aflatoxin B_1, lasiocarpine, and 3'-Me-DAB, similar nucleolar alterations are present in Kupffer cells even though the latter cells do not become malignant. Moreover, although hypo-physectomy inhibits induction of hepatic tumors (Lee and Goodall, 1968) in rats given 3'-Me-DAB 24 h prior to sacrifice, characteristic nucleolar changes occur.

It appears that many ultrastructural changes in nucleoli of rat liver cells are nonspecific and are related to a variety of biochemical alterations in addition to changes in RNA synthesis. Although there is evidence to support the principal importance of nuclear constituents, particulary DNA, in the carcinogenic process, the morphological changes that occur in the nucleus appear to be as nonspecific as those that occur in the cytoplasm.

4. Selected Site-Specific Models of Carcinogenesis

In recent years, the effects of chemical carcinogens on the ultrastructure of cells of various organs other than liver have emerged as reproducible methods for

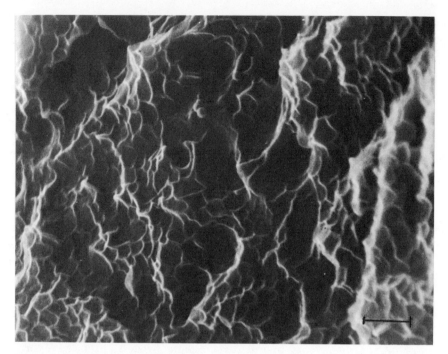

FIGURE 9. Scanning electron micrograph of the luminal surface of a normal superficial cell of the urinary bladder. The normal surface is composed of several microridges. ×12,000. Courtesy of Friedell *et al.* (1977).

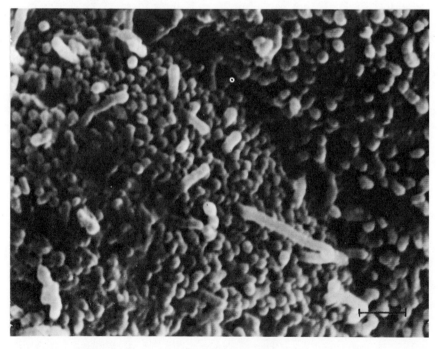

FIGURE 10. Scanning electron micrograph showing pleomorphic microvilli on the luminal surface of a tumor cell from urinary bladder. ×12,000. Courtesy of Friedell *et al.* (1977).

production of malignant tumors in the respective organs. In this section, some examples of interesting alterations in the ultrastructure of the urinary bladder, pancreas, and respiratory tract that occur during carcinogenesis will be discussed briefly.

In the urinary bladder, Friedell *et al.* (1977) and Jabocs *et al.* (1976*a,b*, 1977) found that the appearance of pleomorphic microvilli on the luminal surface of urinary bladder epithelium in rats is correlated with the irreversibility of hyperplastic lesions induced by feeding Fanft (*N*-[4-(5-nitro-2-furyl)-2-thiazolyl]formamide) to test animals. This alteration can be detected by scanning electron microscopy of histologic and cytologic preparations. The authors reported that hyperplastic lesions in surface epithelial cells from animals fed Fanft for 8–10 weeks had numerous pleomorphic microvilli, while cells of hyperplastic lesions in rats fed Fanft for 4–6 weeks had only normal microvilli on their luminal and intercellular surfaces. The authors concluded that pleomorphic microvilli in this model represent a morphological indicator of irreversible but not necessarily progressive proliferative epithelial change. Figures 9 and 10 illustrate the difference in surface appearance of normal and neoplastic superficial epithelium of the urinary bladder as seen by scanning electron microscopy.

These findings were extended to exfoliated cells from rats fed Fanft for 25 weeks followed by a control diet for 35 weeks. Scanning electron microscopy showed pleomorphic microvilli on exfoliated epithelial cells as early as 10 weeks after beginning the carcinogen, and microvilli became increasingly pleomorphic as the bladder lesions progressed to muscle invasion. Accordingly, it appears that, in exfoliated cells, the presence of pleomorphic microvilli are a reliable indicator that the proliferative changes are irreversible. The numerous microvilli of exfoliated tumor cells were in sharp contrast to the peaked microridges or normal superficial exfoliated cells.

Using *N*-methyl-*N*-nitrosourea, dibutylnitrosamine, and other carcinogens, Hicks (1976) demonstrated that the most superficial layer of preneoplastic cells revealed a regular change in the ultrastructure of the cell membrane adjacent to the urine, which did not occur in benign hyperplasia. In some preneoplastic cells, the surface was not only covered by microvilli but the limiting membrane had a glycocalyx that was more complex and structured than that seen in simple, benign hyperplasia. The structured glycocalyx was found on a few cells very early in the stages of preneoplastic growth and in one case within 8 weeks after starting the carcinogen. The number of cells carrying the glycocalyx increased as the hyperplasia progressed. The glycocalyx was observed in frank tumors of rat bladder and in a number of biopsies of human bladder tumors. The author suggested that the unusual glycocalyx may be a marker for malignant transformation in this tissue.

For related reports regarding the appearance of preneoplastic and neoplastic superficial epithelium of the urinary bladder as viewed by scanning and transmission electron microscopy, the reader is referred to the papers by Hicks and Wakefield (1976), Hodges *et al.* (1976), Newman and Hicks (1977), and Kahan *et al.* (1977).

In addition to alterations in the plasma membrane of superficial epithelium of the urinary bladder of rats and humans described above, other ultrastructural alterations in human and rat urinary bladder epithelium in carcinogenesis are of interest. For example, Tatematsu *et al.* (1977) found that in normal bladder epithelium, there is a loose plexus of capillaries beneath the epithelium. They are of relatively uniform diameter, present in low density, and are connected to larger vessels. After 2 weeks' treatment with *N*-butyl-*N*-(4-hydroxybutyl)nitrosamine, the vascularization at 6 weeks became more complex, with tortuous capillaries having a large diameter and numerous long terminal branches. In addition, there were tortuous capillary loops larger than normal. Vascular changes were predominant in bladder cancers after 40 weeks. They were detected by scanning electron microscopy of casts of the bladder.

In a transmission electron microscopic study of experimental tumors in rat bladder and in human bladder cancers, Koss (1977) described poorly formed tight junctions. In addition, there was a suggestion of defective desmosomes.

In view of the increased incidence of cancer of the pancreas among American males, several models for chemical induction of malignant neoplasms of the pancreas, of both acinar and ductal origin, in experimental animals have been developed. While it is not intended to review the extensive literature on this subject, certain salient features of histopathology and ultrastructure of chemically induced pancreatic carcinoma are presented. The subject of experimental carcinogenesis of the pancreas, including specific chemicals, species, histogenesis of the tumors, and related references, have been reviewed succinctly by Reddy *et al.* (1969*d*). One of the early methods for induction of pancreatic malignancy in animals was reported by Reddy *et al.* (1974). Adenocarcinomas developed at 36 weeks in 4 survivors among 24 inbred strain-13 guinea pigs given weekly intragastric *N*-methyl-*N*-nitrosourea at a dose of 10 mg. A transplantable acinar cell carcinoma was induced in a male Fischer rat fed 0.1% nafenopin, a hypolipidemic agent, for 20 months (Reddy and Rao, 1977*b*). It was successfully transplanted into weanling rats. The tumor cells had large nuclei with prominent nucleoli and contained variable numbers of zymogen granules. The ER and Golgi apparatus were prominent. The tumor displayed significant lipase and amylase activity. At the ultrastructural level, there was no difference in the degree of differentiation between subcutaneous and intraperitoneal transplants. Upon further study of the morphological and biochemical characteristics of this tumor (Rao and Reddy, 1979), though only a few zymogen granules were present immediately after the appearance of a palpable tumor transplant, their numbers increased in 20 days or later. In the transplants, mitochondria had well-formed cristae and plasma membranes were closely apposed with distinct intercellular junctions. Isolated cells had irregularly distributed short microvilli and cytoplasmic microfilaments. By scanning electron microscopy, the tumor cells had numerous elongated microvilli in contrast to normal pancreatic cells, which possessed surface microridges or folds. The tumor cells were more susceptible to agglutination by concanavalin A than normal acinar cells; however, if normal isolated pancreatic cells were stimulated with secretin, they too developed increased number of microvilli after 10 min but the change was not associated with enhanced agglutination by concanavalin A. Regarding acinar cells of rat pancreas, there is no correlation between surface microvilli and lectin agglutinability (Reddy *et al.*, 1979*c*).

Pour *et al.* (1974, 1975) have reported ductal and acinar cell pancreatic tumors in hamsters given 2,2′-dihydroxy-di-*N*-propylnitrosamine. This model results in tumors whose morphology and biological behavior are somewhat similar to pancreatic neoplasms in humans. Scanning electron microscopic study of pancreatic tumors induced in hamsters with *N*-nitroso-bis(2-hydroxypropyl)amine disclosed that the luminal cell surfaces in ductal carcinoma cells varied in shape, projected into the lumen to different degrees, and were covered by microvilli of varied length and density (Althoff *et al.*, 1976). Using the same model, Levitt *et al.* (1977) studied the morphogenesis of the ductal carcinomas by transmission electron microscopy. In normal ducts, the lumen was lined by one layer of epithelial cells of uniform height. The luminal cell surfaces in carcinomas were of varying shapes, projected into the lumen to different degrees, and were covered by numerous microvilli. The microvilli had a well-developed glycocalyx (Fig. 11). Adenocarcinoma of the pancreas in rats has been induced with azaserine (Longnecker and Curphey, 1975). By electron microscopy, the most highly differentiated cells in tumor nodules retained the ultrastructural organization and appearance of normal acinar cells. In less-differentiated tumors, there was decreased zymogen production, loss of cell polarity, and loss of acinar pattern.

439

SOME
EFFECTS OF
CARCINOGENS
ON CELL
ORGANELLES

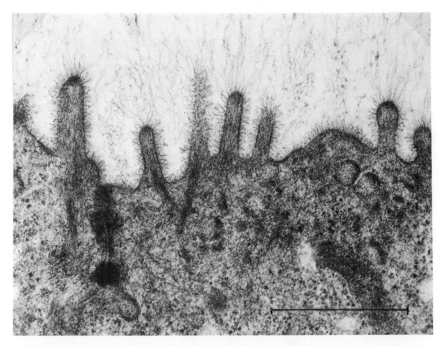

FIGURE 11. Luminal membrane of chemically induced duct carcinoma of the pancreas showing well-developed glycocalyx. ×36,000. Courtesy of Levitt *et al.* (1977).

Even cells with little or no zymogen granules tended to retain moderate amounts of RER and prominent Golgi vesicles. Zymogen granules sometimes had bizarre cylindrical or angular shapes and were smaller than normal. The authors concluded that in this system, the tumors were most likely of acinar cell origin.

Atypical nodules, probably representing preneoplastic acinar cell carcinoma, have also been produced in rats given 4-hydroxyaminoquinoline-1-oxide (Shinozuka *et al.*, 1976). Zymogen granules in the nodules appeared as vesicles of extreme electron lucency similar to those of embryonic pancreas. Some of the granules appeared as empty vacuoles while others contained a pale gray interior.

In view of the high incidence of lung cancer in humans, several experimental models for chemical induction of malignancies of the respiratory tract in laboratory animals have been developed (Saffiotti, 1969; Nettesheim and Griesemer, 1978). A model that has been extensively studied by electron microscopy is that using benzo[*a*]pyrene and ferric oxide in hamsters (Saffiotti *et al.*, 1968). Harris *et al.* (1971) studied the pathogenesis of epithelial hyperplasia and squamous metaplasia in Syrian hamsters given several instillations of benzo[*a*]pyrene and ferric oxide. After 10 intratracheal instillations of the carcinogen, there were wide-spread focal squamous metaplasia and cellular atypia of tracheobronchial epithelium. Ultrastructural examination revealed polygonal cells with no evidence of mucus or ciliated differentiation. Desmosomes with abnormally long

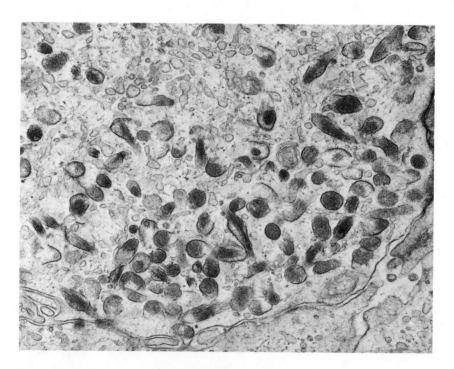

Figure 12. Atypical tracheobronchial epithelium from a hamster given 10 instillations of benzo[*a*]pyrene + ferric oxide. The cytoplasm contains numerous filamentous granules. ×2900. Courtesy of Harris *et al.* (1971).

filaments were present and the cytoplasm contained many lysosomes, few mitochondria, and numerous membrane-bound filamentous granules occurring singly or as dense perinuclear bundles (Fig. 12). These unusual granules were also described by Frasca *et al.* (1968*a*) as occurring infrequently in the bronchial epithelium of normal dogs and frequently in smoking dogs (Frasca *et al.*, 1968*b*). It was suggested that these structures may be abnormal internalized cilia, a secretory product, or degenerating mitochondria. Nucleoli were enlarged, pleomorphic, and some contained microspherules, while others showed micro-segregation (Fig. 13). In summary, the atypical squamous cells produced by benzo[*a*]pyrene+ferric oxide had ultrastructural features similar to those in epithelia of bronchi of smoking dogs and in neoplastic squamous cells in human bronchogenic carcinoma. In a later study (Harris *et al.*, 1972) by light microscopy, squamous metaplasia (without cell atypia) due to vitamin A deficiency was morphologically similar to that caused by the administration of benzo[*a*]pyrene+ ferric oxide. At the ultrastructural level, however, differences were observed. Defects in basement membrane, enlarged nuclei with cytoplasmic invaginations, and pleomorphic nucleoli were restricted to those areas of squamous metaplasia induced by benzo[*a*]pyrene+ferric oxide. Harris *et al.* (1973*a*) also found that after 10 instillations of *N*-methyl-*N*-nitrosourea, the ultrastructural responses in tracheobronchial epithelium of hamsters were similar to those due to benzo[*a*]pyrene+ferric oxide as well as those described in smoking dogs and in

441

SOME
EFFECTS OF
CARCINOGENS
ON CELL
ORGANELLES

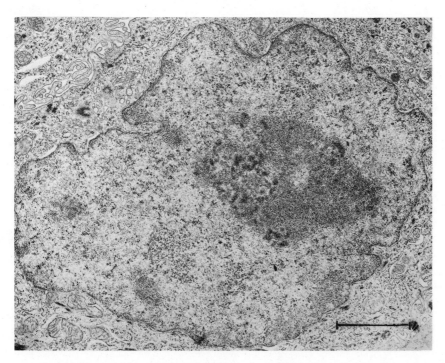

FIGURE 13. Atypical tracheobronchial epithelium from a hamster given 10 instillations of benzo[*a*]pyrene+ferric oxide. There is microsegregation of the nucleus. ×10,900. Courtesy of Harris *et al.* (1971).

human bronchogenic carcinoma. The squamous metaplastic changes induced by N-methyl-N-nitrosourea, like those due to benzo[a]pyrene + ferric oxide, were clearly distinguishable from squamous metaplasia due to simple vitamin A deficiency. Four months after N-methyl-N-nitrosourea, some epithelial cells of tracheobronchial epithelium showed microsegregation. It is of interest that in hamster tracheobronchial epithelium, nucleolar microsegregation occurs after administration of either of two carcinogens, N-methyl-N-nitrosourea or benzó[a]pyrene + ferric oxide, indicating that this alteration is not limited to liver cells.

In tracheobronchial epithelium of hamsters, tritiated benzo[a]pyrene was localized primarily in the heterochromatin as seen by electron autoradiography (Harris *et al.*, 1973b). Human bronchial mucosa has the ability to form metabolites of benzo[a]pyrene that bind to macromolecules, including DNA (Harris *et al.*, 1976).

An additional abnormal spectrum of changes occurs in cilia of hamsters treated with benzo[a]pyrene + ferric oxide (Harris *et al.*, 1974a). These consist of large cilia with multiple axial filaments, aberrant genesis of cilia at the luminal surface and in abnormal locations near the basal lamina. Serial sections showed that some cilia projected into closed intercellular spaces while others projected into adjacent cells. Intracellular cilia were also observed.

ACKNOWLEDGMENTS

The studies from the authors' laboratories were supported in part by Grants CA-5680 and GM-23750 from the United States Public Health Service. We thank the editors and publishers of the *American Journal of Pathology* and of *Cancer Research* for permission to publish Figures 9, 10, 11 and 8, 12, 13, respectively. We thank Lynne Schmutz and Ella Olson for assistance in preparation of the manuscript.

5. References

AGRELO, C., 1978, The effect of carcinogens on the nuclear size of HeLa cells, *Toxicology* **9**:21.

ALLISON, A., 1969, Lysosomes and cancer, in: *Lysosomes in Biology and Pathology*, Vol. 2 (J. L. Dingle and H. Fell, eds.), pp. 178–204, American Elsevier, New York.

ALLISON, A., AND MALLUCCI, L., 1964, Lysosomes in dividing cells, with special reference to lymphocytes, *Lancet* **2**:1371.

ALTHOFF, J., POUR, P., MALICK, L., AND WILSON, R., 1976, Pancreatic neoplasms induced in Syrian golden hamsters. I. Scanning electron microscopic observations, *Am. J. Pathol.* **83**:517.

ANDERSON, H., NEHRING, E., AND WICHSER, W., 1975, Aflatoxin contamination of corn in the field, *J. Agric. Food Chem.* **23**:775.

ANGHILERI, L., HEIDBREDEN, M., WEILER, G., AND DERMIETZEL, R., 1977, Hepatocarcinogenesis by thioacetamide: Correlations of histological and biochemical changes, and possible role of cell injury, *Exp. Cell Biol.* **45**:34.

APFFEL, C., 1978, The endoplasmic reticulum membrane system and malignant neoplasia, in *Progress in Experimental Tumor Research*, Vol. 22 (D. Walbach, ed.), pp. 317–362, Karger, Basel.

ARSTILA, A., AND TRUMP, B., 1972, Ethionine induced alterations in the Golgi apparatus and in the endoplasmic reticulum, *Virchows Arch. B* **10**:344.

BANNASCH, P., 1968, The cytoplasm of hepatocytes during carcinogenesis. Electron and light micro-scopical investigations of the nitrosomorpholine-intoxicated rat liver, *Recent Results Cancer Res.* **19**:1.

BAUER, L., TALUSAN, A., AND MULLER, E., 1972, Ultrastructural changes produced by the carcinogen, aflatoxin B₁, in different tissues, *Virchows Arch. B* **10**:275.

BERG, T., AND CHRISTOFFERSEN, T., 1974, Early changes induced by 2-acetylaminofluorene in lysosomes in rat liver parenchymal cells, *Biochem. Pharmacol.* **23**:3323.

BERNHARD, W., FRAYSSINET, C., LAFARGE, C., AND LEBRETON, E., 1965, Lesions nucleolaires precoces provoquees par l'aflatoxine dans les cellules hepatiques du rat, *C. R. Acad. Sci.* **261**:1785.

BORENFREUND, E., AND HIGGINS, P., 1979, Aggregates of intermediate type filaments in carcinogen-induced cytoplasmic lesions in rat liver cells, *In Vitro* **15**:228 (abstract No. 278).

BRANDES, D., SLOAN, K., ANTON, E., AND BLOEDORN, F., 1967, The effects of X-irradiation on the lysosomes of mouse mammary gland carcinoma, *Cancer Res.* **27**:731.

BUSCH, H., AND SMETANA, K., 1970, *The Nucleolus*, Academic Press, New York.

BUTLER, W., 1966, Early hepatic parenchymal changes induced in the rat by aflatoxin B₁, *Am. J. Pathol.* **49**:113.

BUTLER, W., AND HARD, G., 1976, Chemical carcinogenesis: Early biological responses in induced carcinogenesis in the kidney, in: *The Prediction of Chronic Toxicity from Short Term Studies*, Proceedings of the European Society of Toxicology, Vol. 17 (W. Dundan, B. Leonard, and M. Brunaud, eds.), pp. 34–38, American Elsevier, New York.

BUTLER, W., AND LIJINSKY, W., 1970, Acute toxicity of aflatoxin G₁ to the rat, *J. Pathol.* **102**:209.

BUTLER, W., GREENBLATT, M., AND LIJINSKY, W., 1969, Carcinogenesis in rats by aflatoxins B₁, G₁ and B₂, *Cancer Res.* **29**:2206.

CAMPBELL, T., SINNHUBER, R., LEE, D., WALES, J., AND SALAMAT, L., 1974, Hepatocarcinogenic material in urine specimens from humans consuming aflatoxin, *J. Natl. Cancer Inst.* **52**:1647.

CLIFFORD, J., AND REES, J., 1966, Aflatoxin: A site of action in the rat liver cell, *Nature (London)* **209**:312.

CLOYD, M., AND BIGNER, D., 1977, Surface morphology of normal and neoplastic rat cells, *Am. J. Pathol.* **88**:29.

COLLARD, J., AND TEMMINK, J., 1976, Surface morphology and agglutinability with concanavalin A in normal and transformed murine fibroblasts, *J. Cell Biol.* **68**:101.

DATE, P., GOTHOSKAR, S., AND BHIDE, S., 1976, Effect of partial hepatectomy on tumor incidence and metabolism of mice fed thioacetamide, *J. Natl. Cancer Inst.* **56**:493.

DERENZINI, M., AND MOYNE, G., 1978, The nucleolar origin of certain perichromatin-like granules: A study with alpha-amanitin, *J. Ultrastruct. Res.* **62**:213.

DOBRE, M., MORARU, I., COTUTIU, C., AND MOTOC, F., 1976, Nuclear inclusions and other ultrastructural aspects in the liver of animals treated with N-2-acetylaminofluorene, *Pathol. Eur.* **11**:63.

EMMELOT, P., 1973, Biochemical properties of normal and neoplastic cell surfaces: A review, *Eur. J. Cancer* **9**:319.

EMMELOT, P., AND BENEDETTI, E., 1961, Some observations on the effect of liver carcinogens on the fine structure and function of the endoplasmic reticulum of rat liver, in: *Protein Biosynthesis* (R. Harris, ed.), pp. 99–123, Academic Press, New York.

EPSTEIN, S., ITO, N., MERKOW, L., AND FARBER, E., 1967, Cellular analysis of liver carcinogenesis: The induction of large hyperplastic nodules in the liver with 2-fluorenylacetamide or ethionine and some aspects of their morphology and glycogen metabolism, *Cancer Res.* **27**:1702.

FARBER, E., 1963, Ethionine carcinogenesis, *Adv. Cancer Res.* **7**:383.

FIRMINGER, H., AND MULAY, A., 1952, Histochemical and morphologic differentiation of induced tumors of the liver in rats, *J. Natl. Cancer Inst.* **13**:19.

FLAKS, B., 1970, Changes in the fine structure of rat hepatocytes during the early phases of chronic 2-acetylaminofluorene intoxication, *Chem. Biol. Interact.* **2**:129.

FLAKS, B., 1971, Fine structure of rat hepatocytes during the late phase of chronic 2-acetyl-aminofluorene intoxication, *Chem. Biol. Interact.* **3**:157.

FOUTS, J., AND ROGERS, L., 1965, Morphological changes in the liver accompanying stimulation of microsomal drug metabolizing enzyme activity by phenobarbital, chlordane, benzpyrene or methyl-cholanthrene in rats, *J. Pharmacol. Exp. Ther.* **147**:112.

FRASCA, J., AUERBACH, O., PARKS, V., AND JAMIESON, J., 1968a, Electron microscopic observations of the bronchial epithelium of dogs. I. Control dogs, *Exp. Mol. Pathol.* **9**:363.

FRASCA, J., AUERBACH, O., PARKS, V., AND JAMIESON, J., 1968b, Electron microscopic observations of the bronchial epithelium of dogs. II. Smoking dogs, *Exp. Mol. Pathol.* **9**:380.

443

SOME
EFFECTS OF
CARCINOGENS
ON CELL
ORGANELLES

FRIEDELL, G., JACOBS, J., NAGY, G., AND COHEN, S., 1977, The pathogenesis of bladder cancer, *Am. J. Pathol.* **89**:431.

FRIEND, D., AND FARQUHAR, M., 1967, Functions of coated vesicles during protein absorption in the rat vas deferens, *J. Cell Biol.* **35**:357.

FULLER, G., SPOONCER, W., KING, A., SCHADE, J., AND MACKEY, B., 1977, Survey of aflatoxins in California tree nuts, *J. Am. Oil Chem. Soc.* **54**:231A.

HARRIS, C., SPORN, M., KAUFMAN, D., SMITH, J., BAKER, M., AND SAFFIOTTI, U., 1971, Acute ultrastructural effects of benzo(*a*)pyrene and ferric oxide on the hamster tracheobronchial epithelium, *Cancer Res.* **31**:1977.

HARRIS, C., SPORN, M., KAUFMAN, D., SMITH, J., JACKSON, F., AND SAFFIOTTI, U., 1972, Histogenesis of squamous metaplasia in the hamster tracheal epithelium caused by vitamin A deficiency or benzo[*a*]pyrene–ferric oxide, *J. Natl. Cancer Inst.* **48**:743.

HARRIS, C., KAUFMAN, D., SPORN, M., SMITH, J., JACKSON, F., AND SAFFIOTTI, U., 1973*a*, Ultrastructural effects of *N*-methyl-*N*-nitrosourea on the tracheobronchial epithelium of the Syrian golden hamster, *Int. J. Cancer* **12**:259.

HARRIS, C., KAUFMAN, D., SPORN, M., BOREN, H., JACKSON, F., SMITH, J., PAULEY, J., DEDICK, P., AND SAFFIOTTI, U., 1973*b*, Localization of benzo(*a*)pyrene-^{3}H and alterations in nuclear chromatin caused by benzo(*a*)pyrene–ferric oxide in the hamster respiratory epithelium, *Cancer Res.* **33**:2842.

HARRIS, C., KAUFMAN, D., JACKSON, F., SMITH, J., DEDICK, P., AND SAFFIOTTI, U., 1974*a*, Atypical cilia in the tracheobronchial epithelium of the hamster during respiratory carcinogenesis, *J. Pathol.* **114**:17.

HARRIS, J., PRICE, M., AND WILLISON, M., 1974*b*, A comparative study on rat liver and hepatoma nuclear membranes, *J. Ultrastruct. Res.* **48**:17.

HARRIS, C., FRANK, A., VAN HAAFTEN, C., KAUFMAN, D., CONNOR, R., JACKSON, F., BARRETT, L., McDOWELL, E., AND TRUMP, B., 1976, Binding of [^{3}H]benzo[*a*]pyrene to DNA in cultured human bronchus, *Cancer Res.* **36**:1011.

HAVEL, J., AND KANE, J., 1973, Drugs and lipid metabolism, *Annu. Rev. Pharmacol.* **13**:287.

HERDSON, P., GARVIN, P., AND JENNINGS, R., 1964, Reversible biological and fine structural changes produced in rat liver by a thiohydantoin compound, *Lab. Invest.* **13**:1014.

HERROLD, K., 1969, Aflatoxin induced lesions in Syrian hamsters, *Br. J. Cancer* **23**:655.

HESS, R., STAUBLI, W., AND RIESS, W., 1965, Nature of the hepatomegalic effect produced by ethyl-chlorophenoxy-isobutyrate in the rat, *Nature (London)* **208**:856.

HICKS, R., 1976, Changes in differentiation of the urinary bladder during benign and neoplastic hyperplasia, in *Progress in Differentiation Research* (N. Muller-Berat, C. Rosenfeld, D. Tarin, and D. Viza, eds.), pp. 339–353, North-Holland, Amsterdam.

HICKS, R., AND WAKEFIELD, J., 1976, Membrane changes during urothelial hyperplasia and neoplasia, *Cancer Res.* **36**:2502.

HIRAO, K., MATSUMURA, K., IMAGAWA, A., ENOMOTO, Y., HOSOGI, Y., KANI, T., FUGIKAWA, K., AND ITO, N., 1974, Primary neoplasms in dog liver induced by diethylnitrosamine, *Cancer Res.* **34**:1870.

HODGES, G., HICKS, R., AND SPACEY, G., 1976, Scanning electron microscopy of cell-surface changes in methylnitrosourea (MNU)-treated rat bladders *in vivo* and *in vitro*, *Differentiation* **6**:143.

HRUBAN, Z., SWIFT, H., DUNN, F., AND LEWIS, D., 1965, Effect of β-3-furylalanine on the ultrastructure of the hepatocytes and pancreatic acinar cells, *Lab. Invest.* **14**:70.

JACOBS, J., ARAI, M., COHEN, S., AND FRIEDELL, G., 1976*a*, Early lesions in experimental bladder cancer: Scanning electron microscopy of cell surface markers, *Cancer Res.* **36**:2512.

JACOBS, J., ARAI, M., COHEN, S., AND FRIEDELL, G., 1976*b*, Light and scanning electron microscopy of exfoliated bladder epithelial cells in rats fed *N*-[4-(5-nitro-2-furyl)-2-thiazolyl]formamide, *J. Natl. Cancer Inst.* **57**:63.

JACOBS, J., ARAI, M., COHEN, S., AND FRIEDELL, G., 1977, A long term study of reversible and progressive urinary bladder cancer lesions in rats fed *N*-[4-(5-nitro-2-furyl)-2-thiazolyl]formamide, *Cancer Res.* **37**:2817.

KAHAN, B., RUTZKY, L., KAHAN, A., OYASU, R., WISEMAN, F., AND LeGRUE, S., 1977, Cell surface changes associated with malignant transformation of bladder epithelium *in vitro*, *Cancer Res.* **37**:2866.

KARASAKI, S., 1969, The fine structure of proliferating cells in preneoplastic rat livers during azo-dye carcinogenesis, *J. Cell Biol.* **40**:322.

KETTERER, B., HOLT, S., AND ROSS-MANSELL, P., 1967, The effect of a single intraperitoneal dose of the hepatocarcinogen 4-dimethylaminoazobenzene on the rough-surfaced endoplasmic reticulum of the liver of the rat, *Biochem. J.* **103**:692.

445

SOME
EFFECTS OF
CARCINOGENS
ON CELL
ORGANELLES

KIM, C., KIM, D., AND LEE, Y., 1972, Fine structural changes and autoradiographic studies of rat liver cells induced by aflatoxin B_1 and G_1, *Yonsei Med. J.* **13**:1.

KINGSBURY, J., 1964, *Poisonous Plants of the U.S. and Canada*, pp. 425–435, Prentice–Hall, Englewood Cliffs, N.J.

KOSHIBA, K., THIRUMALACHARY, C., DASKAL, Y., AND BUSCH, H., 1971, Ultrastructural and biochemical studies on ribonucleoprotein particles from isolated nucleoli of thioacetamide-treated rat liver, *Exp. Cell Res.* **68**:235.

KOSS, L., 1977, Some ultrastructural aspects of experimental and human carcinoma of the bladder, *Cancer Res.* **37**:2824.

KRISHNAMACHARI, K., NAGARAJAN, V., BHAT, R., AND TILAK, T., 1975, Hepatitis due to aflatoxicosis: An outbreak in Western India, *Lancet* **1**:1061.

LaFONTAINE, J., AND ALLARD, C., 1964, A light and electron microscope study of the morphological changes induced in rat liver cells by the azo dye 2-Me-DAB, *J. Cell Biol.* **22**:143.

LAZAROW, P., 1978, Rat liver perixosomes catalyze the β-oxidation of fatty acids, *J. Biol. Chem.* **253**:1522.

LEE, K., AND GOODALL, C., 1968, Methylation of ribonucleic acid and deoxyribonucleic acid and tumour induction in livers of hypophysectomized rats treated with dimethylnitrosamine, *Biochem. J.* **106**:767.

LEVITT, M., HARRIS, C., SQUIRE, R., SPRINGER, S., WENK, M., MOLLELO, C., THOMAS, D., KINGSBURY, E., AND NEWKIRK, C., 1977, Experimental pancreatic carcinogenesis. I. Morphogenesis of pancreatic adenocarcinoma in the Syrian golden hamster induced by *N*-nitroso-bis(2-hydroxypropyl)amine, *Am. J. Pathol.* **88**:5.

LILLEHOJ, E., KWOLEK, W., FENNELL, D., AND MILBURN, M., 1975*a*, Aflatoxin incidence and association with bright greenish-yellow fluorescence and insect damage in a limited survey of freshly harvested high-moisture corn, *Cereal Chem.* **52**:403.

LILLEHOJ, E., KWOLEK, W., SHANNON, G., SHOTWELL, O., AND HESSELTINE, C., 1975*b*, Aflatoxin occurrence in 1973 field corn. I. A limited survey in the southeastern U.S., *Cereal Chem.* **52**:603.

LILLEHOJ, E., FENNELL, D., AND KWOLEK, W., 1976, *Aspergillus flavus* and aflatoxin in Iowa corn before harvest, *Science* **193**:495.

LIN, J., LIU, C., AND SVOBODA, D., 1974, Long term effects of aflatoxin B_1 and viral hepatitis on marmoset liver. A prelimanry report, *Lab. Invest.* **30**:267.

LINSELL, C., AND PEERS, F., 1977, Aflatoxin and liver cell cancer, *Trans. R. Soc. Trop. Med. Hyg.* **71**:471.

LONGNECKER, D., AND CURPHEY, T., 1975, Adenocarcinoma of the pancreas in azaserine-treated rats, *Cancer Res.* **35**:2249.

LOUD, A., 1968, A quantitative stereological description of the ultrastructure of normal rat liver parenchymal cells, *J. Cell Biol.* **37**:27.

LOURIA, D., FINKEL, G., SMITH, J., AND BUSE, M., 1974, Aflatoxin-induced tumors in mice, *Sabouraudia* **12**:371.

MAGEE, P., 1963, Cellular injury and chemical carcinogenesis by *N*-nitroso compounds, in: *Cancer Progress*, Vol. 1963 (R. Raven, ed). pp. 56–66, Butterworths, London.

MAGEE, P., AND BARNES, J., 1967, Carcinogenic nitroso compounds, in: *Advances in Cancer Research*, Vol. 10 (A. Hadlow and S. Weinhouse, eds.), pp. 163–246, Academic Press, New York.

MAINI, M., AND STICH, H., 1961, Chromosomes of tumor cells. II. Effects of various liver carcinogens on mitosis of hepatic cells, *J. Natl. Cancer Inst.* **26**:1413.

MASTERS, C., AND HOLMES, R., 1977, Peroxisomes: New aspects of cell physiology and biochemistry, *Physiol. Rev.* **57**:816.

MASTERS, C., AND HOLMES, R., 1979, Peroxisomes—Their metabolic roles in mammalian tissues, *Trends Biochem. Sci.* **4**:233.

MCLEAN, E., 1970, The toxic actions of pyrrolizidine (*Senecio*) alkaloids, *Pharmacol. Rev.* **22**:429.

MELDOLESI, J., CLEMENTI, F., CHIESARA, E., CONTI, F., AND FANTI, A., 1967, Cytoplasmic changes in rat liver after prolonged treatment with low doses of ethionine and adenine, *Lab. Invest.* **17**:265.

MIYAI, K., AND RITCHIE, A., 1970, Natural resolution of hepatic ultrastructural changes induced by DL-ethionine, *Am. J. Pathol.* **61**:211.

MIYAI, K., AND STEINER, J., 1965, Fine structure of interphase liver cell nuclei in subacute ethionine intoxication, *Exp. Mol. Pathol.* **4**:525.

MONNERON, A., 1969, Experimental induction of helical polysomes in adult rat liver, *Lab. Invest.* **20**:178.

MONNERON, A., LIEW, C., AND ALLFREY, V., 1971, Isolation and biological activity of mammalian helical polyribosomes, *J. Mol. Biol.* **57**:335.

MUKHERJEE, T., GUSTAFSSON, R., AFZELIUS, B., AND ARRHENIUS, E., 1963, Effects of carcinogenic amines on amino acid incorporation by liver systems. II. A morphological and biochemical study on the effect of dimethylnitrosamine, Cancer Res. 23:944.

NAIR, V., CASPER, R., SIEGEL, S., AND BAU, D., 1970, Regulation of the diurnal rhythm in hepatic drug metabolism, Fed. Proc. 29:804 (abstract).

NETTESHEIM, P., AND GRIESEMER, R., 1978, Experimental models for studies of respiratory tract carcinogenesis, in: Pathogenesis and Therapy of Lung Cancer (C. Harris, ed.), pp. 75–188, Dekker, New York.

NEWBERNE, P., AND WOGAN, G., 1968, Sequential morphologic changes in aflatoxin B_1 carcinogenesis in the rat, Cancer Res. 28:770.

NEWMAN, J., AND HICKS, R., 1977, Detection of neoplastic and preneoplastic urothelia by combined scanning and transmission electron microscopy of urinary surface on human and rat bladders, Histopathology 1:125.

NICOLSON, G., 1976, Transmembrane control of the receptors on normal and tumor cells. I. Cytoplasmic influence over cell surface components, Biochim. Biophys. Acta 457:57.

NIGAM, V., 1965, Glycogen metabolism in liver during DAB carcinogenesis, Br. J. Cancer 19:912.

NOVIKOFF, A., 1976, The endoplasmic reticulum: A cytochemist's view (a review), Proc. Natl. Acad. Sci. USA 73:2781.

NOVIKOFF, A., AND SHIN, W., 1964, The endoplasmic reticulum in the Golgi zone and its relation to microbodies, Golgi apparatus and autophagic vacuoles in rat liver cells, J. Microsc. (Oxford) 3:187.

NOYES, W., 1975, Aflatoxin-induced changes in human hepatocytes in organ culture, Proc. Am. Assoc. Cancer Res. 16:26.

OKAZAKI, K., SHULL, K., AND FARBER, E., 1968, Effects of ethionine on adenosine triphosphate levels and ionic composition of liver cell nuclei, J. Biol. Chem. 243:4661.

OLASON, D., AND SMUCKLER, E., 1976, Changes in hepatic nuclei induced by acetamide and thioacetamide, Arch. Pathol. Lab. Med. 100:415.

OPIE, E. L., 1944, The pathogenesis of tumors of the liver produced by butter yellow, J. Exp. Med. 80:231.

ORRENIUS, S., AND ERICSSON, J., 1966, On the relationship of liver glucose-6-phosphatase to the proliferation of endoplasmic reticulum in phenobarbital induction, J. Cell Biol. 31:243.

PAUL, J., ROSS, W., AND MONTGOMERY, P., JR., 1971, Ulstrastructural nucleolar segregation and carcinogenicity among the 4-nitroquinoline-1-oxides, J. Natl. Cancer Inst. 47:367.

PEERS, F., GILMAN, G., AND LINSELL, C., 1976, Dietary aflatoxins and human liver cancer. A study in Swaziland, Int. J. Cancer 17:167.

PITOT, H., 1964, Altered template stability: The molecular mark of malignancy? Perspect. Biol. Med. 8:50.

POKROVSKY, A., KRAVCHENKO, L., AND TUTELYAN, V., 1972, Comparative study of the effect of aflatoxin and some antitumour antibiotics on rat liver lysosomes in vivo and in vitro, Biochem. Pharmacol. 21:2489.

PONG, R., AND WOGAN, G., 1970, Time course and dose–response characteristics of aflatoxin B_1 effects on rat liver polymerase and ultrastructure, Cancer Res. 30:294.

PORTER, K., AND BRUNI, C., 1959, An electron microscope study of the early effects of 3'-Me-DAB on rat liver cells, Cancer Res. 19:997.

PORTER, K., PRESCOTT, D., AND FRYE, J., 1973, Changes in surface morphology of Chinese hamster ovary cells during the cell cycle, J. Cell Biol. 57:815.

POUR, P., KRUGER, F., CHEM, D., ALTHOFF, J., CARDESA, A., AND MOHR, U., 1974, Cancer of the pancreas induced in the Syrian golden hamster, Am. J. Pathol. 76:349.

POUR, P., KRUGER, F., ALTHOFF, J., CARDESA, A., AND MOHR, U., 1975, A new approach for induction of pancreatic neoplasms, Cancer Res. 35:2259.

PURCHASE, I., AND VORSTER, L., 1968, Aflatoxin in commercial milk samples, S. Afr. Med. J. 42:219.

RAO, M., AND REDDY, J., 1978, Malignant tumors in rats fed lasiocarpine, Br. J. Cancer 37:289.

RAO, M., AND REDDY, J., 1979, Transplantable acinar cell carcinoma of the rat pancreas. Morphologic and biochemical characterization, Am. J. Pathol. 94:333.

RAO, M., SVOBODA, D., AND REDDY, J., 1974, The ultrastructural effects of aflatoxin B_1 in the rat pancreas, Virchows Arch. B 17:149.

REDDY, J., AND QURESHI, S., 1979, Tumorigenicity of the hypolipidaemic peroxisome proliferator ethyl-α-p-chlorophenoxyisobutyrate (clofibrate) in rats, Br. J. Cancer 40:476.

REDDY, J., AND RAO, M., 1977a, Malignant tumors in rats fed nafenopin, a hepatic peroxisome proliferator, J. Natl. Cancer Inst. 59:1645.

447

SOME
EFFECTS OF
CARCINOGENS
ON CELL
ORGANELLES

REDDY, J., AND RAO, M., 1977*b*, Transplantable pancreatic carcinoma of the rat, *Science* **198**:78.

REDDY, J., AND RAO, M., 1978, Enhancement by Wy-14,643, a hepatic peroxisome proliferator, of diethylnitrosamine-initiated hepatic tumorigenesis in the rat, *Br. J. Cancer* **38**:537.

REDDY, J., AND SVOBODA, D., 1968, The relationship of nucleolar segregation to ribonucleic acid synthesis following the administration of selected hepatocarcinogens, *Lab. Invest.* **19**:132.

REDDY, J., AND SVOBODA, D., 1972, Effect of lasiocarpine on aflatoxin B₁ carcinogenicity in rat liver, *Arch. Pathol.* **93**:55.

REDDY, J., CHIGA, M., AND SVOBODA, D., 1969, Initiation of the division cycle of rat hepatocytes following a single injection of thioacetamide, *Lab. Invest.* **20**:405.

REDDY, J., CHIGA, M., BUNYARATVEJ, S., AND SVOBODA, D., 1970, Microbodies in experimentally altered cells. VIII. CPIB-induced hepatic microbody proliferation in the absence of significant catalase synthesis, *J. Cell Biol.* **44**:226.

REDDY, J., SVOBODA, D., AND RAO, M., 1974, Susceptibility of an inbred strain of guinea pigs to the induction of pancreatic adenocarcinoma by *N*-methyl-*N*-nitrosourea, *J. Natl. Cancer Inst.* **52**:991.

REDDY, J., RAO. M., AND JAGO, M., 1976*a*, Rapid development of hyperplastic nodules and cirrhosis in the liver of rats treated concurrently with thioacetamide and the pyrrolizidine alkaloid lasiocarpine, *Int. J. Cancer* **17**:621.

REDDY, J., RAO, M., AND MOODY, D., 1976*b*, Hepatocellular carcinomas in acatalasemic mice treated with nafenopin, a hypolipidemic peroxisome proliferator, *Cancer Res.* **36**:1211.

REDDY, J., SVOBODA, D., AND RAO, M., 1976*c*, Induction of liver tumors by aflatoxin B₁ in the tree shrew (*Tupaia glis*), a nonhuman primate, *Cancer Res.* **36**:151.

REDDY, J., AZARNOFF, D., AND HIGNITE, C., 1979*a*, Hypolipidaemic hepatic peroxisome proliferators form a novel class of chemical carcinogens, *Nature (London)* **283**:397.

REDDY, J., RAO, M., AZARNOFF, D., AND SELL, S., 1979*b*, Mitogenic and carcinogenic effects of a hypolipidemic peroxisome proliferator, [4-chloro-6-(2,3-xylidino)-2-pyrimidinylthio] acetic acid (Wy-14,643), in rat and mouse liver, *Cancer Res.* **29**:152.

REDDY, J., RAO, M., WARREN, J., AND MINNICK, O., 1979*c*, Concanavalin A agglutinability and surface microvilli of dissociated normal and neoplastic pancreatic acinar cells of the rat, *Exp. Cell Res.* **120**:55.

REDDY, J., SCARPELLI, D., AND RAO, M., 1979*d*, Experimental pancreatic carcinogenesis, in: *Advances in Medical Oncology, Research and Education*, Vol. 9 (N. Thatcher, ed.), pp. 99–109, Pergamon Press, Elmsford, N.Y.

REPORT FROM THE COMMITTEE OF PRINCIPAL INVESTIGATORS, 1978, A cooperative trial in the primary prevention of ischaemic heart disease using clofibrate, *Br. Heart J.* **40**:1069.

RUBIN, E., HUTTERER, F., AND LIEBER, C., 1968, Ethanol increases hepatic smooth endoplasmic reticulum and drug-metabolizing enzymes, *Science* **159**:1469.

RUEBNER, B., MICHAS, C., KANARJAMA, R., AND BANNASCH, P., 1976, Sequential hepatic histologic and histochemical changes produced by diethylnitrosamine in the rhesus monkey, *J. Natl. Cancer Inst.* **57**:1261.

SACHS, L., 1974, Regulation of membrane changes, differentiation, and malignancy in carcinogenesis, *Harvey Lect.* **68**:1.

SAFFIOTTI, U., 1969, Experimental respiratory tract carcinogenesis, in: *Progress in Experimental Tumor Research*, Vol. 11 (F. Homburger, ed.), pp. 302–333, Karger, Basel.

SAFFIOTTI, U., CEFIS, F., AND KOLB, L., 1968, A method for the experimental induction of bronchogenic carcinoma, *Cancer Res.* **28**:104.

SCOTT, P., AND KENNEDY, B., 1975, The analysis of spices and herbs for aflatoxins, *Can. Inst. Food Sci. Technol. J.* **8**:124.

SCOTT, R., AND FURCHT, L., 1976, Membrane pathology of normal and malignant cells—A review, *Human Pathol.* **7**:519.

SHABAD, L., KOLESNICHENKO, T., AND GOLUB, N., 1975, The effect produced by some carcinogenic nitroso compounds on organ cultures from human embryonic lung and kidney tissues, *Int. J. Cancer* **16**:768.

SHANK, R., 1976, The role of aflatoxin in human disease, *Adv. Chem. Ser.* **149**:51.

SHINOZUKA, H., AND ESTES, L., 1977, Activation of intracisternal A particles in mouse liver by diethylnitrosamine, *J. Natl. Cancer Inst.* **58**:1163.

SHINOZUKA, H., AND FARBER, E., 1969, Reformation of nucleoli after ethionine-induced fragmentation in the absence of significant protein synthesis, *J. Cell Biol.* **41**:280.

SHINOZUKA, H., GOLDBLATT, P., AND FARBER, E., 1968, The disorganization of hepatic cell nucleoli induced by ethionine and its reversal by adenine, *J. Cell Biol.* **36**:313.

SHINOZUKA, H., REID, I., SHULL, K., LIANG, H., AND FARBER, E., 1970, Dynamics of liver cell injury and repair. I. Spontaneous reformation of the nucleolus and polyribosomes in the presence of extensive cytoplasmic damage induced by ethionine, *Lab. Invest.* **23**:253.

SHINOZUKA, H., POPP, J., AND KONISHI, Y., 1976, Ultrastructures of atypical acinar cell nodules in rat pancreas induced by 4-hydroxyaminoquinoline-1-oxide, *Lab. Invest.* **34**:501.

SIMARD, A., AND BERNHARD, W., 1966, Le phenomene de la segregation nucleolaire: specificite d'action de certains antimetabolites, *Int. J. Cancer* **1**:463.

SIMARD, A., AND DAOUST, R., 1966, DNA synthesis and neoplastic transformation in rat liver parenchyma, *Cancer Res.* **26**:1665.

SLATER, T., AND GREENBAUM, A., 1965, Changes in lysosomal enzymes in acute experimental liver injury, *Biochem. J.* **96**:484.

SMITH, E., NOSANCHUK, J., SCHNITZER, B., AND SWARM, R., 1968, Fatty inclusions and microcysts, *Arch. Pathol.* **85**:175.

SPORN, M., DINGMAN, C., PHELPS, H., AND WOGAN, G., 1966, Aflatoxin B_1: Binding to DNA *in vitro* and alteration of RNA metabolism *in vivo*, *Science* **151**:1539.

SPRINGER, E., SMITH, H., AND HACKETT, A., 1979, Quantitative ultrastructure of the cytoplasmic organelles of human carcinoma and non-malignant epithelial cell lines, *In Vitro* **15**:228 (abstract No. 279).

STEINER, J., MIYAI, K., AND PHILLIPS, M., 1964, Electron microscopy of membrane-particle arrays in liver cells of ethionine-intoxicated rats, *Am. J. Pathol.* **44**:169.

SUZANGAR, M., EMAMI, A., AND BARNETT, R., 1977, Aflatoxin contamination of village milk in Isfahan, Iran, *Trop. Sci.* **18**:155.

SVOBODA, D., 1964, Fine structure of hepatomas induced in rats with *p*-dimethylaminoazobenzene, *J. Natl. Cancer Inst.* **33**:315.

SVOBODA, D., AND AZARNOFF, D., 1966, Response of hepatic microbodies to a hypolipidemic agent, ethyl chlorophenoxyisobutyrate (CPIB), *J. Cell Biol.* **30**:442.

SVOBODA, D., AND AZARNOFF, D., 1979, Tumors in male rats fed ethyl chlorophenoxyisobutyrate, a hypolipidemic drug, *Cancer Res.* **39**:3419.

SVOBODA, D., AND HIGGINSON, J., 1968, A comparison of ultrastructural changes in rat liver due to chemical carcinogens, *Cancer Res.* **28**:1703.

SVOBODA, D., AND REDDY, J., 1972, Malignant tumors in rats given lasiocarpine, *Cancer Res.* **32**:908.

SVOBODA, D., AND SOGA, J., 1966, Early effects of pyrrolizidine alkaloids on the fine structure of rat liver cells, *Am. J. Pathol.* **48**:347.

SVOBODA, D., GRADY, H., AND HIGGINSON, J., 1966, Aflatoxin B_1 injury in rat and monkey liver, *Am. J. Pathol.* **49**:1023.

SVOBODA, D., REDDY, J., AND BUNYARATVEJ, S., 1971*a*, Hepatic megalocytosis in chronic lasiocarpine poisoning. Some functional studies, *Am. J. Pathol.* **65**:399.

SVOBODA, D., REDDY, J., AND LIU, C., 1971*b*, Multinucleate giant cells in livers of marmosets given aflatoxin B_1, *Arch. Pathol.* **91**:452.

TATEMATSU, M., COHEN, S., FUKISHIMA, S., SHINOHARA, Y., AND ITO, N., 1977, Vascular changes during rat urinary bladder carcinogenesis induced by *N*-butyl-*N*-(4-hydroxybutyl)nitrosamine, *Gann* **68**:127.

TERAO, K., AND NAKANO, M., 1974, Cholangiofibrosis induced by short-term feeding of 3'-methyl-4-(dimethylamino)azobenzene: An electron microscopic observation, *Gann* **65**:249.

TILAK, T., 1975, Induction of cholangiocarcinoma following treatment of a rhesus monkey with aflatoxin, *Food Cosmet. Toxicol.* **13**:247.

TIMME, A., AND FOWLE, L., 1963, Effects of *p*-dimethylaminoazobenzene on the fine structure of rat liver cells, *Nature (London)* **200**:694.

TUITE, J., AND CALDWELL, R., 1971, Infection of corn seed with *Helminthosporium maydis* and other fungi in 1970, *Plant Dis. Rep.* **55**:387.

VAN RENSBURG, S., VAN DER WATT, J., PURCHASE, I., COUTINHO, L., AND MARKHAM, R., 1974, Primary liver cancer rate and aflatoxin intake in a high cancer area, *S. Afr. Med. J.* **48**:2508A.

VESSELINOVITCH, S., MIHAILOVICH, N., WOGAN, G., LOMBARD, L., AND RAO, K., 1972, Aflatoxin B_1, a hepatocarcinogen in the infant mouse, *Cancer Res.* **32**:2289.

VOLMAN, H., 1978, A morphologic and morphometric study of the mitochondria in several hepatoma cell lines and in isolated hepatocytes, *Virchows Arch. B* **26**:249.

WALBORG, E., JR., STARLING, J., DAVIS, E., HIXSON, D., AND ALLISON, J., 1979, Plasma membrane alterations during carcinogenesis, in: *Carcinogens: Identification and Mechanisms of Action* 31st

449

SOME
EFFECTS OF
CARCINOGENS
ON CELL
ORGANELLES

Annual Symposium on Fundamental Cancer Research (A. C. Griffin and C. R. Shaw eds.), pp. 381–398, Raven Press, New York.

WARD, J., SONTAG, J., WEISBURGER, E., AND BROWN, C., 1975, Effect of life-time exposure to aflatoxin B_1 in rats, *J. Natl. Cancer Inst.* **55**:107.

WARREN, J., SIMMON, V., AND REDDY, J., 1980, Properties of hypolipidemic peroxisome proliferators in the lymphocyte [^{3}H]thymidine and *Salmonella* mutagenesis assays, *Cancer Res.* **40**:36.

WEIBEL, E., STAUBLI, W., GNAGI, R., AND HESS, F., 1969, Correlated morphometric and biochemical studies on the liver cell. I. Morphometric model, stereologic methods, and normal morphometric data for rat liver, *J. Cell Biol.* **42**:68.

WEINSTEIN, R., MERK, F., AND ALROY, J., 1976, The structure and function of intercellular junctions in cancer, *Adv. Cancer Res.* **23**:23.

WILLIAMS, D., AND RABIN, B., 1971, Disruption by carcinogens of the hormone dependent association of membranes with polysomes, *Nature (London)* **232**:102.

WILLIAMS, G., AND HULTIN, T., 1973, Ribosomes of mouse liver following administration of dimethyl-nitrosamine, *Cancer Res.* **33**:1796.

WILLINGHAM, M., AND PASTAN, I., 1975, Cyclic AMP modulates microvillus formation and agglutin-ability in transformed and normal mouse fibroblasts, *Proc. Natl. Acad. Sci. USA* **72**:1263.

WILSON, D., AND FLOWERS, R., 1978, Unavoidable low level aflatoxin contamination of peanuts, *J. Am. Oil Chem. Soc.* **55**:111A.

WINSLOW, D., ROSCOE, J., AND ROWLES, P., 1978, Changes in surface morphology associated with ethylnitrosourea-induced malignant transformation of cultured rat brain cells studied by electron microscopy, *Br. J. Exp. Pathol.* **59**:530.

WOGAN, G., AND PAGLIALUNGA, S., 1974, Carcinogenicity of synthetic aflatoxin M_1 in rats, *Food Cosmet. Toxicol.* **12**:381.

WOGAN, G., PAGLIALUNGA, S., AND NEWBERNE, P., 1974, Carcinogenic effects of low dietary levels of aflatoxin B_1 in rats, *Food Cosmet. Toxicol.* **12**:681.

WONG, J., AND HSIEH, D., 1976, Mutagenicity of aflatoxins related to their metabolism and car-cinogenic potential, *Proc. Natl. Acad. Sci. USA* **73**:2241.

YASUZUMI, G., SUGIHARA, R., ITO, N., KONISHI, Y., AND HIASA, Y., 1970, Fine structure of nuclei as revealed by electron microscopy. VII. Hyperplastic liver nodules in rat induced by 3'-methyl-4-dimethylaminoazobenzene, 2-fluorenylacetamide and DL-ethionine, *Exp. Cell Res.* **63**:83.

ZURETTI, M., AND BACCINO, F., 1975, Biochemical and structural changes of rat liver lysosomes by ethionine, *Exp. Mol. Pathol.* **22**:271.

12

Sequential Aspects of Chemical Carcinogenesis: Skin

Isaac Berenblum

1. Origin of the Concept of Sequential Stages of Skin Carcinogenesis

The first indication that experimental carcinogenesis could be augmented by the addition of noncarcinogenic stimuli resulted from scarification of mouse skin combined with, or following, tar painting (Deelman, 1924; Deelman and van Erp, 1926), and later, from combined applications of carcinogenic hydrocarbons with (noncarcinogenic) creosote oil (Sall *et al.*, 1940). But the establishment of sequential stages in carcinogenesis arose by the convergence of two subsequent lines of inquiry.

The primary aim in the one case was to explain why skin papillomas, *induced in the rabbit ear*, tended so often to regress, but also to answer the more basic question of whether such apparently unstable growth was truly neoplastic (Rous and Kidd, 1941; MacKenzie and Rous, 1941; see also Meyenburg and Fritsche, 1943; Friedewald and Rous, 1944*a,b*, 1950). The aim in the other case was to study the nature of the newly discovered cocarcinogenic action of croton oil on *mouse* skin (Berenblum, 1941*a*), and at the more fundamental level, to determine the nature of the functional changes in the tissues during the long latent period of carcinogenesis (Berenblum, 1941*b*; see also Mottram, 1944*a,b*; Berenblum and Shubik, 1947*a,b*, 1949*a,b*; Salaman, 1952).

In the rabbit experiments, papillomas that had regressed could be made to reappear at the identical sites by punching holes in the ear, or by applications

Isaac Berenblum • The Weizmann Institute of Science, Rehovot, Israel.

of turpentine or chloroform. This led Rous and his associates to conclude (1) that foci of tumor cells, no longer visible to the naked eye, remained in a "latent" or dormant state, capable of being "reawakened," and (2) that the induction process and the subsequent growth process involved independent mechanisms—referred to as "initiation" and "promotion."

In the mouse experiments, the cocarcinogen, croton oil, was found capable of enhancing tumor induction when applied *after* a subeffective dose of carcinogenic hydrocarbon, *but not when applied beforehand*. This was taken to mean that the starting of the carcinogenic process and its completion involved separate mechanisms—referred to at the time as "precarcinogenic" and "epicarcinogenic," respectively, with yet a third stage, "metacarcinogenic," responsible for the subsequent transformation of benign papillomas into malignant tumors (Berenblum, 1941b).

Although the two series of experiments were apparently related in the interpretative sense, they did differ in two important respects.

1. In the rabbit experiments, the primary action (initiation) was continued long enough for tumors to appear, while the secondary action (promotion) caused those once regressed to reappear. In the mouse experiments, the primary action (precarcinogenic) was insufficient to produce tumors, while the secondary action (epicarcinogenic) caused visible tumors to appear for the first time.
2. In the rabbit experiments, the secondary action was nonspecific; in the mouse experiments, a specific kind of action (by croton oil) was required, many other skin irritants proving ineffective (see Section 5).

Nevertheless, in the interest of conformity, a single terminology—of initiation and promotion, as proposed by Rous and associates—became accepted for both kinds of effects.

The early studies on sequential stages of skin carcinogenesis, briefly outlined above, have been extensively reviewed by Berenblum (1944, 1954a,b), Saffiotti and Shubik (1963), and Boutwell (1964). For more recent development, see reviews by Hecker (1968, 1971a), Van Duuren (1969, 1976), Berenblum (1969, 1978, 1979), Boutwell (1974, 1978), Stenbäck *et al.* (1974), Yuspa *et al.* (1976a), Van Duuren *et al.* (1978), Scribner and Süss (1978), and Sivak (1979).

2. Quantitative Analysis of the Two-Stage Mechanism

The initiation–promotion hypothesis, as applied to mouse skin, with croton oil as promoting agent, lent itself to quantitative analysis: If tumor induction consisted of an initial transformation of a normal cell into a dormant tumor cell, and if the "dormancy" of the latter had to be overcome by a different kind of action, then the following premises could be formulated and submitted to experimental testing.

1. The initiating phase—if resulting from a cell mutation—should be completed rapidly, while most of the long latent period of carcinogenesis should be taken up with the promoting phase.
2. The total tumor incidence should be determined by the potency of the initiating stimulus, while the speed of action (i.e., the actual latent period) might depend more on the efficiency and persistence of the promoting action.
3. If the conversion, by initiating action, of a normal cell into a dormant tumor cell is essentially an irreversible process—a valid assumption if brought about by a mutation—then a delay in the interval between completion of initiating action and the start of promoting action should not seriously affect the incidence of tumors but merely cause a corresponding delay in their times of appearance.
4. Since promoting action could only operate on cells already transformed by initiating action, reversal of the procedure, i.e., applying the promoting agent before the initiating agent, should be ineffective in producing tumors.

The experimental model for the detailed study of the initiating–promoting system originally involved eight weekly applications of a carcinogenic hydrocarbon followed by twice weekly applications of croton oil for several months (Berenblum, 1941b). Mottram (1944a,b) then introduced a useful simplification by demonstrating that a single application of the carcinogen was sufficient for initiating action. Quantitative analysis of the results thus became easier to interpret. [The use of urethan as a "pure" initiator for skin carcinogenesis (see Section 4) and phorbol esters as promoter (see Section 5) provided further refinements of the technique in later experiments.]

An early attempt to determine the time required for initiating action involved removal of the hydrocarbon with appropriate solvents after brief intervals (followed by standard croton oil treatment). As short a time as 15 min proved adequate (Ball and McCarter, 1960). But since some of the hydrocarbon had by then penetrated the cells, and was thus no longer extractable, the true time of action might have been longer than 15 min. Another approach was to use actinomycin D, as an inhibitor of the initiating phase of skin carcinogenesis, to determine its optimal effect in relation to the time of application of the initiator (Gelboin et al., 1965). Their results [though conflicting with those of others (see Section 7)] led them to conclude that the initiating process involved metabolic changes during one mitotic cycle, which took about a day for completion.

More clear-cut evidence in support of initiating action developing rapidly and occurring in cells actually undergoing mitosis is derived from experiments in which the mitotic rate of the epidermal cells was artificially increased prior to the application of the initiator (Pound and Withers, 1963; Shinozuka and Ritchie, 1967; Hennings et al., 1973; see Section 5). More recently, using colchicine injection, at various intervals prior to initiating action (in order to bring about mitotic arrest), it was possible to narrow down the time of initiating action to the M phase of mitosis (Berenblum and Armuth, 1977). (Others had previously postulated G_1, or S, or G_2 as likely phases during which initiation occurred. Hypothetically, the S phase seems most plausible for simple alkylating agents, as initiators, combining with the DNA of the cell, whereas in the case of initiators of more complex structure reacting with DNA, *followed by defective repair of the induced mutation*, the M phase would more likely be involved.)

In contrast to initiating action, promoting action is a very slow process, requiring long-continued treatment for tumors to develop by the two-stage technique. It should be noted, however, that under certain circumstances, a single application of a carcinogen to mouse skin can cause tumors to develop without supplementary (promoting) action (Mider and Morton, 1939; Law, 1941; Cramer and Stowell, 1943; Terracini *et al.*, 1960). This tends to occur when the application is made during the "resting" phase of the hair cycle (Andreasen and Engelbreth-Holm, 1953; Borum, 1954), and can be attributed to the fact that during the "resting" phase, the hydrocarbon remains for about a week dissolved in the sebum in the hair follicles, and thus has time to act as promoter (at least for a short time) as well as initiator, in contrast to what happens during the "growth" phase of the hair cycle, when there is active sebum secretion, causing the hydrocarbon to be "washed out" within a day or two (Berenblum *et al.*, 1958).

The second of the four premises—that the tumor yield by the two-stage technique should be quantitatively related to the dose of the initiator—was confirmed by using different concentrations of carcinogenic hydrocarbons applied topically (Berenblum and Shubik, 1949a; McCarter *et al.*, 1956; Pyerin and Hecker, 1979; Slaga *et al.*, 1979) or with urethan administered topically (Roe and Salaman, 1954) or systemically (Berenblum and Haran-Ghera, 1957a)—followed in each case by standard croton oil treatment. [That initiating action is only responsible for the *number* of tumors and promoting action *only for their speed of appearance* would seem to be over simplistic, seeing that weak initiators, or low concentrations of potent initiators, followed by standard promoting action, cause *delayed* tumor induction as well as *lower* tumor yield (Slaga *et al.*, 1974a; Scribner and Süss, 1978).]

The irreversible nature of initiating action (the third of the four premises) was likewise confirmed—in this case by testing the two-stage process with varying intervals between the initiating action and the start of promoting action. No falling off in tumor yield resulted in most cases from lengthening the interval, whether the initiator was a carcinogenic hydrocarbon applied topically (Berenblum and Shubik, 1947b; Salaman, 1952; Graffi, 1953; Van Duuren, 1969) or urethan administered systemically (Berenblum and Haran-Ghera, 1957a); also with β-radiation as initiator and 4-nitroquinoline-1-oxide as promoter (Hoshino and Tanooka, 1975). [In a recent experiment by Roe *et al.* (1972), in which the interval between initiation and the start of promotion was as long as 50 weeks, a decrease in tumor yield was observed, the authors conceding, however, that their findings, under such extreme conditions, were not at variance with the postulated irreversibility of "latent tumor cells."]

Support for the fourth premise—that tumors should fail to appear when the sequence of initiating action and promoting action is reversed—was already available in the early results on which the two-stage mechanism was based (Berenblum, 1941*b*), and subsequently confirmed under more varied conditions (see Berenblum and Haran, 1955*a*; Roe, 1959*a*).

455

SEQUENTIAL
ASPECTS OF
CHEMICAL
CAR-
CINOGENESIS:
SKIN

3. Critique of the Two-Stage Hypothesis

The data presented so far strongly support the initiation–promotion hypothesis. This hypothesis has, however, been subjected to criticism from time to time— calling in turn for attempts to meet the objection raised.

The earliest criticism, which questioned the very existence of dormant tumor cells, arose from experiments that suggested vascular and fibrocytic changes in the corium, rather than irreversible changes in the covering epithelium, as being critical for carcinogenesis (Orr, 1934, 1935, 1937). (For contrary evidence, see Ritchie, 1952*a,b*.) Experiments were also described involving reciprocal grafting of carcinogen-treated "initiated" skin to normal sites, and of normal skin to "initiated" site, followed in both cases by croton oil treatment (Billingham *et al.*, 1951; Marchant and Orr, 1953, 1955). Tumors should theoretically have developed preferentially in the skin grafts that had received initiating action prior to transplantation, whereas they arose more frequently at the sites where "initiated" skin had been excised and normal skin grafted in its place. This was interpreted by Orr (1958) to conflict with the notion of dormant tumor cells (though in an earlier publication, he admitted that such postulated dormant tumor cells might have remained behind in the skin appendages). The results could not, in fact, be confirmed by Worst and Bauz (1974), using more modern experimental methods. Moreover, using genetic markers to determine the origin of induced tumors in skin, Lappé (1968, 1969) and Steinmuller (1971) were able to establish that skin tumors were indeed derived from cells carried over in the grafts.

The fact that papillomas in mouse skin produced by the two-stage process tended to regress more commonly than those produced by repeated applications of a carcinogenic hydrocarbon (Shubik, 1950*b*; Saffiotti and Shubik, 1956; Frei and Kingsley, 1968) raised some doubts as to whether the former method of tumor induction was comparable to conventional carcinogenesis. Van Duuren *et al.* (1966), while confirming a high regression rate with crude croton oil as promoter, failed to observe it when using a semipurified, active constituent of croton oil—thus indicating that some unknown anticarcinogen, possibly present in crude croton oil, might have accounted for the regression. [See, however, Stenbäck (1978) on regression of papillomas with 12-*O*-tetradecanoylphorbol-13-acetate as promoter.]

Another disturbing feature was that croton oil possessed some carcinogenic activity of its own (Roe, 1956*b*) and that the tumor incidence could, in some strains of mice, be quite high (Boutwell *et al.*, 1957). Theoretically, croton oil might, in such cases, be acting as a promoting agent *with respect to dormant tumor cells that arose spontaneously*, rather than as a complete carcinogen. Such an eventuality would make it impossible ever to prove the noncarcinogenicity of a "pure" promoter (see Kopelovich *et al.*, 1979). Actually, in practice, the background carcinogenicity of croton oil rarely interferes with the interpretation of results using the two-stage technique.

Alternative explanations of the two-stage phenomenon, e.g., by postulating simple additive or summation effects (see Nakahara, 1961), do not allow for the fact that tumors fail to develop when the two agents, initiator and promoter, are administered in reverse order. The same applies to the theory of multiple random mutations being responsible for the long latent period of carcinogenesis (Charles and Luce-Clausen, 1942; Iversen and Arley, 1950; Fisher and Holomon, 1951; Nordling, 1953; de Waard, 1964; Ashley, 1969; Baum, 1976; Emmelot and Scherer, 1977). (For further discussion on the mechanism of carcinogenic action, and postulated alternative theories, see Sections 10 and 11.)

4. Different Initiators for Skin Carcinogenesis

One of the limitations of the original two-stage technique for mouse skin carcinogenesis was that the initiating action had to depend on the use of a "complete" carcinogen, acting for a very brief period (the potential promoting action not having time to express itself). This complication was eventually eliminated by the discovery that urethan, itself not carcinogenic for skin, could act as a *pure* initiator (Salaman and Roe, 1953; Berenblum and Haran, 1955*b*). It could also be made to function this way when administered systemically, followed by topical applications of croton oil (Haran and Berenblum, 1956; Ritchie, 1957)—as with 2-acetylaminofluorene (Ritchie and Saffiotti, 1955), and with various carcinogenic hydrocarbons (Graffi *et al.*, 1955; Berenblum and Haran-Ghera, 1957*b*; Niskanen and Merenmies, 1960), acting *systemically* as initiators for the skin.

Other initiators for skin carcinogenesis included UV light and β-radiation, certain metabolites of "complete" carcinogens, various alkylating agents, mutagens, etc. The results are summarized in Table 1 (which also lists compounds that failed to act as initiators when tested by the two-stage technique on mouse skin).

5. Different Promoters for Skin Carcinogenesis

The search for promoting agents other than croton oil was dictated by the following considerations: (a) to explain the chemical specificity of croton oil—with high activity of one crude fraction ("croton resin") and inactivity of the residual oil, *though the two had comparable irritant properties for skin* (Berenblum, 1941*b*; see also negative results with many other skin irritants: Berenblum, 1944; Shubik, 1950*a*; Saffiotti and Shubik, 1963; Baroni *et al.*, 1963); (b) the need for pure compounds, to serve as promoters, in trying to determine their mechanism of

457

SEQUENTIAL
ASPECTS OF
CHEMICAL
CAR-
CINOGENESIS:
SKIN

TABLE 1

Agents Tested for Initiating Action in Two-Stage Skin Carcinogenesis[a]

Effective initiators	Negative or borderline initiators
Physical agents	
β-Rays (1, 2)	
Ultraviolet light (3–5)	
"Complete" chemical carcinogens	
Benzo[a]pyrene; 7,12-dimethylbenz[a]anthracene; etc. (6, 7, etc.; see reviews listed in Section 1)	
Non- or weakly acting skin carcinogens	
Benz[a]anthracene (8–10)	Anthracene; phenanthrene; pyrene; anthanthrene (8, 10, 18)
Dibenz[a,c]anthracene; chrysene; benzo[e]pyrene; coronene (9–11)	
Methylchrysenes (12, 13)	
2-Acetylaminofluorene (systemically administered) (15)	2-Acetylaminofluorene (by topical application) (19)
Urethan (16, 17)	Several urethan derivatives (8)
Phenylurethan (18)	4-Dimethylaminoazobenzene (butter yellow) (19)
β-Propiolactone (8, 20, 21)	
Glycidaldehyde; malonaldehyde (both chemically related to β-propiolactone) (21)	
Metabolites of hydrocarbons	
Dihydrodiols of benzo[a]pyrene (22–25)	
Isomeric phenols of benzo[a]pyrene (16)	
Alkylating agents and mutagens (noncarcinogenic for skin), etc.	
Triethylene melamine (8)	Colchicine (8)
Phenylbutyric acid nitrogen mustard (18)	Nitrogen mustard (28) and some derivatives (19)
Dimethyl sulfate; ethylbromoacetate; 2,3-di-chloro-p-dioxane; etc. (27)	Acridine orange; acridine yellow (29, 34)
	15,16-Dihydrocyclopenta[a]phenanthrene-17-one; 1,2,3,4-tetrahydrochrysene-1-one (31)
	Myleran; aminopterin (18, 29)
	8-Azaguanine; 6-mercaptopurine; 2,6-diamino-8-phenylpurine (18)
	5-Bromodeoxyuridine; 5-iododeoxyuridine; [^{3}H]thymidiene (29)
Miscellaneous compounds	
Esters of methanesulfonic acid (32)	Benzocaine, cantharidine; chloral hydrate; coumarin; paraldehyde; phenobarbitone; physostigmine (8)
Chloromononitrobenzenes; chloracetone; β-bromopropionic acid (33)	Acrolein; aspirin; deoxycholic acid; diethyl carbonate; 8-hydroxyquinoline; monosodium inaleic hydrazine; oxalacetic acid; potassium arsenite; vanillin (18)
Aromatic amines and metabolites (34)	Arsenic trioxide; sodium arsenite (37)
N-Methyl-N-nitrosourea (35)	
N-Acetoxy derivatives of N-arylacetamides (36)	

[a] (1) Shubik *et al.* (1953*b*); (2) Hoshino and Tanooka (1975); (3) Epstein and Roth (1968); (4) Pound (1970); (5) Stenbäck (1975); (6) Berenblum (1941*b*); (7) Mottram (1944*b*); (8) Roe and Salaman (1955); (9) Van Duuren *et al.* (1970); (10) Scribner (1973); (11) Van Duuren *et al.* (1968); (12) Hecht *et al.* (1974); (13) Hoffman *et al.* (1974); (14) Hecht *et al.* (1978); (15) Ritchie and Saffiotti (1955); (16) Salaman and Roe (1955); (17) Berenblum and Haran (1955*b*); (18) Salaman and Roe (1956*c*); (19) Salaman and Roe (1953); (20) Colburn and Boutwell (1966); (21) Shamberger *et al.* (1974); (22) Chouroulinkov *et al.* (1976); (23) Slaga *et al.* (1976*b*); (24) Slaga *et al.* (1977); (25) Slaga *et al.* (1979); (26) Slaga *et al* (1978*a*); (27) Van Duuren *et al.* (1974); (28) Berenblum and Shubik (1949*a*); (29) Trainin *et al* (1964); (30) Van Duuren *et al.* (1969); (31) Coombs and Bhatt (1978); (32) Roe (1957); (33) Searle (1966); (34) Mukai and Troll (1969); (35) Waynforth and Magee (1975); (36) Scribner and Slaga (1975); (37) Baroni *et al.* (1963).

action (see Section 11); and (c) because of the possibility of initiation–promotion having relevance to human carcinogenesis (see Bingham *et al.*, 1976; Wynder, 1977).

The variety of compounds capable of acting as promoting agents for mouse skin proved to be quite extensive (see Table 2). On the other hand, a considerable

TABLE 2

Agents Tested for Promoting Action in Two-Stage Skin Carcinogenesis[a]

Effective promoters	Negative or borderline promoters
Physical agents	
Mechanical injury (holes punched in rabbit ear) (1, 2; see Section 1)	
Grenz rays (3)	
"Complete" chemical carcinogens	
Benzo[*a*]pyrene; 7,12-dimethylbenz[*a*]anthracene; etc. (4, 5; see reviews listed in Section 1)	
Non- or weakly acting skin carcinogens	
Dimethylaminostilbene (per os) (6)	
Some petroleum fractions (7)	Acridine; fluorene; phenanthrene (9)
4-Nitroquinoline-1-oxide (8)	Pyrene (10, 11)
Croton oil, etc.; constituents and related compounds	
Crude croton oil (and croton resin) (4, 5, etc.)	Crude croton oil extract lacking croton resin (4)
Euphorbia lattices (12)	
12-*O*-Tetradecanoylphorbol-13-acetate (also known as phorbol-12-myristate-13-acetate) and a number of analogs and derivatives (13, 14; see Table 3)	Phorbol (13, 17); certain other analogs and phorbol derivatives (13, 14; see Table 3)
Some compounds less closely related to phorbol (15, 16; see Fig. 1)	Compounds less closely related to phorbol (15, 16; see Fig. 1)
Straight-chain N-alkanes, alkanols, fatty acids, etc.	
N-Alkanes of medium size (C_{12}–C_{28}), e.g., decane, dodecane, tetradecane (7, 18–20)	Short-chain alkanes, e.g., hexane, octane (19, 20)
N-Alkanols of medium size, e.g., dodecanol (7, 11)	Very-long-chain alkanes (C_{30}–), e.g., squalene (19, 20, 27)
Some long-chain fatty acids, e.g., oleic, lauric (21, 22)	Short-chain alkanols, e.g., hexanol, octanol (19)
Methyl esters of fatty acids (23)	Very-long-chain alkanols, e.g., hexadecanol, octadecanol (19)
"Tween" and "Span" surface-acting agents, e.g., polyoxyethylene sorbiton monostearate (Tween 60) (24–26)	Oleic acid (9, 28; but cf. 21); palmitic acid; stearic acid (21)
	Ricinoleic acid (9)
	Span 20 (7)
Phenolic compounds	
Phenol (29–31)	
Other phenolic compounds (30; see also Tobacco Smoke Condensates below)	
Anthralin (11, 32, 33)	Semiquinones of anthralin (34)
Extracts of tobacco leaf	
Aqueous and other extracts (31, 35, 36)	
Extracts of tobacco smoke condensates	
Crude extracts (37)	
Phenolic fractions (31, 38–40)	
Isolated constituents from such extracts (31)	

TABLE 2 *(cont.)*

459

SEQUENTIAL
ASPECTS OF
CHEMICAL
CAR-
CINOGENESIS:
SKIN

Effective promoters	Negative or borderline promoters
Miscellaneous compounds—conflicting reports	
Acetic acid (41)	Acetic acid (28)
Cantharidin (11, 42)	Cantharidin (28)
Chloroform (in rabbit skin) (1, 2)	Chloroform (in mouse skin) (21)
Iodoacetic acid (impure specimen) (28)	Iodoacetic acid (pure specimen) (7)
Turpentine (in rabbit skin) (2)	Turpentine (in mouse skin) (9, 21, 28)
Miscellaneous compounds—general	
Chloroacetophenone (28)	Arsenic oxide (50); atebrin (10); bromobenzene (30); catechol (11, 30)
Citrus oils (43); oil of sweet orange (44)	Castor oil (9); coumarin (31); emodine (7); estradiol (28)
Fluoro-2,4-dinitrobenzene (45)	"Folliculin" (51); ethylphenylpropionate (7); eugenol (27)
Griseofulvin (per os) (46)	Fumaric acid (7); glyceryl monoricinoleate (9); glycerylphenylpropiolactate (7); hydrogen peroxide (47); monostearine (7); mustard oil (28); podophyllin (28); resorcinol (11)
Paracetic acid; perbenzoic acid; *m*-chloroperbenzoic acid (47)	Urea peroxide (48); scarlet red (28); silver nitrate (7, 9)
Quinone (28)	Various quinones (other than quinone itself) (11, 17, 28, etc.)
Sake (alcoholic beverage) (48)	
Sodium hypochlorite (49)	

[a] (1) Rous and Kidd (1941); (2) MacKenzie and Rous (1941); (3) Epstein (1972); (4) Berenblum (1944*b*); (5) Mottram (1944*b*); (6) Odashima (1962); (7) Saffiotti and Shubik (1963); (8) Hoshino and Tanooka (1975); (9) Shubik (1950*a*); (10) Bernelli-Zazzera (1952); (11) Van Duuren and Goldschmidt (1976); (12) Roe and Peirce (1961); (13) Hecker (1968); (14) Van Duuren (1969); (15) Hecker (1971*b*); (16) Hecker (1978); (17) Armuth and Berenblum (1976); (18) Horton *et al.* (1957); (19) Sicé (1966); (20) Horton *et al.* (1976); (21) Holsti (1959); (22) Arffman and Glavind (1974); (23) Sicé *et al.* (1957); (24) Setälä *et al.* (1954); (25) Setälä (1960); (26) Della Porta *et al.* (1960); (27) Van Duuren (1978); (28) Gwynn and Salaman (1953); (29) Rusch *et al.* (1955); (30) Boutwell and Bosch (1959); (31) Van Duuren *et al.* (1968); (32) Bock and Burns (1963); (33) Yasuhira (1968); (34) Segal *et al.* (1971); (35) Bock (1968); (36) Chortyk and Bock (1976); (37) Gelhorn (1958); (38) Roe *et al.* (1959); (39) Wynder and Hoffmann (1961); (40) Hecht *et al.* (1975); (41) Slaga *et al.* (1975); (42) Hennings and Boutwell (1970); (43) Roe and Peirce (1960); (44) Roe (1959*b*); (45) Bock *et al.* (1969); (46) Barich *et al.* (1962); (47) Bock *et al.* (1975); (48) Kuratsune *et al.* (1971); (49) Hayatsu *et al.* (1971); (50) Baroni *et al.* (1963); (51) Picco *et al.* (1958).

degree of specificity is evident; and particularly well illustrated, among the active compounds, when their potencies of action are taken into account. Some interest was shown, at one time, in the promoting properties of surface-acting lipophilic–hydrophilic substances belonging to the "Tween" and "Span" detergents (Setälä *et al.*, 1954; see Setälä, 1960). These substances require, however, very high concentrations, and frequent applications at short intervals, for effective action; they also possess considerable carcinogenicity of their own (Della Porta *et al.*, 1960). Among the more interesting compounds, possessing strong promoting properties for skin, anthranil (Bock and Burns, 1963; Yasuhira, 1968) deserves special mention.

But by far the most important development in the search for alternative promoting agents was the isolation and identification of the active principle of croton oil. After many unsuccessful (or partially successful) attempts in various laboratories, Hecker and his associates (see reviews by Hecker, 1968, 1971*a*, 1978), and independently Van Duuren and associates (see reviews by Van Duuren, 1969, 1976), succeeded in isolating and characterizing a number of

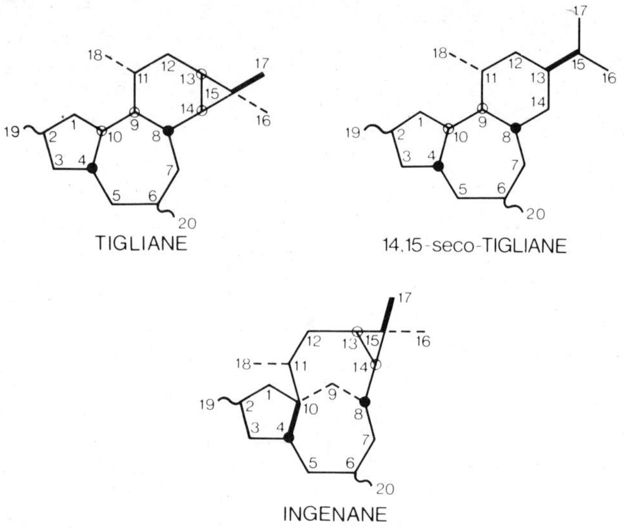

FIGURE 1. Tigliane and other diterpene types, some derivatives of which possess promoting activity.

TABLE 3
Phorbol and Derivatives (Parent Diterpene Tigliane)[a]

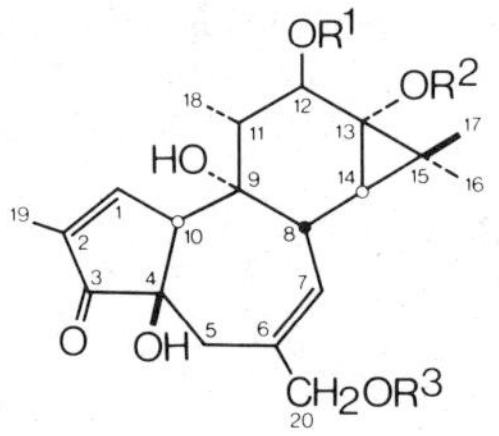

Compound	Promoting activity on mouse skin
Phorbol (unesterified, i.e., $R_1 = R_2 = R_3 = H$)	±
12,13-Diesters of phorbol $R_1 = R_2 =$ acyl, $R_3 = H$)	
12-*O*-Tetradecanoylphorbol-13-acetate (TPA)	++++
Phorbol-12,13-didecanoate	+++
Phorbol-12,13-dibenzoate	+++
Phorbol-12,13-dibutyrate	++
Phorbol-12,13-diacetate	+
4-*O*-Methyl-TPA	±
Phorbol-12-tetradecanoate	−
Phorbol-13-tetradecanoate	++
4α-Phorbol-12,13-didecanoate	−
12,13,20-Triesters of phorbol ($R_1 = R_2 = R_3 =$ acyl)	
Various triesters	−

[a] From Hecker (personal communication).

phorbol diesters with specific fatty acid chains in particular positions in the molecule, as well as providing a number of semisynthetic derivatives (Hecker, 1971*b*, 1978; see Fig. 1 and Table 3). In fact, the most effective promoter for mouse skin proved to be 12-*O*-tetradecanoylphorbol-13-acetate (TPA), also referred to as phorbol myristate acetate, the active constituent of croton oil.

6. Extension of the Two-Stage System in Skin Carcinogenesis

It was already apparent from the early experiments (Berenblum, 1941*b*) that in addition to promoting action, croton oil was capable of encouraging the induced papillomas to become malignant (referred to as "metacarcinogenic" action; see Section 1). This aspect of the problem has since been followed up under varying conditions (see Shubik, 1950*b*; Shubik *et al.*, 1953*a*; Roe, 1956*a,b*; Salaman and Roe, 1956*a,b*; Boutwell *et al.*, 1957; Van Duuren *et al.*, 1966). [The phenomenon is, strictly speaking, a feature of tumor progression (see Foulds, 1954) and therefore "postcarcinogenic" rather than part of the carcinogenic process per se.]

The results of these studies may be summarized as follows.

1. The transition from a benign papilloma to a malignant tumor represents at least one and possibly several irreversible steps (Shubik, 1950*b*; Shubik *et al.*, 1953*a*).
2. These changes usually occur spontaneously—sometimes even after a single application of a carcinogenic hydrocarbon, without subsequent treatment of any kind (see Mider and Morton, 1939; Shubik *et al.*, 1953*a*; Roe, 1956*a*).
3. Since the rate and the extent of progression to malignancy vary from one papilloma to another in the same animal, the process is manifestly determined by a change within the cell, and not through systemic control.
4. Progression to malignancy can, however, be artificially encouraged by additional croton oil treatment (Berenblum, 1941*b*; Roe, 1956*a*) or by its active constituent (Van Duuren *et al.*, 1966), and more effectively by repeated applications of a carcinogenic hydrocarbon or by supplementary treatment by a hydrocarbon *after* the two-stage hydrocarbon–croton oil technique (Shubik, 1950*b*).

As for the initiation–promotion itself, further subdivision has been proposed, based on experimental evidence suggesting (1) that there is a preinitiating phase (Pound and Bell, 1962; Pound and Withers, 1963) and (2) that the promoting phase may itself be made up of two separate stages (Boutwell, 1964). (The term "multistage" is, therefore, commonly used today instead of "two-stage" carcinogenesis.)

The evidence for a preinitiating phase arose from the observation that *with urethan as initiator*, followed by croton oil as promoter, an enhanced tumor response could be elicited when the skin was, in addition, prepainted with croton oil (Pound and Bell, 1962). This did not negate the earlier claim that reversal of the initiation–promotion process failed to cause tumors to appear, since subsequent croton oil treatment was still essential, and since the augmentation also occurred as a result of pretreatment with nonspecific stimuli, such as acetic acid, trichloroacetic acid, xylene, turpentine, or by scarification (Pound and Withers, 1963). Such pretreatment was only effective in relation to urethan as initiator, not with dimethylbenz[a]anthracene (7,12-DMBA), and only slightly so with β-propiolactone as initiator (Hennings et al., 1969). The most plausible explanation of the phenomenon is that initiation requires the cells to be in a state of mitotic division—which is stimulated by all skin irritants, including carcinogenic hydrocarbons (the latter acting at the same time as initiator), but not by urethan—thus requiring additional "preinitiation stimulation," in the latter case, for optimal effects (see Section 2).

The proposal for *two* stages of *promotion* arose from the observation that when 7,12-DMBA as initiator was followed by croton oil for 5 weeks and then by turpentine for a further 5 weeks, the tumor yield was significantly higher than when the 7,12-DMBA was followed by turpentine first and by croton oil afterwards under otherwise identical conditions (Boutwell, 1964). The mechanism of this complex situation is not yet understood. (For speculative considerations in favor of multiple stages of promoting action, see Meyer-Bertenrath, 1969.)

7. Early Studies of Factors Influencing Initiation and Promotion

Many factors influence the outcome of carcinogenic action, both positively (cocarcinogenic) and negatively (anticarcinogenic). These can be further subdivided according to whether their influence is on the carcinogen or on the responding tissue. [For a classification of the various types of cocarcinogenic action, see Berenblum (1969). See also reviews on cocarcinogenesis by Stenbäck et al. (1974) and Sivak (1979), and on anticarcinogenesis by Van Duuren and Melchionne (1969) and Wattenberg (1977, 1978).]

Cocarcinogenic and anticarcinogenic factors *influencing the carcinogen* do so by affecting its rate of absorption into the body, its penetration into the target cells, its metabolic fate, its detoxification and excretion from the body, etc. Such influences can, of course, also operate in connection with the two-stage technique, especially in relation to the initiating phase (which depends on a single, brief action of a relatively small dose of initiator), and perhaps less so in relation to promoting action (which involves oversaturation of the tissue by the promoting agent over a long period of time).

An early example of interference with initiation was inhibition of tumor induction by phenanthrene when added to 7,12-DMBA at the initiating phase (Huh and McCarter, 1960). This was not due to competitive absorption into the target organ, since phenanthrene was found actually to *increase* the amount of 7,12-DMBA absorbed. Hydrocarbons can, however, stimulate the action of hydrolases, which are able to detoxicate carcinogens in the skin (Gelboin and

Blackburn, 1964), as well as in the liver, etc. It may well be that phenanthrene acted in this way. (For further reference to interference with initiating action and its relation to competitive metabolic functions, see Section 10.)

Much more is known about cocarcinogenic and anticarcinogenic factors *affecting tissue response* at the respective stages of skin carcinogenesis.

There is first the genetic angle: Promoting action of croton oil proved to be strictly species specific—operating in the skin of the mouse but not of the rat, guinea pig, or rabbit (Shubik, 1950a)—the effective potency varying even among the different strains of mice (Boutwell, 1964).

Specific inhibitors of carcinogenesis have been found to serve as a useful analytical tool in trying to determine how modifiers of initiation and promotion operate (see also Section 11).

The earliest example of anticarcinogenic action in mouse skin, suspected of operating during the promoting phase (though noted long before the concept of initiation–promotion was formulated), was by sulfur mustard (β,β'-dichloroethylsulfide), which caused pronounced inhibition of tumor induction, *even when the treatment was begun quite late during the course of tarring* (Berenblum, 1929). Using the two-stage technique, the inhibitory effect of sulfur mustard was confirmed, acting during the promoting phase (Van Duuren and Segal, 1976). Furthermore, inhibition also occurred when the sulfur mustard treatment was confined to the interval between initiating and promoting action (De Young *et al.*, 1977b), suggesting that the agent selectively inactivated initiated cells. A similar, though less pronounced, inhibitory effect was observed by acetic acid treatment during the interval between initiation and promotion (Murray, 1978).

Another early example of anticarcinogenic action on mouse skin—by caloric restriction of the diet—was also found to operate during the *promoting* phase (Tannenbaum, 1944). Boutwell and Rusch (1951) were then able definitely to exclude any influence of caloric restriction on the *initiating* phase.

Studies of hormonal influences on carcinogenesis (see Bielschowsky and Horning, 1958; Foulds, 1965; Furth, 1975; Jull, 1976), though mainly directed to internal organs, included some experiments on skin, and a few related to the separate phases of initiation and promotion.

Ritchie *et al.* (1953) found cortisone to cause no more than a slight increase in mitotic rate, and no apparent influence on tumor induction by the 7,12-DMBA–croton oil two-stage technique. Engelbreth-Holm and Absoe-Hanson (1953) did observe some inhibition of tumor induction by cortisone, while definite inhibition during the promoting phase was observed by Boutwell (1964).

In a critical study of the role of adrenal imbalance in skin carcinogenesis, Trainin (1963) administered hydrocortisone during the initiating and promoting phases, respectively, for *excessive* adrenal action and performed adrenalectomy (with subsequent reimplantation of isologous adrenal tissue at the end of the required periods) for *deficient* action. The initiating phase remained unaffected by either form of added treatment, but the promoting phase was strongly inhibited by hydrocortisone and greatly enhanced by adrenalectomy. [See also Belman and Troll (1972) for the influence of other steroid hormones.]

Meites (1958) found that thyroxine, by mouth, caused pronounced inhibition of tumor induction, and thiouracil caused some augmentation when tested in connection with the 7,12-DMBA–croton oil two-stage technique. The results pointed to the effects being on the promoting phase (but there were unfortunately no control groups in which the feeding was confined to the initiating phase).

The choice of inhibitors for the study of the mechanism of initiation and promotion has generally been based on biochemical considerations, e.g., by their metabolic effects on cell replication. Actinomycin D was a case in point, known to interfere with DNA-dependent RNA synthesis in the cell (though admittedly possessing toxic side effects as well).

The influence of actinomycin D on the two-stage system of skin carcinogenesis (Gelboin et al., 1965) seemed at first to indicate specific inhibition of the *initiating* phase, the effect being most pronounced when applied on day 0 or 1 relative to the application of the initiator, but weak when applied 7 days before or 4 days after, and absent when given on day 7 or later. When administered systemically, it had no effect at all. The conclusions drawn from these results were (1) that initiation took place during the mitotic cycle of the cell, (2) that this involved metabolic changes requiring 1 day for completion, and (3) that actinomycin D interfered with this specific metabolic pathway.

The results and conclusions were questioned by others (Hennings and Boutwell, 1967; Van Duuren, 1969), whose experiments (under somewhat different conditions of dosage, etc.) pointed rather to an effect on the promoting phase, inhibition occurring when actinomycin D was applied as late as 30 days after the initiator (Van Duuren, 1969). Some of the effects observed by Gelboin et al. (1965) might have been due to nonspecific, toxic action, causing death of initiated cells, although this was partly answered by later quantitative studies (Bates et al., 1968), using lower doses than originally.

A similar lack of agreement occurred with poly-I·C (a synthetic double-stranded RNA) as inhibitor, Kreibich et al. (1970) claiming that the inhibition was confined to the initiating phase while others (Gelboin and Levy, 1970; Gelboin et al., 1972; Elgjo and Degré, 1973) observed inhibition of the promoting phase. (Poly-I·C has many other properties, including stimulation of cells to synthesize interferon causing resistance to viral replication, and stimulation of cellular and humoral immunity.)

In the light of the widespread belief, at one time, that "immunosurveillance" might be a controlling factor in carcinogenesis (Miller et al., 1963; Grant et al., 1966), it is interesting to note that depression of the immune response by injection of antithymocyte serum at either the initiating or the promoting phase of skin carcinogenesis did not affect the tumor yield or the average latent period (Haran-Ghera and Lurie, 1971), although progression from benign tumors to malignancy was enhanced in the antithymocyte serum-treated groups. [See also the influence of thymectomy on two-state carcinogenesis (Yasuhira, 1969).]

For a further discussion of modifying factors in two-stage carcinogenesis, used as experimental methods of exploring the mechanism of promoting action, see Section 11.

8. *Promoting Action in Tissues Other Than Skin*   465

SEQUENTIAL
ASPECTS OF
CHEMICAL
CAR-
CINOGENESIS:
SKIN

The subject of sequential stages of carcinogenesis in tissues other than skin is dealt with elsewhere in this volume. Here, we are only concerned with it insofar as *skin* initiators and promoters (or compounds closely related to them) happen to act on other tissues as well, e.g., in connection with urethan and with phorbol and some of its derivatives.

The carcinogenicity of urethan for the lung (Nettleship *et al.*, 1943) and for a number of other tissues (see Tannenbaum and Silverstone, 1958; Mirvish, 1968) was recognized before the discovery that it acted as a pure initiator in mouse skin (Salaman and Roe, 1953; Haran and Berenblum, 1956). It was all the more surprising that in relation to radiation leukemogenesis, urethan functioned as a promoter (Berenblum and Trainin, 1960). (Its cocarcinogenic action, when administered concurrently with X-irradiation, had previously been demonstrated by Kawamoto *et al.*, 1958.) Urethan thus seems quite unique—having *initiating* action for one tissue (skin), *promoting* action for another (hematopoietic tissue), and being a *complete carcinogen* for several other tissues.

The role of phorbol and its derivatives presents a somewhat different picture. Phorbol itself was originally thought to be entirely inactive (see Hecker, 1971*a*); later found to possess borderline promoting activity for skin (Baird and Boutwell, 1971; Armuth and Berenblum, 1976); but to be a fairly effective promoter for liver, lung, and mammary gland (Armuth and Berenblum, 1972, 1974); as well as possessing leukemogenic properties when acting alone (Berenblum and Lonai, 1970).

A number of polyfunctional diterpenes (4-*O*-methylphorbol, 12-deoxyphorbol, 4α-phorbol, ingenol, lathyrol, and 6,20-epoxylathyrol), all structurally related to phorbol, were found to be promoters for liver carcinogenesis when tested systemically (Armuth *et al.*, 1979). There was, however, no correlation between their respective promoting or lack of promoting action on skin (applied topically) and such action on the liver (when administered systemically), using appropriate initiators in both cases.

Adaptation of the two-stage technique for transplacental carcinogenesis, with the initiator administered to the pregnant mother and the promoter to the offspring after birth, has yielded positive results (a) for skin carcinogenesis, with croton oil or TPA applications to the young (Bulay and Wattenberg, 1970; Goerttler and Loehrke, 1977; Schweizer *et al.*, 1978); (b) for the forestomach, by feeding TPA to the young (Goerttler *et al.*, 1979); and (c) for internal organs (liver and lung), using injections of phorbol to the young (Armuth and Berenblum, 1979). Positive results for skin were also reported when the initiator was administered to lactating mothers after birth of the young, and TPA applied to the skin of the young, i.e., with transmission of the initiator (or its metabolite) via the milk instead of transplacentally (Goerttler and Loehrke, 1976).

An altogether different, important adaptation of the two-stage technique has been its application to tissue culture (Mondal *et al.*, 1976; Lasne *et al.*, 1977; Kennedy *et al.*, 1978; see also Diamond *et al.*, 1978, and the review by

Chouroulinkov and Lasne, 1978). An interesting aspect of these results was that, in contrast to specific mouse *skin* response, rat and mouse embryo *fibroblasts*, after suitable initiation, proved to be quite sensitive to tumor promotion by TPA.

9. Promoting Action in Other Species

The fact that croton oil (and supposedly its active constituent, TPA) is only effective as a promoter for *mouse* skin, and not for that of the rat, guinea pig, or rabbit (Shubik, 1950a; Saffiotti and Shubik, 1963), seems surprising when one considers that TPA is an effective promoter for *rat* fibroblasts *in vitro* (Lasne *et al.*, 1977) and that the unesterified phorbol can act as a promoting stimulus for mammary tissues in *rat* (Armuth and Berenblum, 1974).

One approach that may resolve the enigma about the specificity of the promoting action of croton oil for mouse skin would be to carry out analogous tests on the skin of other species, *using compounds unrelated to phorbol esters, yet ones known to possess promoting activity for mouse skin.*

While the present review concentrates on *skin* response, one should not overlook the fact that the initiation–promotion principle applies to many tissues and organs in the body, in various species, including humans (see the review by Wynder, 1977). The specificity of croton oil (and of phorbol esters) is therefore somewhat *unique for this group of substances.* Overemphasis on their mode of action might thus provide a distorted picture of the mechanism of promoting action in general (see Section 11).

10. The Mechanism of Initiating Action

That neoplasia might result from a genetic change in the cell nucleus is a very old idea (see Bauer, 1928), generally referred to as "the somatic cell mutation theory of cancer." Though speculative in its original formulation, the theory could account for (1) the irreversibility of the neoplastic change (i.e., the fact that the newly acquired properties are maintained after repeated cell division); (2) the almost infinite variety of tumors; and (3) the fact that each individual tumor tends to "breed true to type." The apparent objection to the theory was that a mutation is virtually instantaneous in its operation, whereas carcinogenesis is one of the slowest biological processes. With the introduction of the two-stage hypothesis, the difficulty could theoretically be overcome, by postulating that only the initiating phase was mutational, while most of the long latent period was taken up with some other (epigenetic) mechanism (see Section 11).

Experimental verification of the mutation concept, as applied to initiating action, did not seem very promising at first (see Berenblum and Shubik, 1949a; Rous, 1959; Trainin *et al.*, 1964); but overwhelming support, from various different directions, soon led to the conviction that a mutational change in the

DNA genome was indeed responsible for the initiating phase of carcinogenesis. Much of the evidence came from experimental findings unrelated to skin response (though not actually conflicting with results obtained in skin, where such information was available). The supporting evidence may be summarized as follows.

1. The ability of most carcinogens, and especially their active metabolites, to bind with DNA (Wheeler, 1962; Dingman and Sporn, 1967; Goshman and Heidelberger, 1967; Warwick, 1969; Brookes, 1975; Sarma *et al.*, 1975; Weinstein *et al.*, 1976; Phillips *et al.*, 1979; but see Chouroulinkov *et al.*, 1979).

2. The fact that, in those cases where compounds possess limited carcinogenic action, i.e., restricted to certain organs, the capacity to bind with DNA *in vivo* is largely confined to, or takes place preferentially in, these particular organs (Magee and Farber, 1962; Prodi *et al.*, 1970; Hawks and Magee, 1974; King *et al.*, 1977; Cooper *et al.*, 1978; Fong *et al.*, 1979). [See, however, Lijinsky and Ross (1969) and Mukai and Troll (1969) for some contradictory evidence.]

3. The fairly good correlation between mutagenic and carcinogenic properties among a wide range of compounds (McCann *et al.*, 1975; Purchase *et al.*, 1976. [But see Rinkus and Legator (1979) for exceptions.]

4. The fact that such correlation with mutagenesis is particularly close for initiators (Colburn and Boutwell, 1966; Jackson and Irving, 1970; Kuroki *et al.*, 1972; Brusick, 1977; Wood *et al.*, 1978), but absent for promoters, such as TPA (Sivak and Van Duuren, 1971; Melmes *et al.*, 1974; McCann *et al.*, 1975; Soper and Evans, 1977).

5. The tendency for the initiating phase of skin carcinogenesis to be inhibited by agents known to interfere with metabolic activation of initiators prior to reaction with DNA (Kinoshita and Gelboin, 1972; Slaga and Boutwell, 1977; Slaga *et al.*, 1978*b*; DiGiovanni *et al.*, 1978; see also Wattenberg, 1978).

When all this is considered in conjunction with the evidence (see Section 2) that the initiating phase develops very rapidly and is virtually irreversible in its potential effects, the idea of a mutational basis for initiating action can now be accepted as fairly well established.

11. The Mechanism of Promoting Action

Accepting tumor initiation as constituting a change in the DNA genome, promoting action—the "awakening" process—might hypothetically operate by derepression of the newly created dormant "tumor" gene, analogous to the control of functional expression in *normal* cell differentiation, as propounded by Jacob and Monod (1961). Such a mechanism has, in fact, been proposed long ago by Pitot and Heidelberger (1963) for *total* carcinogenesis, without necessarily assuming any change in DNA composition. [See also Nery (1976) on "oncogenesis as adaptive ontogenesis."] Derepression of gene function could, however, more logically be attributed to the *promoting* phase of two-stage carcinogenesis (see Boutwell, 1978; Chang *et al.*, 1978).

But if this were the mechanism of promoting action, one would have expected potent promoting agents to show evidence of other forms of derepression as well, by causing many kinds of *divergent* differentiation in *normal* tissues. There is little to suggest this, though examples of deficient or aberrant differentiation of a limited kind have been reported (see Sherbet, 1970; Farber, 1973; Iversen, 1973; Pierce, 1974).

Another hypothesis refers to tumor promotion depending on inhibition of DNA repair (Gaudin *et al.*, 1971, 1972; Soper and Evans, 1977). There is, however, lack of correlation between the capacity for DNA repair and potency of promoting action among the various promoters (Trosko *et al.*, 1975), such repair being also brought about by nonpromoting members of phorbol esters (Langenbach and Kuszynski, 1975). DNA repair may indeed play some part during the interphase between initiation and promotion, or occur during the very early phases of promoting action. It could not, by itself, explain the long latent period of effective promoting action.

A disturbance in the control mechanism of cell division and maturation, through defective chalone action, has been suggested as a possible factor in tumor promotion (Bullough, 1965; Iversen, 1973; Elgjo, 1976). Though attractive in some ways, the idea seems not to have much direct supporting evidence (but see Krieg *et al.*, 1974; Marks, 1976).

Then, there is the evidence that "complete" carcinogens (via their active metabolites) bind covalently with proteins (Abell and Heidelberger, 1962), as well as with nucleic acids (Goshman and Heidelberger, 1967) in skin, as well as in other tissues and organs in the body (see Miller and Miller, 1966). One might, therefore, suppose that protein binding was associated with the promoting phase of carcinogenesis, as against nucleic acid binding being implicated in the initiating phase (Scribner and Boutwell, 1972; Berenblum, 1974). However, there is as yet scant evidence of protein binding by pure promoting agents (Traut *et al.*, 1971).

Beyond such speculations, there is the recent experimental approach of correlating promoting activity, among phorbol esters and related compounds, with some of their other biological properties or "side effects." While such inquiries have a better chance of throwing light on the mechanisms of action, there are certain limitations to the method.

1. A good fit in correlative studies does not necessarily reflect a causative relationship if the number of compounds for testing is small. It may merely be a chance association.
2. Rapidly developing changes that soon pass off are not likely to relate to promoting action, which depends on prolonged treatment, producing its effects months or years later.

3. Since promoting action eventually becomes self-perpetuating (i.e., no longer requiring continuation of the promoting stimulus), a meaningful biological side effect should likewise bring about a *permanent* change. Most of the *reversible* side effects could therefore be ignored.
4. Only those side effects that display the same tissue and species specificity as in connection with promoting action could be considered relevant.

Little attention has so far been paid to these limitations. Among the apparently good fits in the correlative studies, many are, therefore, almost certainly mere chance associations. Some could, however, serve as pointers, for further inquiry by independent methods.

Much attention has been paid to changes in cell division associated with promoting action—based on histological evidence of transient inhibition followed by more sustained increase in mitotic rate, leading to hyperplasia (Dammert, 1961; Frei and Stephens, 1968; Bach and Goerttler, 1971; Slaga *et al.*, 1976*a*; Taper, 1977), and as reflected by increased incorporation of [^{3}H]thymidine (Paul and Hecker, 1969; Hennings and Boutwell, 1970; Baird *et al.*, 1971; Frankfurt and Raitcheva, 1973; Yuspa *et al.*, 1976*b*). The primary object was to detect any correlation between the degree of induced hyperplasia and the potency of promoting action, among the various phorbol esters and other promoters. Yet, it has been evident from the start that no such association existed (Berenblum, 1941*a*, 1944; Shubik, 1950*a*; Gwynn and Salaman, 1953; for more recent evidence see Saffiotti and Shubik, 1963; Raick, 1974; O'Brien *et al.*, 1975; Slaga *et al.*, 1975).

The progressive growth of a tumor is not a function of an *increased* rate of cell division, but the result of a persistent *imbalance* between the rate of cell division and the rate of cell death, i.e., on a *permanent disturbance of growth equilibrium* (Berenblum, 1954*b*). Altered patterns of maturation, differentiation, and other *qualitative* changes in the affected tissue (cf. Glücksmann, 1945; Salaman and Gwynn, 1951; Dammert, 1961; and Major, 1970, for mouse skin response; see also Rovera *et al.*, 1977; Ishii *et al.*, 1978, etc., in tissue culture), rather than stimulation of cell division, might therefore have more relevance to the problem. (For correlation between promoting action and enzymatic changes related to cellular proliferation, see below.)

Somewhat related to the problem of (nonspecific) hyperplasia is that of inflammatory changes in the skin, induced by promoting agents (Janoff *et al.*, 1970; Belman and Troll, 1972). Here, too, a causative association with promoting action would seem unlikely, because of the nonspecific nature of inflammatory response. The fact that certain *anti-inflammatory* agents act as *inhibitors* of tumor promotion (Belman and Troll, 1972; Scribner and Slaga, 1974; Lichti *et al.*, 1977) would seem to support the notion that inflammatory changes do play some sort of role in promoting action—as a modifying factor, though not necessarily in a causative manner.

[The intensity of induced hyperemia in the mouse's ear, following single applications of phorbol esters and related compounds, has been used in one laboratory as a short-term preliminary test for promoting potentialities (Hecker *et al.*, 1966; Hecker, 1971*a*). While apparently useful in a pragmatic sense, limited to this class of compounds, it is unlikely to constitute a relationship in the causative sense (see Driedger and Blumberg, 1979).]

Structural changes in the cytoplasm, as revealed by electron microscopy (Raick, 1973; Komitowski *et al.*, 1977), are difficult to interpret in terms of causal relationship to promoting action, though indicating that the cytoplasm might indeed be the site of such action. Insofar as morphological changes can, in some cases, be related to metabolic derangements, e.g., the observed increase in ribosome accumulation in mouse skin treated with TPA (De Young *et al.*, 1977*a*), they could be indicative of critical involvement.

Reference should also be made to reported changes in membrane stability (possibly resulting in altered permeability), brought about by tumor promoters. While much of the evidence is derived from *in vitro* studies (see Sivak *et al.*, 1969; Kubinski *et al.*, 1973; Wenner *et al.*, 1974), it could have relevance to skin as well (Rohrschneider and Boutwell, 1972; Grimm and Marks, 1974).

This leads one to the subject of biochemical and other functional changes induced by promoting agents, and their possible role in the mechanism of promoting action.

11.1. Stimulation of Synthetic Processes in the Cell

1. Stimulation of DNA synthesis. This has already been dealt with in connection with morphological changes, and is considered to be probably nonspecific with respect to tumor promotion. Minor variations in time relationships (e.g., speed of onset and length of time the effect persists after a single application of the promoter) could hardly be taken as evidence of specificity of action.

2. Stimulation of RNA synthesis. Evidence of such stimulation, shown by increased incorporation of [^{3}H]cytidine, seemed similarly to correlate with the capacity for promoting action, with respect to phorbol and four phorbol derivatives (Baird *et al.*, 1971); but could again reflect a nonspecific effect. [See Hennings and Boutwell (1970) for RNA response to nonpromoting agents.]

3. Stimulation of protein synthesis. Evidence, based on increased incorporation of [^{3}H]leucine, also showed some correlation with promoting activity among the limited group of compounds (Baird *et al.*, 1971), and could likewise represent a nonspecific reflection of cellular proliferation; though increased synthesis of specific proteins, such as histones (Raineri *et al.*, 1973), or of proteins not identifiable in normal skin epithelium (Balmain, 1976), might possibly play a more meaningful role in promoting action.

4. Stimulation of phospholipid synthesis. Such correlation among promoting phorbol esters (Süss *et al.*, 1971; Rohrschneider *et al.*, 1972; Balmain and Hecker, 1974, 1976) is also related to cellular proliferation and, supposedly, nonspecific with respect to promoting action, though some features of the response do seem unusual.

11.2. Effects of Enzymatic Functions in the Cell

471

SEQUENTIAL
ASPECTS OF
CHEMICAL
CAR-
CINOGENESIS:
SKIN

1. Increase in proteinase activity. The increased proteinase activity in mouse skin after treatment with a promoting agent, and the fact that the tumor promoting effect could be interfered with by concurrent treatment with pro- teinase *inhibitors*, has been thought to indicate some sort of correlation, possibly involving a hormonal control (Troll *et al.*, 1970, 1975). It is not clear, however, how increase in proteinase activity could eventually lead to the irreversible change in the tissue resulting from prolonged promoting action.

2. Stimulation of ornithine decarboxylase activity. Of all the metabolic changes in mouse skin following application of promoting agents, the most pronounced observed change is stimulation of ornithine decarboxylase activity (O'Brien *et al.*, 1975; O'Brien, 1976), reaching up to a 400-fold increase after a single application of 17 nmol TPA. [Some augmentation has also been demonstrated in tissue culture (O'Brien and Diamond, 1977). The effect in mouse skin, however, is not confined to treatment with promoting agents, since it has also been observed with nonpromoting irritants (Clark-Lewis and Murray, 1978; Marks *et al.*, 1979).] According to Boutwell and associates (see O'Brien *et al.*, 1975), increased ornithine decarboxylase activity might cause derepression of gene function, also somehow related to prostaglandin synthesis (Verma *et al.*, 1977). The available data, derived from short-term treatment with promoters, point, however, to a *reversible, transitory* derepression, associated with (*nonspecific*) DNA synthesis. [See also Yuspa *et al.* (1976*b*), in relation to *in vitro* effects.] No correlation was found to exist between stimulation of ornithine decar- boxylase activity and changes in cyclic AMP levels in the skin (Mufson *et al.*, 1977).

3. Changes in cyclic nucleotide levels. Though the function of cyclic nucleotides in skin metabolism is not yet fully understood, they seem somehow to be involved in the control of epidermal cell growth and differentiation, possibly related to chalone function (Voorhees *et al.*, 1973). There are several reports of changes in AMP and GMP levels—mainly depression, followed by some enhancement— both after single applications of phorbol esters (Belman and Troll, 1974; Grimm and Marks, 1974; Mufson *et al.*, 1977; Belman *et al.*, 1978) and after multiple applications of TPA following an initiating stimulus (Garte and Belman, 1978). The observed changes are, on the whole, not very pronounced, and their significance, in relation to the mechanism of promoting action, seems ques- tionable.

4. Decrease in histidase activity. After TPA application to the skin of hairless mice, and subsequent extraction of the tissue, a dose-dependent decrease in histidase activity was found in a supernatant fraction (Colburn *et al.*, 1975). The initiators urethan and 7,12-DMBA showed no such effect (though 7,12-DMBA is surely a promoter as well as initiator). The decrease in histidase activity seemed to be associated with DNA synthesis. It is not related to inhibition of general protein synthesis.

11.3. Miscellaneous Side Effects

In addition to mouse skin response, there are many "side effects" of promoting agents, reported in the literature, relating to responses of cells in tissue culture (see Cohen *et al.*, 1977; Weinstein *et al.*, 1977; Diamond *et al.*, 1978; Wilson and Reich, 1979; zur Hausen *et al.*, 1979); also *in vivo*, in relation to carcinogenesis in the liver and other organs; and more remotely, concerning their effects on leukocytes, microorganisms, etc. These come outside the scope of the present review, which deals specifically with skin response.

From the evidence so far available, it is difficult to decide which of the many side effects of promoting agents (in skin or other tissues) are causally involved in the mechanism of promoting action. One thing is certain: they cannot all be relevant! What are clearly needed are some other methods of approach, distinct from correlative studies, as for example using specific inhibitors of promoting action (cf. Van Duuren *et al.*, 1969; Chan *et al.*, 1970; Falk, 1971; Shamberger, 1971; Slaga *et al.*, 1974a, 1978b; Troll *et al.*, 1975; Van Duuren and Segal, 1976; Weeks *et al.*, 1979; see also Section 7), or by analytical procedures relating to modulations of gene expression—i.e., specifically concerned with the "awakening" process (Chang *et al.*, 1978; Kinsella and Radman, 1978), which should eventually give important leads toward the solution of the problem of the mechanism of promoting action.

12. References

ABELL, C. W., AND HEIDELBERGER, C., 1962, Interaction of carcinogenic hydrocarbons with tissues. VIII. Binding of tritium-labeled hydrocarbons to the soluble proteins of mouse skin, *Cancer Res.* **22**:931.

ANDREASEN, E., AND ENGELBRETH-HOLM, J., 1953, On the significance of the mouse hair cycle in experimental carcinogenesis, *Acta Pathol. Microbiol. Scand.* **32**:165.

ARFFMAN, E., AND GLAVIND, J., 1974, Carcinogenicity in mice of some fatty acid methyl esters. 1. Skin application, *Acta Pathol. Microbiol. Scand. Sect. A* **82**:127.

ARMUTH, V., AND BERENBLUM, I., 1972, Systemic promoting action of phorbol in liver and lung carcinogenesis in AKR mice, *Cancer Res.* **32**:2259.

ARMUTH, V., AND BERENBLUM, I., 1974, Promotion of mammary carcinogenesis and leukemogenic action by phorbol in virgin female Wistar rats, *Cancer Res.* **34**:2704.

ARMUTH, V., AND BERENBLUM, I., 1976, Phorbol as a possible promoting agent for skin carcinogenesis, *Z. Krebsforsch.* **85**:79.

ARMUTH, V., AND BERENBLUM, I., 1979, Tritiated thymidine as a broad spectrum initiator in transplacental two-stage carcinogenesis, with phorbol as promoter, *Int. J. Cancer* **24**:355.

ARMUTH, V., BERENBLUM, I., ADOLF, W., OPFERKUCH, H. J., SCHMIDT, R., SORG, B., AND HECKER, E., 1979, Systemic promoting action and leukemogenesis in SWR mice by phorbol and structurally related polyfunctional diterpenes, *J. Cancer Res. Clin. Oncol.* **95**:19.

ASHLEY, D. J. B., 1969, The two "hit" and multiple "hit" theories of carcinogenesis, *Br. J. Cancer* **23**:313.

BACH, H., AND GOERTTLER, K., 1971, Morphologische Untersuchungen zur hyperplasiogenen Wirkung des biologisch aktiven Phorbolesters A_1, *Virchows Arch. B* **8**:196.

BAIRD, W. M., AND BOUTWELL, R. K., 1971, Tumor-promoting activity of phorbol and four diesters of phorbol on mouse skin, *Cancer Res.* **31**:1074.

BAIRD, W. M., SEDGWICK, J. A., AND BOUTWELL, R. K., 1971, Effect of phorbol and four diesters of phorbol on the incorporation of tritiated precursors in DNA, RNA, and proteins in mouse epidermis, *Cancer Res.* **31**:1434.

BALL, J. K., AND McCARTER, J. A., 1960, A study of dose and effect in initiation of skin tumours by a carcinogenic hydrocarbon, *Br. J. Cancer* **14**:577.

BALMAIN, A., 1976, The synthesis of specific proteins in adult mouse epidermis during phases of proliferation and differentiation induced by the tumor promotor TPA, and in basal and differentiating layers of neonatal mouse epidermis, *J. Invest. Dermatol.* **67**:246.

BALMAIN, A., AND HECKER, E., 1974, On the biochemical mechanism of tumorigenesis in mouse skin. VI. Early effects of growth-stimulating phorbol esters on phosphate transport and phospholipid synthesis in mouse epidermis, *Biochim. Biophys. Acta* **362**:457.

BALMAIN, A., AND HECKER, E., 1976, On the biochemical mechanism of tumorigenesis in mouse skin. VII. The effects of tumor promoters on ^{3}H-choline and ^{3}H-glycerol incorporation into mouse epidermal phosphatidylcholine in relation to their effects on ^{3}H-thymidine incorporation into DNA, *Z. Krebsforsch.* **86**:251.

BARICH, L. L., SCHWARZ, J., AND BARICH, D., 1962, Oral griseofulvin: A cocarcinogenic agent to methylcholanthrene-induced cutaneous tumors, *Cancer Res.* **22**:53.

BARONI, C., van ESCH, G. J., AND SAFFIOTTI, U., 1963, Carcinogenesis tests of two inorganic arsenicals, *Arch. Environ. Health* **7**:668.

BATES, R. R., WORTHAM, J. S., COUNTS, W. B., DINGMAN, C. W., AND GELBOIN, H. V., 1968, Inhibition by actinomycin D of DNA synthesis and skin tumorigenesis induced by 7,12-dimethylbenz(a)anthracene, *Cancer Res.* **28**:27.

BAUER, K. H., 1928, Mutationstheorie der Geschwülst-Entstehung, Julius Springer, Berlin.

BAUM, J. W., 1976, Multiple simultaneous event model for radiation carcinogenesis, *Health Phys.* **30**:85.

BELMAN, S., AND TROLL, W., 1972, The inhibition of croton oil-promoted mouse skin tumorigenesis by steroid hormones, *Cancer Res.* **32**:450.

BELMAN, S., AND TROLL, W., 1974, Phorbol-12-myristate-13-acetate effect on cyclic adenosine 3',5'-monophosphate levels in mouse skin and inhibition of phorbol-myristate-acetate-promoted tumorigenesis by theophylline, *Cancer Res.* **34**:3446.

BELMAN, S., TROLL, W., AND GARTE, S. J., 1878, Effect of phorbol myristate acetate on cyclic nucleotide levels in mouse epidermis, *Cancer Res.* **38**:2978.

BERENBLUM, I., 1929, The modifying influence of dichloroethyl sulphide on the induction of tumours in mice by tar, *J. Pathol. Bacteriol.* **32**:425.

BERENBLUM, I., 1941a, The cocarcinogenic action of croton resin, *Cancer Res.* **1**:44.

BERENBLUM, I., 1941b, The mechanism of carcinogenesis: A study of the significance of cocarcinogenic action and related phenomena, *Cancer Res.* **1**:807.

BERENBLUM, I., 1944, Irritation and carcinogenesis, *Arch. Pathol.* **38**:233.

BERENBLUM, I., 1954a, Carcinogenesis and tumor pathogenesis, *Adv. Cancer Res.* **2**:129.

BERENBLUM, I., 1954b, A speculative review: The probable nature of promoting action and its significance in the understanding of the mechanism of carcinogenesis, *Cancer Res.* **14**:471.

BERENBLUM, I., 1968, A re-evaluation of the concept of cocarcinogenesis, *Prog. Exp. Tumor Res.* **11**:21.

BERENBLUM, I., 1974, The two-stage mechanism of carcinogenesis in biochemical terms, in: *The Physiopathology of Cancer*, Vol. 1 (P. Shubik, ed.), p. 393, Karger, Basel.

BERENBLUM, I., 1978, Historical perspective, in: *Carcinogenesis: Mechanisms of Tumor Promotion and Cocarcinogenesis*, Vol. 2 (T. J. Slaga, A. Sivak, and R. K. Boutwell, eds.), p. 1, Raven Press, New York.

BERENBLUM, I., 1979, Theoretical and practical aspects of the two-stage mechanism of carcinogenesis, in: *Carcinogens: Identification and Mechanisms of Action* (A. C. Clark and C. R. Shaw, eds.), p. 25, Raven Press, New York.

BERENBLUM, I., AND ARMUTH, V., 1977, The effect of colchicine injection prior to the initiating phase of two-stage carcinogenesis in mice, *Br. J. Cancer* **23**:615.

BERENBLUM, I., AND HARAN, N., 1955a, The significance of the sequence of initiating and promoting actions in the process of skin carcinogenesis in the mouse, *Br. J. Cancer* **9**:268.

BERENBLUM, I., AND HARAN, N., 1955b, The initiating action of ethyl carbamate (urethane) on mouse skin, *Br. J. Cancer* **9**:453.

BERENBLUM, I., AND HARAN-GHERA, N., 1957a, A quantitative study of the systemic initiating action of urethane (ethyl carbamate) in mouse skin carcinogenesis, *Br. J. Cancer* **11**:77.

473

SEQUENTIAL
ASPECTS OF
CHEMICAL
CAR-
CINOGENESIS:
SKIN

BERENBLUM, I., AND HARAN-GHERA, N., 1957*b*, The induction of the initiating phase of skin carcinogenesis in the mouse by oral administration of 9:10-dimethyl-1:2-benzanthracene, 20-methylcholanthrene, 3:4-benzpyrene, and 1:2:5:6-dibenzanthracene, *Br. J. Cancer* **11**:85.

BERENBLUM, I., AND LONAI, V., 1970, The leukemogenic action of phorbol, *Cancer Res.* **30**:2744.

BERENBLUM, I., AND SHUBIK, P., 1947*a*, The role of croton oil applications, associated with a single painting of a carcinogen, in tumor induction in the mouse's skin, *Br. J. Cancer* **1**:379.

BERENBLUM, I., AND SHUBIK, P., 1947*b*, A new, quantitative approach to the study of the stages of chemical carcinogenesis in the mouse's skin, *Br. J. Cancer* **1**:383.

BERENBLUM, I., AND SHUBIK, P., 1949*a*, An experimental study of the initiating stage of carcinogenesis and a re-evaluation of the somatic cell mutation theory of cancer, *Br. J. Cancer* **3**:109.

BERENBLUM, I., AND SHUBIK, P., 1949*b*, The persistence of latent tumour cells indueced in the mouse's skin by a single application of 9:10-dimethyl-1:2-benzanthracene, *Br. J. Cancer* **3**:384.

BERENBLUM, I., AND TRAININ, N., 1960, Possible two-stage mechanism in experimental leukemogenesis, *Science* **132**:40.

BERENBLUM, I., HARAN-GHERA, N., AND TRAININ, N., 1958, An experimental analysis of the "hair cycle effect" in mouse skin carcinogenesis *Br. J. Cancer* **12**:402.

BERNELLI-ZAZZERA, A., 1952, Contributo alla conoscenza dei fattori co-cancenigeni e del loro meccanismo d'azione sulla cute del topo, *Tumori* **38**:339.

BIELSCHOWSKY, F., AND HORNING, E. S., 1958, Aspects of endocrine carcinogenesis, *Br. Med. Bull.* **14**:106.

BILLINGHAM, R. E., ORR, J. W., AND WOODHOUSE, D. L., 1951, Transplantation of skin components during chemical carcinogenesis with 20-methylcholanthrene, *Br. J. Cancer* **5**:417.

BINGHAM, E., NIEMEIER, R. W., AND REID, J. B., 1976, Multiple factors in carcinogenesis, *Ann. N.Y. Acad. Sci.* **271**:14.

BOCK, F. G., 1968, The nature of tumor-promoting agents in tobacco products, *Cancer Res.* **28**:2362.

BOCK, F. G., AND BURNS, R., 1963, Tumor-promoting properties of anthranil (1,8,9-anthratriol), *J. Natl. Cancer Inst.* **30**:393.

BOCK, F. G., FJELDE, A., FOX, H. W., AND KLEIN, E., 1969, Tumor promotion by 1-fluoro-2,4-dinitrobenzene, a potent skin sensitizer, *Cancer Res.* **29**:179.

BOCK, F. G., MYERS, H. K., AND FOX, H. W., 1975, Cocarcinogenic activity of peroxy compounds, *J. Natl. Cancer Inst.* **55**:1359.

BORUM, K., 1954, The role of the mouse hair cycle in epidermal carcinogenesis, *Acta Pathol. Microbiol. Scand.* **34**:542.

BOUTWELL, R. K., 1964, Some biological aspects of skin carcinogenesis, *Prog. Exp. Tumor Res.* **4**:207.

BOUTWELL, R. K., 1974, The function and mechanism of promoters in carcinogenesis, *CRC Crit. Rev. Toxicol.* **2**:419.

BOUTWELL, R. K., 1978, Biochemical mechanism of tumor promotion, in: *Carcinogenesis: Mechanisms of Tumor Promotion and Cocarcinogenesis*, Vol. 2 (T. J. Slaga, A. Sivak, and R. K. Boutwell, eds.), p. 49, Raven Press, New York.

BOUTWELL, R. K., AND BOSCH, D. K., 1959, The tumor-promoting action of phenol and related compounds, *Cancer Res.* **19**:413.

BOUTWELL, R. K., AND RUSCH, H. P., 1951, The absence of an inhibiting effect of caloric restriction on papilloma formation, *Cancer Res.* **11**:238.

BOUTWELL, R. K., BOSCH, D., AND RUSCH, H. P., 1957, On the role of croton oil in tumor formation, *Cancer Res.* **17**:71.

BROOKES, P., 1975, Covalent interaction of carcinogens with DNA, *Life Sci.* **16**:331.

BRUSICK, D. J., 1977, The genetic properties of beta-propiolactone, *Mutat. Res.* **39**:241.

BULAY, I. M., AND WATTENBERG, L. W., 1970, Carcinogenic effects of subcutaneous administration of benzo(*a*)pyrene during pregnancy in the progeny, *Proc. Soc. Exp. Biol. Med.* **135**:84.

BULLOUGH, W. S., 1965, Mitotic and functional homeostasis: A speculative review, *Cancer Res.* **25**:1683.

CHAN, P. C., GOLDMAN, A., AND WYNDER, E. L., 1970, Hydroxyurea: Suppression of two-stage carcinogenesis in mouse skin, *Science* **168**:130.

CHANG, C.-C., TROSKO, J. E., AND WARREN, S. T., 1978, In vitro assay for tumor promoters and anti-promoters, *J. Environ. Pathol. Toxicol.* **2**:43.

CHARLES, D. R., AND LUCE-CLAUSEN, E. M., 1942, The kinetics of papilloma formation in benzpyrene-treated mice, *Cancer Res.* **2**:261.

CHORTYK, O. T., AND BOCK, F. G., 1976, Tumor-promoting activity of certain extracts of tobacco, *J. Natl. Cancer Inst.* **56**:1041.

475

SEQUENTIAL
ASPECTS OF
CHEMICAL
CAR-
CINOGENESIS:
SKIN

CHOUROULINKOV, I., AND LASNE, C., 1978, Two-stage (initiation–promotion) carcinogenesis *in vivo* and *in vitro*, *Bull. Cancer* **65**:155.

CHOUROULINKOV, I., GENTIL, A., GROVER, P. L., AND SIMS, P., 1976, Tumor-initiation activities on mouse skin of dihydrodiols derived from benzo(*a*)pyrene, *Br. J. Cancer* **34**:523.

CHOUROULINKOV, I., GENTIL, A., TIERNEY, B., GROVER, P. L., AND SIMS, P., 1979, The initiation of tumours on mouse skin by dihydrodiols derived from 7,12-dimethylbenz(*a*)anthracene and 30-methylcholanthrene, *Int. J. Cancer* **24**:455.

CLARK-LEWIS, I., AND MURRAY, A. W., 1978, Tumor promotion and induction of epidermal ornithine decarboxylase activity in mechanically stimulated mouse skin, *Cancer Res.* **38**:494.

COHEN, R., PACIFICI, M., RUBINSTEIN, N., BIEHL, J., AND HOLTZER, H., 1977, Effect of a tumour promoter on myogenesis, *Nature (London)* **266**:538.

COLBURN, N. H., AND BOUTWELL, R. K., 1966, The binding of β-propiolactone to mouse skin *in vivo*. Its correlation with tumor-initiating activity, *Cancer Res.* **26**:1701.

COLBURN, N. H., LAU, S., AND HEAD, R., 1975, Decrease of epidermal histidase activity by tumor-promoting esters, *Cancer Res.* **35**:3154.

COOMBS, M. M., AND BHATT, T. S., 1978, Lack of initiating activity in mutagens which are not carcinogenic, *Br. J. Cancer* **38**:148.

COOPER, H. K., BUECHELER, J., AND KLEIHUES, P., 1978, DNA alkylation in mice with genetically different susceptibilities to 1,2-dimethylhydrazine-induced colon carcinogenesis, *Cancer Res.* **38**:3063.

CRAMER, W., AND STOWELL, R. E., 1943, Skin carcinogenesis by a single application of 20-methylcholanthrene, *Cancer Res.* **3**:36.

DAMMERT, K., 1961, A histological and cytological study of different methods of skin tumorigenesis, *Acta Pathol. Microbiol. Scand.* **53**:33.

DEELMAN, H. T., 1924, Die Entstehung des experimentellen, Teerkresbses und die Bedeutung der Zellenregeneration, *Z. Krebsforsch.* **21**:220.

DEELMAN, H. T., AND VAN ERP, J. P., 1926, Beobachtungen an experimentellen Tumorwachstum, *Z. Krebsforsch.* **24**:86.

DELLA PORTA, G., SHUBIK, P., DAMMERT, K., AND TERRACINI, B., 1960, Role of polyoxyethylene sorbitan monostearate in skin carcinogenesis in mice, *J. Natl. Cancer Inst.* **25**:607.

DE WAARD, R. H., 1964, Coincidence of mutations as a possible cause of malignancy, *Int. J. Radiat. Biol.* **8**:381.

DE YOUNG, L. M., ARGYRIS, T. S., AND GORDON, G. B., 1977*a*, Epidermal ribosome accumulation during two-stage skin tumorigenesis, *Cancer Res.* **37**:388.

DEYOUNG, L. M., MUFSON, R. A., AND BOUTWELL, R. K., 1977*b*, An apparent inactivation of initiated cells by the potent inhibitor of two-stage mouse skin tumorigenesis, bis(2-chloroethyl)sulfide, *Cancer Res.* **37**:4590.

DIAMOND, L., O'BRIEN, T. G., AND ROVERA, G., 1978, Tumor promoters: Effect on proliferation and differentiation of cells in culture, *Life Sci.* **23**:1979.

DIGIOVANNI, J., SLAGA, T. J., VIAJE, A., BERRY, D. L., HARVEY, R. G., AND JUCHAU, M. R., 1978, Effects of 7,8-benzoflavone on skin tumor-initiating activities of various 7- and 12-substituted derivatives of 7,12-dimethylbenz(*a*) anthracene in mice, *J. Natl. Cancer Inst.* **61**:135.

DINGMAN, C. W., AND SPORN, M. B., 1967, The binding of metabolites of aminoazo dyes to rat liver DNA *in vitro*, *Cancer Res.* **27**:938.

DRIEDGER, P. E., AND BLUMBERG, P. M., 1979, Quantitative correlation between *in vitro* and *in vivo* activities of phorbol esters, *Cancer Res.* **39**:714.

ELGJO, K., 1976, Epidermal chalone in experimental skin carcinogenesis, in: *Chalones* (J. C. Hoock, ed.), p. 229, North-Holland/American Elsevier, Amsterdam and New York.

ELGJO, K., AND DEGRÉ, M., 1973, Polyinosinic-polycytidilic acid in two-stage skin carcinogenesis. Effect on epidermal growth parameters and interferon induction in treated mice, *J. Natl. Cancer Inst.* **51**:171.

EMMELOT, P., AND SCHERER, E., 1977, Multi-hit kinetics of tumor formation, with special reference to experimental liver and human lung carcinogenesis and some general conclusions, *Cancer Res.* **37**:1702.

ENGELBRETH-HOLM, J., AND ASBOE-HANSEN, G., 1953, Effect of cortisone on skin carcinogenesis in mice, *Acta Pathol. Microbiol. Scand.* **32**:560.

EPSTEIN, J. H., 1972, Examination of the carcinogenic and cocarcinogenic effects of Grenz radiation, *Cancer Res.* **32**:2625.

EPSTEIN, J. H., AND ROTH, H. L., 1968, Experimental ultraviolet light carcinogenesis: A study of croton oil promoting effects, *J. Invest. Dermatol.* **50**:378.

FALK, H. L., 1971, Anticarcinogenesis—An alternative, *Prog. Exp. Tumor Res.* **14**:105.

FARBER, E., 1973, Carcinogenesis—Cellular evolution as a unifying thread, *Cancer Res.* **33**:2537.

FISHER, J. C., AND HOLOMON, J. H., 1951, A hypothesis for the origin of cancer foci, *Cancer* **4**:916.

FONG, L. Y. Y., LIN, H. J., AND LEE, C. L. H., 1979, Methylation in target and nontarget organs of the rat with methylbenzylnitrosamine and dimethylnitrosamine, *Int. J. Cancer* **23**:679.

FOULDS, L., 1954, The experimental study of tumor progression, *Cancer Res.* **14**:327.

FOULDS, L., 1965, Multiple etiologic factors in neoplastic development, *Cancer Res.* **25**:1339.

FRANKFURT, O. S., AND RAITCHEVA, E., 1973, Fast onset of DNA synthesis stimulated by tumor promoter in mouse epidermis at the initiation stage of carcinogenesis, *J. Natl. Cancer Inst.* **51**:1861.

FREI, J. V., AND KINGSLEY, W. F., 1968, Observations on chemically induced regressing tumors of mouse epidermis, *J. Natl. Cancer Inst.* **41**:1307.

FREI, J. V., AND STEPHENS, P., 1968, The correlation of promotion of tumour growth and of induction of hyperplasia in epidermial two-stage carcinogenesis, *Br. J. Cancer* **22**:83.

FRIEDEWALD, W. F., AND ROUS, P., 1944*a*, The initiating and promoting elements in tumor production: An analysis of the effects of tar, benzpyrene, and methylcholanthrene on rabbit skin, *J. Exp. Med.* **80**:101.

FRIEDEWALD, W. F., AND ROUS, P., 1944*b*, The determining influence of tar, benzpyrene and methylcholanthrene on the character of the benign tumors induced therewith in rabbit skin, *J. Exp. Med.* **80**:127.

FRIEDEWALD, W. F., AND ROUS, P., 1950, The pathogenesis of deferred cancer: A study of the after-effects of methylcholanthrene upon rabbit skin, *J. Exp. Med.* **91**:459.

FURTH, J., 1975, Hormones as etiological agents in neoplasia, in: *Cancer: A Comprehensive Treatise,* Vol. 1 (F. F. Becker, ed.), p. 75, Plenum Press, New York.

GARTE, S. J., AND BELMAN, S., 1978, Effects of multiple phorbol myristate acetate treatments on cyclic nucleotide levels in mouse epidermis, *Biochem. Biophys. Res. Commun.* **84**:489.

GAUDIN, D., GREGG, R. S., AND YIELDING, K. I., 1971, DNA repair inhibition: A possible mechanism of action of co-carcinogens, *Biochem. Biophys. Res. Commun.* **45**:630.

GAUDIN, D., GREGG, R. S., AND YIELDING, K. I., 1972, Inhibition of DNA repair by cocarcinogens, *Biochem. Biophys. Res. Commun.* **48**:945.

GELBOIN, H. V., AND BLACKBURN, N. R., 1964, The stimulatory effect of 3-methylcholanthrene on benzpyrene hydroxylase activity in several rat tissues: Inhibition by actinomycin D and puromycin, *Cancer Res.* **24**:356.

GELBOIN, H. V., AND LEVY, H. B., 1970, Polyinosinic-polycytidylic acid inhibits chemically induced tumorigenesis in mouse skin, *Scince* **167**:205.

GELBOIN, H. V., KLEIN, M., AND BATES, R. R., 1965, Inhibition of mouse skin tumorigenesis by actinomycin D, *Proc. Natl. Acad. Sci. USA* **53**:1353.

GELBOIN, H. V., KINOSHITA, N., AND WIEBEL, F. J., 1972, Microsomal hydrolases: Studies on the mechanism of induction and their role in polycyclic hydrocarbon action, in: *Environment and Cancer,* 24th Annual Symposium on Fundamental Cancer Research, M. D. Anderson Hospital and Tumor Institute, Houston, Williams & Wilkins, Baltimore, p. 214.

GELHORN, A., 1958, The cocarcinogenic activity of cigarette tobacco tar, *Cancer Res.* **18**:510.

GLÜCKSMANN, A., 1945, The histogenesis of benzpyrene-induced epidermal tumors in the mouse, *Cancer Res.* **5**:385.

GOERTTLER, K., AND LOEHRKE, H., 1976, Transmaternal variation of the Berenblum experiment with NMRI mice. Tumour initiation with DMBA via mothers milk followed by promotion with the phorbol ester TPA, *Virchows Arch. A* **370**:97.

GOERTTLER, K., AND LOEHRKE, H., 1977, Diaplacental carcinogenesis: Tumour localization and tumour incidence in NMRI mice after diaplacental initiation with DMBA and urethane and postnatal promotion with the phorbol ester TPA in a modified 2-stage Berenblum/Mottram experiment, *Virchows Arch. A* **376**:117.

GOERTTLER, K., LOEHRKE, H., SCHWEIZER, J., AND HESSE, B., 1979, Systemic two-stage carcinogenesis in the epithelium of the forestomach of mice using 7,12-dimethylbenz(*a*)anthracene as initiator and the phorbol ester 12-*O*-tetradecanoylphorbol-13-acetate as promoter, *Cancer Res.* **39**:1293.

GOSHMAN, I. M., AND HEIDELBERGER, C., 1967, Binding of tritium-labeled hydrocarbons to DNA of mouse skin, *Cancer Res.* **27**:1678.

GRAFFI, A., 1953, Untersuchungen über den Mechanismus der Cancergenese und die Wirkungsweise cancerogener Reize, *Abh. Dtsch. Akad. Wiss. Berlin Kl. Med.* **1**:1 (quoted by Roe *et al.*, 1972).

477

SEQUENTIAL
ASPECTS OF
CHEMICAL
CAR-
CINOGENESIS:
SKIN

GRAFFI, A., SCHARSACH, F., AND HEYER, E., 1955, Zur Frage der Initialwirkung cancerogener Kohlenwasserstoffe auf die Mäusehaut nach intravenöser, intraperitonealer und oraler Applikation, *Naturwissenschaften* **42**:184.

GRANT, G. A., ROE, F. J. C., AND PIKE, M. C., 1966, Effect of neonatal thymectomy on the induction of papillomata and carcinomata by 3,4-benzopyrene in mice, *Nature (London)* **210**:603.

GRIMM, W., AND MARKS, F., 1974, Effect of tumor-promoting phorbol esters on the normal and the isoproterenol-elevated level of adenosine 3',5'-cyclic monophosphate in mouse epidermis in vivo, *Cancer Res.* **34**:3128.

GWYNN, R. H., AND SALAMAN, M. H., 1953, Studies on co-carcinogenesis: SH-reactors and other substances tested for co-carcinogenic action in mouse skin, *Br. J. Cancer* **7**:482.

HARAN, N., AND BERENBLUM, I., 1956, The induction of the initiating phase of carcinogenesis in the mouse by oral administration of urethane (ethyl carbamate), *Br. J. Cancer* **10**:57.

HARAN-GHERA, N., AND LURIE, M., 1971, Effect of heterologous antithymocyte serum on mouse skin tumorigenesis, *J. Natl. Cancer Inst.* **46**:103.

HAWKS, A., AND MAGEE, P. N., 1974, The alkylation of nucleic acids of rat and mouse in vivo by the carcinogen 1,2-dimethylhydrazine, *Br. J. Cancer* **30**:440.

HAYATSU, H., HOSHINO, H., AND KAWAZOE, Y., 1971, Potential cocarcinogenicity of sodium hypochlorite, *Nature (London)* **233**:495.

HECHT, S. S., BONDINELL, W. E., AND HOFFMANN, D., 1974, Chrysene and methylchrysenes: Presence in tobacco smoke and carcinogenicity, *J. Natl. Cancer Inst.* **53**:1121.

HECHT, S. S., THORNE, R. L., MORONPOT, R. R., AND HOFFMANN, D., 1975, A study of tobacco carcinogenesis. XIII. Tumor-promoting subfractions of the weakly acidic fraction, *J. Natl. Cancer Inst.* **55**:1329.

HECHT, S. S., HIROTA, N., LOY, M., AND HOFFMANN, D., 1978, Tumor-initiating activity of fluorinated 5-methylchrysene, *Cancer Res.* **38**:1698.

HECKER, E., 1968, Cocarcinogenic principles from the seed oil of *Croton tiglium* and from other Euphorbiaceae, *Cancer Res.* **28**:2338.

HECKER, E., 1971*a*, Isolation and characterization of the cocarcinogenic principles from croton oil, in: *Methods in Cancer Research*, Vol. 6 (H. Busch, ed.), p. 439, Academic Press, New York.

HECKER, E., 1971*b*, New phorbol esters and related cocarcinogens, in: *Proceedings of the 10th International Cancer Congress*, Houston, Vol. 5, p. 213, Year Book Medical Publishers, Chicago.

HECKER, E., 1978, Structure–activity relationships in diterpene esters irritant and cocarcinogenic to mouse skin, in: *Carcinogenesis: Mechanisms of Tumor Promotion and Cocarcinogenesis*, Vol. 2 (T. J. Slaga, A. Sivak, and R. K. Boutwell, eds.), p. 11, Raven Press, New York.

HECKER, E., IMMICH, H., BRESCH, H., AND SCHAIRER, H. U., 1966, Über die Wirkstoffe des Crotonöl. VI. Entzündungsteste am Mäuseohr, *Z. Krebsforsch.* **68**:366.

HELMES, C. T., HILLESUND, T., AND BOUTWELL, R. K., 1974, The binding of tritium-labeled phorbol esters to the macromolecular constituents of mouse epidermis, *Cancer Res.* **34**:1365.

HENNINGS, H., AND BOUTWELL, R. K., 1967, On the mechanism of inhibition of benign and malignant skin tumors by actinomycin D, *Life Sci.* **6**:173.

HENNINGS, H., AND BOUTWELL, R. K., 1970, Studies on the mechanism of skin tumor promotion, *Cancer Res.* **30**:312.

HENNINGS, H., BOWDEN, G. T., AND BOUTWELL, R. K., 1969, The effect of croton oil pretreatment on skin tumor initiation in mice, *Cancer Res.* **29**:1773.

HENNINGS, H., MICHAEL, D., AND PATTERSON, E., 1973, Enhancement of skin tumorigenesis by a single application of croton oil before and soon after intiation by urethan, *Cancer Res.* **33**:3130.

HOFFMANN, D., BONDINELL, W. E., AND WYNDER, E. L., 1974, Carcinogenicity of methylchrysenes, *Science* **183**:215.

HOLSTI, P., 1959, Tumor promoting effects of some long chain fatty acids in experimental skin carcinogenesis in the mouse, *Acta Pathol. Microbiol. Scand.* **46**:51.

HORTON, A. W., DENMAN, D. T., AND TROSSET, R. P., 1957, Carcinogenesis of the skin. II. The accelerating properties of aliphatic and related hydrocarbons, *Cancer Res.* **17**:758.

HORTON, A. W., ESHLEMAN, D. N., SCHUFF, A. R., AND PERMAN, W. H., 1976, Correlation of cocarcinogenic activity among *n*-alkanes with their physical effects on phospholipid micelles, *J. Natl. Cancer Inst.* **56**:387.

HOSHINO, H., AND TANOOKA, H., 1975, Interval effect of β-irradiation and subsequent 4-nitroquinoline 1-oxide painting on skin tumor induction in mice, *Cancer Res.* **35**:3663.

HUH, T.-V., AND MCCARTER, J. A., 1960, Phenanthrene as an anti-initiating agent, *Br. J. Cancer* **14**:591.

ISHII, D. N., FIBACH, E., YAMASAKI, H., AND WEINSTEIN, I. B., 1978, Tumor promoters inhibit morphological differentiation in cultured mouse neuroblastoma cells, *Science* **200**:556.

IVERSEN, O. H., 1973, Cell proliferation kinetics and carcinogenesis: A review, in: *Proceedings of the 5th International Symposium on Biological Characterization of Human Tumours*, p. 21, Excerpta Medica, Amsterdam.

IVERSEN, S., AND ARLEY, N., 1950, On the mechanism of experimental carcinogenesis, *Acta Pathol. Microbiol. Scand.* **27**:773.

JACKSON, C. D., AND IRVING, C. C., 1970, The binding of N-hydroxy-2-acetylaminofluorene to replicating and nonreplicating DNA in rat liver, *Chem. Biol. Interact.* **2**:261.

JACOB, F., AND MONOD, J., 1961, On the regulation of gene activity, *Cold Spring Harbor Symp. Quant. Biol.* **26**:193.

JANOFF, A., KLASSEN, A., AND TROLL, W., 1970, Local vascular changes by the cocarcinogen, phorbol myristate acetate, *Cancer Res.* **30**:2568.

JULL, J. W., 1976, Endocrine aspects of carcinogenesis, *ACS Monogr.* **173**:52.

KAWAMOTO, S., IDA, N., KIRSCHBAUM, A., AND TAYLOR, G., 1958, Urethan and leukemogenesis in mice, *Cancer Res.* **18**:725.

KENNEDY, A. R., MONDAL, S., HEIDELBERGER, C., AND LITTLE, J. B., 1978, Enhancement of X-ray transformation by 12-tetradecanoyl-phorbol-13-acetate in a cloned line of C3H mouse embryo cells, *Cancer Res.* **38**:439.

KING, H. W. S., OSBORNE, M. R., AND BROOKES, P., 1977, The metabolism and DNA binding of 3-methylcholanthrene, *Int. J. Cancer* **20**:564.

KINOSHITA, N., AND GELBOIN, H. V., 1972, The role of aryl hydrocarbon hydroxylase in 7,12-dimethylbenz(a)anthracene skin tumorigenesis: On the mechanism of 7,8-benzoflavone inhibition of tumorigenesis, *Cancer Res.* **32**:1329.

KINSELLA, A. R., AND RADMAN, M., 1978, Tumor promoter induces sister chromatid exchanges: Relevance to mechanisms of carcinogenesis, *Proc. Natl. Acad. Sci. USA* **75**:6149.

KOMITOWSKI, D., GOERTTLER, K., AND LÖHRKE, H., 1977, Epidermal intercellular relationship during carcinogenesis and cocarcinogenesis by scanning electron microscopy, *Virchows Arch. B* **24**:317.

KOPELOVICH, L., BIAS, N. E., AND HELSON, L., 1979, Tumour promoter alone induces malignant transformation of fibroblasts from humans genetically predisposed to cancer, *Nature (London)* **282**:619.

KREIBICH, G., SÜSS, R., KINZEL, V., AND HECKER, E., 1970, On the biochemical mechanism of tumorigenesis in mouse skin. III. Decrease of tumor yields by poly I/C administered during initiation of skin by an intragastric dose of 7,12-dimethyl-benz(a)anthracene, *Z. Krebsforsch.* **74**:383.

KRIEG, L., KÜHLMANN, I., AND MARKS, F., 1974, Effect of tumor promoting phorbol esters and of acetic acid on mechanisms of controlling DNA synthesis and mitosis (chalones) and on the biosynthesis of histidine-rich protein in mouse epidermis, *Cancer Res.* **34**:3135.

KUBINSKI, H., STRANSTALIEN, M. S., BAIRD, W. M., AND BOUTWELL, R. K., 1973, Interaction of phorbol esters with cellular membranes *in vitro*, *Cancer Res.* **33**:3103.

KURATSUNE, M., KOHCHI, S., HORIE, A., AND NISHIZUMI, M., 1971, Test of alcoholic beverages and ethanol solutions for carcinogenicity and tumor-promoting activity, *Gann* **62**:395.

KUROKI, T., HUBERMAN, E., MARQUARDT, H., SELKIRK, J. K., HEIDELBERGER, C., AND GROVER, P. L., 1972, Binding of K-region epoxides and other derivatives of benz(a) anthracene and dibenz(a,h)anthracene to DNA, RNA, and proteins of transformable cells, *Chem. Biol. Interact.* **4**:389.

LANGENBACH, R., AND KUSZYNSKI, C., 1975, Nonspecific inhibition of DNA repair by promoting and nonpromoting phorbol esters, *J. Natl. Cancer Inst.* **55**:801.

LAPPÉ, M. A., 1968, Evidence for the antigenicity of papillomas induced by 3-methylcholanthrene, *J. Natl. Cancer Inst.* **40**: 823.

LAPPÉ, M. A., 1969, Tumour specific transplantation antigens: Possible origin in premalignant lesions, *Nature (London)* **223**:82.

LASNE, C., GENTIL, A., AND CHOUROULINKOV, I., 1977, Two-stage carcinogenesis with rat embryo cells in tissue culture, *Br. J. Cancer* **35**:722.

LAW, I. W., 1941, Multiple skin tumors in mice following a single painting with 9:10-dimethyl-1:2-benzanthracene, *Am. J. Pathol.* **17**:827.

LICHTI, U., SLAGA, T. H., BEN, T., PATTERSON, E., HENNINGS, H., AND YUSPA, S. H., 1977, Dissociation of tumor-promoter-stimulated ornithine decarboxylase activity and DNA synthesis in mouse epidermis *in vivo* and *in vitro* by fluoccinolene acetonide, a tumor-promoting inhibitor, *Proc. Natl. Acad. Sci. USA* **74**:3908.

LIJINSKY, W., AND ROSS, A. E., 1969, Alkylation of rat liver nucleic acids not related to carcinogenesis by N-nitrosamines, *J. Natl. Cancer Inst.* **42**:1095.

MACKENZIE, I., AND ROUS, P., 1941, The environmental disclosure of latent neoplastic changes in tarred skin, *J. Exp. Med.* **73**:391.

MAGEE, P. N., AND FARBER, E., 1962, Toxic liver injury and carcinogenesis: Methylation of rat-liver nucleic acids by dimethylnitrosamine *in vivo*, *Biochem. J.* **83**:114.

MAJOR, I. R., 1970, Correlation of initial changes in the mouse epidermal cell population with two-stage carcinogenesis—A quantitative study, *Br. J. Cancer* **24**:149.

MARCHANT, J., AND ORR, J. W., 1953, Further attempts to analyse the roles of epidermis and deeper tissues in experimental chemical carcinogenesis by transplantation and other methods, *Br. J. Cancer* **7**:329.

MARCHANT, J., AND ORR, J. W., 1955, A further investigation of the role of skin components in chemical carcinogenesis, *Br. J. Cancer* **9**:128.

MARKS, F., 1976, Epidermal growth control mechanisms, hyperplasia, and tumor promotion in the skin, *Cancer Res.* **36**:2636.

MARKS, F., BERTSCH, S., AND FÜRSTENBERGER, G., 1979, Ornithine decarboxylase activity, cell proliferation, and tumor promotion in mouse skin epidermis *in vivo*, *Cancer Res.* **39**:4183.

McCANN, J., CHOI, E., YAMASAKI, E., AND AMES, B. N., 1975, Detection of carcinogens as mutagens in *Salmonella*-microsome tests: Assay of 300 chemicals, *Proc. Natl. Acad. Sci. USA* **72**(Part I):5139.

McCARTER, J. A., SZERB, J. C., AND THOMPSON, G. E., 1956, The influence of area of skin exposed, duration of exposure, and concentration in determining tumor yield in the skin of the mouse after a single application of a carcinogenic hydrocarbon, *J. Natl. Cancer Inst.* **17**:405.

MEITES, J., 1958, Effects of thyroxine and thiouracil on induction of tumors in mice by 9,10-dimethyl-1,2-benzanthracene and croton oil, *Cancer Res.* **18**:176.

MEYENBURG, H. V., AND FRITSCHE, H., 1943, Experimentelle Untersuchungen zum Thema Präkanzerose bzw Präneoplasie, *Schweiz. Med. Wochenschr.* **73**:201.

MEYER-BERTENRATH, J. G., 1969, Zur Frage eines Zwei-Phasen-Mechanismus der Carcinogenese, *Klin. Wochenschr.* **47**:173.

MIDER, G. B., AND MORTON, J. J., 1939, Skin tumors following a single application of methylcholanthrene in C57 brown mice, *Am. J. Pathol.* **15**:299.

MILLER, E. C., AND MILLER, J. A., 1966, Mechanism of chemical carcinogenesis: Nature of proximate carcinogens and interactions with macromolecules, *Pharmacol. Rev.* **18**:805.

MILLER, J. F. A. P., GRANT, G. A., AND ROE, F. J. C., 1963, Effect of thymectomy on the induction of skin tumours by 3,4-benzopyrene, *Nature (London)* **199**:920.

MIRVISH, S. S., 1968, The carcinogenic action and metabolism of urethan and N-hydroxyurethan, *Adv. Cancer Res.* **11**:1.

MONDAL, S., BRANKOW, D. W., AND HEIDELBERGER, C., 1976, Two-stage chemical oncogenesis in cultures of C3H/10T1/2 cells, *Cancer Res.* **36**:2254.

MOTTRAM, J. C., 1944a, A developing factor in experimental blastogenesis, *J. Pathol. Bacteriol.* **56**:181.

MOTTRAM, J. C., 1944b, A sensitizing factor in experimental blastogenesis, *J. Pathol. Bacteriol.* **56**:391.

MUFSON, R. A., ASTRUP, E. G., SIMSIMAN, R. C., AND BOUTWELL, R. K., 1977, Dissociation of increases in levels of $3':5'$-cyclic AMP and $3':5'$-cyclic GMP from induction of ornithine decarboxylase by tumor promoter 12-O-tetradecanoyl-phorbol-13-acetate in mouse epidermis *in vivo*, *Proc. Natl. Acad. Sci. USA* **74**:657.

MUKAI, F., AND TROLL, W., 1969, The mutagenicity and initiating activity of some aromatic amine metabolites, *Ann. N.Y. Acad. Sci.* **163**:828.

MURRAY, A. W., 1978, Acetic acid pretreatment of initiated epidermis inhibits tumour promotion by a phorbol ester, *Experientia* **34**:1507.

NAKAHARA, W., 1961, Critique of carcinogenic mechanisms, *Prog. Exp. Tumor Res.* **2**:158.

NERY, R., 1976, Carcinogenic mechanisms: A critical review and a suggestion that oncogenesis may be adaptive ontogenesis, *Chem. Biol. Interact.* **12**:145.

NETTLESHIP, A., HENSHAW, P. S., AND MEYER, H. L., 1943, Induction of pulmonary tumors in mice with ethyl carbamate (urethane), *J. Natl. Cancer Inst.* **4**:309.

NISKANEN, E. E., AND MERENMIES, L., 1960, The determining influence of the dose and nature of orally administered carcinogens on mouse skin tumours promoted by Tween 40, *Naturwissenschaften* **47**:46.

NORDLING, C. O., 1953, A new theory on the cancer-inducing mechanism, *Br. J. Cancer* **7**:68.

O'BRIEN, T. G., 1976, The induction of ornithine decarboxylase as an early, possibly obligatory, event in mouse skin carcinogenesis, *Cancer Res.* **36**:2644.

479

SEQUENTIAL
ASPECTS OF
CHEMICAL
CAR-
CINOGENESIS:
SKIN

O'Brien, T. G., and Diamond, L., 1977, Ornithine decarboxylase induction and DNA synthesis in hamster embryo cell cultures treated with tumor-promoting phorbol diesters, *Cancer Res.* **36:**3895.

O'Brien, T. G., Simsiman, R. C., and Boutwell, R. K., 1975, Induction of the polyamine-biosynthetic enzymes in mouse epidermis and their specificity to tumor promotion, *Cancer Res.* **35:**2426.

Odashima, S., 1962, Combined effect of carcinogens with different actions. III. Development of skin cancers in the rat by feeding 4-dimethylaminostilbene following initial painting of 20-methylcholanthrene, *Gann* **53:**269.

Orr, J. W., 1934, The influence of ischaemia on the development of tumours, *Br. J. Exp. Pathol.* **15:**73.

Orr, J. W., 1935, The effect of interference with the vascular supply on the induction of dibenzanthracene tumours, *Br. J. Exp. Pathol.* **16:**121.

Orr, J. W., 1937, The results of vital staining with phenol red during the prgress of carcinogenesis in mice treated with tar, dibenzanthracene and benzpyrene, *J. Pathol. Bacteriol.* **44:**19.

Orr, J. W., 1958, The mechanism of chemical carcinogenesis, with particular reference to the time of development of irreversible changes in the epithelial cells, *Br. Med. Bull.* **14:**99.

Paul, D., and Hecker, E., 1969, On the biochemical mechanism of tumorigenesis in mouse skin. II. Early effects on the biosynthesis of nucleic acids induced by initiating doses of DMBA and by promoting doses of phorbol-12-13-diester TPA, *Z. Krebsforsch.* **73:**149.

Phillips, D. H., Grover, P. L., and Sims, P., 1979, A quantitative determination of the covalent binding of a series of polycyclic hydrocarbons to DNA in mouse skin, *Int. J. Cancer* **23:**201.

Picco, A., Somaglino, W., and Lasi, C., 1958, Richerche sull'azione promovente della follicolina nel duplice meccanismo della carcinogenesi, *Tumori* **44:**173.

Pierce, G. B., 1974, Neoplasms, differentiation and mutations, *Am. J. Pathol.* **77:**103.

Pitot, H. C., and Heidelberger, C., 1963, Metabolic regulatory circuits and carcinogenesis, *Cancer Res.* **23:**1694.

Pound, A. W., 1970, Induced cell proliferation and the initiation of skin tumour formation in mice by ultraviolet light, *Pathology* **2:**269.

Pound, A. W., and Bell, J. R., 1962, The influence of croton oil stimulation on tumour initiation by urethane in mice, *Br. J. Cancer* **16:**690.

Pound, A. W., and Withers, H. R., 1963, The influence of some irritant chemicals and scarification on tumour initiation by urethane in mice, *Br. J. Cancer* **17:**460.

Prodi, G., Rochi, P., and Grilli, S., 1970, *In vivo* interaction of urethan with nucleic acids and protein, *Cancer Res.* **30:**2887.

Purchase, I. F. H., Longstaff, E., Ashby, J., Styles, J. A., Anderson, D., Lefevre, P. A., and Westwood, F. R., 1976, Evaluation of six short therm tests for detecting organic chemical carcinogens and recommendations for their use, *Nature (London)* **264:**624.

Pyerin, W. G., and Hecker, E., 1979, On the biochemical mechanism of tumorigenesis in mouse skin. IX. Interrelation between tumor initiation by 7,12-dimethylbenz(*a*)anthracene and the activities of epidermal arylhydrocarbon monooxygenase and epoxide hydrase, *J. Cancer Res. Clin. Oncol.* **93:**7.

Raick, A. N., 1973, Ultrastructural, histological, and biochemical alterations produced by 12-*O*-tetradecanoyl-phorbol-13-acetate on mouse epidermis and their relevance to skin tumor promotion, *Cancer Res.* **33:**269.

Raick, A. N., 1974, Cell proliferation and promoting action in skin carcinogenesis, *Cancer Res.* **34:**920.

Raineri, R., Simsiman, R. C., and Boutwell, R. K., 1973, Stimulation of the phosphorylation of mouse epidermal histones by tumor-promoting agents, *Cancer Res.* **33:**134.

Rinkus, S. S., and Legator, M. S., 1979, Chemical characterization of 465 known or suspected carcinogens and their correlation with mutagenic activity in the *Salmonella typhimurium* system, *Cancer Res.* **39:**3289.

Ritchie, A. C., 1952*a*, The effect of local injections of adrenalin on epidermal carcinogenesis in the mouse, *J. Natl. Cancer Inst.* **12:**839.

Ritchie, A. C., 1952*b*, The effect of arterial occlusion on epidermal carcinogenesis in the rabbit, *J. Natl. Cancer Inst.* **12:**847.

Ritchie, A. C., 1957, Epidermal carcinogenesis in the mouse by intraperitoneally administered urethane followed by repeated applications of croton oil, *Br. J. Cancer* **11:**206.

Ritchie, A. C., and Saffiotti, U., 1955, Orally administered 2-acetylaminofluorene as an initiator and as a promoter of epidermal carcinogenesis in the mouse, *Cancer Res.* **15:**84.

Ritchie, A. C., Shubik, P., and Leroy, E. P., 1953, The effect of cortisone on the hyperplasia produced in mouse skin by croton oil, *Cancer Res.* **13:**45.

481

SEQUENTIAL
ASPECTS OF
CHEMICAL
CAR-
CINOGENESIS:
SKIN

ROE, F. J. C., 1956a, The development of malignant tumours of mouse skin after "initiating" and "promoting" stimuli. I. The effect of a single application of 9,10-dimethyl-1,2-benzanthracene (DMBA) with and without subsequent treatment with croton oil, *Br. J. Cancer* **10**:61.

ROE, F. J. C., 1956b, The development of malignant tumours of mouse skin after "initiating" and "promoting" stimuli. III. The carcinogenic action of croton oil, *Br. J. Cancer* **10**:72.

ROE, F. J. C., 1957, Tumor initiation in mouse skin by certain esters of methanesulfonic acid, *Cancer Res.* **17**:64.

ROE, F. J. C., 1959a, The effect of applying croton oil before a single application of 9,10-dimethyl-1,2-benzanthracene (DMBA), *Br. J. Cancer* **18**:87.

ROE, F. J. C., 1959b, Oil of sweet orange: A possible role in carcinogenesis, *Br. J. Cancer* **13**:92.

ROE, F. J. C., AND PEIRCE, W. E. H., 1960, Tumor promotion by citrus oils: Tumors of the skin and urethral orifice in mice, *J. Natl. Cancer Inst.* **24**:1389.

ROE, F. J. C., AND PEIRCE, W. E. H., 1961, Tumor promotion by euphorbia lattices, *Cancer Res.* **21**:338.

ROE, F. J. C., AND SALAMAN, M. H., 1954, A quantitative study of the power and persistence of the tumor-initiating effect of ethyl carbamate (urethane) on mouse skin, *Br. J. Cancer* **8**:666.

ROE, F. J. C., AND SALAMAN, M. H., 1955, Further studies on incomplete carcinogenesis: Triethylene melamine (T.E.M.), 1,2-benzanthracene and β-propiolactone as initiators of skin tumour formation in the mouse, *Br. J. Cancer* **9**:177.

ROE, F. J. C., SALAMAN, M. H., COHEN, J., AND BURGAN, J. G., 1959, Incomplete carcinogens in cigarette smoke condensate: Tumor-promotion by a phenolic fraction, *Br. J. Cancer* **12**:623.

ROE, F. J. C., CARTER, R. L., MITCHLEY, B. C. V., PETO, R., AND HECKER, E., 1972, On the persistence of tumour initiation and the acceleration of tumour progression in mouse skin tumorigenesis, *Int. J. Cancer* **9**:264.

ROHRSCHNEIDER, L. R., AND BOUTWELL, R. K., 1972, Phorbol esters, fatty acids and tumour promotion, *Nature New Biol.* **243**:213.

ROHRSCHNEIDER, L. R., O'BRIEN, D. H., AND BOUTWELL, R. K., 1972, The stimulation of phospholid metabolism in mouse skin following phorbol ester treatment, *Biochim. Biophys. Acta* **280**:57.

ROUS, P., 1959, Surmise and fact on the nature of cancer, *Nature (London)* **183**:1357.

ROUS, P., AND KIDD, J. G., 1941, Conditional neoplasms and subthreshold neoplastic states, *J. Exp. Med.* **73**:365.

ROVERA, G., O'BRIEN, T. G., AND DIAMOND, L., 1977, Tumor promoters inhibit spontaneous differentiation of Friend erythroleukemia cells in culture, *Proc. Natl. Acad. Sci. USA* **74**:2894.

RUSCH, H. P., BOSCH, D., AND BOUTWELL, R. K., 1955, The influence of irritants on mitotic activity and tumor formation in mouse epidermis, *Acta Unio Int. Contra Cancrum* **11**:699.

SAFFIOTTI, U., AND SHUBIK, P., 1956, The effects of low concentrations in epidermal carcinogenesis: A comparison with promoting agents, *J. Natl. Cancer Inst.* **16**:961.

SAFFIOTTI, U., AND SHUBIK, P., 1963, Studies on promoting action in skin carcinogenesis, *Natl. Cancer Inst. Monogr.* **10**:489.

SALAMAN, M. H., 1952, The latent period of co-carcinogenesis, *Br. J. Cancer* **6**:155.

SALAMAN, M. H., AND GWYNN, R. H., 1951, The histology of co-carcinogenesis in mouse skin, *Br. J. Cancer* **5**:252.

SALAMAN, M. H., AND ROE, F. J. C., 1953, Incomplete carcinogens: Ethyl carbamate (urethane) as an initiator of skin tumour formation in the mouse, *Br. J. Cancer* **7**:472.

SALAMAN, M. H., AND ROE, F. J. C., 1956a, The development of malignant tumours of mouse skin after "initiating" and "promoting" stimuli. II. The influence of alternate applications of croton oil on malignant tumour-production by repeated applications of dilute 9,10-dimethyl-1,2-benzanthracene (DMBA), *Br. J. Cancer* **10**:70.

SALAMAN, M. H., AND ROE, F. J. C., 1956b, The development of malignant tumours of mouse skin after "initiating" and "promoting" stimuli. IV. Comparison of the effects of single and divided doses of 9,10-dimethyl-1,2-benzanthracene (DMBA), *Br. J. Cancer* **10**:79.

SALAMAN, M. H., AND ROE, F. J. C., 1956c, Further tests for tumour-initiating activity: N,N-Di-(20-chloroethyl)-p-aminophenylbutyric acid (CB1348) as an initiator of skin tumour formation in the mouse, *Br. J. Cancer* **10**:363.

SALL, R. D., SHEAR, M. J., LEITER, J., AND PERRAULT, A., 1940, Studies in carcinogenesis. XII. Effect of the basic fraction of creosote oil on the production of tumors in mice by chemical carcinogens, *J. Natl. Cancer Inst.* **1**:45.

SARMA, D. S. R., RAJALAKSHMI, S., AND FARBER, E., 1975, Chemical carcinogenesis. Interactions of carcinogens with nucleic acids, in: *Cancer: A Comprehensive Treatise*, Vol. 1 (F. F. Becker, ed.), p. 235, Plenum Press, New York.

SCHWEIZER, J., LOEHRKE, H., AND GOERTTLER, K., 1978, Transmaternal modification of the Berenblum/Mottram experiment in mice, *Bull. Cancer* **65**:265.

SCRIBNER, J. D., 1973, Tumor initiation by apparently noncarcinogenic polycyclic aromatic hydrocarbons, *J. Natl. Cancer Inst.* **50**:1717.

SCRIBNER, J. D., AND BOUTWELL, R. K., 1972, Inflammation and tumor promotion: Selective protein induction in mouse by tumor promoters, *Eur. J. Cancer* **8**:617.

SCRIBNER, J. D., AND SLAGA, T. J., 1974, Influence of nonsteroid anti-inflammatory agents on protein synthesis and hyperplasia caused by a tumor promoter, *J. Natl. Cancer Inst.* **52**:1865.

SCRIBNER, J. D., AND SLAGA, T. J., 1975, Tumor initiation by *N*-acetoxy derivatives of *N*-arylacetamides, *J. Natl. Cancer Inst.* **54**:491.

SCRIBNER, J. D., AND SÜSS, R., 1978, Tumor initiation and promotion, *Int. Rev. Exp. Pathol.* **18**:137.

SEARLE, C. E., 1966, Tumor initiatory activity of some chloromononitrobenzenes and other compounds, *Cancer Res.* **26**:12.

SEGAL, A., KATZ, C., AND VAN DUUREN, B. L., 1971, Structure and tumor-promoting activity of anthranil (1,8-dihydroxy-9-anthrone) and related compounds, *J. Med. Chem.* **14**:1152.

SETÄLÄ, K., 1960, Progress in carcinogenesis, tumor-enhancing factors: A bioassay of skin tumor formation, *Prog. Exp. Tumor Res.* **1**:225.

SETÄLÄ, K., SETÄLÄ, H., AND HOLSTI, P., 1954, A new physicochemically well-defined group of tumor-promoting (cocarcinogenic) agents for mouse skin, *Science* **120**:1075.

SHAMBERGER, R. J., 1971, Inhibitory effect of vitamin A on carcinogenesis, *J. Natl. Cancer Inst.* **47**:667.

SHAMBERGER, R. J., ANDREONE, T. L., AND WILLIS, C. E., 1974, Antioxidants and cancer. IV. Initiating activity of malonaldehyde as a carcinogen, *J. Natl. Cancer Inst.* **53**:1771.

SHERBET, G. V., 1970, Epigenetic processes and their relevance to the study of neoplasia, *Adv. Cancer Res.* **13**:97.

SHINOZUKA, J. D., AND RITCHIE, A. C., 1967, Pretreatment with croton oil, DNA synthesis, and carcinogenesis by carcinogen followed by croton oil, *Int. J. Cancer* **2**:77.

SHUBIK, P., 1950*a*, Studies on the promoting phase in the stages of carcinogenesis in mice, rats, rabbits, and guinea pigs, *Cancer Res.* **10**:13.

SHUBIK, P., 1950*b*, The growth potentialities of induced skin tumors in mice: The effect of different methods of chemical carcinogenesis, *Cancer Res.* **10**:713.

SHUBIK, P., BASERGA, R., AND RITCHIE, A. C., 1953*a*, The life and progression of induced skin tumors in mice, *Br. J. Cancer* **7**:342.

SHUBIK, P., GOLDFARB, A. R., RITCHIE, A. C., AND LISCO, H., 1953*b*, Latent carcinogenic action of beta-irradiation on mouse epidermis, *Nature (London)* **171**:934.

SICÉ, J., 1966, Tumor-promoting activity of *n*-alkanes and 1-alkanols, *Toxicol. Appl. Pharmacol.* **9**:70.

SICÉ, J., SHUBIK, P., AND FELDMAN, R., 1957, Epithelial tumors induced by normal paraffins and derivatives, *Int. Congr. Occup. Health* **3**:266.

SIVAK, A., 1979, Cocarcinogenesis, *Biochim. Biophys. Acta* **560**:67.

SIVAK, A., AND VAN DUUREN, B. L., 1971, Cellular interactions of phorbol myristate acetate in tumor promotion *Chem. Biol. Interact.* **3**:401.

SIVAK, A., RAY, F., AND VAN DUUREN, B. L., 1969, Phorbol ester tumor-promoting agents and membrane stability, *Cancer Res.* **29**:624.

SLAGA, T. J., AND BOUTWELL, R. K., 1977, Inhibition of tumor-initiating ability of the potent carcinogen 7,12-dimethylbenz(*a*)anthracene by the weak tumor initiator 1,2,3,4-dibenzanthracene, *Cancer Res.* **37**:128.

SLAGA, T. J., BOWDEN, G. T., SCRIBNER, J. D., AND BOUTWELL, R. K., 1974*a*, Dose–response studies on the ability of 7,12-dimethylbenz(*a*)anthracene and benz(*a*)anthracene to initiate skin tumors, *J. Natl. Cancer Inst.* **53**:1337.

SLAGA, T. J., BOWDEN, G. T., AND BOUTWELL, R. K., 1975, Acetic acid, a potent stimulator of mouse epidermal macromolecular synthesis and hyperplasia, but with weak tumor-promoting ability, *J. Natl. Cancer Inst.* **55**:983.

SLAGA, T. J., SCRIBNER, J. D., THOMPSON, S., AND VIAJE, A., 1976*a*, Epidermal cell proliferation and promoting ability of phorbol esters, *J. Natl. Cancer Inst.* **57**:1145.

SLAGA, T. J., VIAJE, A., BERRY, D. L., BRACKEN, W., BUTY, S. G., AND SCRIBNER, J. D., 1976*b*, Skin tumor initiating ability of benzo(*a*)pyrene 4,5-7,8- and 7,8-diol-9,10-epoxides, and 7,8-diol, *Cancer Lett.* **2**:115.

SLAGA, T. J., BRACKEN, W. M., VIAJE, A., LEVIN, W., YAGI, H., JERINA, D. M., AND CONNEY, A. H., 1977, Comparison of the tumor-initiating activities of benzo(*a*)pyrene arene oxides and diol-epoxides, *Cancer Res.* **37**:4130.

483

SEQUENTIAL
ASPECTS OF
CHEMICAL
CAR-
CINOGENESIS:
SKIN

SLAGA, T. J., BRACKEN, W. M., DRESNER, S., LEVIN, W., YAGI, H., JERINA, D. M., AND CONNEY, A. H., 1978a, Skin tumor-initiating activities of the twelve isomeric phenols of benzo(a)pyrene, *Cancer Res.* **38**:678.

SLAGA, T. J., VIAJE, A., BUTY, S. G., AND BRACKEN, W. M., 1978b, Dibenz(a,c)anthracene: A potent inhibitor of skin-tumor initiation by 7,12-dimethylbenz(a) anthracene, *Res. Commun. Chem. Pathol. Pharmacol.* **19**:477.

SLAGA, T. J., BRACKEN, W. M., GLEASON, G., LEVIN, W., YAGI, H., JERINA, D. M., AND CONNEY, A. H., 1979, Marked differences in the skin tumor-initiating activity of the optical enantiomers of the diastereomeric benzo(a)pyrene 7,8-diol-9,10-epoxides, *Cancer Res.* **39**:67.

SOPER, C. J., AND EVANS, F. J., 1977, Investigations into the mode of action of cocarcinogen 12-O-tetradecanoylphorbol-13-acetate using auxotrophic bacteria, *Cancer Res.* **34**:2487.

STEINMULLER, D., 1971, A reinvestigation of epidermal transplantation during chemical carcinogenesis, *Cancer Res.* **31**:2080.

STENBÄCK, F., 1975, Studies on the modifying effect of ultraviolet radiation on chemical skin carcinogenesis, *J. Invest. Dermatol.* **64**:253.

STENBÄCK, F., 1978, Tumor persistence and regression in skin carcinogenesis. An experimental study, *Z. Krebsforsch.* **91**:249.

STENBÄCK, F., GARCIA, H., AND SHUBIK, P., 1974, Present status of the concept of promoting action and cocarcinogenesis in skin, in: *The Physiopathology of Cancer*, 3rd ed., Vol. 1, p. 155, Karger, Basel.

SÜSS, R., KINZEL, V., AND KREIBICH, G., 1971, Cocarcinogenic croton oil fraction A₁ stimulates lipid synthesis in cell culture, *Experientia* **27**:46.

TANNENBAUM, A., 1944, The dependence of the genesis of induced skin tumors on the caloric intake during different stages of carcinogenesis, *Cancer Res.* **4**:673.

TANNENBAUM, A., AND SILVERSTONE, H., 1958, Urethan (ethyl carbamate) as a multipotential carcinogen, *Cancer Res.* **18**:1225.

TAPER, H. S., 1977, Induction of the deficient acid DNAse activity in mouse interfollicular epidermis by croton oil as a possible tumor promoting mechanism, *Z. Krebsforsch.* **90**:197.

TERRACINI, B., SHUBIK, P., AND DELLA PORTA, G., 1960, A study of skin carcinogenesis in the mouse with single applications of 9,10-dimethyl-1,2-benzanthracene of different dosages, *Cancer Res.* **20**:1538.

TRAININ, N., 1963, Adrenal imbalance in mouse skin carcinogenesis, *Cancer Res.* **23**:415.

TRAININ, N., KAYE, A. M., AND BERENBLUM, I., 1964, Influence of mutagens on the initiation of skin carcinogenesis, *Biochem. Pharmacol.* **13**:263.

TRAUT, M., KREIBICH, G., AND HECKER, E., 1971, Über die Proteinbildung carcinogener Kohlwasserstoffe und cocarcinogener Phorbolester, in: *Aktuelle Probleme aus dem Gebiet der Cancerologie*, Vol. 3 (H. Lettré and G. Wagner, eds.), p. 91, Springer, Berlin.

TROLL, W., KLASSEN, A., AND JANOFF, A., 1970, Tumorigenesis in mouse skin. Inhibition by synthetic inhibitors of proteases, *Science* **169**:1211.

TROLL, W., ROSSMAN, T., KATZ, J., AND LEVITZ, M., 1975, Proteinases in tumor promotion and hormone action, in: *Proteases and Biological Control* (E. Reich, D. B. Ritkin, and E. Shaw, eds.), p. 977, Cold Spring Harbor Laboratory, Cold Spring Harbor, N.Y.

TROSKO, J. E., YAGER, J. D., JR., BOWDEN, G. T., AND BUTCHER, F. R., 1975, The effects of several croton oil constituents on two types of DNA repair and cyclic nucleotide levels in mammalian cells in vitro, *Chem. Biol. Interact.* **11**:191.

VAN DUUREN, B. L., 1969, Tumor-promoting agents in two-stage carcinogenesis, *Prog. Exp. Tumor Res.* **11**:31.

VAN DUUREN, B. L., 1976, Tumor-promoting and co-carcinogenic agents in chemical carcinogenesis, *ACS Monogr.* **173**:24.

VAN DUUREN, B. L., 1978, Structural prognostication of carcinogenicity and tumorenhancing activity in various chemicals, in: *Prevention and Detection of Cancer*, Part 1, Vol. 2 (H. E. Nieburg, ed.), p. 207, Dekker, New York.

VAN DUUREN, B. L., AND GOLDSCHMIDT, B. M., 1976, Cocarcinogenic and tumor-promoting agents in tobacco carcinogenesis, *J. Natl. Cancer Inst.* **56**:1237.

VAN DUUREN, B. L., AND MELCHIONNE, S., 1969, Inhibition of tumorigenesis, *Prog. Exp. Tumor Res.* **12**:55.

VAN DUUREN, B. L., AND SEGAL, A., 1976, Inhibition of two-stage carcinogenesis in mouse skin by bis(2-chloroethyl)sulfide, *Cancer Res.* **36**:1025.

VAN DUUREN, B. L., LANGSETH, L., SIVAK, A., AND ORRIS, L., 1966, The tumor-enhancing principles of *Croton tiglium* L. II. A comparative study, *Cancer Res.* **26**:1729.

Van Duuren, B. L., Sivak, A., Langseth, L., Goldschmidt, B. M., and Segal, A., 1968, Initiators and promoters in tobacco carcinogenesis, *Natl. Cancer Inst. Monogr.* **28:**173.

Van Duuren, B. L., Sivak, A., Katz, C., and Melchionne, S., 1969, Inhibition of tumor induction in two-stage carcinogenesis on mouse skin, *Cancer Res.* **29:**947.

Van Duuren, B. L., Sivak, A., Goldschmidt, B. M., Katz, C., and Melchionne, S., 1970, Initiating activity of aromatic hydrocarbons in two-stage carcinogenesis, *J. Natl. Cancer Inst.* **44:**1167.

Van Duuren, B. L., Goldschmidt, B. M., Katz, C., Seidman, I., and Paul, J. S., 1974, Carcinogenic activity of alkylating agents, *J. Natl. Cancer Inst.* **53:**695.

Van Duuren, B. L., Witz, G., and Goldschmidt, B. M., 1978, Structure–activity relationships of tumor promoters and cocarcinogens and phorbol myristate acetate and related esters with plasma membranes, in: *Carcinogenesis: Mechanisms of Tumor Promotion and Cocarcinogenesis*, Vol. 2 (T. J. Slaga, A. Sivak, and R. K. Boutwell, eds.)., p. 491, Raven Press, New York.

Verma, A. K., Rice, H. M., and Boutwell, R. K., 1977, Prostaglandins and skin tumor promotion: Inhibition of tumor-promoter-induced ornithine decarboxylase activity in epidermis by inhibitors of prostaglandin synthesis, *Biochem. Biophys. Res. Commun.* **79:**1160.

Voorhees, J. J., Duell, E. A., Bass, L. J., and Harrell, E., 1973, Role of cyclic AMP in the control of epidermal cell growth and differentiation, *Natl. Cancer Inst. Monogr.* **38:**47.

Warwick, G. P., 1969, The covalent binding of metabolites of 4-dimethylaminoazobenzene to liver nucleic acids *in vivo*, in: *Physico-chemical Mechanisms of Carcinogenesis*, Vol. 1 (E. D. Bergmann and R. Pullman, eds.), p. 218, The Israel Academy of Science and Humanities, Jerusalem.

Wattenberg, L. W., 1977, Inhibitors of chemical carcinogenesis, *Adv. Cancer Res.* **26:**197.

Wattenberg, L. W., 1978, Inhibition of chemical carcinogenesis, *J. Natl. Cancer Inst.* **60:**11.

Waynforth, H. B., and Magee, P. N., 1975, The effect of various doses and schedules of administration of *N*-methyl-*N*-nitrosourea, with and without croton oil promotion, on skin papilloma production in BALB/c mice, *Gann Monogr. Cancer Res.* **17:**439.

Weeks, C. E., Slaga, T. L., Hennings, H., Gleason, G. L., and Bracken, W. M., 1979, Inhibition of phorbol ester-induced tumor promotion in mice by vitamin A analog and anti-inflammatory steroids, *J. Natl. Cancer Inst.* **63:**401.

Weinstein, I. B., Jeffrey, A. M., Jennette, K. W., Blobstein, S. H., Harvey, R. G., Harris, C., Autrop, H., Kasai, H., and Nakanishi, K., 1976, Benzo(*a*)pyrene diol epoxides as intermediates in nucleic acid binding *in vitro* and *in vivo*, *Science* **193:**592.

Weinstein, I. B., Wigler, M., and Pietropaolo, C., 1977, The action of tumor-promoting agents in cell culture, in: *Cold Spring Harbor Conference on Cell Proliferation* **4:**751.

Wenner, C. E., Hackney, J., Kimelberg, H. K., and Mayhew, E., 1974, Membrane effects of phorbol esters, *Cancer Res.* **34:**1731.

Wheeler, G. P., 1962, Studies related to the mechanisms of action of cytotoxic alkylating agents. A Review, *Cancer Res.* **22:**651.

Wilson, E. L., and Reich, E., 1979, Modulation of plasminogen activator synthesis in chick embryo fibroblasts by cyclic nucleotides and phorbol myristate acetate, *Cancer Res.* **39:**1579.

Wood, A. W., Chang, R. L., Levin, W., Thomas, P. E., Ryan, D., Stoming, T. A., Thakker, D. R., Jerina, D. M., and Conney, A. H., 1978, Metabolic activation of 3-methylcholanthrene and its metabolites to products mutagenic to bacterial and mammalian cells, *Cancer Res.* **38:**3398.

Worst, P. K. M., and Bauz, R., 1974, Skin transplantation in the study of chemical carcinogenesis. II. Iso- and autografting of skin from mice intragastrically initiated with 9,12-dimethyl-1,2-benzanthracene with and without subsequent application of the promoting agent TPA, *Z. Krebsforsch.* **82:**285.

Wynder, E. L., 1977, Nutritional carcinogenesis, *Ann. N.Y. Acad. Sci.* **300:**360.

Wynder, E. L., and Hoffmann, D., 1961, A study of tobacco carcinogenesis. VIII. The role of the acidic fractions as promoters, *Cancer* **14:**1306.

Yasuhira, K., 1968, Skin papilloma production by anthranil painting after urethan initiation in mice, *Gann* **59:**187.

Yasuhira, K., 1969, Suspicious influence of thymectomy on skin papilloma induction, *Gann* **60:**57.

Yuspa, S. H., Hennings, H., and Saffiotti, U., 1976a, Cutaneous chemical carcinogenesis: Past, present and future, *J. Invest. Dermatol.* **67:**199.

Yuspa, S. H., Lichti, U., Ben, T., Patterson, E., Hennings, H., Slaga, T. J., Colburn, N., and Kelsey, W., 1976b, Phorbol esters stimulate DNA synthesis and ornithine decarboxylase activity in mouse epidermal cell cultures, *Nature (London)* **262:**402.

zur Hausen, H., Bornkamm, G. W., Schmidt, R., and Hecker, E., 1979, Tumor initiators and promoters in the induction of Epstein–Barr virus, *Proc. Natl. Acad. Sci. USA* **76:**782.

13

Sequential Events in Chemical Carcinogenesis

Emmanuel Farber

1. Introduction

1.1. Multistep Nature of Carcinogenesis

It has become increasingly evident that the vast majority of if not all cancers develop slowly as a multistep process in which discrete focal new cell populations appear sequentially as possible precursor lesions for the next step (Foulds, 1969, 1975; Farber, 1973a; Farber and Cameron, 1980; Farber and Sporn, 1976; Medline and Farber, 1980). The multistep patterns appear to occur in most known instances of cancer induced by chemicals and radiations and by some viruses (Foulds, 1975; Farber and Cameron, 1980; Peto, 1977). The field has been reviewed by Foulds (1969, 1975) in extenso and more recently by Farber and Cameron (1980) and there is no need for an additional comprehensive review at this time. However, it does appear to be appropriate to consider analytically and critically some of the component processes in chemical carcinogenesis and to discuss some emerging general principles that seem to be pertinent to the further study of mechanisms of cancer development with chemicals.

Research in experimental animals during the past three decades has repeatedly confirmed the apparent "two-stage" induction of skin neoplasia in mice and rabbits and has extended it in principle to other organs or tissues, such as the liver, mammary gland, colon, urinary bladder, etc. (Pitot, 1979; Farber and Cameron, 1980). Also, research in humans has confirmed the occurrence of atypical hyperplasia, dysplasia, and carcinoma-*in situ* in several sites as "precancerous lesions" and as possible steps toward cancer (e.g., Koss, 1975).

EMMANUEL FARBER • Departments of Pathology and Biochemistry, University of Toronto, Toronto, Ontario, Canada.

However, the critical properties of each of the different cell populations that relate to their roles in cancer development and the manner in which the two aspects of carcinogenesis, the experimental and the human, fit together into some biologically meaningful pattern or patterns remain essentially unknown (e.g., Smets, 1980).

The designation "two-stage" is clearly a convenient way of indicating the usual number of *manipulations* performed by the investigator, i.e., it is *operational*, and is not in any way indicative of the actual number of steps that the skin or any other tissue undergoes during cancer development, since we can identify many more than two steps in every instance of a so-called "two-stage" system (Foulds, 1975; Farber and Cameron, 1980). Even a superficial view reveals that multiple focal proliferations of cells in target tissues or organs are common early features of the carcinogenic process. Nodules in solid organs and papillomas, polyps, or other exophytic focal proliferations on surfaces as well as more diffuse local hyperplasias appear during cancer development with chemicals. These in turn act as sites for subsequent focal changes that form the nidus for further proliferative lesions in the preneoplastic and premalignant phases of cancer development. The genesis, properties, options, and fates of each of such sequential cell populations and their roles, *if any*, in the evolution toward cancer are among the most important problems in the carcinogenic process if understanding and novel approaches for control are legimate topics of importance in chemical carcinogenesis. These will constitute a major portion of this article.

1.2. The Strategy of Chemical Carcinogenesis

If the process of carcinogenesis with chemicals is characterized by a number of focal or discrete cell proliferations, each of which is at increased risk for the development of the next change in a rare cell ("a rare event," Farber and Cameron, 1980), then the suggestion for this basic theme, rare events (presumptive mutations) separated by periods of selection (Fig. 1), is an old one going back many decades and restated anew in every generation (e.g., see Cairns, 1975; Farber, 1980; Farber and Cameron, 1980; Nowell, 1976). How can this formulation be reconciled with a "two-stage" operation? This poses no problem when examined from the point of view of the properties of the new cell populations that appear in sequence. As emphasized previously (Farber, 1973b, 1980; Farber and Cameron, 1980), initiated cells in several systems do not acquire any measurable autonomy or independence with respect to growth and therefore require an appropriate differential selection for their development into papillomas, nodules, or other initial focal proliferations. However, once the second rare event occurs in one or more such focal proliferations, the system becomes "self-generating" and is no longer environment dependent for progression (see Farber, 1980). Thus, the "two-stage" designation relates only to the need for at least two operational or environmental influences in order to induce some autonomy of growth or at least some change that makes further evolution independent of the need for an additional identifiable environmental stimulus.

487

SEQUENTIAL
EVENTS IN
CHEMICAL
CAR-
CINOGENESIS

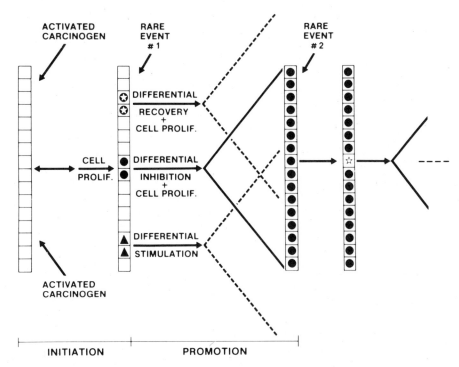

FIGURE 1. Diagrammatic representation of initiation and promotion, as viewed with the rare event–selection hypothesis. The different symbols represent different types of functionally altered hepatocytes. Although only three general types of initiated cells are included (✪, ●, ▲), it is possible that many more types may be induced by an initiating dose of a carcinogen. Conceivably, only some types can be promoted or selected by environments appropriate to each particular tissue or organ. According to this hypothesis, amplification (or expansion) of appropriately altered hepatocytes is the first prerequisite of promotion in the liver.

In other words, at least two manipulations are usually required to induce the first neoplastic step (Fig. 2).

The challenges then become: how many such rare event–selection sequences are necessary for cancer development in any tissue? What is the physiological nature of each one that enables a selection to be made? What are the selecting forces at each step and how can they be modulated? What forces generate the slow movement toward cancer and how can these forces be diverted? Such questions form another legitimate group in the study of mechanisms of carcinogenesis and will be addressed as part of this review.

2. Agents and Processes in the Analysis of Carcinogenesis

Given the increasing success that has been achieved in the identification and characterization of cancer-inducing chemicals beginning in the 1920s, the study of chemical carcinogenesis has been dominated to a large and expanding degree by the principle that the understanding of the chemical and physical properties

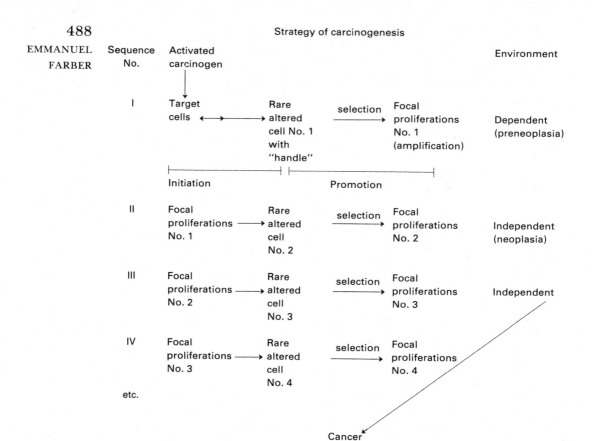

FIGURE 2. Proposed sequences of rare events–selection (promotion) initiated by exposure to an appropriate dose of a carcinogen coupled with cell proliferation. The number of sequences leading to cancer is unknown. The first sequence (initiation–promotion) is environment dependent. All subsequent ones would appear to be self-generating.

of chemical carcinogens and of their immediate interactions with target and other tissues will lead to the elucidation of carcinogenic processes. With the discovery of promoting agents and the clarification of the chemistry of some of the materials most active for skin, such as croton oil, this reductionist approach concentrating on agents was extended to postinitiation phenomena. No one who is familiar with the successes in the areas of chemistry and biochemistry of initiators and promoters can take exception to this scientific approach *as a first step*. However, the increasing study of the *responses of living cells and tissues* to a wide variety of toxic or potentially toxic agents at both the biochemical and the biological levels of organization over the past few decades has made it eminently evident that the living organism is by no means a passive object for change.

On the contrary, it is a very dynamic partner in any interaction between agent and target tissue. In fact, as emphasized a few years ago (Farber, 1973a), a cell is "the smallest *integrating* unit in biology: a pseudointelligent computer that receives, screens, changes, reacts to and adapts to a host of environmental signals, all of this activity apparently designed, through evolution, for cell survival and

489
SEQUENTIAL
EVENTS IN
CHEMICAL
CAR-
CINOGENESIS

host survival." In other words, it is unlikely that we will be very successful in developing a rational understanding of cancer induction by concentrating our focus on the agents alone. An increasing interest and study of the *different processes* that constitute carcinogenesis, *as processes*, would seem to be a prerequisite for elucidation of its essential nature. Although investigators pay passing lip service to this approach in chemical carcinogenesis, relatively little scientific attention is devoted to this type of study. This narrow approach to the study of toxic responses, i.e., to the "toxic components in toxicology," is not unique to research workers in chemical carcinogenesis but remains the dominant scientific philosophy in toxicology generally.

There are at least two practical consequences of this simplistic view of chemical carcinogenesis. The first is the naive conviction that "cleaning up our environment" is all that will be necessary to control the bulk of cancer in any population. Although the removal of identifiable hazards, such as those generated during cigarette smoking or in the workshop, must be of high priority in any battle with cancer, there is no proof that some of the major forms of cancer in any geographic location (e.g., cancer of the colon, breast, and uterus in North America) lend themselves to this approach. Also, in the case of promoters that usually require prolonged exposure, it is questionable whether the "environmental approach" is adequate to cope with the problem effectively.

The second concerns the scientific attitude to research in chemical carcinogenesis. It has been pointed out sporadically that the response patterns of living tissues to carcinogens are by no means unique to this group of toxic agents. Rather, it seems to be more reasonable to view the carcinogenic process from a broader perspective of evolution and adaptation generally (Coggin and Anderson, 1974; Farber and Cameron, 1980; Haddow, 1972; Prehn, 1976). Since the tags we place on chemicals are not a recognizable medium of communication at the cellular level, are we narrowing our perspective too much by the literal use of terms such as "carcinogen"? It is very likely that most if not all the changes induced in target cells by "carcinogens" have no direct relevance to cancer but are a reflection of more general response patterns to injury at the molecular as well as cellular levels. In this context, it is critical to know whether the changes in cells seen on exposure to known chemical carcinogens have any direct relevance to the behavior of an ultimate population of malignant neoplastic cells or do such changes at each step simply increase the probability for the occurrence of subsequent steps that progressively move toward cancer and that have a greater mechanistic relationship to malignancy as they evolve? If this latter view has any validity and usefulness, do these different cell populations, especially the early ones, play a functional role in the adaptation of the organism to a hazardous environment (e.g., Farber and Cameron, 1980)?

It is noteworthy that there is a major discrepancy between the number and apparent diversity of immediate *chemical and biochemical* effects of different carcinogens, promoters, and other modulators of carcinogenesis such as vitamin A analogs and the number of immediate *biological* endpoints of the exposure to such agents. For example, chemical carcinogens induce a wide array of discrete chemical changes in the DNA in target cells (Rajalakshmi *et al.*, this volume), yet the first observable biological endpoints, a nodule, a papilloma, a polyp, etc., are virtually indistinguishable when induced by quite different carcinogens. The same is true in principle for later focal lesions and for the cancers that appear ultimately. In other words, the response patterns to carcinogens (and to other potentially toxic agents) are often very similar if not identical in appearance and behavior, even when induced by agents of widely divergent chemical and physical properties. This indicates the existence of a sort of biological direction to the cellular response to many toxic agents, including carcinogens. Thus, a large diverse array of agents added to a system or organism often generates a common pattern of response. This lack of correspondence between *diversity of input* and *commonality of output* poses a major problem for interpretation in a complex process such as carcinogenesis and emphasizes the necessity to develop models in which one can measure and relate input and output for each step. In at least two well-defined systems for chemical carcinogenesis, the skin and the liver, such a close correlation is becoming feasible (e.g., see Farber and Cameron, 1980) and should be encouraged maximally.

3. The First Sequence: Initiation–Promotion

Cancer development with chemicals can begin with a brief exposure (a few hours or days) to an activated form of a carcinogen and the chemical need not be present as such ever again, as far as can be determined. This is valid not only in the skin, which was the first tissue in which this was demonstrated clearly, but also in liver, colon, mammary gland, urinary bladder, kidney, brain, and other organs or tissues (Berenblum, 1975; Berenblum, 1978; Farber and Cameron, 1980; Pitot, 1979; Scribner and Süss, 1978). The brief exposure to the chemical induces neither a cancer cell nor a neoplastic cell but rather some cell that can be differentially stimulated to produce a focal proliferation. By "neoplastic" is meant a cell that can proliferate without the need for an added or known stimulus for growth, i.e., a cell that has acquired some degree of autonomy.

The existence of an initiated state cannot be detected *per se* but makes itself evident only when some promoting or selecting environment is created, i.e., by the occurrence of subsequent focal proliferation. Thus, the concept of initiation is intricately bound up with the subsequent appearance of discrete proliferative lesions.

The separation of this first sequence, initiation–promotion, is justified because of its dependence on the environment for its appearance. With a single exposure to an initiating dose of a carcinogen, the further history is closely dependent upon the imposition of a suitable promoting environment. This can be created by a "pure" promoter or by further exposure to a carcinogen. In the former case, repeated exposure over a relatively long period (weeks to months in rats or mice) is usually required. In the latter case, a briefer exposure to an active carcinogen may suffice.

This first sequence generates a new cell population that is at risk for a second 491
SEQUENTIAL
EVENTS IN
CHEMICAL
CAR-
CINOGENESIS "rare event" from which a second new population can develop. The occurrence of this new focal change in a rare cell and its amplification by selection or differential growth seems to be no longer environment dependent but appears to be self-generating. Because of this relative autonomy, at least with respect to added exogenous agents, we consider this second rare event as the beginning of "neoplasia" and everything preceding this change as "preneoplasia." The subsequent steps are poorly understood and are discussed in Section 4 (Fig. 2).

3.1. Initiation

3.1.1. Definition

Operationally, initiation can be defined as some change in the target tissue or organ, induced by a brief exposure to a carcinogen, that may ultimately lead to cancer under the appropriate environment. Such a definition is not very useful analytically, since it does not indicate any currently exploitable property.

A more useful definition is as follows: *initiation is a change in a target tissue or organ induced by exposure to a carcinogen that can be promoted or selected to develop focal proliferations, one or more of which can act as sites of origin for the ultimate development of malignant neoplasia.* Such a definition would appear to be valid in those tissues in which the process has been studied in some detail, such as skin, liver, mammary gland, urinary bladder, pancreas, and perhaps colon and stomach (see Foulds, 1969, 1975; Farber and Cameron, 1980). Implicit in this definition is some alteration in single cells or groups of cells that enable them to act as initial sites that can be promoted or selected. However, it is singularly devoid of even a hint of the "functional or biological nature" of the altered cells. What allows them to develop focal proliferations (e.g., papillomas in the skin, islands or foci and nodules in solid organs such as liver, kidney, pancreas, etc., "polyps" in the gastrointestinal tract, etc.)? If they had acquired some degree of autonomy of growth control and were programmed normally for continual cell proliferation (e.g., skin, colon, etc.), focal proliferation would not be unexpected. However, loss of growth control does not appear to have been acquired at this early stage in carcinogenesis in any system so far studied. With doses of carcinogens that are just sufficient for initiation, no further progressive change can be seen without promotion or selection, even in tissues that are undergoing continual cell proliferation. *In vitro* culture of initiated organs or tissues has so far failed to show any selective growth of presumptive initiated cells (see Farber and Cameron, 1980, for review of the literature). Also, in the few studies reported, transplantation of such lesions has been singularly unsuccessful with rare exceptions.

3.1.2. Generation and Properties

Initiation is at least a *two-step process*—the induction of one or more biochemical changes or lesions followed by a round of cell proliferation. The multistep nature of initiation has been suspected for several sites for some years but has been shown *in vivo* only for liver (see Farber, 1980, for references). It is difficult to demonstrate any role for cell proliferation in tissues in which cell proliferation is a continuing property, such as in skin, colon, fetal, and postnatal tissues.

The possible or probable roles of metabolic activation of most carcinogens, the interactions of activated moieties of carcinogens with DNA and other cellular macromolecules, and the repair of "damage" to DNA are detailed in other chapters (9 and 10) and will not be discussed further here, except to reemphasize their importance.

However, it is now apparent from the experience with carcinogenesis in the liver that the chemical or biochemical lesions generated by the interactions of ultimate carcinogens with cellular constituents such as DNA are not sufficient to initiate liver cancer development in the absence of a round of cell proliferation. This is evident both with cancer (see Craddock, 1976, for references) and with initiation (see Scherer and Emmelot, 1975; Pitot, 1979; Farber, 1980) as endpoints. The cell proliferation can be generated by some primary mitogenic stimulus such as partial hepatectomy or a chemical mitogen (Cayama *et al.*, 1978) or as a response to cell death (Ying *et al.*, 1979a).

The mechanistic role of cell proliferation in initiation is not known. A common hypothesis invokes DNA synthesis as fixing a damage in a daughter strand. Other possibilities, however, such as different susceptibilities of cells through differences in activation or inactivation, unusual availability of susceptible regions of DNA at different times during the S phase, or alterations in the repair processes at selected times in the cell cycle need to be considered. For example, recent, as yet unpublished work by Sarma and co-workers (Ying, Cayama, Columbano, and Sarma, personal communication) indicates that the loss of O^6-methylguanine from liver DNA generated from 1,2-dimethylhydrazine, N-methyl-N-nitrosourea, or dimethylnitrosamine is severely inhibited during liver regeneration following partial hepatectomy. It has been suggested that this methylated base may be an important altered product in DNA for carcinogenesis with methylating carcinogens (see Pegg, 1977).

With both the Scherer–Emmelot model (Scherer, Steward, and Emmelot, 1977) and our model (Cayama *et al.*, 1978; Ying *et al.*, 1979a,b; Tsuda *et al.*, 1980) of liver carcinogenesis, cell proliferation to be effective must occur within 36–48 h after the administration of the carcinogen (diethylnitrosamine, N-methyl-N-nitrosourea, 1,2-dimethylhydrazine, benzo[*a*]pyrene, dimethylnitrosamine). Although maximal degrees of initiation occur when the carcinogen is given after partial hepatectomy, the latter is effective but less so if it follows the administration of the carcinogen by about 36–40 h. These newer developments offer more rapid and probably more selective approaches to the correlation of types of biochemical lesions with initiation of liver carcinogenesis (see Pegg, 1977).

A property of an initiated state of considerable importance is its relative irreversibility. Not only skin but also liver, urinary bladder, and other tissues show this property (Farber and Cameron, 1980; Pitot, 1979; Solt *et al.*, 1980). This is most easily explained in terms of a permanent damage in DNA, such as a mutation in a structural or more likely a regulatory segment (e.g., Burnet, 1978). However, until the evidence for this is no longer circumstantial and until the molecular nature of the irreversible steps in normal development and differentiation is understood, we prefer to denote such an event in a descriptive manner as a "rare event" (Farber and Cameron, 1980).

The lack of a major degree of reversibility of the initiated state indicates that the very early carcinogen-induced altered cells are not recognized by the host in a manner that enables the host to destroy them. This places in serious doubt the validity of the concept of immune surveillance at an early stage in chemical carcinogenesis as has been proposed for host control of cancer development (Thomas, 1959; see Stutman, 1975).

If the initiation process in the liver or elsewhere involves an occasional single or rare target cell, as is probable (e.g., Scherer and Hoffmann, 1971; Solt *et al.*, 1977; Iannaconne *et al.*, 1978), such isolated cells have yet to be characterized as to phenotype or genotype, since they have not been seen. Although many markers appear after the proliferation of the initiated cells, it is not known what role the cell proliferation plays in their appearance.

3.1.3. Essential Nature of Initiated Cells

With respect to *the* key functional property of any initiated cell population, *the ability to be stimulated to form a focal area of proliferation*, this problem has yet to be broached in most systems. Despite the 50 years or so of interest in chemical carcinogenesis in the skin, no insight has been generated into the property or properties that are useful in the differential response of the initiated skin cells to a promoting environment.

In the liver, three properties of initiated cells early in their possible evolution to cancer have received emphasis. The first, the appearance of enzyme deficiencies or excesses or other biochemical changes, has been used to identify putative preneoplastic hepatocytes (see Farber and Cameron, 1980; Emmelot and Scherer, 1980) (see Section 3.2.3b). However, so far, no hypothesis has appeared implicating any one or more of such changes in the mechanism of focal proliferation. They remain largely as convenient indices of alteration with no mechanistic implication. Also, no such marker so far described is present in every focal collection of preneoplastic hepatocytes (Scherer and Emmelot, 1975; Pugh and Goldfarb, 1978; Sirica *et al.*, 1978; Farber *et al.*, 1979; Ogawa *et al.*, 1980). The second property, resistance to the inhibitory effects of a carcinogen on cell proliferation has been postulated and shown to be *one type* of *initiated cell* in which a mechanism for selective cell proliferation (promotion) can be formulated (Solt and Farber, 1976). This new approach has enabled many questions to be posed concerning the early steps in chemical carcinogenesis (e.g., see Farber, 1979, 1980; Farber and Cameron, 1980). More recently, a third functional property has been proposed—retention of response to mitogens by the initiated cell and loss of such response by the surrounding cells (Ohde *et al.*, 1979*a, b*). As with the second property, this can be readily used as a model for a mechanism of promotion (see Section 3.2).

In this context, it is attractive to consider that many different types of initiated cells may be induced by exposure to an active carcinogen (Fig. 1) and that the nature of the cells selected or "promoted" may be a property of the promoting or selecting environment. Conceivably, each target organ or tissue for a carcinogen might well have a spectrum of types of potentially initiated cells but the cells selected or promoted may reflect the mechanism of promotion appropriate for that particular tissue or organ (see Section 3.2). Since a round of cell proliferation seems to be an essential step for initiation, the only cells that are targets for the initiating effect of a carcinogen would be those that are cycling or those that enter the cycle before repair of the critical molecular lesions is complete.

Thus, initiation of chemical and some other forms of carcinogenesis can be viewed as the *induction* of altered cells that can be *selected* by an environment appropriate for those cells and for the tissue or organ in which they are induced.

Whether some or all initiated cells have, in addition to a "handle" for selection, properties that relate directly or intimately to cancer cells remains unknown. At one extreme is the hypothesis that the initiation process does nothing relevant to cancer other than allow a rare cell or group of cells to develop into a focal proliferative lesion and that all subsequent steps related to cancer are acquired at later times. At the other extreme is the hypothesis that the initiating dose of a carcinogen imparts some more direct cancer-related property or properties to the initiated cells and that such properties play a role in determining which of the many preneoplastic lesions progress to cancer. The obvious challenge to cancer research is to devise experimental approaches to test these hypotheses.

Prehn (1976) and others have periodically suggested that a carcinogen or carcinogenic stimulus might not *induce* an altered cell during initiation but rather might encourage the selection of a preformed cell already present in the target tissue. Since promoting agents or environments for the skin or liver often do not lead to the appearance of preneoplastic or neoplastic lesions in the absence of an initiating exposure to a carcinogen, it does not appear likely that initiated or altered cells exist preformed in most models of carcinogenesis. In the many studies on skin and in the increasing number on liver, exposure to a carcinogen under "initiating conditions" is a prerequisite for carcinogenesis except in a rare strain of susceptible animals (see Boutwell, 1964, 1974; Peraino *et al.*, 1978; Pitot *et al.*, 1978; Scherer and Emmelot, 1976; Solt and Farber, 1976; Solt *et al.*, 1977). However, the unusual susceptibility of a rare preformed cell to the inducing or initiating effects of carcinogens cannot be ruled in or out with the currently available methods of cell analysis in tissues. A negative conclusion concerning the selection of a preformed altered cell by a carcinogen *in vitro* has been reached by Heidelberger (1973).

Thus, in several different systems, it appears that exposure to a carcinogen under initiating conditions *induces* rather than *selects* altered target cells, although an unusual or rare susceptibility of some preformed cells to such an inducing effect has not been ruled out. If, as seems probable, many different types of initiated cells may be induced by exposure to an activated carcinogen, the

existence of a small population of preformed cells that are peculiarly programmed for susceptibility becomes much less likely.

495

SEQUENTIAL
EVENTS IN
CHEMICAL
CAR-
CINOGENESIS

In the liver, the initiated resistant cell that can be selected in the Solt–Farber
model appears to be randomly distributed without any apparent predilection
for one or other zones of the liver acinus (Solt *et al.*, 1977). This plus other
considerations (see Farber and Cameron, 1980) make it highly unlikely that the
target cell in the liver for carcinogens is a hypothetical stem cell. Whether such
hypothetical stem cells exist and are targets in many other tissues remains
unknown. In those tissues in which a reserve of proliferating cells are considered
to be stem cells (e.g., bone marrow, skin?), it is unknown whether such cells are
peculiarly susceptible to the initiating effects of a carcinogen. Naturally in such
tissues, if a round of cell proliferation is obligatory for initiation, as is very
probable, the replicating cells would be the exclusive targets in carcinogenesis.

3.2. The Process of Promotion or Selection

3.2.1. Definition

Operationally, the term "promotion" is often used for the process whereby
"neoplastic development," "tumor formation," or "cancer development" is accelerated or encouraged in a tissue that has been exposed for a relatively brief
period to an initiating dose of a carcinogen. As with the term "initiation," this
type of definition is not very useful for any stepwise analysis of carcinogenesis,
since it does not include limits to endpoints and incorporates in a vague manner
both early and late steps in the multistep process of cancer development.

A more useful definition is as follows: *promotion is the process whereby an initiated
tissue or organ develops focal proliferations, one or more of which may act as precursors
for subsequent steps in the carcinogenic process.* The definition appears to be valid
at least in the skin and the liver, two sites in which the sequential analysis of
cancer development is the most advanced. This definition limits promotion to
a single biological phenomenon and to one that may be quantitated using at
least three parameters—number, size, and rate of appearance. This definition
also implies that an essential element of promotion is the *selective stimulation* of
only a very small proportion of the cell population in the original target tissue.
In other words, a promoting environment supplies the *motive force for the proliferation of initiated cells in a selective fashion.*

3.2.2. Properties

In the skin and in one model in the liver, "*the resistant cell model*" (Solt *et al.*,
1977; Farber, 1980), the application of a strong promoter or promoting environment produces, as a very early phenomenon, focal proliferations, the number
of which is proportional to the dose of the initiating carcinogen used. In the
liver model, a single relatively brief period (2–3 weeks) of focal proliferation,
resulting in the appearance of liver cell nodules (hyperplastic nodules), is

sufficient to set in motion the remainder of the process leading to liver cell cancer in about 70–80% of the animals (Solt *et al.*, 1977; Cayama and Solt, 1980). In one or very few nodules, new focal cellular proliferations appear that generate "nodules within nodules," and this process seems to repeat itself until obvious malignant hepatocellular carcinoma appears. Thus, the termination of the promoting operation occurs long before the second rare event appears, i.e., an external promoting environment is only necessary for a relatively brief period during the preneoplastic phase of carcinogenesis (see Farber and Cameron, 1980).

In the skin, even with very potent promoters such as some of the phorbol esters, repeated application is necessary before focal proliferations (papillomas) become easily recognized. However, as has been repeatedly reported (see Farber and Cameron, 1980), the application of the promoter can terminate *before* the appearance of the next obvious tissue change, focal alterations in one or a few papillomas ("rare event" number 2) (see Shubik *et al.*, 1953; Foulds, 1975; Burns *et al.*, 1978; Farber and Cameron, 1980).

In other models of liver carcinogenesis (e.g., Peraino *et al.*, 1978; Pitot *et al.*, 1978) and of carcinogenesis in other organs (e.g., Pitot, 1979; Farber and Cameron, 1980), the promoting environment has been imposed for many months and the minimal time for adequate promotion has yet to be reported.

The demonstration of a "material continuity" (Foulds, 1975; Farber and Cameron, 1980) or a physical or cellular link between initiated cells and presumed subsequent steps in the stepwise evolution to cancer is an absolute prerequisite for any model for the study of the sequential events in carcinogenesis (see Section 5) and this is lacking in most models.

In the skin, the focal proliferations appearing during promotion have classically been called "tumors" or papillomas. Similarly, in the liver the focal proliferations or hyperplastic nodules have been designated by some authors as adenomas (e.g., Sasaki and Yoshida, 1935) or more recently neoplastic nodules (Squire and Levitt, 1975). Since the vast majority of the so-called papillomas and adenomas or neoplastic nodules undergo regression or maturation (remodeling) on termination of the promoting environment, we consider their designation as benign neoplasms as inappropriate. As long as persistence or continued proliferation is environment dependent and reversible, we consider the focal proliferations to be largely hyperplastic in nature and not neoplastic. Thus, it appears reasonable to designate the lesions that appear prior to rare event number 2 as *preneoplastic* and essentially *hyperplastic*.

3.2.3. Essential Nature and Possible Mechanisms

According to this formulation, promotion consists, at a minimum, of the expansion or amplification of carcinogen-induced initiated cells to form focal proliferations, one or more of which develop further changes that may lead to cancer. Thus, an essential feature of promotion is the creation of a mitogenic environment that imposes a differential effect on initiated cells vis-à-vis the surrounding cells.

If the first carcinogen-induced initiated cells have not acquired any autonomy of growth or proliferation, as appears to be the case, how can such cells be encouraged to produce focal proliferations? At least three possible biological mechanisms of promotion come to mind:

497
SEQUENTIAL
EVENTS IN
CHEMICAL
CAR-
CINOGENESIS

a. Differential inhibition (e.g., Solt and Farber, 1976).
b. Differential stimulation (e.g., Ohde *et al.*, 1979*a,b*).
c. Differential recovery.

a. Differential inhibition. If a general stimulus for cell proliferation (e.g., a promoter) is applied, and cell proliferation is inhibited in the surrounding cells but not in the initiated ones, a focal proliferation of the initiated cells would be expected. Such an overall biological mechanism could well lead to nodules or papillary growths. If the stimulus is reasonably intensive and if the inhibition is marked, rapid proliferation of initiated cells would be anticipated. This appears to be the overall mechanism occurring in the "resistant cell model" of liver carcinogenesis (Solt and Farber, 1976).

Since most carcinogens inhibit cell proliferation and/or DNA synthesis to a greater degree in many uninitiated cells than in preneoplastic or neoplastic cells (see Farber, 1979, for references), differential inhibition is a likely phenomenon in at least some tissues or organs that are exposed to carcinogens continuously or even intermittently for a relatively long period. Chronic exposure to carcinogens is commonly seen in most instances of cancer in nature.

b. Differential stimulation. This has been proposed as the overall mechanism for liver cancer induction by at least two xenobiotic enzyme inducers, α-hexachlorocyclohexane and cyproterone acetate (Ohde *et al.*, 1979*a,b*). These compounds are mitogenic for hepatocytes. However, the uninitiated hepatocytes lose their response after one or a few cell cycles while the initiated cells continue to respond, thus generating nodules.

c. Differential recovery. Differential recovery is a proposed biological mechanism for some systems in which both the initiated cells and the surrounding cells respond equally but the initiated cells fail to return to the resting condition as quickly or as completely as do the surrounding cells. This delay or block in reovery is seen in liver hyperplastic foci and nodules (see Farber, 1980) and might well be a property of other initiated cells also. Conceivably, the active phorbol esters or other effective skin promoters might operate through such an overall mechanism.

Since each one of these three suggested mechanisms would probably operate through different biochemical or molecular mechanisms, it would appear to be important to establish the overall phenomenon before focusing on one or more molecular hypotheses.

Another critical question concerning promotion is whether focal or differential cell proliferation is sufficient to set in motion the train of events leading to cancer or whether additional effects of carcinogens or of promoting environments, such as gene activation, or other biochemical cellular modulations in the amplified or expanded initiated cells are required. In other words, is *amplification of an initiated cell population sufficient* or is *amplification plus modulation* essential?

To my knowledge, this crucial question has not been posed experimentally, since the assumption is generally made that modulation (gene activation?) is needed for progression and evolution to cancer. This prejudgment seems both unscientific and unjustified. This is particularly evident when one realizes that the amplified initiated cell population does not progress to cancer en masse but rather appears almost certainly to provide a population at higher risk for the next rare event (number 2, Farber and Cameron, 1980) (see Section 3.2.4).

3.2.4. Fate and Options for Focal Proliferations

It is well known that the majority of papillomas in the skin induced by a phorbol ester after application of a single dose of a carcinogen undergo regression with only a minority persisting (e.g., see Boutwell, 1964, 1974; Burns *et al.*, 1978). A similar phenomenon has been seen in the liver and urinary bladder (see Farber and Cameron, 1980) and possibly in the colon (DeCosse *et al.*, 1975).

In the liver and in the skin, at least two populations of focal proliferations (nodules and papillomas) have been identified—a majority that regress or mature (remodel) and a minority that persist. Subsequent focal cellular changes have been found in an occasional persistent nodule or papilloma.

In the liver, new insights are appearing from studies on the resistant cell hypothesis (Enomoto and Farber, 1980; Ogawa *et al.*, 1980; Solt *et al.*, 1980). Since a sequence of early preneoplastic hepatocyte lesions can be followed, it is becoming apparent that there are at least *three focal lesions* that can be distinguished. The very smallest foci, composed of only a few cells (perhaps up to 8 or 16 cells), are generally low in epoxide hydrolase activity. These small lesions persist for long segments of the animal's life span and do not seem to undergo any remarkable change in appearance. This is also the experience of Scherer and Emmelot (1975), Sirica *et al.* (1978), and Peraino *et al.* (1978). When livers containing these very early foci are selected (or promoted), the foci rapidly grow into nodules within a matter of days (Solt *et al.*, 1977). When still microscopic, the enlarging foci now become much more active for epoxide hydrolase. When these reach a size of about 1 mm or so within 2–3 weeks, they retain their activity of epoxide hydrolase and now show one of two overall fates. The majority (90–94%) undergo remodeling toward normal-appearing liver with the gain of negative markers and the loss of positive ones (see Ogawa *et al.*, 1980). The rate of remodeling is quite variable, some nodules showing a rapid change (1 month or so) and others a slow change (a few months) and the majority falling in between. A small minority, about 6–10%, show no remodeling but persist as white unremodeled nodules. Basophilic nodules and ultimately metastasizing hepatocellular carcinoma can be seen arising inside a few such nodules. The remodeling nodules show few if any hepatocytes labeled with thymidine while the persistent nodules regularly show labeled hepatocytes.

Thus, it appears that more refined steps may be identified early in carcinogenesis with the use of a much better synchronized system. Because of the intensity of the selection pressure (the promoting environment), all the responding resistant hepatocytes behave pretty much in unison, producing a moving cohort up to the time of the appearance of the visible hyperplastic nodule. If the selection pressure is continued beyond the brief period now used (2 weeks), the nodules become larger and easily separated from the surrounding liver.

499
SEQUENTIAL
EVENTS IN
CHEMICAL
CAR-
CINOGENESIS

For biochemical, metabolic, and dynamic biological studies, grossly visible lesions that are synchronized are essential. Most of the models of liver carcinogenesis do not generate such lesions and therefore are not particularly useful for these types of studies. This is regretable, since the limitations that exist in a model that requires microscopic examination for analysis are serious.

Another desirable property of models of carcinogenesis is the clear-cut evidence that each proposed lesion is truly a step in a proposed sequence. This requires that a physical link be established between the different populations. This is readily shown in the papilloma in the mouse skin in which further progression to cancer can be seen. In the liver, only the resistant cell model has shown this sequence: resistant initiated cell → focus → nodule → metastasizing hepatocellular carcinoma (Solt *et al.*, 1977).

However, in no system has it been possible to study in any detail the steps between the putative preneoplastic lesion, the nodule of the papilloma, and the ultimate malignancy (see Section 4).

3.3. *Naturally Occurring Promotion or Selection*

There is a strong suspicion on the part of some investigators that many tissues or organs create a "physiological" promoting or selecting environment. The most provocative evidence in this respect relates to carcinogenesis in the colon or the urinary tract. In each of these locations, diversion of the normal stream of movement of contents has been found to lead to a decreased incidence of neoplasia with known carcinogens (e.g., Navarrete and Spjut, 1967; Gennaro *et al.*, 1973; Oyasu *et al.*, 1980). Also there exist in the literature many examples in which cancer can be induced by a single exposure to a large dose of carcinogen, a situation that might well be dependent upon an interplay between a "physiological" promotion and the appropriate metabolic and structural changes in a target organ or tissue. For the liver, the continual exposure to many compounds from the intestine and for the skin, exposure to ultraviolet light could be playing a selecting role in carcinogenesis.

4. *Subsequent Sequences: Progression*

As already indicated, there is considerable evidence that one or more of the focal proliferations appearing during promotion or selection are the sites of further change in one or a few cells. These few cells seem to have acquired some autonomy, since they apparently proliferate without the evident need for an external influence. It is believed that this process of appearance of rare change (rare event)–selection repeat itself until the organism dies with advanced malignant neoplasia (Fig. 2).

In humans, one consistently sees in many organs several types of putative precancerous lesions, such as atypical hyperplasia, dysplasia, and carcinoma-*in situ* (see Foulds, 1975; Farber and Cameron, 1980). These lesions appear to occur at later times in carcinogenesis than do the focal proliferations discussed above. How these sets of lesions relate to each other and to altered biological behavior of cells during *in vitro* transformation (e.g., atypical growth, growth in soft agar, acquisition of infinite capacity for growth, etc.) is not clear and remains potentially a very fruitful area for study (see Farber and Cameron, 1980). In the human and to some degree in the experimental models, disturbances in normal maturation or differentiation, such as in squamous epithelia, are commonly seen. The possible role of such a disturbance in biochemical programming remains a challenge to the experimentalist.

The development of models for the sequential analysis of the early changes in the carcinogenic process is most encouraging. However, since these changes are environment dependent, and the later ones seem not to be, it may be more difficult to develop synchronized models for the later steps in the process (see Section 5).

In the liver and in the skin in experimental animals and in many sites in humans, it has been shown that presumptive precancerous lesions or even cancerous lesions can arise in an area of focal proliferation characteristic of the early sequence in the neoplastic process. This has been reported many times in the skin. In the liver, frankly malignant lesions or histologically atypical nodules have been found to arise in hyperplastic nodules induced by ethionine, aramite, diethylnitrosamine, or 3'-methyl-4-dimethylaminoazobenzene (Popper *et al.*, 1960; Farber, 1963; Epstein *et al.*, 1967; Goldfarb, 1973; *Solt et al.*, 1977). Thus, clearly the suggested role of some of the early focal lesions as possible precursors of cancer is well grounded. Any suggested sequence that bypasses or omits the hyperplastic nodule, the papilloma, or similar analogous lesions as *one site of origin of cancer* ignores this unequivocal evidence (e.g., Williams, 1980).

Of course, great caution must be used in assigning an *exclusive role* as cancer precursor to the preneoplastic focal proliferation. Over the years, investigators have brought forth evidence that cancer can arise in at least some organs (skin, colon, liver, etc.) without the occurrence of focal proliferations as precursor lesions. It is certainly very possible that cancer can develop through different sequences (see Farber and Cameron, 1980). However, if such proposed sequences are to be studied and analyzed in detail, appropriate *analyzable* models must be developed. To date, very few if any models that can be subjected to critical analysis via hypothesis testing have been reported. An obvious problem in model design that makes a negative finding uninterpretable is the fact that new focal proliferations always grow more quickly than their precursors. Naturally, under these conditions, any proliferating cell population very often destroys rapidly its precursor population. Thus, the absence of a visible precursor at any moment in time does *not* establish that such a precursor did not exist. Clearly, a large expanded precursor population, such as a nodule, is necessary in most instances, in order to observe a new population arising in an older one. This serious experimental complication has been overlooked in many studies that claim the absence of a precursor for any cell population acting as a step in a sequence leading to cancer.

A critical issue that has not yet been analyzed is the basis for the difference between the majority of focal populations that undergo some form of regression or remodeling and the minority that persist. In turn, are all the persisting nodules capable of acting as sites for further steps to cancer or is this population also heterogeneous in this respect? With respect to regression versus persistence, is this built in at the time of initiation or is it simply a reflection of the intensity of a continuing environment that favors persistence by stimulating cell proliferation? If the latter is valid, the degree of persistence is the result of a stochastic phenomenon and not predetermined by exposure to the carcinogen.

With regard to the question of equivalence or otherwise of all persisting lesions, conceivably they may *all* be capable of acting as precursors for cancer but the rates are different and the animal succumbs to one cancer before others appear.

Clearly, this is one of the most important questions concerning the role of preneoplastic lesions in the evolution to cancer.

5. Overview

It is evident from this brief discussion and from more extensive reviews (e.g., Foulds, 1969, 1975; Farber and Cameron, 1980) that cancer in many sites often arises as a stepwise multistep process. This conclusion can no longer be contested.

However, the models or systems available to study the genesis, properties, options, and fates of each of such sequential cell populations as steps in the development of cancer and their roles if any in the evolution toward cancer are still not well developed. For the early changes, the skin and liver remain the best models. However, no model yet exists for the study of any possible sequence of events beginning with a persistent focal proliferation and ending in some aspect of malignant neoplasia. In almost every instance, the different steps that occur run together in a manner that does not enable the identification and analysis of any discrete link in this chain. In our view, the main reason for this is the "self-generating" nature of this apparently "environment-independent" segment of the carcinogenic process. Also, in every model used, the number of early preneoplastic lesions is far larger by a factor of 10^2 to 10^3 than the number of cancers ultimately seen. This is a serious limitation to the sequential analysis of cancer development. It would be highly desirable to develop a model in which the number of early, middle, and late lesions equals the number of cancers.

Only in such a model could one be certain that one is studying the carcinogenic process. The available liver and skin models may allow this refinement even now.

Up to now, we have been content to act to a large degree primarily as *naturalists*, observing nature as it appears with only a minimum of experimental manipulation of the process. While essential at the beginning of the study of any biological phenomenon, such an approach cannot hope to elucidate in a factual way any process, except the simplest and most elementary of biological phenomenon.

This lesson was clearly presented in the exciting developments of our current understanding of skin carcinogenesis in the 1930–1950 decades. During this period, the *experimental* or *in vivo manipulative* approach proved itself. Yet somehow, even today, this lesson has gone unheeded except in rare instances in an occasional study of carcinogenesis in liver, urinary bladder, mammary gland, and connective tissue.

It appears that increasing emphasis has been and is being placed on *in vitro* systems as the major hope. These have shown interesting and in a few instances exciting developments. Yet, only in a few combined *in vivo–in vitro* approaches have they opened up new insights into cancer development as it occurs in an intact animal or human (see Farber and Cameron, 1980, for references). Although the study of transformation *in vitro* with chemicals is a legitimate endeavor in basic biological science, there consistently appears a desire or a compulsion to relate the findings to the intact organism. Given the high reactivity of activated carcinogens with DNA and many other cellular constituents, given the extreme diversity of biological effects of active promoters such as some of the phorbol esters, given the absence of the highly restrictive homeostatic system in the intact organism that limits severely what actually happens, and given the plasticity and adaptability of cells and cell systems when removed from the severe restrictions of the homeostatic forces *in vivo*, there exists a reasonable probability that any biological phenomenon studied *in vitro* may not have a close relevance to the phenomena of cancer development *in vivo*. Therefore, a close interplay between *in vitro* and *in vivo* studies would appear to be an important prerequisite for the analysis of carcinogenesis. For example, it is clearly evident that perhaps as much as 50 or 60% of the time taken for epithelial cancer development with chemicals involves altered or initiated cells that show no ability to escape from the rigid growth control in normal tissues. It is in this segment of the process that promotion by external agents or manipulations exerts its major influence. *In vitro*, this period of no autonomous growth is largely bypassed. How does one relate the *in vitro* to the *in vivo*?

Another aspect that needs some discussion is the need for systems that require *many different manipulations* if the multistep process of carcinogenesis is to be dissected into its component steps. This principle is elementary and yet seems to be ignored by a significant number of investigators studying the carcinogenic process with chemicals. The more manipulations required to propel the system toward cancer, the more analyzable the model.

As mentioned in Section 3.2.4, if a model is designed or is being used for metabolic or for dynamic biological approaches to the analysis of the sequence of changes, some way to obtain discrete cell populations synchronized with respect to the step involved must be developed. The newer cell sorters may be useful, despite the relatively small numbers of cells involved, if suitable markers can be identified. An alternative approach is to manipulate the experimental system so as to augment or amplify the cell population under study (see Farber, 1973*b*).

A highly desirable property of a model is a testable hypothesis. By the latter is meant a proposal, based on a rational analysis, that can be subjected to a clear-cut experimental test. Unfortunately, cancer, including carcinogenesis, has been the subject of enormous speculative activity for many decades. In the early years, when the scientific technology and knowledge were meager, few alternatives to speculation were present. Given the current state of scientific technology, realistic hypothesis testing, rather than grandiose speculation, would seem to be very appropriate.

Hypothesis testing is needed at different levels of biological organization. Yet, this seems to be hampered by the early acceptance of concepts based on minimal or no data. To cite but two examples: (a) The concept of loss of growth control dominates current views of initiation and promotion. Yet, even a casual examination of its foundation is anything but convincing (e.g., see Farber and Cameron, 1980). (b) A commonly expressed view is that cancer development with chemicals requires "multiple hits" by the carcinogen on the cells that might evolve into cancer (e.g., Scherer and Emmelot, 1979; Emmelot and Scherer, 1980). Although several "rare events" (Farber and Cameron, 1980) are very likely necessary for the ultimate development of cancer, there is no clear-cut evidence that these need be induced by a carcinogen. For example, in the three instances in which a likely precursor population, the skin papilloma, was exposed to a carcinogen, no influence of the carcinogen on the development of cancer was observed in two (Mottram, 1945; Henderson and Rous, 1964). While the paucity of experimental data does not allow any conclusion at this time, it would be premature to conclude that another "hit" by a carcinogen is influencing in a major way the evolution of a papilloma to a carcinoma. At least two other possibilities must be considered. The first, the most radical, would propose that the carcinogen gives *no* information to a cell that relates directly to cancer but merely induces a cell that can be selectively amplified by a promoting environment. The second, less radical, would propose that the postinitiation effects of carcinogens are largely if not entirely related to the promoting effects of the carcinogen, i.e., in selectively encouraging the growth of the initiated cells by effects on the surrounding cells. Clearly, scientific analysis demands that such notions be entertained and tested.

Until a more critical view of the possibilities is used, it is unlikely that novel approaches to the analysis of early steps in the carcinogenic process will be developed.

Despite these criticisms and limitations, it appears that cancer research is approaching a more critical view of each step in the process whereby cancer occurs with chemicals. Given the complexity of *any* single malignant neoplasm from any point of view—morphologic, biochemical, immunologic, biological—it appears unlikely that the problem of the essential nature or natures of any malignant cell population can be solved by exclusive emphasis on the cancer cell. More likely, an historical approach, with emphasis on the stepwise sequence of cellular, biological, biochemical, molecular, and immunologic changes leading to cancer, coupled with a focused study on cancer cell populations, would be more appropriate from the current perspective.

Acknowledgments

The author's research included in this review was supported by research grants from the National Cancer Institute of Canada, the National Cancer Institute, National Institutes of Health (CA-21157), and the Medical Research Council of Canada (MA 5994).

I would like to express my appreciation to Hélène Robitaille for the willing assistance given during the preparation of this manuscript.

6. References

BERENBLUM, I., 1975, Sequential aspects of chemical carcinogenesis in skin, in: *Cancer: A Comprehensive Treatise*, Vol. 1 (F. F. Becker, ed.), pp. 323–344, Plenum Press, New York.

BERENBLUM, I., 1978, Established principles and unresolved problems in carcinogenesis, *J. Natl. Cancer Inst.* **60:**723.

BOUTWELL, R. K., 1964, Some biological aspects of skin carcinogenesis, *Prog. Exp. Tumor Res.* **4:**207.

BOUTWELL, R. K., 1974, The function and mechanism of action of promoters of carcinogenesis, *CRC Crit. Rev. Toxicol.* **2:**418.

BURNET, F. M., 1978, Cancer: Somatic–genetic considerations, *Adv. Cancer Res.* **28:**1.

BURNS, F. J., VANDERLAAN, M., SNYDER, E., AND ALBERT, R. E., 1978, Induction and progression kinetics of mouse skin papillomas, in: *Carcinogenesis: Mechanisms of Tumor Promotion and Cocarcinogenesis*, Vol. 2 (T. J. Slaga, A. Sivak, and R. K. Boutwell, eds.), p. 91, Raven Press, New York.

CAIRNS, J., 1975, Mutation, selection and the natural history of cancer, *Nature (London)* **255:**197.

CAYAMA, E., AND SOLT, D. B., 1980, Promoting effect of 2-acetylaminofluorene plus liver mitogenic stimulus on hepatocarcinogenesis induced by methylnitrosourea or diethylnitrosamine, *Proc. Am. Assoc. Cancer Res.* **21:**73.

CAYAMA, E., TSUDA, H., SARMA, D. S. R., AND FARBER, E., 1978, Initiation of chemical carcinogenesis requires cell proliferation, *Nature (London)* **275:**60.

COGGIN, J. H., AND ANDERSON, N. G., 1974, Cancer differentiation and embryonic antigens: Some central problems, *Adv. Cancer Res.* **19:**105.

CRADDOCK, V. M., 1976, Cell proliferation and experimental liver cancer, in: *Liver Cell Cancer* (H. M. Cameron, D. A. Linsell, and G. P. Warwick, eds.), pp. 153–201, Elsevier, Amsterdam.

DeCOSSE, J. J., ADAMS, M. B., KUZMA, J. F., LoGERBO, P., AND CONDON, R. E., 1975, Effect of ascorbic acid on rectal polyps of patients with familial polyposis, *Surgery* **78:**608.

EMMELOT, P., AND SCHERER, E., 1980, The first relevant cell stage in rat liver carcinogenesis. A quantitative approach, *Biochim. Biophys. Acta* **605:**247.

ENOMOTO, K., AND FARBER, E., 1980, Immunohistochemical study of epoxide hydratase (EH) activity in rat liver during chemical carcinogenesis, *Proc. Am. Assoc. Cancer Res.* **21:**82.

EPSTEIN, S., ITO, N., MERKOW, L., AND FARBER, E., 1967, Cellular analysis of liver carcinogenesis. The induction of large hyperplastic nodules in the liver with 2-fluorenylacetamide or ethionine and some aspects of their morphology and glycogen metabolism, *Cancer Res.* **27:**1702.

FARBER, E., 1963, Ethionine carcinogenesis, *Adv. Cancer Res.* **7:**383.

505

SEQUENTIAL
EVENTS IN
CHEMICAL
CAR-
CINOGENESIS

FARBER, E., 1973a, Carcinogenesis—Cellular evolution as a unifying thread: Presidential address, *Cancer Res.* **33**:2537.

FARBER, E., 1973b, Hyperplastic liver nodules, *Methods Cancer Res.* **7**:345.

FARBER, E., 1979, Reaction of liver to carcinogens—A new analyical approach, in: *Toxic Liver Injury* (E. Farber and M. M. Fisher, eds.), pp. 445–467, Dekker, New York.

FARBER, E., 1980, The sequential analysis of liver cancer induction, *Biochim. Biophys. Acta* **605**:149.

FARBER, E., AND CAMERON, R., 1980, Sequential analysis of cancer development, *Adv. Cancer Res.* **31**:125.

FARBER, E., AND SPORN, M. B. (eds.), 1976, Early lesions and the development of epithelial cancer, *Cancer Res.* **36**:2675.

FARBER, E., CAMERON, R. G., LAISHES, B., LIN, J.-L., MEDLINE, A., OGAWA, K., AND SOLT, D. B., 1979, Physiological and molecular markers during carcinogenesis, in: *Carcinogens: Identification and Mechanisms of Action* (A. C. Clark and C. R. Shaw, eds.), pp. 319–335, Raven Press, New York.

FOULDS, L., 1969, 1975, *Neoplastic Development*, Volumes 1 and 2, Academic Press, New York.

GENNARO, A. R., VILLANEUVA, R., SUKONTHAMAN, Y., VATHANOPHAS, V., AND ROSEMOND, G. P., 1973, Chemical carcinogenesis in transposed intestinal segments, *Cancer Res.* **33**:536.

GOLDFARB, S., 1973, A morphological and histochemical study of carcinogenesis of the liver in rats fed 3'-methyl-4-dimethylaminoazobenzene, *Cancer Res.* **33**:1119.

HADDOW, A., 1972, Molecular repair, wound healing and carcinogenesis: Tumor production a possible overhealing?, *Adv. Cancer Res.* **16**:181.

HEIDELBERGER, C., 1973, Chemical oncogenesis in culture, *Adv. Cancer Res.* **18**:317.

HENDERSON, J. S., AND ROUS, P., 1964, Further experiments in the causes of sequential neoplastic changes. The effects of 20-methylcholanthrene on transplanted epidermal mouse papillomas and the derivative carcinomas, *J. Exp. Med.* **120**:197.

IANNACONNE, P. M., GARDNER, R. L., AND HARRIS, H., 1978, The cellular origin of chemically induce tumor, *J. Cell Sci.* **29**:249.

KOSS, L. G., 1975, Precancerous lesions, in: *Persons at High Risk of Cancer* (J. F. Fraumeni, Jr., ed.), pp. 85–101, Academic Press, New York.

MEDLINE, A., AND FARBER, E., 1980, Multi-step theory of neoplasia, *Recent Adv. Histopathol.* **11**:in press.

MOTTRAM, J. C., 1945, The change from benign to malignant in chemically induced warts in mice, *Br. J. Exp. Pathol.* **26**:1.

NAVARRETE, A., AND SPJUT, H. J., 1967, Effect of colostomy on experimentally produced neoplasms of the colon of the rat, *Cancer* **20**:1466.

NOWELL, P. C., 1976, The clonal evolution of tumor cell populations, *Science* **194**:23.

OGAWA, K., SOLT, D. B., AND FARBER, E., 1980, Phenotypic diversity as an early property of putative preneoplastic hepatocyte populations in liver carcinogenesis, *Cancer Res.* **40**:725.

OHDE, G., SCHULTE-HERMANN, R., AND SCHUPPLER, J., 1979a, Proliferation of preneoplastic cells and tumor formation in rat liver: Promotion by inducers of growth and monooxygenases, Deutsche Pharmakologische Gesellschaft, abstract 20th spring meeting, Mainz, PR 18, abstract No. 71.

OHDE, G., SCHUPPLER, J., SCHULTE-HERMANN, R., AND KEIGER, H., 1979b, Proliferation of rat liver cells in preneoplastic nodules after stimulation of liver growth by xenobiotic inducer, *Arch. Toxicol. Suppl.* **2**:451.

OYASU, R., HIRAO, Y., AND IZUMI, K., 1980, Promotion by urine of urinary bladder carcinogenesis, *Proc. Am. Assoc. Cancer Res.* **21**:70.

PEGG, A. E., 1977, Formation and metabolism of alkylated nucleosides: Possible role in carcinogenesis by nitroso compounds and alkylating agents, *Adv. Cancer Res.* **25**:195.

PERAINO, C., FRY, R. J. M., AND GRUBE, D. D., 1978, Drug-induced enhancement of hepatic tumorigenesis, in: *Carcinogenesis: Mechanisms of Tumor Promotion and Cocarcinogenesis*, Vol. 2 (T. J. Slaga, A. Sivak, and R. K. Boutwell, eds.), p. 421, Raven Press, New York.

PETO, R., 1977, Epidemiology, multistage models and short-term mutagenicity tests, in: *Origins of Human Cancer* (H. H. Hiatt, J. D. Watson, and J. A. Winsten, eds.), pp. 1403–1428, Cold Spring Harbor Laboratory, Cold Spring Harbor, N.Y.

PITOT, H. C., 1979, Biological and enzymatic events in chemical carcinogenesis, *Annu. Rev. Med.* **30**:25.

PITOT, H. C., BARSNESS, L., AND KITAGAWA, T., 1978, Stages in the process of hepatocarcinogenesis in rat liver, in: *Carcinogenesis: Mechanisms of Tumor Promotion and Cocarcinogenesis*, Vol. 2 (T. J. Slaga, A. Sivak, and R. K. Boutwell, eds.), p. 433, Raven Press, New York.

POPPER, H., STERNBERG, S. S., OSER, B. L., AND OSER, M., 1960, The carcinogenic effect of aramite in rats. A study of hepatic nodules, *Cancer* **13**:1035.

PREHN, R. T., 1976, Tumor progression and homeostasis, *Adv. Cancer Res.* **23**:203.

PUGH, T., AND GOLDFARB, S., 1978, Quantitative histochemical and autoradiographic studies of hepatocarcinogenesis in rats fed 2-acetylaminofluorene, *Cancer Res.* **38**:4450.

SASAKI, T., AND YOSHIDA, T., 1935, Experimentelle Erzeugung des Lebercarcinoms durch Fütterung mit *o*-amidoazotulol, *Arch. Pathol. Anat. Allg. Pathol.* **295**:175.

SCHERER, E., AND EMMELOT, P., 1975, Foci of altered liver cells induced by a single dose of diethylnitrosamine and partial hepatectomy: Their contribution to hepatocarcinogenesis in the rat, *Eur. J. Cancer* **11**:145.

SCHERER, E., AND EMMELOT, P., 1976, Kinetics of induction and growth of enzyme-deficient islands involved in hepatocarcinogenesis, *Cancer Res.* **36**:2544.

SCHERER, E., AND EMMELOT, P., 1979, Multihit kinetics of tumor cell formations and risk assessment of low doses of carcinogen, in: *Carcinogens: Identification and Mechanisms of Action* (A. C. Clark and C. R. Shaw, eds.), pp. 337–364, Raven Press, New York.

SCHERER, E., AND HOFFMANN, M., 1971, Probable clonal genesis of cellular islands induced in rat liver by diethylnitrosamine, *Eur. J. Cancer* **7**:369.

SCHERER, E., STEWARD, A. P., AND EMMELOT, P., 1977, Kinetics of formation of O^6-ethylguanine and its removal from liver DNA of rats receiving diethylnitrosamine, *Chem. Biol. Interact.* **19**:1.

SCRIBNER, J. D., AND SÜSS, R., 1978, Tumor initiation and promotion, *Int. Rev. Exp. Pathol.* **18**:137.

SHUBIK, P., BASEGA, R., AND RITCHIE, A. C., 1953, The life and progression of individual skin tumours in mice, *Br. J. Cancer* **7**:342.

SIRICA, A. E., BARSNESS, L., GODSWORTHY, T., AND PITOT, H. C., 1978, Definition of stages during hepatocarcinogenesis in the rat: Potential application to the evaluation of initiating and promoting agents in the environment, *J. Environ. Pathol. Toxicol.* **2**:21.

SMETS, L. A., 1980, Cell transformation as a model for tumor induction and neoplastic growth, *Biochim. Biophys. Acta* **605**:93.

SOLT, D. B., AND FARBER, E., 1976, A new principle for the analysis of chemical carcinogenesis, *Nature (London)* **263**:701.

SOLT, D., MEDLINE, A., AND FARBER, E., 1977, Rapid emergence of carcinogen-induced hyperplastic lesions in a new model for the sequential analysis of liver carcinogenesis, *Am. J. Pathol.* **88**:595.

SOLT, D. B., CAYAMA, E., SARMA, D. S. R., AND FARBER, E., 1980, Persistence of resistant putative preneoplastic hepatocytes induced by *N*-nitrosodiethylamine or *N*-methyl-*N*-nitrosourea, *Cancer Res.* **40**:1112.

SQUIRE, R. A., AND LEVITT, M. H., 1975, Report of a workshop on classification of specific hepatocellular lesions in rats, *Cancer Res.* **25**:3214.

STUTMAN, O., 1975, Immunodepression and malignancy, *Adv. Cancer Res.* **22**:261.

THOMAS, L., 1959, Discussion, in: *Cellular and Humoral Aspects of Hypersensitivity* (H. S. Lawrence, ed.), pp. 529–532, Harper & Row, New York.

TSUDA, H., LEE, G., AND FARBER, E., 1980, The induction of resistant hepatocytes as a new principle for a possible short term *in vivo* test for carcinogens, *Cancer Res.* **40**:1157.

WILLIAMS, G. M., 1980, The pathogenesis of rat liver cancer caused by chemical carcinogens, *Biochim. Biophys. Acta* **605**:167.

YING, T. S., SARMA, D. S. R., AND FARBER, E., 1979a, Role of liver cell necrosis in the induction of preneoplastic lesions, *Proc. Am. Assoc. Cancer Res.* **20**:14.

YING, T. S., SARMA, D. S. R., AND FARBER, E., 1979b, Induction of presumptive preneoplastic lesions in rat liver by a single dose of 1,2-dimethylhydrazine, *Chem. Biol. Interact.* **28**:363.

14

Neoantigen Expression in Chemical Carcinogenesis

Robert W. Baldwin and Michael R. Price

1. Introduction

Neoplastic transformation induced by chemical carcinogens results in the expression in transformed cells of antigens that are not present in their normal cell counterpart, at least in the adult host. In early studies with chemically induced tumors (Foley, 1953; Baldwin, 1955; Prehn and Main, 1957), neoantigens were defined by their capacity to elicit immunity to transplanted tumor and were termed "tumor-specific transplantation antigens." It is now evident that immune responses are elicited against these antigens in the autochthonous host, and considerable effort has been directed to resolve their role as a limiting (or enhancing) component of chemical carcinogenesis. It is appropriate to refer to these classical neoantigens, which are characterized by an immunological specificity that is unique to individual tumors, as "tumor-associated rejection antigens" (the term "tumor-specific" has been avoided here since recent experiments have raised the possibility that these antigens may be induced in nontransformed cells and so cannot be viewed as specific markers of malignancy).

Following the development of transplanted tumor models in syngeneic hosts for studying tumor immune reactions, *in vitro* methods have been introduced for detecting cellular and humoral immune responses to tumor-associated antigens. Techniques such as the measurement of antibody binding to viable tumor cells or the *in vitro* assay of serum antibody and sensitized cell-mediated cytotoxicity against tumor cells, are by definition detecting antigens expressed at the cell surface. Moreover, the specificities of these reactions are frequently identical to

Robert W. Baldwin and Michael R. Price • Cancer Research Campaign Laboratories, University of Nottingham, Nottingham, England

508

ROBERT W.
BALDWIN
AND
MICHAEL R.
PRICE

those of the tumor rejection antigens. Even so, it is preferable to refer to the neoantigens detected by *in vitro* assay as "tumor-associated surface antigens" since their identity as rejection antigens is in most cases not established.

During the past few years, it has been realized that chemically induced tumors may express a diversity of neoantigens in addition to the classical rejection antigens. These include antigens inducing limited immunoprotection against a number of tumors and often the nature and specificity of these are unknown, so that their description as "common tumor-associated antigens" is appropriate. In some instances, these have been distinguished from another class of common antigen that again may function as a rejection antigen, this being the reexpressed embryonic antigen or oncodevelopmental antigen. Almost all of these antigens are immunogenic in the autochthonous host as well as in the syngeneic recipient of transplanted tumor, so that they have the potential at least to elicit reactions that modify tumor growth. However, to what extent these antigens function as targets for immunosurveillance is unknown. Also, it is now an open question as to whether their expression is confined exclusively to the transformed cell, although they may be regarded as valuable markers for studying transformation events in chemical carcinogenesis.

2. Neoantigens on Chemically Induced Tumors

2.1. Tumor-Associated Neoantigens

Considerable effort in the past 25 years has been devoted to characterizing tumor-associated rejection antigens and common tumor-associated antigens that operate to promote reactions leading to the control of progressive neoplastic growth and possibly to the ultimate destruction of tumor cells (Table 1). It has been possible to evaluate the contribution of these components to tumor immunity only by detailed examination of a range of chemically induced tumors and by design of highly controlled experimental procedures using syngeneic hosts for tumor transplantation tests. The expression of tumor-associated surface antigens in several tumor models has also been characterized both by the phenomena that they evoke *in vivo* and by the *in vitro* analyses of cell-mediated and humoral immune reactions in tumor-immune or tumor-bearing hosts. In a number of instances, these antigenic components have been isolated as purified, solubilized preparations, and it is now feasible to define not only their nature and characteristics as cell-surface membrane-associated products, but also their role in the transformation of cells by chemical carcinogens.

2.1.1. Polycyclic Hydrocarbons

Early studies by Foley (1953), Baldwin (1955), and Prehn and Main (1957) using transplanted 3-methylcholanthrene (3-MC)-induced sarcomas in the rat or mouse showed that by appropriate manipulation of the progressively growing tumor (surgical excision or ligation of tumor blood supply), the treated animals were subsequently resistant to challenge with viable cells of the same tumor. Comparably, animals treated with tumor cells attenuated by irradiation (Révész, 1960; Klein *et al.*, 1960) or cytotoxic drugs (Apffel *et al.*, 1966) developed the capacity to reject cells of the immunizing 3-MC-induced sarcoma. In these studies, many of the tumors were found to be strongly immunogenic, and immunized animals were frequently protected against large numbers of viable sarcoma cells or even grafts of tumor tissue. Additionally, with sarcomas induced by 3-MC and other polycyclic hydrocarbons (Table 1), the state of immunity conferred exhibited a high degree of specificity, and protection was only evident against the transplanted tumor to which the animal had previously been exposed, and not against other tumors, even though these may have been induced by the same carcinogen (reviewed by Baldwin, 1973). This is exemplified by the studies of Basombrío (1970), who demonstrated only a single instance of cross-reactivity among a series of 25 murine sarcomas that were examined in a crisscross fashion or by multiple immunization.

509
NEOANTIGEN
EXPRESSION
IN CHEMICAL
CAR-
CINOGENESIS

More recently, the specificity of these responses has been challenged, particularly in experiments in which graded doses of 3-MC-induced murine sarcomas have been employed to challenge immunized mice, and reactions against both individually specific tumor-associated antigens and common tumor-associated antigens have been revealed (Leffell and Coggin, 1977; Hellström *et al.*, 1978). In the past, it has been suggested that such cross-reacting rejection-type antigens may represent contamination with endogenous virus (e.g., Holmes *et al.*, 1971), although in studies with 3-MC-induced murine sarcomas, Hellström *et al.* (1978) concluded that while endogenous murine leukemia viral antigens may increase the immunogenicity of common antigens, cross-protection could not completely be attributed to viral structures. However, Basombrío (1978) has emphasized that in tests designed to define tumor antigenic profiles, it is important to exclude not only the possibility of virus contamination, but also minor histocompatibility differences that may be introduced if tumors have been imported from another laboratory. Variability due to this latter problem may be discounted by the demonstration of skin graft exchange and negative responses to normal tissues.

The expression of common tumor-associated antigens would appear to be not restricted to sarcomas induced by 3-MC since they have been detected in protection tests with 3-MC-induced squamous cell carcinomas of the skin (Economou *et al.*, 1977) and lung (Jamasbi and Nettesheim, 1977). Also, Taranger *et al.* (1972*a,b*) found that mice immunized with a pool of 3-MC-induced bladder papilloma tissue developed fewer papillomas after subsequent implantation of a pellet of 3-MC in the bladder. In later studies, however, Wahl *et al.* (1974) determined that 3-MC-induced bladder sarcomas and carcinomas in mice displayed individually distinct tumor-associated rejection antigens in classical tumor transplant rejection tests.

Apart from the above examples of cross-protection and early experiments by Reiner and Southam (1967, 1969) who reported that immunization with a pool of 3-MC-induced murine sarcomas in some instances produced protection against

510

ROBERT W.
BALDWIN
AND
MICHAEL R.
PRICE

TABLE 1

Expression of Tumor-Associated Antigens on Chemically Induced Tumors

Carcinogen	Tumor type	Species	Tumor-associated rejection antigen	Tumor-associated surface antigen	Common tumor-associated antigen	Onco-developmental antigen
Polycyclic hydrocarbons						
3-Methylcholanthrene	Fibrosarcoma	Mouse	+	+	+	+
		Rat	+	+		+
		Guinea pig	+	+	+	
	Mammary carcinoma	Mouse	+			
		Rat	+			
	Squamous cell carcinoma	Mouse			+	
	Respiratory tract carcinoma	Rat			+	
	Lymphoma	Mouse	+			
	Bladder carcinoma/papilloma	Mouse	+		+	
		Rat			+	
	Bladder sarcoma	Mouse	+			
	Skin carcinoma/papilloma	Mouse	+			
	In vitro transformed prostate cells	Mouse	+	+		
	3T3 cells transformed *in vitro* and maintained *in vivo*	Mouse	+			
	Normal fibroblasts, transformed and maintained *in vitro* and *in vivo*	Mouse	+			+
Dibenz[a,h]anthracene	Sarcoma	Mouse	+			
		Guinea pig	+			
7,12-Dimethylbenz[a]anthracene	Sarcoma	Mouse	+	+		+
		Guinea pig	+	+		+
	Epithelioma	Mouse	+		+	
	Respiratory tract carcinoma	Rat				+

511

NEOANTIGEN
EXPRESSION
IN CHEMICAL
CAR-
CINOGENESIS

Carcinogen	Tumor	Species				
Benzo[a]pyrene	Sarcoma	Mouse	+		+	+
	Respiratory tract carcinoma	Rat	+		+	+
Dibenzo[a,i]pyrene	Sarcoma	Rat	+			+
Aminoazo dyes						
4-Dimethylaminoazobenzene	Hepatoma	Rat	+	+		
3'-Methyl-4-dimethylaminoazobenzene	Hepatoma	Rat	+	+		
o-Aminoazotoluene	Hepatoma	Mouse	+	+		
5-[[l-(Dimethylamino)-phenyl]azo]-quinoline	Hepatoma	Rat	+	+		
Aromatic amines						
N-2-Fluorenylacetamide	Mammary carcinoma	Rat	+	+		+
	Hepatoma	Rat	+	+		+
	Ear duct carcinoma	Rat	+	+		
Alkylnitrosamines						
Diethylnitrosamine	Hepatoma	Rat	+	+		+
	Hepatoma	Guinea pig	+	+		
N-Butyl-N-(4-hydroxybutyl)-nitrosamine	Bladder carcinoma	Rat	+			
N-Methyl-N-nitrosourea	Brain glioma	Rat	+			
Ethylnitrosourea	Glioma	Rat	+			
	Schwannoma	Rat	+			
N-Methyl-N-nitrosourethan	Colon carcinoma	Mouse	+	+	+	+
N-Methyl-N'-nitroso-N-nitrosoguanidine	In vitro transformed prostate cells	Mouse		+	+	+
	Colon carcinoma	Rat	+			
Hydrazine						
1,2-Dimethylhydrazine	Colon carcinoma	Mouse	+		+	+
	Colon carcinoma	Rat	+			
Miscellaneous						
Urethan	Pulmonary adenoma	Mouse	+	+		+
Mineral oil	Plasmacytoma	Mouse	+	+		
Plastic film	Sarcoma	Mouse	+	+		

512

ROBERT W.
BALDWIN
AND
MICHAEL R.
PRICE

other sarcomas not included in the immunizing pool, rejection antigens on many polycyclic hydrocarbon-induced tumors are generally characterized by their polymorphism. As shown in Table 1, these systems include squamous cell carcinomas (Pasternak et al., 1964; Tuffrey and Batchelor, 1964) and sarcomas (Pasternak, 1963; Oettgen et al., 1968) induced by 7,12-dimethyl-benz[a]anthracene, together with sarcomas induced by dibenz[a,h]anthracene (Prehn, 1960; Morton et al., 1965), benzo[a]pyrene (Delorme and Alexander, 1964; Globerson and Feldman, 1964), and dibenzo[a,i]pyrene (Old et al., 1962).

While sarcomas induced by 3-MC are in most cases consistently immunogenic, there is a species variability with respect to the number of viable cells that treated animals are able to reject. Thus, challenge inocula with up to 6 g of viable tumor tissue may be rejected by guinea pigs immunized by implantation of X-irradiated sarcoma tissue (Oettgen et al., 1968), whereas transplantation resistance in the rat or mouse may be overcome by much smaller challenges with between 10^6 and 10^8 viable sarcoma cells. The maximum number of cells rejected is not necessarily the best guide to describe the immunogenicity of a tumor since this will be influenced by several complex factors such as the method of immunization and the minimum number of cells required for growth in all untreated animals (TD_{100}). The 3-MC-induced sarcoma Meth A, for instance, is considered to be one of the most highly immunogenic of the chemically induced murine tumors as demonstrated by resistance against challenge of 2×10^4 cells (approximately $100 \times TD_{100}$) following immunization with a single dose of 10^5 X-irradiated tumor cells (Law et al., 1978; Price et al., 1979b). The immunogenicity of 3-MC-induced sarcomas within a species is also subject to variability (Baldwin, 1955; Old et al., 1962; Johnson, 1968; Takeda, 1969; Bartlett, 1972), and an inverse relationship between the latency period of induction and immunogenic potential has been reported (Old et al., 1962; Johnson, 1968). One interpretation of this is that tumors with long latent periods of induction are subject to immunoselection with the consequence that they tend to be less immunogenic than those of short latency (Prehn, 1967). However, Bartlett (1972) determined that early appearing murine sarcomas showed a wide range of immunogenicities, and in the rat, sarcomas of different latent period and induced by different doses of 3-MC had quantitatively similar immunogenicities (Baldwin et al., 1979). Thus, while host immunoselection may be a contributory factor modifying the immunogenicity of tumors, it is evident that antigenic variability is a real effect in chemical carcinogenesis.

A well-developed cellular response to tumor-associated rejection antigens is viewed to be necessary for tumor rejection responses to be effective. This has been clearly established in studies showing that sensitized lymphoid cells have the capacity to adoptively transfer immunity to normal recipients (Hellström and Hellström, 1969), and in neutralization tests, specific inhibition of tumor growth was observed in mice inoculated with mixtures of tumor cells and sensitized lymph node cells (Klein et al., 1960; Borberg et al., 1972) or peritoneal exudate cells (Old et al., 1962). In addition, the specificity of these cellular responses has been confirmed by delayed-type hypersensitivity reactions elicited by tumor cells or cell extracts from sarcomas induced by 3-MC and polycyclic hydrocarbons in guinea pigs (Oettgen *et al.*, 1968; Suter *et al.*, 1972) and in mice using the radioisotopic footpad assay (Minami *et al.*, 1979). Complimentary to these *in vivo* investigations has been the use of tests such as the inhibition of macrophage migration (Halliday and Webb, 1969; Halliday, 1971; Suter *et al.*, 1972), leukocyte adherence inhibition (Halliday and Miller, 1972), and macrophage electrophoretic mobility assay (Bubeník *et al.*, 1978), each of which has been employed to evaluate tumor-specific immune reactions to 3-MC-induced sarcomas in mice and guinea pigs.

The direct demonstration of cytotoxic activity of lymphoid cells from immune donors for cultured tumor target cells has been reported in a number of studies using colony inhibition and microcytotoxicity tests (Hellström *et al.*, 1968, 1970; Baldwin and Moore, 1971; Cohen *et al.*, 1972; Zöller *et al.*, 1975). While close parallels were established in the specificity of the cytotoxicity of sensitized lymphoid cells *in vitro* and tumor-associated rejection antigens, the results of these tests require reevaluation since there has been increasing recognition of the reactivity of natural killer (NK) cells as an effector mechanism in addition to that provided by specifically immune T cells, which were presumed to be the mediators of cytotoxicity in these tests (Herberman and Holden, 1978; Baldwin, 1977; Herberman *et al.*, 1979). However, although NK cells have revealed themselves to be highly cytotoxic against selected tumors in *in vitro* cytotoxicity tests, a fundamental issue still to be resolved is whether they can actually mediate *in vivo* resistance against tumor growth.

Further evidence demonstrating the occurrence and confirming the specificity of surface antigens on 3-MC-induced sarcomas in the mouse and rat comes from analyses of humoral antibody reactions with these tumors. Thus, serum either from mice immunized by surgical excision of tumor (Hellström *et al.*, 1968) or from rats treated with γ-irradiated tumor grafts (Baldwin and Moore, 1971) inhibited the capacity of cultured sarcoma cells to form colonies, whereas normal serum and serum from donors immunized against other tumors were without effect. Similar findings have also been obtained in tests employing the microcytotoxicity assay of Takasugi and Klein (1970) to detect complement-dependent cytotoxic antibody in the serum of mice immunized against transplanted 3-MC-induced sarcomas (Bloom, 1970; Bloom and Hildemann, 1970; DeLeo *et al.*, 1977, 1978). In the most extensive analysis of this kind, DeLeo *et al.* (1977, 1978) have studied the specificity of surface antigens associated with the 3-MC-induced sarcoma, Meth A. While this type of serological approach for typing tumor-associated antigens would appear to be most promising, with chemically induced murine tumors, murine leukemia virus (MuLV) and its antigens are frequently expressed (Old and Boyse, 1965; Whitmore *et al.*, 1971; Grant *et al.*, 1974*b*), and normal mouse serum often contains antibodies against MuLV antigens (Old and Stockert, 1977). Nevertheless, with the Meth A sarcoma, DeLeo *et al.* (1977, 1978) confirmed the individually distinct tumor-specific reactivity of syngeneic anti-Meth A serum for Meth A sarcoma cells, and in direct tests and absorption assays, the possibility that this reactivity was directed against MuLV antigens was

514

ROBERT W.
BALDWIN
AND
MICHAEL R.
PRICE

eliminated. A fascinating aspect of this system is that the specifically cytotoxic serum used in these studies also contains an antibody that precipitates a common tumor-associated protein, p53, in experiments using a variety of tumors metabolically labeled with $[^{35}S]$methionine and solubilized with detergent prior to performing the immunoprecipitation procedure (DeLeo *et al.*, 1979). The significance of this finding is as yet unknown although clearly the identification of a common transformation-related antigen is of immense interest.

Individually distinct tumor-associated surface antigens have been detected using the indirect membrane immunofluorescence technique to identify antibody in syngeneic immune serum binding to 3-MC-induced sarcoma cells in the mouse (Lejneva *et al.*, 1965) and rat (Baldwin *et al.*, 1971*a,c*, 1972*a*), and in the latter studies, a total of 122 combinations between a panel of 26 tumor-immune sera and 8 transplanted sarcomas were tested with conclusive evidence of cross-reactivity occurring between only one pair of tumors. In order to introduce a quantitative aspect to antibody binding assays, radioisotopic antiglobulin reagents (Harder and McKhann, 1968; Burdick *et al.*, 1973) and more recently, labeled protein A (the F_c reactive protein from *Staphylococcus aureus*; Brown *et al.*, 1977, 1978; Cleveland *et al.*, 1979) have been employed to demonstrate antibodies reactive with tumor-associated surface antigens. Again, the major class of antigen demonstrated was an individually distinct surface antigen, although in one investigation common tumor-associated antigens were detected (Cleveland *et al.*, 1979). These were found to emerge on tumor cells with increasing passage in culture, leading the authors to the conclusion that only primary- or secondary-passage tumor cells should be employed in tests to define antigenic profiles.

2.1.2. Aminoazo Dyes

Tumor-associated rejection antigens expressed on aminoazo dye-induced hepatomas in mice (Müller, 1968) and rats (Gordon, 1965; Baldwin and Barker, 1967*a*) were initially demonstrated by the induction of immunity to transplanted tumor cells in syngeneic animals. Two major features displayed by rat hepatomas induced by 4-dimethylaminoazobenzene (DAB) are that the tumors are consistently immunogenic so that immunized animals are able to reject up to 5×10^5 to 10^6 viable tumor cells and that each tumor expresses an individually distinct tumor rejection antigen (reviewed by Baldwin, 1973). The individual specificity of these antigens is further exemplified in tests showing that cross-protection was only rarely observed using cell lines established from separate primary hepatoma nodules from a single animal as evaluated in conventional tumor transplant rejection tests or in Winn assays using sensitized peritoneal lymphoid cells (Ishidate, 1974). Antigenic homogeneity of one of the tumors was further demonstrated with four clonal sublines of different chromosomal structure (Ishidate, 1974).

With respect to the expression of an individually distinct tumor-associated rejection antigen, it is evident that there is a direct parallel between these hepatomas and many of the 3-MC-induced sarcomas already discussed (Table

1). However, it should be noted that with several 3-MC-induced sarcomas particularly in the mouse and guinea pig, it is possible to isolate tumor-rejection-inducing activity in cell-membrane fractions or solubilized tumor extracts (reviewed by Baldwin and Price, 1975; see also Pellis *et al.*, 1974; Pellis and Kahan, 1975; Law and Appella, 1975; Bubeník *et al.*, 1978; Law *et al.*, 1978; Sikora *et al.*, 1979), whereas this has not been achieved with the rat hepatomas (Price and Baldwin, 1974a,b; Price *et al.*, 1978, 1979e). A number of experiments were thus performed in order to elucidate the factors that influence the immunogenicity of rat hepatomas and to define the necessary conditions under which tumor-associated rejection antigens may function effectively. In the first study, immunizing inocula of γ-irradiated rat hepatoma cells were exposed to glutaraldehyde at concentrations that did not inactivate a number of serologically defined surface antigens, and it was determined that this then abolished their capacity to induce protection to tumor cell challenge (Price *et al.*, 1979a,c). Second, mild heat treatment of irradiated cells ($\geq 41^\circ$C for 30 min) also destroyed their immunoprotective capacity (Dennick *et al.*, 1979). Impairment of the immunogenic character of irradiated hepatoma cells in these ways was correlated with the loss in residual metabolic activity possessed by the irradiated cells. It was concluded that for optimal immunoprotection, this requirement for a residual metabolic activity in the cellular immunogen emphasized that the mode of presentation was critical since the treatments employed may also modify the microenvironment of membrane antigens as well as influencing the cells' biosynthetic apparatus. Expenditure of metabolic energy is required to maintain the spatial configuration of many surface membrane proteins and glycoproteins via their transmembrane interaction with microfilaments, microtubules, and other cytoskeletal elements (Nicolson, 1976). Thus, the method of presentation of antigen directs the immune system along certain pathways which, using the endpoint assay of viable tumor cell challenge, may be revealed as rejection or possibly enhancement of tumor outgrowth. It is attractive to invoke that macrophages play a key role in establishing these responses and to propose that the form in which the antigen is presented determines the manner of antigen processing. Early tests to explore this possibility have demonstrated that tumor-specific immunity can be transferred to normal rats by inoculation of adherent peritoneal exudate cells that have been primed *in vivo* for 24 h with irradiated tumor cells, so clearly these cells may play an important and perhaps central role in the generation of tumor transplant immunity.

Conversely, when the same treatments of light glutaraldehyde fixation or mild heating of irradiated cells were applied to the 3-MC-induced sarcoma, Meth A, there was no loss in their immunogenicity, again emphasizing the basic difference between these tumor models (Price *et al.*, 1979b). The minimum essential conditions for revealing immunoprotection against the rat hepatoma are that at least 10^7 irradiated hepatoma cells are required to induce resistance against a challenge of 10^3 viable cells (ratio of immunizing:challenge cells 10^4:1), whereas with the Meth A sarcoma, a single injection of 10^5 attenuated cells protects against 2×10^4 tumor cells (ratio of immunizing:challenge cells 5:1). This wide discrepancy in

515
NEOANTIGEN
EXPRESSION
IN CHEMICAL
CAR-
CINOGENESIS

516

ROBERT W.
BALDWIN
AND
MICHAEL R.
PRICE

the efficacy of immunization suggests that there is a qualitative difference in the tumor-associated rejection antigens expressed on the rat and mouse tumors since it is highly unlikely that such a marked difference in immunogenic character could be accounted for by quantitative considerations alone, e.g., number of antigenic determinants per cell (Price et al., 1979b).

The expression of individually distinct tumor-associated surface antigens on DAB-induced rat hepatomas was confirmed in an extensive study showing that serum from immune donors only reacts in membrane immunofluorescence tests with surface antigens of cells derived from the immunizing tumor (Baldwin and Barker, 1967b; Baldwin et al., 1971a,b,c, 1972a). Clearly, however, fluorescence techniques requiring visual assessment of results have a number of practical disadvantages, and there is a need for more quantitative and objective assays for the demonstration of tumor-specific antibodies. Complement-dependent cytotoxicity tests have proved to be relatively insensitive in detecting syngeneic immune antibodies against rat hepatomas in short-term ^{51}Cr release tests although this approach has been employed for the demonstration of IgM antibody in tumor-bearer, but not hyperimmune sera (Price, 1978; Price and Baldwin, 1977a; Price et al., 1979d). To what extent this may be attributed to an autoimmune response remains to be established (Lando et al., 1977).

The radioisotopic antiglobulin test using dispersed tumor cell suspensions offers a number of advantages over other commonly employed assays for the demonstration of serum antibodies such as cytotoxicity or membrane immunofluorescence (Williams, 1977). Studies using this test with either freshly prepared hepatoma cells from trypsinized tumor or tissue cultured tumor cells have shown that it is possible to reveal tumor-specific antibody binding reactions with syngeneic sera diluted from 1/10 to 1/50, suggesting that the radioisotopic antiglobulin test is of the order of 10 to 50 times more sensitive than the previously employed indirect membrane immunofluorescence assay (Al-Sheikly et al., 1980).

A major problem associated with the DAB-induced rat hepatoma model relates to the question as to whether the antigenic targets for these serological reactions can also be identified as the tumor-associated rejection antigens. The tumor-specific antigens defined serologically have been isolated in membrane fractions or as solubilized tumor membrane glycoproteins and while these materials may induce specific antibody formation in treated rats, no protection is afforded against challenge with viable hepatoma cells (Price and Baldwin, 1974a,b; Price et al., 1978, 1979e). The mode of antigen presentation has already been invoked as playing an important role, although recent tests have established that solubilized hepatoma-specific antigens may also induce resistance to tumor transplants in rats that have been pretreated before immunization with cyclophosphamide (Price et al., 1980a). The interpretation of these findings is that antigen immunization probably results in the preferential induction of suppressor lymphoid cell populations and that cyclophosphamide pretreatment prevents the proliferation of suppressor precursors. Although similar observations have been made with 3-MC-induced rat sarcomas (Minami et al., 1979), further tests are required to establish fully that the determinant inducing tumor rejection is that one recog-

nized by antibody in syngeneic immune sera. However, it should now be possible
to resolve this point using immunoadsorbent-purified antigens (i.e., serologically
defined antigen preparations) in immunization experiments with cyclophos-
phamide-treated animals.

517
NEOANTIGEN
EXPRESSION
IN CHEMICAL
CAR-
CINOGENESIS

2.1.3. Aromatic Amines

Although aromatic amines constitute a major class of chemical carcinogens, only
the immunological properties of tumors induced by N-2-fluorenylacetamide
(FAA) have been analyzed in detail. Even though FAA-induced hepatic tumors
and hyperplastic nodules express abnormal antigens including the so-called
preneoplastic antigen, defined using heterologous antisera (Isojima *et al.*, 1969;
Farber, 1973, 1976; Griffin and Kizer, 1978), this class of tumor appears to be
nonimmunogenic or at best weakly immunogenic in tumor transplant rejection
tests (Baldwin and Embleton, 1969, 1971; Wepsic *et al.*, 1976; Tracey *et al.*, 1978).
For example, by excision of growing tumor or by implantation of irradiated
tumor grafts, only 2 of 11 FAA-induced mammary carcinomas showed resistance
to further challenge with viable tumor cells (Baldwin and Embleton, 1969). In
other tests, it was possible to prevent the growth of a nonimmunogenic FAA-
induced mammary carcinoma by contacting the challenge inoculum with Bacillus
Calmette-Guérin (BCG) or its methanol extraction residue (Hopper *et al.*, 1975),
although these procedures did not lead to the development of tumor-specific
immunity against further challenge as is demonstrable with other immunogenic
carcinogen-induced tumors (Baldwin and Pimm, 1978; Hopper *et al.*, 1975). In
another series of experiments, tumor transplantation resistance could be induced
only against 3 of 10 FAA-induced rat hepatomas and 1 of 3 ear duct carcinomas
(Baldwin and Embleton, 1971). Compared to the 3-MC-induced rat sarcomas
or DAB-induced rat hepatomas, the degree of resistance elicited in these tests
was low, as reflected by the maximum number of tumor cells (10^3 to 10^5) rejected
by immunized rats (Baldwin and Embleton, 1969, 1971).

  Variability in the expression of tumor-associated rejection antigens on FAA-
induced tumors is clearly demonstrated in these studies, and this is in accord
with the conclusions of a number of investigations showing variability in
immunogenicity. None of these tumor transplant rejection tests can establish
conclusively whether some tumors are totally deficient in rejection antigens, and
it may be possible to conduct more precise analyses using sensitive *in vitro* assays
of cell-mediated and humoral immune reactions. In this respect, however,
tumor-specific antibody was detected by membrane immunofluorescence tests
in sera from rats immunized against the few weakly immunogenic rat tumors
(Baldwin and Embleton, 1971). These immune sera reacted only with the surface
of cells of the immunizing tumor, showing a close correlation with tumor
immunogenicity. Furthermore, sera taken from rats similarly treated with cells
displaying no significant tumor rejection antigens did not react positively in
membrane immunofluorescence tests. In contrast, in assays of cell-mediated
immunity using lymph nodes from rats bearing FAA-induced tumors, the

518

ROBERT W.
BALDWIN
AND
MICHAEL R.
PRICE

reactions observed exhibited a greater complexity, although evidence was obtained to suggest the involvement of sensitization to oncodevelopmental antigens (Baldwin and Embleton, 1974). Such findings exemplify an inherent difficulty of these systems in that the *in vitro* assays of cell-mediated immunity may not necessarily be detecting the same neoantigens functional in transplant rejection tests (Klein, 1973; Baldwin, 1976).

2.1.4. Alkylnitrosamines

Diethylnitrosamine (DEN)-induced hepatomas in strain-2 guinea pigs are significantly immunogenic, immunity to syngeneic transplanted tumor being induced by excision of tumor grafts or by intradermal or intramuscular injection of subthreshold cell doses such that progressive growth is prevented (Zbar *et al.*, 1969). These tumors have been studied by Rapp and his associates as models for immunotherapy (Zbar *et al.*, 1971, 1972*a,b*; Bartlett and Zbar, 1972) since growth can be suppressed by injecting hepatoma cells in admixture with BCG. Regression of hepatoma–BCG mixed inocula leads to suppression of tumor transplanted simultaneously at another site, and in addition, direct intratumoral injection of BCG into an established tumor graft suppresses its development and limits metastatic spread to the draining lymph nodes.

The adoptive transfer of immunity by peritoneal exudate cells from guinea pigs immunized with DEN-induced hepatomas results in a marked cell-mediated immune response, this being detected either by suppression of tumor growth or by the production of delayed hypersensitivity reactions (Kronman *et al.*, 1969; Wepsic *et al.*, 1970; Zbar *et al.*, 1970). The specificity of these reactions has indicated that the rejection antigens expressed by these hepatomas are individually distinct, and heterologous antisera prepared against intact tumor cells have, after appropriate absorption, been rendered monospecific, reacting in complement fixation (Leonard *et al.*, 1972) and membrane immunofluorescence tests (Leonard, 1973) only with cells of the homologous tumor. In the rat, DEN-induced hepatomas are also immunogenic, and syngeneic animals treated with γ-irradiated tumor grafts are resistant to challenge with cells of the immunizing tumor (Baldwin and Embleton, 1971). No extensive analyses of cellular and humoral responses to these tumors are as yet available, although serum from rats immunized against one hepatoma has been found to contain antibody weakly reacting in immunofluorescence tests with cells of the homologous tumor (Baldwin and Embleton, 1971). In contrast, DEN-induced murine pulmonary adenocarcinomas do not exhibit significant immunogenicity, and protection against challenge with as few as 2×10^4 tumor cells was not induced in mice immunized with irradiated tumor grafts (Pasternak *et al.*, 1966).

More recently, there has been increased interest in neurogenic tumors induced by more complex nitroso compounds (Table 1). Individually specific tumor-associated rejection antigens have been detected in tumor transplant rejection tests in rats with a brain gliosarcoma (Tracey *et al.*, 1978), a mixed glioma, and a neurinoma of the peripheral nervous system (Cornain *et al.*, 1975). However, the latter authors reported that spleen cells from rats bearing these tumors were cross-reactive in *in vitro* cytotoxicity tests (perhaps indicative of common tumor-associated antigens or probably NK cell activity), but it was possible to reveal specific cytotoxicity reactions to each tumor after carbonyl iron treatment of spleen cells, passage through a nylon wool column, and removal of C3-receptor-positive cells (Cornain *et al.*, 1975). Similar individually distinct reactions against a proportion of N-nitrosourea-induced rat brain gliomas have been observed using fluorescent antibody techniques or in complement-dependent cytotoxicity assays, and it was concluded that these findings confirmed variability in antigen expression (Stavrou *et al.*, 1978). Finally, it should be noted that tumor-associated antigens have been demonstrated on one line of mouse prostate cells transformed *in vitro* by nitrosoguanidine, these findings being compatible with the antigenicity of the same line transformed by 3-MC (Embleton and Heidelberger, 1972).

519

NEOANTIGEN
EXPRESSION
IN CHEMICAL
CAR-
CINOGENESIS

2.1.5. Hydrazines

The importance of gastrointestinal tumors induced by dimethylhydrazine (DMH) as an appropriate model for human colon cancer has previously been reported (Haase *et al.*, 1973), and indeed, a rat tumor antigen similar to human carcino-embryonic antigen has been described (Abeyounis and Milgrom, 1976). Primary adenocarcinomas of the colon and small bowel, induced in rats by DMH or nitrosoguanidine, have been diagnosed and followed during their growth and after treatment by repeated double-contrast large-bowel roentgenograms (Steele *et al.*, 1975b). In addition, antitumor immune responses were monitored serially and correlated with tumor development, emphasizing the relevance of these tumors to human cancer.

Various *in vitro* assays of immunogenicity and immunosensitivity have identified several cell-surface antigens associated specifically with these bowel adenocarcinomas. These include antigens described as "private" or individually distinct, common or "tissue type specific," and "widespread" as well as gut-specific oncodevelopmental antigens (Steele and Sjögren, 1974, 1977; Steele *et al.*, 1975a; Sjögren and Steele, 1975a,b).

Probably the most significant class of antigen expressed by these tumors in the rat belongs to the group of common tumor-associated antigens that are restricted to tumors of the same histological type, since these may induce limited immunoprotection in cross test combinations of colon tumors (Steele and Sjögren, 1977). Furthermore, from the evidence available, it was concluded that these determinants may not simply represent derepressed fetal antigens. This type of antigen has also been implicated in experiments designed to examine the role of immune surveillance against primary DMH-induced colon carcinomas in rats, and the tests supported the concept that immune surveillance against neoplasia depends on the T-lymphocyte response (although the authors recognized that other explanations could not be excluded) (Bansal *et al.*, 1978).

In mice, DMH-induced colon carcinomas have been examined for the expression of tumor-associated rejection antigens and common tumor-associated

520

ROBERT W.
BALDWIN
AND
MICHAEL R.
PRICE

antigens in tumor transplant rejection tests; in contrast to the studies with rat tumors, no significant cross-protection between these tumors was demonstrated (Belnap *et al.*, 1979). Nevertheless, using an ^{125}I-protein A binding assay for detecting antibodies to cell-surface antigens, a tumor-associated antigen(s) was identified that was shared with other carcinogen-induced tumors and that was not related to contaminating MuLV antigens or fetal determinants (Cleveland *et al.*, 1979).

2.2. Neoantigen Expression on Cells Transformed in Vitro by Chemical Carcinogens

An important approach in studying chemical carcinogenesis has been the induction and maintenance of cells transformed *in vitro* following exposure to carcinogens. These systems have an advantage for immunological studies over tumors induced *in vivo* in that they permit the study of neoantigen expression under conditions where host immunoselection cannot modify this effect. Tumor-associated rejection antigens have been detected on 3-MC-transformed C3H mouse fibroblasts (Mondal *et al.*, 1970, 1971). In these studies, 11 of 17 transformed lines produced "challenge protection" following surgical removal of subcutaneous growth derived from these cells. Similarly, 3T3 cells treated with 3-MC and maintained *in vivo* in the immunologically protected confines of Millipore chambers were immunogenic, eliciting tumor rejection responses in syngeneic mice (Basombrío and Prehn, 1972*b,c*). The *in vitro* transformed cells, like tumors induced *in vivo*, express individually distinct antigens, so that when specificity tests were carried out, there was no cross-protection and mice immunized against one cell line did not reject another, even though the same carcinogen was used for transformation (Mondal *et al.*, 1970). In this study, two transformed lines derived from separate colonies in the same culture dish were also studied, and still the progeny of these cells were immunologically distinct. Tumors developing from cells transformed by 3-MC in diffusion chambers also express highly distinctive tumor-associated rejection antigens, and in this case the transformed cells were the progeny of a single normal parental cell (Basombrío and Prehn, 1972*b,c*).

Individually distinct cell-surface antigens similar to tumor-associated rejection antigens have also been identified by *in vitro* tests including antibody binding, as detected by membrane immunofluorescence, and lymphocyte cytotoxicity on *in vitro* transformed cells (Embleton and Heidelberger, 1972, 1975). Multiple transformed lines derived from cloned mouse prostate or embryo cells treated *in vitro* with several polycyclic hydrocarbons, including 3-MC, expressed highly characteristic cell-surface antigens. For instance, in one series, over 100 cross-tests were carried out between different carcinogen-transformed mouse prostate cell lines and only a single cross-reacting pair was identified (Embleton and Heidelberger, 1972). These tests, particularly those involving tumor rejection, establish that different chemically transformed progeny of a single parent clone have highly distinctive antigens. It is not likely, therefore, that tumor-associated

521

NEOANTIGEN
EXPRESSION
IN CHEMICAL
CAR-
CINOGENESIS

antigens appear, as suggested by Burnet (1970*a,b*), by selection following carcinogen treatment of a preexisting clone within the normal cell population. The argument here was that such clones might escape attention of the immune system of the host in the normal state by virtue of their small numbers, but clonal amplification following malignant transformation would result in their recognition as a population antigenically different from the surrounding normal cells.

On the contrary, there are several features that emphasize that the carcinogen plays a crucial role in determining the immunogenicity of the transformed cell. Fibroblast cell lines transformed spontaneously *in vitro* in Millipore chambers were almost always devoid of immunogenicity as defined by their capacity to induce "tumor" rejection responses (Parmiani *et al.*, 1971). Likewise, no tumor-rejection-inducing activity was detected with spontaneously transformed cells derived from mouse prostate cells (Embleton and Heidelberger, 1972). Although these findings further reinforce the view that expression of these highly distinctive neoantigens is not an essential requirement for malignancy, their expression was closely associated with the malignant phenotype (Embleton and Baldwin, 1980). For example, transformed murine cells modified to less malignant growth characteristics by 5-fluorodeoxyuridine treatment or growth on glutaraldehyde-fixed normal cell monolayers had lower tumor-rejection-inducing activities (Mondal *et al.*, 1971).

Epithelial cells derived from adult rat liver have been reported to undergo malignant transformation following *in vitro* treatment with chemical carcinogens including nitrosamines and aminoazo dyes (Williams *et al.*, 1973; Montesano *et al.*, 1973; Borenfreund *et al.*, 1975; Williams, 1979). The possibility of early antigenic changes during transformation of rat liver cells was suggested by the findings that cells treated *in vitro* with N-methyl-N-nitrosourea, 3'-methyl-DAB, or aflatoxin B elicited antibody responses in syngeneic rats (Iype *et al.*, 1973). Moreover, rabbit antisera prepared against rat liver cells transformed *in vitro* by chemical carcinogens were reported to be able to detect abnormal antigens on the transformed cells (Yokota *et al.*, 1978). It should be stressed, however, that none of these studies have conclusively demonstrated cell-surface antigens with specificities similar to those detected by tumor rejection or *in vitro* tests on carcinogen-induced hepatocellular carcinomas (Baldwin, 1973; Embleton, 1979). Moreover, it has been questioned whether the published studies even detect tumor-associated antigens (Embleton, 1979). This is emphasized by the finding that antisera prepared in syngeneic rats against cultured rat liver cells detect fetal calf serum components incorporated into cell membranes from the culture medium (Embleton and Iype, 1978). This type of effect has been reported in other studies with both rat and human tumor cells (Irie *et al.*, 1974; Phillips and Perdue, 1977).

2.3. Antigenic Heterogeneity of Tumor Cells in Carcinogen-Induced Tumors

Almost all human tumors and transplanted animal tumors appear to be monoclonal as suggested by their stable phenotypes and verified by cytogenetic and

522

ROBERT W.
BALDWIN
AND
MICHAEL R.
PRICE

isoenzyme studies (Fialkow, 1976, 1979). From this type of evidence, Greaves (1979) argued that while multiple cells might be influenced by a carcinogen, controls in maturation and proliferation lead to a single cell selection at the *onset of malignancy.* Comparably, Nowell (1976) concluded that even though a large number of cells may be affected by a carcinogen, the macroscopic tumor usually represents the progeny of a single cell, or at most a few cells, this being based on the view that other neoplastic or preneoplastic cells in exposed tissue do not successfully proliferate or are destroyed before progression to tumor formation.

In fact, evidence is mounting that tumors are heterogeneous in neoplastic cell composition. This point is emphasized by studies showing that multiple independent sublines can be derived from a tumor, by selective procedures with specific growth characteristics. For example, clones of cells have been derived from the B16 melanoma with varying capabilities to form pulmonary growths following intravenous injection (Fidler and Kripke, 1977; Poste and Fidler, 1980). Sublines with modified metastatic potential or preferential organ specificity have similarly been isolated from a number of experimental animal tumors including a UV-induced murine fibrosarcoma and a 3-MC-induced murine fibrosarcoma (Kerbel, 1979*b*; Kripke *et al.*, 1978; Brunson *et al.*, 1978; Tao and Burger, 1977).

Since tumor-associated rejection antigens expressed on carcinogen-induced tumors are highly polymorphic, and in most instances stable cell-surface products (see Section 2.1), the analysis of these antigenic specificities represents a direct approach for determining the heterogeneity or otherwise of malignant cells within the primary tumor. This approach was first used by Prehn (1970), who established tumor lines with tissue taken from discrete poles of primary 3-MC-induced sarcomas and determined the specificity of the tumor rejection response induced by each tumor. This study identified one of nine sarcomas in which immunization of syngeneic mice with tumor from a subline established from one pole of the primary did not induce protection with tumor established with tissue taken from a separate part of the primary. These observations were interpreted in favor of tumor cell heterogeneity in 3-MC-induced primary sarcomas, although others (Möller and Möller, 1976) used the data to support the view that *most* tumors were monoclonal. By using a similar approach in studying primary 3-MC-induced rat sarcomas, it was shown that a more substantial proportion (3/7) of the tumors contained malignant cells exhibiting rejection antigens with different specificities (Pimm *et al.*, 1980). This study, therefore, provides conclusive evidence that 3-MC-induced sarcomas are not monoclonal. In support of this view, the multicellular origin of 3-MC-induced murine sarcomas has been established also by studies on the expression of variants of the X-linked enzyme phosphoglycerate kinase (PGK-1) in mice with X-chromosome inactivation mosaicism (Reddy and Fialkow, 1979). Since only one of the two X chromosomes is active in XX somatic cells, a female heterozygous at the X-linked PGK enzyme locus for the usual *Pgk*-1^b gene and the variant *Pgk*-1^a has two populations of cells, synthesizing either type A or type B isoenzymes (Nielsen and Chapman, 1977). Both enzyme types are found in normal tissue from mosaic mice. Since a tumor developing from a single cell will express only one of the

PGK enzyme types, the finding that most tissue fragments from 3-MC-induced sarcomas exhibit both isoenzyme phenotypes indicates multicellular origin.

523

NEOANTIGEN
EXPRESSION
IN CHEMICAL
CAR-
CINOGENESIS

The question as to whether tumors induced with other carcinogens, especially at low doses, show similar polyclonal properties has to be resolved, but there is no compelling reason why this should not be so. These developments, therefore, have considerable importance in understanding tumor progression (Kerbel, 1979a). One view (Nowell, 1976), based on the monoclonal origin of most tumors, argues that tumors have an inherent instability, which results in the tumor continually throwing out mutant cells, some of which may have a selective advantage. These then become the progenitors of new clones that eventually predominate. The result is the evolution of an increasingly malignant and autonomous tumor that is not subject to most normal constraints, including immunological ones imposed by the host (Kerbel, 1979a). If, however, primary tumors contain multiple neoplastic cell clones, either because the initial tumor is multicellular in origin or because it contains multiple primaries that coalesce to form a single growth, this will add a further complexity in understanding the progression of the tumor.

This is illustrated by studies on the antigenic characteristics of primary 3-MC-induced sarcomas and secondary regrowths developing following surgical removal of the primary tumor (Pimm and Baldwin, 1977). Primary sarcomas induced by subcutaneous injection of 3-MC were surgically removed and established as tumor lines by transplantation into syngeneic rats. The primary tumor hosts were then kept until secondary tumors developed at the site of the primary (50–100 days), and these were also established as transplanted tumor lines. By studying the immunizing capacity of tumor derived from the primary and recurrent tumor, it was established that each expressed a tumor-associated rejection antigen with characteristic individually distinct specificity.

These experiments indicate that the primary and secondary sarcomas arose by amplification of separate and possibly multiple populations of 3-MC-transformed cells. This could result in a number of ways.

1. Expansion of residual tumor remaining following surgical resection of the primary; this is comparable to selection of separate tumor cell populations taken from opposite poles of primary 3-MC-induced sarcomas (Prehn, 1970; Pimm *et al.*, 1980).

2. 3-MC may affect many cells either simultaneously or sequentially through exposure to persisting carcinogen metabolites, but the resulting tumor represents the progeny of at most a few cells. The tumor-excision tests then suggest that transformed cells were present that progress to form a tumor only after removal of the primary. This also implies that the transformed cells may have been in a dormant state, perhaps through negative feedback effects initiated by a dominant clone. These "dormant" cell populations then acquire the potential for growth, either following removal of the dominant cells in the primary following its surgical excision or through other environmental changes, which may be immunological or physiological, triggered by surgical trauma (Haddow, 1974).

524

ROBERT W.
BALDWIN
AND
MICHAEL R.
PRICE

3. New tumors may arise after removal of the primary sarcomas, these being induced by residual carcinogen. This may be a less likely interpretation in view of the long latent period of the primary tumors (200–300 days) and the rapid outgrowth of the postsurgical growths (50–100 days). But residual 3-MC or metabolites can be detected by their fluorescence properties in subcutaneous tissue around the site of primary sarcomas (Pimm *et al.*, 1980), and again the carcinogenic response may be influenced by the trauma resulting from surgical removal of the primary tumor (Haddow, 1974).

2.4. Nature of Tumor-Associated Neoantigens

In a number of investigations it has been necessary to resort to degradative procedures to solubilize tumor-associated antigens from chemically induced tumors, and the use of reagents such as papain infers that the antigenic determinants are expressed on integral membrane proteins or glycoproteins (for references, see Baldwin and Price, 1975; Price and Baldwin, 1977*b*). Comparably, the widely used 3 M KCl extraction procedure was initially developed for the solubilization of membrane-protein-retaining histocompatibility antigens, the proposed release mechanism being that 3 M KCl treatment reduced the structure of ordered water at the cell surface, thus liberating water-soluble membrane protein from the lipid bilayer (Reisfeld and Kahan, 1970, 1972). Alternatively, 3 M KCl treatment may solubilize membrane-associated proteins by proteolysis since, first, the solubilization of HLA antigens by 3 M KCl was largely prevented by the inclusion of proteolytic enzyme inhibitors (Mann, 1972). Second, long incubation periods (14–18 h) are required for maximum antigen release, and the chaotropic action of hypertonic salt would be expected to be complete within a shorter period of time. Thus, it was concluded that the presence of hypertonic salt together with cells or homogenates augmented the action of soluble and possibly membrane-bound proteolytic enzymes. Although the 3 M KCl extraction procedure has been extensively used for antigen solubilization from both experimental animal and human tumors, this alone gives little information regarding antigen expression and its likely chemical nature, and unless other facts are known about the subcellular localization of antigen, it is not even possible to state categorically that these determinants were originally membrane-associated. However, in some instances, hypertonic salt treatment of tumor cell membranes, rather than cells or homogenates that contain soluble autolytic enzymes, has proved successful in the solubilization of tumor antigens. For example, using a DEN-induced guinea pig hepatoma, 3 M KCl extraction of purified plasma membranes released an antigen that elicited delayed cutaneous hypersensitivity responses in syngeneic immune animals (Leonard *et al.*, 1975). The antigenic material was excluded from Sephadex G-200 gel filtration columns. When high salt treatment was applied to intact hepatoma cells, however, tumor antigen eluted in the included volume of these columns (Meltzer *et al.*, 1971; Leonard *et al.*, 1972). These findings therefore emphasize that several factors may be operative in accomplishing antigen solubilization by hypertonic salt extraction. Similar difficulties in interpretation have been encountered in attempting to purify tumor-associated surface antigens from 3 M KCl extracts of 3-MC-induced sarcomas in the rat (Price *et al.*, 1979*e*). In this case, antigenic activity isolated from immunoadsorbent columns containing immobilized syngeneic immune serum antibodies was found to elute in the excluded volume of Sephadex G-200 columns. There were variations between separate partially purified antigen preparations particularly with respect to molecular size analysis by SDS poly-acrylamide gel electrophoresis, and it was concluded that this material probably represented macromolecular aggregates (Price *et al.*, 1979*e*).

Recently, a number of attempts have been reported to render soluble, membrane-associated tumor antigens from chemically induced tumors using detergents, the advantage being that the antigen is solubilized in an undegraded form. But those methods have severe disadvantages such that antigenic activity may be lost presumably by causing irreversible conformation changes. However, detergent binding studies have revealed selective binding to the hydrophobic portion of membrane proteins while leaving the hydrophilic domain relatively free (Robinson and Tanford, 1975). Since the latter part is not buried within the lipid bilayer, it would be anticipated that this portion would also carry the antigenic determinant to be exposed to the extracellular environment. Therefore, it is likely that detergent extraction may prove effective in solubilizing membrane antigens and leaving their activity intact. Indeed, solubilization of 3-MC-induced murine-sarcoma-specific antigens capable of eliciting tumor rejection responses has been accomplished using sodium deoxycholate (Sikora *et al.*, 1979) or NP-40 (Natori *et al.*, 1977, 1978; Law *et al.*, 1978). There is a discrepancy in the results of these studies since the former workers demonstrated that the antigens solubilized by deoxycholate would bind to wheat germ agglutinin coupled to Sepharose 4B, whereas Law and his group determined that tumor-rejection-inducing activity was present in both wheat germ agglutinin-bound and -unbound fractions (Law *et al.*, 1978). However, in both investigations, antigenic activity passed through columns containing immobilized *Lens culinaris* lectin (Sikora *et al.*, 1979; Law *et al.*, 1978).

In tests with DAB-induced hepatomas and 3-MC-induced sarcomas in the rat, deoxycholate extraction of subcellular membranes was not so successful in liberating antigen capable of inducing tumor resistance in immunoprotection tests (Price *et al.*, 1979*e*). However, with one hepatoma, D23, there was some indication of positive antibody reactivity in treated rats. Although these findings suggest that deoxycholate was not particularly effective in solubilizing rat tumor-associated antigens, they also exemplify the general intractability of these membrane components.

Many of the above findings are consistent with the view that tumor-associated antigens on chemically induced tumors are expressed on integral membrane proteins or glycoproteins. Studies of azo dye-induced hepatomas and 3-MC-induced sarcomas in the rat are also in accord with this proposal, and the following results lend further support to this concept.

526

ROBERT W.
BALDWIN
AND
MICHAEL R.
PRICE

1. Tumor-associated surface antigenic activity is retained in purified plasma membrane preparations but has not been detected in soluble cytoplasmic protein fractions or on tumor nuclei (Price and Baldwin, 1974a,b).

2. For the solubilization of tumor-associated antigens, it is necessary to resort to limited papain digestion of tumor cells or membranes, and 3 M KCl extraction of tumor homogenates (Baldwin et al., 1973, 1978; Bowen and Baldwin, 1979a,b; Harris et al., 1973; Preston and Price, 1977; Price and Baldwin, 1977b; Price et al., 1978, 1979e; Hannant et al., 1979, 1980).

3. Antigenic activity may be enriched in soluble fractions by ion-exchange chromatography or by gel filtration. Using the latter technique, papain solubilized rat hepatoma antigens elute with a molecular weight of about 55,000 (Baldwin et al., 1973, 1978; Price et al., 1979e).

4. Antigenic activity is retained on and can be eluted from Sepharose–concanavalin A, indicative of the presence of glucosyl and/or mannosyl residues in the isolated fractions (Bowen and Baldwin, 1979a; Hannant et al., 1980).

5. Tumor-associated surface antigens are retained on and can be eluted with 3 M NaSCN from immunoadsorbent columns containing immobilized Ig fractions from syngeneic hyperimmune sera, and this single procedure allows considerable purification of antigenic activity to be rapidly achieved in a single step (Preston and Price, 1977; Price et al., 1979e; Hannant et al., 1980).

Attempts to develop cell-free radioimmunoassays for these antigens have generally been unsuccessful although coprecipitation tests using radioiodinated antigen preparations and absorbed heteroantisera were capable of detecting a component(s) showing individually distinct tumor specificity in investigations employing 3-MC-induced sarcomas in the mouse (Natori et al., 1978) or rat (Price et al., 1979e). One of the major problems in this type of study has been to retain the capacity of radiolabeled antigens to rebind with antibodies in syngeneic immune sera, and recent tests have established that immunoadsorbent-purified hepatoma-associated antigens have a lowered affinity for syngeneic antibodies as compared to their unlabeled counterparts (Price et al., 1979a; Hannant et al., 1979, 1980). This particular antigen preparation was labeled with ^{125}I-coupled tyrosine using a carbodiimide reagent since antigens labeled with radioactive iodine using the chloramine-T procedure were completely inactivated. However, for optimal retention of serological reactivity (as assessed by the rebinding of antigen to specific immunoadsorbents or in double-antibody coprecipitation tests), it was found necessary to protect the antigenic determinant by radiolabeling antigens when bound to the immunoadsorbent, followed by elution from the solid phase upon completion of the reaction (Hannant et al., 1980). It was noted in these studies that the mild oxidizing agent chloramine-T appears to be particularly deleterious to these antigens, which might imply that tyrosine is a component of or a residue in the immediate environment of the antigenic determinant itself, although further investigations are required to substantiate this proposal.

527
NEOANTIGEN
EXPRESSION
IN CHEMICAL
CAR-
CINOGENESIS

2.5. Relationship between Tumor-Associated Neoantigens and Histocompatibility Antigens

Genetic products of the major histocompatibility complex (MHC) code for cell-surface antigens involved in allograft rejection. In addition, it has been determined that products of different regions of the MHC function in the control of immune responses by regulating both cooperative and cytotoxic interactions (Klein, 1975; Katz and Benacerraf, 1975). Murine T-cell-mediated cytotoxicity against virus-infected (Doherty et al., 1976; Zinkernagel and Doherty, 1977; Collavo et al., 1979) or chemically modified (Shearer et al., 1977; Shearer and Schmitt-Verhulst, 1977) cells requires homology at the K and/or D region of the H-2 complex between sensitizing effector and target cells, a phenomenon termed "H-2 restriction." However, to what extent products of the MHC are involved in T-cell-mediated immunity against tumor cells is unknown, although a number of investigators have accumulated evidence to suggest that there may be a relationship between tumor-associated antigens and histocompatibility antigens. Indeed, this has been suspected for a number of years since reports have indicated that a reciprocal relationship exists between the expression of tumor antigens on histocompatibility antigens on both chemically induced (Haywood and McKhann, 1971) and virus-induced (Ting and Herberman, 1971; Cikes et al., 1973) tumors. Parmiani recently summarized the possible relationships between these two antigen classes—tumor-associated antigenic activity may be expressed on the following: (a) alien histocompatibility antigens, (b) alien minor histocompatibility antigens, (c) modified histocompatibility antigens, (d) a complex with histocompatibility antigens, (e) a complex with β-2-microglobulin, (f) a modified normal nonhistocompatibility antigen structure (reported by Price et al., 1980b). There would appear to be no unifying hypothesis to account for the relationship between tumor antigens and histocompatibility antigens, so that the various proposals are best considered as separate issues.

In a number of studies with tumors of different etiologies, it has been concluded that H-2 specificities not normally associated with the strain of origin are expressed (Martin et al., 1973; Invernizzi and Parmiani, 1975; Parmiani and Invernizzi, 1975; Garrido et al., 1976; Wrathmell et al., 1976; Schirrmacher and Robinson, 1979; Parmiani et al., 1979), suggesting originally that H-2 antigens cross-reacted with tumor-associated rejection antigens and may even be identical products. This latter proposal, however, is now considered to be unlikely. For example, Klein and Klein (1975) determined that hybrid cells derived from the fusion of the TA3Ha ascites sarcoma (H-2^a) and a 3-MC-induced sarcoma in A.SW mice (MSWBS-H-2^s) were immunogenic in the syngeneic A.SW host. Previously, it was shown that chromosome No. 17 (the genetic determinant of the H-2 complex) of one parental strain, or the other, can be removed from the

528

ROBERT W.
BALDWIN
AND
MICHAEL R.
PRICE

hybrid by selection in the opposite parental strain. In this case, therefore, it was possible to select hybrids deficient in H-2^a or H-2^s and these still showed immunogenicity albeit at a weaker level when compared with the unselected hybrid. From this it was concluded that the genetic determinant of the tumor-associated rejection antigen was not localized on chromosome 17, but that a proper balance of this chromosome is required for the full expression of immunogenicity in this system (Klein and Klein, 1975). Another approach was taken by Carbone et al. (1978); in a comparative study of cultured and transplanted variants of a tumor, they found that the cultured cells tended to lose serologically defined alien H-2 antigens expressed on the transplanted tumor, whereas both variants equally expressed a tumor-associated rejection antigen as assessed in transplantation tests. Further evidence establishing a nonidentity between tumor antigens and H-2 molecules has been more directly obtained by the demonstration that tumor-associated rejection activity may be separated from histocompatibility antigens (Law et al., 1978; Rogers et al., 1978; Appella et al., 1978; Alaba et al., 1979; Sikora et al., 1979) or alien histocompatibility antigens (Law et al., 1980) by chromatographic fractionation of solubilized tumor membranes. However, the significance of alien histocompatibility antigens associated with tumors in controlling and directing immune responses, as well as contributing to the immunogenicity and imposing selective pressures on growth of syngeneic tumors, has been considered in detail elsewhere (Sondel and Bach, 1980).

Thomson et al. (1976, 1979) have developed the concept that antigens associated with 3-MC-induced sarcomas in rats and even some human tumors have a noncovalently linked β-2-microglobulin subunit analogous to H-2 and HLA molecules. However, in tests with DAB-induced rat hepatomas, this could not be confirmed (Bowen and Baldwin, 1979a), although tumor-associated antigens expressed on these tumors were putatively identified as modified minor alloantigen as defined by their reactivity with various syngeneic and allogeneic antisera (Bowen and Baldwin, 1975, 1979b). In accordance with these findings, Germain et al. (1975) demonstrated that exposure of murine P815 mastocytoma cells to alloantiserum protected them from the cytotoxic action of syngeneic immune lymphoid cells.

Clearly, the significance of the possible relationships between tumor-associated neoantigens and products of the MHC needs to be further evaluated. It is, however, worth emphasizing that the expression of histocompatibility antigens and other defined normal products may play an important role not only in phenomena such as genetic restriction of T-cell-mediated cytolysis but also may influence the immunogenicity of tumors. Taking one example, tumor rejection studies with five different lines of a strain-1 guinea pig leukemia (L2C) in syngeneic animals showed that the four lines carrying the Ia antigen possessed a tumor-associated rejection antigen (Forni et al., 1976). The one Ia-negative leukemia did not appear to have a tumor-associated rejection antigen against which immunity could be induced. However, immunization with an Ia-positive L2C leukemia elicited protection against the Ia-negative line. This implies that the Ia-negative line does have a tumor antigenic component that is an appropriate receptor for immune attack but that alone is nonimmunogenic. The data are also consistent with the requirement of Ia for immunogenicity, but the nature of the tumor antigen–Ia antigen relationship remains to be elucidated.

529

NEOANTIGEN
EXPRESSION
IN CHEMICAL
CAR-
CINOGENESIS

2.6. Oncodevelopmental Antigens

Interest in oncodevelopmental antigens has stemmed largely from the early work of Abelev *et al.* (1963), who reported that a fetal protein (termed "α-fetoprotein"), present in the serum of newborn but not adult mice, was also secreted into the circulation by *o*-aminoazotoluene-induced hepatomas (for reviews on α-fetoprotein, see Abelev *et al.*, 1979; Sell and Becker, 1978; Hirai, 1979). The expression of fetal characteristics in neoplasia occurs through a process of derepression of dormant genes, and other fetal components produced by malignant cells include hormones (Odell and Wolfson, 1975; Jeffcoate and Rees, 1978), enzymes (Weinhouse, 1972; Singer, 1979), and placental proteins (Rosen *et al.*, 1975). In addition, oncodevelopmental antigens that are immunogenic in the autochthonous tumor-bearing host or syngeneic recipient of transplanted tumor or fetal tissues have been demonstrated on a variety of carcinogen-induced tumors (reviewed by Baldwin *et al.*, 1974*a*; Coggin and Anderson, 1974; Lausch and Rapp, 1974; Coggin and Ambrose, 1979; Rees *et al.*, 1979).

The phase-specific expression of oncodevelopmental antigens at certain stages of embryogenesis, but disappearing before or at parturition, supports the view that these determinants arise through derepression of gene products. This is exemplified by studies with a variety of chemically induced rat tumors, wherein serum or lymphoid cells from multiparous donors reactive with cell-surface antigens on these tumors also reacted with 14- to 15-day-old fetal cells but not with cells obtained at early or later stages of fetal development or with cells from normal adult tissues (Baldwin and Vose, 1974; Baldwin *et al.*, 1974*a*). Similarly, phase-specific oncodevelopmental antigens are associated with 9- to 10-day-old fetuses in hamsters (Coggin *et al.*, 1970, 1971; Ambrose *et al.*, 1971). As in the rat, these antigens are not normally expressed on older hamster embryos, although they may be demonstrated following exposure of third-trimester fetal cells to trypsin (Girardi and Reppucci, 1972).

In the mouse, the phase-specific expression of fetal antigens has been demonstrated by showing that cytotoxic lymphocytes, reactive against oncodevelopmental antigens, were generated by *in vitro* culture of normal adult spleen cells with 14- to 15-day-old fetal mouse liver cells, cocultivation for 4–5 days being optimal for the production of cytotoxic effector cells (Chism *et al.*, 1975, 1976). In cold target inhibition tests, liver cells from 14- to 15-day-old fetuses, but not 13- or 16-day-old fetuses, inhibited the cytotoxicity of sensitized lymphocytes for radiolabeled syngeneic tumor target cells (Chism *et al.*, 1976). A note of caution here is suggested by the work of Parker *et al.* (1977), who determined that after *in vitro* culture, normal adult fibroblasts may express oncodevelopmental

530

ROBERT W.
BALDWIN
AND
MICHAEL R.
PRICE

antigens, indicating that cultured normal adult cells may represent an inappropriate control in the study of oncodevelopmental antigens.

Oncodevelopmental antigens that are immunogenic in syngeneic animals were originally demonstrated serologically by the membrane immunofluorescence reactivity of multiparous sera for SV40-transformed hamster cells (Duff and Rapp, 1970). Subsequently, in extensive membrane immunofluorescence studies using a range of DAB-induced hepatomas and 3-MC-induced sarcomas in the rat, it was found that a proportion of multiparous rat sera reacted positively with these tumors compared with the effects of age-matched virgin female controls (Baldwin *et al.*, 1972*a,b*, 1974*a*). In further membrane immunofluorescence tests with these tumors and also a number of spontaneously arising sarcomas and mammary carcinomas and FAA-induced mammary carcinomas, the discriminatory activity of individual multiparous rat serum samples with different tumors was consistent with the view that the specificity of oncodevelopmental antigens may be complex and not entirely cross-reactive between tumors of different histological types (Rees *et al.*, 1979). Other studies have attempted to identify the specificity of these determinants. For example, in investigations of rat colon carcinomas induced by DMH or *N*-methyl-*N'*-nitro-*N*-nitrosoguanidine, oncodevelopmental antigens were detected that exhibited widespread and organ-related specificity (Steele and Sjögren, 1974). Furthermore, it was possible to separate these antigenic specificities in a series of experiments involving the formation and dissociation of immune complexes (Steele *et al.*, 1975*a*; Baldwin and Price, 1976).

Humoral responses in the tumor-bearing host have been found in other studies to be directed against oncodevelopmental antigens. Martin *et al.* (1976) have speculated that the membrane immunofluorescence reactivity of sera from rats bearing DMH-induced colon carcinomas for cultured tumor cells may be directed against fetal antigens, and cross-reactive, tissue-type-specific antigens were associated with both primary and transplanted tumors. Comparably, Nelson *et al.* (1977) detected antibody against oncodevelopmental antigens in the serum of rats treated with DMH at least 2 months before roentgenologic diagnosis of tumor.

In tests using 3-MC-induced murine sarcomas, it has been found that even though such tumors may express individually distinct tumor-associated surface antigens (Cleveland *et al.*, 1979) and to not display cross-reactivity in tumor transplant rejection tests (Parker and Rosenberg, 1977), tumor-bearer serum may exhibit cross-reactivity in complement-dependent cytotoxicity assays, and these responses may be eliminated by absorption with fetal cells (Parker and Rosenberg, 1977). This type of finding is analogous to results obtained in an analysis of the antigenic targets against which rat tumor-bearer lymphoid-cell-mediated cytotoxic responses are directed. In this case, the cross-reactive *in vitro* cytotoxicity of tumor-bearer lymph node or spleen cells was found to be directed against both the individually distinct tumor-associated surface antigens and cross-reactive oncodevelopmental antigens (Zöller *et al.*, 1975, 1976, 1977), although in this study the contribution of NK cells was not assessed.

Another important class of transformed cell upon which oncodevelopmental antigens have been demonstrated includes those induced *in vitro* by treatment of normal cultured cells with chemical carcinogens. Murine fibroblasts transformed by 3-MC or 7,12-dimethylbenz[*a*]anthracene (7,12-DMBA) express oncodevelopmental antigens detectable by membrane immunofluorescence staining of viable cells in suspension by multiparous mouse serum (Embleton and Heidelberger, 1975). As in comparable studies with tumors induced *in vivo*, multiparous sera showed reactivity for many of the lines examined, and these findings further emphasize the possibility that the appearance of fetal antigens of one type or another may be a characteristic feature of neoplastic change.

A number of other assays have been employed for the demonstration of oncodevelopmental antigens. Hellström *et al.* (1976) used a leukocyte adherence inhibition test in an analysis of 3-MC-induced murine sarcomas and bladder carcinomas, and in extensive population studies it was concluded that the technique was suitable for identifying oncodevelopmental antigens. This assay, together with the macrophage electrophoretic mobility test and leukocyte migration inhibition technique, was also employed by Pasternak *et al.* (1979, 1980), who were able to detect oncodevelopmental antigens associated with both experimental and human tumors. It should be noted that in this study, murine fetal antigen preparations cross-reacted with determinants to which human cancer patients were sensitized, suggesting that there may be interspecies cross-reactivity in oncodevelopmental antigen expression.

The effects of preimmunization with fetal tissues or cells on the development of immunity as evidenced by rejection of transplanted tumor have received extensive investigation. In a number of reports, immunization with syngeneic or allogeneic fetal tissue has been successful in inducing resistance against challenge with viable tumor cells (reviewed by Rees *et al.*, 1979; Coggin and Ambrose, 1979). In contrast, other studies have failed to demonstrate tumor immunity in animals sensitized to fetal tissue, and in certain instances, tumor enhancement has been reported.

Prehn (1967) initially presented limited evidence indicating the development of weak immunity to urethan-induced tumors in mice immunized with 10-day-old fetal tissue, although further evaluation of the immunogenicity of fetal material failed to confirm these early observations (Basombrío and Prehn, 1972*a*). Following these investigations, the tumor rejection response against a number of carcinogen-induced tumors in embryo-sensitized animals has been the subject of several reports (Bendich *et al.*, 1973; Le Mevel and Wells, 1973; Ménard *et al.*, 1973; Castro *et al.*, 1973; Grant *et al.*, 1974*a*; Ting and Grant, 1976). In most cases, X-irradiated fetal tissue or cells were employed for immunization since nonirradiated cells may rapidly mature into tissue devoid of fetal antigens (Coggin and Anderson, 1974; Coggin and Ambrose, 1979). Nevertheless, in extensive studies in this laboratory, immunoprotection against viable tumor cell challenge administered via the subcutaneous, intraperitoneal, and intrapleural routes was not observed in rats sensitized against fetal materials using several procedures including multiple inoculations of γ-irradiated embryo cells, excision

532

ROBERT W.
BALDWIN
AND
MICHAEL R.
PRICE

of developing embryoma, and multiparity (Baldwin *et al.,* 1974*b*; Shah *et al.,* 1976). However, weak immunity to pulmonary tumor growth was observed in treated rats challenged intravenously with tumor cells (Rees *et al.,* 1975*b*).

Reasons for the failure of oncodevelopmental antigens to elicit immunoprotection against tumor challenge in a number of model systems are as yet not clearly resolved. Several explanations have been put forward to account for the experimental observations including the proposal that there may be qualitative or quantitative differences in the immune response to oncodevelopmental antigens and the classical tumor-associated rejection antigens (Rees *et al.,* 1979). Tumor cells may induce immunological escape mechanisms to evade rejection either by stimulating lymphoid cells capable of suppressing rejection responses or as a direct result of products released from the tumor cell that in turn are capable of neutralizing host effector cells (Rees *et al.,* 1974, 1975*a*, 1979). Indeed, evidence has been advanced to suggest that α-fetoprotein induces suppressor T lymphocytes with a capacity to abrogate helper T-cell function *in vitro* (Murgita *et al.,* 1977). The instability of oncodevelopmental antigens at the cell surface may make them inappropriate receptors for immune attack. This may further be reflected in differences in the rate of antigen turnover and shedding from the developing tumor, which may have important consequences on the immunogenicity of oncodevelopmental antigens (Price and Baldwin, 1977*b*). Alternatively, oncodevelopmental antigens may be depleted from the cell surface by modulation or redistribution following interaction with antibody (Ortaldo *et al.,* 1974; Gooding, 1976). Thus, the reduced availability of surface antigenic determinants may provide the tumor with an escape from immune destruction.

Despite these reservations concerning the immunogenicity of oncodevelopmental antigens, it should be emphasized that they appear to be associated with numerous types of chemically induced tumors (Table 1), and thus they should be regarded as valuable potential markers for studying transformation-related events.

2.7. Neoantigen Expression in Chemical Carcinogenesis

The expression of neoantigens is not an obligatory component of carcinogen-induced neoplastic transformation, since as already described (Section 2.1.3)

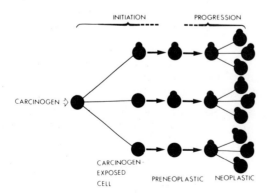

FIGURE 1. Tumor-specific antigen expression in carcinogenesis.

tumor-associated rejection antigens cannot be demonstrated on some tumors, e.g., FAA-induced hepatocellular carcinomas and mammary carcinomas. But when expressed, tumor antigens appear to be related to the malignant phenotype, and so the question of when these cell-surface components appear in the carcinogenic process becomes important. Three possible pathways leading to their expression have been postulated (Embleton and Baldwin, 1980), and these are represented diagrammatically in Fig. 1.

533

NEOANTIGEN
EXPRESSION
IN CHEMICAL
CAR-
CINOGENESIS

1. Neoantigens appear as a consequence of early interactions of carcinogen with target cells and persist through all stages of carcinogenesis to the malignant phenotype.

2. Neoantigen expression does not occur until the initiated cell is converted to the preneoplastic cell. Once expressed, this characteristic is maintained through to the malignant stage.

3. Neoantigens only become expressed at the stage when malignant cell clones develop.

2.7.1. Neoantigen Expression as a Response to Carcinogen

Transplantation tests with 3-MC-induced murine skin papillomas established that each papilloma expressed individually distinct rejection antigens. Moreover, these papilloma-associated antigens persisted through progression to the malignant state, being detected on skin carcinomas derived from individual papilloma lines (Lappé, 1969). These early studies support the view that neoantigen expression is more closely allied to carcinogen-induced responses than to cellular changes associated with progression to the malignant phenotype. This is further emphasized by studies on the immunogenicity of mouse mammary tumors arising from hyperplastic alveolar nodule (HAN) outgrowth lines (Ruppert et al., 1978). Tumors developing following treatment of hormone-induced HANs with 7,12-DMBA or 3-MC were weakly immunogenic as defined by tumor transplantation resistance assays. Also, the frequency of immunogenic tumors (40–50%) was comparable to that demonstrated with tumors arising spontaneously with hormone-induced HANs. In comparison, tumors arising from HANs *initially* induced with 7,12-DMBA were highly immunogenic with individually distinct tumor-associated rejection antigens, suggesting that the degree of immunogenicity of a tumor depends on events occurring during transformation of normal cells to the "hyperplastic" state rather than subsequent progression to a frank neoplastic tumor. This is compatible with the hypothesis already discussed (Section 2.3) that carcinogen treatment may influence many cells, but the emergence of one or a few clones of neoplastic cells results in the development of tumors expressing individually distinct tumor-associated rejection antigens.

The concept that neoantigen expression occurs as an early consequence of carcinogen–cell interactions is further emphasized by studies on the immunogenicity of cells treated for short periods with 3-MC (Embleton and Baldwin, 1979). In this approach, antisera were prepared by immunizing syngeneic rats with

534

ROBERT W.
BALDWIN
AND
MICHAEL R.
PRICE

embryo cells treated *in vitro* for 18 h with 3-MC under conditions adequate for carcinogen metabolism. These antisera were then shown to react in membrane immunofluorescence tests with cells derived from a proportion of the 3-MC-induced sarcomas tested. Eight reproducibly positive reactions were obtained in 60 test combinations derived from 3 anti-3-MC-treated embryo sera and 34 target tumors. Seven of these reactions were obtained with 3-MC-induced sarcomas, the other positive reaction occurring with an aminoazo dye-induced hepatocellular carcinoma. In comparison, antisera raised to embryo cells treated with acetone (the solvent used for 3-MC administration) were completely negative.

If it is considered that neoantigen expression in chemically induced tumors is related to some aspect of carcinogen–cell interactions, then it might be expected that the immunogenicity of a tumor is related to the initiating dose of carcinogen. The evidence on this point is still very limited and contradictory. For example, Prehn (1975), studying murine sarcomas induced by 3-MC implanted in pellets, suggested that tumor immunogenicity may be related to the dose of carcinogen used for their induction. No such correlation was observed, however, when comparing the immunogenicities of sarcomas induced in rats with 3-MC administered in trioctanoin (Baldwin *et al.*, 1979; Pimm *et al.*, 1980), but when one considers the number of variables including rate of carcinogen metabolism and the influences of carcinogen on cell survival, it is hardly surprising that widely different effects may be obtained. A more controlled approach to this problem would be provided by studying the immunogenicity of tumors derived from cells treated *in vitro* with graded doses of carcinogen, but this type of investigation has not yet been reported.

2.7.2. Neoantigen Expression in Relation to Tumor Progression

The studies discussed in the previous section with carcinogen-induced skin papillomas and mammary gland hyperplastic nodules suggest that neoantigens appear early in the carcinogenic process. But the related feature of changes in neoantigen expression during later stages in carcinogenesis, particularly where rapid outgrowth and/or metastasis occur, remains to be elucidated. This is outstandingly important, however, since the early concept of tumor progression (Foulds, 1965) involving stepwise and sometimes permanent changes in the properties of neoplastic cells have been applied to several experimental systems including skin, liver, and mammary carcinogenesis (Pitot, 1979). In this case the question is not whether neoantigens expressed in premalignant tissues persist through to the malignant phase, but whether these changes are accompanied either by the appearance of new antigens or even by the deletion of some components which may modify tumor cell development. The direct analysis of these situations has not been evaluated because of the limited number of experimental systems. There are, however, several investigations revealing antigenic differences between metastatic variants from the parental tumor line derived from 3-MC-induced tumors (Sugarbaker and Cohen, 1972; Faraci, 1974; Kerbel,

1979b). Furthermore, it has been shown that pulmonary and renal metastases derived from a primary 3-MC-induced sarcoma-bearing rat expressed tumor-associated rejection antigens different from those on the primary tumor (Pimm et al., 1980).

2.7.3. Origin of Tumor-Associated Neoantigens

Several hypotheses have been proposed to account for neoantigen expression on carcinogen-induced tumors (Embleton and Baldwin, 1980). One possibility is that they are products of genes that exist in the genome of all normal cells, being repressed under normal circumstances. Then, as a consequence of carcinogen-induced malignant transformation, the relevant genes become derepressed, leading to their products being expressed at the cell surface and so recognized as tumor antigens (oncodevelopmental antigens, alien histocompatibility antigens, etc.). Alternatively, these genes may be normally expressed in a minority of cell lineages in the organism, perhaps at specific stages of differentiation, and become stabilized by malignant transformation (Greaves, 1979). Both these postulates infer that tumor antigens are normal cell products being expressed inappropriately in time or tissue.

The converse of the above concept is that tumor antigens are new cell products coded for by carcinogen-modified genes, or by modified epigenetic control mechanisms governing gene expression. Most chemical carcinogens react with, and damage, DNA, producing various effects such as base displacement, base substitution, and frameshifts (Lawley, 1980; Roberts, 1980). These modifications could produce new or modified cistrons coding for new products, or perhaps more likely, introducing profound modifications in normal products. The antigenic specificities (or nonantigenicity) resulting from carcinogen-induced transformation may then depend on the type of DNA lesion produced. For example, antibody binding of antisera against FAA–DNA conjugates with DNA modified in vitro with FAA derivatives has identified conformational changes in DNA (Sage et al., 1979). Since hepatic tumors induced in rats with FAA do not express tumor rejection antigens, whereas those induced by aminoazo dyes are immunogenic, further studies with antisera to DAB–DNA conjugates may reveal differences in the mode of DNA binding of these carcinogens (Heidelberger, 1975; Drinkwater et al., 1978; Miller et al., 1979).

2.7.4. Immunological Intervention in Chemical Carcinogenesis

The finding that neoantigens appear early in cells exposed to chemical carcinogens suggests that some form of immunological manipulation may be able to inhibit tumor induction. This was originally developed in terms of T-lymphocyte-mediated immunity, since the original concept of immune surveillance as proposed by Burnet and extended by Thomas (Burnet, 1970b) postulated that one function of the immune system is to eliminate or prevent the proliferation of nascent malignant cells. Criticisms of this concept have been advanced based on a number of studies, but particularly those showing that the incidence

536

ROBERT W.
BALDWIN
AND
MICHAEL R.
PRICE

of tumors, either naturally arising or carcinogen induced, is very closely similar in congenitally athymic mice as in normal mice (Stutman, 1975). Therefore, most approaches to modulating chemical carcinogenesis have been developed using nonspecific immunomodulating agents such as bacterial immunoadjuvants. The function of these agents is quite diverse including stimulation of specific tumor-immune responses as well as natural immunity involving NK cells and activated macrophages (Milas and Scott, 1977; Baldwin and Pimm, 1978; Baldwin and Byers, 1979). The approach is emphasized by studies showing that intravenous injection of *Corynebacterium parvum* starting before a single intramuscular injection of 3-MC significantly inhibited the number and rate of sarcoma development (Woodruff and Speedy, 1978). Furthermore, injection of BCG into the subcutaneous site of 3-MC injection limited tumor induction. In this case the response may have been due to the local influx of macrophages, which eliminated carcinogen-damaged cells and even eliminated carcinogen. However, systemic treatment with BCG has been shown to influence local tumor development as evidence by a reduction in skin papilloma incidence following initiation with 7,12-DMBA and promotion with croton oil (Schinitsky *et al.*, 1973).

3. Conclusions and Perspectives

Undoubtedly the "individually distinct" neoantigens on carcinogen-induced tumors are of utmost importance, both as markers for studying changes in cell-surface characteristics in carcinogenesis and as targets for immunomodulation of the carcinogenic response.

There is compelling evidence to suggest that the expression of these highly polymorphic neoantigens results from direct or indirect interaction of carcinogen with cells. However, this neoantigen expression need not necessarily be related to the malignant phenotype. This is emphasized by the detection of "abnormal" antigens on 3-MC-treated rat embryo cells (Embleton and Baldwin, 1979). Similarly, neoantigens have been induced on cells of a spontaneous rat mammary carcinoma following 3-MC treatment (Reeve, Embleton, and Baldwin, unpublished findings). This postulate that neoantigen expression is related to cellular interactions with carcinogen now requires further evaluation. In this context it may be that the analysis of neoantigen expression will provide a probe for specifying the mode of binding of carcinogen to DNA. This approach then would complement the mutagenesis tests in defining the significance of reactions of metabolically activated carcinogen metabolites to nucleophilic sites in cells (Miller, 1979).

Further consideration of the relationship between carcinogen–cell interactions and neoantigen expression has been restricted until recently by the limited advances made in characterizing these cell-surface membrane components. Characterization of tumor antigens following their release and solubilization from tumor cells has now been achieved with several systems, and relatively homogeneous products have been prepared from a number of tumors. The purity of these products in terms of tumor antigen content is still far from desirable, but the development of monoclonal antibodies to tumor-associated antigens should rapidly improve isolation procedures by the use of immunoadsorbent techniques. This approach, in which antibody-producing cells are fused with mouse myeloma cells to yield hybrid cells secreting specific antibody molecules, is still in its infancy. The potential of the approach is emphasized, however, by recent studies establishing that monoclonal antibodies can be produced to neoantigens on rodent tumors (Gunn *et al.*, 1980; Lennox *et al.*, 1980).

537
NEOANTIGEN
EXPRESSION
IN CHEMICAL
CAR-
CINOGENESIS

Finally, the concept that some form of immunostimulation therapy can be used to limit chemical carcinogenesis has to be reevaluated. The original arguments that most neoplastic cells are destroyed by an immunosurveillance network have not received continued support primarily because of the observations on tumor incidence in normal and immune-deprived hosts. The criticisms have, however, principally applied to the *natural* role of T-lymphocyte-mediated responses. It is now recognized that several nonspecific components of the cell-mediated immune response including activated macrophages and NK cells may contribute to the control of tumor growth. Also, it may be that stimulation of specific T-cell responses either alone or in concert with an enhanced natural immunity (macrophage/NK cells) will modify the carcinogenic response.

ACKNOWLEDGMENT

This work was supported by grants from the Cancer Research Campaign.

4. References

ABELEV, G. I., PEROVA, S. D., KHRAMKOVA, N. I., POSTNIKOVA, A. A., AND IRLIN, I. S., 1963, Production of embryonal α-globulin by transplantable mouse hepatomas, *Transplantation* 1:174.

ABELEV, G. I., ENGELHARDT, N. V., AND ELGORT, D. A., 1979, Immunochemical and immunohistochemical micromethods in the study of tumor-associated embryonic antigens, *Methods Cancer Res.* 18:1.

ABEYOUNIS, C. J., AND MILGROM, F., 1976, A thermostable antigen characteristic for carcinogen-induced rat intestinal tumors, *J. Immunol.* 116:30.

ALABA, O., ROGERS, M. J., AND LAW, L. W., 1979, Rauscher leukemia virus-induced tumor antigens: Complete separation from gp70, p30 and H-2, *Int. J. Cancer* 24:608.

AL-SHEIKLY, A. W., EMBLETON, M. J., AND PRICE, M. R., 1980, Detection of tumor specific antigens and alloantigens using a radioisotopic antiglobulin assay, in: *Biology of the Cancer Cell* (K. Letnansky, ed.), pp. 121–126, Kugler, Amsterdam.

AMBROSE, K. R., ANDERSON, N. G., AND COGGIN, J. H., 1971, Interruption of SV40 oncogenesis with human foetal antigen, *Nature (London)* 233:194.

APFFEL, C. A., ARNASON, B. G., AND PETERS, J. H., 1966, Induction of tumor immunity with tumor cells treated with iodoacetate, *Nature (London)* 209:694.

APPELLA, E., DUBOIS, G. C., NATORI, T., ROGERS, M. J., AND LAW, L. W., 1978, Histocompatibility antigens and tumor-specific transplantation antigens of methylcholanthrene-induced sarcomas,

538

ROBERT W.
BALDWIN
AND
MICHAEL R.
PRICE

in: *Biological Markers of Neoplasia: Basic and Applied Aspects* (R. W. Ruddon, ed.), pp. 213–225, Elsevier, New York.

BALDWIN, R. W., 1955, Immunity to methylcholanthrene-induced tumours in inbred rats following atrophy and regression of implanted tumors, *Br. J. Cancer* **9**:652.

BALDWIN, R. W., 1973, Immunological aspects of chemical carcinogenesis, *Adv. Cancer Res.* **18**:1.

BALDWIN, R. W., 1976, Role of immunosurveillance against chemically induced rat tumors, *Transplant. Rev.* **28**:62.

BALDWIN, R. W., 1977, Natural cell mediated immunity: Immune surveillance revisited, *Nature (London)* **270**:557.

BALDWIN, R. W., AND BARKER, C. R., 1967*a*, Tumor-specific antigenicity of aminoazo-dye-induced rat hepatomas, *Int. J. Cancer* **2**:355.

BALDWIN, R. W., AND BARKER, C. R., 1967*b*, Demonstration of tumour-specific humoral antibody against aminoazo-dye-induced rat hepatomata, *Br. J. Cancer* **21**:793.

BALDWIN, R. W., AND BYERS, V. S., 1979, Immunoregulation by bacterial organisms and their role in the immunotherapy of cancer, *Springer Semin. Immunopathol.* **2**:79.

BALDWIN, R. W., AND EMBLETON, M. J., 1969, Immunology of 2-acetylaminofluorene-induced rat mammary adenocarcinomas, *Int. J. Cancer* **4**:47.

BALDWIN, R. W., AND EMBLETON, M. J., 1971, Tumor-specific antigens in 2-acetylaminofluorene-induced rat hepatomas and related tumors, *Isr. J. Med. Sci.* **7**:144.

BALDWIN, R. W., AND EMBLETON, M. J., 1974, Neoantigens on spontaneous and carcinogen-induced rat tumours defined by *in vitro* lymphocytotoxicity, *Int. J. Cancer* **13**:433.

BALDWIN, R. W., AND MOORE, M., 1971, Tumour-specific antigens and tumour-host interactions, in: *Immunological Tolerance to Tissue Antigens* (N. W. Nisbet and M. W. Elves, eds.), pp. 299–313, Orthopaedic Hospital, Oswestry, England.

BALDWIN, R. W., AND PIMM, M. V., 1978, BCG in tumor immunotherapy, *Adv. Cancer Res.* **28**:91.

BALDWIN, R. W., AND PRICE, M. R., 1975, Neoantigen expression in chemical carcinogenesis, in: *Cancer: A Comprehensive Treatise*, Vol. 1 (F. F. Becker, ed.), pp. 353–383, Plenum Press, New York.

BALDWIN, R. W., AND PRICE, M. R., 1976, Immunobiology of rat neoplasia, *Ann. N. Y. Acad. Sci.* **276**:3.

BALDWIN, R. W., AND VOSE, B. M., 1974, The expression of a phase specific foetal antigen on rat embryo cells, *Transplantation* **18**:525.

BALDWIN, R. W., BARKER, C. R., EMBLETON, M. J., GLAVES, D., MOORE, M., AND PIMM, M. V., 1971*a*, Demonstration of cell-surface antigens on chemically induced tumors, *Ann. N. Y. Acad. Sci.* **177**:268.

BALDWIN, R. W., GLAVES, D., HARRIS, J. R., AND PRICE, M. R., 1971*b*, Tumor-specific antigens associated with aminoazo-dye-induced rat hepatomas, *Transplant. Proc.* **3**:1189.

BALDWIN, R. W., GLAVES, D., AND PIMM, M. V., 1971*c*, Tumor-associated antigens as expressions of chemically-induced neoplasia and their involvement in tumor-host interactions, in: *Progress in Immunology* (B. Amos, ed.), pp. 907–920, Academic Press, New York.

BALDWIN, R. W., GLAVES, D., PIMM, M. V., AND VOSE, B. M., 1972*a*, Tumour specific and embryonic antigen expression on chemically induced rat tumours, *Ann. Inst. Pasteur (Paris)* **122**:715.

BALDWIN, R. W., GLAVES, D., AND VOSE, B. M., 1972*b*, Embryonic antigen expression in chemically induced rat hepatomas and sarcomas, *Int. J. Cancer* **10**:233.

BALDWIN, R. W., HARRIS, J. R., AND PRICE, M. R., 1973, Fractionation of plasma membrane-associated tumour specific antigen from an aminoazo dye-induced rat hepatoma, *Int. J. Cancer* **11**:385.

BALDWIN, R. W., EMBLETON, M. J., PRICE, M. R., AND VOSE, B. M., 1974*a*, Embryonic antigen expression on experimental rat tumours, *Transplant. Rev.* **20**:77.

BALDWIN, R. W., GLAVES, D., AND VOSE, B. M., 1974*b*, Immunogenicity of embryonic antigens associated with chemically-induced rat tumours, *Int. J. Cancer* **13**:135.

BALDWIN, R. W., PRICE, M. R., AND MOORE, V. E., 1978, Biochemical and immunological characterization of tumor specific antigens on chemically induced rat tumors, in: *Biological Markers of Neoplasia: Basic and Applied Aspects* (R. W. Ruddon, ed.), pp. 11–24, Elsevier, New York.

BALDWIN, R. W., EMBLETON, M. J., AND PIMM, M. V., 1979, Neoantigens in chemical carcinogenesis, in: *Carcinogens: Identification and Mechanisms of Action* (A. C. Griffin and C. R. Shaw, eds.), pp. 365–379, Raven Press, New York.

BANSAL, S. C., MARK, R., BANSAL, B. R., AND RHOADS, J. E., 1978, Immunologic surveillance against chemically induced primary colon carcinoma in rats, *J. Natl. Cancer Inst.* **60**:667.

BARTLETT, G. L., 1972, Effect of host immunity on the antigenic strength of primary tumors, *J. Natl. Cancer Inst.* **49**:493.

BARTLETT, G. L., AND ZBAR, B., 1972, Tumor-specific vaccine containing *Mycobacterium bovis* and tumor cells: Safety and efficiency, *J. Natl. Cancer Inst.* **48**:1709.

539

NEOANTIGEN
EXPRESSION
IN CHEMICAL
CAR-
CINOGENESIS

BASOMBRÍO, M. A., 1970, Search for common antigenicities among twenty-five sarcomas induced by methylcholanthrene, *Cancer Res.* **30:**2458.

BASOMBRÍO, M. A., 1978, Letter to the Editor, *Cancer Res.* **38:**3568.

BASOMBRÍO, M. A., AND PREHN, R. T., 1972a, Search for common antigenicities between embryonic and tumoral tissue, *Medicina (Buenos Aires)* **32:**42.

BASOMBRÍO, M. A., AND PREHN, R. T., 1972b, Antigenic diversity of tumors chemically induced within the progeny of a single cell, *Int. J. Cancer* **10:**1.

BASOMBRÍO, M. A., AND PREHN, R. T., 1972c, Studies on the basis for diversity and time of appearance of antigens in chemically induced tumors, *Natl. Cancer Inst. Monogr.* **35:**117.

BELNAP, L. P., CLEVELAND, P. H., COLMERAUER, M. E. M., BARONE, R. M., AND PILCH, Y. H., 1979, Immunogenicity of chemically induced murine colon cancers, *Cancer Res.* **39:**1174.

BENDICH, A., BORENFREUND, E., AND STONEHILL, E. H., 1973, Protection of adult mice against tumor challenge by immunization with irradiated adult skin or embryo cells, *J. Immunol.* **111:**284.

BLOOM, E. T., 1970, Quantitative detection of cytotoxic antibodies against tumor-specific antigens of murine sarcomas induced by 3-methylcholanthrene, *J. Natl. Cancer Inst.* **45:**443.

BLOOM, E. T., AND HILDEMANN, W. H., 1970, Mechanisms of tumor-specific enhancement versus resistance toward a methylcholanthrene-induced murine sarcoma, *Transplantation* **10:**321.

BORBERG, H., OETTGEN, H. F., CHOUDRY, K., AND BEATTIE, E. J., 1972, Inhibition of established transplants of chemically induced sarcomas in syngeneic mice by lymphocytes from immunized donors, *Int. J. Cancer* **10:**539.

BORENFREUND, E., HIGGINS, P. J., STEINGLASS, M., AND BENDICH, A., 1975, Properties and malignant transformation of established rat liver parenchymal cells in culture, *J. Natl. Cancer Inst.* **55:**375.

BOWEN, J. G., AND BALDWIN, R. W., 1975, Tumour-specific antigen related to rat histocompatibility antigens, *Nature (London)* **258:**75.

BOWEN, J. G., AND BALDWIN, R. W., 1979a, Tumour antigens and alloantigens. 1. Cross-reactivity of a rat tumour specific antigen with normal alloantigens of the host strain, *Int. J. Cancer* **23:**826.

BOWEN, J. G., AND BALDWIN, R. W., 1979b, Tumour antigens and alloantigens. II. Lack of association of rat hepatoma D23 specific antigen with β-2-microglobulin, *Int. J. Cancer* **23:**833.

BROWN, J. P., KLITZMAN, J. M., AND HELLSTRÖM, K. E., 1977, A microassay for antibody binding to tumor cell surface antigens using ^{125}I-labeled protein A from *Staphylococcus aureus, J. Immunol. Methods* **15:**57.

BROWN, J. P., KLITZMAN, J. M., HELLSTRÖM, I., NOWINSKI, R. C., AND HELLSTRÖM, K. E., 1978, Antibody response of mice to chemically induced tumors, *Proc. Natl. Acad. Sci. USA* **74:**955.

BRUNSON, K. W., BEATTIE, G., AND NICHOLSON, G. L., 1978, Selection and altered properties of brain-colonising metastatic melanoma, *Nature (London)* **272:**543.

BUBENÍK, J., INDROVÁ, M., NEMČKOVÁ, Š., MALKOVSKÝ, M., VON BROEN, B., PÁLEK, V., AND ANDERLÍKOVÁ, J., 1978, Solubilized tumour-associated antigens of methylcholanthrene-induced mouse sarcomas. Comparative studies by *in vitro* sensitization of lymph-node cells, macrophage electrophoretic mobility assay and transplantation tests, *Int. J. Cancer* **21:**348.

BURDICK, J. F., COHEN, A. M., AND WELLS, S. A., 1973, A simplified isotopic antiglobulin assay: Detection of tumor-cell antigens, *J. Natl. Cancer Inst.* **50:**285.

BURNET, F. M., 1970a, A certain symmetry: Histocompatibility antigens compared with immunocyte receptors, *Nature (London)* **226:**123.

BURNET, F. M., 1970b, *Immunological Surveillance*, Pergamon Press, Oxford.

CARBONE, G., INVERNIZZI, G., MESCHINI, A., AND PARMIANI, G., 1978, *In vitro* and *in vivo* expression of original and foreign H-2 antigens and of the tumor-associated transplantation antigen of a murine fibrosarcoma, *Int. J. Cancer* **21:**85.

CASTRO, J. E., LANCE, E. M., MEDAWAR, P. B., ZANELLI, J., AND HUNT, R., 1973, Foetal antigens and cancer, *Nature (London)* **243:**225.

CHISM, S., BURTON, R., AND WARNER, N. L., 1975, Lymphocyte activation *in vitro* to murine onco-foetal antigens, *Nature (London)* **257:**594.

CHISM, S., BURTON, R., AND WARNER, N. L., 1976, *In vitro* induction of tumorspecific immunity. II. Activation of cytotoxic lymphocytes to murine oncofetal antigens, *J. Natl. Cancer Inst.* **57:**377.

CIKES, M., FRIBERG, S. AND KLEIN, G., 1973, Progressive loss of H-2 antigens with concomitant increase of cell surface antigen(s) determined by Moloney leukemia virus in cultured murine lymphomas, *J. Natl. Cancer Inst.* **50:**347.

CLEVELAND, P. H., BELNAP, L. P., KNOTTS, F. B., NAYAK, S. K., BAIRD, S. M., AND PILCH, Y. H., 1979, Tumor-associated antigens of chemically-induced murine tumors: The emergence of MuLV and fetal antigens after serial passage in culture, *Int. J. Cancer* **23:**380.

540

ROBERT W.
BALDWIN
AND
MICHAEL R.
PRICE

COGGIN, J. H., AND AMBROSE, K. R., 1979, Embryonic and fetal determinants on virally and chemically induced tumors, *Methods Cancer Res.* **18**:371.

COGGIN, J. H., AND ANDERSON, N. G., 1974, Cancer differentiation and embryonic antigens: Some central problems, *Adv. Cancer Res.* **19**:106.

COGGIN, J. H., AMBROSE, K. R., AND ANDERSON, N. G., 1970, Fetal antigen capable of inducing transplantation immunity against SV40 hamster tumor cells, *J. Immunol.* **105**:524.

COGGIN, J. H., AMBROSE, K. R., BELLOMY, B. B., AND ANDERSON, N. G., 1971, Tumor immunity in hamsters immunized with fetal tissues, *J. Immunol.* **107**:526.

COHEN, A. M., MILLAR, R. C., AND KETCHAM, A. S., 1972, Host immunity to a growing transplanted methylcholanthrene-induced guinea pig sarcoma, *Cancer Res.* **32**:2421.

COLLAVO, D., BIASI, G., ZANOVELLO, P., CHIECO-BIANCHI, L., AND COLOMBATTI, A., 1979, Role of the H-2 complex in the T-cell-mediated cytotoxicity to Moloney murine sarcoma virus (M-MSV)-induced tumors, in: *Current Trends in Tumor Immunology* (S. Ferrone, S. Gorini, R. B. Herberman, and R. A. Reisfeld, eds.), pp. 309–322, Garland STPM Press, New York.

CORNAIN, S., CARNAUD, D., SILVERMAN, D., KLEIN, E., AND RAJEWSKY, M. F., 1975, Spleen-cell reactivity against transplanted neurogenic rat tumors induced by ethylnitrosourea: Uncovering of tumor specificity after removal of complement-receptor-bearing lymphocytes, *Int. J. Cancer* **16**:301.

DELEO, A. B., SHIKU, H., TAKAHASHI, T., JOHN, M., AND OLD, L. J., 1977, Cell surface antigens of chemically-induced sarcomas in the mouse, *J. Exp. Med.* **146**:720.

DELEO, A. B., SHIKU, H., TAKAHASHI, T., AND OLD, L. J., 1978, Serological definition of cell surface antigens of chemically induced sarcomas of inbred mice, in: *Biological Markers of Neoplasia: Basic and Applied Aspects* (R. W. Ruddon, ed.), pp. 25–34, Elsevier, New York.

DELEO, A. B., JAY, G., APPELLA, E., DUBOIS, G. C., LAW, L. W., AND OLD, L. J., 1979, Detection of a transformation-related antigen in chemically induced sarcomas and other transformed cells of the mouse, *Proc. Natl. Acad. Sci. USA* **76**:2420.

DELORME, E. J. AND ALEXANDER, P., 1964, Treatment of primary fibrosarcoma in the rat with immune lymphocytes, *Lancet* **1**:117.

DENNICK, R. G., PRICE, M. R., AND BALDWIN, R. W., 1979, Modification of the immunogenicity and antigenicity of rat hepatoma cells. II. Mild heat treatment, *Br. J. Cancer* **39**:630.

DOHERTY, P. C., BLANDEN, R. V., AND ZINKERNAGEL, R. M., 1976, Specificity of virus-immune effector T cells for H-2K or H-2D compatible reactions: Implications for H-antigen diversity, *Transplant. Rev.* **29**:89.

DRINKWATER, N. R., MILLER, J. A., MILLER, E. C., AND YANG, N.-C., 1978, Covalent intercalative binding to DNA in relation to the mutagenicity of hydrocarbon epoxides and *N*-acetoxy-2-acetyl-aminofluorene, *Cancer Res.* **38**:3247.

DUFF, R., AND RAPP, F., 1970, Reactions of serum from pregnant hamsters with surface of cells transformed by SV40, *J. Immunol.* **105**:521.

ECONOMOU, G., TAKEIKI, N., AND BOONE, C., 1977, Common tumor rejection antigens in methyl-cholanthrene-induced squamous cell carcinomas in mice detected by tumor protection and a radioisotopic footpad assay, *Cancer Res.* **37**:37.

EMBLETON, M. J., 1979, Antigenic changes associated with liver carcinogenesis, *J. Toxicol. Environ. Health* **5**:453.

EMBLETON, M. J., AND BALDWIN, R. W., 1979, Tumour-related antigen specificities associated with 3-methylcholanthrene-treated rat embryo cells, *Int. J. Cancer* **23**:840.

EMBLETON, M. J., AND BALDWIN, R. W., 1980, Antigenic changes in chemical carcinogenesis, *Br. Med. Bull.* **36**:83.

EMBLETON, M. J., AND HEIDELBERGER, C., 1972, Antigenicity of clones of mouse prostate cells transformed *in vitro*, *Int. J. Cancer* **9**:8.

EMBLETON, M. J., AND HEIDELBERGER, C., 1975, Neoantigens on chemically transformed clones C3H mouse embryo cells, *Cancer Res.* **35**:2049.

EMBLETON, M. J., AND IYPE, P. T., 1978, Surface antigens on rat liver epithelial cells grown in medium containing foetal bovine serum, *Br. J. Cancer* **38**:456.

FARACI, R. P., 1974, *In vitro* demonstration of altered antigenicity of metastases from a primary methylcholanthrene-induced sarcoma, *Surgery* **76**:469.

FARBER, E., 1973, Hyperplastic liver nodules, *Methods Cancer Res.* **7**:345.

FARBER, E., 1976, The pathology of experimental liver cell cancer in: *Liver Cell Cancer* (H. M. Cameron, D. A. Linsell, and G. P. Warwick, eds.), pp. 243–277, Elsevier, Amsterdam.

FIALKOW, P. J., 1976, Clonal origin of human tumors, *Biochim. Biophys. Acta* **458**:283.

FIALKOW, P. J., 1979, Clonal origin of human tumors, *Annu. Rev. Med.* **30**:135.

FIDLER, I. J., AND KRIPKE, M. L., 1977, Metastasis results from pre-existing variant cells within a malignant tumor, *Science* **197**:893.

FOLEY, E. J., 1953, Antigenic properties of methylcholanthrene-induced tumors in mice of the strain of origin, *Cancer Res.* **13**:835.

FORNI, G., SHEVACH, E. M., AND GREEN, I., 1976, Mutant lines of guinea pig L2C leukemia, *J. Exp. Med.* **143**:1067.

FOULDS, L., 1965, Multiple etiologic factors in neoplastic development, *Cancer Res.* **25**:1339.

GARRIDO, F., SCHIRRMACHER, V., AND FESTENSTEIN, H., 1976, H-2-like specificities of foreign haplotypes appearing on a mouse sarcoma after vaccinia virus infection, *Nature (London)* **259**:228.

GERMAIN, R. W., DORE, N. F., AND BENACERRAF, B., 1975, Inhibition of T-lymphocyte mediated tumor-specific lysis by alloantisera directed against the H-2 serological specificities of the tumor, *J. Exp. Med.* **142**:1023.

GIRARDI, A. J., AND REPPUCCI, P., 1972, The relationship of hamster fetal antigen to SV40 tumor-specific transplantation antigen, in: *Embryonic and Fetal Antigens in Cancer*, Vol. 2 (N. G. Anderson, J. S. Coggin, E. Cole, and J. W. Holleman, eds.), pp. 167–170, USAEC, Oak Ridge.

GLOBERSON, A., AND FELDMAN, M., 1964, Antigenic specificity of benzo[a]pyrene-induced sarcomas, *J. Natl. Cancer Inst.* **32**:1229.

GOODING, L. R., 1976, Expression of early fetal antigens on transformed mouse cells, *Cancer Res.* **36**:3499.

GORDON, J., 1965, Isoantigenicity of liver tumours induced by an azo dye, *Br. J. Cancer* **19**:387.

GRANT, J. P., LANDISCH, S., AND WELLS, S. A., 1974a, Immunologic similarities between fetal cell antigens and tumor cell antigens in guinea pigs, *Cancer* **33**:376.

GRANT, J. P., BIGNER, D. D., FISCHINGER, P. J., AND BOLOGNESI, D. P., 1974b, Expression of murine leukemia virus structural antigens on the surface of chemically induced murine sarcomas, *Proc. Natl. Acad. Sci. USA* **71**:5037.

GREAVES, M. F., 1979, Tumour markers, phenotypes and maturation arrest in malignancy: A cell selection hypothesis, in: *Tumour Markers: Impact and Prospects* (E. Boelsma and Ph. Rümke, eds.), pp. 201–211, Elsevier, Amsterdam.

GRIFFIN, M., AND KIZER, D. E., 1978, Purification and quantitation of preneoplastic antigen from hyperplastic nodules and normal liver, *Cancer Res.* **38**:1136.

GUNN, B., EMBLETON, M. J., MIDDLE, J. G., AND BALDWIN, R. W., 1980, Monoclonal antibody against a naturally occurring rat mammary carcinoma, *Int. J. Cancer* **26**:325.

HAASE, P., COWEN, D. M., KNOWLES, J. C., AND COOPER, E. H., 1973, Evaluation of dimethylhydrazine-induced tumours in mice as a model system for colorectal cancer, *Br. J. Cancer* **28**:530.

HADDOW, A., 1974, Molecular repair, wound healing and carcinogenesis: Tumor production a possible overhealing? *Adv. Cancer Res.* **16**:181.

HALLIDAY, W. J., 1971, Blocking effect of serum frum tumor-bearing animals on macrophage migration inhibition with tumor antigens, *J. Immunol.* **106**:855.

HALLIDAY, W. J., AND MILLER, S., 1972, Leukocyte adherence inhibition: A simple test for cell-mediated tumour immunity and serum blocking factors, *Int. J. Cancer* **8**:477.

HALLIDAY, W. J., AND WEBB, M., 1969, Delayed hypersensitivity to chemically induced tumors in mice and correlation with an *in vitro* test, *J. Natl. Cancer Inst.* **43**:141.

HANNANT, D., BOWEN, J. G., DENNICK, R. G., PRICE, M. R., AND BALDWIN, R. W., 1979, Purification of tumour specific antigens—Problems of affinity, avidity and resolution, in: *Affinity Chromatography and Molecular Interactions*, Vol. 86 (J. M. Egly, ed.), p. 477, INSERM, Paris.

HANNANT, D., BOWEN, J. G., PRICE, M. R., AND BALDWIN, R. W., 1980, Radioiodination of rat hepatoma specific antigens and retention of serological reactivity, *Br. J. Cancer*, **41**:716.

HARDER, F. H., AND McKHANN, C. F., 1968, Demonstration of cellular antigens on sarcoma cells by an indirect ^{125}I-labelled antibody technique, *J. Natl. Cancer Inst.* **40**:231.

HARRIS, J. R., PRICE, M. R., AND BALDWIN, R. W., 1973, The purification of membrane-associated tumour antigens by preparative polyacrylamide gel electrophoresis, *Biochim. Biophys. Acta* **311**:600.

HAYWOOD, G. R., AND McKHANN, C. F., 1971, Antigenic specificities on murine sarcoma cells, *J. Exp. Med.* **133**:1171.

HEIDELBERGER, C., 1975, Chemical carcinogenesis, *Annu. Rev. Biochem.* **44**:79.

HELLSTRÖM, I., HELLSTRÖM, K. E., AND PIERCE, G. E., 1968, *In vitro* studies of immune reactions against autochthonous and syngeneic mouse tumors induced by methylcholanthrene and plastic discs, *Int. J. Cancer* **3**:467.

541

NEOANTIGEN
EXPRESSION
IN CHEMICAL
CAR-
CINOGENESIS

542

ROBERT W.
BALDWIN
AND
MICHAEL R.
PRICE

HELLSTRÖM, I., HELLSTRÖM, K. E., AND SHANTZ, G., 1976, Demonstration of tumor-associated immunity with a leukocyte adherence inhibition (LAI) assay, *Int. J. Cancer* **18**:354.

HELLSTRÖM, K. E., AND HELLSTRÖM, I., 1969, Cellular immunity against tumor antigens, *Adv. Cancer Res.* **12**:167.

HELLSTRÖM, K. E., HELLSTRÖM, I., AND BROWN, J. P., 1978, Unique and common tumor-specific transplantation antigens of chemically induced mouse sarcomas, *Int. J. Cancer* **21**:317.

HERBERMAN, R. B., AND HOLDEN, H. T., 1978, Natural cell-mediated immunity, *Adv. Cancer Res.* **27**:305.

HERBERMAN, R. B., KAY, H. D., BONNARD, G. D., ORTALDO, J. R., FAGNANI, R., DJEU, J. Y., AND HOLDEN, H. T., 1979, Characteristics of effector cells of natural and antibody-dependent cytotoxicity and factors affecting their expression, in: *Current Trends in Tumor Immunology* (S. Ferrone, S. Gorini, R. B. Herberman, and R. A. Reisfeld, eds.), pp. 61–70, Garland STPM Press, New York.

HIRAI, H., 1979, Model systems of AFP and CEA expression, *Methods Cancer Res.* **18**:39.

HOLMES, E. C., MORTON, D. L., SCHIDLOWSKY, G., AND TRAHAN, E., 1971, Cross-reacting tumor-specific transplantation antigens in methylcholanthrene-induced guinea pig sarcomas, *J. Natl. Cancer Inst.* **46**:693.

HOPPER, D., PIMM, M. V., AND BALDWIN, R. W., 1975, Methanol extraction residue of BCG in the treatment of transplanted rat tumours, *Br. J. Cancer* **31**:176.

INVERNIZZI, G., AND PARMIANI, G., 1975, Tumour-associated transplantation antigens of chemically induced sarcomata cross-reacting with allogeneic histocompatibility antigens, *Nature (London)* **254**:713.

IRIE, R. F., IRIE, K., AND MORTON, D. L., 1974, Natural antibody in human serum to a neoantigen in human cultured cells growing in fetal bovine serum, *J. Natl. Cancer Inst.* **52**:1051.

ISHIDATE, M., 1974, Antigen specificity of different cell lines of rat ascites hepatoma originating in the same individual, *Gann Monogr. Cancer Res.* **16**:195.

ISOJIMA, S., YAGI, Y., AND PRESSMAN, D., 1969, Antigens common to rat hepatomas induced with 2-acetylaminofluorene, *Cancer Res.* **29**:140.

IYPE, P. T., BALDWIN, R. W., AND GLAVES, D., 1973, Cell surface antigenic changes induced in normal adult rat liver cells by carcinogen treatment *in vitro*, *Br. J. Cancer* **27**:128.

JAMASBI, R. J., AND NETTESHEIM, P., 1977, Demonstration of cross-reacting tumor rejection antigens in chemically induced respiratory tract carcinomas in rats, *Cancer Res.* **37**:4059.

JEFFCOATE, W. J., AND REES, L. H., 1978, Adrenocorticotropin and related peptides in non-endocrine tumors, *Curr. Top. Exp. Endocrinol.* **3**:57.

JOHNSON, S., 1968, The effect of thymectomy and of the dose of 3-methylcholanthrene on the induction and antigenic properties of sarcomas in C57 Bl mice, *Br. J. Cancer* **22**:93.

KATZ, D. H., AND BENACERRAF, B., 1975, The function and interrelationship of T cell receptors, Ir genes and other histocompatibility gene products, *Transplant. Rev.* **22**:175.

KERBEL, R. S., 1979*a*, Implications of immunological heterogeneity of tumours, *Nature (London)* **280**:358.

KERBEL, R. S., 1979*b*, Immunologic studies of membrane mutants of a highly metastatic murine tumor, *Am. J. Pathol.* **97**:609.

KLEIN, G., 1973, Tumor immunology, *Transplant. Proc.* **5**:31.

KLEIN, G., AND KLEIN, E., 1975, Are methylcholanthrene-induced sarcoma-associated, rejection inducing (TSTA) antigens, modified forms of H-2 or linked determinants?, *Int. J. Cancer* **15**:879.

KLEIN, G., SJÖGREN, H. O., KLEIN, E., AND HELLSTRÖM, K. E., 1960, Demonstration of resistance against methylcholanthrene-induced sarcomas in the primary autochthonous host, *Cancer Res.* **20**:1561.

KLEIN, J., 1975, *Biology of the Mouse Histocompatibility-2 Complex*, Springer, Berlin.

KRIPKE, M. L., GRAYS, E., AND FIDLER, I. J., 1978, Metastatic heterogeneity of cells from an ultraviolet light-induced murine fibrosarcoma of recent origin, *Cancer Res.* **38**:2962.

KRONMAN, B. S., RAPP, H. J., AND BORSOS, T., 1969, Tumor-specific antigens: Detection by local transfer of delayed skin hypersensitivity, *J. Natl. Cancer Inst.* **43**:869.

LANDO, P., BLOMBERG, F., RAFTELL, M., BERZINS, K., AND PERLMANN, P., 1977, Complement dependent cytotoxicity against hepatoma cells mediated by IgM antibodies in the serum from tumor bearing rats, *Scand. J. Immunol.* **6**:1081.

LAPPÉ, M. A., 1969, Tumour specific transplantation antigens: Possible origin in pre-malignant lesions, *Nature (London)* **223**:82.

LAUSCH, R. N., AND RAPP, R., 1974, Tumor-specific antigens and re-expression of fetal antigens in mammalian cells, *Prog. Exp. Tumor Res.* **19**:45.

LAW, L. W., AND APPELLA, E., 1975, Studies of soluble transplantation antigens and tumor antigens, in: *Cancer: A Comprehensive Treatise*, Vol. 4 (F. F. Becker, ed.), pp. 135–157, Plenum Press, New York.

LAW, L. W., APPELLA, E., AND DUBOIS, G. C., 1978, Immunogenic properties of solubilized, partially purified tumor rejection antigen (TSTA) from a chemically induced sarcoma, in: *Biological Markers of Neoplasia: Basic and Applied Aspects* (R. W. Ruddon, ed.), pp. 35–43, Elsevier, New York.

LAW, L. W., DUBOIS, G. C., ROGERS, M. J., APPELLA, E., PIEROTTI, M. A., AND PARMIANI, G., 1980, Tumor rejection activity of antigens isolated from membranes of a methylcholanthrene-induced sarcoma, C-1, bearing alien H-2 antigens, *Transplant. Proc.* **7:**46.

LAWLEY, P. D., 1980, DNA as a target of alkylating carcinogens, *Br. Med. Bull.* **36:**19.

LEFFELL, M. S., AND COGGIN, J. H., 1977, Common transplantation antigens on methylcholanthrene-induced murine sarcomas detected by three assays of tumor rejection, *Cancer Res.* **37:**4112.

LEJNEVA, O. M., ZILBER, L. A., AND IEVLEVA, E. S., 1965, Humoral antibodies to methylcholanthrene sarcomata detected by a fluorescent technique, *Nature (London)* **206:**1163.

LE MEVEL, B. P., AND WELLS, S. A., 1973, Foetal antigens cross-reactive with tumor-specific transplantation antigens, *Nature New Biol.* **244:**183.

LENNOX, E., COHN, J., AND LOWE, T., 1980, Syngeneic monoclonal antibodies to a methylcholanthrene-induced mouse sarcoma, *Transplant. Proc.* **7:**95.

LEONARD, E. J., 1973, Cell surface antigen movement: Induction in hepatoma cells by antitumor antibody, *J. Immunol.* **110:**1167.

LEONARD, E. J., MELTZER, M. S., BORSOS, T., AND RAPP, H. J., 1972, Properties of soluble tumor-specific antigen solubilized by hypertonic potassium chloride, *Natl. Cancer Inst. Monogr.* **35:**129.

LEONARD, E. J., RICHARDSON, A. K., HARDY, A. S., AND RAPP, H. J., 1975, Extraction of tumor-specific antigen from cells and plasma membranes of line-10 hepatoma, *J. Natl. Cancer Inst.* **55:**73.

MANN, D. L., 1972, The effect of enzyme inhibitors on the solubilization of HL-A antigens with 3M KCl, *Transplantation* **14:**398.

MARTIN, F., MARTIN, M., LAGNEAU, A., BORCLES, M., AND KNOBELS, S., 1976, Circulating antibodies in rats bearing grafted colon carcinoma, *Cancer Res.* **36:**3039.

MARTIN, W. J., ESBER, E., COTTON, W. G., AND RICE, J. M., 1973, Derepression of alloantigens in malignancy. Evidence for tumor susceptibility alloantigens and for possible self-reactivity of lymphoid cells active in the microcytotoxicity assay, *Br. J. Cancer Suppl.* **28:**48.

MELTZER, M. S., LEONARD, E. J., RAPP, H. J., AND BORSOS, T., 1971, Tumor-specific antigen solubilized by hypertonic potassium chloride, *J. Natl. Cancer Inst.* **47:**703.

MÉNARD, S., COLNAGHI, M. I., AND DELLA PORTA, G., 1973, *In vitro* demonstration of tumor-specific common antigens and embryonal antigens in murine fibrosarcomas induced by 7,12-dimethyl-benz[a]anthracene, *Cancer Res.* **33:**478.

MILAS, L., AND SCOTT, M. T., 1977, Antitumor activity of *Corynebacterium parvum*, *Adv. Cancer Res.* **26:**257.

MILLER, E. C., KADLUBAR, F. F., MILLER, J. A., PITOT, H. C., AND DRINKWATER, N. R., 1979, The N-hydroxy metabolites of N-methyl-4-aminoazobenzene and related dyes as proximate carcinogens in the rat and mouse, *Cancer Res.* **39:**3411.

MILLER, J. A., 1979, Remarks on chemicals and chemical carcinogenesis, in: *Carcinogens: Identification and Mechanisms of Action* (A. C. Griffin and C. R. Shaw, eds.), pp. 455–459, Raven Press, New York.

MINAMI, A., MIZUSHIMA, Y., TAKEICHI, N., HOSOKAWA, M., AND KOBAYASHI, H., 1979, Dissociation of anti-tumor immune responses in rats immunized with solubilized tumor-associated antigens from a methylcholanthrene induced fibrosarcoma, *Int. J. Cancer* **23:**358.

MÖLLER, G., AND MÖLLER, E., 1976, The concept of immunological surveillance against neoplasia, *Transplant. Rev.* **28:**3.

MONDAL, S., IYPE, P. T., GRIESBACH, L. M., AND HEIDELBERGER, C., 1970, Antigenicity of cells derived from mouse prostate after malignancy transformation *in vitro* by carcinogenic hydrocarbons, *Cancer Res.* **30:**1593.

MONDAL, S., EMBLETON, M. J., MARQUARDT, H., AND HEIDELBERGER, C., 1971, Production of variants of decreased malignancy and antigenicity from clones transformed *in vitro* by methylcholanthrene, *Int. J. Cancer* **8:**410.

MONTESANO, R., SAINT-VINCENT, L., AND TOMATIS, L., 1973, Malignant transformation *in vitro* of rat liver cells by dimethylnitrosamine and N-methyl-N'-nitro-N-nitrosoguanidine, *Br. J. Cancer* **28:**215.

543

NEOANTIGEN
EXPRESSION
IN CHEMICAL
CAR-
CINOGENESIS

544

ROBERT W.
BALDWIN
AND
MICHAEL R.
PRICE

MORTON, D. L., GOLDMAN, L., AND WOOD, D., 1965, Tumor specific antigenicity of methylcholanthrene (MCA) and dibenzanthracene (DBA) induced sarcomas of inbred guinea pigs, *Fed. Proc. Fed. Am. Soc. Exp. Biol.* **24:**684.

MÜLLER, M., 1968, Versuche zur Erzeugung einer Transplantationsimmunität gegen *o*-Aminoazotoluol-Hepatome bei syngenen und F_1 Hybrid-Mäusen, *Arch. Geschwulstforsch.* **31:**235.

MURGITA, R. A., GOIDL, E. A., KONTIANEN, S., AND WIGZELL, H., 1977, α-Fetoprotein induces suppressor T cells *in vitro*, *Nature (London)* **267:**257.

NATORI, T., LAW, L. W., AND APPELLA, E., 1977, Biological and biochemical properties of Nonidet P-40-solubilized and partially purified tumor-specific antigens of the transplantation type from plasma membranes of a methylcholanthrene-induced sarcoma, *Cancer Res.* **37:**3406.

NATORI, T., LAW, L. W., AND APPELLA, E., 1978, Immunochemical evidence of a tumor-specific surface antigen obtained by detergent solubilization of the membranes of a chemically induced sarcoma, Meth. A, *Cancer Res.* **38:**359.

NELSON, K. A., SJÖGREN, H. O., AND ROSENGREN, J. E., 1977, Detection of antibodies to embryonic antigens in sera of multiparous or colon tumor-bearing rats by a new indirect immunofluorescence assay, *Int. J. Cancer* **20:**227.

NICOLSON, G. L., 1976, Transmembrane control of the receptors on normal and tumour cells. II. Surface changes associated with transformation and malignancy, *Biochim. Biophys. Acta* **458:**1.

NIELSEN, J. T., AND CHAPMAN, V. W., 1977, Electrophoretic variation for X-chromosome-linked phosphoglycerate kinase (PCK-1) in the mouse, *Genetics* **87:**319.

NOWELL, P. C., 1976, The clonal evolution of tumor cell populations, *Science* **194:**23.

ODELL, W. D., AND WOLFSON, A., 1975, Ectopic hormone secretion by tumors, in: *Cancer: A Comprehensive Treatise*, Vol. 3 (F. F. Becker, ed.), pp. 81–119, Plenum Press, New York.

OETTGEN, H. F., OLD, L. J., MCLEAN, E. P., AND CARSWELL, E. A., 1968, Delayed hypersensitivity and transplantation immunity elicited by soluble antigens of chemically induced tumours in inbred guinea pigs, *Nature (London)* **220:**295.

OLD, L. J., AND BOYSE, E. A., 1965, Antigens of tumors and leukemias induced by viruses, *Fed. Proc. Fed. Am. Soc. Exp. Biol.* **24:**1009.

OLD, L. J., AND STOCKERT, E., 1977, Immunogenetics of cell surface antigens of mouse leukemia, *Annu. Rev. Genet.* **11:**127.

OLD, L. J., BOYSE, E. A., CLARKE, D. A., AND CARSWELL, E. A., 1962, Antigenic properties of chemically induced tumors, *Ann. N.Y. Acad. Sci.* **101:**80.

ORTALDO, J. R., TING, C. C., AND HERBERMAN, R. B., 1974, Modulation of fetal antigen(s) in mouse leukemia cells, *Cancer Res.* **34:**1366.

PARKER, G. A., AND ROSENBERG, S. A., 1977, Cross-reacting antigens in chemically induced sarcomas are fetal determinants, *J. Immunol.* **118:**1590.

PARKER, G. A., HYATT, C., AND ROSENBERG, S. A., 1977, Normal adult murine cells in tissue culture express fetal antigens, *Transplantation* **23:**161.

PARMIANI, G., AND INVERNIZZI, G., 1975, Alien histocompatibility determinants on the cell surface of sarcomas induced by methylcholanthrene, *Int. J. Cancer* **16:**756.

PARMIANI, G., COLNAGHI, M. I., AND DELLA PORTA, G., 1971, Immunodepression during urethane and *N*-nitrosomethylurea leukaemogenesis in mice, *Br. J. Cancer* **25:**354.

PARMIANI, G., BALLINARI, D., CARBONE, G., INVERNIZZI, G., AND PIEROTTI, M. A., 1979, Tumor-associated transplantation antigens and alien H-2 antigens on chemically induced sarcomas, in: *Current Trends in Tumor Immunology* (S. Ferrone, S. Gorini, R. B. Herberman, and R. A. Reisfeld, eds.), pp. 323–333, Garland STPM Press, New York.

PASTERNAK, G., 1963, Die unterschiedliche Reaktionsfähigkeit zweier Mäuseinzuchstämme gegen spezifische Antigene transplantabler Carcinogentumoren, *Acta Biol. Med. Ger.* **10:**572.

PASTERNAK, G., GRAFFI, A., HOFFMANN, F., AND HORN, K.-H., 1964, Resistance against carcinomas of the skin induced by dimethylbenzanthracene (DMBA) in mice of the strain XVII/*Bln*, *Nature (London)* **203:**307.

PASTERNAK, G., HOFFMANN, F., AND GRAFFI, A., 1966, Growth of diethylnitrosamine-induced lung tumours in syngeneic mice specifically pre-treated with X-ray killed tumour tissue, *Folia Biol. (Prague)* **12:**299.

PASTERNAK, G., VON BROEN, B., SCHLOTT, B., ALBRECHT, S., GRYSCHEK, G., REINHÖFER, J., AND THUY, L. T., 1979, Lymphocyte reactivity in animal and human tumor systems to fetal antigens as detected by MEM, LAI and LMI techniques, in: *Cell Electrophoresis: Clinical Application and Methodology* (A. W. Preece and D. Sabolovic, eds.), pp. 225–234, Elsevier, Amsterdam.

545

NEOANTIGEN
EXPRESSION
IN CHEMICAL
CAR-
CINOGENESIS

PASTERNAK, G., SCHLOTT, B., ALBRECHT, S., GRYSCHEK, G., REINHÖFER, J. AND VON BROEN, B., 1980, Cellular immune reactions to foetal extracts in patients with malignant tumours, in: *Biology of the Cancer Cell* (K. Letnansky, ed.), pp. 173–178, Kugler, Amsterdam.

PELLIS, N. R., AND KAHAN, B. D., 1975, Specific tumor immunity induced with soluble materials: Restricted range of antigen dose and of challenge tumor load for immunoprotection, *J. Immunol.* **115**:1717.

PELLIS, N. R., TOM, B. J., AND KAHAN, B. D., 1974, Tumor-specific and allospecific immunogenicity of soluble extracts from chemically induced murine sarcomas, *J. Immunol.* **113**:708.

PHILLIPS, E. R., AND PERDUE, J. F., 1977, Immunological identification of fetal calf serum-derived proteins on the surfaces of cultured transformed and untransformed rat cells, *Int. J. Cancer* **20**:798.

PIMM, M. V., AND BALDWIN, R. W., 1977, Antigenic differences between primary methylcholanthrene-induced rat sarcomas and post-surgical recurrences, *Int. J. Cancer* **20**:37.

PIMM, M. V., EMBLETON, M. J., AND BALDWIN, R. W., 1980, Multiple antigenic specificities within primary 3-methylcholanthrene-induced rat sarcomas and metastases, *Int. J. Cancer* **25**:621.

PITOT, H. C., 1979, Biological and enzymatic events in chemical carcinogenesis, *Annu. Rev. Med.* **30**:25.

POSTE, G., AND FIDLER, I. J., 1980, The pathogenesis of cancer metastasis, *Nature (London)* **283**:139.

PREHN, R. T., 1960, Tumor-specific immunity to transplanted dibenz[*a,h*]anthracene-induced sarcomas, *Cancer Res.* **20**:1614.

PREHN, R. T., 1967, The significance of tumor-distinctive histocompatibility antigens, in: *Cross Reacting Antigens and Neoantigens* (J. J. Trentin, ed.), pp. 105–117, Williams & Wilkins, Baltimore.

PREHN, R. T., 1970, Analysis of antigenic heterogeneity within individual 3-methylcholanthrene-induced mouse sarcomas, *J. Natl. Cancer Inst.* **45**:1039.

PREHN, R. T., 1975, Relationship of tumor immunogenicity to concentration of the oncogen, *J. Natl. Cancer Inst.* **55**:189.

PREHN, R. T., AND MAIN, J. M., 1957, Immunity to methylcholanthrene-induced sarcomas, *J. Natl. Cancer Inst.* **18**:769.

PRESTON, V. E., AND PRICE, M. R., 1977, Partial purification of a plasma membrane-associated tumour-specific antigen from a rat sarcoma by using immunoadsorbent column chromatography, *Biochem. Soc. Trans.* **5**:123.

PRICE, M. R., 1978, A microassay for the detection of tumour-specific complement dependent serum cytotoxicity against a chemically induced rat hepatoma, *Transplantation* **25**:224.

PRICE, M. R., AND BALDWIN, R. W., 1974*a*, Preparation of aminoazo dye-induced rat hepatoma membrane fractions retaining tumour specific antigen, *Br. J. Cancer* **30**:382.

PRICE, M. R., AND BALDWIN, R. W., 1974*b*, Immunogenic properties of rat hepatoma subcellular fractions, *Br. J. Cancer* **30**:394.

PRICE, M. R., AND BALDWIN, R. W., 1977*a*, Tumour-specific complement-dependent serum cytotoxicity against a chemically-induced rat hepatoma, *Int. J. Cancer* **20**:284.

PRICE, M. R., AND BALDWIN, R. W., 1977*b*, Shedding of tumor cell surface antigens, in: *Dynamic Aspects of Cell Surface Organization* (G. Poste and G. L. Nicolson, eds.), pp. 423–471, Elsevier, Amsterdam.

PRICE, M. R., PRESTON, V. E., ROBINS, R. A., ZÖLLER, M., AND BALDWIN, R. W., 1978, Induction of immunity to chemically-induced tumours by cellular or soluble antigens, *Cancer Immunol. Immunother.* **3**:247.

PRICE, M. R., DENNICK, R. G., HANNANT, D., AND AL-SHEIKLY, A. W. A. R., 1979*a*, Detection, isolation and immunogenicity of rat tumour antigens, in: *Cell Electrophoresis: Clinical Application and Methodology* (A. W. Preece and D. Sablovic, eds.), pp. 247–254, Elsevier, Amsterdam.

PRICE, M. R., DENNICK, R. G., AND LAW, L. W., 1979*b*, Effect of heat and glutaraldehyde upon the immunogenicity of Meth A sarcoma cells, *Br. J. Cancer* **40**:663.

PRICE, M. R., DENNICK, R. G., ROBINS, R. A., AND BALDWIN, R. W., 1979*c*, Modification of the immunogenicity and antigenicity of rat hepatoma cells. I. Cell-surface stabilization with glutaraldehyde, *Br. J. Cancer* **39**:621.

PRICE, M. R., HÖFFKEN, K., AND BALDWIN, R. W., 1979*d*, Activity of syngeneic complement for revealing antibody-induced cytotoxicity against a rat hepatoma, *Transplantation* **28**:140.

PRICE, M. R., MOORE, V. E., AND BALDWIN, R. W., 1979*e*, Biochemical aspects of tumor-specific antigens, in: *Current Trends in Tumor Immunology* (S. Ferrone, S. Gorini, R. B. Herberman, and R. A. Reisfeld, eds.), pp. 187–209, Garland STPM Press, New York.

PRICE, M. R., HANNANT, D., BOWEN, J. G., AND BALDWIN, R. W., 1980*a*, Suppressor cells in rats immunized against solubilized hepatoma specific antigens, *Br. J. Cancer* **42**:176.

546

ROBERT W.
BALDWIN
AND
MICHAEL R.
PRICE

PRICE, M. R., HANNANT, D., EMBLETON, M. J., AND BALDWIN, R. W., 1980b, Detection and isolation of tumour associated antigens; ICREW Workshop Report, *Br. J. Cancer* **41**:843.

REDDY, A. L., AND FIALKOW, P. J., 1979, Multicellular origin of fibrosarcomas in mice induced by the chemical carcinogen 3-methylcholanthrene, *J. Exp. Med.* **150**:878.

REES, R. C., PRICE, M. R., BALDWIN, R. W., AND SHAH, L. P., 1974, Inhibition of rat lymph node cell cytotoxicity by hepatoma-associated embryonic antigen, *Nature (London)* **252**:751.

REES, R. C., PRICE, M. R., SHAH, L. P., AND BALDWIN, R. W., 1975a, Detection of hepatoma-associated embryonic antigen in tumour-bearer serum, *Transplantation* **19**:424.

REES, R. C., SHAH, L. P., AND BALDWIN, R. W., 1975b, Inhibition of pulmonary tumour development in rats sensitised to rat embryonic tissue, *Nature (London)* **255**:329.

REES, R. C., PRICE, M. R., AND BALDWIN, R. W., 1979, Oncodevelopmental antigen expression in chemical carcinogenesis, *Methods Cancer Res.* **18**:99.

REINER, J., AND SOUTHAM, C. M., 1967, Evidence of common antigenic properties in chemically induced sarcomas of mice, *Cancer Res.* **27**:1243.

REINER, J., AND SOUTHAM, C. M., 1969, Further evidence of common antigenic properties in chemically induced sarcomas of mice, *Cancer Res.* **29**:1814.

REISFELD, R. A., AND KAHAN, B. D., 1970, Biological and chemical characterization of human histocompatibility antigens, *Fed. Proc. Fed. Am. Soc. Exp. Biol.* **29**:2034.

REISFELD, R. A., AND KAHAN, B. D., 1972, Markers of biological individuality, *Sci. Am.* **226**(6):28.

RÉVÉSZ, L., 1960, Detection of antigenic differences in isologous host-tumor systems by pretreatment with heavily irradiated tumor cells, *Cancer Res.* **20**:443.

ROBERTS, J. J., 1980, Carcinogen-induced DNA damage and its repair, *Br. Med. Bull.* **36**:25.

ROBINSON, N. C., AND TANFORD, C., 1975, The binding of deoxycholate, Triton X-100, sodium dodecyl sulfate, and phosphatidylcholine vesicles to cytochrome b_5 *Biochemistry* **14**:369.

ROGERS, M. J., LAW, L. W., AND APPELLA, E., 1978, Separation of the tumor rejection antigen (TSTA) from the major viral structural proteins associated with the membrane of an R-MuLV-induced leukemia, in: *Biological Markers of Neoplasia: Basic and Applied Aspects* (R. W. Ruddon, ed.), pp. 53–62, Elsevier, New York.

ROSEN, S. W., WEINTRAUB, B. D., VAITUKAITIS, B. D., SUSSMAN, H. H., HERSHMAN, J. M., AND MUGGIA, F. M., 1975, Placental proteins and their sub units as tumor markers, *Ann. Intern. Med.* **82**:71.

RUPPERT, B., WEI, W., MEDINA, D., AND HEPPNER, G. M., 1978, Effect of chemical carcinogen treatment on the immunogenicity of mouse mammary tumors arising from hyperplastic alveolar nodule outgrowth lines, *J. Natl. Cancer Inst.* **61**:1165.

SAGE, E., SPODHEIM-MAURIZOT, M., RIO, P., LENG, M., AND FUCHS, R. P. P., 1979, Discrimination by antibodies between local defects in DNA induced by 2-aminofluorene derivatives, *FEBS Lett.* **108**:66.

SCHINITSKY, M. R., HYMAN, L. R., BLAZKOVEC, A. A., AND BURKHOLDER, P. M., 1973, *Bacillus Calmette-Guérin* vaccination and skin tumor promotion, *Cancer Res.* **33**:659.

SCHIRRMACHER, V., AND ROBINSON, P., 1979, Differences between normal cells and tumor cells in their expression of certain H-2 determinants, in: *Current Trends in Tumor Immunology* (S. Ferrone, S. Gorini, R. B. Herberman, and R. A. Reisfeld, eds.), pp. 335–346, Garland STPM Press, New York.

SELL, S., AND BECKER, F. F., 1978, Alpha-fetoprotein, *J. Natl. Cancer Inst.* **60**:19.

SHAH, L. P., REES, R. C., AND BALDWIN, R. W., 1976, Tumour rejection in rats sensitized to embryonic tissue. I. Rejection of tumour cells implanted subcutaneously and detection of cytotoxic lymphoid cells, *Br. J. Cancer* **33**:577.

SHEARER, G. M., AND SCHMITT-VERHULST, A. M., 1977, Major histocompatibility complex restricted cell-mediated immunity, *Adv. Immunol.* **25**:55.

SHEARER, G. M., SCHMITT-VERHULST, A. M., AND REHN, T. G., 1977, Significance of the major histocompatibility complex as assessed by T-cell-mediated lympholysis involving syngeneic stimulating cells, *Contemp. Top. Immunobiol.* **7**:221.

SIKORA, K., KOCH, G., BRENNER, S., AND LENNOX, E., 1979, Partial purification of tumour-specific transplantation antigens from methylcholanthrene-induced murine sarcomas by immobilized lectins, *Br. J. Cancer* **40**:831.

SINGER, R. M., 1979, Fetal isoenzyme modulation in human tumor xenografts, *Methods Cancer Res.* **18**:169.

SJÖGREN, H. O., AND STEELE, G., 1975a, Colon carcinoma antigens in the rat, *Ann. N.Y. Acad. Sci.* **259**:404.

547

NEOANTIGEN
EXPRESSION
IN CHEMICAL
CAR-
CINOGENESIS

SJÖGREN, H. O., AND STEELE, G., 1975*b*, The immunology of large bowel carcinoma in a rat model, *Cancer* **36**:2469.

SONDEL, P. M., AND BACH, F. H., 1980, The alienation of tumor immunity: Alien driven diversity and alien selected escape, *Transplant. Proc.* **7**:211.

STAVROU, D., ANZIL, A. P., AND ELLING, H., 1978, Tumor specific fluorescent and complement-dependent cytotoxic antibodies in the serum of rats with chemically induced brain gliomas, *Acta Neuropathol. (Berlin)* **43**:111.

STEELE, G., AND SJÖGREN, H. O., 1974, Embryonic antigens associated with chemically induced colon carcinomas in rats, *Int. J. Cancer* **14**:435.

STEELE, G., AND SJÖRGREN, H. O., 1977, Cell surface antigens in a rat colon cancer model: Correlation with inhibition of tumor growth, *Surgery* **82**:164.

STEELE, G., SJÖGREN, H. O., AND PRICE, M. R., 1975*a*, Tumor-associated and embryonic antigens in soluble fractions of a chemically-induced rat colon carcinoma, *Int. J. Cancer* **16**:33.

STEELE, G., SJÖGREN, H. O., ROSENGREN, J. E., LINDSTRÖM, C., LARSON, A., AND LEANDOER, L., 1975*b*, Sequential studies of serum blocking activity in rats bearing chemically induced primary bowel tumors, *J. Natl. Cancer Inst.* **54**:959.

STUTMAN, O., 1975, Immunodepression and malignancy, *Adv. Cancer Res.* **22**:261.

SUGARBAKER, E. V., AND COHEN, A. M., 1972, Altered antigenicity in spontaneous pulmonary metastases from an antigenic murine sarcoma, *Surgery* **72**:155.

SUTER, L., BLOOM, B. R., WADSWORTH, E. M., AND OETTGEN, H. F., 1972, Use of the macrophage migration inhibition test to monitor fractionation of soluble antigens of chemically induced sarcomas of inbred guinea pigs, *J. Immunol.* **109**:766.

TAKASUGI, M., AND KLEIN, E., 1970, A microassay for cell-mediated immunity, *Transplantation* **9**:219.

TAKEDA, K., 1969, *Immunology of Cancer*, Hokkaido University, Sapporo, Japan.

TAO, T.-W., AND BURGER, M. M., 1977, Non-metastasising variants selected from metastasising melanoma cells, *Nature (London)* **270**:437.

TARANGER, L. A., CHAPMAN, W. H., HELLSTRÖM, I., AND HELLSTRÖM, K. E., 1972*a*, Immunological studies on urinary bladder tumors of rats and mice, *Science* **176**:1337.

TARANGER, L. A., HELLSTRÖM, I., CHAPMAN, W. H., AND HELLSTRÖM, K. E., 1972*b*, *In vitro* demonstration of common tumor antigens in mouse and rat bladder carcinomas, *Proc. Am. Assoc. Cancer Res.* **13**:56.

THOMSON, D. M. P., GOLD, P., FREEDMAN, S. O., AND SHUSTER, J., 1976, The isolation and characterization of tumor-specific antigens of rodent and human tumors, *Cancer Res.* **36**:3518.

THOMSON, D. M. P., TATARYN, D. N., O'CONNOR, R., RAUCH, J., FRIEDLANDER, P., GOLD, P., AND SHUSTER, J., 1979, Evidence for the expression of human tumorspecific antigens associated with β-2 microglobulin in human cancer and in some colon adenomas and benign breast lesions, *Cancer Res.* **39**:604.

TING, C. C., AND GRANT, J. P., 1976, Humoral antibody response and tumor transplantation resistance elicited by fetal tissues in mice, *J. Natl. Cancer Inst.* **56**:401.

TING, C. C., AND HERBERMAN, R. B., 1971, Inverse relationship of polyoma tumorspecific cell surface antigen to H-2 histocompatibility antigens, *Nature New Biol.* **232**:118.

TRACEY, R. S., WEPSIC, H. T., ALAIMO, J., AND MORRIS, H. P., 1978, Growth of transplanted rat tumors following administration of cell-free tumor antigens, *Cancer Res.* **38**:1208.

TUFFREY, M. A., AND BATCHELOR, J. R., 1964, Tumour specific immunity against murine epitheliomas induced with 9,10-dimethyl-1,2-benzanthracene, *Nature (London)* **204**:349.

WAHL, D. V., CHAPMAN, W. H., HELLSTRÖM, I., AND HELLSTRÖM, K. E., 1974, Transplantation immunity to individually unique antigens of chemically induced bladder tumors in mice, *Int. J. Cancer* **14**:114.

WEINHOUSE, S., 1972, Glycolysis, respiration, and anomalous gene expression in experimental hepatomas: G. H. A. Clowes Memorial Lecture, *Cancer Res.* **32**:2007.

WEPSIC, H. T., ZBAR, B., RAPP, H. J., AND BORSOS, T., 1970, Systemic transfer of tumor immunity: Delayed hypersensitivity and suppression of tumor growth, *J. Natl. Cancer Inst.* **44**:955.

WEPSIC, H. T., NICKEL, R., AND ALAIMO, J., 1976, Characterization of growth properties and demonstration of the tumor-specific transplantation antigens of Morris hepatomas, *Cancer Res.* **35**:246.

WHITMORE, C. E., SALERNO, R. A., RABSTEIN, L. S., HUEBNER, R. J., AND TURNER, H. C., 1971, RNA tumor-virus antigen expression in chemically induced tumors. Virus-genome-specified common antigens detected by complement fixation in mouse tumors induced by 3-methylcholanthrene, *J. Natl. Cancer Inst.* **47**:1255.

548

ROBERT W.
BALDWIN
AND
MICHAEL R.
PRICE

WILLIAMS, A. F., 1977, Differentiation antigens of the lymphocyte cell surface, *Contemp. Top. Mol. Immunol.* **6**:83.

WILLIAMS, G. M., 1979, Liver cell culture systems for the study of hepatocarcinogenesis, in: *Advances in Medical Oncology, Research and Education*, Vol. 1 (G. P. Margison, ed.), pp. 273–293, Pergamon Press, Oxford.

WILLIAMS, G. M., ELLIOTT, J. M., AND WEISBURGER, J. H., 1973, Carcinoma after malignant conversion *in vitro* of epithelial-like cells from rat liver following exposure to chemical carcinogens, *Cancer Res.* **33**:606.

WOODRUFF, M., AND SPEEDY, G., 1978, Inhibition of chemical carcinogenesis by *Corynebacterium parvum*, *Proc. R. Soc. London Ser. B* **201**:209.

WRATHMELL, A. B., GAUCI, C. L., AND ALEXANDER, P., 1976, Cross-reactivity of an alloantigen present on normal cells with the tumour-specific transplantation type antigen of the acute myeloid leukaemia (SAL) of rats, *Br. J. Cancer* **33**:187.

YOKOTA, T., SIZARET, P., AND MARTEL, N., 1978, Tumor-specific antigens on rat liver cells transformed *in vitro* by chemical carcinogens, *J. Natl. Cancer Inst.* **60**:125.

ZBAR, B., WEPSIC, H. T., RAPP, H. J., BORSOS, T., KRONMAN, B. S., AND CHURCHILL, W. H., 1969, Antigenic specificity of hepatomas induced in strain-2 guinea pigs by diethlynitrosamine, *J. Natl. Cancer Inst.* **43**:833.

ZBAR, B., WEPSIC, H. T., RAPP, H. J., STEWART, L. C., AND BORSOS, T., 1970, Two-step mechanism of tumor graft rejection in syngeneic guinea pigs. II. Initiation of reaction by a cell fraction containing lymphocytes and neutrophils, *J. Natl. Cancer Inst.* **44**:701.

ZBAR, B., BERNSTEIN, I. D., AND RAPP, H. J., 1971, Suppression of tumor growth at the site of infection with living *bacillus Calmette Guérin*, *J. Natl. Cancer Inst.* **46**:831.

ZBAR, B., BERNSTEIN, I. D., BARTLETT, G. L., HANNA, G., AND RAPP, H. J., 1972a, Immunotherapy of cancer: Regression of intradermal tumors and prevention of growth of lymph node metastases after intralesional injection of living *Mycobacterium bovis*, *J. Natl. Cancer Inst.* **49**:119.

ZBAR, B., RAPP, H. J., AND RIBI, E. E., 1972b, Tumor suppression by cell walls of *Mycobacterium bovis* attached to oil droplets, *J. Natl. Cancer Inst.* **48**:831.

ZINKERNAGEL, R. M., AND DOHERTY, P. C., 1977, Major transplantation antigens, viruses, and specificity of surveillance T cells, *Contemp. Top. Immunobiol.* **7**:179.

ZÖLLER, M., PRICE, M. R., AND BALDWIN, R. W., 1975, Cell-mediated cytotoxicity to chemically induced rat tumours, *Int. J. Cancer* **16**:593.

ZÖLLER, M., PRICE, M. R., AND BALDWIN, R. W., 1976, Inhibition of cell-mediated cytotoxicity to chemically induced rat tumours by soluble tumour and embryo cell extracts, *Int. J. Cancer* **17**:129.

ZÖLLER, M., PRICE, M. R., AND BALDWIN, R. W., 1977, Evaluation of ^{51}Cr release for detecting cell-mediated cytotoxic responses to solid chemically-induced rat tumours, *Br. J. Cancer* **35**:834.

Physical Carcinogenesis

Physical Carcinogenesis: Radiation—History and Sources

ARTHUR C. UPTON

1. Introduction

More than half a century has elapsed since the carcinogenic effects of radiation were first recorded. Study of such effects has since received continuing impetus from the early and expanding uses of radiation in diagnosis and therapy, and from the far-reaching applications of nuclear technology in science, medicine, and industry. In historical perspective, the effects of radiation have received greater study than those of any other physical agent of comparable environmental significance. As such, our experience with radiation is applicable to the study and control of other environmental carcinogens.

It is beyond the scope of this report to review in detail the vast literature on biological and carcinogenic effects of radiation. An attempt will be made herein merely to survey those historical aspects which are of major relevance to the accompanying chapters on carcinogenesis.

2. Types of Radiations

Carcinogenic activity has been documented for radiations of the electromagnetic spectrum (Fig. 1) and for corpuscular, or particulate, radiations. Of the electromagnetic radiations, only ultraviolet radiations and the ionizing radiations

ARTHUR C. UPTON ● Health Sciences Center, State University of New York at Stony Brook, Stony Brook, New York.

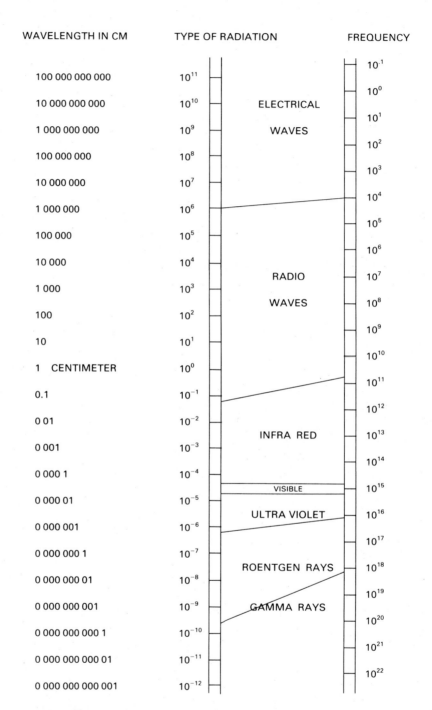

FIGURE 1. The electromagnetic spectrum, showing wavelength and frequency of the different bands. From Glasser (1944).

(γ-rays, X-rays) are known to possess carcinogenic properties, whereas corpuscular radiations (α-particles, β-particles, protons, neutrons), which are also ionizing, have been found to be carcinogenic in every case investigated.

As is discussed elsewhere, the carcinogenic effects of ultraviolet radiation (Urbach, this volume) and of the ionizing radiations (Kellerer and Rossi, this volume; Storer, this volume) are attributed to their production of physicochemical changes in critical macromolecular constituents (e.g., DNA) of cells in which they are absorbed. Only small amounts of energy need be involved, the lethal dose of ionizing radiation for mammals being of the order of 10^{-3} cal/g, deposited randomly in discrete events averaging about 60 eV each (Hutchinson and Rauth, 1962). Although the biological effects of radiation cannot be defined fully as yet at the molecular level, knowledge of the effects of radiation on DNA has advanced rapidly, and it is now known that effects on DNA may be influenced profoundly by biological repair processes. Among the changes in DNA attributable to ultraviolet irradiation, formation of pyrimidine dimers is considered to be foremost in importance, while the changes in DNA attributable to ionizing radiation include base alteration, base destruction, sugar–phosphate bond cleavage, chain breakage (single-strand and double-strand), crosslinking of strands (intrastrand and interstrand), and degradation (Kanazir, 1969). Double-strand breaks, which are thought to constitute roughly 7–10% of all the breaks induced by X-irradiation in mammalian cells, are estimated to require approximately 600 eV per break (Corry and Cole, 1968), compared to 44 eV per break for single-strand breaks (Lehman and Ormerod, 1970). Either type of strand break may, if repaired incorrectly, lead to more complicated changes in the affected DNA, including base-pair alterations and deletions such as have been implicated in radiation mutagenesis (Malling and De Serres, 1969).

It is now amply clear that the induction of a mutagenic or carcinogenic effect in DNA must be viewed as the end result of a sequence of reactions, the outcome of which may depend as much on the influence of repair mechanisms as on the nature of the primary lesion itself (Fox and Lajtha, 1973). At least three types of DNA repair have been noted in bacteria: (1) photoenzymatic repair, (2) excision repair, and (3) postreplication (recombinational) repair (United Nations, 1972; Fox and Lajtha, 1973). Excision repair, through which pyrimidine dimers are removed from affected DNA, is deficient in many patients suffering from xeroderma pigmentosum, the deficiency itself presumably accounting for their photosensitivity (see Urbach, this volume). This type of repair also varies in effectiveness among different mammalian cell lines. Photoenzymatic repair has not been found in mammals other than marsupials. Because both types of repair involve enzyme systems that are affected by genetic, physiological, metabolic, and environmental factors (Fox and Lajtha, 1973), their role in mutagenesis and carcinogenesis can be characterized only in a general way. Further complicating assessment of their role is our uncertainty concerning the relationship between the DNA in mammalian cells and its associated nucleoprotein, which also appears to undergo alteration and repair following irradiation (United Nations, 1972; Fox and Lajtha, 1973).

3. Sources and Levels of Radiation in the Environment

ARTHUR C.
UPTON

Man has evolved in the continuous presence of radiations, which vary with altitude, latitude, and other environmental factors (Bener, 1969; Stair, 1969; National Academy of Sciences, 1972; United Nations, 1972; Urbach, this volume). The levels of ionizing radiation received by the general population from various sources are summarized in Table 1. From inspection of the table, it is evident that

TABLE 1

Estimated Average Annual Whole-Body Dose Rates in the United States (1970)

Source	Average dose rate[a] (mrem/yr)
Environmental	
Natural	
Cosmic rays	44
Terrestrial radiation	
External	40
Internal (mostly from ^{40}K)	18
Subtotal	102
Global fallout	4
Nuclear power	0.003
SUBTOTAL	106
Medical	
Diagnostic	72[b]
Radiopharmaceuticals	1
SUBTOTAL	73
Occupational	0.8
Miscellaneous	2
TOTAL	182

From NAS–NRC (1972).

[a] The numbers shown are average values only. For given segments of the population, dose rates considerably greater than those may be experienced.
[b] Based on the abdominal dose.

the major source of exposure to manmade radiation is the use of X-rays in medical diagnosis. Other manmade sources contribute as yet only such a minute percentage to the overall exposure that even though they may be expected to increase in magnitude within the foreseeable future, their total importance is likely to remain relatively small (National Academy of Sciences, 1972; United Nations, 1972).

4. *Historical Developments in Carcinogenesis by Ionizing Radiation*   555

PHYSICAL
CAR-
CINOGENESIS:
RADIATION—
HISTORY AND
SOURCES

4.1. Observations in Humans

Study of radiation carcinogenesis in human populations is complicated by several difficulties: (1) Cancer is sufficiently rare that large populations must be studied to define the incidence of neoplasms at any one site, few populations being large enough or exposed to high enough doses to yield quantitative dose-incidence data for specific malignancies. (2) Even in such populations, the latent period intervening between irradiation and the appearance of neoplasms is so long that it hampers the follow-up of exposed individuals and the evaluation of their absorbed dose. (3) Because of the length of the latent period, none of the irradiated populations investigated to date has been followed long enough to disclose the cumulative lifetime effects of radiation on the incidence of cancer. (4) Many of the existing dose–incidence data have been derived from patients exposed to radiation for medical purposes, in whom the effects of radiation are complicated by effects of other forms of treatment or by effects of the underlying disease itself. (5) Some of the existing data are based on effects of internally deposited radionuclides, interpretation of which is complicated by variations of the radiation dose in space and time. (6) The natural incidence of cancer varies so widely from one organ to another and under the influence of so many variables (e.g., genetic background, age, sex, geographic location, diet, socioeconomic factors) that dose–incidence data derived from one population may not be strictly applicable to another.

4.1.1. Early Radiologists and Radiation Workers

The first neoplasm attributed to radiation was an epidermoid carcinoma on the hand of a radiologist (Frieben, 1902), followed by dozens of similar cases in ensuing decades, owing in part to the practice among pioneer radiographers of exposing their hands repeatedly in focusing their primitive fluoroscopic equipment. The manifestations of injury in such victims commonly began with reddening and blistering of the skin, often within weeks after exposure. Whether or not exposure was then discontinued, the lesions frequently remained painful and were accompanied by paresthesia, anesthesia, throbbing, and tenderness. Within a few years, they were characteristically followed by atrophy of the epidermis and development of keratoses from which malignant cells frequently extended into the dermis. Many of the carcinomas arising in this way were multiple and occurred on both hands. Within 15 yr after Roentgen's discovery of the X-ray, 94 cases of skin cancer had been attributed to radiation among physicians, X-ray technicians, and radium handlers in America, England, and Germany (Hesse, 1911). The neoplasms were predominantly squamous cell and basal cell carcinomas but also included fibrosarcomas (Furth and Lorenz, 1954). Because the development of such tumors characteristically required a long induction period (averaging 10–39 yr), with radiation dermatitis preceding the appearance of the tumors themselves, it was generally thought that tumor induction would not occur unless preceded by gross radiation damage to the skin (see Furth and Lorenz, 1954). Although tumors have since been reported to follow irradiation in normal-appearing skin (see International Commission on Radiological Protection, 1969), they have ceased to be an occupational disease of radiologists. Radiodermatitis and skin cancer may continue to occur, however, among those using radiation equipment without adequate safeguards (Mohs, 1952).

The induction of leukemia by ionizing radiation was also first tentatively reported because of clustering of 5 cases of leukemia in pioneer radiation workers (von Jagie *et al.*, 1911). Since then, the leukemogenic action of ionizing radiation has been amply confirmed by epidemiological studies in radiation workers and in other irradiated populations, over 200 cases of "radiation-induced" leukemia appearing in the world literature between 1911 and 1959 (Cronkite *et al.*, 1960).

4.1.2. Dial Painters

The induction of bone tumors by radiation was first observed in dial painters (see Martland, 1931; Looney, 1958) who had ingested radium in applying luminous paint to clock and watch dials, through the practice of pointing their brushes between their lips. In addition to osteosarcomas, such victims showed an excess of fibrosarcomas and carcinomas of paranasal and mastoid sinuses (Aub *et al.*, 1952; Marinelli, 1958; Looney, 1958). The development of the tumors was usually preceded by radiation osteitis, characterized by coarsening of trabeculae and necrosis of bone, with rarefaction, formation of atypical osseous tissue, and localized calcification (Aub *et al.*, 1952; Looney, 1958). The latent period for induction of the tumors varied inversely with the radium content of the skeleton, being as short as 10 yr in patients with 6–50 μg of radium and more than 25 yr in those with smaller radium burdens (Evans, 1966). The incidence of bone tumors has been interpreted to vary roughly as the square of the terminal concentration of radium in the skeleton, exceeding 20% at levels of 5 μCi or more, but with no evidence of tumor induction at levels of less than 0.5 μCi (National Academy of Sciences, 1972; United Nations, 1972). Interpretation of the dose–incidence relation is complicated by the inhomogeneity of the radiation dose in space and time, the radium being localized in hot spots, and the amount present in the skeleton at the time the tumors have been detected being only a small percentage of that present earlier.

4.1.3. Miners of Radioactive Ore

Carcinoma of the lung, long known to be an occupational disability of pitchblend miners in Saxony and Bohemia, has only recently been attributed to irradiation by radon in this population (Weller, 1956). U.S. uranium miners have likewise shown an excess of pulmonary carcinomas, varying with the duration and intensity of their exposure, even after correction for such variables as age, cigarette smoking, "heredity, urbanization, self-selection, diagnostic accuracy, prior hard-rock mining, nonradioactive-ore constituents, including silica dust" (Lundin *et al.*, 1971). A comparable excess of bronchial carcinoma has been noted in other hard-rock miners who are similarly exposed to radon and its radioactive disintegration products (National Academy of Sciences, 1972; United Nations, 1972).

The duration of exposure among affected U.S. uranium miners averages 15–20 yr; however, the cumulative dose responsible for tumorigenesis in any given individual cannot be estimated precisely, owing to the following sources of uncertainty: (1) The miners received their irradiation primarily from inhaling radon and its radioactive disintegration products present in the atmosphere of the mines in concentrations which were measured only infrequently within the 2500 mines in question. (2) The concentration of radioactivity in the air of a given mine varied from time to time and from one part of the mine to another, depending on operating conditions, ventilation, meteorological factors, the quality of the ore being extracted, and other variables. (3) The dose of radiation delivered by the radon and its radioactive decay products varied from one region of the respiratory tract to another, depending on the extent to which the radionuclides were adsorbed to aerosols, dust, or other particulates, and on the physiochemical properties of the inhaled atmosphere and any aerosols or particulates it may have contained. (4) The radiation dose received from a given level of total radioactivity—expressed in "working level" (WL) units or "working level months" (WLM)—varied, depending on the relative proportions of radon and its several radioactive decay products which were inhaled and subsequently cleared from the lung. (5) The dose of radiation delivered to the cancer-forming cells may be expected to have varied, depending on (a) the identity of the cells in question (which is uncertain, although such cells are generally presumed to be the basal cells of the bronchial epithelium), (b) the thickness of the bronchial epithelium and overlying mucous layers in different segments of the respiratory tract (which may vary in the presence of bronchitis or other inflammation), and (c) the rate of clearance of adsorbed radioactive particulates. (6) The fraction of the total dose that was responsible for tumor induction in a given miner cannot be distinguished from that part of his dose which he received after his tumor had been elicited and which was to that extent superfluous. (7) Most miners worked in more than one mine during their careers, often intermittently and irregularly, receiving a considerable fraction of their total cumulative radiation exposure in hard-rock mines other than uranium mines. (8) The radiation received by the miners consisted of a complex mixture of γ-rays, β-radiations, and α-particles, the relative contributions of which cannot be assessed precisely, owing in part to uncertainty about the relative biological effectiveness of the α-particles. (9) Most of the miners were cigarette smokers, necessitating correction for the known carcinogenic effects of smoking (Lundin *et al.*, 1969; National Academy of Sciences, 1972; United Nations, 1972), and the data have suggested that the combined effects of smoking and irradiation exceeded those to be expected from simple additivity of the effects of each factor alone (Lundin *et al.*, 1969).

4.1.4. Patients Exposed to Radiation for Medical Purposes

A number of patients exposed to large doses of radiation delivered therapeutically to various regions of the body have been evaluated for subsequent changes in cancer incidence. These populations include (1) patients given X-ray therapy to the mediastinum in infancy for enlargment of the thymus or other conditions, in whom an excess of thyroid tumors, leukemias, osteochondromas, salivary gland tumors, and other neoplams in irradiated sites has been observed (Hempelmann, 1969; National Academy of Sciences, 1972); (2) patients given X-ray therapy to the spine for ankylosing spondylitis, in whom an excess of leukemias and tumors in certain irradiated sites (e.g., lung, bone, pharnx, pancreas, stomach) has been observed (Court Brown and Doll, 1957, 1965); (3) patients sterilized by pelvic X-irradiation for treatment of menorrhagia, in whom an excess of leukemias and gastrointestinal tumors has been observed (see Pochin, 1972; National Academy of Sciences, 1972); (4) patients treated with X-rays for various nonneoplastic disorders, in whom solid tumors (chiefly sarcomas) have been observed to arise subsequently at the site of irradiation Cade, 1957); (5) patients treated with phosphorus-32 for polycythemia vera, in whom an excess of leukemias has been observed (see Wald *et al.*, 1962: National Academy of Sciences, 1972); (6) patients treated with radium-226 for ankylosing spondylitis or tuberculosis of the skeleton, in whom an excess of osteosarcomas and osteochondromas has been observed (Spiess and Mays, 1970); (7) patients given X-ray therapy to the mammary gland for postpartum mastitis, in whom an excess of carcinomas of the breast has been observed (National Academy of Sciences, 1972); (8) patients treated with iodine-131 for adenocarcinoma of the thyroid gland, in whom an excess of leukemias has been observed (Pochin, 1969); and (9) patients treated for various other conditions in whom an excess of malignancies has been observed (National Academy of Sciences, 1972; United Nations, 1972).

Certain groups of patients exposed to radiation for diagnostic examination have also revealed an excess of some types of cancer, e.g. (1) women subjected to repeated fluoroscopic examination of the lung in the treatment of pulmonary tuberculosis, who have been observed to show an excess of carcinoma of the breast (Mackenzie, 1965; Myrden and Hiltz, 1969); (2) children exposed prenatally in the diagnosic examination of their mothers, who have been found to show an excess incidence of leukemia and other childhood malignancies (Stewart *et al.*, 1958; MacMahon and Hutchison, 1964; National Academy of Sciences, 1972); (3) patients injected intravascularly with thorium oxide (thorotrast) for angiographic examination, who have shown an increased incidence of leukemia, hemangioendotheliomas of the liver, and certain other tumors (de Silva Horta *et al.*, 1965); and (4) patients examined radiographically for various other conditions (National Academy of Sciences, 1972).

4.1.5. Japanese Atomic Bomb Survivors

The incidence of leukemia in Japanese atomic bomb survivors appeared to become elevated within 5 yr after irradiation and to remain elevated to a lesser degree 25 yr later (Ishimaru *et al.*, 1971; National Academy of Sciences, 1972; United Nations, 1972). As in other irradiated human populations, the leukemias included all types except the chronic lymphocytic type (National Academy of Sciences, 1972). The data for Hiroshima implied a linear dose–incidence relationship, whereas the data for Nagasaki implied a sigmoid dose–incidence relationship, differences which are consistent with experiments on leukemia induction in mice, in view of the differences in the relative proportions of fast neutrons and γ-rays received in the two cities, fast neutrons predominating at Hiroshima but making a negligible contribution to the dose in Nagasaki (National Academy of Sciences, 1972).

The incidence of malignancies other than leukemia became elevated in the survivors after a latency substantially longer than the latency for leukemias (National Academy of Sciences, 1972). The neoplasms appearing in excess include thyroid carcinomas, carcinomas of the breast, bronchial carcinomas, and tumors of gastrointestinal organs (National Academy of Sciences, 1972).

Dose–induction data, although preliminary, imply that susceptibility to the induction of cancer was higher in children than in those who were irradiated as adults (Jablon and Kato, 1970; National Academy of Sciences, 1972).

4.1.6. Marshallese Exposed to Fallout

Among natives of the Marshall Islands who were accidentally exposed to nuclear fallout from a weapon test in 1954, the incidence of thyroid nodules increased from zero to more than 80% between 8 and 16 yr after exposure in those who were heavily irradiated at less than 10 yr of age (Conard *et al.*, 1970). In some victims, the development of tumors was associated with hypothyroidism. The dose to the thyroid in such cases was estimated to approximate 700–1400 rads from internally deposited radioiodine and 175 rads from external γ-rays. Less than 10% of persons exposed at ages older than 10 yr developed tumors, and no tumors were observed in unexposed controls.

4.2. Observations in Experimental Animals

Within less than a decade after the first observations of radiation-induced cancer in humans, studies on the experimental induction of tumors in laboratory animals were reported (Table 2). Since then, neoplasms of virtually every type have been induced experimentally. The early literature on the subject has been reviewed by Lacassagne (1945*a,b*), Brues (1951), and Furth and Lorenz (1954). More recent reviews have been published by Casarett (1965), Upton (1967), and the United Nations (1972).

From experimental studies on radiation carcinogenesis, the following conclusions can be made: (1) Neoplasms of virtually any type can be induced, given appropriate conditions of irradiation and animals of suitable susceptibility. (2) Irradiation may influence the pathogenesis of neoplasia through a variety of

TABLE 2

Early Experiments on Radiation Carcinogenesis

Author	Date	Radiation or isotope	Species	Type of tumor
Marie *et al.*	1910	X-ray	Rat	Sarcoma, spindle-celled
Marie *et al.*	1912	X-ray	Rat	Sarcoma, spindle-celled
Lazarus-Barlow	1918	Ra	Mouse, rat	Carcinoma of skin
Bloch	1923	X-ray	Rabbit	Carcinoma
Bloch	1924	X-ray	Rabbit	Carcinoma
Goebel and Gérard	1925	X-ray	Guinea pig	Sarcoma, polymorphous
Daels	1925	Ra	Mouse, rat	Sarcoma, spindle-celled
Jonkhoff	1927	X-ray	Mouse	Carcinoma-sarcoma
Lacassagne and Vinzent	1929	X-ray	Rabbit	Fibrosarcoma, osteosarcoma, rhabdomyosarcoma
Schürch	1930	X-ray	Rabbit	Carcinoma
Daels and Biltris	1931	Ra	Rat	Sarcoma of cranium, kidney, spleen
Daels and Biltris	1931	Ra	Guinea pig	Sarcoma of cranium, kidney, spleen
Daels and Biltris	1937	Ra	Chicken	Carcinoma of biliary tract, osteosarcoma
Schürch and Uehlinger	1931	Ra	Rabbit	Sarcoma of bone, liver, spleen
Uehlinger and Schürch	1935–1947	Ra, Ms-Th	Rabbit	Sarcoma of bone, liver, spleen
Sabin *et al.*	1932	Ra, Ms-Th	Rabbit	Osteosarcoma
Lacassagne	1933	X-ray	Rabbit	Sarcoma, spindle-celled, myxosarcoma
Petrov and Krotkina	1933	Ra	Guinea pig	Carcinoma of biliary tract
Sedginidse	1933	X-ray	Mouse	Carcinoma, spindle-celled
Ludin	1934	X-ray	Rabbit	Chondrosarcoma

From Lacassagne (1945*a,b*), Furth and Lorenz (1954), and Upton (1968).

changes, some of which involve direct effects on the tumor-forming cells themselves, and others indirect effects on distant cells or organs (Cole and Nowell, 1965; Upton, 1967). (3) In certain experimentally induced neoplasms, oncogenic viruses may be implicated, but the nature of their role and their general significance for radiation carcinogenesis remain to be disclosed (Upton, 1967; United Nations, 1972). (4) The dose–effect relation for carcinogenesis is not precisely known for any neoplasm over a wide range of dose, dose rate, and linear energy transfer (LET); however, radiations of higher LET, such as α-particles and fast neutrons, are generally more effective than radiations of low LET, such as X-rays and γ-rays, and their effectiveness is less dependent on dose and dose rate (Upton, 1967; United Nations, 1972). (5) The process of neoplasia involves a series of alterations, some of which may precede conception and any of which may conceivably be caused by radiation; hence the dose required for inducing cancer in a given individual may be postulated to depend on the extent to which mechanisms other than radiation contribute to the process. (6) The dose–incidence relation in experimental animals is generally curvilinear, with the following features: (a) in the high dose region, the incidence tends to reach a plateau or to decline with increasing dose, presumably because of excessive injury (Upton, 1967; United Nations, 1972); (b) in the intermediate dose region, the incidence tends to rise more steeply with increasing dose than at lower or higher dose levels; (c) with decreasing dose and dose rate, the curve tends to become shallower, at least in the case of low-LET radiation.

From the foregoing, the cancer biologist is tempted to infer that at low dose levels (1) "initiating" effects of radiation predominate, which are to some extent reversible in incipient stages; (2) these effects may be magnified by other types of effects ("enhancing," "promoting," etc.) at intermediate dose levels; and (3) both types of carcinogenic effects fail to be expressed fully at high dose levels, because of side-effects or excessive injury.

5. Evolution of Radiation Protection Standards

Although it was recognized within months after Roentgen's discovery of the X-ray in 1895 that this form of radiation could cause serious injury to the skin and deeper tissues (Table 3), the first organized efforts to promote radiation safety standards were those of the Roentgen Society in 1916 (Morgan, 1967).

In 1921, the newly formed British X-Ray and Radium Protection Committee considered establishing a maximum tolerance dose, to be defined in terms of a reproducible biological standard and to be expressed insofar as possible in physical units (Stone, 1959). In 1928, the International Committee on Radiological Protection (ICRP) was established, and 1 yr later the Advisory Committee on X-Ray and Radium Protection was formed in the United States, under the sponsorship of leading radiological organizations. In 1931, this committee recommended a tolerance dose of 0.2 R/day (measured in air), which was endorsed in 1934 by IRCP. Two years later, the United States committee reduced

TABLE 3

Early Reports of Radiation Injury Following Discovery of X-Rays by Roentgen in 1895

Date	Type of injury	Reported by
1896	Dermatitis of hands	Grubbé
1896	Smarting of eyes	Edison
1896	Epilation	Daniel
1897	Constitutional symptoms	Walsh
1899	Degeneration of blood vessels	Gassman
1902	Cancer in X-ray ulcer	Frieben
1903	Bone growth inhibited	Perthes
1903	Sterilization produced	Albers-Schonberg
1904	Blood changes produced	Milchner and Mosse
1906	Bone marrow changes demonstrated	Warthin
1911	Leukemia in five radiation workers	Jagie
1912	Anemia in two X-ray workers	Bélére

From Stone (1959).

its recommended tolerance level to 0.1 R/day, in order to conform more closely with the tolerance level in Europe, where the dose was customarily measured on the skin, thus including backscatter, rather than in air as was customary in the United States, and to compensate for the growing prevalence of 200-kv X-ray machines and the resulting increase in the percentage of the surface dose penetrating to deeper parts of the body (Stone, 1959).

Selection of the tolerance level of 0.1 R/day, as opposed to higher or lower levels, was based on study of the occupational exposures of people who had worked with radiation for many years without detectable injury. The number of such people was relatively small, however, and the estimation of their exposure levels highly uncertain. With the advent of nuclear fission, and expansion in the number of radiation workers, it became increasingly important to establish a more reliable tolerance dose, without unnecessarily restricting the development of atomic energy and allied fields. The ensuing stepwise reduction of the maximum permissible dose (Tables 4 and 5) occurred not because of newly documented evidence of injury at previous tolerance levels, but because new knowledge about the effects of low-level radiation implied a need for greater margins of safety.

The large-scale atmospheric testing of nuclear weapons in the 1950s caused growing concern about the hazards of radioactive fallout to the general public. As a result of this concern, a number of national and international groups were formed to consider the risks of low-level irradiation to the general population. In 1955, the United States National Academy of Sciences–National Research Council (NAS–NRC) established a Committee on the Biological Effects of Atomic Radiation, which made a thorough study of the hazards of radiation (see NAS–NRC, 1956, 1960). Similar studies were carried out by the Medical Research Council in England (1956, 1960), and by the United Nations Scientific Committee on the Effects of Atomic Radiation (see United Nations, 1958, 1962, 1964, 1966, 1969). In 1959, the U.S. Congress established the Federal Radiation Council (FRC) (see Palmiter and Tompkins, 1965); this council, in contrast to the aforementioned

563

PHYSICAL
CAR-
CINOGENESIS:
RADIATION—
HISTORY AND
SOURCES

TABLE 4
Some Historical Highlights in the Evolution of Radiation Protection Standards

1902	Rollins established photographic indication of "safe" intensity
1921	British X-Ray and Radium Protection Committee considered "establishing a maximum tolerance dose"
1925	First attempt was made by Mutscheller to define a "tolerance dose"
1931	U.S. Advisory Committee on X-Ray and Radium Protection recommended a dose limit of 0.2 R/day
1936	U.S. Advisory Committee on X-Ray and Radium Protection reduced dose limit to 0.1 R/day
1950	International Commission on Radiological Protection recommended a dose limit of 0.3 R/wk
1956	International Commission on Radiological Protection recommended an occupational dose limit of 5 R/yr
1956	National Academy of Sciences recommended 10 R/30 yr for gonadal dose limit of general population
1960	Federal Radiation Council Recommended 5 R/yr dose limit for radiation workers and 0.17 R/yr dose limit for general population, exclusive of natural background and medical radiation

From Stone (1959) and Upton (1969).

TABLE 5
Historical Sequence of Reductions in Maximum Permissible Doses for Radiation Workers

Exposure period	Maximum permissible doses (R)			
	1931–1936	1936–1948	1948–1956	1956
Per day	0.2	0.1	0.05	
Per 6-day week	1.2	0.6	0.3	0.3
Per 50-wk year	60	15	15	5
Per decade	600	300	150	50
Up to age 60	2400	1200	600	200

From Stone (1957).

groups which had no statutory authority, was mandated to advise the President on radiation matters affecting health. Although legislative responsibility for the regulation of radiation health remained with the states, the Federal Radiation Council was designated as the policy-forming body to advise in the recommendation of radiation standards for all federal agencies.

In its first report (1960), the Federal Radiation Council stated its philosophy about radiation protection policy as follows:

> There is a particular uncertainty with respect to the biological effects at very low doses and dose rates. It is not prudent, therefore, to assume that there is a level of radiation exposure below which there is absolute certainty that no effect may occur.
>
> This consideration, in addition to the adoption of the conservative hypothesis of a linear relation between biological effect and the amount of dose, determines our basic approach to the formulation of radiation protection guides.

Fundamentally, setting basic radiation protection standards involves passing judgment on the extent of the possible health hazards society is willing to accept in order to realize the known benefits of radiation.

There should not be any man-made radiation without the expectation of benefit resulting from such exposure.

The safety standards established by the Federal Radiation Council conformed with the recommendations of the ICRP and the NCRP in stipulating that occupational exposure of the whole body and the most radiosensitive organs of the body (the bone marrow, lens of the eye, and gonads) should not deliver a cumulative dose (in rems) exceeding 5 times the age of the worker (in years) beyond 18 (Table 6). A worker aged 28, for example, would be allowed a

TABLE 6
Radiation Protection Guides

Type of exposure	Duration or condition of exposure	Maximum permissible dose (rems)
Exposure of radiation worker		
Whole body, head and trunk, active blood-forming organs, gonads, or lens of eye	Accumulated dose	5 times number of years beyond age 18
	13 wk	3
Skin of whole body and thyroid	Year	30
	13 wk	10
Hands and forearms, feet and ankles	Year	75
	13 wk	25
Bone	Body Burden	0.1 μg of radium–226 or its biological equivalent
Other organs	Year	15
	13 wk	5
Exposure of general population		
Individual	Year	0.5 (whole body)
Average	30 yr	5 (gonads)

From FRC Report No. 1 (1960).

cumulative total dose of up to 50 rems. A larger dose was considered permissible to a part of the body, such as the thyroid or the skin, since it was presumed to entail less risk than exposure of the whole body or its more radiosensitive organs. The radiation guide for bone was based largely on accumulated knowledge of the effects of internally deposited radium. For the public as opposed to the radiation worker, the protection standards were more conservative, and exposure of the gonads was regarded as the most important consideration. An average gonad dose of only 5 rems per generation (or 30 yr) was specified as the maximum permissible limit because it was thought that this level, which amounted to roughly a doubling of the natural background radiation level, would affect the mutation

565

PHYSICAL
CAR-
CINOGENESIS:
RADIATION—
HISTORY AND
SOURCES

rate only slightly and would not therefore involve serious genetic risk (see NAS–NRC, 1960; ICRP, 1966, United Nations, 1966).

Since publication of the first report of the Federal Radiation Council, epidemiological studies of irradiated populations have disclosed greater evidence of carcinogenic effects of irradiation at low dose levels than had been suspected. As a result of this new evidence, risk estimates imply the possibility that the risk of cancer associated with low-level radiation may be comparable in magnitude to the risk of genetic effects (NAS–NRC, 1972), i.e., that up to 1–2% of the natural cancer incidence may be attributable to background radiation (NAS–NRC, 1972). It is considered increasingly important, therefore, that the dose to the individual, as well as the average dose to the population, be kept as low as is practicable (NAS–NRC, 1972).

Since the average gonadal dose to the population from medical exposure nearly equals that from natural background (Table 1), growing attention is being given to limitation of the doses involved in medical and dental practice (NAS–NRC, 1972). Methods for reducing the dose to the patient from medical exposure include (1) reduction of the number of radiographs per patient with avoidance of all unnecessary exposure, (2) reduction of the duration and intensity of exposure per radiograph, (3) use of radiography in preference to fluoroscopy whenever possible, (4) reduction of field size to a minimum, (5) shielding of tissues outside the field to be examined, especially the gonads, (6) proper training of staff engaged in radiological examinations, and (7) proper calibration and optimal operation of radiological apparatus (IRCP, 1960).

6. References

AUB, J. C., EVANS, R. D., HEMPELMANN, L. H., AND MARTLAND, H. S., 1952, The late effects of internally-deposited radioactive materials in man, *Medicine* **31(3)**:221–329.

BENER, P., 1969, Spectral intensity of natural ultraviolet radiation and its dependence on various parameters, in: *The Biologic Effects of Ultraviolet Radiation* (F. Urbach, ed.), pp. 351–358, Pergamon Press, New York.

BRUES, A. M., 1951, Carcinogenic effects of radiation, *Advan. Biol. Med. Phys.* **2**:171–191.

CADE, S., 1957, Radiation induced cancer in man, *Brit. J. Radiol.* **30**:393–402.

CASARETT, G. W., 1965, Experimental radiation carcinogenesis, *Prog. Exp. Tumor Res.* **7**:82.

COLE L. J., AND NOWELL, P. C., 1965, Radiation carcinogenesis: The Sequence of events, *Science* **150**:1782.

CONARD, R. A., DOBYNS, B. M., AND SUTOW, W. W., 1970, Thyroid neoplasia as a late effect of acute exposure to radioactive iodines in fallout, *JAMA* **214**:316–324.

CORRY, P. M., AND COLE, A., 1968, Radiation-induced double strand scission of the DNA mammalian metaphase chromosomes, *Radiation Res.* **36**:528–543.

COURT BROWN, W. M., AND DOLL, R., 1957, *Leukemia and Aplastic Anemia in Patients Irradiated for Ankylosing Spondylitis*, Medical Research Special Report Series, No. 295, H.M.S.O., London.

COURT BROWN, W. M., AND DOLL, R., 1965, Mortality from cancer and other causes after radiotherapy for ankylosing spondylitis, *Brit. Med. J.* **2**:1327–1332.

CRONKITE, E. P., MOLONEY, W., AND BOND, V. P., 1960, Radiation leukemogenesis, an analysis of the problem, *Am. J. Med.* **5**:673–682.

DE SILVA HORTA, J., ABBAT, J. D., CAYOLLA DA MOTTA, L. A. R. C., AND RORIZ, M. L., 1965, Malignancy and other late effects following administration of thorotrast, *Lancet* **2**:201.

EVANS, R. D., 1966, The effects of skeletally deposited alpha-ray emitters in man, *Brit. J. Radiol.* **39:**881–895.

FEDERAL RADIATION COUNCIL, 1960, *Report No. 1: Background Material for the Development of Radiation Protection Standards*, Government Printing Office, Washington, D.C.

FOX, B. W., AND LAJTHA, L. G., 1973, Radiation damage and repair, *Brit. Med. Bull.* **29:**16–22.

FRIEBEN, A., 1902, Demonstration lines cancroids des rechten Handrückens, das sich nach lang-dauernder Einwirkung von Röntgenstrahlen entwickelt hatte, *Fortschr. Geb. Röntgenstr.* **6:**106.

FRUTH, J., AND LORENZ, E., 1954, Carcinogenesis by ionizing radiations, in: *Radiation Biology*, Vol. 1 (A. Hollaender, ed.), pp. 1145–1201, McGraw-Hill, New York.

GLASSER, O., 1944, Radiation spectrum, in: *Medical Physics* (O. Glasser, ed.), p. 1969, Year Book Publishers, Chicago.

HEMPELMANN, L. H., 1969, Risk of thyroid neoplasms after irradiation in childhood, *Science* **160:**159–163.

HESSE, O., 1911, *Symptomalologie, Pathogenese und Therapie des Röntgenkarzinoms*, J. A. Barth, Leipzig.

HUTCHINSON, F., AND RAUTH, A. M., 1962, The characteristics of the energy loss of spectrum for fast electrons which are important in radiation biology, *Radiation Res.* **16:**598.

INTERNATIONAL COMMISSION ON RADIOLOGICAL PROTECTION, 1960, *Report of Committee III: Protection Against X-Rays up to Energies of 3 Mev and Beta- and Gamma-Rays from Sealed Sources*, Pergamon Press, New York.

INTERNATIONAL COMMISSION ON RADIOLOGICAL PROTECTION, 1966, The evaluation of risks from radiation, *Health Phys.* **12:**239–302.

INTERNATIONAL COMMISSION ON RADIOLOGICAL PROTECTION, 1969, *Publication 14: Radiosensitivity and Spatial Distribution of Dose*, Reports prepared by Two Task Groups of Committee 1 of the International Commission on Radiological Protection, Pergamon Press, New York.

ISHIMARU, T., HOSHIMO, T., ICHIMARU, M., OKADA, A., TOMIYASU, T., TSUCHIMOTO, T., AND YAMAMOTO, T., 1971, Leukemia in atomic bomb survivors, Hiroshima and Nagasaki, 1 October 1950–30 September, 1966, *Radiation Res.* **45:**216–233.

JABLON, S., AND KATO, H., 1970, Childhood cancer in relation to prenatal exposure to A-bomb radiation, *Lancet* **2:**1000–1003.

KANAZIR, D. T., 1969, Radiation-induced alterations in the structure of deoxyribonucleic acid and their biological consequences, in: *Progress in Nucleic Acid Research and Molecular Biology*, Vol. 9, pp. 117–122, Academic Press, New York.

LACASSAGNE, A., 1945a, Les cancers produits par les rayonnements corpusculaires; mécanisme présumable de la cancerisation par les rayons, in *Actualities Scientifiques et Industrielles*, No. 981, Hermann et Cie, Paris.

LACASSAGNE, A., 1945b, Les cancers produits par les rayonnements électromagnétiques, in *Actualités Scientifiques et Industrielles*, No. 975, Hermann et Cie, Paris.

LEHMAN, A. R., AND ORMEROD, M. G., 1970, The replication of DNA in murine lymphoma cells (L5178Y). 1. Rate of replication, *Biochim. Biophys. Acta* **204:**128–143.

LOONEY, W. B., 1958, Effects of radium in man, *Science* **127:**630–633.

LUNDIN, F. E., LLOYD, J. W., SMITH, E. M., ARCHER, V. E., AND HOLADAY, D. A., 1969, Mortality of uranium miners in relation to radiation exposure, hard rock mining, and cigarette smoking—1950 through September, 1967, *Health Phys.* **16:**571–578.

LUNDIN, F. E., JR., WAGONER, J. K., AND ARCHER, V. E., 1971, *Radon Daughter Exposure and Respiratory Cancer: Quantitative and Temporal Aspects*, NIOSH–HIEHS Joint Monograph No. 1, U.S. Public Health Service, Bethesda, Md.

MACKENZIE, I., 1965, Breast cancer following multiple fluoroscopies. *Brit. J. Cancer* **19:**1–8.

MACMAHON, B., AND HUTCHISON, G. B., 1964, Prenatal X-ray and childhood cancer: A review, *Acta Unio Int. Contra Cancrum* **20:**1172–1174.

MALLING, H. V., AND DE SERRES, E. J., 1969, Identification of the spectrums of X-ray-induced intragenic alterations at the molecular level in *Neurospora crassa*, *Jap. J. Genet.* **44:**61 (Suppl. 2).

MARINELLI, L. D., 1958, Radioactivity and the human skeleton, *Am. J. Roentgenol.* **80:**729–739.

MARTLAND, H. S., 1931, The occurrence of malignancy in radioactive persons: A general review of data gathered in the study of the radium dial painters, with special reference to the occurrence of osteogenic sarcoma and the interrelationship of certain blood diseases, *Am. J. Cancer* **15:**2435–2516.

MEDICAL RESEARCH COUNCIL, 1956, *The Hazards to Man of Nuclear and Allied Radiations*, H.M.S.O., London.

567

PHYSICAL
CAR-
CINOGENESIS:
RADIATION—
HISTORY AND
SOURCES

MEDICAL RESEARCH COUNCIL, 1960, *The Hazards to Man of Nuclear and Allied Radiations: A Second Report to the Medical Research Council*, H.M.S.O., London.

MOHS, T. B., 1952, Roentgen-ray cancer of the hands of dentists, *J. Am. Dent. Assoc.* **45:**160–164.

MORGAN, K. Z., 1967, History of damage and protection from ionizing radiation, in *Principles of Radiation Protection: A Textbook of Health Physics* (K. Z. Morgan and J. E. Turner, eds.), pp. 1–75, Wiley, New York.

MYRDEN, J. A., AND HILTZ, J. E., 1969, Breast cancer following multiple fluoroscopies during artificial pneumothorax treatment of pulmonary tuberculosis, *Canad. Med. Assoc. J.* **100:**1032–1034.

NATIONAL ACADEMY OF SCIENCES–NATIONAL RESEARCH COUNCIL, 1956, *The Biological Effects of Atomic Radiation: Summary Reports*, Washington, D.C.

NATIONAL ACADEMY OF SCIENCES–NATIONAL RESEARCH COUNCIL, 1960, *The Biological Effects of Atomic Radiation: Summary Reports*, Washington, D.C.

NATIONAL ACADEMY OF SCIENCES–NATIONAL RESEARCH COUNCIL, 1972, *The Effects on Populations of Exposure to Low Levels of Ionizing Radiation*, Report of the Advisory Committee on the Biological Effects of Ionizing Radiations, Washington, D.C.

PALMITER, C. C., AND TOMPKINS, P. C., 1965, Guides, standards, and regulations from the Federation Radiation Council point of view, *Health Phys.* **2:**865–868.

POCHIN, E. E., 1969, Long-term hazards of radioiodine treatment of thyroid cancer in: *Thyroid Cancer*, UICC Monograph Series, Vol. 12, pp. 293–304, Springer, Berlin.

POCHIN, E. E., 1972, Frequency of induction of malignancies in man by ionizing radiation, in: *Encyclopedia of Medical Radiology* (A. Zuppinger and O. Hug, eds.), pp. 341–355, Springer, Berlin.

SPIESS, H., AND MAYS, C. W., 1970, Bone cancers induced by 224 ra (Th X) in children and adults, *Health Phys.* **19:**713–720.

STAIR, R., 1969, Measurement of natural ultraviolet radiation: Historical and general introduction, in: *The Biologic Effects of Ultraviolet Radiation* (F. Urbach, ed.), pp. 377–390, Pergamon Press, New York.

STEWART, A., WEBB, J., AND HEWITT, D. A., 1958, A survey of childhood malignancies, *Brit. Med. J.* **1:**1495–1508.

STONE, R. S., 1957, Common sense in radiation protection applied to clinical practice, *Am. J. Roentgenol. Radium Ther. Nuclear Med.* **78:**993–999.

STONE, R. S., 1959, Maximum permissible exposure standards, in: *Protection in Diagnostic Radiology*, Rutgers University Press, New Brunswick, N.J.

UNITED NATIONS, 1958, *Report of the United Nations Scientific Committee on the Effects of Atomic Radiation*, General Assembly, Official Records: 13th Session, Suppl. No. 17 (A/3838), New York.

UNITED NATIONS, 1962, *Report of the United Nations Scientific Committee on the Effects of Atomic Radiation*, General Assembly, Official Records: 17th Session, Suppl. No. 16 (A/5216), New York.

UNITED NATIONS, 1964, *Report of the United Nations Scientific Committee on the Effects of Atomic Radiation*, General Assembly, Official Records: 19th Session Suppl. No. 14 (A/5814), New York.

UNITED NATIONS, 1966, *Report of the United Nations Scientific Committee on the Effects of Atomic Radiation*, General Assembly, Official Records: 21st Session, Suppl. No. 14 (A/6314), New York.

UNITED NATIONS, 1969, *Report of the United Nations Scientific Committee on the Effects of Atomic Radiation*, Official Records of the General Assembly, 24th Session, Suppl. No. 13 (A/7613), New York.

UNITED NATIONS, 1972, *Ionizing Radiation: Levels and Effects, A Report of the United Nations Scientific Committee on the Effects of Atomic Radiation*, General Assembly, Official Records: 27th Session, Suppl. No. 25 (A/8725), New York.

UPTON, A. C., 1967, Comparative observations on radiation carcinogenesis in man and animals, in: *Carcinogenesis: A Broad Critique* pp. 631–675, University of Texas, M. D. Anderson Hospital and Tumor Institute, Williams and Wilkins, Baltimore.

UPTON, A. C., 1968, Radiation carcinogenesis, in: *Methods in Cancer Research*, Vol. IV (H. Busch, ed.), pp. 53–82, Academic Press, New York.

VON JAGIE, N., SCWARZ, G., AND VON SIENBENROCK, L., 1911, Blutbefunde bei Rontgenologon, *Berl. Klin. Wschr.* **48:**1220–1222.

WALD, N., THOMA, G. E., JR., AND BROWN, G., 1962, Hematologic manifestations of radiation exposure in man, in: *Progress in Hematology*, Vol. 3, pp. 1–52, Grune and Stratton, New York.

WELLER, C. V., 1956, *Causal Factors in Cancer of the Lung*, pp. 43–47, Thomas, Springfield, Ill.

16

Biophysical Aspects of Radiation Carcinogenesis

ALBRECHT M. KELLERER AND HARALD H. ROSSI

1. Introduction

Although radiation carcinogenesis was recognized some 75 years ago, we still know little about the mechanisms involved. Because of its profoundly important theoretical and practical aspects, the subject has been very extensively studied, but most of the information obtained has been of a phenomenological nature. It seems unlikely that a complete step-by-step description of radiogenic cancer induction will be possible in the foreseeable future. Merely the first purely physical process—that of energy deposition by charged particles—is highly complex and difficult to quantitate. There is every reason to believe that the ensuing physicochemical, biochemical, intracellular, intercellular, and systemic processes are at least as complex and that many of them are unknown at this time.

Between the two extremes of a purely descriptive treatment of a phenomenon and the detailed knowledge of the causal chain of events responsible for it can be intermediate levels of understanding. Sometimes these can be based on generally observed or otherwise deduced basic features that permit the formulation of basic kinetics. This in turn can furnish clues concerning its mechanism. An example of this kind of understanding are the laws of Mendelian genetics, which formulated the basic laws of inheritance before the underlying cytogenetic and molecular mechanisms were recognized.

ALBRECHT M. KELLERER ● Institut für Medizinische Strahlenkunde, University of Würzburg, Würzburg, Federal Republic of Germany.
HARALD H. ROSSI ● Radiological Research Laboratory, Department of Radiology, Cancer Center/Institute of Cancer Research, Columbia University College of Physicians and Surgeons, New York, New York.

570

ALBRECHT M.
KELLERER
AND
HARALD H.
ROSSI

The application of radiation biophysics can provide certain limited insights of this kind to the subject of radiation carcinogenesis. This approach is comparatively recent and has not been widely adopted. It remains in a state of continuing development, as indicated by substantial modifications in this chapter as compared with its version in the previous edition. However, this reflects further development rather than change and the basic conclusions drawn previously are confirmed and extended rather than altered.

Since the arguments are based on energy deposition in irradiated tissues and especially on the stochastic nature of this process, it is necessary that its principal features be considered. However, the presentation is condensed and simplified. General literature references have been provided for more exhaustive study.

2. Interaction of Radiation and Matter

2.1. Mechanisms

Radiation is termed "ionizing" when its interactions are so energetic that they remove electrons from the atoms that constitute the irradiated matter. In the case of many materials—including tissues—this leads to permanent changes that are produced with far greater efficiency than is obtained with radiations that merely induce electronic or molecular excitations.

In nearly all cases of practical interest, ionization occurs through the agency of electrically charged particles that may be high-speed electrons or nuclear constituents such as protons and α-particles. These are *charged particle radiations* that may originate in external or internal sources or may be generated inside the irradiated matter by *uncharged particle radiations*. The latter include high-frequency electromagnetic quanta (or photons) such as X- and γ-rays and electrically neutral particles such as neutrons.

Although the energies of ionizing particles can vary by an enormous factor of at least 10^{20}, the energies of principal practical importance range roughly from 0.1 to 10 MeV. In this energy interval, the range of directly ionizing particles is generally much less than the dimensions of the human body or even the dimensions of organs of small animals. Consequently, irradiation by charged particles arising from external sources is of limited significance, but it is important in the case of radioactive substances that are deposited within the irradiated tissues by physiological processes. Examples include location of ingested or injected radium in bone and concentrations of radioactive iodine isotopes in the thyroid. With a few exceptions (such as the presence of water containing tritium, the radioactive isotope of hydrogen), internal irradiations tend to be quite nonuniform. More or less uniform irradiation of organs of whole animals usually occurs when the more penetrating indirectly ionizing radiations are applied.

It may be useful to provide numerical indications of the degree of penetration of some of these radiations. Figure 1 depicts the mean free path, λ, and its reciprocal, the linear *absorption coefficient*, μ, in water for protons and neutrons

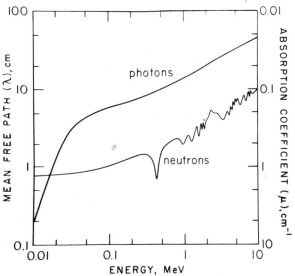

571

BIOPHYSICAL
ASPECTS OF
RADIATION
CAR-
CINOGENESIS

FIGURE 1. Mean free path, $\lambda(E)$, and absorption coefficient, $\mu(E)$, as a function of energy for photons and neutrons in water.

of energies between 10 keV and 10 MeV; μ is defined by the equation

$$N = N_0 e^{-\mu d} \qquad (1)$$

where N_0 is the number of incident particles and N is the number of particles that arrive at a depth d. The *mean free path* (or *attenuation length*), λ, is equal to $1/\mu$. When d is equal to $1/\mu$, the fraction of particles that have not interacted is e^{-1}, which is approximately 0.37. For example, μ for 1-MeV photons is approximately 0.07/cm, which means that a thickness of about 1/0.07 or approximately 14 cm of water will transmit 37% of incident 1-MeV photons without interactions.

It must be noted that these curves cannot be used to derive immediately the energy deposition as a function of depth in the irradiated material because in many instances the interactions lead to the production of secondary radiations that have appreciable penetration of their own, with the result that more energy arrives at any given depth than merely that carried by the primary radiation. In the case of photons, the three principal types of interaction reflected in Fig. 1 are the *photoelectric effect*, the *Compton effect*, and *pair* (and to some extent *triplet*) *production*. The first of these processes is of importance only at the low end of the energy scale and results in the ejection of a photoelectron and of fluorescent radiation, both of which are locally absorbed. Pair production, which occurs only at the upper end of the energy scale, results in the generation of an electron–positron pair. Following the annihilation of the positron, about 1 MeV of the original photon energy appears as the shared energy of two new photons that have appreciable penetration. The main section of the photon curve in Fig. 1 is due to the Compton effect, in which varying fractions of the incident photon energy appear in the form of scattered photons, particularly near the low end of the energy scale.

ALBRECHT M.
KELLERER
AND
HARALD H.
ROSSI

In the case of neutrons, by far the most important reaction responsible for the shape of the curve in Fig. 1 is *elastic scattering* (principally by hydrogen), in which the neutron can retain a substantial fraction of its energy. Thus, also in this case appreciable radiation energy can penetrate beyond the site where primary radiation has been absorbed.

To illustrate the far more restricted penetration of charged-particle radiations, the range of perhaps the two most important charged particles in radiobiology, the electron and the proton, is shown in Fig. 2. In contrast to the uncharged-particle radiations, which tend to be absorbed exponentially and cannot be characterized by a well-defined range of penetration, charged particles have as a rule a reasonably well-defined distance of penetration.

The principal process determining the range of charged particles is electronic collision. The electrons of atoms located in the vicinity of the particle trajectory are subject to electrical impulses that excite them, or eject them from their parent atom with varying energy. To a good first approximation, the interaction is proportional to the square of the charge of the incident particle and inversely proportional to the square of its velocity. Both the electron and the proton carry unit charge, but because of its far greater mass a proton moves much more slowly than an electron of equal energy. This results in a much higher rate of energy loss and consequently a much shorter range for the proton.

The rate of energy loss of charged particles is known as the *linear energy transfer* (LET), and it is usually specified in terms of kiloelectron volts per micrometer in the medium of interest (usually water or tissue). Figure 3 shows the LET in water of electrons and protons as a function of their energy.

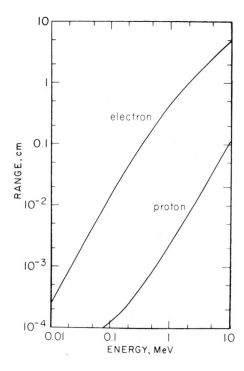

FIGURE 2. Range of electrons and protons in water as a function of energy (ICRU, 1970).

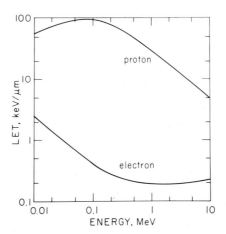

FIGURE 3. Linear energy transfer, LET, for electrons and protons in water as a function of their energy (ICRU, 1970).

573
BIOPHYSICAL
ASPECTS OF
RADIATION
CAR-
CINOGENESIS

The LET is only an average characterizing a complicated process. The electrons resulting from ionizing collisions are ejected with initial kinetic energies that generally have a very wide range (and highly skewed) distribution. The term *δ-rays* is applied to these electrons if their energy is sufficient such that they can in turn ionize, and there may be several generations of such secondaries produced. The track of an ionizing particle therefore, consists of *primary ionizations* produced in close proximity to the geometrical trajectory and *secondary ionizations* that surround this path up to highly variable distances. This pattern has been referred to as the *inchoate energy distribution,* and the locations where the primary and secondary particles undergo energy losses are termed *transfer points* (Kellerer

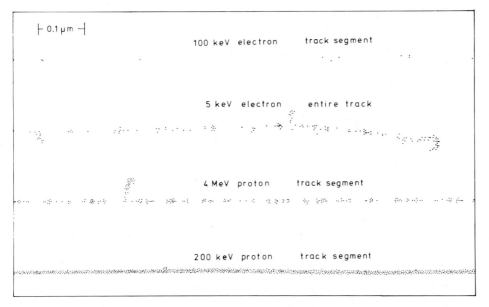

FIGURE 4. Two-dimensional projections of track segments in tissue of electrons and protons of different energies. The dots represent ionizations; the lateral extension of the track core is somewhat enlarged in the diagrams in order to resolve the individual energy transfers. The length of the track segments is 1 μm, i.e., a fraction of the dimension of the nucleus of a mammalian cell.

574

ALBRECHT M.
KELLERER
AND
HARALD H.
ROSSI

and Chmelevsky, 1975). Figure 4 gives two-dimensional projections of the inchoate energy distributions generated in small sections of the trajectories of charged particles of different LET.

2.2. Dosimetry

The physical quantity that is of central importance in radiobiology is the *absorbed dose, D*, which is defined as

$$D = E/m \tag{2}$$

where E is the energy deposited in a volume element and m is the mass contained in the volume element. E is proportional to the product of the number of charged particles traversing the element and to their LET. It should be noted that this statement as well as the definition [equation (2)] hold only if the number of particles that deposit E is large since D is the mean or expectation value of the specific energy (defined below).

In the case of uncharged-particle radiation, the absorbed dose evidently depends on the fraction of the incident energy that is transformed into kinetic energy of charged particles. A useful quantity in this connection is the *kerma,* which is the kinetic energy of charged particles released per unit mass in a specified material (here usually tissue). Figure 5 shows this quantity per unit fluence (number of uncharged particles per unit cross-sectional area) for photons and neutrons. In irradiated matter, kerma and the absorbed dose frequently have nearly the same numerical value. The equality exists if the range of charged particles is short compared to the attenuation length of uncharged particles. In this condition, the energy absorbed per unit mass at most locations in the medium

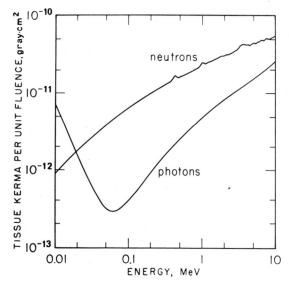

FIGURE 5. Tissue kerma per unit fluence for photons and neutrons as a function of energy. Based on Bach and Caswell (1968).

is nearly the same as the kinetic energy of the charged particles released. This
is the condition known as *radiation equilibrium*. It does not obtain when the
absorption of uncharged-particle radiations is comparable to that of the charged-
particle radiations or when one is near interfaces of different materials. For
example, in the case of X-irradiation, soft tissues in proximity to bone receive a
higher dose than those more distant due to the greater electron emission from
the irradiated bone, while the tissue kerma does not depend on the nature of
any material that may surround the point of interest.

575
BIOPHYSICAL
ASPECTS OF
RADIATION
CAR-
CINOGENESIS

Under well-defined conditions, absorbed doses can be measured and often
also calculated within an accuracy of a few percent. However, in some instances,
and in particular those relating to human carcinogenesis, doses must often be
determined retrospectively on the basis of incomplete information. Under these
conditions, major uncertainties arise.

According to the widely accepted Système International d'Unités (SI), the
quotient of energy by mass when expressed in base units is square meters per
second squared. An acceptable and more usual formulation is in terms of joules
per kilogram. In radiological physics this unit has been given the special name
gray (Gy). Until a few years ago and during the current interim period (which
is to end in a few years), the *rad* has been the unit of absorbed dose and quantities
of the same dimension (such as kerma). One rad (100 ergs/g) is equal to 0.01 Gy.

2.3. Microdosimetry

Many radiobiological phenomena and at least one type of radiation carcinogenesis (see Section 5) are due to tissue response to radiation injury.
However, in all instances individual cells are injured randomly, and consequently
the energy absorbed by individual cells is a relevant quantity. It appears to be
established that virtually all of the radiation sensitivity of the eukaryotic cell
resides in its nucleus, and it is quite probable that the ultimate target is DNA.
The biological effect of ionizing radiations is therefore determined by energy
concentrations in domains of subcellular dimensions.

As explained above, radiation energy is deposited by discrete, directly ionizing
particles. Its concentration is therefore subject to statistical fluctuations. These
fluctuations can be appreciable in small volumes for doses that are sufficiently
large to produce marked biological effects. Consider, for example, a region with
a diameter of 1 μm in tissue that receives an absorbed dose of 1 Gy. In the case
of γ-rays, the mean number of electrons traversing this volume is more than
10; in the case of fast neutrons, the frequency of particle traversals is only of
the order of 1/10. Any radiation effects are, of course, determined by the energy
actually deposited, and it is plain that this can differ greatly from the *mean* or
expectation value that is represented by the absorbed dose. In the example just
quoted, there is no neutron secondary and therefore no energy deposition in 9
out of 10 cases, but in the remaining one the energy density is typically 10 times
larger than the absorbed dose. Such fluctuations are the principal subject of
microdosimetry.

576

ALBRECHT M.
KELLERER
AND
HARALD H.
ROSSI

The central variable in microdosimetry is the *specific energy*, z, which is defined as

$$z = \Delta E / \Delta m \qquad (3)$$

where ΔE is the energy actually deposited in the region of mass, Δm.

Unlike the absorbed dose, the specific energy is a *stochastic* quantity that has a range of values in uniformly irradiated matter. The variability of z is expressed by the probability distribution $f(z)$, which represents the probability that the specific energy is equal to z. The width of this distribution depends on three factors:

1. The mass Δm of the region. Strictly speaking, this involves both the size and the shape of the region, but as a rule, shape is of secondary importance and it is usually assumed that the volume is at least approximately spherical and that it can therefore be characterized by its *diameter, d.*
2. The absorbed dose.
3. The LET of the charged particles traversing Δm.

The influence of these factors is illustrated in Figs. 6 and 7, which are logarithmic representations of $f(z)$ vs. z for various absorbed doses of ^{60}Co γ-rays and 5.7-MeV neutrons for spheres having diameters of 0.5 or 12 μm. Neutrons of energy 5.7 MeV are somewhat more energetic and therefore less densely ionizing than fission neutrons. The average LET is higher for natural α-emitters and lower for more energetic neutrons. Electrons produced by ^{60}Co γ-rays have minimal LET; in the case of X-rays, the LET is somewhat greater.

The curves in Figs. 6 and 7 have common characteristics. At high doses the number of particles is large, particularly for γ-radiation and the larger diameter. Consequently, statistical fluctuations are small and z is unlikely to differ from D. As the dose is reduced, fluctuations become greater because the number of particle traversals is correspondingly lessened. At low doses, a distribution is observed that has a shape largely independent of dose but an amplitude proportional to dose. This occurs when the average number of events is less than 1. In this case, one is dealing with the energy-deposition spectrum generated by single particles (indicated by the broken lines in Figs. 6 and 7). A reduction of dose merely results in a decrease of the amplitude of the spectrum with the remainder of the distribution appearing at $z = 0$ (which is not shown on these logarithmic graphs).

Microdosimetric distributions are determined experimentally with spherical gas-filled proportional counters. It is sufficient to obtain the energy-deposition spectra generated by individual particles; the other distributions can then be readily computed.

Figure 8 permits a comparison of single-event spectra for different radiations in a spherical tissue region of diameter 1 μm, and illustrates in more quantitative terms than Fig. 4 the extremely broad range of event sizes that can be produced by the sparsely ionizing fast electrons, on the one hand, and the slow, heavy neutron recoils, on the other hand.

577

BIOPHYSICAL
ASPECTS OF
RADIATION
CAR-
CINOGENESIS

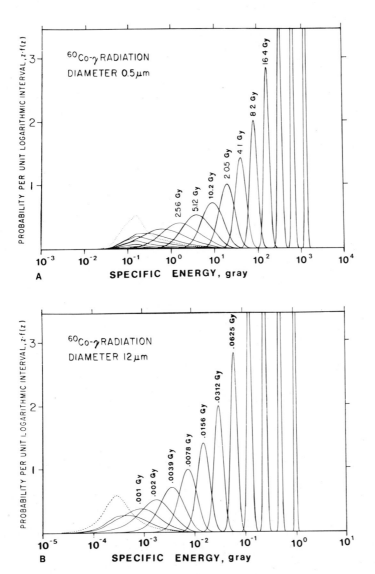

FIGURE 6. Probability per unit logarithmic interval of specific energy, z, at various doses of ^{60}Co γ-rays in a spherical tissue region of diameter (a) 0.5 μm and (b) 12 μm. The distributions of the increments of z produced in single events are given as broken lines.

For any distribution, $f(z)$, the mean value of z is defined by

$$\bar{z} = \int_0^\infty zf(z)\, dz \tag{4}$$

In Figs. 6 and 7, it is evident that $\bar{z}$ is equal to D at high doses. Although the shape of the distribution for finite energy losses does not change with decreasing dose when only single events are of importance, the decreasing

578

ALBRECHT M.
KELLERER
AND
HARALD H.
ROSSI

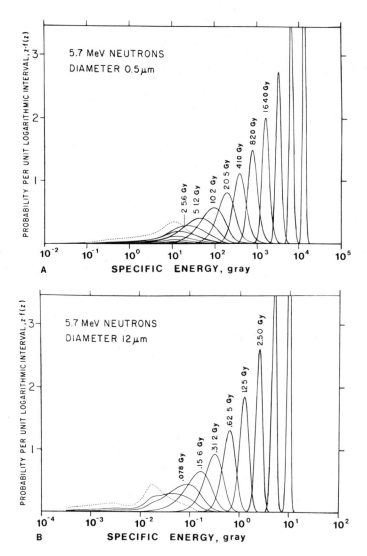

FIGURE 7. Probability per unit logarithmic interval of specific energy, z, at various doses of 5.7-MeV neutrons in a spherical tissue region of diameter (a) 0.5 μm and (b) 12 μm. The distributions of the increments of z produced in single events are given as broken lines.

frequency of events and the corresponding increase of instances in which there is no event result in equality between $\bar{z}$ and D at all doses.

It can be assumed that the biological effect of radiation on the cell is due to deposition of energy in one or several sensitive sites. Consider one of these sites and denote the probability of it being affected by $E(z)$. Any dose D then produces corresponding distributions $f(z)$ and $E(D)$. The effect produced by this dose is given by

$$E(D) = \int_0^\infty E(z)f(z) \, dz \tag{5}$$

579

BIOPHYSICAL
ASPECTS OF
RADIATION
CAR-
CINOGENESIS

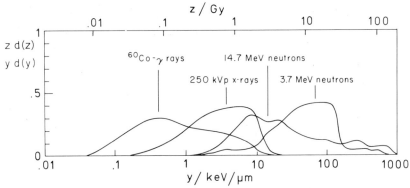

FIGURE 8. Probabilities of event sizes per unit logarithmic interval of linear energy y or specific energy z for different radiations in a spherical tissue region of 1-μm diameter.

Comparison of equations (4) and (5) indicates that if

$$E(z) = kz \qquad (6)$$

i.e., if the effect probability is proportional to z, then

$$E(D) = k\bar{z} = kD \qquad (7)$$

Thus, $\bar{z}$ and therefore also the absorbed dose are meaningful averages of specific energy if the effect probabilities are proportional to z. As will be seen in the next section, most, if not all, somatic radiation effects on higher organisms are characterized by a dependence that is proportional not to z but rather to z^2. This statement applies in particular to the few instances where the induction of malignancies by ionizing radiation could be studied in adequate detail. This nonlinear dependence is the ultimate reason for the need to employ microdosimetry in the analysis of the primary steps in radiation carcinogenesis.

The assumption that cellular injury or death is due to energy concentration in one or several sites in the cell is a reasonable first approximation that will largely be employed in the following discussions. It appears, however, that a more realistic picture is one in which the radiation-sensitive material in the cell (presumably the nuclear DNA) is distributed in a highly nonuniform pattern throughout a larger volume (presumably the nucleus). This pattern has been termed the *matrix*. As will be explained below, there are strong indications that the lesions responsible for cellular impairment are due to the combination of pairs of altered molecular configurations in the matrix. Since the combination probability of such pairs may be expected to depend on their separation, it is essential for any theoretical analysis to know the distance distribution of pairs of transfer points in the irradiated medium. The *proximity function*, $t(x)$, has been developed for this purpose. According to its definition, $t(x)\, dx$ is the mean energy deposited by the same particle at a distance x to $x + dx$ from randomly selected energy transfers in the medium. Figure 9 gives $t(x)$ for neutrons of

580

ALBRECHT M.
KELLERER
AND
HARALD H.
ROSSI

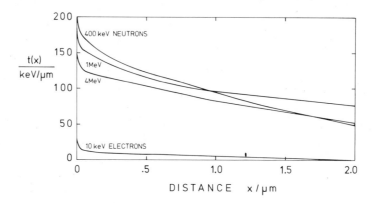

FIGURE 9. Computed proximity functions $t(x)$ for neutrons (F. Zieker, personal communication) and for 10-keV electrons (Chmelevsky *et al.*, 1980).

different energies and for 10-keV electrons, i.e., for inchoate distributions of the type illustrated in Fig. 4.

3. General Stochastic Considerations

3.1. The Linear Dose–Effect Relation at Small Doses

There is a well-known distinction in radiobiology between effects due to injury of individual cells and effects due to the collective response of irradiated cells. It is, however, also important to determine whether the response of a given cell is independent of the irradiation of other entities (cells, medium, etc.). When this independence exists, the cell may be termed *autonomous*. In the following, cells will be understood to be autonomous if not stated otherwise.

As has been pointed out in the preceding section, the absorbed dose determines only the mean value of the specific energy absorbed in microscopic volumes which may widely deviate from this mean value. It has also been concluded in the preceding section that the statistical fluctuations in energy deposition play no role if the cellular damage is proportional to the specific energy, z; in this case, the average effect observed at a given absorbed dose is proportional to this absorbed dose.

In all effects on higher organisms, one finds, however, that densely ionizing radiations are more effective than sparsely ionizing radiations, such as X- or γ-rays. All commonly employed ionizing radiations work by the same primary physical processes, namely by electronic excitations and by ionizations. The unequal biological effectiveness of different types of ionizing radiations can therefore only be explained by the different spatial distributions of absorbed energy on a microscopic scale. Specifically, the increased biological effectiveness of densely ionizing radiations must be due to the high local concentration of absorbed energy near the tracks of heavy charged particles. Accordingly, one concludes that the dependence of cellular damage on specific energy, z, is steeper than linear. The actual form of the nonlinear dependence, $E(z)$, will be considered later. One can, however, draw certain important conclusions that follow from microdosimetry and are valid regardless of the actual form of $E(z)$. Such conclusions will be dealt with in the remainder of this section.

581

BIOPHYSICAL
ASPECTS OF
RADIATION
CAR-
CINOGENESIS

One general conclusion that follows from microdosimetry is that in the limit of small absorbed doses, the average cellular effect is always proportional to dose. Such a linear relation between observed cellular effect and absorbed dose must be expected regardless of the dependence of cellular effect on specific energy; it is due to the fact that even at the smallest doses, finite amounts of energy are deposited in a cell when this cell is traversed by a charged particle. The energy deposited in such single events does not depend on the dose; accordingly, the effect in those cells that are traversed by a charged particle does not change with decreasing dose. The only change that occurs with decreasing absorbed dose is the decrease in the fraction of cells that are subject to an event of energy deposition. This can be treated quantitatively, and microdosimetry can furnish conclusions as to the range of absorbed doses in which the statement applies for different radiation qualities.

The effect probability $E(D)$ at a given dose D is equal to the sum of all products of the probabilities for various numbers ν of events (charged-particle traversals) in the sensitive sites and the effect probabilities E_ν under the condition that ν events occur:

$$E(D) = \sum_{\nu=1}^{\infty} p_\nu E_\nu \tag{8}$$

The equation is written in the form that does not include the spontaneous incidence, E_0; i.e., it is assumed that $E(D)$ is corrected for the spontaneous incidence and that the latter need therefore not be considered.

Because energy-deposition events are by definition statistically independent, their number follows Poisson statistics; i.e., the probability p_ν that exactly ν events occur is

$$p_\nu = e^{\phi D} (\phi D)^\nu / \nu! \tag{9}$$

The term ϕD is the mean number of events per site. Event frequencies, ϕ, for various radiation qualities and site sizes will be given below.

It will in the present context not be necessary to evaluate equation (8) in its complete form. Instead, it will be sufficient to consider the case of small event frequencies, ϕD, which occurs at small doses especially of densely ionizing radiations.

In order to evaluate the case where the number, ϕD, of events is small compared to 1, equation (9) can be expanded into a power series. Because it is assumed that $D \ll 1$, the term $e^{\phi D}$ can be set equal to 1, and with this simplification one obtains

$$E(D) = E_1 \phi D + E_2 (\phi D)^2 / 2 + \cdots \tag{10}$$

where E_1 is the probability for the effect if exactly one event has taken place

582

ALBRECHT M.
KELLERER
AND
HARALD H.
ROSSI

and E_2 is the effect probability if two events have taken place. The probability E_2 will normally exceed E_1, but if ϕD is sufficiently small, the quadratic term and higher terms can be neglected in comparison with the linear term.

A possible objection to this conclusion is that E_1 may be zero while E_2 is not zero; i.e., one could assume that the effect cannot be produced by a single charged particle, while it can be produced by two particles. However, this assumption is inconsistent with microdosimetric evidence. It has been found that for both sparsely and densely ionizing radiations, there is a broad distribution of the increments of specific energy produced in single events. There is always a probability, although it may be small, that the same amount of energy deposited in two events can also be deposited in one event. One can therefore quite generally state that in the limiting case of small absorbed doses, the cellular effect is proportional to dose. If, as pointed out above, the spontaneous incidence is eliminated by subtraction from the observed effect, one has the simple linear relation

$$E(D) = E_1 \phi D \quad \text{for} \quad D \ll 1 \tag{11}$$

This relation implies that in the action of ionizing radiation on autonomous cells there is no threshold as far as absorbed dose is concerned. The probability E_1 may be small if one deals with sparsely ionizing radiation, but ultimately in the limiting case of very small absorbed doses the effect must be proportional to dose. It is important to realize that this is the case whether there is or is not a threshold in the dependence of the cellular effect on specific energy z. The absence of a threshold with regard to absorbed dose is merely due to the fact that even at the smallest doses some of the cells receive relatively large amounts of energy when they are traversed by a single charged particle.

The preceding considerations apply only to objects that are small enough that at the lowest doses of practical interest, the number of absorption events is small. That this is the case for cells or subcellular units but not for multicellular organisms can be seen from the following example. The exposure to environmental radioactivity and to cosmic radiation leads to absorbed doses of the order of 1 mGy/year. This background exposure corresponds to a large number of events for a multicellular organism. For man, several charged-particle traversals occur per second. For a smaller animal, such as a mouse, a few events may occur per minute. For a single mammalian cell, however, only a few events per year will occur, and if one considers only the nucleus of the cell, less than one event per year will take place. These are the frequencies that result mainly from sparsely ionizing radiations, such as the γ-component of the environmental radiation or the relativistic mesons from the cosmic radiation. If one were to consider the densely ionizing radiation, event frequencies would be considerably lower.

Table 1 gives event frequencies per gray for microscopic regions of various diameters and for different qualities. The largest region included corresponds to the typical size of a mammalian cell. Various radiobiological studies have shown that for most cellular effects, only energy deposition within the cell nucleus

TABLE 1

583
BIOPHYSICAL
ASPECTS OF
RADIATION
CAR-
CINOGENESIS

Event Frequencies (ϕ) per Gray in Spherical Tissue Regions Exposed to Different Radiations

Diameter of critical region, d (μm)	^{60}Co γ-rays	Type of radiation		
		Neutrons		
		0.43 MeV	5.7 MeV	15 MeV
12	2×10^{-1}	5.5×10^{-3}	5.1×10^{-3}	6.1×10^{-3}
5	3.6×10^{-2}	4.2×10^{-4}	8.6×10^{-4}	1.1×10^{-3}
2	5.8×10^{-3}	3.9×10^{-5}	1.2×10^{-4}	1.6×10^{-4}
1	1.2×10^{-3}	8×10^{-6}	3.2×10^{-5}	3.8×10^{-5}
0.5	1.7×10^{-4}	2×10^{-6}	7.3×10^{-6}	9×10^{-6}

is relevant; therefore, a region of 5-μm diameter, which corresponds approximately to the cell nucleus, is included in Table 1. In Section 4, evidence will be given that for most effects in eukaryotic cells, the effective site diameter is somewhat less than the size of the nucleus; smaller diameters are therefore also of interest.

One can generally state that the linear component in the dose–effect relation must be dominant whenever the event frequencies are substantially below 1; i.e., if the absorbed dose is considerably smaller than $1/\phi$. This defines the dose region in which proportionality between effect and absorbed dose can be assumed. For the whole cell, the value of $1/\phi$ is approximately 0.5 and 20 mGy for γ-rays and 5.7-MeV neutrons, respectively. If one considers only the nucleus of the cell as the sensitive region, the values of $1/\phi$ are approximately 3 and 240 mGy for these two radiation qualities. As mentioned earlier, a recent analysis (see Section 4) has shown that the actual sensitive sites in the cell are somewhat smaller than the cellular nucleus, and one deals therefore with even larger values of $1/\phi$. It is a very important result for all considerations regarding radiation protection that below about 1 mGy, and for densely ionizing radiations at considerably higher doses, a linear relation must hold if one deals with effects on autonomous cells. As pointed out, this is because even at the smallest doses appreciable amounts of energy are deposited in those cells that are subject to an event of energy deposition. The mean specific energy produced in a single event in the cell or in its sensitive site is equal to the reciprocal, $1/\phi$, of the event frequency; i.e., one deals with doses of about 1 mGy in the nucleus of the cell for sparsely ionizing radiations and with a few tenths of a gray for densely ionizing radiations, such as neutrons. In Section 4, it will be shown that the effective event size produced in single events is even higher because the relevant average of the specific energy produced in single events is larger than the frequency average, which corresponds to the values of ϕ.

3.2. Dose–Effect Relation and the Number of Absorption Events

The considerations in this section are of a more abstract nature and require a certain amount of mathematical formalism. The essential result that links the

584
ALBRECHT M.
KELLERER
AND
HARALD H.
ROSSI

logarithmic slope of the dose–effect relation with the number of absorption events in the cell can, however, be understood and applied without detailed knowledge of the mathematical derivation. This derivation is therefore given in the Appendix, and only the main conclusions are discussed in this section. A practical application of the result will be dealt with in Section 5. For the purpose of the present discussion, rigorous definitions of some of the quantities involved are necessary.

The considerations in the preceding section are valid regardless whether the effect, E, is considered as the probability for a quantal effect, i.e., an effect that either takes place or does not take place in the cell, or whether it is considered as the average value within the irradiated cellular population of a gradual effect. The following considerations will be restricted to the former case; i.e., only the occurrence or nonoccurrence of certain cellular effects will be considered. The coefficients $E(D)$, $E(z)$, and E_ν therefore represent probabilities and can only take values between 0 and 1. Examples of such quantal effects, which include the survival of irradiated cells or the occurrence of certain cytogenetic alterations, are of great practical importance in quantitative radiobiology. Another example is transformation of irradiated cells, which underlies carcinogenesis. This latter case will be further discussed in Section 5.1.

It is also necessary to provide a clarification of various terms that can be applied to the geometrical configuration of the radiosensitive elements in the cell. As already stated, the space occupied by this material is termed the *matrix*. The matrix must be assumed to have a complex shape and it seems indeed likely that it does not form a connected body. The term *gross sensitive volume* (gsv) (Rossi, 1964) has been employed for that part of the cell that contains the matrix. A more specific definition is that the gsv is the smallest convex volume containing the matrix. However, in many cases it is sufficiently accurate to consider the gsv to be either the smallest sphere that meets this condition or to simply consider the nucleus to be the gsv.

The concept of a *sensitive site* has frequently been invoked in biophysical models of radiation-induced cytogenetic alteration such as chromosome aberrations (e.g., see Lea, 1946; Wolf, 1954; Savage, 1970); however, it is not confined to radiation effects on chromosome structure. In the next section it will be shown that various effects on eukaryotic cells can be adequately understood if one postulates sites that are somewhat smaller than the cell nucleus and that are affected with a probability dependent on the square of the energy actually deposited in these sites. In such considerations it is not necessarily implied that the cell contains only one of these sites, but it is merely implied that the response of the cell can often be interpreted in terms of the energy concentration in volumes that are smaller than the gsv. The radius or a mean diameter of a site is thus the average distance over which individual energy deposits interact, although the site does not have physical reality.

In the following, a slightly different concept will be used, namely that of a *critical region*. The reason for introducing yet another term is that it will be convenient in the following considerations to deal with a reference volume that contains all the sensitive structures of the cell but may be even larger than the gross sensitive region itself. The concept is useful, first, because it can be applied to a population of irradiated cells that are not all equal or are not all in the same stage of the generation cycle. In such an inhomogeneous population, the gross sensitive region and its size may vary from cell to cell; however, their critical region can be chosen in such a way that it is equal for all irradiated cells. Furthermore, it is convenient to obtain certain conservative estimates in the absence of precise knowledge concerning the gross sensitive region; this can be done by equating the critical region either with the cell nucleus or with the whole cell.

Another concept that has to be further explained is that of an *energy-deposition event* (for brevity, *event*). This is defined (ICRU, 1980) as energy deposition by a charged particle or by a charged particle together with its associated secondary particles in the region of interest. Two ionizing particles that pass the region are counted as separate events only if they are statistically independent. Usually, for example in the case of neutron irradiation, one can identify an absorption event with the appearance of a charged particle in the reference region.

These definitions are of interest in connection with an important theorem concerning the number of absorption events in the cell and the slope of the dose–effect curves in a logarithmic representation of effect probability as a function of absorbed dose.

Assume that c is the slope of the dose–effect relation in a logarithmic representation*; then

$$c = \frac{d \ln E(D)}{d \ln D} \tag{12}$$

where $E(D)$ is the effect probability at dose D; it is assumed that this probability is corrected for spontaneous incidence, which need therefore not be considered.

It can be shown, and the detailed derivation is given in the Appendix, that the slope c is equal to the difference of the mean event number, n_E, in the critical region of those cells that show the effect and the mean event number, n, in the critical region of the cells throughout the exposed population regardless of whether they show the effect or not:

$$c = n_E - n \tag{13}$$

This equation holds at any value of absorbed dose. The relation remains valid if a critical region larger than the actual gsv is considered. The sole condition is that energy deposition outside the critical region does not affect the cell. As pointed out above, it is often sufficient to identify the critical region with the nucleus of the cell. It is also important to note that biological variability, e.g., the variation of sensitivity throughout the cellular population, does not invalidate the result.

---

* It should be noted that a (fully) logarithmic graph is different from the semilogarithmic plots that are usually employed to display the (log of) cell survival as a function of absorbed dose.

586

ALBRECHT M.
KELLERER
AND
HARALD H.
ROSSI

The theorem is fundamental for the application of microdosimetry to the analysis of dose–effect relations. If, for certain values of the absorbed dose, the effect probability $E(D)$ and the slope c of the dose–effect curve in logarithmic representation are known, one can derive the minimum size of the critical structure. Although n_E, the frequency of traversals in the affected cells, may not be known, it is evident from equation (13) that it cannot be less than c. One can therefore ask how large the sensitive structure must be so that at the dose D the cell is traversed by at least c charged particles with a probability $E(D)$. The answer is given by microdosimetric data for various radiation qualities and for different sizes of the critical region. In this way, one can derive lower limits for the dimensions of the sensitive structures in the cell and for the interaction distances of elementary lesions in the cell.

Equation (13) contains as a limiting case a statement that is of significance to the analysis of dose–effect curves at very small doses. The relation implies that in the region of small doses, the slope c of the effect curve in the logarithmic representation is equal to the order of the reaction kinetics that determine the effect. In the limit where the absorbed dose D (and consequently n) approaches 0, this fact may appear obvious. According to the considerations in the previous section, it is to be expected that at least in the case of radiation action on autonomous cells, first-order kinetics apply at low doses; this corresponds to a value of $c = 1$ when $n \ll 1$.

In connection with basic aspects of radiation carcinogenesis, it is of interest to determine whether c can in fact be less than 1. The degree to which this can occur is limited by the fact that n_E cannot be less than 1 since the number of absorption events in affected cells must be at least 1. Consequently,

$$c > 1 - \phi D \qquad (14)$$

This inequality follows directly from the more general relation expressed in equation (13).

Studies performed by Vogel (1969) and by Shellabarger *et al.* (1974, 1980) on the induction by neutrons of mammary tumors in Sprague–Dawley rats show that in the range of very small doses, the logarithmic slope c of the dose–effect curve is considerably less than 1. This fact will be further discussed in Section 5 and it will be concluded that in these experiments the observed tumor frequencies in the irradiated animals cannot merely reflect the action of radiation on autonomous cells that give rise to the observed tumors without mutual interaction or interference.

4. The Quadratic Dependence of the Cellular Effect on Specific Energy

4.1. Dose–Effect Relations

It has been pointed out in the preceding sections that the dependence, $E(z)$, of the cellular effect on specific energy is not identical to the observed dependence,

$E(D)$, of the cellular effect on absorbed dose. This would be the case only if the cellular damage was a linear function of specific energy. In the preceding section general statements have been derived that are valid regardless of the actual form of the dependence of effect on specific energy. Particularly, it has been pointed out that at very low doses, the cellular effect must always be linearly related to absorbed dose. It has also been possible to derive a relation that connects the mean number of charged particles traversing the affected and unaffected cells with the slope of the dose–effect curve in the logarithmic representation. In the present section, the actual dependence of cellular effect on specific energy will be analyzed. It will be seen that dose–effect relations, as well as relative biological effectiveness (RBE)–effect relations for higher organisms, point to a quadratic dependence of the primary cellular damage on specific energy.

587
BIOPHYSICAL
ASPECTS OF
RADIATION
CAR-
CINOGENESIS

As far as the production of two-break chromosome aberrations is concerned, a quadratic dependence of the yield of the observed effect on energy deposited in sensitive cells had been postulated as early as in the works of Sax (1938, 1941) and in numerous other studies, particularly those by Lea (1946). In this case, the quadratic dependence is merely due to the fact that two-break chromosome aberrations are assumed to result from the interaction of two "chromosome breaks." The yield of breaks is assumed to be proportional to energy absorbed in the cell, and the average number of breaks per cell is therefore simply proportional to dose. Statistical fluctuations in energy deposition in the cell are, however, highly relevant if the probability for the production of a two-break aberration depends on the square of the concentration of breaks in the cell. A two-break aberration can result from two breaks that are produced in the same charged-particle track, or it can result from the interaction of two breaks produced by independent particle tracks. In the former case, one expects a linear relation to absorbed dose; in the latter case, one expects a quadratic dependence on absorbed dose. For densely ionizing radiations, such as neutrons or α-particles, the increments of specific energy produced in the critical sites of the cell are so large that the linear component is dominant. For sparsely ionizing radiations, such as X- or γ-rays, on the other hand, the ionization density in the charged-particle tracks is so low that neighboring breaks are usually produced by independent particle tracks. One must therefore expect the quadratic component to be dominant in the latter case. This characteristic difference between densely ionizing radiation and sparsely ionizing radiation has been borne out by experimental results.

While the quadratic dependence of the yield of the chromosome aberrations on absorbed dose is approximately valid for sparsely ionizing radiation, it must be concluded from microdosimetric data that at very small doses the dose–effect relation must be linear even for such radiations. Until recently, it has not been possible to assess the magnitude of this linear component because of limitations in the statistical accuracy of the experimental data. However, work performed in different laboratories (see Brewen et al., 1973; Schmid et al., 1973; Brenot et al., 1973) with X-rays and with fast electrons has indeed shown a linear relation at small doses of X-rays and a quadratic dependence only at somewhat higher

588
ALBRECHT M.
KELLERER
AND
HARALD H.
ROSSI

doses. These studies thus confirm the predictions made on general micro-dosimetric principles. As will be shown, the relative contributions of the linear and quadratic components can be accounted for on the basis of microdosimetric data. In the following it will be seen that such considerations apply also to other radiation effects on eukaryotes. Furthermore, the quantitative relation of the site diameter, the radiation quality, and the ratio between linear and quadratic components of the cellular damage will be discussed.

Figure 10 illustrates dose–effect relations for the yield of pink mutations in *Tradescantia* (Sparrow *et al.*, 1972). Curves are given for 430-keV neutrons and for X-rays. For the purpose of the present discussion, the saturation and the ultimate decline of the yield in the range of higher doses will not be considered. This latter effect may be connected to cell killing, but as a study on the transformation of cells *in vitro* (Borek and Hall, 1973; see Section 5.1) has indicated, it may involve a complex interrelation between the observed cellular alterations and cell killing.

It should be pointed out that a logarithmic representation has been used for these curves in order to represent the experimental data in the range of low doses and small observed yields of mutations with sufficient accuracy. The logarithmic representation has the further advantage that proportionality of the effect to a power, n, of the absorbed dose expresses itself in the slope, n, of the effect curve. In their initial parts, both the curve for neutrons and the curve for X-rays have the slope 1; i.e., effect and absorbed dose are proportional in both cases. The slope of the X-ray curve approaches the value 2 at somewhat higher

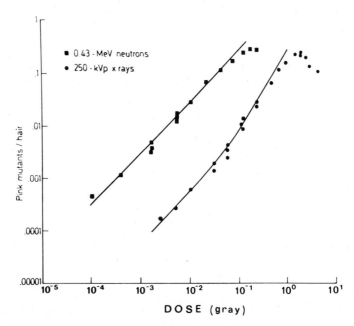

FIGURE 10. Induction of pink mutant cells in the stamen hairs of *Tradescantia* by X-rays and 430-keV neutrons (Sparrow *et al.*, 1972). The spontaneous incidence is subtracted from the observed values.

doses, and the observations are therefore consistent with the statement that in an intermediate dose range, the yield of mutations produced by X-rays is proportional to the square of the absorbed dose. The accuracy with which the linear component in the dose–effect curve for X-rays has been established in this experiment is due to the fact that this particular experimental system permits the scoring of extremely large numbers of irradiated cells in the stamen hairs of *Tradescantia*.

While the example given in Fig. 10 supports the general conclusions drawn from microdosimetric consideration, it remains to be seen whether these results are also quantitatively in agreement with predictions based on microdosimetry. For this reason the quadratic dependency of cellular damage on specific energy and the resulting dose–effect relation will be analyzed in detail.

If one assumes that the degree of cellular damage or the probability for a certain effect in the cell is proportional to the square of specific energy

$$E(z) = kz^2 \tag{15}$$

then the average effects observed at a certain absorbed dose are obtained by averaging the square of the specific energy in the sensitive sites of the cells over its distribution throughout the irradiation population:

$$E(D) = k \int_0^\infty z^2 f(z) dz \tag{16}$$

It can be shown [see Kellerer and Rossi (1972) for the mathematical details] that the integral in equation (16) has a simple solution. One finds that this integral, which is the expectation value of z^2, is equal to the square of the absorbed dose plus the product of absorbed dose and the energy average, ζ, of the increments of specific energy produced in single events in the site:

$$\bar{z}^2 = \int_0^\infty z^2 f(z)\, dz = \zeta D + D^2 \tag{17}$$

Accordingly, one has

$$E(D) = k(\zeta D + D^2) \tag{18}$$

The ratio of the linear component to the quadratic component is therefore equal to the ratio ζ/D of the characteristic increment ζ of specific energy to the absorbed dose. If the absorbed dose is larger than ζ, the quadratic component dominates; if the absorbed dose is equal to ζ, both components are equal. The value of ζ is determined by the size of the site and by the type of the ionizing radiation. It is largest for smallest site diameters, and it is considerably larger for densely ionizing radiation than for sparsely ionizing radiation, such as γ- or X-rays.

590

ALBRECHT M.
KELLERER
AND
HARALD H.
ROSSI

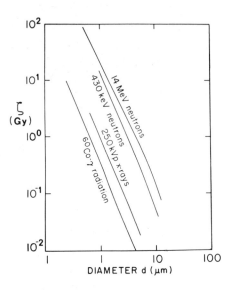

FIGURE 11. Energy mean, ζ, of the specific energy produced in single events by different radiation qualities in spherical tissue regions of diameter d.

The value of ζ for different radiation qualities as a function of the diameter for the reference volume is shown in Fig. 11. These values are obtained from experimental microdosimetric determinations as well as from theoretical calculations. In the example represented in Fig. 10, one finds that for X-rays the linear component is equal to the quadratic component at a dose of approximately 0.1 Gy. According to Fig. 11, the value of 0.1 Gy for ζ corresponds to a site diameter of approximately 2 μm. According to the microdosimetric determinations, the quantity ζ for neutrons should be approximately 35 times larger than for X-rays, and the initial part of the neutron curve in Fig. 10 is, in fact, shifted vertically by about this factor relative to the initial part of the X-ray curve.

The analysis of dose–effect relations for two-break chromosome aberrations (Kellerer and Rossi, 1972; Schmid *et al.*, 1973; Brenot *et al.*, 1973) has led to somewhat larger values of ζ, namely values that correspond to site diameters of approximately 1 μm.

Survival curves for mammalian cells *in vitro* can, to a good approximation, be represented by an exponential that contains a linear and a quadratic term in dose:

$$S(D) = S_0 \, e^{-k(\zeta D + D^2)} \tag{19}$$

where $S(D)$ is the survival at dose D and S_0 is the survival at zero dose. If one uses this equation, which has earlier been invoked by Sinclair (1968), one obtains values that also correspond to site diameters of one to several micrometers for cells in S phase. For cells in G_1 and G_2 and in mitosis, the initial linear component is more pronounced, and the values of ζ therefore correspond to smaller site diameters of only a fraction of a micrometer. Whether this latter observation corresponds to a more condensed state of the DNA in these stages of the generation cycle of the cell [see observations of Dewey *et al.* (1972) and earlier results by Cole (1967)] or whether the initial linear component in the survival curve is partly due to a type of cellular damage that is linearly related to specific energy in the sensitive sites of the cell remains an open question.

The theory of dual radiation action attributes the quadratic dependence of biological effects on specific energy to a mechanism in which the former are due to the production of *lesions* that are produced by the interaction of pairs of *sublesions*. Sublesions are presumably alterations of DNA that are produced at a rate that is proportional to specific energy, and they can combine over a distance that is equal to the mean diameter of the site. It may be expected that the interaction probability for a pair of sublesions depends on their initial separation, and this has in fact been shown in *molecular ion experiments* (see Rossi, 1979; Colvett and Rohrig, 1979; Bird, 1979; Kellerer *et al.*, 1980). In these studies pairs of charged particles traverse the cell at varying separation and it is found that the linear portion of the dose–effect curve decreases markedly if the mean separation of the particles is increased. The experiments disclose a highly skewed dependence of sublesion combination on initial separation and support the conclusion that the "site" is in fact the entire nucleus.

Additional complications are that the biological effectiveness cannot indefinitely increase with energy concentration and that for very heavily ionizing particles, energy is wasted in individual cells, leading to a saturation effect that results in declining effectiveness per unit of dose. Another very likely, and possibly related, phenomenon is that the production of sublesions also depends on energy concentration in distances that are of the order of nanometers. Yet another effect is diffusion of energy from the inchoate distribution prior to the induction of sublesions.

The treatment given above in terms of the site model does not take account of the manner in which a given amount of energy is distributed in a fixed nominal interaction volume. In view of these complicating factors, it must be considered to be an approximation. It is, however, often adequate and also didactically useful. It should also be noted that more realistic treatments merely change the physical interpretation of the factors k and ζ in equation (18). None of the complications cited above cause any change of the basic dependence of $E(D)$ on two terms that respectively are linear and quadratic in absorbed dose.

4.2. Dose–RBE Relations

It has already been pointed out that the theoretical considerations based on microdosimetry must be restricted to autonomous cells. Thus, equation (19) represents a survival curve based on the assumption that the survival probability of cells in tissue cultures decreases exponentially with the mean number of lesions in the cells. The same assumption is also justified for effects other than cell death, particularly for somatic mutations and genetic effects in general.

It can, however, not be assumed that such comparatively simple kinetics obtain in radiation carcinogenesis, which is a highly complex process. The dose–effect curves for the induction of cancers in experimental animals can have a great variety of shapes, and an example will be given in Section 5 of an instance where it can be proven that tumors do not arise simply as a result of radiation-induced transformations of autonomous cells.

592

ALBRECHT M.
KELLERER
AND
HARALD H.
ROSSI

Although the dose–effect curve is usually the most important quantitative expression of radiobiological effects, another important relation is the dependence of RBE on dose. The RBE of radiation A relative to radiation B is defined as D_B/D_A, where D_B and D_A are respectively the absorbed doses of the two radiations that produce the same biological effect. The RBE is usually found to depend on the degree of effect and therefore on the absorbed dose of either radiation. This dependence is not only of theoretical interest, but also of considerable pragmatic importance because it is vital to any attempts to evaluate late radiation effects. This will in Section 5.3 be shown for the observation on A-bomb survivors in Hiroshima and Nagasaki. The bomb that exploded over Nagasaki released γ-radiation, but almost no neutron radiation whereas at Hiroshima the neutron component was significant in terms of absorbed dose and very likely dominant in terms of biological effect.

The importance of the dose–RBE relation arises from the possibility that it may be the same for autonomous cells and for interacting cell systems. This may be expected to be the case if the interaction process is the same regardless of the quality of the radiation that caused the primary cellular damage. It would appear that this condition is met, or at least adequately approximated, in many instances.

In the following example, neutrons and X-rays will be used, but the considerations are equally valid for any two types of radiation. From the quadratic dependence of cellular damage on specific energy, one derives the condition for equal effectiveness of X-rays and neutrons:

$$k(\zeta_X D_X + D_X^2) = k(\zeta_n D_n + D_n^2) \tag{20}$$

where ζ_X and ζ_n are values of ζ for X-rays and neutrons, and D_X and D_n are the absorbed doses for X-rays and neutrons. Since the RBE of neutrons relative to X-rays is defined as the ratio of the X-ray dose to the equivalent neutron dose,

$$\text{RBE} = D_X/D_n \tag{21}$$

one can express the RBE as a function of either the X-ray dose or the neutron dose. In the following, the RBE of neutrons will be expressed as a function of the neutron dose. Inserting equation (21) into equation (20), one obtains

$$\zeta_X \cdot \text{RBE} \cdot D_n + \text{RBE}^2 \cdot D_n^2 = \zeta_n D_n + D_n^2 \tag{22}$$

or

$$\text{RBE} = \frac{2(\zeta_n + D_n)}{\zeta_X + [\zeta_X^2 + 4(\zeta_n + D_n)D_n]^{1/2}} \tag{23}$$

This relation is shown in Fig. 12 for various values of ζ_n/ζ_X. It is easy to identify certain general characteristics of the dependence of RBE on dose. At very low doses the linear components are dominant both for neutrons and for X-rays,

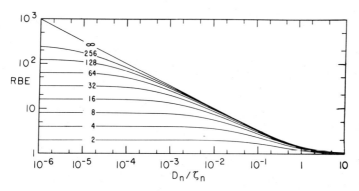

FIGURE 12. Relation between RBE and neutron dose (D_n) according to equation (23). The neutron dose is given in multiples of ζ_n; the parameter of the curves is ζ_n/ζ_X.

593
BIOPHYSICAL
ASPECTS OF
RADIATION
CAR-
CINOGENESIS

and RBE must then have a constant value equal to the ratio ζ_n/ζ_X of the ζ values for neutrons and for X-rays. This plateau of RBE corresponds to the region in the example of Fig. 10 where the initial part of the X-ray curve runs parallel to the neutron curve. In the range of intermediate doses one can neglect the linear component for X-rays, while the linear component for neutrons is still dominant. In this case the RBE of neutrons is inversely proportional to the square root of the neutron dose; in a logarithmic plot of RBE vs. neutron dose, one obtains curves of slope $-1/2$. At the high doses, finally, one should expect that RBE tends toward the value 1. It is, however, often not easy to obtain meaningful biological data with neutrons at doses large enough that the linear component can be neglected.

The dose–RBE relation expected on the basis of a quadratic dependence of primary cellular damage on specific energy has been compared with the experimental observations for a wide spectrum of radiation effects on mammalian cells. Figure 13 is a compilation of such results for neutrons having an energy of 0.43 MeV and for fission neutrons that have about the same effective energy. One must draw the general conclusion that in the intermediate dose range in which the available data are most complete, the observed dose–RBE relations are in agreement with the dependence theoretically predicted. In the example of the mutations in *Tradescantia*, it has been possible to find the plateau of the values of RBE at low doses, and this value agrees with microdosimetric data. It is not surprising that relatively little data are available in the range of extremely small doses, as few experimental systems permit the necessary statistical accuracy at small doses. However, it is remarkable that in two experimental systems, namely in the lens opacification studies and in the system for induction of mammary tumors in the rat, extremely high values of the RBE of neutrons have been found at low doses. These values exceed the predictions made on the basis of microdosimetric data, and they may be taken as evidence that, in addition to the quadratic dependence of the effect on energy concentration over regions of the order of magnitude of one to several micrometers' diameter, one deals with the already mentioned differences in effectiveness of sublesion production. This

594

ALBRECHT M.
KELLERER
AND
HARALD H.
ROSSI

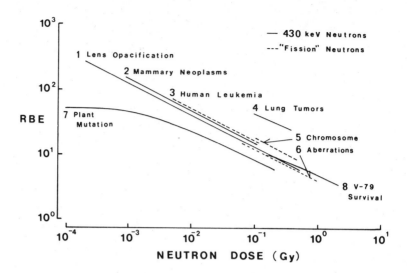

FIGURE 13. Logarithmic plot of the RBE of low-energy neutrons vs. neutron dose. (1) Bateman *et al.* (1972); (2) Shellabarger *et al.* (1974); (3) Rossi (1977); (4) Ullrich *et al.* (1979); (5) Awa (1975); (6) Biola *et al.* (1971); (7) Sparrow *et al.* (1972); (8) Hall *et al.* (1973).

implies a dependence of the effectiveness of ionizing radiation on the distribution of energy in regions of the order of only a few nanometers. Formally, this would correspond to a dependence of the coefficients k in equation (18) on radiation quality.

The induction of mammary tumors by neutrons and X-rays and the study of leukemia incidence after neutron irradiation and exposure to γ-rays will be discussed in the next section. As an example of a dose–RBE relation that extends over an extremely wide range of doses, the studies on the opacification of the murine lens may be considered. Figure 14 contains this relation together with its 95% confidence limits. One should note that the inverse relationship between the RBE of neutrons and the square root of the neutron dose extends over more than 4 orders of magnitude of the neutron dose in this example. These results obtained in a multicellular system are therefore in good agreement with the

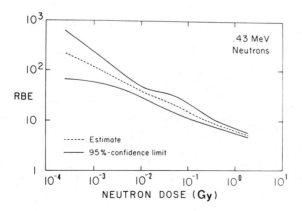

FIGURE 14. RBE of 430-keV neutrons relative to X-rays for the induction of lens opacification in the mouse (Bateman *et al.*, 1972; Kellerer and Brenot, 1973).

various other observations supporting the assumption that the primary cellular damage is proportional to the square of the specific energy in sites of the order of one to several micrometers.

5. Applications to Radiation Carcinogenesis

Many of the subjects covered in the preceding sections are of relatively recent origin. In particular, the theory of dual radiation action was developed only a few years ago and is, as are many concepts of microdosimetry, subject to further development. Practical applications are still few in number since few radiation carcinogenesis studies are broad enough to permit a detailed analysis of dose–effect relations and of their dependence on radiation quality. However, in the few instances where data relating to radiation carcinogenesis were analyzed, they could be interpreted in terms of the theory and they have also lead to other results. In the case of mammary neoplasms in the rat, it could be deduced that the observed incidence depends not only on lesions in autonomous cells, but is codetermined by radiation-induced changes in several cells or in tissue. Furthermore, in an analysis of data on the induction of human leukemia, conclusions were reached that are of importance to risk estimates.

The findings on the induction of mammary neoplasms demonstrate a complexity of the process of radiation carcinogenesis that is also reflected in the variety of often complicated dose–effect relations observed in other experimental animal studies. In at least some instances radiation does not cause cancer by mere transformation of individual cells that subsequently proliferate regardless of any radiation injury to other cells. One is thus not dealing with the relatively simple autonomous response of a single cell. Consequently, theoretical predictions cannot be made with respect to the dose–effect relations, although for reasons given above it may be expected that the theoretical dose–RBE relations should apply. However, even in the transformation of what would appear to be autonomous cells, the theoretical dose–effect relation is at least markedly modified by processes that are at this point only poorly understood.

5.1. Transformation

While the development of radiogenic cancer cannot be fully accounted for if only isolated cells are considered, it appears plausible that it is initiated by changes (probably cytogenetic) in individual cells, and this kind of change may well be exhibited by cells in culture that can be scored as having undergone an *oncogenic transformation* by their altered morphology. Cells in tissue culture ordinarily grow in an orderly manner and in a single layer until they are subject to contact inhibition. However, fresh explants of embryonic fibroblasts, as well as a few established cell lines, can produce transformed clones when exposed to chemical and physical agents. This change can be readily recognized by a densely stained,

596

ALBRECHT M.
KELLERER
AND
HARALD H.
ROSSI

piled-up appearance and by the random crisscross pattern of cells at the periphery of the clone. Cells from such clones satisfy many of the criteria of malignancy and produce fibrosarcomas when injected in large numbers into immunosuppressed animals.

It was shown by Borek and Sachs (1966) that transformations can be induced by radiation in cultures of explants of hamster embryo cells. The dose–effect curves for X- and neutron irradiations are shown in Fig. 15 (Borek *et al.*, 1978). It should be noted that in this logarithmic representation, the ordinate represents the fraction of observed clones that are transformed; it thus represents the transformation frequency in cells that survived the irradiation. The decline of the X-ray curve at high doses cannot, therefore, be explained as simply due to killing of transformed cells by high doses. It would appear that one must be dealing with differences in sensitivity to killing. These may be either a greater sensitivity of those cell types in the (heterogeneous) population that can be transformed, or cells containing the lesions responsible for transformation are more sensitive than those that do not.

There are considerable difficulties in the assay of transformations. The maximum fraction of clones that can be transformed is less than 1%, and at low doses the fraction of transformed cells is much smaller. The resultant statistical uncertainties can accommodate a wide range of curve shapes. The straight lines drawn through the rising portions in Fig. 15 are certainly not inconsistent with the data. However, there are two considerations that indicate that even in this dose range one is dealing with complex mechanisms that may be responsible for a more complicated curve shape. Fractionation at doses of less than 1.5 Gy results in an unusual *increase* in effect, and a complex shape has in fact been demonstrated in another transforming cell system.

Miller *et al.* (1979) in experiments on transformable mouse fibroblasts ($10T\frac{1}{2}$ cells) obtained the dose–effect relations shown in Fig. 16, wherein what appear

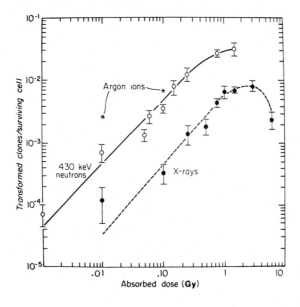

FIGURE 15. Dose–response curves for cell transformation by X-rays, neutrons, and argon ions. The data *points* plotted are the means of replicate experiments, and the error *bars* represent the S.E. or the error expected from the number of clones counted, whichever was larger (Borek *et al.*, 1978).

597

BIOPHYSICAL
ASPECTS OF
RADIATION
CAR-
CINOGENESIS

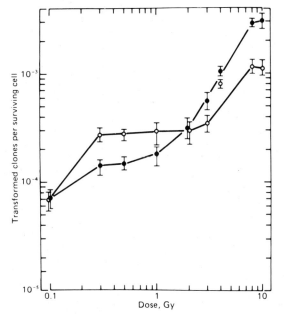

FIGURE 16. Pooled data from many experiments for the transformation rate for single (●) and split (○) doses of X-rays. The time interval between split doses was 5 h (Miller *et al.*, 1979).

to be linear and quadratic rises are separated by a plateau in which the transformation rate per surviving cell changes little over a threefold range of dose. An additional peculiarity is that fractionation of the dose into two increments separated by 5 h decreases the transformation rate at high doses, but increases it at low doses. The same dependence was found for the hamster embryo system by Borek (1979), and in mouse 3T3 cells by Little and Terzaghi (1976).

The fractionation effect shown in Fig. 17 can be accounted for by the simple assumption that there is no interaction between doses given in different fractions. In terms of dual radiation action, this means that sublesions produced by the first fraction are eliminated (probably by repair processes) before the second fraction is applied. In this case the effect of a fractionated dose, D, should be twice the effect of a single dose, $D/2$. This means that when the curve rises

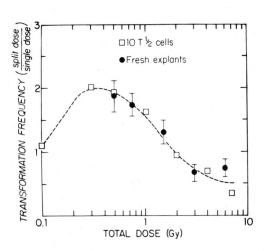

FIGURE 17. Comparison of the data for C3H/10T$\frac{1}{2}$ cells and fresh explants of hamster embryo cells. The ratio of the transformation frequencies for split and single doses is plotted as a function of total dose (Miller *et al.*, 1979).

598

ALBRECHT M.
KELLERER
AND
HARALD H.
ROSSI

linearly, fractionation should not change the number of transformations observed, that in the quadratically rising portion fractionation should lessen the transformation rate, and that at zero slope (the plateau) fractionation should double the rate. The data are in substantial agreement with this algorithm, which is equivalent to the requirement that either of the curves results from a 45° shift of the other on a logarithmic plot.

Although the fractionation effects can thus be explained on the basis of the unusual shape of the dose–effect curve, the reason for this shape is not obvious. It would appear that the linear and quadratic components of dual radiation action instead of adding in the usual way are separated because the linear component is saturating before the quadratic component is significant; the quadratic component then levels out as well at high doses. In a homogeneous cell population, the implied saturation cannot be due to a reduction of the cells available for transformation because the curve levels first at a low frequency ($\sim 10^{-4}$) and subsequently rises by more than a decade.

It is evident from microdosimetric considerations that the initial portion of the curve must be due to transformations produced by individual electrons with a frequency of about 10^{-6} per cell, but there is no reason evident why this process should stop after only about 1 cell in 10,000 has been transformed. A possible explanation is competition between transformation and other effects for available sublesions. If dual radiation action is to be a general mechanism, it follows that the nature of any radiation effect induced depends on the identity of the sublesions that form the relevant lesions. It would seem entirely possible that a given sublesion may contribute to the formation of lesions associated with various effects depending on the nature of the other sublesions. This would seem particularly plausible if the radiation-induced lesion is considered to be a rearrangement of substantially linear DNA molecules that result when the four terminations produced by two double-strand breaks (sublesions) rejoin in an altered pairing.

If this hypothesis is correct, the initial portion of the curve can be interpreted to indicate that single electrons can in an initial step produce a pair of initial sublesions (and the lesions resulting from their combination) causing transformation. While the number of cells so affected increases linearly with dose, subsequent electron events cause a much more copious production of sublesions which are more likely partners for either of the two initial sublesions. The second part of the curve can then be interpreted to correspond to a process in which the two critical sublesions are produced by separate electrons and competition operates against each of them. This qualitative explanation would appear to account for observations, but a numerical justification has yet to be provided.

5.2. Mammary Neoplasms in the Sprague–Dawley Rat

Bond *et al.* (1960) and Shellabarger *et al.* (1969, 1974) discovered that moderate doses of γ- or X-rays produce a high incidence of mammary neoplasms in rats of the Sprague–Dawley strain. The majority of the tumors are not malignant (fibroadenomas), but an appreciable proportion are adenocarcinomas. It was found that the incidence of these neoplasms is approximately proportional to the γ- or X-ray dose up to a few gray, where the incidence curve flattens and finally declines when doses in excess of 5 Gy are applied. This is a phenomenon common in radiation carcinogenesis. It was also concluded that the effect is not *abscopal*, i.e., it requires irradiation of that part of the tissue where the neoplasms are to arise, and it was moreover demonstrated that the effect can be produced by *in vitro* irradiation of excised mammary tissue when it is subsequently grafted onto unirradiated animals.

Vogel (1969) as well as Shellabarger *et al.* (1974) investigated the effectiveness of neutrons for this phenomenon and found it to be high in relation to that of γ- or X-rays, particularly at low levels of incidence. On the basis of this experience and in view of the microdosimetric considerations that have been described in the preceding section, a large-scale experiment was performed by Shellabarger *et al.* (1980) employing 0.43-MeV neutrons down to doses as low as 1 mGy. This experiment is of particular interest to the analysis of dose–effect relations at small doses and for the understanding of the RBE of neutrons vs. X-rays. It will therefore be described in some detail.

Groups of Sprague–Dawley rats received, at age 60 days, a single dose of neutrons or X-rays. The neutron doses were 1, 4, 16, or 64 mGy; the X-ray doses were 0.28, 0.56, or 0.85 Gy. Subsequent to irradiation, the animals were examined for mammary neoplasms; when neoplasms were noted, they were removed surgically and the animals were returned to the experiment.

A conventional analysis based on the *total incidence* of neoplasms throughout life without correction for mortality leads to the dose–effect curves of Fig. 18. It must be noted that the dose scales for neutrons (upper scale) and for X-rays (lower scale) differ by a factor of 10; the dose ratio for equal effect is therefore 10 times larger than would appear from the graph. One deduces from these dose–effect relations RBE values for the neutrons of 100 or more at small doses

599

BIOPHYSICAL
ASPECTS OF
RADIATION
CAR-
CINOGENESIS

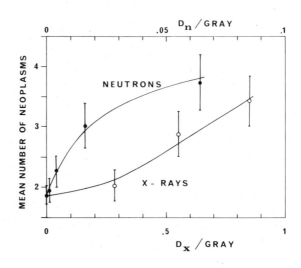

FIGURE 18. Mean number of mammary neoplasms throughout life per animal in Sprague–Dawley rats irradiated by 400-keV neutrons or X-rays. The scales for the neutron dose and the X-ray dose differ by a factor of 10 (Shellabarger *et al.*, 1980).

ALBRECHT M.
KELLERER
AND
HARALD H.
ROSSI

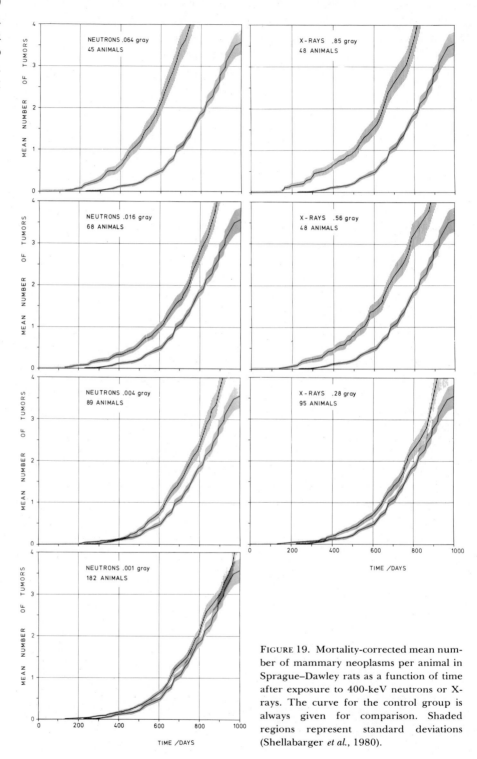

FIGURE 19. Mortality-corrected mean number of mammary neoplasms per animal in Sprague–Dawley rats as a function of time after exposure to 400-keV neutrons or X-rays. The curve for the control group is always given for comparison. Shaded regions represent standard deviations (Shellabarger *et al.*, 1980).

and still in excess of 10 at higher neutron doses of the order of 0.1 Gy. Furthermore, it is striking that the dose–effect relation for neutrons is *sublinear*, i.e., that
a graph relating effect to dose has negative curvature.

The general characteristics of these observations are readily apparent from
the simple analysis based only on total incidence; however, it is desirable to
consider also the more rigorous actuarial analysis that indicates the actual time
course of the appearance of radiation-induced neoplasms and that permits the
identification of possible qualitative differences in the effect produced by
neutrons and by X-rays.

A suitable quantity in the numerical analysis is the *cumulative tumor rate* that
can also be considered as the mortality-corrected mean number of tumors per
animal as a function of time after irradiation. Figure 19 gives the time course
of the cumulative tumor rate for all mammary neoplasms in the different
irradiated groups. The shaded areas correspond to the standard deviations, and
the lower curve repeats in each plot the time course for the unirradiated controls.

It is apparent from these data that Sprague–Dawley rats are subject to a high
spontaneous rate of mammary neoplasms during the later phases of their life.
It is also apparent that the effect of irradiation can be described as a forward
shift of the spontaneous occurrence in time. A point of particular interest is that
a single dose of 1 mGy of neutrons produces a significantly increased incidence
or, alternatively expressed, a significantly earlier occurrence of neoplasms. The
time shift for this very low neutron dose is readily recognized to be approximately
30–40 days. The high RBE values of neutrons versus X-rays at low doses are
also evident.

It is one of the major assumptions of the theory that, beginning with the
production of elementary lesions, the series of steps leading to the effect under
observation is the same regardless of the radiation type involved. The validity
of this assumption is difficult to assess. However, one necessary (also certainly
not sufficient) condition is that the time course of incidence be the same. The
curves in Fig. 19 suggest no systematic differences in the time course of incidence
for neutrons and for X-rays. All the curves are well in agreement with the
assumption that the spontaneous incidence is merely shifted forward in time. A
more systematic analysis indicates that the cumulative tumor rate, $R(t)$, i.e., the
mortality-corrected mean number of tumors per animal, can be represented by
the equation

$$R(t) = 7.5 \times 10^{-10} [(t - \Delta t)/\text{day}]^{3.3} \qquad (24)$$

for all times t exceeding a *latent time* Δt that depends on absorbed dose. One
concludes that there is no evidence of characteristic differences between the
neutron- and the X-ray-induced effects. This is further supported by the analysis
of the relative frequency of different types of neoplasms produced by different
radiations. For the control group, one obtains the value $\Delta t = 106$ days. For the
group exposed to 1 mGy of neutrons, $\Delta t = 142$ days; this corresponds to a forward
shift of the incidence of neoplasms by 36 days. The time shifts for all doses are
plotted in Fig. 21 together with other dose–effect relations.

602

ALBRECHT M.
KELLERER
AND
HARALD H.
ROSSI

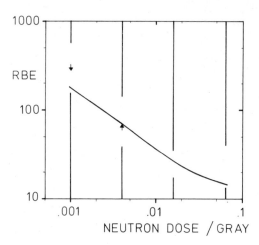

FIGURE 20. Dose dependence of the RBE of 400-keV neutrons for the induction of mammary neoplasms in Sprague–Dawley rats. Vertical bars indicate the ranges of RBE that are excluded on a level of statistical significance exceeding 95%; arrows represent differences with lower level of significance. The solid curve is an estimate consistent with the different types of dose–effect relations that can be constructed (Shellabarger *et al.*, 1980).

The experimental data indicate clearly the high RBE values of neutrons at low doses, but the actual dependence of RBE on neutron dose has to be deduced by a more detailed analysis. The result of such an analysis is shown in Fig. 20. This shows the dependence of RBE on neutron dose together with confidence limits of this dependence obtained by nonparametric comparison of groups of animals exposed to different doses of neutron or γ-rays. The vertical bars cover those ranges of RBE that can be excluded with statistical certainty exceeding 95%. The analysis is based on the data in the experiment of Shellabarger *et al.* (1980), but also on earlier results obtained by Bond *et al.* (1960) with γ-rays. Details of the nonparametric procedure to obtain the curve are described by Kellerer and Brenot (1973). The RBE–dose dependence and the very large RBE values are in general agreement with the theoretical considerations and are also consistent with the earlier experimental results in the lens opacification studies. However, the RBE values at low neutron doses exceed, as stated in Section 4.2, the predictions made on the basis of microsimetric data; and the data also indicate that RBE may level out at high neutron doses at values larger than unity. As stated earlier, this may reflect the increased effectiveness in sublesion production.

The information presented thus far corroborates the postulates of the theory. However, there is another aspect of the results that is of significance with regard to the mechanisms of tumor induction. The RBE–dose relation shown in Fig. 18 puts certain constraints on the dose–effect relations both for X-rays and for neutrons, although it does not determine their shapes. As pointed out, the data in Fig. 18 indicate a dependence that may be approximately linear for X-rays while it is *sublinear* for neutrons. However, Fig. 18 is based on data that are not corrected for mortality and it represents only one of many possible ways to construct dose–effect relations. It is therefore desirable to ascertain the findings by comparing the dose–effect relations constructed in different ways. Such dose–effect relations are given in logarithmic form in Fig. 21. In this presentation straight lines correspond to proportionality of the effect to a power of the

603

BIOPHYSICAL
ASPECTS OF
RADIATION
CAR-
CINOGENESIS

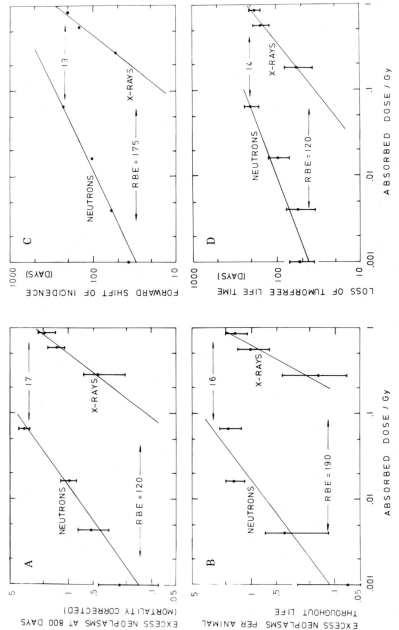

FIGURE 21. Dose–effect relations constructed in different ways for the induction of mammary neoplasms in Sprague–Dawley rats by 400-keV neutrons and X-rays. The straight lines in the logarithmic representation are rough fits to the data, and the estimated RBE values at the lowest and highest neutron doses correspond to these lines. Vertical bars are standard deviations. (Data from Shellabarger *et al.*, 1980.) (A) Total excess incidence of mammary neoplasms per animal; this corresponds to the data in Fig. 18. (B) Mortality-corrected excess incidence of mammary neoplasms per animal at day 800 postirradiation. (C) Estimated forward shift of the occurrence of mammary neoplasms due to irradiation. (D) Average loss of tumor-free life of the animals due to irradiation.

604

ALBRECHT M.
KELLERER
AND
HARALD H.
ROSSI

absorbed dose; the slope of the line is numerically equal to the power of the absorbed dose.

Panel A gives the data from Fig. 18, i.e., the uncorrected total incidence. Panel B gives the mortality-corrected excess number of neoplasms at day 800 after irradiation. Panel C gives the forward shifts in time that are listed in Table 1, and Panel D gives the average loss of tumor-free life span of the animals. It is evident that all of these various ways of constructing dose–effect relations lead to dose exponents for neutrons that are substantially below 1 and may be equal to 0.5. For X-rays the data may be consistent with proportionality to absorbed dose, i.e., with a dose exponent of 1. The solid lines through the data are rough fits that indicate the general character of the dose–effect relations. The RBE values estimated from these relations at the highest and lowest neutron doses are indicated in the individual panels. Although there are differences due to statistical uncertainties, it is apparent even from these rough fits, regardless of the details of the analysis, that one obtains sublinear dose–effect relations for neutrons and large RBE values at small neutron doses.

It had already been concluded in an earlier analysis (Rossi and Kellerer, 1972) that the sublinearity of the incidence of neoplasms versus neutron dose extends to doses that are so low that multiple traversals of cells are highly improbable. As mentioned earlier, the average number of particles traversing a cell nucleus is of the order of 1 for a neutron dose of 250 mGy. The lowest dose used in these experiments was 1 mGy where only 1 in about 250 cell nuclei experiences a traversal by a neutron secondary, i.e., where the mean number n of events per nucleus is roughly 0.004. If one considers the whole cell, the mean number n of events at 1 mGy of 430-keV neutrons is about 0.05. In Section 3.2 it has been concluded that, in a logarithmic plot of the effect probability (corrected for control incidence) versus dose, the slope of the resulting curve cannot be smaller than $(1 - n)$ if one deals with autonomous cells. Because in the present experiment the slope is considerably less, one must conclude that the observed incidence is determined not only by transformations of individual cells, but also by radiation-induced processes in adjacent cells or by dose-dependent changes at the tissue level. The observed decrease of the yield of neoplasms per unit dose cannot, at any rate, be due to a depletion of a critical cell population. At this time, no further statement can be made, but one may consider factors such as virus release by damaged cells with some local saturation or an induced increase of immune reactions even at low doses of the order of 1 mGy.

The induction of mammary neoplasms in the Sprague–Dawley rats offers a remarkable illustration of the considerations given in the earlier theoretical sections. This is, however, at present the only study that permits a detailed analysis that includes the dose–effect relations, the RBE–dose dependence, and the time dependence of the induction of neoplasms by sparsely and densely ionizing radiations. It is, therefore, important to ascertain that these findings are not merely specific to the Sprague–Dawley rat with their high spontaneous incidence of mostly benign mammary neoplasms.

Shellabarger (private communication) has recently performed a further
experiment on the induction of mammary neoplasms by X-rays and 430-keV
neutrons in rats of the ACI strain that exhibit a low spontaneous incidence of
mammary neoplasms, but show a pronounced incidence of adenocarcinomas
after treatment with the synthetical hormone diethylstilbestrol (DES).

605

BIOPHYSICAL
ASPECTS OF
RADIATION
CAR-
CINOGENESIS

Data for non-DES-treated animals have been obtained at neutron doses
between 0.045 and 0.36 Gy, and the neutron–RBE values in this dose range are
somewhat in excess of 10, both for fibroadenomas and for adenofibromas. This
is, as seen from Fig. 20, consistent with the data for the Sprague–Dawley rats.

For the DES-treated animals data have been obtained for neutron doses
between 0.01 and 0.09 Gy. One deals in this case exclusively with adenocarcinomas, and the incidence is high even for the unirradiated animals. The RBE
shows the expected decrease with neutron dose, but at a specified neutron dose
the RBE values exceed those obtained for the Sprague–Dawley rats. An RBE of
about 200 is obtained at a neutron dose of 0.01 Gy. There is at present no
explanation why the neutron RBE is markedly enhanced in this experiment that
involves the synergism of DES and ionizing radiation. However, the observation
is of obvious importance.

A further significant result is that the DES-treated animals show a dose–
response relation for neutrons that is as clearly sublinear as the dose–response
of the Sprague–Dawley rats.

Apart from its biophysical implications, the sublinear dose–response is important from the standpoint of risk estimates for small doses. It could lead to an
increased effect if a dose is split into two parts separated by a time interval that
is long enough that the effects of the two doses are independent and simply
additive. If such a possibility exists for low doses of densely ionizing radiations,
it becomes doubtful whether linear extrapolations from observations at high
dose rates and high doses to low dose rates and low doses are always conservative.

The analogy to the split-dose experiments with cell transformations will be
noted (Borek and Hall, 1974). However, these experiments were performed at
high doses and with sparsely ionizing radiation. An increased effect of lower
dose rates with densely ionizing radiation has been found in the induction of
osteosarcomas in α-irradiated mice (Müller et al., 1978), and it has earlier been
demonstrated for the induction of osteosarcomas in patients subjected to injections of short lived radium-224 (Spiess and Mays, 1973). However, the doses
were relatively high in these instances.

Various other examples can be given that indicate the variety and complexity
of dose–effect relations for radiation carcinogenesis. For one case, namely the
high spontaneous frequency of reticulum cell sarcomas in RFM mice, it has
actually been shown that sparsely ionizing radiation causes a substantial decrease
of the incidence (Ullrich and Storer, 1979); this appears to be not a real decrease
of the neoplastic response, but a shift toward an increased incidence of thymic
lymphoma. Another, contrasting example of a well-established dose dependence
is the induction of ovarian tumors in mice by γ-radiation (Yuhas, 1974). In this
case a purely quadratic dose dependence has been established for absorbed doses

606

ALBRECHT M.
KELLERER
AND
HARALD H.
ROSSI

down to 0.2 Gy, and a marked recovery effect is found with decreasing dose rates.

Finally, one may mention studies by Ullrich *et al.* (1979) on the induction of lung tumors in RFM mice by X-rays and fission neutrons. These observations are interesting because a threshold-type dose–effect relation is found for X-rays and a dose relation with positive curvature is obtained for neutrons. However, even in this case the RBE–dose dependence agrees with the inverse relation between RBE and the square root of the neutron dose.

In view of the complexities of the dose–effect relations, it is unlikely that general statements can be made on the dose dependence for radiogenic cancer in man. However, it also appears that the inverse relation between RBE and the square root of the neutron dose remains valid. This will be considered for the most important set of human epidemiological data for late somatic effects.

5.3. Radiation Leukemogenesis

The epidemiological data on the induction of cancer by ionizing radiation are commonly so limited that it is impossible to determine the shape of the dose–effect curve with even moderate confidence. The data cannot usually be shown to be inconsistent with a variety of relations including a simple straight line. It has, therefore, often been decided to adopt the "linear hypothesis," i.e., the assumption that the risk is proportional to dose. It is generally agreed that this is a "prudent" assumption in that it is likely to lead to overestimates rather than underestimates. This belief is, at least in part, due to findings of experimental radiobiology. Curves relating cancer incidence in animals to dose can, as shown in Section 5.2, have a variety of shapes, but at least in the case of low-LET radiations, one usually observes a positive curvature at low doses.

The acceptance of linearity permits the formulation of various concepts employed in radiation protection. Thus, the *population dose* (usually measured in *man-rem*) has been defined as the sum of the doses received by persons in a given group, and it is assumed that within wide limits the total number of cancers induced by a given population dose will be the same regardless of the distribution of individual doses in the population. The assumption of linearity is commonly applied to both low- and high-LET radiations with the implied further assumption that the RBE is a constant. It should be noted that this constancy is assumed not only for the low doses of interest to radiation protection, but also for the much higher doses where the significant effect frequencies are observed, which determine the slope of the linear relations derived.

The postulate that the RBE is independent of dose at moderate or high doses (of the order of 1 Gy) is obviously at variance with theoretical considerations and with experimental data on nonhuman systems. It seems plausible that man should not be an exception and that risk estimates based on constant RBE must either overestimate the hazard of low-LET radiation or underestimate the hazard of high-LET radiation. A determination on whether this is so is of fundamental importance to radiation protection.

The first attempt at such an analysis employed data on leukemia mortality. Among the various types of cancer that can be induced by radiation, leukemia has the highest potential utility for statistical analysis because it is one of the most frequently induced malignancies and because its natural incidence is relatively low.

The most important sources of information on radiation-induced leukemia are the data obtained from studies on survivors of the Japanese cities exposed to nuclear weapons at the end of World War II. Not only are the populations involved far larger than those in other studies, but special efforts have also been made by the Atomic Bomb Casualty Commission to achieve maximum follow-up, to select optimum control populations, and to determine as accurately as possible the doses received by individuals.

The most important aspect of these observations is, however, that they were obtained for two types of radiations. In Hiroshima, a substantial neutron dose was delivered that was primarily responsible for the biological effects observed. In Nagasaki, the relative neutron dose was very low and virtually negligible at greater distances from the epicenter of the explosion (Ishimaru *et al.*, 1971). The availability of data for both neutron and γ-radiation thus provides an opportunity to address the question of whether the dose dependence of RBE regularly found in other systems can be shown to apply also to human leukemia.

Earlier assessments of the Japanese leukemia data were based on "dose" (also "T-65 dose" or "air dose"), which is actually the tissue kerma in free air (see Section 2). The fraction of this kerma that was due to neutrons varied somewhat with distance from the epicenter, but for the population of interest, it was between 20 and 25% at Hiroshima and essentially negligible at Nagasaki.

An early analysis (Rossi and Kellerer, 1974) first addressed the question whether the effectiveness of radiation at Hiroshima compared with that at Nagasaki was the same at all levels of leukemia mortality. Since the comparison is based on R_H, the kerma ratio, rather than the ratio of absorbed doses in the bone marrow, it does not constitute a determination of the RBE (which will be shown to be much higher). However, the ratio between dose and kerma does not depend on either of these quantities, and consequently, the dependence of RBE on dose is a multiple of the dependence of R_H on kerma.

Utilizing the nonparametric techniques discussed in the previous section, the relation depicted in Fig. 22 is obtained.* Although the most crucial of the limits (the lower bound at 10 rads) is established with 86% rather than 95% significance, this value seems sufficiently large, particularly in view of the conservative assumptions made. It may thus be concluded that the neutron RBE for human leukemia, like that for virtually all other somatic effects investigated, increases with decreasing level of effect.

---

* In this as well as in the other analysis, the information for the highest kerma level at Nagasaki and the two highest kerma levels at Hiroshima has been ignored, for two reasons. One is that survivors in these categories must represent a highly selected and uncertain group because LD_{50} levels are approached or even exceeded. The other reason is that, in accord with all other experience with radiation carcinogenesis, it must be expected that the dose–effect curve should at such high doses saturate or even decrease.

608

ALBRECHT M.
KELLERER
AND
HARALD H.
ROSSI

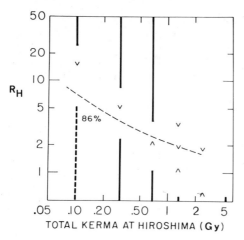

R_H

86%

.05   .10   .20   .50   1   2   5
TOTAL KERMA AT HIROSHIMA (Gy)

FIGURE 22. Relative biological effectiveness of the radiation in Hiroshima for the induction of leukemia compared to that in Nagasaki as a function of kerma in Hiroshima (Rossi and Kellerer, 1974). The solid bars indicate those values that can be excluded with 95% confidence; the broken bar indicates a level of confidence of 86%. The broken curve is the result of a least-squares fit.

While this finding is of interest, it is of course even more desirable to determine the shapes of the dose–effect relations. In particular, the very important question arises of whether, as in the case of mammary neoplasms, the neutron dose–effect relation rises with a power of the dose that is less than 1 or whether the power is 1 or exceeds 1. Linear extrapolations would in the former case underestimate the neutron hazard, but in the latter case overestimate the γ-ray hazard.

In order to gain information on this point, it was assumed that for both cities the dose–effect can be approximated by

$$I(K) = I_0 + aK + bK^2 \tag{25}$$

where I is the incidence and I_0 its control level, K is the total kerma, and a and b are constants. Utilizing a statistical treatment described elsewhere (Kellerer and Brenot, 1974), it was established that for Hiroshima the quadratic component has to be rejected and only a linear component need be assumed. For Nagasaki, the least-squares estimate of a turned out to be negative, and only the quadratic component was considered in the further analysis. It thus appears that at Hiroshima, where the biological effect of the neutrons was dominant (because of their higher RBE), radiation induced leukemia at a rate proportional to kerma, while at Nagasaki, where neutrons could be all but neglected, the leukemia mortality increased with the square of kerma.

In a final step, a more accurate treatment was utilized by assuming that in both cities the incidence could be expressed by

$$I = I_0 + aK_n + bK_\gamma^2 \tag{26}$$

where K_n and K_γ are the kermas of neutrons and γ-rays and the parameters I_0, a, and b are the same for both cities. The least-squares fit obtained on this basis is shown in Fig. 23a and b together with the observed mortalities and their standard deviations.

When the factors relating marrow dose to kerma became available (Kerr, 1978), it was possible to derive the leukemia mortality to dose of neutrons or

609

BIOPHYSICAL
ASPECTS OF
RADIATION
CAR-
CINOGENESIS

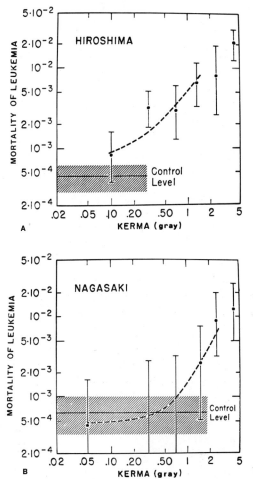

FIGURE 23. Mortality of leukemia for the period from October 1950 to September 1966 vs. kerma at Hiroshima (Rossi and Kellerer, 1974). The bars represent 95% confidence ranges; the shaded area is the 95% confidence region for the unirradiated population of the city. The broken curve is the result of a least-squares fit.

γ-radiation. These are about 8.5×10^{-2}/Gy for neutrons and 3×10^{-3}/Gy^2 for γ-radiation. These relations are shown in Fig. 24. It should be noted that they apply for doses that are less than about 1 Gy and more than about 0.1 and 0.01 Gy, respectively, of γ- and neutron radiations. It should also be noted that they apply to the mortality from all types of leukemia. It has been claimed (Mole, 1975) that there are different RBE relations for different types of leukemia.

Employing a different, somewhat simpler approach, Rossi and Mays (1978) essentially confirmed these findings. They are also, at least in part, supported by others (Jablon, 1979; Ishimaru et al., 1979), and there is now increasing acceptance of the opinion that the risk of leukemia is substantially proportional to neutron dose and that it increases at least approximately as the square of the dose of low-LET radiation.

The induction of other types of neoplasms in the atomic bomb survivors has been too low to permit an accurate analysis. Significant conclusions, however, are possible if mortality from malignant neoplasms is considered in toto. Figure 25, based on a survey by Beebe et al. (1977), details the mortality per year as a

610

ALBRECHT M.
KELLERER
AND
HARALD H.
ROSSI

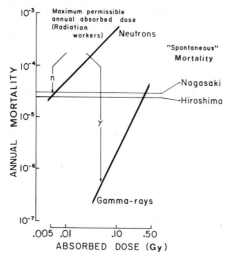

FIGURE 24. Annual mortality of leukemia vs. absorbed dose to the bone marrow as deduced from the Japanese data. The graph also shows the "natural" mortality at Hiroshima and Nagasaki and the maximum permissible annual absorbed doses for radiation workers (Rossi, 1977).

function of kerma in Hiroshima and Nagasaki. The straight line fitted to the data from Hiroshima ignores again the two highest kerma points, as it is difficult to account for selection effects in the survivors and resulting uncertainties in the dose estimates at these high exposure levels that include a substantial neutron component. Furthermore, it should be noticed that the curves are fitted to different control values in the two cities, and that the assumption of a common control value would lead to markedly increased RBE values for the radiation in Hiroshima compared to that in Nagasaki.

High RBE values are indicated by the data in Fig. 25 even without a rigorous analysis. However, using information on the relation between kerma and absorbed doses for neutron and γ-radiation (Jones, 1977), an estimate of the radiation-induced annual mortality from all malignant neoplasms from 1950 to 1974 is

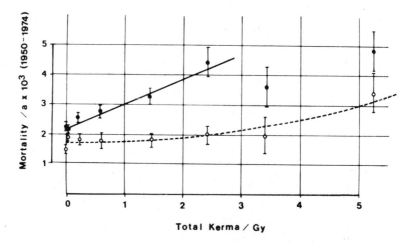

FIGURE 25. Annual mortality from all malignant neoplasms (averaged over 24 years) in individuals exposed to various values of total kerma at Hiroshima and Nagasaki.

1.3 × 10^{-2}(D_n/Gy) and 1.7 × 10^{-4}(D_γ/Gy)^2, where D_n is the neutron dose to the
bone marrow and D_γ the γ-ray dose.

Various uncertainties limit the reliability of the numerical risk estimates. In any case, these estimates should not be applied to low-LET absorbed doses of 10 mGy or less, as a more refined statistical analysis or an augmentation of the observations to a broader sample of the exposed population might disclose a linear component in the data from Nagasaki. However, despite its statistical limitations the information contained in Fig. 25 is of high pragmatic and fundamental interest.

The pragmatic conclusion is that the relation between mortality due to cancer in general and dose of high-LET radiation is substantially linear at doses in the range from roughly 10 mGy to 100 mGy, but the relation is nonlinear for doses of low-LET radiation that range from perhaps 50 mGy up to several gray. It follows that risk estimates for low-LET radiation obtained by linear extrapolation from high doses are too high. It also follows that while the hazard from low-LET radiation is thus likely to be less than given by most current risk estimates, the hazard of neutron radiation is greater than implied by a Q (quality factor) of 10.

The basic scientific conclusion is that data on human cancer are consistent with the theory of dual radiation action. Radiation carcinogenesis is therefore very likely to be a process initiated by lesions that in turn are due to the interaction of pairs of sublesions. It seems reasonable to speculate that these sublesions are double-strand breaks of DNA, but any further or more assured notions must await the availability of additional pertinent information.

6. Appendix

In the following, a formal derivation will be given of the theorem that is expressed in equation (13) of Section 3.2. As exemplified in Section 5.1, this theorem can be utilized to decide whether an observed dose–effect relation is compatible or incompatible with the assumption that the effect is due to independent alterations in individual cells.

Let E_ν be the probability of observing the effect in a cell after exactly ν energy-deposition events have occurred. As pointed out earlier, an event is energy transfer to the critical region of the cell by a charged particle and/or its secondaries. The cells are assumed to belong to an irradiated population in which no interaction of cellular damage occurs; i.e., energy deposition in one cell does not influence the effect probability for another cell.

Energy-deposition events are by definition statistically independent; their number is therefore distributed according to Poisson statistics. According to equation (8), the effect probability at dose D is

$$E(D) = \sum_{\nu=1}^{\infty} p_\nu E_\nu = \sum_{\nu=1}^{\infty} \left[e^{-\phi D}(\phi D)^\nu / \nu! \right] E_\nu \qquad (A1)$$

611
BIOPHYSICAL
ASPECTS OF
RADIATION
CAR-
CINOGENESIS

612

ALBRECHT M.
KELLERER
AND
HARALD H.
ROSSI

It is important to note that this equation holds even for an inhomogeneous population. The sole condition is that the critical regions for the individual cells are chosen to be of equal size. Without this condition, Poisson statistics would not apply. Since the critical regions can be larger than the sensitive sites of the cells or even than the cells themselves, the condition of equality of critical regions can always be met even for a population of unequal cells. It is, furthermore essential to note that the coefficients E_ν do not depend on absorbed dose. This is the case because, by definition, energy deposition outside the critical region does not influence the fate of the cell; the effect is determined solely by the number of events taking place within the critical region and by the amount of energy imparted by these events.

The slope of the dose–effect relation in the logarithmic representation is

$$c = \frac{d \ln E}{d \ln D} = \frac{D}{E} \frac{dE}{dD} \tag{A2}$$

If one inserts equation (A1) into this expression, one obtains

$$c = \frac{D}{E(D)} \sum_{\nu=1}^{\infty} E_\nu e^{-\phi D} \left[\frac{(\phi D)^{\nu-1}}{(\nu-1)!} \phi - \phi \frac{(\phi D)^\nu}{\nu!} \right]$$

$$= \frac{\sum_{\nu=1}^{\infty} E_\nu e^{-\phi D}[(\phi D)^\nu / \nu!](\nu - \phi D)}{\sum_{\nu=1}^{\infty} E_\nu e^{-\phi D}[(\phi D)^\nu / \nu!]} \tag{A3}$$

$$= \frac{\sum_{\nu=1}^{\infty} \nu p_\nu E_\nu}{\sum_{\nu=1}^{\infty} p_\nu E_\nu} - \phi D$$

The term

$$\pi_\nu = \frac{p_\nu E_\nu}{\sum_{\nu=1}^{\infty} p_\nu E_\nu} \tag{A4}$$

can be understood as a conditional probability, namely as the fraction of cells with exactly ν events among those cells that are affected. From equations (A3) and (A4),

$$c = \sum_{\nu=1}^{\infty} \nu \pi_\nu - \phi D \tag{A5}$$

This form of the equation for the logarithmic slope of the dose–effect curves has a highly interesting interpretation. The sum $\Sigma_{\nu=1}^{\infty} \nu \pi_\nu$ is the mean number of events in those cells that show the effect; one can symbolize this mean value by $\bar{n}_E$. On the other hand, the mean number of absorption events throughout the cell population, regardless of whether the cells will show the effect or not, is equal to ϕD; this latter quantity can, therefore, be symbolized as $\bar{n}$. Thus, the difference of the mean event numbers in those cells that show the effect and in the cells throughout the population is equal to the slope of the dose–effect curve in the logarithmic representation at the particular value of the absorbed dose considered. This is the theorem discussed in Sections 3 and 5:

$$c = \bar{n}_{\mathrm{E}} - \bar{n} \tag{A6}$$

A somewhat more general formulation of the relation can be found elsewhere (Kellerer and Hug, 1972).

ACKNOWLEDGMENTS

This investigation was supported by Contract DE-AC02-78EVO4733 from the Department of Energy and by Grant CA-12536 to the Radiological Research Laboratory/Department of Radiology, and by Grant CA-13696 to the Cancer Center/Institute of Cancer Research, awarded by the National Cancer Institute, DHHS.

7. References

Awa, A. A., 1975, Chromosome aberrations in somatic cells, *J. Radiat. Res. Suppl.* **16**:122–131.

Bach, R. L., and Caswell, R. S., 1968, Energy transfer to matter by neutrons, *Radiat. Res.* **35**:1–25.

Bateman, J. L., Rossi, H. H., Kellerer, A. M., Robinson, C. V., and Bond, V. P., 1972, Dose dependence of fast neutron RBE for lens opacification in mice, *Radiat. Res.* **51**:381–390.

Beebe, G., Kato, H., and Land, C. (eds.), 1977, *Mortality Experience of Atomic Bomb Survivors 1950–1974: Life Span Study 8*, Radiation Effects Research Foundation, Technical Report, pp. 1–77.

Biola, M. T., Lego, R., Ducatez, G., and Bourguignon, M., 1971, *Formation de Chromosomes Dicentrique dans les Lymphocytes Humains Soumis in Vitro à un Flux de Rayonnement Mixte (Gamma, Neutrons)*, pp. 633–645, IAEA, Vienna.

Bird, R. P., 1979, Biophysical studies with spatially correlated ions. 3. Cell survival studies using diatomic deuterium, *Radiat. Res.* **78**:210–233.

Bond, V. P., Cronkite, E. P., Lippincott, S. W., and Shellabarger, C. J., 1960, Studies on radiation induced mammary gland neoplasia in the rat, *Radiat. Res.* **12**:276–285.

Borek, C., 1979, Neoplastic transformation following split doses of x-rays, *Br. J. Radiol.* 50:845–846.

Borek, C., and Hall, E. J., 1973, Transformation of mammalian cells *in vitro* by low doses of x-rays, *Nature (London)* **244**:450–453.

Borek, C., and Hall, E. J., 1974, Effect of split doses of x-rays on neoplastic transformation of single cells, *Nature (London)* **252**:499–501.

Borek, C., and Sachs, L., 1966, *In vitro* transformation by x-irradiation, *Nature (London)* **210**:276–278.

Borek, C., Hall, E. J., and Rossi, H. H., 1978, Malignant transformation in cultured hamster embryo cells produced by X-rays, 430 keV monoenergetic neutrons, and heavy ions, *Cancer Res.* **38**:2997–3005.

Brenot, J., Chemtob, M., Chmelevsky, D., Fache, P. Parmentier, N., Soulie, R., Biola, M. T., Haag, J., Lego, R., Bourguignon, M., Courant, D., Dacher, J., and Ducatez, G., 1973, Aberrations chromosomiques et microdosimétrie, in: *Proceedings of the IV Symposium of Microdosimetry*, Verbania, Euratom, Brussels.

Brewen, J. G., Preston, R. J., Jones, K. P., and Gosslee, D. D., 1973, Genetic hazards of ionizing radiations: Cytogenetic extrapolations from mouse to man, *Mutat. Res.* **17**:245–254.

614

ALBRECHT M. KELLERER AND HARALD H. ROSSI

CHMELEVSKY, D., KELLERER, A. M., TERRISOL, M., AND PATAN, J. P., 1980, Proximity functions for electrons up to 10 keV, *Radiat. Res.* **84:**219–238.

COLE, A., 1967, Chromosome structure, in: *Theoretical and Experimental Biophysics*, Vol. I (A. Cole, ed.), Dekker, New York.

COLVETT, R. D., AND ROHRIG, N., 1979, Biophysical studies with spatially correlated ions. 2. Multiple scattering, experimental facility, and dosimetry, *Radiat. Res.* **78:**192–209.

DEWEY, W. C., NOEL, J. S., AND DETTOR, C. M., 1972, Changes in radiosensitivity and dispersion of chromatin during the cell cycle of synchronous Chinese hamster cells, *Radiat. Res.* **52:**373–394.

HALL, E. J., ROSSI, H. H., KELLERER, A. M., GOODMAN, L. J., AND MARINO, S., 1973, Radio-biological studies with monoenergetic neutrons, *Radiat. Res.* **54:**431–443.

ICRU, 1970, *Report 16: Linear Energy Transfer*, International Commission on Radiation Units and Measurements, Washington, D.C.

ICRU, 1971, *Report 19: Radiation Quantities and Units*, International Commission on Radiation Units and Measurements, Washington, D.C.

ISHIMARU, T., HOSHINO, T., ICHIMARU, M., OKADA, H., TOMIYASU, T., AND TSUCHIMOTO, T., 1971, Leukemia in atomic bomb survivors, Hiroshima and Nagasaki, 1 October 1950–30 September 1966, *Radiat. Res.* **45:**216–233.

ISHIMARU, T., OTAKE, M., AND ICHIMARU, M. 1979, Dose response relationship of neutrons and γ rays to leukemia incidence among atomic bomb survivors in Hiroshima and Nagasaki by type of leukemia, 1950–1971, *Radiat. Res.* **77:**377–394.

JABLON, S., 1979, Comments on "Leukemia Risk from Neutrons" by H. H. Rossi and C. W. Mays, *Health Phys.* **36:**205–206.

JONES, T. D., 1977, CHORD operators for cell-survival models and insult assessment to active bone marrow, *Radiat. Res.* **71:**269–283.

KELLERER, A. M., AND BRENOT, J., 1973, Nonparametric determinations of modifying factors in radiation action, *Radiat. Res.* **55:**28–39.

KELLERER, A. M., AND BRENOT, J., 1974, On the statistical evaluation of dose–response functions, *Radiat. Environ. Biophys.* **11:**1–13.

KELLERER, A. M., AND CHMELEVSKY, D., 1975, Concepts of microdosimetry. I. Quantities, *Radiat. Environ. Biophys.* **12:**61–69.

KELLERER, A. M., AND HUG, O., 1972, Theory of dose–effect relations, in: *Encyclopedia of Medical Radiology*, Vol. II/3, pp. 1–42, Springer, New York.

KELLERER, A. M., AND ROSSI, H. H., 1972, The theory of dual radiation action, *Curr. Top. Radiat. Res.* **8:**85–158.

KELLERER, A. M., LAM, Y. M., AND ROSSI, H. H., 1980, Biophysical studies with spatially correlated ions. IV. Analysis of cell survival data for diatomic deuterium, *Radiat. Res.* **83:**511–528.

KERR, G. D., 1978, Organ Dose Estimates for the Japanese Atomic Bomb Survivors, Oak Ridge National Laboratory Draft Technical Report 5436, Oak Ridge, Tennessee.

LEA, D. E., 1946, *Actions of Radiations on Living Cells*, Cambridge University Press, Cambridge.

LITTLE, J. B., AND TERZAGHI, M., 1976, Oncogenic transformation *in vitro* after split dose x-irradiation, *Int. J. Radiat. Biol.* **29:**583–587.

MILLER, R., HALL, E. J., AND ROSSI, H. H., 1979, Oncogenic transformation of mammalian cells *in vitro* with split doses of x-rays, *Proc. Natl. Acad. Sci. USA* **76:**5755–5758.

MOLE, R. H., 1975, Ionizing radiation as a carcinogen, *Br. J. Radiol.* **48:**157.

MÜLLER, W. A., GOSSNER, W., HUG, O., AND LUZ, A., 1978, Late effects after incorporation of the short lived α emitters ^{224}Ra and ^{227}Th in mice, *Health Phys.* **35:**33–56.

ROSSI, H. H., 1964, Correlations of radiation quality and biological effect, *Ann. N.Y. Acad. Sci.* **114:**4–15.

ROSSI, H. H., 1977, The effects of small doses of ionizing radiation: Fundamental biophysical characteristics, *Radiat. Res.* **71:**1–8.

ROSSI, H. H., 1979, Biophysical studies with spatially correlated ions. 1. Background and theoretical considerations, *Radiat. Res.* **78:**185–191.

ROSSI, H. H., AND KELLERER, A. M., 1972, Radiation carcinogenesis at low doses, *Science* **175:**200–202.

ROSSI, H. H., AND KELLERER, A. M., 1974, The validity of risk estimates of leukemia incidence based on Japanese data, *Radiat. Res.* **58:**131–140.

ROSSI, H. H., AND MAYS, C. W., 1978, Leukemia risk from neutrons, *Health Phys.* **34:**353–360.

SAVAGE, J. R. K., 1970, Sites of radiation induced chromosome exchanges, *Curr. Top. Radiat. Res.* **6:**131–194.

615

BIOPHYSICAL
ASPECTS OF
RADIATION
CAR-
CINOGENESIS

SAX, K., 1938, Chromosome aberrations induced by x-rays, *Genetics* **23**:494–516.

SAX, K., 1941, Types and frequencies of chromosomal aberrations induced by x-rays, *Cold Spring Harbor Symp. Quant. Biol.* **9**:93.

SCHMID, E., RIMPL, G., AND BAUCHINGER, M., 1973, Dose–response relation of chromosome aberrations in human lymphocytes after *in vitro* irradiation with 3 MeV electrons, *Radiat. Res.* **57**:228–238.

SHELLABARGER, C. J., BOND, V. P., CRONKITE, E. P., AND APONTE, G. E., 1969, Relationship of dose of total-body ^{60}Co radiation to incidence of mammary neoplasia in female rats, in: *Radiation-Induced Cancer*, IAEA-SM-118/9.

SHELLABARGER, C. J., KELLERER, A. M., ROSSI, H. H., GOODMAN, L. J., BROWN, R. D., MILLS, R. E., RAO, A. R., SHANLEY, J. P., AND BOND, V. P., 1974, Rat mammary carcinogenesis following neutron or x-irradiation, in: *Biological Effects of Neutron Irradiation*, IAEA, Vienna.

SHELLABARGER, C., CHMELEVSKY, D., AND KELLERER, A. M., 1980, Induction of mammary neoplasms in the Sprague–Dawley rat by 430 keV neutrons and x-rays, *J. Natl. Cancer Inst.* **64**:821–833.

SINCLAIR, W. K., 1968, The shape of radiation survival curves of mammalian cells cultured *in vitro*, in: *Biophysical Aspects of Radiation Quality*, IAEA, Vienna.

SPARROW, A. H., UNDERBRINK, A. G., AND ROSSI, H. H., 1972, Mutations induced in *Tradescantia* by small doses of x-rays and neutrons: Analysis of dose–response curves, *Science* **176**:916–918.

SPIESS, H., AND MAYS, C. W., 1973, Protraction effect on bone sarcoma induction of ^{224}Ra in children and adults, in: *Radionuclide Carcinogenesis*, AEC Symposium Series 29, CONF-720505, pp. 437–450, National Technical Information Service, Springfield, Va.

ULLRICH, R. L., AND STORER, J. B., 1979, Influence of γ irradiation on the development of neoplastic disease in mice. I. Reticular tissue tumors, *Radiat. Res.* **80**:303–316.

ULLRICH, R. L., JERNIGAN, M. C., AND ADAMS, L. M., 1979, Induction of lung tumors in RFM mice after localized exposures to X-rays or neutrons, *Radiat. Res.* **80**:464–473.

VOGEL, H. H., 1969, Mammary gland neoplasms after fission neutron irradiation, *Nature (London)* **222**:1279–1281.

WOLF, S., 1954, Delay of chromosome rejoining in *Vicia faba* induced by irradiation, *Nature (London)* **173**:501–502.

YUHAS, J. M., 1974, Recovery from radiation–carcinogenic injury to the mouse ovary, *Radiat. Res.* **60**:321–322.

8. Selected General References

Section 2

ATTIX, F. H., AND ROESCH, W. C., 1968, *Radiation Dosimetry*, Vol. I, Academic Press, New York.

HINE, G. J., AND BROWNELL, G. K., 1956, *Radiation Dosimetry*, Academic Press, New York.

ICRU, 1970, *Report 16: Linear Energy Transfer*, International Commission on Radiation Units and and Measurements, Washington, D.C.

ICRU, 1980, *Report 33: Radiation Quantities and Units*, International Commission on Radiation Units and Measurements, Washington, D.C.

KELLERER, A. M., AND CHMELEVSKY, D., 1975, Concepts of microdosimetry. I. Quantities, *Radiat. Environ. Biophys.* **12**:61–69.

KELLERER, A. M., AND CHMELEVSKY, D., 1975, Concepts of microdosimetry. II. Probability distributions of the microdosimetric variables, *Radiat. Environ. Biophys.* **12**:205–216.

KELLERER, A. M., AND CHMELEVSKY, D., 1975, Concepts of microdosimetry. III. Mean values of the microdosimetric distributions, *Radiat. Environ. Biophys.* **12**:321–335.

KELLERER, A. M., AND CHMELEVSKY, D., 1975, Criteria for the applicability of LET, *Radiat. Res.* **63**:226–234.

ROSSI, H. H., 1967, Energy distribution in the absorption of radiation, *Adv. Biol. Med. Phys.* **11**:27–85.

WHYTE, G. N., 1959, *Principles of Radiation Dosimetry*, Wiley, New York.

Section 3

ELKIND, M., AND WHITMORE, G., 1967, *The Radiobiology of Cultured Mammalian Cells*, Gordon & Breach, London.

616

ALBRECHT M.
KELLERER
AND
HARALD H.
ROSSI

FISZ, M., 1965, *Probability Theory and Mathematical Statistics*, Wiley, New York.

HUG, O., AND KELLERER, A. M., 1966, *Stochastik der Strahlenwirkung*, Springer, New York.

KELLERER, A. M., AND HUG, O., 1972, Theory of dose–effect relations, in: *Encyclopedia of Medical Radiology*, Vol. II/3, pp. 1–42, Springer, New York.

ZIMMER, K. G., 1961, *Studies on Quantitative Radiation Biology*, Oliver & Boyd, London.

Section 4

KELLERER, A. M., AND ROSSI, H. H., 1972, The theory of dual radiation action, *Curr. Top. Radiat. Res.* **8:**85–158.

KELLERER, A. M., AND ROSSI, H. H., 1978, A generalized formulation of dual radiation action, *Radiat. Res.* **75:**471–488.

LEA, D. E., 1946, *Actions of Radiations on Living Cells*, Cambridge University Press, Cambridge.

ROSSI, H. H., 1970, The effects of small doses of ionizing radiation, *Phys. Med. Biol.* **15:**255–262.

SAVAGE, J. R. K., 1970, Sites of radiation induced chromosome exchanges, *Curr. Top. Radiat. Res.* **6:**131–194.

Section 5

NATIONAL ACADEMY OF SCIENCES–NATIONAL RESEARCH COUNCIL, 1980, *The Effects on Populations of Exposure to Low Levels of Ionizing Radiation*, Washington, D.C.

U.S. ATOMIC ENERGY COMMISSION, 1973, *Radionuclide Carcinogenesis*, US-AEC Symposium Series 29, CONF-720505, National Technical Information Service, Springfield, Va.

UNITED NATIONS, 1977, *Sources and Effects of Ionizing Radiation*, New York.

17

Ultraviolet Radiation: Interaction with Biological Molecules

FREDERICK URBACH

1. Introduction

Solar radiation is a very important element in our environment and yet, because of its ubiquity, the wide scope of its chemical and biological effects is often not fully appreciated. That solar energy fixation makes life possible is a generally known fact. It is not so generally appreciated that many of the effects of solar radiation are detrimental. Most people are aware that a painful sunburn can be caused by excessive exposure to the sun, and that colors fade and materials age in the sun. There also are more subtle effects of sunlight on living cells, including the production of mutations and the development of skin cancer following sufficient chronic exposure to sunlight.

Recent work has shown that plant and animal cells are able to repair radiation-induced genetic damage. Evidently, plants and animals have evolved in such a way as to be able to protect themselves from the detrimental radiations of the sun, while at the same time allowing themselves to receive the benefit of other portions of the solar spectrum. The situation is one of balance: sunlight is necessary for life, yet in excess it is harmful.

The short-wave portion of the solar spectrum is potentially very detrimental to plant and animal cells. A small amount of ozone in the atmosphere filters out these harmful wavelengths of ultraviolet light and thus prevents most such

FREDERICK URBACH • Temple University School of Medicine, Skin and Cancer Hospital, Philadelphia, Pennsylvania.

radiation from reaching the surface of the earth. The formation of this ozone shield in geological time was most likely a prerequisite for the evolution of terrestrial life. However, even in the presence of this ozone layer, a biologically significant amount of ultraviolet radiation does reach the surface of the earth.

Ample evidence indicates that the sun's illumination possesses carcinogenic activity. Many geographic and population studies correlate fair skin plus degree and intensity of sun exposure with skin cancer (Segi, 1963; Urbach *et al.*, 1972). Controlled experiments in animals have proven that ultraviolet (UV) radiation can be carcinogenic [multiple exposures lead to cancer (Blum, 1959)] as well as a tumor initiator [a high dose of UV radiation followed by promotion with chemical cocarcinogens (Epstein, 1966; Pound, 1970)]. The observation that reduced ability to repair UV-induced damage of cells occurs in patients genetically predisposed to an extremely high incidence of skin cancer has stimulated great interest among investigators dealing with the etiology of cancer (Cleaver, 1968, 1970).

2. Effects of Ultraviolet Radiation on Biological Systems

The first observation of UV effects on living systems dates back to 1877, when Downes and Blunt reported that bacteria were inactivated by light. A large variety of UV effects on many cell types and organisms were reported in the next 50 years, but the early work suffered from a lack of appreciation of the necessity for controlling the wavelengths of the light as well as from a lack of understanding of the importance of the physiological state of the biological system before, during, and after the radiation. Gates discovered that the relative effectiveness of different wavelengths in killing bacteria paralleled the absorption spectrum of nucleic acid. The chemical basis for some of the deleterious effects of UV on nucleic acids did not become evident until the late 1940s. The most recent discovery of Beukers and Berends (1960) of UV-induced thymine dimers in DNA stimulated a resurgence of interest in UV photobiology.

It has now become apparent that in addition to thymine dimers there are many other types of photoproducts produced in the nucleic acid of cells, and some of these have been isolated and characterized (Smith and Hanawalt, 1969). In a number of cases, their relative biological importance has also been determined.

One area in which photobiology has been particularly useful has been in the study of cellular repair mechanisms per se: not merely to learn more about mechanisms of recovery from light-induced damage, but also to understand the broader aspects of the mechanisms that may operate to protect cells from many of the hazards of their natural environment.

Among the major effects of UV radiation on biological systems are inhibition of cell division, inactivation of enzymes, induction of mutation, and killing of cells and tissues.

ULTRAVIOLET
RADIATION:
INTERACTION
WITH
BIOLOGICAL
MOLECULES

Some of the biological effects of UV radiation can now be explained in terms of specific chemical and physical changes produced in DNA. Structural defects are produced in DNA by chemical mutagens and by radiations. This defective DNA may be repaired by cellular enzyme systems and thus serves as the substrate for repair enzymes (see below). Although our knowledge of the possible types of induced structural changes is far from complete, it may be useful to discuss briefly the most frequently formed products whose actions are best understood. Some structural defects can disrupt the continuity of the molecule, while others interfere with replication or transcription by changing hydrogen bonding. Single-strand breaks and DNA–DNA crosslinks are induced by UV, but these usually occur only at high doses, so that their practical importance is questionable (Smith, 1966). Pyrimidine hydrates do not seem to be formed efficiently in double-stranded DNA, but are formed in single-stranded DNA and may be of possible importance in the induction of mutations (Smith, 1966). The cyclobutane-type dimers formed by pyrimidines (separately and as mixed dimers) are chemically the most stable and well-defined lesions readily produced by UV in DNA (Beukers and Berends, 1960; Smith and Hanawalt, 1969). Dimers can also be formed between thymine and cytosine, or between cytosine pairs alone (Setlow *et al.*, 1965). Their formation involves linking the 5,6-unsaturated bonds to form a cyclobutane ring and must distort the phosphodiester backbone of the twin helix in the vicinity of each dimer. In bacteria, a UV dose of 1 erg/mm^2 will produce about six pyrimidine dimers in a DNA molecule containing 10^7 nucleotides. This is the approximate number of nucleotides in the genome of *Escherichia coli* (Cairns, 1963). The biological importance of this type of dimer has been demonstrated in certain situations (Cleaver, 1968), but this type of photoproduct is not formed in DNA under all conditions and thus other types of photoproducts must also be of significance. Under certain conditions, DNA can crosslink with protein (Smith, 1966). One chemical mechanism for this crosslinking may involve the attachment of amino acid residues through their SH or OH groups to the 5- or 6-carbon of cytosine and thymine.

The sensitivity of DNA to alteration by UV can be changed by a variety of factors, notably changes in the environment of physical state, or change in base composition. The effects of near-UV radiation (>300 nm) on nucleic acids have been actively explored owing to the fact that wavelengths in this region of the spectrum are components of terrestrial sunlight. From an *in vivo* study of the photoreactivity of thymine in HeLa cell DNA, it has been concluded that ring-saturated photoproducts of the thymine glycol type are formed in comparable amounts to thymine dimers on irradiation at 313 nm (Hariharan and Cerutti, 1977). Light of this wavelength has also been used to study the photochemistry of DNA containing iodinated cytosine (Rahn and Stafford, 1979). Pyrimidine adducts in DNA are photolysed to unknown products by wavelengths in the range 310–340 nm. The biological consequences of the pyrimidine adducts remain unclear, but it appears that either they and their photolysis products are not lethal or that both are lethal but are susceptible to repair under certain conditions (Patrick, 1977).

Finally, the biological importance of any given photochemical alteration of nucleic acid depends on whether or not it is formed under a particular set of experimental conditions, and, if formed, whether the biological system can repair the lesion (Smith and Hanawalt, 1969).

4. Photochemistry of Proteins

UV irradiation of proteins results in the formation of both low- and high-molecular-weight products. In the presence of oxygen, high-molecular-weight aggregates begin to decompose and thus the protein solubility increases. Irradiated proteins are much more susceptible to enzymatic digestion.

Two different theories of the mechanism of UV inactivation of enzymes have evolved over a period of years. One holds that the alteration of any amino acid residue causes inactivation of an enzyme (McLaren and Sugar, 1964). The other theory states that enzyme inactivation is the consequence of disruption of specific cysteine residues and of hydrogen bonds responsible for the spatial integrity of the active center of the enzyme (Augenstein and Riley, 1967).

5. Photoinactivation of Cells and Tissues

As might be expected, application of the knowledge of the photochemistry of DNA and proteins to interpretation of effects on metabolizing, living cells is fraught with great difficulty. Living cells have a variety of mechanisms specifically designed for dealing with potentially injurious events and exhibit different sensitivities to the same stimulus at different stages in the growth cycle. DNA is the principal target for most injurious effects of photons on growing cells. Damage to a single nucleotide may kill a cell, or result in a nonlethal mutation, or may not be detectable by any biological assay. Most of the insight into photobiological events has been obtained from studies of bacteria, particularly *E. coli* and a variety of more or less sensitive mutants of this organism (for review, see Howard-Flanders, 1968; Smith and Hanawalt, 1969). In recent years, viruses have become a most useful biological tool for photobiological investigations. Extensive studies have been made on bacteriophages and plant and animal viruses (Luria, 1955; McLaren and Sugar, 1964).

Effects of light become even much more complex in large eukaryotic cells or in multicellular organisms. Such systems have much more redundancy of genetic information, so that inactivation of a particular gene may not be consequential. The nuclei are shielded by the surrounding cytoplasm or even by light-absorbing materials (pigments, chitin, etc.), and there are fewer critical functions necessary for survival of a particular cell.

As in microorganisms, the major effect in mammalian cells is a more or less marked and long-lasting inhibition of DNA synthesis. The rate of synthesis can be estimated by incorporating tritiated thymidine into the DNA.

As regards the effects of UV radiation on the chromosomes of mammalian cells, several types of lesions were described long ago including breaks and rearrangement. A review has been published by Rauth (1970). These lesions have been studied (among others) in Chinese hamster cells and human lymphocytes. Chromosome lesions are generally produced by a low dose of UV radiation. Their production is enzyme dependent and is related to repair mechanisms (Bender *et al.*, 1973). They do not necessarily appear after the first division (Parrington, 1972). As the lesions can be photoreactivated, they are probably produced by pyrimidine dimers (Griggs and Bender, 1973). Rommelaere *et al.* (1973) discovered another widespread type of lesion in the form of sister chromatid exchanges, the frequency of which increased greatly after UV irradiation. This parameter has been shown to be extremely sensitive (Ikushima and Wolff, 1974), and thus is valuable in detecting very low doses of UV radiation, although it is not specific to that agent.

UV and X-ray irradiation exert a synergistic effect on the frequency of chromosome breaks in human lymphocytes (Holmberg and Jonasson, 1974). The UV sensitivity of eukaryotic cells varies during the mitotic cycle, the cells being more resistant in metaphase and telophase. In such cells, selective irradiation of parts of the cell has provided much useful information, e.g., that, as expected, irradiation of the nucleus is more deleterious to survival of the cell than irradiation of the cytoplasm (Giese, 1964).

6. DNA Repair

Since biologically important amounts of UV radiation reach earth, and must have done so since the beginning of evolution, mechanisms must have arisen very early in biological time to protect cells and to aid in the recovery from the damaging effects of photons.

In recent years, three major kinds of recovery have been described:

1. The damaged molecule or part of a molecule can be restored to its functional state *in situ*. This is accomplished either by an enzymatic mechanism or by "decay" of the damage to some innocuous form.
2. The damaged part can be removed and replaced with undamaged material to restore normal function.
3. The damage may remain unrepaired, but the cell may either bypass or ignore the damage.

Because of the importance of the sequence of events necessary for appropriate biological replication and normal function of DNA molecules, conditions favorable to survival of a cell usually require that any molecular repair process be completed within some narrowly defined period of time to be effective. Furthermore, the type of recovery as well as the extent of recovery will depend on the nature of the molecule that has been damaged.

A large number of different repair mechanisms have been described to date, and other kinds are being discovered with increasing frequency as new methods for photoinjury and analysis of repair are studied. An excellent review of presently known repair mechanisms can be found in Smith and Hanawalt (1969) and in the proceedings of a symposium on molecular and cellular repair processes (Beers *et al.*, 1972).

Here, only the most important and best-studied repair processes will be described.

7. Enzyme-Catalyzed Photoreactivation

Enzyme-catalyzed photoreactivation is the best-known form of *in situ* repair. In this system, illumination with visible light facilitates the direct repair *in situ* of photoproducts produced by absorption of UV photons in DNA. It has been clearly shown that most nonmammalian cells contain an enzyme system that splits pyrimidine dimers, thus restoring a normal DNA strand *in situ.* The enzyme binds specifically to UV-irradiated DNA to form a complex that is stable in the dark. If the complex is illuminated with long UV (330 nm or longer) or visible light, it separates into the active enzyme and a repaired DNA that can no longer bind to the enzyme. Illuminating the enzyme or the damaged DNA prior to complex formation has no effect on UV damage repair (Kelner, 1953, 1969).

The photoreactivation mechanism is of greatest importance for the survival of plants and small animals (such as insects) in the field, accounting for the capability of such cells to survive in tropical and mountainous areas. However, photoreactivation has been shown to exist in human leukocytes (Sutherland, 1974). In mammals, this enzyme is probably not expressed or is masked by other more effective mechanisms.

8. Excision Repair

The studies of Setlow (1968) provided the first experimental evidence leading to a model for repair of UV damage in the dark. A repair mechanism was postulated in which defective regions in one of the two DNA strands could be excised and subsequently replaced with normal nucleotides, utilizing the complementary base-pairing information in the intact strand. This mechanism (Fig. 1), which has come to be known as "cut and patch," has turned out to be of widespread significance for the repair of a variety of structural defects of DNA.

623

ULTRAVIOLET
RADIATION:
INTERACTION
WITH
BIOLOGICAL
MOLECULES

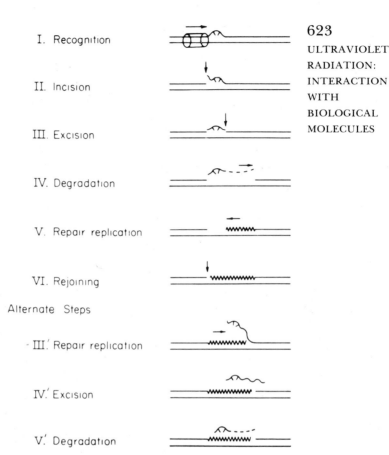

FIGURE 1. Schematic representation of the postulated steps in the excision repair of damaged DNA. Steps I through VI illustrate the "cut and patch" sequence. An initial incision in the damaged strand is followed by local degradation before the resynthesis of the region has begun. In the alternative "patch and cut" model, the resynthesis step III begins immediately after the incision step II and the excision of the damaged region occurs when repair replication is complete. In either model, the final step (VI) involves a rejoining of the repaired section to the contiguous DNA of the original parental strand. From Smith and Hanawalt (1969) with permission.

Excision repair involves (Smith and Hanawalt, 1969) the following:

1. *Recognition.* This system is capable of recognizing a variety of structural defects in DNA, including those that do not involve pyrimidines and those not due to UV effects (usually caused by alkylating agents, etc.). The exact nature of the recognition mechanism is not known.
2. *Incision.* Following recognition of DNA damage, a single-strand break near the damage point must be produced. This is most likely done by an enzymatic process.
3. *Excision and repair replication.* These processes may occur as separate steps or concurrently. It is thought that the known enzymes exonuclease III and DNA polymerase may be responsible for these steps.
4. *Rejoining.* Completion of the repair process requires rejoining of the repaired segment to the continuous DNA strand. Polynucleotide ligase may well be the enzyme responsible for this step.

Evidence for excision repair mechanisms has been found in microorganisms, viruses, and mammalian cells (Lieberman and Forbes, 1973).

The observation of Howard-Flanders (1968) that double-mutant strains of *E. coli*, deficient in both excision and recombination, were more sensitive to UV than either of the single-mutant strains alone suggested the existence of a dark repair mechanism other than "cut and patch." The nature of DNA synthesis on unrepaired templates is not yet clear, but studies in various mutant strains of bacteria support the presence of at least one and perhaps more than one dark repair system in addition to the excision repair mode.

Numerous authors have shown by various biochemical methods that synthesis of DNA of relatively low molecular weight takes place immediately after irradiation, and that a short time afterwards this newly formed DNA is of normal molecular weight (Painter, 1975).

The dimers prevent replication from being carried out continuously. Replication probably occurs between the dimers that have not yet been excised, leaving gaps in the new strands opposite each dimer of the parental strand (Lehmann, 1972). The mechanism by which replication fills the gaps has not yet been properly elucidated, nor has the degree to which the replication is error-free. It is probable that at least part of the repair is inaccurate as a result of errors of replication opposite a lesion. Depending on the degree of accuracy, either repair is total or a lesion persists that may lead to death, mutation, or carcinogenesis.

It is important to note that the known DNA repair systems in bacteria are under genetic control and that genetic loci control the extent of DNA degradation and may control gene products needed for the correct functioning of the repair enzymes. The finding by Cleaver and Carter (1973) of a genetic defect of excision repair in a heritable disease in man (xeroderma pigmentosum) and the fact that variants of this disorder involve different abilities to repair UV damage to the cells are of considerable importance for the hypothesis that heritable characteristics may be involved in the liability for cancer production in man.

10. Ultraviolet Light, DNA Repair, and Carcinogenesis

Since the end of the 19th century, when the earliest suggestions were made that frequent and prolonged exposure to sunlight is the cause of skin cancer (Unna, 1894; Dubreuilh, 1896; Shield, 1899), substantial experimental, epidemiological, and clinical observations have changed these earlier suspicions to virtual certainty (Blum, 1959; Urbach, 1966; Gordon *et al.*, 1972).

The evidence for the assumption that exposure to sunlight, particularly the mid-UV component, is an essential and major factor in the development of most human skin cancers can be briefly summarized as follows:

1. Skin cancer appears on those parts of the body most exposed to sunlight, particularly the head, neck, arms, and hands (Silverstone and Gordon, 1966).

625

ULTRAVIOLET
RADIATION:
INTERACTION
WITH
BIOLOGICAL
MOLECULES

2. Squamous cell carcinoma in particular (and basal cell carcinoma to a lesser degree) occurs primarily on skin sites most heavily exposed to solar radiation (Urbach, 1966).

3. There is a greater prevalence of skin cancer in outdoor workers (Blum, 1959), and in a particular community a greater frequency of skin cancer (and occasionally the only incidence of skin cancer) is found in those who have spent the longest periods outdoors (Urbach et al., 1972; O'Brien et al., 1970).

4. For similar types of skin, skin cancer increases fairly rapidly with decrease in latitude, particularly in the middle latitudes (mid 50s to low 20s). This tendency is not shown for any other cancer except malignant melanoma (Dorn, 1944; Blum, 1959; Gordon et al., 1972).

5. Susceptible racial types, particularly those of Celtic origin, are more prone to skin cancer than other whites, and especially to multiple lesions. The characteristic skin has little pigment, or scattered freckles, and susceptible individuals seem more often to have fair hair and blue or gray eyes and to sunburn easily, severely, and often (O'Brien et al., 1970; Gellin et al., 1966; Silverstone and Searle, 1970; Urbach et al., 1972).

6. In extensive, carefully controlled experiments with UV on animal (primarily mouse) skin, it has been shown without any doubt that skin cancer is produced by repeated exposure to wavelengths between 320 and 250 nm, with the range 320–280 nm being most effective (Findlay, 1928; Blum, 1959; Epstein, 1966). Tumors have also been induced by massive single doses of UV (Hsu et al., 1975), and tumor cells have been initiated by a single, modest UV exposure and promoted into cancers by chemical substances (Epstein, 1966; Pound, 1970).

Despite these and numerous other biological and biochemical studies, the pathogenetic mechanism of UV carcinogenesis on the cellular level remains obscure. Basic data about the molecular effect of UV on DNA had not helped until pyrimidine dimer formation, excision, and repair by unscheduled DNA replication were demonstrated in mammalian cells in vitro (Evans and Norman, 1968) and in vivo (Epstein et al., 1968) and in cultured cells from skin-cancer-prone patients (Cleaver, 1968). This last observation resulted in a flurry of research activity because the possible implication of unrepaired DNA damage in cancer production hit a responsive chord—a "Zeitgeist" phenomenon. However, xeroderma pigmentosum variants were soon discovered in which excision repair systems were apparently normal, although the patients were as exquisitely cancer prone as those showing little or no DNA repair (Cleaver and Carter, 1973).

Excision repair is now known to occur after damage with both carcinogenic and noncarcinogenic agents (Roberts, 1972) as well as in the skin of humans and mice (Epstein et al., 1971), rat liver and kidney, rabbit brain, UV-induced squamous cell carcinoma of hairless mouse skin (Lieberman and Forbes, 1973), and human tumor cell suspensions (Norman et al., 1972). It is thus clear that a great variety of mammalian cells and at least some malignant cells have excision repair capacity.

In addition to the well-documented capability of UV radiation to induce cancer of the skin in humans and mice, Setlow (personal communication, 1973) has been able to show that *in vitro* UV-irradiated fish liver cells, reinjected into isogeneic recipients, give rise to tumors. The tumor induction is UV dose dependent, and illumination of the irradiated cells with visible light before injection markedly reduces tumor production. Since fish cells possess the photo-reactivating enzyme, these data imply that pyrimidine dimers induced in cellular DNA by UV are related to the development of the tumors.

The available evidence suggests that injury to DNA is somehow related to carcinogenesis. In view of the evidence that DNA damage encourages mutagenesis in cells, this is a tenable assumption. However, in mouse skin and in most cancer patients, the DNA repair systems seem to be capable of repairing UV damage; thus, lack of DNA repair cannot be the basis of most skin cancers. An elegant experiment of Zajdela and Latarjet (1973) suggests a possible reason for this dilemma. They painted a solution of caffeine, a potent inhibitor of DNA repair, on the skin of mice during irradiation with UV. The caffeine-treated skin developed fewer skin cancers than an unpainted control area on the same animal.

Epstein *et al.* (1971) and Zajdela and Latarjet (1973) suggest that the production of skin cancer by UV is initiated by repair of DNA, allowing the cell to survive, yet leaving in place or even favoring subsequent errors in DNA replication, resulting in a greater likelihood of malignant change. Further experiments are needed to sort out the mechanisms involved and the relative contribution of DNA damage and DNA repair to carcinogenesis.

11. References

AUGENSTEIN, L., AND RILEY, P., 1967, The inactivation of enzymes by UV light: The effect of environment of cystine disruption by UV light, *Photochem. Photobiol.* **6**:423.

BEERS, R. F., JR., HERRIOTT, R., AND TILGHMAN, R. C. (eds.), 1972, *Molecular and Cellular Repair Processes*, Johns Hopkins Press, Baltimore.

BENDER, M. A., GRIGGS, H. G., AND WALKER, P. L., 1973, Mechanisms of chromosomal aberration production. I. Aberration induction by ultraviolet light, *Mutat. Res.* **20**:387–402.

BEUKERS, R., AND BERENDS, W., 1960, Isolation and identification of the irradiation product of thymine, *Biochim. Biophys. Acta* **41**:550–551.

BLUM, H. F., 1959, *Carcinogenesis by Ultraviolet Light*, Princeton University Press, Princeton, N.J.

CAIRNS, J., 1963, The chromosome of *Escherichia coli*, *Cold Spring Harbor Symp. Quant. Biol.* **28**:43–46.

CLEAVER, J. E., 1968, Defective repair replication of DNA in xeroderma pigmentosum, *Nature (London)* **218**:652.

CLEAVER, J. E., 1970, DNA damage and repair in light sensitive human skin disease, *J. Invest. Dermatol.* **54**:181.

CLEAVER, J. E., AND CARTER, P. M., 1973, Xeroderma pigmentosum: Influence of temperature on DNA repair, *J. Invest. Dermatol.* **60**:29–32.

DORN, H. F., 1944, Illness from cancer in the United States, *U.S. Public Health Rep.* **59**:33–48, 65–77, 97–115.

Dubreuilh, W., 1896, Des Hyperkeratoses Circonscriptes, *Ann. Dermatol. Syphiligr.* (Ser. 3) **7**:1158–1204.

Epstein, J. H., 1966, Ultraviolet light carcinogenesis, in: *Advances in Biology of Skin*, Vol. VII (W. Montagna and R. L. Dobson, eds.), Pergamon Press, Oxford.

Epstein, J. H., Fukuyama, K., and Epstein, W. L., 1968, UVL induced stimulation of DNA synthesis in hairless mouse epidermis, *J. Invest. Dermatol.* **51**:445.

Epstein, W. L., Fukuyama, K., and Epstein, J. H., 1971, UV light, DNA repair and skin carcinogenesis in man, *Fed. Proc.* **30**:1766–1771.

Evans, R. G., and Norman, A., 1968, Unscheduled incorporation of thymidine in ultraviolet irradiated human lymphocytes, *Radiat. Res.* **36**:287.

Findlay, G. M., 1928, Ultraviolet light and skin cancer, *Lancet* **215**:1070–1073.

Gellin, G. A., Kopf, A. W., and Garfinkel, L., 1966, Basal cell epithelioma: A controlled study of associated factors, in: *Advances in Biology of Skin*, Vol. VII (W. Montagna and R. L. Dobson, eds.), Pergamon Press, Oxford.

Giese, A. C., 1964, Studies on UV radiation action upon animal cells, in: *Photophysiology*, Vol. 2 (A. C. Giese, ed.), p. 203ff, Academic Press, New York.

Gordon, D., Silverstone, H., and Smithhurst, B. A., 1972, The epidemiology of skin cancer in Australia, in: *Melanoma and Skin Cancer* (W. H. McCarthy, ed.), NSW Government Printer, Sydney, Australia.

Griggs, H. C., and Bender, M. A., 1973, Photoreactivation of ultraviolet induced chromosomal aberrations, *Science* **179**:86–88.

Hariharan, P. V., and Cerutti, P. A., 1977, Formation of products of the 5,6-dihydroxydihydrothymine type by ultraviolet light in HeLa cells, *Biochemistry* **16**:2791–2795.

Holmberg, M., and Jonasson, J., 1974, Synergistic effect of X-ray and UV irradiation on the frequency of chromosome breakage in human lymphocytes, *Mutat. Res.* **23**:213–221.

Howard-Flanders, P., 1968, DNA repair, *Am. Rev. Biochem.* **37**:175–199.

Hsu, J., Forbes, P. D., Harber, L. C., and Lakow, E., 1975, Induction of skin tumors in hairless mice by a single exposure to ultraviolet radiation, *Photochem. Photobiol.* **21**:185–188.

Ikushima, T., and Wolff, S., 1974, UV-induced chromatid aberrations in cultured Chinese hamster cells after one, two, or three rounds of DNA replication, *Mutat. Res.* **22**:193–201.

Kelner, A., 1953, Growth, respiration and nucleic acid synthesis in UV-irradiated and in photoreactivated *E. coli*, *J. Bacteriol.* **65**:252–262.

Kelner, A., 1969, Biological aspects of UV damage, photoreactivation and other repair systems in micro-organisms, in: *The Biologic Effects of UV Radiation* (F. Urbach, ed.), Pergamon Press, Oxford.

Latarjet, R., and Zajdela, F., 1974, The inhibiting effect of caffeine on the induction of skin cancer by UV in the mouse, *Compt. Rend. Acad. Sci.* **277**:1073–1076.

Lehmann, A. R., 1972, Postreplication repair of DNA in ultraviolet-irradiated mammalian cells, *Mol. Biol.* **66**:319–337.

Lieberman, M. W., and Forbes, P. D., 1973, Demonstration of DNA repair in normal and neoplastic tissues after treatment with proximate chemical carcinogens and UV radiation, *Nature New Biol.* **241**:199–201.

Luria, S. E., 1955, Radiation and viruses, in: *Radiation Biology*, Vol. 2 (A. Hollander, ed.), p. 333ff, McGraw–Hill, New York.

McLaren, A. D., and Sugar, D., 1964, *Photochemistry of Proteins and Nucleic Acids*, Pergamon Press, Oxford.

Norman, H., Ottoman, R. E., Chan, P., and Kilsak, I., 1972, Unscheduled DNA synthesis, *Mutat. Res.* **15**:358.

O'Beirn, S. F., Judge, P., Urbach, F., MacCon, C. F., and Martin, F., 1970, The prevalence of skin cancer in County Galway, Ireland, in: *Proceedings of the 6th National Cancer Conference*, pp. 489–500, Lippincott, Philadelphia.

Painter, R. B., 1975, Repair in mammalian cells: Overview, in: *Molecular Mechanisms for Repair of DNA* (P. C. Hanawalt and R. B. Setlow, eds.), pp. 595–600, Plenum Press, New York.

Parrington, J. M., 1972, Ultraviolet-induced chromosome aberration and mitotic delay in human fibroblast cells, *Cytogenetics* **11**:117–131.

Patrick, M. H., 1977, Studies on thymine-derived UV photoproducts in DNA. I. Formation and biological role of pyrimidine adducts in DNA, *Photochem. Photobiol.* **25**:357–372.

Pound, A. W., 1970, Induced cell proliferation and the initiation of skin tumor formation in mice by ultraviolet light, *Pathology* **2**:269–275.

627

ULTRAVIOLET
RADIATION:
INTERACTION
WITH
BIOLOGICAL
MOLECULES

RAHN, R. O., AND STAFFORD, R. S., 1979, Photochemistry of DNA containing iodinated cytosine, *Photochem. Photobiol.* **30:**449–454.

RAUTH, A. M., 1970, Effects of ultraviolet light on mammalian cells in culture, *Curr. Top. Radiat. Res.* **6:**195–248.

ROBERTS, J. J., 1972, in: *Molecular and Cellular Repair Processes* (R. F. Beers, R. Herriott, and R. Tilghman, eds.), p. 238ff, Johns Hopkins Press, Baltimore.

ROMMELAERE, J., SUSSKIND, M., AND ERRERA, M., 1973, Chromosome and chromatid exchanges in Chinese hamster cells, *Chromosoma* **41:**243–257.

SEGI, M., 1963, World incidence and distribution of skin cancer, in: *Monograph No. 10, National Cancer Institute* (F. Urbach and H. L. Stewart, eds.), Government Printing Office, Washington, D.C.

SETLOW, R. B., 1968, The photochemistry, photobiology, and repair of polynucleotides, *Prog. Nucleic Acid Res. Mol. Biol.* **8:**257ff.

SETLOW, R. B., CARRIER, W. L., AND BOLLUM, F. J., 1965, Pyrimidine dimers in the UV-irradiated poly dI:dC, *Proc. Natl. Acad. Sci. USA* **53:**1111–1118.

SHIELD, A. M., 1899, A remarkable case of multiple growths of the skin caused by exposure to the sun, *Lancet* **1:**22–23.

SILVERSTONE, H., AND GORDON, D., 1966, Regional studies in skin cancer, 2nd report: Wet tropical and sub-tropical coast of Queensland, *Med. J. Austr.* **2:**733–740.

SILVERSTONE, H., AND SEARLE, J. H. A., 1970, The epidemiology of skin cancer in Queensland: The influence of phenotype and environment, *Br. J. Cancer* **24:**235–252.

SMITH, K. C., 1966, Physical and chemical changes induced in nucleic acids by UV light, *Radiat. Res. Suppl.* **6:**54–79.

SMITH, K. C., AND HANAWALT, P. C., 1969, *Molecular Photobiology,* Academic Press, New York.

SUTHERLAND, B. M., 1974, Photoreactivating enzyme from human leukocytes, *Nature (London)* **248:**109–112.

UNNA, P. G., 1894, *Die Histopathologie der Hautkrankheiten,* A. Hirschwald, Berlin.

URBACH, F., 1966, Ultraviolet radiation and skin cancer in man, in: *Advances in Biology of Skin,* Vol. VII (W. Montagna and R. L. Dobson, eds.), Pergamon Press, Oxford.

URBACH, F., ROSE, D. B., AND BONNEM, M., 1972, Genetic and environmental interactions in skin carcinogenesis, in: *Environment and Cancer,* pp. 335–371, Williams & Wilkins, Baltimore.

18

Radiation Carcinogenesis

1. Introduction

Ionizing radiation in sufficiently high dosage acts as a complete carcinogen in that it serves as both initiator and promoter. Further, cancers can be induced in nearly any tissue or organ of man or experimental animals by the proper choice of radiation dose and exposure schedule. Principal interest in radiation as an environmental carcinogen is not at very high dosage levels, however, since relatively few individuals receive such high dosages and in most cases where they do the radiation is received as localized treatment for a malignant tumor. Additionally, radiation delivered to the entire body, as is usually the case for environmental exposure, is acutely fatal (within weeks) at doses higher than a few hundred rads. For these reasons, the major goal of studies on radiation as a carcinogen is the determination of its cancerogenic effectiveness in the extremely low to moderate dosage range. Because radiation can be easily delivered in precisely measured quantities and because it is a fairly potent carcinogen, it has also been widely used as an experimental tool in cancer research.

Information on the effects of radiation on man has been obtained from a variety of sources. These include persons or populations receiving (1) occupational exposure (radiologists and uranium miners), (2) accidental exposure, (3) therapeutic exposure, (4) diagnostic exposure (X-rays or radioisotopes), and (5) wartime exposure (Hiroshima and Nagasaki). Summary information and an evaluation of the data so far obtained from these sources have been recently summarized in the 1972 reports of the United Nations Scientific Committee on the Effects of Atomic Radiation (UNSCEAR Report) and the NAS-NRC Advisory Committee on the Biological Effects of Ionizing Radiations (BEIR Report).

JOHN B. STORER ● Biology Division, Oak Ridge National Laboratory, Oak Ridge, Tennessee. Research sponsored by the U.S. Atomic Energy Commission under contract with the Union Carbide Corporation.

Information from experimental animals has been accumulating for over 70 yr, although at a greatly accelerated rate over the past 25 yr. Because of this rapid proliferation of information, any review of the subject that deals with specific conclusions is likely to become obsolete rapidly. General principles emerging from animal experimentation are likely to stand the test of further research, however, and for this reason emphasis in this chapter is on principles rather than specific details.

2. Tissue Sensitivity

2.1. Man

As indicated earlier, cancer of nearly any tissue can be induced by the proper choice of radiation dose and treatment schedule. The question, then, is not whether some tissues are absolutely refractory to carcinogenic effects but whether there are differences in sensitivity to the induction of cancer. There is ample evidence at the present time to conclude that human tissues do indeed show a very wide range in susceptibility to radiation-induced cancers. This conclusion is based on published studies of all the exposed populations enumerated earlier but leans most heavily on data from the two largest populations, namely the survivors of the atomic bombings in Japan as reported by the Atomic Bomb Casualty Commission (ABCC) and the patients with ankylosing spondylitis treated with therapeutic radiation in Great Britain as reported by Court Brown and Doll (1965).

A number of scientific committees have studied this question and have attempted to classify various tissues according to relative sensitivity. These committees include the United Nations Scientific Committee on the Effects of Atomic Radiation (1972), the NAS-NRC Advisory Committee on the Biological Effects of Ionizing Radiations (1972), and a task group for the International Commission on Radiological Protection (ICRP) (1969). These groups, although basing their conclusions on essentially the same data reached slightly different conclusions. In turn, the conclusions I have reached are also somewhat different. The reason for these differences is that each individual or committee attempting to classify relative sensitivity must make judgments on the following points. First, is there consistency between and among the various studies with respect to the induction of a particular type of tumor? For example, if a slight excess incidence of cancer of a particular type is found in one irradiated population but not in any of the others, then the suspicion of a chance sampling variation arises, particularly if the positive population has a small sample size. Second, are the control data adequate to reach the conclusion of a radiation-induced excess of cases? This consideration is particularly important in studies on cancer incidence following therapeutic radiation, where the patient population is already ill with a disease which might itself be associated with an increased cancer risk. Third, is the number of cases sufficient to conclude that there is a significant excess of a particular cancer? An observed incidence of one case when the expected number

is 0.21 yields a relative risk of 4.8* but does not inspire much confidence in the
validity of the risk estimate. Finally, is the observed increased incidence of cancer
likely due to factors other than ionizing radiation? It is virtually impossible to
match perfectly between control and irradiated populations such factors
as economic status, medical history, personal habits, occupation, and dietary
preferences, all of which could contribute to predilection to the development of
cancer.

While there is an impressive amount of data on radiation carcinogenesis in
human populations, the data are inadequate for most types of cancer to permit a
clear-cut classification of tissue sensitivities. For this reason, any such classification
(with the exception of a few tissues) must be tentative and reflect the best
judgment of the reviewer or the reviewing committee. Fortunately, it seems
unlikely that the data will be improved in view of the widespread awareness of the
hazards of unnecessary radiation exposure.

2.1.1. Leukemia

Myeloid leukemia and the acute leukemias are probably the most easily induced of
all radiation-induced neoplasms. All studies in which the sample sizes were
sufficiently large, the radiation doses were higher than about 50 rads, and an
appreciable fraction of the body was irradiated have shown an excess of leukemia
over the control group (Seltser and Sartwell, 1965; Court Brown and Doll, 1965;
Doll and Smith, 1968; Ishimaru et al., 1971).

There have also been a number of reports of an association between in utero
exposure to diagnostic X-rays and an increased risk of leukemia. In these cases,
the radiation doses were very small, amounting only to a few rads. Because the
evidence is somewhat conflicting, these studies will be considered in more detail in
Section 6 under the heading of "host factors."

Unlike solid tumors of other tissues, where the latent period between exposure
and development of the tumor may be very long (and the period of increased risk
perhaps also correspondingly long), the leukemias occur early, show a high
incidence, and then fall to close to the control incidence. Perhaps the best source
of information on the human leukemias is the population of Japanese exposed to
radiation from the atomic bomb (Ishimaru et al., 1971; Jablon and Kato, 1972). By
5 yr after their exposure, they showed a significantly increased leukemia incidence in the higher-dose groups. This increase was sustained for several years, but
by 25 yr after exposure the incidence had fallen to close to control values. Barring
an unanticipated second wave of leukemias, then, the data are essentially
complete for this disease in the ABCC studies. For this reason, it is not premature
to try to evaluate the shape of the dose–response curve, and this will be done in a
later section. Briefly, the Hiroshima survivors who were exposed to a mixture of
neutrons and γ-rays showed an increased leukemia incidence at doses of 50 rads

---

* This example is taken from Table 2-1, p. 164, of the Report of the NAS-NRC Advisory Committee on
the Biological Effects of Ionizing Radiations (NAS-NRC, 1972).

and above. In Nagasaki, where the exposure was to γ-rays, no increase was detectable at doses below about 100 rads, although the sample size was about one-half that of Hiroshima.

In contrast to the acute and myeloid leukemias, other neoplasms of reticular tissues, such as chronic lymphatic leukemia and Hodgkin's disease, are resistant to radiation induction.

2.1.2. Cancer of the Thyroid

The other relatively easily induced tumor in human populations is cancer of the thyroid, particularly when the radiation is delivered to juveniles. It should be noted that, in contrast to leukemia, thyroid cancer is relatively infrequently fatal. Roughly 10–20% of the cases are fatal depending on age at onset. In general, those cancers occurring late in life tend to be more malignant. For these reasons, it is necessary to establish incidence rates (preferably confirmed by biopsy) for thyroid cancers rather than to depend on death rates. This requirement makes it more difficult to determine precisely the relationship between radiation dose and response.

The principal populations studied to date have been persons receiving therapeutic radiation (usually as infants) for thymic enlargement (Hempelmann et al., 1967), the Marshallese people inadvertently exposed to fallout radiation (Conard et al., 1970), and the survivors of the Japanese bombings (Wood et al., 1969). These studies indicate that at doses in excess of about 50 rads there is a significantly elevated risk of thyroid neoplasms. In one of the studies of children irradiated for thymic enlargement, the dose to the thyroid was estimated at less than 30 rads (Pifer et al., 1968). Over an observation period of about 30 yr, there was a slight but not statistically significant increase in thyroid cancer. Benign tumors appeared to be significantly increased, but the validity of this conclusion is questionable because of the great uncertainty in estimating the frequency of benign lesions in the control population. The duration of the period of elevated risk is not known, and studies such as those at ABCC cannot be considered complete at the present time.

Interestingly, patients receiving very large doses of radiation from [131]I (5000–10,000 rads) do not show an increased incidence of thyroid cancer. Presumably these high doses kill the thyroid cells, and neoplasms cannot develop (Conard et al., 1970).

2.1.3. Cancer of the Breast

Breast cancer can also be induced by radiation exposure, but in contrast to leukemias and thyroid cancer, where an excess incidence has been reported following relatively small radiation doses, higher doses (in excess of about 100 rads) are required for its induction. Wanebo et al. (1968a) reported the incidence in women periodically examined in the Adult Health Study at the ABCC. This group consists of a subsample of the much larger Life Span Study, but because of the repeated medical examinations it is possible to ascertain incidence of a disease, whereas the Life Span Study detects mortality from various diseases. At radiation doses in excess of 90 rads, the incidence was significantly increased, although the total number of cases was small. This observation was subsequently verified by mortality data from the Life Span Study (Jablon and Kato, 1972). A significant increase in mortality was seen only in the period of more than 20 yr after exposure, reflecting the slow time course of the fatal progression of the disease.

Independent verification of susceptibility of the breast to radiation-induced cancer is provided by earlier studies of women exposed to repeated fluoroscopic examinations in the course of treatment of tuberculosis by pneumothorax (Mackenzie, 1965; Myrden and Hiltz, 1969) and by studies of women treated with X-rays for acute postpartum mastitis (Mettler *et al.*, 1969). In both studies, there was a significant excess incidence of breast cancer. The radiation doses are not very well known in the fluoroscopy cases, but at least some of the women must have received very large doses since they showed evidence of severe radioder-matitis. The majority of the women must have received at least several hundred roentgens based on the output of the machine, number of fluoroscopies, and exposure time for each procedure. In the series treated for mastitis, the tumor incidence was about twice that found in the general population. The radiation doses ranged from about 100 to 600 rads, with a mean dose to the irradiated breast (most patients received unilateral radiation) of about 350 rads.

On the basis of these studies, it is concluded that the breast is moderately sensitive to the induction of cancer by radiation.

2.1.4. Cancer of the Lung

Evidence that the lung is moderately sensitive to cancer induction is provided principally from studies of uranium miners occupationally exposed to radon and radon daughters, the patients treated for ankylosing spondylitis by X-rays, and the studies at the ABCC. However, there are difficulties in the interpretation of all these studies, that make quantitative conclusions difficult. First of all, cancer of the lung is common and its incidence is known to be affected by such variables as smoking habits and urban as opposed to rural living. Additionally, the incidence rate in various populations has been changing rapidly, making it difficult to interpret the effect of an additional variable such as radiation exposure.

There is no question that uranium miners whose lungs were occupationally exposed to α-particle radiation from radon and radon daughters showed an increased incidence of lung cancer (Lundin *et al.*, 1971). Further, those believed to be more heavily exposed showed a higher incidence. The difficulty is that the radiation dosages are not at all well known. Estimates of dose are based on work histories and on infrequent determinations of the radon content in air samples obtained in the mines. Continuous monitoring of work areas was not practiced. It is known that radon concentrations vary greatly by location within the same mine and that there are large temporal variations in concentrations at the same location within a mine. Attempts have been made to estimate the extent of exposure of the miners, but these are at best only rough approximations. α-Particles are densely ionizing (they have a high value for linear energy transfer or LET) and, in general, densely ionizing radiations are biologically more effective on a dose-for-dose basis than lightly ionizing radiations such as X- or γ-rays. This point is of importance when we consider the data for the Japanese since the people in Hiroshima were exposed to radiation with a large component of neutrons, which also have a high LET.

In the patients treated for ankylosing spondylitis, the relative risk of developing lung cancer was approximately twice that in the general population (Court Brown and Doll, 1965). The average dose to the lung of these patients has recently been reestimated as about 400 rads (BEIR Report, NAS-NRC, 1972). There is some uneasiness about accepting this incidence figure at face value, however, for the following reasons. The patient population was ill with a seriously debilitating disease. Medications and treatments other than radiation were undoubtedly administered. The smoking habits of the patients may very well have differed from those of the general population, and, finally, the disease interferes with free motion of the rib cage. This interference could conceivably affect the clearance rate of inhaled materials from the lung and thus contribute to susceptibility to cancer.

Perhaps the best population in which to evaluate carcinogenic effect is the Japanese survivors (Beebe *et al.*, 1971; Wanebo *et al.*, 1968b; Jablon and Kato, 1972), but even here there are serious problems. The segment of the population in Hiroshima which received significant radiation exposure (part of which was at high LET) showed about twice the risk of cancer than did those receiving negligible exposures (median dose of 0 rads). This control group itself and the group "not-in-city" at the time of the bombing both showed consistently higher rates than the general population of Japan. Further, the significantly irradiated population in Nagasaki (low LET radiation) did not show an excess risk over those negligibly exposed.

Tuberculous patients in Israel who presumably were exposed to more diagnostic radiation from fluoroscopy than the general population have been reported to show an increased risk of lung cancer (Steinitz, 1965). Radiation doses are not known, however, nor have other variables been evaluated, such as the primary disease itself, which might lead to an increased cancer risk. It is interesting that excessive lung cancer risk in the patients repeatedly fluoroscoped in connection with pnemothorax treatment of tuberculosis was not reported.

In view of the above uncertainties, it seems fair to conclude that the lung is probably moderately sensitive to radiation-induced cancer, but precise quantitative relationships remain to be established.

2.1.5. Salivary Gland Tumors

Salivary gland tumors are relatively rare, and few have been reported as being radiation induced. On the basis of the available evidence, however, it is concluded that the salivary gland is moderately sensitive to cancer induction. Belsky *et al.*

(1972) have reported from the ABCC on 30 cases in their study population. Of these, three occurred in patients exposed to more than 300 rads, whereas the expected number in this group was 0.4. This difference is statistically significant.

Supporting evidence of radiation-induced salivary gland tumors is found in the studies on children irradiated for thymic enlargement (Hempelmann *et al.*, 1967) and in other patients receiving radiation to areas which included the salivary glands (Saenger *et al.*, 1960; Hazen *et al.*, 1966).

2.1.6. Skin

Cancer of the skin was a frequent sequela to exposure to very large doses of radiation received by earlier X-ray workers who were unaware of the hazards of radiation exposure. These cancers usually arise in areas of chronic radiation dermatitis, and X-ray doses must have been well in excess of 1000 rads. In the two largest populations studied to date, namely the spondylitics (Court Brown and Doll, 1965) and the Japanese survivors (Johnson *et al.*, 1969), no excess of skin cancer has been found even at doses of several hundred rads. Initially it appeared that skin cancer in children treated with 450–805 rads for ringworm of the scalp might be increased (Albert and Omran, 1968; Schulz and Albert, 1968). According to the BEIR Report (NAS-NRC, 1972), a recent reevaluation of the data by Albert indicates no significant effect.

In view of the fact that skin cancer is induced only by very high doses, we conclude that this tissue is relatively resistant to radiation-induced cancer.

2.1.7. Bone

Like skin, bone is resistant to cancer induction, even though a large number of radiation-induced sarcomas have been reported. These tumors have occurred principally in persons with internally deposited radium and mesothorium as a result of occupational exposure (radium dial painters) or therapeutic administration for various diseases including bone tuberculosis and ankylosing spondylitis (Evans *et al.*, 1969, 1972; Spiess and Mays, 1970, 1971). The radium isotopes selectively localize near the cells of interest. In general, bone cancers have not been seen at doses below about 500 rads, and the great majority have occurred at doses well in excess of a 1000 rads. Since, as pointed out earlier, the α-particle radiation from these isotopes has a high LET and therefore would be expected to be appreciably more effective than X- or γ-radiation, it is apparent that bone must be relatively resistant to cancer induction.

Studies of the two principal populations exposed to an external source of penetrating radiation where the dosimetry problem is much less complex support this conclusion. No excess bone cancers have been found in the Japanese survivors (Yamamoto and Wakabayaski, 1968). Five bone cancers were found in the spondylitic patients treated with X-rays, whereas only 1.1 were expected at control rates (Court Brown and Doll, 1965). However, many of these patients received well over 1000 rads to the spine, and this small number of excess cases is therefore not unexpected.

Bone tumors have been reported in other patients receiving radiotherapy, but again the radiation doses to bone were very high (Bloch, 1962).

2.1.8. Stomach

Court Brown and Doll (1965) reported an excess number of cases of gastric cancer in the spondylitics treated with X-rays. In the Japanese survivors, however, no evidence of an increased incidence has been found (Yamamoto *et al.*, 1970). Because of the lack of independent confirming evidence from the various other study populations, it is concluded that the stomach is relatively resistant to radiation-induced cancer and that the excess in the spondylitics may be related either to their primary disease or to its treatment by other medications.

2.1.9. Other Tissues

There have been reports of excess cancers of other specific tissues in some of the irradiated populations. These sites include the pancreas, larynx, pharynx, and esophagus. Other studies have been unable to confirm these reports, and it is concluded therefore that the tissues other than those specifically discussed in earlier paragraphs are probably relatively resistant.

Cancers of these other types occur sufficiently infrequently that it is a common practice to pool them in a category of "all other cancers." When such pooling is done, it is often possible to demonstrate an excess over the control population. Because the excess risk is usually small, however, amounting to considerably less than the risk for leukemia, it follows that each individual site or tissue must be relatively resistant.

The classification of tissues into rough categories of relative sensitivity is shown in Table 1. These classifications must be considered as approximate and subject to

TABLE 1
Relative Sensitivity of Various Human Tissues to the Induction of Radiogenic Cancer

High sensitivity	Moderate sensitivity	Low sensitivity
Myelopoietic tissue (Acute leukemia and myeloid leukemia)	Breast	Skin
Thyroid	Lung	Bone
	Salivary gland	Stomach
		Other tissues (including other lymphomas)

change as the period of follow-up of the various irradiation populations is increased. It is conceivable that some cancers have a very long latent period (in excess of 25 yr) and that they will show a dramatic increase as follow-up continues. This possibility seems unlikely, and if latency is very much greater than 25 yr it may exceed the normal remaining life expectancy of many members of the irradiated populations and therefore never become manifest.

There is a pronounced lack of uniformity of tissue sensitivities to cancer induction among the various species of experimental animals or even within strains of the same species. In general, most animals, like man, are sensitive to the induction of leukemia. There seem to be special sensitivities to many other tumor types. Some lines of rats are exquisitely sensitive to mammary tumor induction (Shellabarger *et al.*, 1969). Mice are very sensitive to ovarian tumors (Furth *et al.*, 1959), and burros seem resistant to any type of tumor (Brown *et al.*, 1965). For these reasons, it is not possible to classify precisely the relative tissue sensitivities for experimental animals as a whole. The important point to determine is whether animals behave like man in the sense of showing marked variations in susceptibility without regard to whether there is precise correspondence in terms of specific tumor types. This appears to be the case for all species so far studied.

No attempt will be made to tabulate and summarize the very extensive literature on experimental animals. Instead, we will consider a single large experiment in one mouse strain which clearly establishes that there are differences in sensitivity. The data shown in Table 2 are from an experiment initiated in the Oak Ridge National Laboratory by Upton and his colleagues and completed by me and my colleagues. The experiment is now complete, but the data are not yet completely analyzed. Certain conclusions can be drawn, however, and these form the basis of the following discussion. A total of 12,000 female mice of the RFM/Un strain were irradiated at the age of 10 wk with γ-rays. Doses ranged from 10 to 400 rads. A total of 4000 mice served as unirradiated controls, giving a total sample size of 16,000. The mice were then set aside to live out their lives. Over 97% were autopsied, and of these about 40% were subjected to histological examination. There was excellent correspondence between tumor diagnoses based on gross autopsy and those verified histologically.

In Table 2, the tissues classified as highly sensitive were those where a significant increase in tumor incidence over control values was seen at 25 rads. (No significant increase in any tumor type occurred at 10 rads in a group of about 3000 mice.) The column headed "moderate sensitivity" refers to tumors showing a significant increase at 50–150 rads, and the "resistant" category includes tumors showing either no increase at any dose or an increase only at doses greater than 150 rads.

TABLE 2

Relative Tissue Sensitivities in RFM Female Mice to the Induction of Radiogenic Cancer

High sensitivity	Moderate sensitivity	Low sensitivity
Thymus	Pituitary	Bone
Ovary	Uterus	Skin
	Breast	Stomach
	Myelopoietic tissue (myeloid leukemia)	Liver
	Lung	Gastrointestinal tract
	Harderian gland	Other tissues

Unlike man, female mice of this strain are susceptible to the induction of endocrine-associated tumors (ovary, pituitary, uterus), but like man the various tissues show a wide range of sensitivity. It would be unreasonable to expect that the mouse (or dog, monkey, rat, or burro) would show a precise one-to-one correspondence of tissue sensitivity to cancer induction. There is excellent agreement, however, in terms of the general principle that all tissues are not equally radiosensitive.

3. Dose–Response Relationships

There are two rather divergent philosophies of approach to the problem of the relationship of radiation dose to the probability of tumor induction. These approaches might be characterized as administrative and scientific. The administrative approach has been used by those concerned with health protection. In order to insure that hazards are not underestimated, this approach assumes that any amount of radiation exposure, no matter how small, is potentially deleterious. Further, it is assumed that the risk is directly proportional to dose; i.e., twice the dose yields twice the risk. These two assumptions lead to the so-called linear no-threshold hypothesis. In support of this hypothesis, the argument is often made that since data from human populations are not sufficiently precise to exclude a linear relationship with a great deal of confidence (the level usually unspecified), the hypothesis should be accepted. Since many other relationships such as quadratic, sigmoid, and higher polynomials also cannot be excluded, this does not constitute an adequate evaluation of the most likely true dose–response curve.

Two other assumptions are usually made in the administrative approach, even though they conflict with a considerable body of scientific evidence. These assumptions are that there is no effect of dose rate and that the relative biological effectiveness (RBE) of densely ionizing radiations is constant regardless of dosage level. Taken altogether, these various assumptions result in a system having both the virtue of conservatism (it is unlikely that risks are underestimated) and a simplified method of bookkeeping (weighting factors for total dose, dose rate, and variable RBE need not be applied).

The scientific approach, unencumbered with the thorny problems of health protection or the serious consequences of underestimating risk, seeks to establish the true functional relationship of dose and response. It is important to establish this relationship since, by knowing the true functional form, it is possible to draw inferences about the nature of the carcinogenic mechanisms and factors involved in the expression of neoplasms.

3.1. Theoretical Considerations

The initiating cellular change in radiation carcinogenesis must result directly or indirectly from ionizations produced in the cell. The change itself almost surely is in the informational content of the cell, whether somatic mutation, viral activation, or whatever. If a single ionizing event is adequate to produce the change and if, further, the change itself is sufficient to produce cancer uninfluenced by host factors or promoting effects, then the dose–response relationship should be linear, with no dose rate effect at least in a restricted dosage range. Further, if the initiating change is a somatic mutation, one would expect all tissues to be roughly equally sensitive to cancer induction since it is unlikely that there are major differences in resistance to mutation in the various tissues.

If, on the other hand, host factors such as immune competence, endocrine function, cellular proliferation rate, and level of repair enzymes play a predominant role in whether the transformed cells ultimately produce neoplasms, it is difficult to visualize a linear relationship. Most quantitative biological characteristics in populations show an approximately normal or log normal distribution. Presumably a characteristic such as the immune competence of individuals within a population would show a similar distribution, as would other host characteristics which might influence the induction of cancer. In this case, a sigmoid rather than a linear dose–response curve would be anticipated. To obtain a linear relationship under these circumstances would require a rectangular distribution of the relevant host factor in the population. Such distributions must be extremely rare in biological materials. For radiation-induced skin tumors in rats (Burns *et al.*, 1968), kidney tumors in rats (Maldague, 1969), and osteogenic sarcomas in patients exposed to internally deposited radium (Evans *et al.*, 1969), a sigmoid relationship adequately fits the data over a restricted dosage range. The relationship breaks down at very high doses, where either cell killing or intercurrent mortality from other cancers reduces the cancer incidence.

There are other cases where variability in host factors appears to play a relatively minor role in determining the outcome of radiation exposure. These cases would include the induction of mammary cancers in rats (Shellabarger *et al.*, 1969) and thymic lymphomas in mice (Storer, 1973). If the dose–response relationship is truly sigmoid, the "tail" at the low dose end is very short and the incidence rises rapidly at low to moderate doses. For intermediate cases, the dose–response curve may represent a complex interaction between the curve for induction of the initiating event and the population distribution of relevant host factors. In those cases where host factors or promoting factors play a significant role, it is likely that the dose–response curve deviates from simple linearity, with less effectiveness per rad at the low dose end.

Even if induction of the initiating event is of overriding importance, as it may be in very sensitive tissues, it can be argued on physical grounds that the dose–response curve for low LET radiation cannot be linear. If a single ionizing event in the cell initiates the neoplastic change, then low LET radiation delivered at very low dose rates should be at least as effective as low LET radiation at high dose rates. The reason for this is that at very low rates the vast majority of ionizations are of the single-hit variety. The fact is that in nearly all (perhaps all) cases adequately studied, low dose rate radiation is less effective than high dose rate radiation (e.g., see Upton *et al.*, 1970). At moderate to high doses of low LET radiation, a large fraction of the cells are subjected to multiple ionizing events (two or more hits) within a brief time span. Since exposure under these circumstances is more effective than under conditions of low dose rates, multiple ionizing events in the cell must be more efficient in inducing the neoplastic change. This argument is supported by studies of high LET radiations, such as neutrons, where fewer cells are "hit" per unit dose but those that are hit receive multiple ionizing events. This is true whether the radiation is delivered at low rates or at high rates because of the nature of the ionizing tracks. Neutrons tend to show effects that are very much less dependent on dose rate than low LET radiations. Further, on a dose-for-dose basis they are more effective than X- or γ-rays (Upton *et al.*, 1970). These observations argue strongly that multiple event injury is usually required to produce the neoplastic change. If this were not the case, then high LET radiations would be less effective than low LET radiations because most of their ionizations would be wasted.

If we accept the hypothesis of multiple ionizations being required for neoplastic change, then the dose–response curve for low LET radiations at high dose rates cannot be linear. The reason is that at low total doses most of the events will be of the single-hit variety, and as the dose increases an increasing number of multiple hits will occur. With high LET radiation, on the other hand, the relationship will be linear since the proportion of multiple hits does not vary with dose. These physical considerations lead to the prediction that the RBE for neutrons should vary with dose, being higher at low doses than at high doses. This prediction has not been adequately tested for cancer induction, although the data from the Japanese survivors (see UNSCEAR Report, United Nations, 1972) are compatible with this prediction. In a wide variety of other experimental test systems, it has been demonstrated that RBE does indeed vary with dose and in the way predicted (see Kellerer and Rossi, 1972).

A final complication in the theoretical prediction of dose–response curves is the role of cell killing by radiation. In one respect, cell transformation and cell killing are working at cross purposes since transformed cells that are killed cannot produce cancers. It is unlikely that the curves for these two responses are identical or even similar, leading to problems in prediction. It is known that cell-killing curves for mammalian cells and low LET radiation are not linear. What effect this would have on the composite curve for cancer yield is not clear. Cell killing may also act in the opposite direction by serving as a promoting agent if the stimulus to proliferation of transformed cells originates from the killing of other cells in the tissue. In this case, the dose–cancer relationship should be concave because of the low efficiency of cell killing at low doses.

In view of all the factors discussed above, it would seem little short of miraculous if the true dose–response curve for cancer induction by X- or γ-rays turns out to be the administratively convenient simple linearity. It is more likely that different relationships will be found for different tumors and different radiation qualities, with the majority of cases being sigmoid or concave (which could represent one end of a sigmoid) particularly for low LET radiation.

There are only two populations and two tumor types where the information is adequate to make it worthwhile considering the dose–response curves, namely, leukemia in the Japanese survivors (Ishimaru *et al.*, 1971) and bone tumors in the persons exposed to internally deposited radium (Evans *et al.*, 1969; Spiess and Mays, 1970, 1971).

As indicated earlier, barring an unexpected second wave of leukemia, the data are essentially complete for this disease in the Japanese. For Hiroshima, the increase in incidence appears to increase linearly with dose. For Nagasaki, the relationship appears sigmoid or curvilinear upward at the lower dose end, with no excess at doses less than 100 rads. A simple linear relationship cannot be excluded on statistical grounds for either population. The difference may very well be real, however, and possible explanations for it should be considered.

The chief radiobiological difference between the two populations is that those in Hiroshima received a mixture of neutrons and γ-rays while those in Nagasaki received essentially γ-rays. If an RBE of 5 is assigned to the neutron component of the Hiroshima radiation, the two dose–response relationships come into much closer alignment (Ishimaru *et al.*, 1971). If a variable RBE, ranging from 10 at the lowest doses to 1 at the high doses is applied, the correspondence of the curves is improved further (UNSCEAR Report, United Nations, 1972). If it is assumed the neutrons show a linear dose–response relationship, which is reasonable from the data, then it follows that the γ-ray line is curvilinear upward. A similar conclusion has been reached by Rossi and Kellerer (this volume) using a different method of analysis.

The other population, where the period of follow-up has been sufficiently long and the incidence of tumors sufficiently high to justify an analysis of the shape of the dose–response curve, consists of persons carrying appreciable skeletal burdens of radium isotopes. The group which has been studied the longest is comprised of persons in the United States who ingested radium in the course of painting luminous instrument dials ("radium dial painters") and patients who ingested nostrums containing radium for a variety of diseases. These exposures occurred in the early part of the century. The period of intake of radium was quite variable, but since the radium isotopes avidly deposit in bone the radiation exposure has been continuous. The complex problem of dosimetry has been and continues to be actively studied and for our purposes can be considered reasonably accurate. There are, of course, inhomogeneities in dose from one part of the skeleton to another and very pronounced variations within a bone. The usual method of expressing dose is to average the energy absorption over the entire skeleton and sum the dose received over the relevant period of exposure.

A plot of the incidence of bone tumors as a function of dose yields two very distinct regions (Evans *et al.*, 1969, 1972). At doses below about 1000 rads, no bone tumors have been observed. At doses above 1000 rads, there is a high incidence of tumors (roughly 30%), but the incidence does not increase with further increases in dose. The function best describing the relationship is a sigmoid curve with a precipitously rising segment in the region between about 900 and 1200 rads. The radiation from radium and its decay products is principally α-particles. If, as is generally agreed, this high LET radiation has a high RBE, it is obvious that bone is relatively refractory to tumor induction and massive doses of low LET radiation such as X- or γ-rays would be required for a major increase in tumor incidence.

A more recent study from Germany on patients treated for tuberculosis (principally of the bone) or ankylosing spondylitis in the period 1946–1951 indicates tumor induction at considerably lower total doses (Spiess and Mays, 1970, 1971). A sigmoid dose–response curve appears to describe the relationship adequately, however. There are two major differences between this and the U.S. study. In the German series, many of the patients were treated as juveniles and the authors have been able to demonstrate a greater sensitivity of juveniles to bone tumor indication. The second difference is that the German patients were treated with nearly pure ^{224}Ra, while in the U.S. series the exposure was principally to ^{226}Ra or ^{228}Ra (mesothorium). Because of the short half-life of ^{224}Ra, most of the radiation dose is absorbed near the surface of bone and in actively growing sites. This inhomogeneity results in far higher doses to the relevant cells at risk than would be suggested by averaging over the entire skeletal mass. For this reason, it is likely that ^{224}Ra and ^{226}Ra are about equally cancerogenic at the microdosimetry level and the apparent greater effectiveness of the ^{224}Ra at the macrodosimetry level is spurious.

It was indicated earlier that the high LET neutron component of the radiation in Hiroshima may very well have yielded a linear dose–response curve for leukemia induction. On the other hand, an even higher LET from α-particles appeared to yield a sigmoid curve for bone tumor induction in the dial painters. How can this apparent paradox be resolved? In the first place, there is no *a priori* reason to believe that the dose–response curves for the induction of all tumors should necessarily have the same shape. Different curves would be expected if host factors were involved unequally in the induction of different tumors. For example, if the initiating cellular change is of overriding importance in the induction of leukemia and host defense or promoting factors are of little importance, then a high LET radiation might very well yield a linear relationship since the probability of producing the initiating event should be proportional to dose. On the other hand, host factors may be of great importance in the induction of bone sarcomas and a sigmoid curve result. This would be particularly true if cell killing and tissue regeneration serve as promoting agents for these two tumor types. Lymphopoietic and myelopoietic cells are very sensitive to cell killing, and significant numbers are killed at low doses. Bone cells are considerably more resistant. It it were necessary to kill a sufficient number of bone cells so that extensive regeneration and remodeling of bone had to occur before the promoting effect was manifest, then the observed sigmoid curve could result.

Despite the very large number of studies conducted on the effects of ionizing radiation on experimental animals, there are only a limited number suitable for examination of the shape of the dose–response curve for cancer induction. There are a number of reasons for this relative paucity of data. In many cases, end points other than cancer incidence were looked for and careful necropsies were not performed. When external sources of radiation have been employed, it has been a common practice to perform total-body exposures. This limits the size of the dose that can be used, and further, in the case of mice in particular, there tends to be a "swamping" effect of a high incidence of early-occurring lymphomas and leukemias which preclude the development of later-occurring solid tumors. Unless sample sizes are very large, too few solid tumors of specific sites are seen to evaluate dose and response. Another common problem has been the failure of the investigator to provide data corrected for competing causes of death (see UNSCEAR Report, United Nations, 1972). At high radiation doses, there may actually be an apparent decrease in the incidence of late-occurring tumors, which is an artifact arising from the depletion of the population by incidence of earlier-occurring diseases such as thymic lymphoma so that few of the initial population remain at risk for developing the late tumor. Correction procedures to circumvent this problem are available (for example, Hoel and Walburg, 1972), but only recently has the need for their use been widely recognized.

Some of the most useful studies have been those which employ partial-body or single-organ irradiation. High doses can be achieved and the complication of competing risks is greatly reduced. Partial-body exposure has been achieved by either feeding or injecting radioisotopes that selectively localize in specific tissues or by shielding much of the body from radiation from external sources. When low LET radiations have been used, the majority of studies have shown dose–response curves that are curvilinear upward or a sigmoid relationship. Mays and Lloyd (1972a) have reviewed the incidence of bone sarcomas in a wide variety of species exposed to ^{90}Sr (a low LET bone-seeking isotope). In all cases, a curvilinear relationship gave the best fit. In the larger studies, a linear, no-threshold fit could be convincingly rejected.

External irradiation to limited areas of the skin of rats (Burns *et al.*, 1968) resulted in sigmoid dose–response curves over a portion of the dose range. When the optimally carcinogenic dose was exceeded, the incidence decreased significantly. A similar effect has been reported for renal cancers in rats (Maldague, 1969). The reason for the decline is undoubtedly cell killing. If an organ is completely ablated by radiation, it obviously cannot undergo neoplastic change.

In test systems showing a high sensitivity to tumor induction, the dose–response relationship may appear linear in the low dose range. For example, female Sprague-Dawley rats are exquisitely sensitive to the induction of mammary tumors, and a linear relationship at the low dose end followed by a plateau at higher doses describes the data (Shellabarger *et al.*, 1969). Similarly, in the as yet unreported studies in Oak Ridge that were referred to earlier, the incidence of thymic lymphoma appears linear in a restricted dose range beginning at 25 rads. Extrapolation of the line back to 0 dose predicts reasonably well the control incidence. If a large sample had not been irradiated at 10 rads, a conclusion that the dose–response curve is linear would have been justified. However, the 10-rad group showed no increase in thymic lymphomas, and it appears that the relationship is probably sigmoid with a very short tail in the low dose region. This points up the difficulty in choosing among various alternative curves for tumors that are easily induced. Very large samples are required and even then the choice of one function over another may be tenuous.

On a dose-for-dose basis, high LET radiations are more effective carcinogens than low LET radiations. Most animal studies at high LET values have been conducted using internally deposited α-emitters such as radium or plutonium (both bone seekers). Except for the case of neutrons, it is extremely difficult to use external sources of high LET radiation. The mass and charge of the particles (protons, α-particles, and heavier ions) that yield densely ionizing tracks makes them very poorly penetrating except at very high energies. Once they are accelerated to high enough energies to become penetrating, they give up most of their energy in tissue at low LET. There are exceptions, but the necessary hardware for external sources of high LET radiation is not commonly available. Neutrons, because of their lack of charge, penetrate reasonably well, and their interactions in tissue yield a high proportion of high LET radiation. The difficulty is that partial-body or single-organ exposure is extremely difficult because the beam cannot be focused (neutrons are uncharged) and body shielding is extraordinarily difficult. Most, if not all, neutron studies therefore have utilized total-body radiation with the attendant problem of restricted dose range and a "swamping" effect of easily induced tumors.

The studies with internally deposited α-emitters have yielded two types of dose–response curves for the induction of bone tumors, namely linear and curvilinear upward (see review by Mays and Lloyd, 1972b). The principal species studied have been mice and beagle dogs. Within each species both types of curves have been found, so the effect is not species specific. Curiously, the same investigators (Finkel and Biskis, 1962; Finkel et al., 1969), using the same mouse strain, found both types of curve depending on the choice of isotope (Mays and Lloyd, 1972b). In the studies with dogs, the sample sizes are too small and the follow-up is insufficiently long to choose either type of function with confidence. It is concluded that high LET radiation yields dose–response curves that are more nearly linear than those for low LET radiation, but the data are inadequate to determine which, if any, functional form is characteristic.

One unusual characteristic of the dose–response curve for any tumor type so far studied over a sufficiently wide dose range is that the incidence plateaus in the higher dose range. This indicates that even in genetically homogeneous populations such as mice there are individuals apparently refractory to induction of the cancer, suggesting that host factors that are not genetically determined may play a role in determining whether the malignancy becomes manifest.

In the summary, the true form of most dose–response curves for cancer induction is probably sigmoid (the curvilinear form representing one tail of the distribution). For easily induced tumors, where host factors may play a minor role in the outcome, it is extremely difficult to distinguish between linearity and a rapidly rising sigmoid with a very short "tail" at the low dose end. Very large sample sizes are required and the benefits to be derived by such a distinction may not be worth the bother.

4. Threshold or Minimum Effective Doses

Most experienced investigators agree that it is a futile exercise to attempt to establish the dose of radiation or any other known carcinogen below which there is absolutely no increased probability of developing cancer. There are a number of reasons why this is so. The first of these has to do with proving a negative effect, something much more difficult than proving a positive effect. If, for example, one conducted a meticulously controlled study in 10,000 or 100,000 animals exposed to, say, 5 rads and found precisely the same number (or even fewer) cancers in the treated group as in an equal-sized control group, one could still not conclude that at 5 rads there is absolutely no possibility of increased risk. Suppose one found no cancers of a particular type in either group (an unlikely possibility, as will be shown below). The value of 0 in 10,000 still has a statistically calculable upper confidence limit which is greater than zero. One might then feel confident that with a certain probability the risk does not exceed this upper limit, but zero risk could not be assumed. To complicate matters further, radiation does not produce unique cancers that are identifiable as being radiation induced. It simply changes the overall incidence of naturally occurring cancers (or perhaps cancers induced by other agents). For this reason, there is always a variable background "noise" level in the population which reduces the statistical certainty that the radiation risk does not exceed some specified value. The unanswerable argument can also be raised that in a heterogeneous population such as man there may be a uniquely sensitive population subset that will respond at doses which are ineffective in the majority of the population.

While it is virtually impossible to demonstrate empirically that there is an absolute threshold, there is an alternative approach which suggests that for certain tumors there may be a "practical" threshold (Evans et al., 1969). This approach is based on the fact that for many tumors the latent period, i.e., the time between radiation exposure and appearance of the tumor, increases as the dose decreases. This appears to be the case for radiogenic bone sarcomas in the dial painters (Evans et al., 1969) and for a number of different types of tumors in experimental animals (Furth et al., 1959; Upton, 1964; Hulse, 1967; Burns et al., 1968; Dougherty and Mays, 1969; Hug et al., 1969; Shellabarger et al., 1969; Nilsson, 1970). If one extrapolates to low doses, the latent period may exceed the remaining life expectancy and a practical threshold is therefore predicted. The difficulty with this approach is that it requires extrapolation beyond the range of dosages where reasonably good data exist into the low dosage region of statistical uncertainty, and the same objections can be raised as with predictions of absolute thresholds. Nevertheless, if risk estimates in the low dose range can be made by extrapolations from data at high doses (BEIR Report, NAS-NRC, 1972), it would seem equally valid (or invalid) to predict practical thresholds by the same procedure.

In summary, the preferred approach to more realistic risk estimates at low doses is not to attempt to demonstrate thresholds but to elucidate the most likely shape of the dose–response curves by as many independent lines of evidence as possible. Examples of such independent lines of approach include empirical studies, studies of RBE as a function of dose, evaluation of latency with dose, and research on mechanisms of cancer induction including the role of host factors.

5. Physical Factors

5.1. Dose Rate

There are no data on the effectiveness of low LET radiation delivered at low rates over long periods of time to human populations. All the studied populations, including those receiving multiple fractionated exposures, received the radiation at high rates. On physical grounds, it would not be expected that fractionated exposure would be the equivalent of continuous low rate exposure unless the dose per fraction was very small. The reason for this has to do with the likelihood of two or more ionizing events occurring in the target of interest in a brief time interval. At low dose rates, most of the injury will be of the single-hit variety. Multiple very small doses would also yield the same type of injury. The only human population in which doses per fraction and multiplicity of fractions would be expected to simulate continuous exposure is the occupationally exposed radiologists. Radiologists practising in the United States in the earlier part of this century indeed showed an excess of leukemia and other tumors (Seltser and Sartwell, 1965). The problem is that their radiation doses are not at all well known and there must have been major inhomogeneities of dose. Braestrup (1957) attempted to estimate their dosages based on the type of equipment employed and work practices. He has estimated an average dose of 2000 rads accumulated over many years. It can be calculated that the excess risk of leukemia in this group (relative risk of 2.5) amounts to considerably less than what would be expected from 200 rads of high dose rate exposure. Because of the great uncertainties in dose estimates and factors associated with the radiation quality, this line of evidence can be considered only as suggestive of a much lessened effectiveness of protracted exposure.

The dial painters and the patients treated with radium received their exposure continuously over a long period of time. There is no comparable group, however, that received a single brief exposure for comparison. Further, in experimental studies, high LET radiations have been shown to exert their effects relatively independently of dose rate, presumably because the majority of injury is of the multiple ionizing event type and dose rate does not affect the proportion of this type of injury with high LET radiations. It must be concluded that there are no suitable studies to evaluate the dose rate effect on carcinogenesis in man.

With very few exceptions, studies on experimental animals have shown that low LET radiation delivered at low dose rate is far less effective in producing cancer than the same total dose given at high dose rates. This general rule also applies to mutation induction.

Grahn and Sacher have systematically investigated the effects of dose rate on survival time and have shown that the lower rates are less effective by a factor of at least 5 (see review by Grahn *et al.*, 1972) in shortening longevity. Since in the low total dose domain life shortening was entirely explainable on the basis of tumor induction, it follows that the cancerogenic effect is reduced at low rates. Leukemias and ovarian tumors, both of which are easily induced in mice, show a lower incidence at low dose rates than at high dose rates (Upton *et al.*, 1970).

One problem in interpreting some of the experimental studies is that no correction procedures have been applied to the incidence figures. If the animals exposed at low rates survive longer than those at high rates, the observed final incidence of tumors might be the same or even higher at low rates. This could result from the animals being at risk longer or more animals being at risk in the critical period, and uncorrected values can therefore be misleading. This problem is discussed in detail by UNSCEAR (United Nations, 1972).

One notable exception to the rule of lessened effectiveness at low rates is the report by Shellabarger and Brown (1972) that the incidence of benign mammary tumors in Sprague-Dawley rats was the same whether γ-radiation was delivered at 0.03 R/min or at 10 R/min. The incidence of carcinomas was lower at the lower rate. This test system is an unusual one in many respects and apparently does not represent the general case.

Many of the reported studies have compared the effectiveness of only two dose rates, and the difference between them is often not great. Further, the lower rate is often not very low. Yuhas (1973) is currently studying the relative effectiveness in mice of γ-rays at eight different dose rates ranging from 1 rad/day to 100 rads/min. Terminated exposures are used so as to reduce the amount of wasted radiation. Four total doses are being used. A preliminary analysis shows that for some tumors the highest dose rate is not always the most effective but the lowest dose rate is always the least effective. Thus there appears to be an optimum rate for the induction of certain tumors which lies in the moderately high dose range. Some of the confusion in the literature may result from investigators not choosing low enough dose rates for making comparisons.

It is not possible to assign a single value to the effectiveness factor for low dose rate exposures with much confidence. Most studies suggest that such exposures are perhaps one-fifth to one-tenth as effective as high dose rate exposures, depending on the end point. On physical grounds, one would expect low dose rates to yield more nearly linear dose–response curves because the injury is primarily single hit and the probability of such injury should be proportional to dose. If host factors do not intervene, the effectiveness factor might then vary with dose in much the manner the RBE of neutrons varies with dose. At very low doses, the effectiveness might approximate that for high dose rates, with a progressive divergence as dose increases until some limiting value is reached. This speculation presupposes nonlinearity of response at high rates and a closer approximation to linearity at low rates. For purposes of risk estimation, linearity is assumed at high rates (BEIR Report, NAS-NRC, 1972), which would lead to a constant factor for relative effectiveness at low rates if linearity is also assumed at low rates. While committees concerned with health protection assume an effectiveness factor of unity (no effect of dose rate), the experimental studies indicate that radiation is far less effective when delivered at low rates.

5.2. Radiation Quality

In general, high LET radiations such as neutrons and α-particles are more effective than low LET radiations such as X- and γ-rays. The precise value of the RBE appears to vary with total dose, dose rate, and biological end point. The data from human populations are not adequate to sort out the contribution of each of these variables, but the data are at least consistent with the general conclusion. Better concordance of the dose–response curves for leukemia induction in Nagasaki and Hiroshima is obtained if the neutron component of the radiation at Hiroshima is assigned an RBE of 5 (Ishimaru *et al.*, 1971). The concordance is further improved if a sliding scale of RBEs ranging from 10 to 1, depending on the total dose, is applied (UNSCEAR Report, United Nations, 1972). For other tumors as well, the agreement between the data from the Japanese populations and those from other populations is improved by using an RBE of 5 for neutrons (BEIR Report, NAS-NRC, 1972). The data are not adequate, however, to reach a firm conclusion that the RBE is precisely 5. It could range from 1 to 10.

In the case of lung cancer in uranium miners exposed to α-particles from radon and radon daughters, the risk estimates agree better with those from populations exposed to low LET radiations if an RBE of 10 is applied to the estimated α-particle dose BEIR Report, NAS,-NRC, 1972).

It is difficult to assign an RBE to the radiation received by the radium dial painters and patients receiving radium internally because of the lack of a suitable comparison group. An RBE of 10, however, is not inconsistent with the fragmentary data from other groups.

Evidence from animals and plants strongly supports the concept that the RBE of neutrons increases with decreasing dose (see Kellerer and Rossi, 1972, for a summary). Unfortunately, data are as yet limited with respect to the RBE in carcinogenesis, although fragmentary data are consistent with this conclusion (UNSCEAR Report, United Nations, 1972).

It was pointed out earlier that high LET radiations tend to exert their effect relatively independently of dose rate (Upton, 1964; Upton *et al.*, 1970). Since this is the case and since low LET radiation is less effective at low dose rates, it follows that the apparent RBE for high LET radiation will increase at low dose rates, not because these radiations are more effective, but because the baseline low LET radiation is less effective.

5.3. Internal Emitters vs. External Exposure

There is no evidence to suggest and no reason to believe that a cell or tissue can distinguish whether the ionizing energy it absorbs originated from radionuclides within the body or from an external radiation source. If the tissue dosages and dose rates are similar, then one would expect similar results. With few exceptions, however, it is difficult to simulate the dose distribution from an internal emitter with external sources. The reason is that the various isotopes are differentially taken up by various tissues, resulting in marked macroscopic differences in dose as well as microdosimetric differences. Despite the problems in dosimetry, studies with internal emitters have provided some of the most useful experimental data in radiation carcinogenesis since very large doses can be delivered to the organs showing a high affinity for the isotope. This gets the tumor incidence up out of the background range and dose–response relationships can be examined. Similar studies could be conducted using external beams by selective organ irradiation, but it would be most difficult to accomplish other than a brief high dose rate exposure.

5.4. Total-Body Exposure vs. Partial-Body Exposure

With the exception of the Japanese survivors and children receiving radiation exposure while *in utero*, the human populations studied to date received essentially partial-body irradiation. From these studies, certain general principles have emerged. The risk of induction of solid tumor at any specified site is increased only if the site is included in the radiation field. In the case of leukemia, it is necessary only to irradiate a certain fraction (as yet unspecified) of the bone marrow to increase the risk. Further, if the dose to this fraction of the marrow is averaged over the entire marrow, the leukemia risk is about the same as if the entire marrow had received this average dose. The exception to this conclusion occurs when a very limited part of the marrow receives a very high dose. Presumably in this case there is sufficient cell killing to preclude leukemic transformation. An apparent example of this effect is provided by the study on women treated intensively with radiation for cancer of the uterine cervix. Despite a high average marrow dose, there was no evidence of an increase in leukemia (Hutchison, 1968). Data are not adequate to determine whether the risk of a tumor at a particular site is greater if a specified dose is delivered to the entire body or only to the particular site of interest. If generalized host factors such as immune competence are involved in determining the outcome, it might be expected that whole-body radiation would be more effective.

As indicated in the preceding section, studies of carcinogenesis with internally deposited radionuclides are usually studies on partial-body irradiation. Not unexpectedly, tumors occur in the tissues and organs where the isotopes concentrate. Similarly, in studies with external beams, cancers occur only in the areas included in the radiation field. The situation is not as clear-cut in the case of leukemia. In contrast to the case in man, shielding of a portion of the marrow of mice greatly reduces the incidence of leukemia (see review by Upton and Cosgrove, 1968). This may result from a greater mobility of stem cells in the mouse and a consequent greater ability to repopulate irradiated areas with normal cells. It could also mean that the immune state is of more importance in mouse than in man. This could be particularly true if viral action plays a greater role in the mouse. As in man, the data are not adequate to determine whether a total-body dose is more effective in producing solid tumors of specific sites than radiation restricted to that site. Despite the experimental problems associated with this approach, particularly in mice where total-body doses can be delivered that are insufficient to produce more than a small increase in a limited number of cancer types, it should be possible to resolve this point.

6. Host Factors

Persons exposed to radiation as juveniles have a higher risk of leukemia and most other cancers than do persons exposed as adults. This conclusion seems amply supported by the data of Jablon and Kato (1972) for the Japanese survivors and of Spiess and Mays (1970, 1971) for patients treated with radium. The precise factor by which the risk is increased probably varies with tumor type and is difficult to estimate. It is probably highest for thyroid cancer since adults seem relatively refractory to induction of this cancer while children are quite sensitive. For osteogenic sarcomas, leukemia, and some other tumors the risk may be higher by about a factor of 2.

There have also been reports suggesting an extreme sensitivity of the human fetus to the induction of leukemia and perhaps other types of tumors (Stewart *et al.*, 1958; MacMahon and Hutchison, 1964; MacMahon, 1962; Gibson *et al.*, 1968; Stewart and Kneale, 1970; Bross and Natarajan, 1972). If the reported association between diagnostic radiation exposure and the likelihood of developing leukemia represents a causal relationship, prenatal radiation sensitivity must be astonishing since a dose of a few rads at most would increase leukemia incidence by about 50%. These reports are based on retrospective studies in which children dying from leukemia are usually identified from a tumor registry. The cases are then matched with suitable normal controls and an attempt is made to determine whether there is a difference in the previous histories of the two groups with respect to some specified variable or variables. This type of approach has been very useful in epidemiology since the study can be done reasonably quickly and the enormous sample sizes needed for prospective studies (discussed later) are not required. Studies on radiation as a possible etiological agent vary, of course, in the method

of selecting the control group and in the ascertainment of whether radiation has
been delivered. In a typical study, the investigator might find that 15% of the mothers of leukemic children had received diagnostic radiation (usually pelvimetry) during the relevant pregnancy, while only 10% of the mothers of control children had been so exposed, this leads to a relative risk estimate of 15/10 or 1.5.

Stewart *et al.* (1958), who appear to have been the first to report the association between *in utero* exposure and childhood cancer, initially examined the history of other factors as well and identified some (history of reproductive wastage, childhood infections) that other workers (Gibson *et al.*, 1968) subsequently confirmed as being positively associated with leukemia risk. In later reports by Stewart and her colleagues (Stewart, 1961; Stewart and Kneale, 1968, 1970), the other factors were ignored and emphasis was placed on radiation as the most likely etiological agent. It is interesting that in a study predating Stewart's, Manning and Carroll (1957) did not consider radiation history but did determine that a history of allergies leads to an increased estimate of risk. This has also been confirmed subsequently (Bross and Natarajan, 1972).

Following these early reports, a large number of studies were conducted ro attempt to confirm or refute the reported association of radiation and leukemia. Relative risk estimates, ranging from 0.42 (Lewis, 1960) to 1.72 (Kaplan, 1958), were reported, but most of these studies were conducted on a relatively modest scale. MacMahon (1962) undertook a reasonably large-scale study of the problem that differed from the earlier studies in that he used hospital records rather than interviews to determine whether radiation exposures had been given. He found a relative risk of about 1.4. MacMahon and Hutchison (1964) reviewed the earlier studies and concluded that the pooled data from all studies to that time gave a weighted best estimate of relative risk of 1.4. In 1968, Gibson *et al.* reported on a very large-scale study of this problem. They identified four factors as being associated with an increased risk of leukemia. These were a history of (1) *in utero* radiation, (2) preconception radiation to either parent, (3) reproductive wastage (earlier stillbirths or abortions), and (4) childhood viral disease. When each was considered singly and in the absence of any of the others, the risk estimates were greatly reduced. for example, if there was only a history of *in utero* radiation and none of the other factors, the relative risk was only 1.06. It was only when the variables were combined that the risk estimates increased, with a maximum risk in the group having a history of all four factors. Bross and Natarajan (1972) have recently reanalyzed the same data and reported somewhat higher risk estimates.

For establishing cause and effect rather than identifying an association, prospective studies are preferred. In prospective studies, a population exposed to the factor and a control population are first identified and then the determination is made of what subsequently happened with respect to the incidence of the disease in question. Such studies are enormously difficult in the case of a rare disease like leukemia because of the very large sample sizes required. Three such studies have been made in the case of children receiving *in utero* radiation. Court Brown *et al.* (1960) studied a population of about 40,000 such children. Based on the incidence of leukemia in the general population, they expected an incidence of 10.5 cases in their treated population but observed only 9. Griem *et al.* (1967) studied about 1000 cases in which women were subjected to routine X-ray pelvimetry (and thus there was no selection which might bias the results) and found no leukemia, but, of course, the population size was quite small. Diamond (1968) evaluated leukemia incidence in a population of 20,000 irradiated children and 40,000 controls. He found an increase of the disease in the irradiated white segment of the population but a decrease in blacks. Thus the three prospective studies were negative, but the sample sizes were probably not large enough to detect less than a 40 or 50% increase in risk.

More recently, Stewart and Kneale (1970) reported a linear increase in relative risk of cancer with the number of X-ray films taken (radiation dose). From this, they estimated the excess cancer risk at 572 cases per million per rad of exposure. Jablon and Kato (1970) examined the validity of this estimate in light of the Japanese experience. About 1300 Japanese children received significant *in utero* exposure at the time of the bombing. Although the number is small, the product of number of people times the average dose is large, about 35,000 man-rads. (If a linear, no-threshold relationship is assumed, the expected number of cases can be calculated from the product of people times dose or man-rads. Thus the expected number of cases is the same if 1 million people are exposed to 1 rad or if 10,000 people are exposed to 100 rads. This can lead to some unusual conclusions if the dose–response curve is clearly non-linear as in the case of epilation; e.g., see Evans *et al.*, 1972.) From Stewart and Kneale's estimate, about 20 cases of cancer in the Japanese children would have been expected. No cases of leukemia were observed. Only one case of cancer of any type (liver) was seen in this population, while the expectation at national rates was about 0.75.

In view of the above uncertainties and particularly in view of the fact that leukemia induction may result from the complex interplay of a number of factors, it is concluded that the question of extreme sensitivity of parental children to leukemia induction by radiation remains unresolved. Certainly risk estimates based on the available evidence are very tenuous at best.

Juvenile experimental animals, particularly mice, are, like man, more susceptible to a number of radiogenic neoplasms (Kaplan, 1948; Upton *et al.*, 1960; Lindop and Rotblat, 1962). In contrast to the suggested very high susceptibility of prenatal children, the fetal stages in animals do not show increased sensitivity and in some cases have appeared to be refractory (Upton *et al.*, 1960; Upton, 1964; Upton *et al.*, 1966; Rugh *et al.*, 1966; Warren and Gates, 1969). When very old animals (mice) are irradiated, they do not show an increased tumor incidence (Storer, 1973), probably because the latent period exceeds the remaining life expectancy. This lack of effect is probably also true for man but is ignored if the period of follow-up is short (due to death from other causes).

7. Relationship to Spontaneous Incidence Rate

Radiation either could induce an absolute number of new tumors independent of the spontaneous incidence rate or could act multiplicatively with the spontaneous rate. In the former case, the appropriate method of expressing risk would be the "absolute" risk; i.e., a specified dose of radiation would be expected to yield some number of tumors independently of whether the spontaneous incidence is high or low. If, on the other hand, radiation acts multiplicatively and the increase in number of cases depends on natural incidence, then the "relative" risk is the proper expression. The difference in these two concepts is of more than trivial significance. For administrative convenience, one would hope that the absolute risk concept is correct because then risk estimates would be independent of race, geography, epoch, and presence or absence of cocarcinogenic factors. Nature rarely takes cognizance of administrative convenience, however, and it seems likely that for some tumors, at least, the relative risk may be proper. This could depend on what factors are involved in the so-called natural incidence.

Data from human populations are inadequate to choose between these two alternatives and both methods are used in risk estimates, although perhaps the majority of epidemiologists use the relative risk because of convenience. The issue could perhaps be resolved by animal experimentation, although at the present time experimental data are also inadequate for the evaluation.

8. Effect on Longevity

It has long been believed by many investigators that radiation causes a nonspecific life shortening that might be the equivalent of premature or accelerated aging. This is formally equivalent to an increased mortality rate, particularly at later ages. Dublin and Spiegelman (1948) reported a mortality ratio of 1.3 for U.S. radiologists compared to other physicians. In 1956, Warren estimated a loss of longevity in radiologists practicing before 1942 of about 5 yr. Seltser and Sartwell (1965) reexamined this question and found excess mortality from all causes in the radiologists as compared to ophthalmologists-otolaryngologists. Court Brown and Doll (1958), however, did not find such an effect in British radiologists, but possibly their radiation exposures were lower because of differences in safety practices. Court Brown and Doll (1965) found excess mortality from a variety of causes in the irradiated spondylitics. Since the excess incidence of cancer and leukemia in the U.S. radiologists and in the spondylitics did not account for the loss of longevity, this seemed good evidence of nonspecific life shortening, a conclusion in apparently good agreement with studies in many species of experimental animals.

More recently, Jablon and Kato (1972) in a report on the mortality experience at ABCC through 1970 in persons exposed to more than 200 rads did not find excess mortality for several categories of disease including cerebrovascular disease and circulatory disease, two very common causes of death. Mortality from leukemia and from other cancers was significantly increased, as was death from all causes (which includes neoplasms). Deaths from all diseases except neoplasms were increased slightly (mortality ratio of 1.12) but nothing like the extent of the increase for neoplasms. Thus the concept of nonspecific life shortening in man is called into serious question.

Based on studies in mice where careful autopsies were performed, Walburg and Cosgrove (1970), Grahn *et al.* (1972), and Storer (1973) have concluded that in the low to moderate dose range, the loss of longevity in mice can be accounted for solely on the basis of increased tumor incidence. At higher doses, particularly in female mice, there is a component of life shortening that has not yet been accounted for (Storer, 1973), but it seems likely that it results from specific radiogenic diseases as yet unrecognized rather than an across-the-board premature aging.

9. Interactions with Other Agents

When studies on the interaction of radiation with chemical, physical, or biological agents are undertaken, there are myriad (almost infinite) possible combinations and permutations of agents, dosages, and treatment schedules. This is perhaps the reason that interest in studying such interactions has been limited. A classic example of a synergistic effect in human populations is provided by studies on lung cancer in uranium miners. Nearly every case of lung cancer occurred in cigarette smokers (see review by Bair, 1970). Examples of experimental studies of interactions are provided by the reports of Shubik *et al.* (1953), Upton *et al.* (1961), Lindsay and Chaikoff (1964), Lindop and Rotblat (1966), Berenblum *et al.* (1968), Cole and Foley (1969), Telles *et al.* (1969), Segaloff and Maxfield (1971), Epstein (1972), and Shellabarger and Straub (1972). In general, the two-stage concept of cancer induction, namely initiation and promotion, as advanced by Berenblum (1941) seems to apply reasonably well to these interaction studies (see Berenblum, this volume). Radiation at sufficiently high doses is a complete carcinogen in that it serves as both initiator and promotor. There are a number of strong chemical carcinogens that act the same way. When large doses of radiation are combined with high doses of a strong carcinogen, it would be expected that no particular synergism would be obtained and the resulting tumor yield would be that predicted by independent action. This was found to be the case in a study by Shellabarger and Straub (1972) in which breast tumors in rats were induced by neutrons combined with methylcholanthrene. If initiating doses of radiation are combined with a promoting agent such as croton oil or urethan, one would predict synergism, and such effects have been reported (Shubik *et al.*, 1953; Cole and Foley, 1969). There are problems in interpreting much of the existing experimental data because it is not always clear that the sequence of administration of the agents was optimal, full dose–response curves are rarely run, and in cases of fatal tumors the data are usually not corrected for competing risks. It is probably possible to predict the outcome of combining radiation and other agents based on the characteristics of each agent (if these are adequately known) and the dose level used. However, such predictions have not been adequately tested.

The mechanism by which ionizing radiation induces tumors remains obscure, although increasing evidence is accumulating which implicates a number of variables. In certain murine tumors, the activation or release of oncogenic viruses must play a major role. For man, however, there is no good evidence that an effect mediated through viruses occurs. In recent years, there has been intensive investigation of the role of the immune system in carcinogenesis. Since radiation is a potent immunosuppressor, it is apparent that this could be a factor in radiation carcinogenesis. Radiation effects on the immune system have been extensively reviewed in the recent UNSCEAR Report (United Nations, 1972). The concept that somatic cell mutations are the initiating change in cancer induction is widely supported, but direct experimental proof remains elusive. Many carcinogens are also potent mutagens, which supports but does not prove the somatic mutation hypothesis. Endocrine imbalances are almost certainly involved in the induction of some tumors of experimental animals, particularly female mice.

One thing that confounds the interpretation of experiments in the general areas mentioned above is the role of cell killing and subsequent increased rate of cellular proliferation. For example, immunosuppression is attained only by killing immunocompetent cells, and it may be significant that the principal induced tumors in immunosuppressed patients are reticulum cell sarcomas. Radiation may activate latent endogenous viruses, but cellular proliferation is apparently necessary for amplification of the effect. Carcinogens are capable of cell killing or at least inhibition of mitosis, both of which lead to a later increase in cellular proliferation. Potent mutagens are also capable of cell killing, and mutational change is very likely a major mechanism of cell death. A cancer-producing endocrine imbalance in irradiated female mice apparently results from killing of the very sensitive oocytes. In view of these considerations, it seems likely that cell killing plays a primary role in radiation carcinogenesis even though the intermediate steps (immune suppression, viral amplification, endocrine effects, etc.) may be varied.

11. References

ALBERT, R. E., AND OMRAN, A. R., 1968, Follow-up study of patients treated by X-ray epilation for tinea capitis. 1. Population characteristics, post-treatment illnesses, and mortality experience, *Arch. Environ. Health* **17**:899.

BAIR, W. J., 1970, Inhalation of radionuclides and carcinogenesis, in: *Inhalation Carcinogenesis* (P. Nettesheim, M. G. Hanna, Jr., and J. R. Gilbert, eds.), pp. 77–97, USAEC Division of Technical Information, Symposium Series 18, National Technical Information Service, Springfield, Va., CONF–691001.

BEEBE, G. W., KATO, H., AND LAND, C. E., 1971, Studies on the mortality of A-bomb survivors. 4. Mortality and radiation dose, 1950–1966, *Radiation Res.* **48**:613.

BELSKY, J. L., TACHIKAWA, K., CIHAK, R. W., AND YAMOMOTO, T., 1972, Salivary gland tumors in atomic bomb survivors, Hiroshima–Nagasaki, 1957 to 1970, *JAMA* **219**:864.

BERENBLUM, I., 1941, The mechanism of carcinogenesis: A study of the significance of carcinogenic action and related phenomena, *Cancer Res.* **1**:807.

BERENBLUM, I., CHEN, L., AND TRAININ, N., 1968, A quantitative study of the leukemogenic action of whole-body x-irradiation and urethane, *Israel J. Med. Sci.* **4:**1159.

BLOCH, C., 1962, Osteogenic sarcoma: Report of a case and review of literature, *Am. J. Roentgenol.* **87:**1157.

BRAESTRUP, C. B., 1957, Past and present radiation exposure to radiologists from the point of view of life expectancy, *Am. J. Roentgenol.* **78:**988.

BROSS, I. D. J., AND NATARAJAN, N., 1972, Leukemia from low level radiation, *New Engl. J. Med.* **287:**107.

BROWN, D. G., JOHNSON, D. F., AND CROSS, F. H., 1965, Late Effects observed in burros surviving external whole-body gamma irradiation, *Radiation Res.* **25:**574.

BURNS, F. J., ALBERT, R. E., AND HEIMBACH, R. D., 1968, RBE for skin tumors and hair follicle damage in the rat following irradiation with alpha particles and electrons, *Radiation Res.* **36:**225.

COLE, L. J., AND FOLEY, W. A., 1969, Modification of urethan–lung tumor incidence by low x-radiation doses, cortisone and transfusion of isogenic lymphocytes, *Radiation Res.* **39:**391.

CONRAD, R. A., DOBYNS, B. M., AND SUTOW, W. W., 1970, Thyroid neoplasia as late effect of exposure to radioactive iodine in fallout, *JAMA* **214:**316.

COURT BROWN, W. M., AND DOLL, R., 1958, Expectation of life and mortality from cancer among British radiologists, *Brit. Med. J.* **2:**181.

COURT BROWN, W. M., AND DOLL, R., 1965, Mortality from cancer and other causes after radiotherapy for ankylosing spondylitis, *Brit. Med. J.* **2:**1327.

COURT BROWN, W. M., DOLL, R., AND HILL, A. B., 1960, Incidence of leukemia after exposure to diagnostic radiation *in utero, Brit. Med. J.* **2:**1539.

DIAMOND, E. L., 1968, Unpublished studies. Cited by Kessler, I. I., and Lilienfeld, A. M., 1969, Perspectives in the epidemiology of leukemia, in: *Advances in Cancer Research*, Vol. 12 (G. Klein and S. Weinhouse, eds.), pp. 225–302, Academic Press, New York.

DOLL, R., AND SMITH, P. G., 1968, The long-term effects of x irradiation in patients treated for metropathia haemorrhagica, *Brit. J. Radiol.* **41:**362.

DOUGHERTY, T. F., AND MAYS, C. W., 1969, Bone cancer induced by internally-deposited emitters in beagles, in: *Radiation-Induced Cancer*, pp. 361–367, IAEA, Vienna.

DUBLIN, L. I., AND SPIEGELMAN, M., 1948, Mortality of medical specialists 1938–1942, *JAMA* **137:**1519.

EPSTEIN, J. H., 1972, Examination of the carcinogenic and cocarcinogenic effects of Grenz radiation, *Cancer Res.* **32:**2625.

EVANS, R. D., KEANE, A. T., KOLENKOW, R. J., NEAL, W. R., AND SHANAHAN, M. M., 1969, Radiogenic tumors in the radium and mesothorium cases studied at M.I.T., in: *Delayed Effects of Bone-Seeking Radionuclides* (C. W. Mays, W. S. S. Jee, R. D. Lloyd, B. J. Stover, J. H. Dougherty, and G. N. Taylor, eds.), pp. 157–194, University of Utah Press, Salt Lake City.

EVANS, R. D., KEANE, A. T., AND SHANAHAN, M. M., 1972, Radiogenic effects in man of long-term skeletal alpha-irradiation, in: *Radiobiology of Plutonium* (B. J. Stover and W. S. S. Jee, eds.), pp. 431–468, The J. W. Press, Salt Lake City.

FINKEL, M. P., AND BISKIS, B. O., 1962, Toxicity of plutonium in mice, *Health Phys.* **8:**565.

FINKEL, M. P., BISKIS, B. O., AND JINKINS, P. B., 1969, Toxicity of radium-226 in mice, in: *Radiation-Induced Cancer*, pp. 369–391, IAEA, Vienna.

FURTH, J., UPTON, A. C., AND KIMBALL, A. W., 1959, Late pathologic effects of atomic detonation and their pathogenesis, *Radiation Res. Suppl.* **1:**243.

GIBSON, R. W., BROSS, I. D. J., GRAHAM, S., LILIENFELD, A. M., SCHUMAN, L. M., LEVIN, M. L., AND DOWD, J. E., 1968, Leukemia in children exposed to multiple risk factors, *New Engl. J. Med.* **279:**906.

GRAHN, D., FRY, R. J. M., AND LEA, R. A., 1972, Analysis of survival and cause of death statistics for mice under single and duration-of-life gamma irradiation, in: *Life Sciences and Space Research*, Vol. X (A. C. Strickland, ed.), Akademie-Verlag, Berlin.

GRIEM, M. D., MEIER, P., AND DOBBEN, G. D., 1967, Analysis of the morbidity and mortality of children irradiated in fetal life, *Radiology* **88:**347.

HAZEN, R. W., PIFER, J. W., TAYOOKA, T., LIVENGOOD, J., AND HEMPELMANN, L. H., 1966, Neoplasms following irradiation of the head, *Cancer Res.* **26:**305.

HEMPELMANN, L. H., PIFER, J. W., BURKE, G. W., TERRY, R., AND AMES, W. R., 1967, Neoplasms in persons treated with X-rays in infancy for thymic enlargement: A report of third follow-up survey, *J. Natl. Cancer Inst.* **38:**317.

HOEL, D. G., AND WALBURG, H. E., JR., 1972, Statistical analysis of survival experiments, *J. Natl. Cancer Inst.* **49:**361.

HUG, O., GÖSSNER, W., MÜLLER, W. A., LUZ, A., AND HINDRINGER, B., 1969, Production of osteosarcomas in mice and rats by incorporation of radium-224, in: *Radiation-Induced Cancer*, pp. 393–409, IAEA, Vienna.

HULSE, E. V., 1967, Incidence and pathogenesis of skin tumors in mice irradiated with single external doses of low energy beta particles, *Brit. J. Cancer* **21**:531.

HUTCHISON, G. B., 1968, Leukemia in patients with cancer of the cervix uteri treated with radiation: A report covering the first 5 years of an international study, *J. Natl. Cancer Inst.* **40**:951.

International Commission on Radiological Protection, 1969, *Publication 14: Radiosensitivity and Spatial Distribution of Dose*, Pergamon Press, Oxford.

ISHIMARU, T., HOSHINO, T., ICHIMARU, M., OKADA, H., TOMIYASU, T., TSUCHIMOTO, T., AND YAMAMOTO, T., 1971, Leukemia in atomic bomb survivors, Hiroshima and Nagasaki, 1 October 1950–30 September 1966, *Radiation Res.* **45**:216.

JABLON, S., AND KATO, H., 1970, Childhood cancer in relation to prenatal exposure to atomic-bomb radiation, *Lancet* **2**:1000.

JABLON, S., AND KATO, H., 1972, Studies of the mortality of a-bomb survivors. 5. Radiation dose and mortality, 1950–1970, *Radiation Res.* **50**:649.

JOHNSON, M. L. T., LAND, C. E., GREGORY, P. B., TAURA, T., AND MILTON, R. C., 1969, *Effects of Ionizing Radiation on the Skin, Hiroshima–Nagasaki*, ABCC TR 20–69.

KAPLAN, H. S., 1948, Influence of age on susceptibility of mice to the development of lymphoid after irradiation, *J. Natl. Cancer Inst.* **9**:55.

KAPLAN, H. S., 1958, An evaluation of the somatic and genetic hazards of the medical uses of radiation, *Am. J. Roentgenol.* **80**:696.

KELLERER, A. M., AND ROSSI, H. H., 1972, The theory of dual radiation action, *Curr. Topics Radiation Res. Quart.* **8**:85.

LEWIS, T. L. T., 1960, Leukemia in childhood after antenatal exposure to X-rays, *Brit. Med. J.* **2**:1551.

LINDOP, P. J., AND ROTBLAT, J., 1962, The age factor in the susceptibility of man and animals to radiation, I. The age factor in radiation sensitivity in mice, *Brit. J. Radiol.* **35**:23.

LINDOP, P. J., AND ROTBLAT, J., 1966, Induction of lung tumors by the action of radiation and urethane, *Nature (Lond.)* **210**:1392.

LINDSAY, S., AND CHAIKOFF, 1964, The effects of irradiation on the thyroid gland with particular reference to the induction of thyroid neoplasms: A review, *Cancer Res.* **24**:1099.

LUNDIN, F. E., JR., WAGONER, J. K., AND ARCHER, V. E., 1971, *Radon Daughter Exposure and respiratory Cancer: Quantitative and Temporal Aspects*, Report from the epidemiological study of United States uranium miners, NIOSH-NIEHS Joint Monograph No. 1., U.S. Public Health Service, National Technical Information Service, Springfield, Va., P.B. 204–871.

MACKENZIE, I., 1965, Breast cancer following multiple fluoroscopies, *Brit. J. Cancer* **19**:1.

MACMAHON, B., 1962, Prenatal x ray exposure and childhood cancer, *J. Natl. Cancer Inst.* **28**:1173.

MACMAHON, B., AND HUTCHISON, G. B., 1964, Prenatal x-ray and childhood cancer: A review, *Acta Unio. Int. Contra Cancrum* **20**:1172.

MALDAGUE, P., 1969, Comparative study of experimentally induced cancer of the kidney in mice and rats with x-rays, in: *Radiation-Induced Cancer*, pp. 439–458, IAEA, Vienna.

MANNING, M. D., AND CARROLL, B. E., 1957, Some epidemiological aspects of leukemia in children, *J. Natl. Cancer Inst.* **19**:1087.

MAYS, C. W., AND LLOYD, R. D., 1972a, Bone sarcoma risk from ^{90}Sr, in: *Biomedical Implications of Radiostrontium Exposure* (M. Goldman and L. K. Bustad, eds.), pp. 352–370, USAEC Division of Technical Information, Symposium Series 25, National Technical Information Service, Springfield, Va., CONF–710201.

MAYS, C. W., AND LLOYD, R. D., 1972b, Bone sarcoma incidence vs. alpha particle dose, in: *Radiobiology of Plutonium* (B. J. Stover and W. S. S. Jee, eds.), pp. 409–430, The J. W. Press, Salt Lake City.

METTLER, F. A., HEMPELMANN, L. H., DUTTON, A. M., PIFER, J. W., TOYOOKA, E. T., AND AMES, W. R., 1969, Breast neoplasms in women treated with X-rays for acute post-partum mastitis: A pilot study, *J. Natl. Cancer Inst.* **43**:803.

MYRDEN, J. A., AND HILTZ, J. E., 1969, Breast cancer following multiple fluoroscopies during artificial pneumothorax treatment of pulmonary tuberculosis, *Canad. Med. Assoc. J.* **100**:1032.

NATIONAL ACADEMY OF SCIENCES–NATIONAL RESEARCH COUNCIL, 1972, *The Effects on Populations of Exposure to Low Levels of Ionizing Radiation*, Report of the Advisory Committee on the Biological Effects of Ionizing Radiations, Washington, D.C.

NILSSON, A., 1970, Pathologic effects of different doses of radiostrontium in mice: Dose effect relationship in ^{90}Sr-induced bone tumors, *Acta Radiol. Ther. Phys. Biol.* **9**:155.

PIFER, J. W., HEMPELMANN, L. H., DODGE, H. J., AND HODGES, F. J., II, 1968, Neoplasms in the Ann Arbor series of thymus irradiated children; a second survey, *Am. J. Roentgenol. Radium Ther. Nuclear Med.* **103**:13.

RUGH, R., DUHAMEL, L., AND SKAREDOFF, L., 1966, Relation of embryonic and fetal x irradiation to life time average weights and tumor incidence in mice, *Proc. Soc. Exp. Biol. Med.* **121**:714.

SAENGER, E. L., SILVERMAN, F. N., STERLING, T. D., AND TURNER, M. E., 1960, Neoplasia following therapeutic irradiation for benign conditions in childhood, *Radiology* **74**:889.

SAENGER, E. I., SILVERMAN, F. N., STERLING, T. D., AND TURNER, M. E., 1960, Neoplasia following therapeutic irradiation for benign conditions in childhood, *Radiology* **74**:889.

SCHULZ, R. J., AND ALBERT, R. E., 1968, III. Dose to organs of the head from the X-ray treatment of tinea capitis, *Arch. Environ. Health* **17**:935.

SEGALOFF, A., AND MAXFIELD, W. S., 1971, The synergism between radiation and estrogen in the production of mammary cancer in the rat, *Cancer Res.* **31**:168.

SELTSER, R., AND SARTWELL, P. E., 1965, The influence of occupational exposure to radiation on the mortality of American radiologists and other medical specialists, *Am. J. Epidemiol.* **81**:2.

SHELLABARGER, C. J., AND BROWN, R. D., 1972, Rat mammary neoplasia following ^{60}Co irradiation at 0.03 R or 10 R per minute, *Radiation Res.* **51**:493.

SHELLABARGER, C. J., AND STRAUB, R., 1972, Effect of 3-methylcholanthrene and fission neutron irradiation, given singly or combined, on rat mammary carcinogenesis, *J. Natl. Cancer Inst.* **48**:185.

SHELLABARGER, C. J., BOND, V. P., CRONKITE, E. P., AND APONTE, G. E., 1969, Relationship of dose of total-body ^{60}Co radiation to incidence of mammary neoplasia in female rats, in: *Radiation-Induced Cancer*, pp. 161–172, IAEA, Vienna.

SHUBIK, P., GOLDFARB, A. R., RITCHIE, A. C., AND LISCO, H., 1953, Latent carcinogenic action of beta-irradiation on mouse epidermis, *Nature (Lond.)* **171**:934.

SPIESS, H., AND MAYS, C. W., 1970, Bone cancers induced by ^{224}Ra(ThX) in children and adults, *Health Phys.* **19**:713.

SPIESS, H., AND MAYS, C. W., 1971, Erratum, *Health Phys.* **20**:543.

STEINITZ, R., 1965, Pulmonary tuberculosis and carcinoma of the lung, *Am. Rev. Resp. Dis.* **92**:758.

STEWART, A., 1961, Aetiology of childhood malignancies, *Brit. Med. J.* **1**:452.

STEWART, A., AND KNEALE, G. W., 1968, Changes in the cancer risk associated with obstetric radiography, *Lancet* **1**:104.

STEWART, A., AND KNEALE, G. W., 1970, Radiation dose effects in relation to obstetric X-rays and childhood cancers, *Lancet* **1**:1185.

STEWART, A., WEBB, J., AND HEWITT, D., 1958, A survey of childhood malignancies, *Brit. Med. J.* **1**:1495.

STORER, J. B., 1973, Unpublished data.

TELLES, N. C., WARD, B. C., WILLENSKY, E. A., AND JESSUP, G. L., 1969, Radiation–ethionine carcinogenesis, in: *Radiation-Induced Cancer*, pp. 233–245, IAEA, Vienna.

UNITED NATIONS, 1972, *Ionizing Radiation: Levels and Effects*, Vol. II: *Effects*, Report of the United Nations Scientific Committee on the Effects of Atomic Radiation, United Nations, New York.

UPTON, A. C., 1964, Comparative aspects of carcinogenesis by ionizing radiation, *Natl. Cancer Inst. Monogr.* **14**:221.

UPTON, A. C., AND COSGROVE, G. E., 1968, Radiation induced leukemia, in: *Experimental Leukemia* (M. Rich, ed.), pp. 131–158, Appleton-Century-Crofts, New York.

UPTON, A. C., ODELL, T. T., JR., AND SNIFFEN, E. P., 1960, Influence of age at time of irradiation on induction of leukemia and ovarian tumors in RF mice, *Proc. Soc. Exp. Biol. Med.* **104**:769.

UPTON, A. C., WOLFF, F. F., AND SNIFFEN, E. P., 1961, Leukemogenic effect of myleran on the mouse thymus, *Proc. Soc. Exp. Biol. Med.* **108**:464.

UPTON, A. C., JENKINS, V. K., AND CONKLIN, J. W., 1964, Myeloid leukemia in the mouse, *Ann. N.Y. Acad. Sci.* **114(1)**:189.

UPTON, A. C., CONKLIN, J. W., AND POPP, R. A., 1966, Influence of age at irradiation on susceptibility to radiation-induced life-shortening in RF mice, in: *Radiation and Ageing* (P. J. Lindop and G. A. Sacher, eds.), pp. 337–344, Taylor & Francis, London.

UPTON, A. C., RANDOLPH, M. L., AND CONKLIN, J. W., 1970, Late effects of fast neutrons and gamma-rays in mice as influenced by the dose rate of irradiation: Induction of neoplasia, *Radiation Res.* **41**:467.

WALBURG, H. E., JR., AND COSGROVE, G. E., 1970, Life shortening and cause of death in irradiated germ free mice, in: *Proceedings of the First European Symposium on Late Effects of Radiation* (P. Metalli, ed.), pp. 51–67, Comitato Nazionale Energia Nucleare, Roma.

WANEBO, C. K., JOHNSON, K. G., SATO, K., AND THORSLUND, T. W., 1968a, Breast cancer after exposure to the atomic bombings of Hiroshima and Nagasaki, *New Engl. J. Med.* **279**:667.

WANEBO, C. K., JOHNSON, K. G., SATO, K., AND THORSLUND, T. W., 1968b, Lung cancer following atomic radiation, *Am. Rev. Resp. Dis.* **98**:778.

WARREN, S., 1956, Longevity and causes of death from irradiation in physicians, *JAMA* **162**:464.

WARREN, S., AND GATES, O., 1969, Effects of continuous irradiation of mice from conception to weaning, in: *Radiation Biology of the Fetal and Juvenile Mammal* (M. R. Sikov and D. D. Mahlum, eds.), pp. 419–437, USAEC Technical Information Division, Symposium Series 17, National Technical Information Service, Springfield, Va., CONF–690501.

WOOD, J. W., TAMAGAKI, H., NERIISKI, S., SATO, T., SHELDON, W. F., ARCHER, P. G., HAMILTON, H. B., AND JOHNSON, K. G., 1969, Thyroid carcinoma in atomic bomb survivors Hiroshima and Nagasaki, *Am. J. Epidemiol.* **89**:4.

YAMAMOTO, T., AND WAKABAYASKI, T., 1968, *Bone Tumors Among the Atomic Bomb Survivors of Hiroshima and Nagasaki*, ABCC TR 26–68.

YAMAMOTO, T., KATO, H., ISHIDA, K., TAHARA, E., AND MCGREGOR, D. H., 1970, Gastric carcinoma in fixed population, Hiroshima and Nagasaki, *Gann* **61**:473.

YUHAS, J. M., 1973, Personal communication.

19

Cancer Associated with Asbestosis, Schistosomiasis, Foreign Bodies, and Scars

K. GERHARD BRAND

1. Introduction

The cancers discussed in this chapter have a common attribute: they emerge from areas of chronic fibrotic tissue reactions in response to injury or permanently embedded foreign bodies. For several pragmatic reasons, however, it has not been customary to view these cancers as a group. Histopathologically they fall into different classes. Clinically they afflict different organs and thus are dealt with by different medical specialties. Even more importantly, their prevention rests on diverse epidemiological or technological approaches. In keeping with the objectives of this Treatise, which aims for overview and biological comprehension, it seems appropriate to emphasize the group relationship of these cancers and to amalgamate the pieces of information that each contributes toward recognition and deeper understanding of the carcinogenic forces involved.

2. Cancer Associated with Asbestos and Other Fibers

An etiologic connection between asbestosis and cancer can no longer be disputed. One out of five asbestos workers dies from cancer of the lung; in another 10% the pleura, peritoneum, larynx, pharnyx, or the alimentary tract is afflicted. The

K. GERHARD BRAND • Department of Microbiology, University of Minnesota Medical School, Minneapolis, Minnesota.

time of latency from first exposure until detection of the cancer is between 20 and 40 years. Consequently, cancers of these organs appear in asbestos workers at a significantly earlier age than in the population at large.

2.1. Cancer Types and Organs Involved

A neoplasm that in almost all cases results from asbestos exposure is the *mesothelioma*. It develops in the pleura and less frequently in the peritoneum. Until a few decades ago this tumor was rarely seen. Today it is virtually indicative of past exposure to asbestos, especially crocidolite. However, a quantitative correlation does not seem to exist between the amount of fibers taken up and the probability of mesothelioma development. Many patients have been reported whose exposure had been minimal and of short duration (Chen and Mottet, 1978). There is an increased incidence of mesotheliomas in residential areas around asbestos plants relative to the prevailing wind direction in the region (Newhouse and Thompson, 1965). Also, family members of asbestos workers are at a high risk most likely due to asbestos dust brought into the house on the clothing (Anderson *et al.*, 1976). Furthermore, many mesotheliomas are presently being encountered without verification of asbestos exposure. This increase in the general population is believed to be due to widespread, low-level fiber contamination of air, water, as well as beverages, especially those sterilized by filtration through asbestos filters.

Mesotheliomas are tumors with weak malignancy in the pathological sense. They have little tendency to grow invasively and to metastasize. Nevertheless, in advanced stages cure cannot be expected. The tumor expands locally along the pleural spaces and eventually encases the lungs, leading to fatal respiratory insufficiency. It originates in areas of chronic foreign body (FB) reaction that may be minimal in response to few tissue-embedded fibers. The neoplastic originator cells are derived from the mesothelial lining of the serous membranes. The histological appearance of the tumors is variable. Spindle-shaped or pleomorphic cells predominate, often in mixture. Giant cells, osteogenic foci, or tubulopapillary surface structures add to the picture. The variability makes it occasionally difficult to reach a clear pathological diagnosis (Kannerstein and Churg, 1977). Therefore, some cases may be missed, others falsely recorded. Nevertheless, the significant increase of mesotheliomas in recent decades stands as an indisputable fact.

Bronchogenic carcinomas are likewise frequently seen in connection with asbestosis of the lungs. The age of these patients at the time of cancer onset is significantly lower than for bronchogenic carcinomas in the general population (Martischnig *et al.*, 1977). Furthermore, the incidence is much higher for women who have been exposed to asbestos than for nonexposed women. Tobacco smoking has been recognized as a decisive cocarcinogenic factor. Asbestosis in smokers leads to bronchogenic carcinoma nearly 10 times more frequently than in nonsmokers (Selikoff *et al.*, 1968). Such a correlation does not exist regarding mesotheliomas.

Asbestos-associated bronchogenic carcinomas are characterized by a predilection of the lower lobes and a higher degree of parenchymatous fibrosis (Kannerstein and Churg, 1972). However, the extent of the fibrotic tissue reaction does not correlate quantitatively with the probability of either bronchogenic carcinoma or mesothelioma development. Even minimal or short-term exposure that may not result in any demonstrable asbestosis seems to favor development of these cancer types (Martischnig *et al.*, 1977; Warnock and Churg, 1975).

663

ASBESTOSIS,
SCHISTO-
SOMIASIS,
FOREIGN
BODIES,
AND SCARS

Another possible sequel of asbestos exposure is *cancer of the upper airways,* especially of the larynx or pharynx. Again, smoking has a decisively enhancing influence (Shettigara and Morgan, 1975; Stell and McGill, 1973). Furthermore, a significantly higher mortality from *cancers of the stomach, colon, and rectum* (Selikoff, 1974) has been recorded in asbestos workers. Presumably, the fibers reach those areas with swallowed sputum or contaminated food and beverages.

2.2. Asbestos Cancer in Experimental Animals

Tumors can readily be induced in rats and mice with any of the important industrial kinds of asbestos by intrapleural or intraperitoneal injection. Usually, mesotheliomas are obtained that are histopathologically indistinguishable from those of humans (Martischnig *et al.*, 1977; Stanton and Wrench, 1972; Wagner and Berry, 1969). However, fibro-, rhabdomyo-, and osteosarcomas have also been described. The latency is 1 to 2 years, as compared to 20 to 40 years in humans. Generally, but not always (Pott *et al.*, 1976), considerable fibrosis precedes tumor appearance. Realizing that direct injection of fibers poorly corresponds to the natural mode of fiber uptake in humans, methods were devised whereby the fibers were introduced into the animals through inhalation or intratracheal instillation. With high doses administered over extended time periods, various tumor types, similar to those observed in humans, were regularly obtained; when small doses were given over brief periods, mesotheliomas developed only occasionally (Wagner *et al.*, 1974).

2.3. Cancer from Other Kinds of Fibers

In animal experiments, not only asbestos fibers but also fibers made of glass and numerous other materials were found to induce tumors. This prompted epidemiological investigations on workers who had had occupational contact with such materials. An increased incidence of carcinomas of the mouth, nose, and sinuses was registered for workers in the textile industry who had regularly inhaled *wool and cotton dust.* A high rate of general respiratory diseases, but so far not of cancers, was seen in *glass fiber* workers. Since this is a relatively young industry, the long-term effects of massively inhaled glass fibers may not yet have become apparent. Workers in the *talc* industry were found to develop cancer of the lung and pleura at a higher than normal rate. This, however, seems to be due to contamination of crude talc with asbestos fibers (Pott *et al.*, 1976).

In this context it may be mentioned that deposits of natural substances have also been incriminated (Bischoff, 1963; Bischoff and Bryson, 1964). For example, *cholesterol crystals* are often present in the walls of dermoid cysts, in lung scars, and in the gallbladder mucosa when there is a tendency to stone formation. Cancers are known to arise not infrequently in these pathological situations.

2.4. Factors Determining or Influencing Fiber Carcinogenesis

Individual predisposition and species susceptibility. An increased incidence of neoplasias, particularly in the gastrointestinal tract, has been reported for families of mesothelioma patients (Vianna and Polan, 1978). Thus, a genetically determined predisposition cannot be overlooked. On the other hand, pathophysiological peculiarities may also account for inherent differences between individuals regarding the probability of cancer developing in response to asbestos exposure. Especially the following possible factors come to mind: the ability of the respiratory system to trap fibers in the upper airways and to eliminate them by ciliary transport and expectoration before they can invade the tissue; the capacity of phagocytes to prevent fibers from settling and accumulating in critical tissue areas (Chen and Mottet, 1978); the degree of FB-reactive fibrosis, which in some individuals (e.g., those with a tendency to keloid formation) may be pronounced. Adding further factors such as age, physical condition, nutritional status, etc., it appears plausible that individuals with equal exposure do not only show different degrees of clinical asbestosis, but also differ in susceptibility to neoplasia.

When different *kinds of asbestos* are epidemiologically compared, the highest cancer risk is associated with exposure to crocidolite. However, these differences are not observed in animal experiments upon introduction of the fibers by injection. The reason for this discrepancy may be seen in the physical nature of the fibers. Whereas the extremely thin and perfectly straight fibers of crocidolite asbestos pass freely through the upper airways when inhaled, the thicker or curly fibers of chrysotile, amosite, and others are largely intercepted and expelled (Timbrell *et al.*, 1971). Alternatively (Gross and DeTreville, 1970; Harington, 1973; Webster, 1973), it was suggested that chemical cocarcinogens may be present on some asbestos materials and not on others. This may explain the observation that crocidolites from different mining regions possess different carcinogenic potentials (Webster, 1973). However, crocidolites vary also in fiber length and thickness, which is more likely the decisive factor of carcinogenicity as the following information indicates.

Fiber shape and dimensions. Animal experiments have shown (Pott and Friedrichs, 1972; Stanton and Wrench, 1972; Stanton *et al.*, 1977) that straight, rigid, nondegradable fibers of any kind are carcinogenic provided that the length exceeds $8\mu m$ and the diameter is below $1.5~\mu m$. Up to a length of $200~\mu m$ they reach the alveoli when inhaled; if they are shorter than $8~\mu m$ they will be effectively phagocytosed and dispersed in the regional lymph nodes.

Chrysotile shows low carcinogenicity upon inhalation. Due to their thickness and spiral shape, the fibers are trapped and expectorated. However, when directly injected into animals, chrysotile is as carcinogenic as crocidolite, because once in the tissue it gradually splits lengthwise into thinner fibers.

Tobacco smoking favors the development of bronchogenic and laryngeal carcinomas in asbestosis patients and experimental animals (Kannerstein and Churg, 1977; Martischnig *et al.*, 1977; Selikoff *et al.*, 1968; Shelton *et al.*, 1963). It may actually be considered the decisive carcinogenic factor in those cases that have minimal or short-term asbestos exposure and exhibit few if any signs of clinical asbestosis. On the other hand, smoking does not influence the incidence of mesotheliomas. The autochthonous carcinogenic property of asbestos remains, therefore, indisputable. The fiber load, however, becomes critically important in connection with smoking. Large amounts cause asbestosis, mesotheliomas, and bronchial carcinomas in both smokers and nonsmokers; small amounts may not lead to overt asbestosis, but they cause bronchogenic and laryngeal carcinomas in smokers and mesotheliomas in both groups. Thus, it appears that asbestos and tobacco are independent carcinogens. They may affect a susceptible cell synergistically. Or the epidemiological data may reflect a summation of independent asbestos and tobacco cancers. According to the data, bronchogenic carcinomas occur 10 times more frequently in non-asbestos-exposed smokers and 100 times more frequently in asbestos-exposed smokers than in non-asbestos-exposed nonsmokers.

Smoking may further contribute to the carcinogenic process indirectly. By paralyzing and ultimately destroying bronchial cilia, it impairs the elimination of inhaled dust particles. It also causes interstitial fibrosis of the lung parenchyma, thus accelerating and enhancing the development of asbestosis.

2.5. Preneoplastic Events

Asbestosis, the fibrotic tissue reaction against foreign particles, conspicuously precedes cancer appearance in most cases. Attempts to correlate the extent of fibrosis and the number of embedded fibers have remained unsatisfactory for several reasons. Besides individual differences in connective tissue reactivity, it is difficult to quantitate the fibers. They can be demonstrated in the tissue as "ferruginous bodies." This pleomorphic structure is composed of a proteinaceous coat and a core that contains iron. The iron is probably derived from erythrocytes, the coat from macrophages that have disintegrated after unsuccessful attempts to phagocytose the fibers. However, since fibers of any material give rise to these structures, their demonstration is not specific for asbestos. Moreover, the rate of fibers converting to ferruginous bodies varies. In humans it is probably not more than 1% (Gaensler and Addington, 1969).

Pathologically, asbestosis of the lung parenchyma is characterized by diffuse interstitial fibrosis with obliteration of alveolar segments. Most carcinomas arise directly from these fibrotic areas. In the pleura, the massive asbestotic fibrosis is preceded by small blue-white nodules, the so-called "milky spots." They appear within a few years following asbestos exposure and consist of macrophages, histiocytes, and lymphocytes. They are highly vascularized by capillaries and

665

ASBESTOSIS,
SCHISTO-
SOMIASIS,
FOREIGN
BODIES,
AND SCARS

often contain numerous asbestos fibers. The later mesotheliomas seem to emerge at these specific sites. Other early alterations of the pleura occur in the form of "pleural plaques." In these small fibrotic spots, which gradually hyalinize and calcify, asbestos fibers are usually not demonstrable and mesotheliomas rarely arise.

Numerous *animal experiments* have provided further insights into the events of fiber-induced preneoplasia.

In order to study the response of the bronchial and alveolar linings, lungs of rats were washed following *inhalation or intratracheal instillation* of chrysotile (Jaurand *et al.*, 1978; Tetley *et al.*, 1976). Macrophages in the wash fluid showed abnormal morphology and lipid metabolism. Lysosomal enzymes, especially lipases, were increased. So was the level of surfactant, a substance that protects cellular membranes by decreasing surface tension.

In the tissue itself, macrophages and giant cells accumulate. They are filled with asbestos fibers and hemosiderin of destroyed erythrocytes. At this stage, macrophages seem to secrete specific substances that stimulate fibroblastic activity, collagen production, and fibrosis (Heppleston and Styles, 1967). However, the life span of the macrophages is not noticeably shortened. Following their death and disintegration, ferruginous bodies are left behind.

Transport of fibers into deeper tissue regions is mediated by macrophages. It occurs stepwise and, hence, rather slowly (Kanazawa *et al.*, 1970). It takes about 2 years, i.e., the whole life span of a rat, before milky spots appear in the pleura.

Because of the relatively short life span of rats and mice, the late stages of asbestos preneoplasia were inaccessible for study by inhalation experiments. Therefore, *injection experiments* were performed, which bypassed the early stages of fiber phagocytosis and dissemination. Not only asbestos fibers but also glass fibers with corresponding dimensions were investigated and yielded essentially the same results (Stanton *et al.*, 1977). They caused an immediate exudative-cellular FB reaction with incomplete phagocytosis. Fibrotic conversion ensued soon and extensively. In contrast, glass fibers less than 8μm in length were successfully phagocytosed and transported to regional lymph nodes. Neither fibrosis nor tumors developed. The same outcome was observed when glass fibers thicker than 3 μm were injected. The correlation between fibrosis and tumorigenicity was striking. Large ovoid mesothelial cells with abnormal hyperchromatic nuclei and increased mitotic index (possibly the originator cells of mesotheliomas) were seen to sprout out directly from the thickened fibrotic pleura (Jagatic *et al.*, 1967).

The above results were obtained mainly in rats. Since guinea pigs are highly resistant to tumor induction by fibers (Pott and Friedrichs, 1972), it was of interest to compare the two species (Davis, 1970). In guinea pigs, the acute stage of the cellular FB reaction persists for a much longer time. Macrophages and giant cells remain continuously active, and fibers liberated after the death of macrophages are immediately rephagocytosed. Fibrosis develops sluggishly and trails that of rats by 1 to 2 years. Even more pronounced are the species differences with regard to ferruginous bodies. In rats they do not form at all (Gross and DeTreville, 1967), but in guinea pigs they are regularly found (Wagner, 1963). Since formation of ferruginous bodies is a function of macrophages, one may suspect that macrophage activity impedes tumor development. This conjecture finds support in recent studies on FB tumorigenesis (see Section 5.5). Consistent with these relationships are the observations in humans, a species that is highly prone to asbestos carcinogenesis: predictably, less than 1% of asbestos fibers taken up appear as ferruginous bodies (Gaensler and Addington, 1969).

Other experiments concerned the question of how asbestos inhalation leads to abdominal cancer. Apparently, fibers may reach the abdomen by lymphogenic or hematogenous dissemination (Kanazawa *et al.*, 1970), as well as with swallowed sputum (Jacobs *et al.*, 1978).

2.6. Effect of Asbestos Fibers on Cells in Culture

Chrysotile proved to be the kind of asbestos most damaging to cultured fibroblasts and macrophages, which constitute the primary defense cells in the pathogenesis of pneumoconioses. Aging of the cells is accelerated (Beck *et al.*, 1971; Richards *et al.*, 1974), accompanied by vacuolization and flattening, lipid reduction, and disruption of lysosomes (Davies *et al.*, 1974) with loss of hydrolytic enzymes such as lactic acid dehydrogenase, lactase, and acid phosphatase (Miller, 1978). The crucial damage seems to occur on cell membranes. Since long, pointed fibers cannot be taken in completely by the cell, their ends stick out and keep leaks permanently open. This condition is nevertheless not immediately lethal, and for some time the cell is still able to function.

This mechanical theory of asbestos cytotoxicity is at odds with the fact that crocidolite causes less damage to cultured cells, in comparison to chrysotile, although its fibers are even straighter and thinner. Therefore, the presence in chrysotile of a chemical component with *in vitro* cytotoxicity, possibly magnesium, is being discussed (Beck *et al.*, 1971).

Of great relevance appears to be the *in vitro* observation that exhausted macrophages upon phagocytosis of nondegradable particles secrete substances that stimulate fibroblasts to synthesize and deposit collagen (Burrell and Anderson, 1973; Heppleston and Styles, 1967).

3. Cancer Associated with Schistosomiasis

A causal relationship between *Schistosoma haematobium* infection and cancer of the urinary bladder is indicated by several pieces of evidence.

Epidemiology. The frequency of bladder cancer is significantly increased in endemic areas of *Schistosoma haematobium*. In Egypt, where a large segment of the rural population is known to be infected, carcinoma of the bladder ranks first among all types of cancers recorded in males. Regionally, there is a correlation between the occurrence of bladder cancer and the prevalence of diffuse schistosomal bladder calcifications as detected by X-ray screening of the general population (Gelfand, 1972).

Cancer age and estimation of cancer latency. The incidence of bladder cancer in schistosomiasis patients peaks between the ages of 30 and 50 years, whereas bladder cancer without underlying schistosomiasis is rarely encountered before the age of 50.

Schistosomal infection is commonly contracted in endemic areas during childhood. The hematuria of advanced schistosomiasis usually commences during the second decade of life. Accordingly, it can be surmised that the latency of schistosomiasis-associated bladder cancer ranges between 20 and 30 years.

Anatomical site. Schistosomiasis-associated carcinomas may be found throughout the bladder, often at multiple sites, but especially in the posterior wall. It appears significant that they are rarely located in the trigone, which is a frequent site of nonschistosomiasis cancers.

Macroscopic appearance. Bladder carcinomas in schistosomiasis have in about 80% of the cases a nodular, fungating appearance, often with a firm, solid, keratinized surface; verrucous or papillary growth is rarely observed (Elsebai, 1977). In contrast, most nonschistosomiasis cancers of the bladder present as papillary lesions with soft, friable, highly vascularized surfaces.

Histopathology. The great majority of schistosomiasis cancers (75%) are squamous carcinomas, often with marked keratinization; transitional cell carcinomas are found in only about 20% and adenocarcinomas in 5% (Elsebai, 1977). This is in striking contrast to nonschistosomiasis carcinomas, which are of the transitional cell type in over 95%.

Metastasibility. Unlike the transitional cell carcinomas that predominate in the nonschistosomiasis cases, a relatively low tendency to metastasize is initially observed in squamous schistosomiasis carcinomas. Pelvic lymph node involvement can be documented in only 20 to 30% of such cases at the time of primary surgery (Elsebai, 1977). Nevertheless, regrowth originating from the pelvic region occurs in many cases after radical cystectomy despite thorough dissection of pelvic lymph nodes. At this advanced stage, development of metastases in the bones, lung, liver, etc. must be expected as a rule.

Attempts to produce cancer *experimentally in primate or nonprimate animals* by incorporating schistosomal eggs or by inducing schistosomal infection have as yet been unsuccessful (Al-Hussein and MacDonald, 1967; Kuntz *et al.*, 1978).

The precancer tissue reactions around schistosomal eggs. Eggs are released from adult worms lodging in the venules of the vesical and pelvic plexuses. On their way toward the mucosal surface of the bladder, many of the eggs get permanently stuck in the muscular layers of the submucosa either singly or clustered. The tissue reaction against trapped eggs is generally that of a nonspecific chronic FB reaction (Gazayerli *et al.*, 1971) and shows no tendency to resolve because of the poor biodegradability of the egg shells. Yet, the eggs cannot be regarded as entirely inert. By means of immunofluorescence, it was demonstrated that soluble material with specific antigenicity is released from young, viable ova through submicroscopic pores in the shells (Boros and Warren, 1970). This probably explains the histopathological observation of periovular micronecroses during the initial phase of the disease. But soon the necrogenic virulence of the soluble egg material vanishes, apparently due to specific intervention by cell-mediated immune mechanisms (Boros and Warren, 1970; Lichtenberg *et al.*, 1971). The tissue now reacts more proliferatively with an influx of macrophages, giant cells, lymphocytes, and especially eosinophils. The result is the formation of the classical "bilharzial granulomas" or "pseudotubercles," which are about 1 to 2 mm in diameter. The granulomas tend to coalesce into larger nodules and further expand into polyps, warty papillomas, or plateaulike masses containing numerous ova. Papillomatous folds are usually encrusted by concretions of uric acid and oxalates, later augmented by phosphatic deposits. The transitional epithelial mucosa in the affected areas may become atrophic in some spots, but generally shows hyperplasia in that it both thickens and grows downward into the tunica propria. Squamous metaplasia with hyperkeratosis, resembling leukoplacic patches, is very frequently seen. Especially these latter changes may represent the precursor events that lead to cancer after many more years. Indeed, the squamous nature of the metaplastic changes seems to foretell the characteristic histopathology of most later carcinomas.

With time, the dead ova calcify and the FB-reactive tissue becomes predominantly fibrotic due to pronounced fibroblastic proliferation and collagen formation. The vascular network thins out as capillaries and small vessels obliterate. The resulting ischemia may cause epithelial atrophy, visible as "sandy patches" over fibrotic plaques especially in the trigone. Even frank mucosal necrosis may occur leading to ulcerations with the egg-laden muscularis as the base. It should be noted, however, that schistosomal carcinomas have never been seen to originate from sandy patches or ulcers (Elsebai, 1977).

The end stage of the fibrotic tissue reaction in schistosomiasis is cicatrization, which causes severe contracture of the bladder and strictures of the urethra and ureters. Extensive calcifications throughout the bladder wall are readily detectable on X-ray examination. Secondary bacterial infections of the bladder and the hydronephrotic kidneys are now a common and usually terminal complication. This then is also the time when the incidence curve of carcinomas begins to rise.

4. Scar-Associated Cancer

The discussion of both asbestos and schistosomiasis cancers pointed to tissue fibrosis as a circumstance conspicuously linked to preneoplastic development. This association is further strengthened by numerous reports of scar-related cancer (reviewed among others by Bischoff and Bryson, 1964; Cruickshank *et al.*, 1963; Dunham, 1972; Johnston and Miles, 1973; Ju, 1966; Ott, 1970; Raeburn and Spencer, 1957; Strauss *et al.*, 1963; Treves and Pack, 1930).

After latencies of several decades, sarcomas were seen to arise from scars caused by bullet wounds, surgical operations, or amputations. Carcinomas, frequently of the epidermoid type, developed from deep burn scars and chronic fistulas of the bones (osteitis fibrosa), Morbus Paget, or chronic osteomyelitis. The average latency is approximately 30 years. Colitis ulcerosa leads in about 6% of the cases to carcinoma of the colon. The latency from onset of colitis symptoms until discovery of the cancer usually lasts more than 10 years and averages around 15 years, regardless of age. Most significantly, the cancers arise in colon segments that show maximum degrees of fibrosis and stricture (Aylett, 1958; Dukes, 1958). Thorough histological studies of cancerous mammary tissues revealed in many cases a local association of cancer origin and tissue scars. These had resulted from accidental injuries or surgical trauma, including biopsies and abscess incisions (Freund *et al.*, 1976). It is also known that women with fibrocystic anomalies of the mammary glands are at considerable risk of developing mammary cancer (Davis *et al.*, 1964). Furthermore, primary carcinoma of the liver must be expected to occur in 8.5% of patients with cirrhosis and in 20% of patients with hemochromatosis. In both diseases, the liver parenchyma is progressively replaced by fibrotic connective tissue during the preneoplastic period.

A vast amount of literature (reviewed among others by Auerbach *et al.*, 1979; Raeburn and Spencer, 1957; Ripstein *et al.*, 1968; Spain, 1957; Strauss *et al.*, 1963) has accumulated concerning pulmonary cancers arising from tuberculous granulomas, cavities, or calcified foci, as well as from chronic fibrotic pneumonitis, bronchiectasis, or infarcts. Autopsies between 1970 and 1975 indicated in 16% of all lung cancers an association with scars. Peripheral bronchioloalveolar adenocarcinomas were recorded more often (70–85%) than bronchogenic squamous cell carcinomas (10–18%). The ratio is significant because, overall, the latter type of carcinomas accounts for well over 50% of lung cancers. Another important finding comes from epidemiological investigations, which show that tobacco smoking has no influence on the frequency of scar-related lung cancers (Auerbach *et al.*, 1979).

Studies were carried out to establish the causes of lung scars that led to neoplasia and to describe their pathological appearance (Auerbach *et al.*, 1979; Raeburn and Spencer, 1957). Three categories were distinguished. (1) Solitary or multiple nodules, less than 1 cm in diameter. They were characterized by a dense core of packed collagen fibers and often contained inclusions of anthracotic pigment or cholesterol crystals. Bronchiolar hyperplasia was noted peripherally. Tuberculosis and other necrotizing processes were incriminated as the causes. (2) Larger scars, several centimeters in diameter, and usually located close to the pleura. Peripheral bronchiolar hyperplasia was pronounced, as in the first category, with fibroadenomatous or squamous features. Causes included parenchymatous inflammations and atelectases. (3) Typical scars resulting from pulmonary infarcts. In older studies, such scars were rarely found to be linked to lung cancer, probably because of the high mortality or low life expectancy of patients suffering from conditions that led to pulmonary infarcts or embolism. Over the years, the prognosis of these diseases has greatly improved, and consequently the frequency of chronic lung scars from infarctions is on the rise. Accordingly, the relative frequency of scars from inflammatory processes such as tuberculosis declines. This probably explains why presently more than half of the scar-related cancers of the lung can be traced back to infarction scars and no longer to tuberculous scars as was the case two decades ago.

ASBESTOSIS,
SCHISTO-
SOMIASIS,
FOREIGN
BODIES,
AND SCARS

5. Cancer Associated with Tissue-Embedded Foreign Bodies

5.1. In Humans

Nondegradable FBs acquired by accident or implanted for medical reasons cause chronic tissue reactions that are characterized by scarlike fibrotic encapsulation of the FBs. In accordance with the preceding discussion, it comes as no surprise that such tissue conditions likewise lead to neoplasms in humans and animals. Numerous human cases have been reported and reviewed (Bischoff and Bryson, 1964; Bischoff, 1972; Bowers and Radlauer, 1969; Burns *et al.*, 1972; Dalinka *et al.*, 1969; Herrmann *et al.*, 1971; O'Connell *et al.*, 1976; Ott, 1970; Raeburn and Spencer, 1957; Siddons and McArthur, 1952; Strauss *et al.*, 1963; Thompson and Entin, 1969; Zafiracopoulos and Rouskas, 1974; and others). Especially noteworthy is the finding that any kind of nondegradable foreign material, be it metal or plastic, can lead to cancer at virtually any organ site.

Sarcomas were seen in association with subcutaneous shrapnel pieces or rifle bullets, with bone plates, screws, or nails, with metal pieces in the brain, bone splinters following fractures, plastic plombage in the lung, and recently with vascular protheses. Corresponding to the tissue of cancer origin, predominantly fibro-, chondro-, and meningosarcomas were recorded. The latencies ranged between 10 and 50 years.

FB-associated carcinomas were also found, among them lung carcinomas at sites of chronically embedded shrapnel pieces, as well as laryngeal carcinomas at sites of embedded fish bones or bone splinters. Mammary carcinomas developed in association with cardiac pacemakers that had been implanted between the gland and the major pectoral muscle. Plastic surgery of the breast by means of Silastic polymer to correct fibrocystic deformities has also led to carcinomas. Here it must be remembered, however, that mammary fibrocystic disease itself poses an increased risk of mammary cancer.

5.2. Experimental FB Tumorigenesis in Animals

Carcinogenicity of implanted nondegradable materials in animals was reported by several independent investigators at first as a merely incidental observation. Subsequently, however, the subject was systematically studied and a vast body of literature has accumulated. The results have been reviewed periodically (Bischoff, 1972; Bischoff and Bryson, 1964; Brand and Brand, 1980*a*; Brand *et al.*, 1975, 1976*b*; Carter, 1970; Ott, 1970). These monographs should be consulted for detailed references relative to the following discussion points.

Species differences in tumor frequency. Especially rats and mice, but also dogs, are found to be susceptible to FB tumorigenesis, in contrast to guinea pigs, chickens, and hamsters.

A comparative tumor induction study on numerous inbred and hybrid mouse strains revealed pronounced *differences in tumor frequency and latency which are genetically determined* (Brand *et al.*, 1977). The observed differences do not correspond with those reported for chemical or viral tumor induction.

A marked *influence of sex* on tumor frequency and latency was seen in studies involving female, male, and gonadectomized animals of different mouse strains (Brand *et al.*, 1977; Michelich and Brand, 1980). However, the effect varied between strains even to the point of inversion. Hence, the findings cannot be explained on an endocrinological basis alone.

The *age of the animals* at the time of FB implantation is inconsequential. This conclusion is based on the fact that cumulative tumor incidence curves of old and young animal groups have identical slopes. Yet, shorter latencies are generally recorded for groups of older animals due to curtailment of observation time, which causes tumors with inherently longer latencies to be missed.

Nutrition rich in protein lowers tumor frequency and prolongs latency. However, no difference is seen in animals on normal and low-protein diets.

Experimental FB sarcomas, like those in humans, appear in a great variety of *histopathological types* including fibromyxo-, hemangio-, rhadomyo-, reticulo-, osteogenic, and less frequently other sarcomas. They can be grouped according to the degree of anaplasticity: (1) well-differentiated sarcomas with low mitotic rate and minimal pleomorphism, usually containing some collagen; (2) spindle cell sarcomas with slightly higher mitotic rate and greater pleomorphism, containing little or no collagen; (3) anaplastic invasive round cell sarcomas with areas of necrosis and hemorrhage, and with high mitotic rate and hyperchromatic nuclei; (4) anaplastic sarcomas as in (3), but with numerous multinucleated cells. Most tumors fall into categories 3 and 4.

Electron microscopic studies showed that FB sarcoma cells of mice are characterized by nonbranching microfilaments, about 60 Å in width. They are scattered diffusely throughout the cytoplasmic matrix or are arranged in perinuclear or cytoplasmic bundles. Extracellularly, they form irregular deposits resembling basal laminae. Ample numbers of lysosomes are also regularly evident. Smooth-surfaced endoplasmic reticulum is restricted to the Golgi region. In many but not all tumors, and most abundantly in hemangiosarcomas, intercellular junctions of the adherens type are seen manifested as electron densities along the cytoplasmic surface of adjacent cell membranes.

Specifically in sarcomas with higher degrees of anaplasticity, rough endoplasmic reticulum is seen as short irregular profiles, often with dilated cisternae. Large numbers of polyribosomelike structures are always present, nuclear pockets or blebs only occasionally. Mitochondria are numerous and often swollen or filled with dense myelinlike configurations. Cells of highly anaplastic sarcomas may contain large cytoplasmic masses of microfilaments.

Tumors of low anaplasticity are comprised primarily of stellate or elongated cells with fewer mitochondria, fewer polyribosomelike structures, and longer profiles of rough endoplasmic reticulum.

Tumor growth, invasiveness, metastasibility, transplantability. Whereas tumors of the histopathological classes 1 and 2 may remain encapsulated and noninvasive for some time, most FB sarcomas grow rapidly and cause death of the animals within a few weeks by spreading invasively and destructively. Therefore, metastases are rarely seen in mice. On the other hand, lack of metastasibility seems generally characteristic of murine cancers. All FB sarcomas of mice are transplantable to isogeneic recipients. When kept in serial transplantation passages, the tumors may gain in malignancy as expressed by degree of histological anaplasticity, growth rate, invasiveness, and metastasibility. They may even become transplantable to allogeneic recipients.

Karyological aberrations regarding both chromosome number and morphology are a regular feature of murine FB sarcomas. Most karyotypes are found in the hyperdiploid or in the hypo- to hypertetraploid ranges, but so far no singular chromosomal characteristic has been identified as class-specific for these sarcomas. A tendency to tetraploidy is generally seen in anaplastic tumors containing multinucleated cells or cells with excessively enlarged nuclei.

In contrast to tumors induced by chemicals or viruses, *tumor-specific transplantation antigens* are lacking or extremely weak in FB sarcomas of mice. Even in immunosuppressed animals, i.e., in the absence of immune surveillance forces, no such antigens emerge (Michelich *et al.*, 1977). Moreover, normal transplantation antigens are often lost not only in established FB sarcomas but already in preneoplastic cells many months before the stage of autonomous tumor growth is reached. Here then is a striking example of a cancer completely unsusceptible to immune surveillance.

Oncogenic viruses have been searched for in murine FB sarcomas without convincing results. While intracisternal type A particles and immature type C particles were occasionally visualized, the findings were irregular, inconsistent, and without specific correlation to the process of FB tumorigenesis. Biochemical and enzymological studies likewise remained negative.

5.3. Specific Properties of Tumorigenic Implant Materials

The question of whether *chemical or physical factors* are responsible for tumorigenesis has been resolved unequivocally. Materials of any kind and chemical composition cause tumors in animals provided they possess smooth continuous surfaces and are nondegradable *in vivo*. In powdered, perforated, or porous form, the same materials lose their tumorigenicity.

Size and shape of implants are decisive determinants of tumorigenicity. When single, near-quadratic rectangles of different sizes are compared, a linear correlation between surface area and tumor frequency becomes apparent. When multiple pieces are implanted, the tumor frequency corresponds to the total surface area; tumor latency, however, is prolonged, indicating that the latter parameter is affected by the size of the individual implants.

Despite equal size and shape, different implant materials may still show pronounced differences in tumor frequency and latency as a result of specific *physicochemical surface properties*. These include electrostatic, hydrophilic, ionic, and other properties. Most influential, however, is the smoothness of the surface and its resistance to erosion. Tumor frequency markedly decreases and latency is prolonged when materials with roughened surface are used.

5.4. Investigations on the Origin of FB-Sarcomas

The FB reaction of the tissue obviously occupies a central position in the preneoplastic process. Within 2 weeks after implanting a plastic disk subcutaneously in a mouse, granulocytes and monocytic macrophage-type cells infiltrate the site. The latter also settle on the implant surface and form a monolayer with numerous binucleated and mitotic cells. A few polymorphonuclear leukocytes, fibroblastlike cells, and thin elongated spindle cells resembling smooth muscle cells may be interspersed. Already at this stage a very thin coherent membrane begins to develop around the implant consisting of fibroblasts and collagen fibers. Blood capillaries sprout into the area from the periphery. Fibroblasts, arranged like an epithelial layer, cover the inner side of the membrane, which remains separated from the macrophage monolayer on the implant surface by a fine capillary space. During the following weeks, the membrane thickens due to fibroblastic proliferation and collagen deposition. It thus becomes relatively less cellular and enters into a stage of stagnancy and quiescence approximately by the third month. It is then macroscopically discernible as a firm capsule around the implant. At the ultrastructural level, macrophages no longer show morphological signs of phagocytic activity. Specifically, the mitochondria and lysosomes are now sparse and poorly differentiated.

The tumorigenic FB reaction consists apparently of two morphologic-functional components: (1) the acute cellular reaction, with phagocytically active macrophages dominating; and (2) dormancy of macrophages and fibrotic encapsulation of the implant. Experimental interference with this course of the FB reaction affects the tumorigenic process significantly. Initiation and maintenance of acute inflammation or application of phagocytosable substances at the implant site prolong tumor latency by several months. The same effect is achieved by mechanically roughening the implant surfaces or by continuous application of cortisone. Under such circumstances the acute stage of the FB reaction is protracted as indicated by the presence of granulocytes and active macrophages, particularly giant cells, as well as by dense vascularization and minimal fibrosis.

From these findings it was inferred that a correlation exists between macrophage inactivity and fibrosis on the one hand and the process of FB tumorigenesis on the other. Further observations point in the same direction. Animal species with a low incidence of FB sarcomas differ fundamentally from mice in FB reactivity. Chickens produce only very thin capsules around implants;

in guinea pigs the fibrotic capsules regress after a few months. In humans, fibrotic scar formation proceeds much slower than in mice. Also, differences of tumorigenicity of various implant materials correlate with the degrees of fibrosis evoked. Cellophane, for example, is both more fibrogenic and more tumorigenic than polystyrene and especially glass. Similar observations were made with implants of different polyelectrolyte composition or different degrees of hydrophilia. Because of their shape, concave buttonlike implants result in more extensive fibrosis and also more tumors. Intraperitoneal implants give rise to sarcomas only when they become fixed and encapsulated by fibrotic adhesions.

The apparent relationship between chronic FB reaction and tumorigenesis prompted many investigators to *search for preneoplastic foci in FB-reactive tissues* by morphological and biochemical means. Six to twelve months after FB implantation in mice or rats, i.e., during the stage of fully developed chronic fibrosis, nests of proliferating atypical fibroblasts were regularly detected. These areas were histochemically characterized by abnormal distribution of mucopolysaccharides and mucoproteins. Therefore, they were suspected of being "presarcomatous" lesions. However, it was not possible to demonstrate in serial studies further maturation and transition to overt sarcomas. On the contrary, the abnormal foci usually resolved completely while new ones appeared at other locations. Hence, this phenomenon does not seem to reflect specifically the presarcomatous developments, but rather the dynamics of a normal chronic FB reaction with focal acute reexacerbations.

Recent progress in the elucidation of the tumorigenic process was made by employing a method that evolved from the *detection of presarcoma cells on implant surfaces*. In the basic experiment, rigid films made of various plastics or glass were subcutaneously implanted in CBA/H or CBA/H-T6 mice. These two substrains are histocompatible but distinguishable on the basis of the T6 marker chromosomes. After various time intervals the implants were excised and cut into smaller segments. Each piece was transplanted to an animal of the opposite subline. Resulting tumors were grown *in vitro* for chromosome analysis to confirm the first implant carrier as the animal from which the tumor cells originated. The following information was obtained by this approach.

Clonal tumor origin. Tumors developing from transplanted segments of the same original implant proved to be identical or closely related ("homologous") in all measurable parameters such as duration of tumor latency, aberration of chromosome number and morphology, histophathological type, degree of anaplasticity, growth behavior, and generation time in culture and animal passages. Obviously, the homologous tumors were derived from the same clone of preneoplastic cells. The specific tumor characteristics must have been predetermined in every clonal cell at the time of film cutting and transplantation. It was inferred (a) that preneoplastic cell clones arise from single "parent cells" and (b) that the carcinogenic initiation event occurs in the parent cell, thereby creating the specific determinants of later tumor characteristics.

Nonuniformity of the carcinogenic initiation events. Homologous FB tumors of common clonal derivation have equal or almost equal latencies. Apparently, the duration of latency is predetermined by the carcinogenic initiation event in the parent cell. If one presupposes that FB carcinogenesis was in each case initiated by one and the same specific molecular event, the observed latency times should form a normal distribution curve. This is not so. Latency distribution curves of FB tumors produced under uniform experimental conditions show regularly six to seven peaks suggesting the existence of six or seven statistical subpopulations of latencies, each with its own normal distribution curve (Brand *et al.*, 1976a). Since latency is determined by and thus representative of the initiation event, as many kinds of events must be expected as there are latency classes. In other words, initiation of FB carcinogenesis is probably not due to a uniform molecular occurrence. Rather, carcinogenic initiation and determination may be brought about by diverse intracellular events or defects.

Surface dependency of clonal preneoplastic cells. Segments of FB-reactive tissue capsules transferred to recipient animals do not usually lead to tumors unless a fresh FB piece is laid into the capsule pocket (Fig. 1). The capsule-derived sarcomas were occasionally heterologous with the implant-derived tumors. These findings are important in several respects. (1) They prove that preneoplastic cells reside not only on the implant surface but in the FB-reactive tissue as well. (2) More than one preneoplastic cell clone can arise in an FB reaction. Since the clones differ in their inherent tumor latency, the clone with the shortest latency prevails; thus, individual tumors are of monoclonal origin. (3) Most important is the finding that in the absence of the FB the tumorigenic process cannot reach completion. Further experiments did indeed show that preneoplastic cells

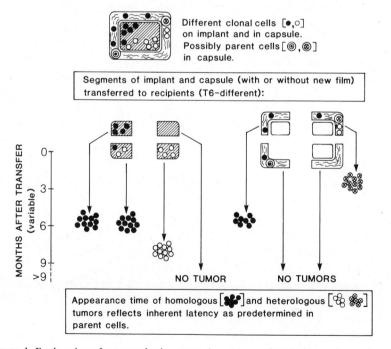

FIGURE 1. Exploration of preneoplastic events. A summary of typical experimental results.

have to establish physical contact with the implant surface for at least 1 to 2 months in order to acquire neoplastic autonomy. There are rare exceptions to this requirement. If the implant is removed from the tissue capsule during the advanced stage of FB reaction, i.e., 6 to 12 months postimplantation, sarcomas may develop nevertheless from the empty capsule. This exceptional occurrence can be explained in several ways. During the removal of the implant, mature early sarcoma cells may have been rubbed off mechanically and stayed behind in the empty capsule pocket. Or the fibrotic capsule tissue did not resolve, but hardened to form a permanent scar, possibly incorporating mineral deposits or calcifications. Such tissue conditions may conceivably provide a similar surface effect on preneoplastic cells as the implant itself.

Identification of the cell type of tumor origin (Fig. 2). Since macrophages predominate in the tumorigenic FB reaction, they were first suspected of being the source of FB sarcomas. This possibility found support in the hypothesis that macrophages can convert into collagen-producing fibroblasts (Kouri and Ancheta, 1972; Maximow, 1927; McDougal and Azar, 1972). However, experimental evidence excluded macrophages from consideration. Studies on mouse radiation chimeras showed that FB sarcomas do not stem from bone marrow-derived cells, and hence not from macrophages, which are blood-borne (Volkman and Gowans, 1965). Morphological, ultrastructural, and *in vitro* studies excluded also the fibroblasts, but incriminated mesenchymal stem cells of the microvasculature, such as pericytes, endothelial cells, or their precursors. This cell type is known to possess pluripotentiality, thus accounting for the variety of sarcoma types seen. Occasionally, mixed tumors were observed, e.g., fibromyxo- or fibrohemangiosarcomas; chromosomal analyses confirmed that either compartment originated from the same preneoplastic cell clone, i.e., from the same parent cell. Most significantly, certain ultrastructural features of FB sarcomas were compatible with cells of the vascular system and less so with fibroblasts. These included especially (1) the presence of a pericellular, periodic acid–Schiff-positive, argyrophilic, and filamentous substance resembling basal lamina; (2) sparsity of collagen; and (3) prominent cytoplasmic accumulations of 60-Å microfilaments.

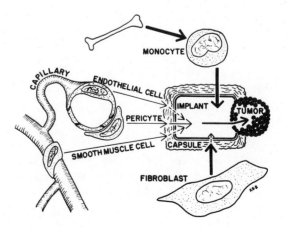

FIGURE 2. Cell types involved in FB reaction and in FB tumorigenesis. From Johnson *et al.* (1973) with permission of *Cancer Research.*

The nature of the tumor originator cell type was unveiled more directly through cell culture experiments. It was found that the preneoplastic clonal cells can be isolated *in vitro* from implant and capsule segments. After single-cell cloning, they can be expanded to pure populations. Light and electron microscopic studies on these cells revealed that they appear phenotypically and sequentially in two morphological types: first as compact, spindly cells, often in beadlike arrangement and resembling pericytes, and later as flat, pavementlike cells in patches resembling endothelium.

The number of preneoplastic cells and clones in tumorigenic FB reactions was estimated in two ways. The first approach was based on the finding that subcutaneous implantation of one $0.2 \times 7 \times 15$-mm plastic film into CBA/H mice caused sarcomas in 80% of the test animals, implantation of one $0.2 \times 15 \times 22$-mm film in 95%. Tumor-negative implant/capsule complexes were transplanted for continued observation to young CBA/H-T6 animals before the original implant carriers died of old age. No CBA/H tumors were recorded during the lifetime of the recipients. Hence, it could be assumed that preneoplastic cells indeed had not emerged. In this situation it was statistically permissible to apply the Poisson distribution to the data. The most probable number (MPN) of preneoplastic parent cells was computed as 1 in animals that had received one 7×15-mm film, and as 3 in animals with one 15×22 mm film. These calculations were confirmed by more direct "counting" experiments. Films were implanted in mice, then excised, cut, and prepared in such a way that cell areas as small as 2×2 mm remained on the segments. These were transferred to recipients. The frequency of heterologous sarcomas indicated the number of different parent cells and clones on the implant at the time of cutting and transfer.

These investigations led to the general conclusion that the number of preneoplastic parent cells is extremely small relative to the multitude of cells mobilized or newly generated in an FB reaction. Furthermore, there is a linear relationship between the implant surface area and the MPN of tumorigenic parent cells, provided other variables are held constant, e.g., animal strain, kind of material, surface characteristics, etc.

The appearance time and location of preneoplastic parent cells and clones (Table 1) were determined by transplantation of implant segments as well as FB-reactive tissue segments, with new FB pieces inserted, throughout the preneoplastic period. The first preneoplastic cells are demonstrable in 30% of the animals within 4 weeks, and in 80% of the animals within 8 weeks postimplantation in the FB-reactive tissue, but not on the implant surfaces. Clones develop instantly and expand at first strictly inside the tissue. Only by the sixth to seventh month postimplantation, rarely earlier, can preneoplastic cells be detected on implant surfaces.

When implants with roughened surfaces are comparatively tested, the appearance of preneoplastic parent cells is delayed by approximately 6 months while the MPN remains unchanged. Consequently, tumor latency is prolonged, but the tumor incidence is as high as in experiments with smooth-surfaced implants.

679

ASBESTOSIS,
SCHISTO-
SOMIASIS,
FOREIGN
BODIES,
AND SCARS

TABLE 1

Appearance and Maturation of Preneoplastic Cells in FB-Reactive Tissue and on the Implant Surface Relative to Time Postimplantation and Course of the FB Reaction[a]

Months following implantation	Morphological criteria of the FB reaction	Location of preneoplastic cells[b]
1–2	Tissue: Acute cellular infiltration and proliferation (macrophages; few granulocytes and fibroblasts). Outgrowth of capillaries. Implant surface: Macrophages, giant cells, patches of granulocytes.	
2–3	Tissue: Decreasing cell density, relative increase of fibroblasts. Collagen production. Implant surface: Macrophages, giant cells.	
3–7	Tissue deposition of collagen. Obliteration of capillaries. Phagocytic inactivity of macrophages. Implant surface: Inactive macrophages. Fewer giant cells.	
5 to over 30	No further change.	

[a] Modified after Brand and Brand (1980a) with permission of *Zentralblatt fuer Bakteriologie, Parasitienkunde, Infektionskrankheiten und Hygiene.*
[b] ⊚, Preneoplastic parent cells; O, preneoplastic clonal cells; ●, tumor cells.

The experimental exploration of FB tumorigenesis led to the conclusion that the process passes through a *sequence of essential developmental stages.* These are expressed by the morphological, ultrastructural, and functional tissue and cell changes already described. Furthermore, it was found that the preneoplastic cells can be cultured *in vitro* with gradually increasing ease. Apparently, the threshold of proliferative response lowers as the cells mature toward neoplastic autonomy.

The first stage of FB tumorigenesis is characterized by the acute FB reaction. Preneoplastic cells can be detected only indirectly by *in vivo* transfer, not by *in vitro* culture, and only in the FB-reactive tissue, not on the implant surface.

During the second stage, macrophages take on an inactive and quiescent appearance. The FB-reactive tissue around the implant develops into a well-demarcated fibrotic capsule. Blood capillaries begin to obliterate, especially in the central layers of the capsule. Preneoplastic clonal cells can be demonstrated within and outside the capsule by *in vivo* transfer and occasionally by *in vitro* culture, but still not on the implant surface. If the whole FB/capsule complex is excised and transplanted to a recipient animal, tumor latency is shortened by 1 to 2 months, possibly due to acceleration of both fibrosis and vascular obliteration in the capsule.

The third stage begins with the appearance of preneoplastic clonal cells on the implant surface. The chronic fibrotic FB reaction is now fully developed. The preneoplastic cells can easily be cultured *in vitro* from both the capsule and the FB surface.

During the fourth stage, those preneoplastic cells that are attached to the implant surface undergo the final maturation step toward neoplastic autonomy. Clonal sister cells that have remained in the capsule tissue do not advance beyond the maturation point reached in stage three.

During the fifth stage, mature autonomous neoplastic cells detach from the implant surface and begin uncontrollable sarcomatous proliferation.

When plastics with roughened surfaces are used, the acute cellular FB reaction in stage one is markedly protracted. Successful demonstration of preneoplastic cells and appearance of tumors are delayed by several months.

Glass implants, in comparison to smooth plastic implants of equal size, cause less vigorous acute FB reactions. Possibly for this reason, fewer parent cells are counted and tumor incidence is lower. Subsequently during stage two, the tissue capsules remain thinner and fibrosis appears unobtrusive. This may cause the pace of preneoplastic cell maturation to slow during stages two and three so that tumor latencies lengthen.

5.5. Experimental FB Tumorigenesis: Key Findings and Theoretical Deductions

The five preneoplastic stages described reflect three cellular phases of carcinogenic development: (1) the initiation event during stage one; (2) surface-independent maturation during stages two and three; (3) surface-dependent maturation during stage four.

The carcinogenic initiation event occurs during the early FB reaction, possibly when the acute macrophage-dominated inflammation converts into fibrosis. By this time a dense capillary network has developed from vascular stem cells where the initiation event is assumed to occur. Subsequently, the subacute fibrotic tissue transition causes many blood capillaries to obliterate. Under these circumstances, the early preneoplastic vascular cells may escape the controlling forces that normally govern a homeostatic tissue environment.

As the experiments have clearly shown, the initiation event does not come about through direct action of the FB on a susceptible cell. This is fundamentally in contrast to such cell-invasive agents as chemical carcinogens, oncoviruses, or radiation. The carcinogenic FB is neither biochemically active nor can it exert even passively a physical effect on the cells since no direct contact is established at the time when the initiation event occurs. Hence, one must consider either a spontaneous intracellular event or one that is caused by a concomitant extraneous agent. In the experimental mouse model, a spontaneous event appears most likely because the MPN of preneoplastic parent cells, i.e., the frequency of initiation events, correlates with implant size, which in turn determines the extent of the FB reaction. Obviously, the larger the number of FB-reactive proliferating cells, the greater are the chances of spontaneous intracellular errors.

Regarding the nature of the spontaneous intracellular initiation event, hardly any clue has been found so far. General hypotheses of carcinogenesis presently discussed would suggest among others gene mutations, activation of indigenous viral genomes, misdirected epigenetic differentiation, or chromosomal aberrations. Especially the latter have been studied in FB-induced murine sarcomas. However, no specific defect patterns have been reported as yet.

Surface-independent maturation. According to a widely accepted hypothesis, preneoplastic "maturation" is viewed as a progressive cellular evolution whereby a sequence of discrete mutational changes brings the cells stepwise closer to neoplastic autonomy. In the case of FB tumorigenesis, this concept cannot claim validity. Here, it is a singular event that not only decides the neoplastic destination, but already specifies the characteristics of the later cancer.

The neoplastic determinants are suppressed for the duration of tumor latency. Release does not occur abruptly but stepwise as indicated by the observation that preneoplastic clonal cells can be cultured *in vitro* with gradually increasing facility.

The suppressor mechanism is regulated by an intracellular timer that must have been set by the initiation event, because latency is terminated in each clonal cell at the same time.

Another relevant observation was made on *in vitro* cultures of preneoplastic clonal cells. When such cells were reimplanted into animals, tumor latency was prolonged by the length of the *in vitro* period. In other words, preneoplastic maturation was arrested while the cells were in culture. Since their proliferation in culture is much more rapid than *in vivo*, it must be concluded that preneoplastic maturation does not relate to the number of cell divisions but is dependent on other factors provided only *in vivo*.

Factors that promote FB tumorigenesis *in vivo* seem to be connected with the state of macrophage inactivity and fibrosis. Experimental interference with these tissue conditions drastically affects the tumorigenic process. While interrelationships between macrophage function and fibrosis have been verified (Heppleston and Styles, 1967; Leibovich and Ross, 1975, 1976), the tumor-promoting mechanism remains to be explored at the functional and molecular level.

Surface-dependent maturation. In the fibrotic capsule, the preneoplastic cells reach a certain stage of maturation. However, the final step to neoplastic autonomy is accomplished only when the cells attach themselves to the FB surface. Occasionally, firm scars, calcium deposits, or osseous metaplasia can exert the same surface effect. Experimentally, it was shown that the surface properties of the foreign material have little influence on the preneoplastic maturation at this stage. When preneoplastic clonal cells, which had proceeded to stage three, were seeded on glass disks or on smooth or roughened plastic disks and then implanted in animals, tumor growth commenced at the same time. This is in contrast to the earlier stages of FB tumorigenesis, when surface properties of implants have a decisive influence on the pace of preneoplastic development.

The cell membrane is the obvious structure directly affected by surface attachment. Various consequences must be expected. Paucity of physiological ions in the attachment zone may alter membrane potential and molecular interactions (Andrade, 1973; Warren, 1974). The arrangement of macromolecules and the distribution patterns of specific functional loci may be disturbed (Barnett *et al.*, 1974; Berlin *et al.*, 1974). Essential intercellular contacts and communication may be interrupted (Loewenstein, 1979). The latter aspect was investigated by implantation of Millipore filters. Only those with pore sizes below 0.2 μm proved tumorigenic.

Whatever happens at the cell membrane level, it generates a signal ordering the hereditary apparatus of the cell to express the neoplastic properties that have been predetermined by the initiation event. Only by being hereditary can the information be passed through generations of preneoplastic and cancer cells.

The role of the FB in the tumorigenic process as analyzed in the preceding paragraphs is threefold, yet in each phase it is a passive one. The FB does not directly induce the carcinogenic initiation event; all it does is stimulate cell proliferation, thereby increasing the likelihood of spontaneous carcinogenic errors in labile stem cells of the microvasculature. By its continued presence, the nondegradable FB exhausts the macrophages and forces the reactive tissue into chronic fibrosis. In this state, a specific promotional effect is exerted on preneoplastic cell maturation. Finally, the FB provides a firm surface for cell attachment. The effect on the cell membrane and its intracellular consequences are the last prerequisite for neoplastic autonomy.

Previous hypotheses of FB tumorigenesis shall not be discussed here in detail. The interested reader is referred to the monographs cited before. Suffice it to say that none of the earlier hypotheses can comprehensively account for all crucial aspects of FB tumorigenesis although they may relate to one or the other of the preneoplastic stages. For example, hypotheses that incriminate direct interactions between the FB surface and cells as the cause of FB sarcomas may relate to the stage of surface-dependent maturation, but certainly not to the preceding stages. Likewise, hypotheses that focus on the chronic fibrotic FB reaction and the presumed sequels such as anoxia, lack of nutrients, accumulation of carcinogenic metabolites, etc., can neither explain initiation, which occurs well before completion of hypovascular tissue fibrosis, nor surface-dependent maturation.

6. *Asbestos, Schistosomiasis, Foreign Body, and Scar Cancers of Humans in the Light of Experimental Foreign Body Tumorigenesis*

The group relationship of these cancers is apparent in view of the etiologic involvement of FBs and/or tissue fibrosis. Several new facets have been added to our understanding from the results of experimental FB tumorigenesis in mice. However, several inconsistencies have become visible as well, and thus complicate the unifying concept.

6.1. Common Mechanism of Preneoplastic Promotion Indicated by Macrophage
Inactivity and Tissue Fibrosis

683

ASBESTOSIS,
SCHISTO-
SOMIASIS,
FOREIGN
BODIES,
AND SCARS

6.1. Common Mechanism of Preneoplastic Promotion Indicated by Macrophage Inactivity and Tissue Fibrosis

Good quantitative correlation was observed between fibrosis and promotional force when tumors were induced in mice or rats by intrapleural instillation of asbestos fibers or subcutaneous implantation of FBs. Experimental interference with fibrotic development affected tumor latency significantly.

Preneoplastic fibrosis was demonstrated as an essential feature in every cancer type of this group and even in certain chemically induced tumors (Carter *et al.*, 1970; Shurgin and Becker, 1974). However, the correlation between fibrosis and carcinogenic promotion does not hold up in every case of human asbestos cancer. Many bronchogenic carcinomas and occasional mesotheliomas have developed despite minimal exposure to asbestos and in the absence of pronounced fibrotic tissue alterations (Chen and Mottet, 1978). Also, the form of fibrosis seems to be of importance. Focal or nodular manifestations as in silicosis, berylliosis, or anthracosis usually do not lead to cancer, in contrast to the diffuse form of fibrosis in asbestosis and schistosomiasis. Possibly, the promotional effect is not directly related to fibrosis, but is caused by antecedent factors that partake in chronic inflammation and may, in fact, themselves be the inducers of the fibrotic tissue conversion. Products given off by macrophages or other inflammatory cells, especially when in a state of chronic exhaustion and functional paralysis, are prime suspects (Davis, 1970; Johnson *et al.*, 1972). Support comes from experimental findings on mice chronically infected with lactate dehydrogenase virus, which is known to reside in the macrophage population. The infected cells are not only unimpaired in their viability, but they are even stimulated in some of their physiological functions. In such animals, the latency of FB sarcomas is significantly prolonged as compared to noninfected control animals (Brinton-Darnell and Brand, 1977). On the same hypothetical basis, the cancer-promoting influence of tobacco smoking may be explainable, at least partly, since macrophages are severely affected by it. Taking everything together, it appears that the state of fibrosis is not so much a primary element, but rather a result and indicator of the factors that promote the development of these cancers.

6.2. Different Cell Types of Tumor Origin

The tumors of this group show fundamental histological differences. In the case of murine FB sarcomas, the differences can satisfactorily be explained by the pluripotentiality of the originator cell type. The same explanation may apply to the histological differences among asbestos mesotheliomas, but hardly to the group as a whole. The occurrence of both carcinomas and sarcomas, which descend respectively from epithelium and mesenchyme, makes a common cell type most unlikely. Schistosomiasis cancer presumably originates from the transitional epithelium of the bladder, bronchogenic carcinomas from bronchial epithelium, mesotheliomas from the pluripotential mesenchymal surface cells of the serous membranes. FB and scar sarcomas of humans may develop from mesenchymal stem cells of the microvasculature, as do the experimental FB sarcomas of mice. Histologically, they cover the same spectrum, but electron micrographs that could answer the question conclusively are not available.

6.3. Nonuniformity of Initiation Events

There is a general agreement that the neoplastic state reflects a disturbance of cellular growth control. Undoubtedly, the cell must be equipped with a very complex multifactorial system to serve such growth-related regulatory tasks as membrane transport functions, intercellular communications, biosynthetic processes preparatory to cell division, special differentiated cell functions in response to specific demands, and so on. Numerous molecular reactions and switching mechanisms must be in operation at the genetic, epigenetic, and regulatory levels with feedback loops to maintain continuous checks and balances. A single hereditary error in any of numerous sensitive points may lead to irreversible disorder of growth control. The nature of such errors may vary as well. They may occur in the form of structural defects, biomolecular losses, additions, or translocations; they may be spontaneous or caused by extraneous agents; they may result from genetic or epigenetic interference by viruses or viral genomes. The experimental demonstration of distinct latency classes in FB tumorigenesis and other forms of carcinogenesis (Brand *et al.*, 1976*a*; Iversen *et al.*, 1968; Turusov *et al.*, 1971) may indeed reflect diversity regarding both location and nature of the carcinogenic molecular aberrations.

The rare occurrence of FB sarcomas in humans, as compared to mice, suggests that species differences exist regarding susceptibility of vascular stem cells to carcinogenic initiation events. Other cell types, e.g., mesothelial cells, do not show such a species difference. This conclusion is derived from the fact that the incidence of mesotheliomas upon asbestos exposure is about equal in humans and mice. The latency differs, however; but this is explained by the different modes of fiber acquisition. In humans, it occurs very gradually by inhalation of minute doses, followed by a slow transport of the fibers through the lung to the pleura. In mouse experiments, large doses must be inserted directly into the pleura space, otherwise few if any mesotheliomas develop during the lifetime of the animal.

The carcinogenic initiation event in murine FB tumorigenesis may relate to spontaneous karyological aberrations. Genomic and regulatory instability supposedly constitutes an inherent property of stem cells and regenerative cells. It has been suggested that pluripotentiality and differentiability are being preserved beyond embryogenesis by exempting those cells from chromosome stabilization, which is effected in differentiated cells by irreversible DNA methylation or deamination (Scarano, 1971). The price to be paid for pluripotentiality could well be an increased susceptibility to spontaneous errors at the chromosomal and subchromosomal levels (German, 1973). This thesis is supported by the finding that fully differentiated cell types (e.g., mouse fibroblasts) show much greater chromosomal stability in culture (Brand, unpublished). However, contrary to some other experimental cancer models, no specific karyological aberrations have been identified so far in murine FB tumorigenesis. The etiological relationship at the level of the initiation event, therefore, remains questionable.

In experimental FB tumorigenesis, the inititiation event was shown to occur within a few weeks following FB implantation, long before fibrosis is pronounced. In asbestos and schistosomiasis cancers, the FB material accumulates gradually in the tissue. Consequently, the chronic FB reaction develops and expands much more slowly and the initiation event may coincide with or even follow fibrotic tissue changes. Taking schistosomiasis carcinogenesis as an example, spontaneous defects may occur early in epithelial cells while they are engaged in repair activities responding to the continuous tissue damage by penetrating worm eggs. Or, the initiation events may occur during the stages of advanced diffuse cicatrization which must be expected to interfere with normal induction signals essential for the guidance of epithelial differentiation and maintenance of tissue structure. This would conform with the marked metaplastic distortions and displacements of epithelium especially in the areas of fibrosis (Spain, 1957). Epithelial cells, separated from their normal matrix and occupied with misdirected regenerative efforts, may be particularly prone to spontaneous errors at the growth regulation level. In the case of sarcomas, spontaneous initiation events may likewise have occurred under such circumstances (Raeburn and Spencer, 1957; Ripstein *et al.*, 1968).

Besides spontaneous intracellular events, various possibilities of extraneous cancer induction must be taken into consideration as well. In asbestos carcinogenesis, it may be due to direct mechanical damage of cell membranes by the fibers (Pott and Friedrichs, 1972). But also carcinogenic chemicals or metabolites have access to potential cancer originator cells. Fibrotic blockage of blood and lymph vessels as a result of chronic FB reaction or scar formation could lead to accumulation of carcinogens by inhibiting their transport or catabolism (Elsebai, 1977; Freund *et al.*, 1976; Ripstein *et al.*, 1968). Concerning the origin of schistosomiasis cancer, renally excreted carcinogens such as nitrosamines are regarded by some authors as factors of major importance (Elsebai, 1977; Hicks *et al.*, 1977). However, especially apparent is the possible role of chemical carcinogens in asbestos cancer. A direct vehicle function of asbestos fibers, which are known to possess a remarkable absorptive affinity for chemical contaminants (Harington, 1973), is under continued investigation, but uptake of carcinogens by inhalation seems of far greater importance. This is suggested especially by the influence of cigarette smoking on the incidence of bronchogenic and laryngeal carcinomas in asbestos-exposed individuals (Selikoff *et al.*, 1968; Shettigara and Morgan, 1975). The role of tobacco is most likely chemical in nature. Although smoking also causes paralysis of ciliary motility and stimulates interstitial fibrosis, these factors have at most minor importance. Otherwise, mesothelioma incidence should as well be positively affected by smoking. This is not so, obviously for the reason that mesothelial cells of the pleura are not directly accessible to carcinogenic inhalants. The frequency of pulmonary scar carcinomas is likewise independent of smoking. This seems to indicate that in scar carcinogenesis the initiation events do not take place in epithelial cells lining the bronchial or alveolar surfaces, but rather in nonventilated areas of the scarred or atelectatic parenchyma. In this situation, the carcinogenic initiation event is more likely spontaneous in nature; conceivably, it may be induced by diagnostic, therapeutic, or accidental radiation.

6.4. The Question of Immune Surveillance

As was experimentally shown, there is no basis for immune defense against FB sarcomas because they lack tumor-specific transplantation antigens. However, in view of the possibility that chemical carcinogens may initiate asbestos, schistosomiasis, and scar cancers, emergence of tumor-specific antigens and thus a basis for immune defense could be expected in such cases.

6.5. Resume: The Common and the Differing Attributes

No uniformity exists regarding the intracellular carcinogenic initiation processes, the inducing agents or events, or the cell types of cancer origin. Differences are seen not only between the etiologic subgroups, i.e., asbestos, schistosomiasis, FB, and scar cancers, but also among tumors within subgroups. This was demonstrated experimentally on FB tumors of mice, and is also apparent among asbestos cancers of humans.

FBs never act as direct primary inducers of carcinogenesis. In fact, they are dispensable, as in the case of scar cancers. However, by their presence in the tissue they force FB-reactive cells to proliferate and thus enhance the probability of carcinogenic initiation events.

Presumably, common among these cancers is the preneoplastic promotion process, which is morphologically characterized by macrophage inactivity and diffuse tissue fibrosis. The FBs have an important role during this phase in that they create and maintain those chronic tissue conditions that underly preneoplastic promotion.

7. Prevention

7.1. Asbestos Cancer

Avoidance or reduction of asbestos exposure is seen as the most important preventive measure. However, complete elimination of asbestos or similar fibers is obviously not feasible in industrialized countries. Therefore, attempts have been made to set safety limits of exposure. Unfortunately, such attempts have been thwarted by the observation that minimal dosages can still lead to cancer. Therefore, attempts are under way by industry to develop artificial noncarcinogenic fibers.

The role of tobacco smoking is acknowledged, but it should be realized that general carcinogenic air pollutants may have the same effect. Ionizing radiation, especially in the form of diagnostic or therapeutic X-rays, must also be considered as potential inducers in asbestos-exposed persons. Therefore, every effort should be made to discourage these persons from smoking, to keep them away from areas of chemical air pollution, and to exercise special caution in applying X-irradiation.

7.2. Scar Cancer

The same general recommendations as given for the prevention of asbestos cancer apply here.

7.3. Schistosomiasis Cancer

Prevention of schistosomal infection is the only reasonable way of preventing this cancer. Thus, the problem is an extremely complex one involving parasitological, zoological, epidemiological, ecological, and most importantly sociological aspects.

7.4. FB Cancer

A substantial number of FB-associated cancers have been reported in the literature. However, considering the total number of present implant carriers in the world, the risk of acquiring such a cancer appears to be small. On the other hand, many modern implant systems have been developed only recently. Hence, most implants have been in place for a limited number of years whereas latencies of FB cancers reportedly reach 50 and more years. Two approaches were used to assess the risk more precisely (Brand and Brand, 1980b).

In the first study, case reports were collected and evaluated with special attention to the recorded latencies. The FBs were either accidentally acquired, e.g., during World War I, or they were implanted for medical reasons. It was found that well over 25% of the cancers appeared within 15 years, 50% within 25 years. The present upsurge of medical and cosmetic implantations began during the late 1950s and early 1960s, i.e., about 20 years ago. It can be estimated that during those early years the number of implantations worldwide reached into the hundreds of thousands. Since at least 25% of the implant-associated cancers should have emerged by now, one would expect tens of thousands of cases to have occurred if the incidence in humans approached 100% as it does in experimental rats and mice. However, as relatively few cases have been reported in recent years, the likelihood of implant-associated tumors in humans is minimal, although obviously not zero.

The second study was carried out on human tissue specimens of chronic FB reactions against a variety of implants that had been *in situ* for up to 19 years.

Employing histological and cell culture methods, which had been developed and proven successful in mice, attempts were made to identify specific precancer cells in the human tissues. No abnormal, clonally aneuploid cells resembling the precancer cells of murine FB reactions were detected in any of the specimens. Hence, the rarity of human FB cancers can satisfactorily be explained by the rare emergence of precancer cells in human FB reactions.

Despite those favorable observations and results, the possibility of neoplasms arising in association with implants, however remote, must not be dismissed, and measures of prevention should be considered in individual cases. FBs acquired by accident should be removed if feasible. The same recommendation applies to medical devices that have served their purpose. Medically unnecessary implantations should be avoided, especially those of cosmetic nature unless psychiatrically indicated. In conformance with experimental findings discussed in preceding sections, the size of implants should be kept to a minimum. The surfaces should be discontinuous, if possible, or textured. Nets, sponges, or ceramics are preferable over solid materials with smooth surfaces. Most importantly, implant carriers must not be lost to follow-up, but should regularly be reexamined not only to assure proper implant function, but also to exclude tissue changes indicative of abnormal growth.

8. References

AL-HUSSEIN, M., AND MACDONALD, D. F., 1967, Lack of urothelial topical tumorigenicity of *Schistosoma* ova in mice, *Cancer Res.* **27**:228–229.

ANDERSON, H. A., LILIS, R., DAUM, S. M., FISHBEIN, A. S., AND SELIKOFF, I. J., 1976, Household-contact asbestos neoplastic risk, *Ann. N.Y. Acad. Sci.* **271**:311–323.

ANDRADE, J. D., 1973, Interfacial phenomena and biomaterials, *Med. Instrum.* (*Baltimore*) **7**:110–120.

AUERBACH, O., GARFINKEL, L., AND PARKS, V. R., 1979, Scar cancer of the lung. Increase over a 21 year period, *Cancer* **43**:636–642.

AYLETT, S., 1958, Malignant tumors of the colon, in: *Cancer*, Vol. 4 (R. W. Raven, ed.), pp. 86–102, Butterworths, London.

BARNETT, R. E., FURCHT, L. T., AND SCOTT, R. E., 1974, Differences in membrane fluidity and structure in contact-inhibited and transformed cells, *Proc. Natl. Acad. Sci. USA* **71**:1992–1994.

BECK, E. G., HOLT, P. F., AND NASRALLAH, E. T., 1971, Effects of chrysotile and acid-treated chrysotile on macrophage cultures, *Br. J. Ind. Med.* **28**:179–185.

BERLIN, R. D., OLIVER, J. M., UKENA, T. E., AND YIN, H. H., 1974, Control of cell surface topography, *Nature* (*London*) **247**:45–46.

BISCHOFF, F., 1963, Carcinogenesis through cholesterol and derivatives, *Prog. Exp. Tumor Res.* **3**:412–444.

BISCHOFF, F., 1972, Organic polymer biocompatibility and toxicology, *Clin. Chem.* (New York) **18**:869–894.

BISCHOFF, F., AND BRYSON, G., 1964, Carcinogenesis through solid state surfaces, *Prog. Exp. Tumor Res.* **5**:85–133.

BOROS, D. L., AND WARREN, K. S., 1970, Delayed hypersensitivity-type granuloma formation and dermal reaction induced and elicited by a soluble factor isolated from *Schistosoma mansoni* eggs, *J. Exp. Med.* **132**:488–507.

BOWERS, D. G., JR., AND RADLAUER, C. B., 1969, Breast cancer after prophylactic subcutaneous mastectomies and reconstruction with Silastic prostheses, *Plast. Reconstr. Surg.* **44**:541–544.

BRAND, I., BUOEN, L. C., AND BRAND, K. G., 1977, Foreign body tumors of mice: Strain and sex differences in latency and incidence, *J. Natl. Cancer Inst.* **58**:1443–1447.

Brand, K. G., and Brand, I., 1980a, Untersuchungen und Literaturstudien zum Krebsproblem, *Zentralbl. Bakteriol. Parasitenkd. Infektionskr. Hyg. Abt. 1 Orig. Reihe B* **171:**1–17, 359–387, and 544–573.

Brand, K. G., and Brand, I., 1980b, Risk assessment of carcinogenesis at implantation sites, *Plast. Reconstr. Surg.* **66:**591–594.

Brand, K. G., Buoen, L. C., Johnson, K. H., and Brand, I., 1975, Etiological factors, stages, and the role of the foreign body in foreign body tumorigenesis: A review, *Cancer Res.* **35:**279–286.

Brand, K. G., Buoen, L. C., and Brand, I., 1967a, Multiphasic incidence of foreign body-induced sarcomas, *Cancer Res.* **36:**3681–3683.

Brand, K. G., Johnson, K. H., and Buoen, L. C., 1976b, Foreign body tumorigenesis, *CRC Crit. Rev. Toxicol.* **4:**353–394.

Brinton-Darnell, M., and Brand, I., 1977, Delayed foreign body-tumorigenesis in mice infected with lactate dehydrogenase-elevating virus, *J. Natl. Cancer Inst.* **59:**1027–1029.

Burns, W. A., Kanhouwa, S., Tillman, L., Saini, N., and Herrmann, J. B., 1972, Fibrosarcoma occurring at the site of a plastic vascular graft, *Cancer* **29:**66–72.

Burrell, R., and Anderson, M., 1973, The induction of fibrogenesis by silica-treated alveolar macrophages, *Environ. Res.* **6:**389–394.

Carter, R. L., 1970, Induced subcutaneous sarcomata: Their development and critical appraisal, in: *Metabolic Aspects of Food Safety* (F. J. C. Roe, ed.), pp. 569–591, Blackwell, Oxford.

Carter, R. L., Birbeck, M. S. C., and Roberts, J. D. B., 1970, Development of injection-site sarcomata in rats: A study of the early reactive changes evoked by a carcinogenic nitrosoquinoline compound, *Br. J. Cancer* **24:**300–311.

Chen, W., and Mottet, N. K., 1978, Malignant mesothelioma with minimal asbestos exposure, *Hum. Pathol.* **9:**253–258.

Cruickshank, A. H., McConnell, E. M., and Miller, D. G., 1963, Malignancy in scars, chronic ulcers, and sinuses, *J. Clin. Pathol.* **16:**573–580.

Dalinka, M. K., Rockett, J. F., and Kurth, R. J., 1969, Carcinoma of the breast following simple mastectomy and mammoplasty, *Radiology* **93:**914.

Davies, P., Allison, A. C., Ackerman, J., Butterfield, A., and Williams, S., 1974, Asbestos induces selective release of lysosomal enzymes from mononuclear phagocytes, *Nature (London)* **251:**423–425.

Davis, H. H., Simons, M., and Davis, J. B., 1964, Cystic disease of the breast: Relationship to carcinoma, *Cancer* **17:**957–978.

Davis, J. M. G., 1970, The long term fibrogenic effects of chrysotile and crocidolite asbestos dust injected into the pleural cavity of experimental animals, *Br. J. Exp. Pathol.* **51:**617–627.

Dukes, C. E., 1958, Malignant tumors of the colon, rectum, and anus, in: *Cancer*, Vol. 2 (R. W. Raven, ed.), pp. 134–153, Butterworths, London.

Dunham, L. J., 1972, Cancer in man at site of prior benign lesion of skin or mucous membrane: A review, *Cancer Res.* **32:**1359–1374.

Elsebai, I., 1977, Parasites in the etiology of cancer—Bilharziasis and bladder cancer, *CA-Cancer J. Clin.* **27:**100–106.

Freund, H., Brian, S., Laufer, N., and Eyal, Z., 1976, Breast cancer arising in surgical scars, *J. Surg. Oncol.* **8:**477–480.

Gaensler, E. A., and Addington, W. W., 1969, Asbestos or ferruginous bodies, *N. Engl. J. Med.* **280:**488–492.

Gazayerli, M., Khalil, H. A., and Gazayerli, I. M., 1971, Schistosomiasis hematobium (urogenic bilharziasis), in: *Pathology of Protozoal and Helminthic Diseases* (R. A. Marcial-Rojas, ed.), pp. 434–449, Williams & Wilkins, Baltimore.

Gelfand, M., 1972, Schistosomiasis: A clinical account, *Trop. Doct.* **2:**3–8.

German, J., 1973, Oncogenic implications of chromosomal instability, *Hosp. Pract.* **8:**93–104.

Gross, P., and DeTreville, R. T. P., 1967, Experimental asbestosis: Studies on the progressiveness of the pulmonary fibrosis caused by chrysotile dust, *Arch. Environ. Health* **15:**638–649.

Gross, P., and DeTreville, R. T. P., 1970, Studies on the carcinogenic effects of asbestos dust, in: *Pneumoconiosis, Proceedings of the International Conference, Johannesburg, 1969*, pp. 220–224.

Harington, J. S., 1973, Chemical factors (including trace elements) as etiological mechanisms, in: *Biological Effects of Asbestosis* (P. Bogovski, V. Timbrell, J. C. Gilson, and J. C. Wagner, eds.), pp. 304–311, IARC Scientific Publication 8, Lyon, France.

689

ASBESTOSIS,
SCHISTO-
SOMIASIS,
FOREIGN
BODIES,
AND SCARS

HEPPLESTON, A. G., AND STYLES, J. A., 1967, Activity of a macrophage factor in collagen formation by silica, *Nature (London)* **214:**521–522.

HERRMANN, J. B., KANHOUWA, S., KELLEY, R. J., AND BURNS, W. A., 1971, Fibrosarcoma of the thigh associated with a prosthetic vascular graft, *N. Engl. J. Med.* **284:**91.

HICKS, R. M., JAMES, C., WEBBE, G., AND NELSON, G. S., 1977, *Schistosoma haematobium* and bladder cancer, *Trans. R. Soc. Trop. Med. Hyg.* **71:**288.

IVERSEN, U., IVERSEN, O. H., AND BJERKNES, R., 1968, A comparison of the tumourigenic effect of five graded doses of 3-methyl-cholanthrene applied to the skin of hairless mice at intervals of 3 or 14 days, *Acta Pathol. Microbiol. Scand.* **73:**502–520.

JACOBS, R., HUMPHREYS, J., DODGSON, K. S., AND RICHARDS, R. J., 1978, Light and electron microscope studies of the rat digestive tract following prolonged and short-term ingestion of chrysotile asbestos, *Br. J. Exp. Pathol.* **59:**443–453.

JAGATIC, J., RUBNITZ, M. E., GODWIN, M. C., AND WEISKOPF, W., 1967, Tissue response to intraperitoneal asbestos with preliminary report of acute toxicity of heat-treated asbestos in mice, *Environ. Res.* **1:**217–230.

JAURAND, M. C., BIGNON, J., GAUDICHET, A., MAGNE, L., AND OBLIN, A., 1978, Biological effects of chrysotile after SO_2 sorption. II. Effects on alveolar macrophages and red blood cells, *Environ. Res.* **17:**216–227.

JOHNSON, K. H., GHOBRIAL, H. K. G., BUOEN, L. C., BRAND, I., AND BRAND, K. G., 1972, Foreign body tumorigenesis in mice: Ultrastructure of the preneoplastic tissue reactions, *J. Natl. Cancer Inst.* **49:**1311–1319.

JOHNSON, K. H., GHOBRIAL, H. K. G., BUOEN, L. C., BRAND, I., AND BRAND, K. G., 1973, Nonfibroblastic origin of foreign body sarcomas implicated by histologic and electron microscopic studies, *Cancer Res.* **33:**3139–3154.

JOHNSTON, R. M., AND MILES, J. S., 1973, Sarcomas arising from chronic osteomyelitic sinuses, *J. Bone Joint Surg.* **55:**162–168.

JU, D. M. C., 1966, Fibrosarcoma arising in surgical scars, *Plast. Reconstr. Surg.* **38:**429–437.

KANAZAWA, K., BIRBECK, M. S. C., CARTER, R. L., AND ROE, F. J. C., 1970, Migration of asbestos fibres from subcutaneous injection sites in mice, *Br. J. Cancer* **24:**96–106.

KANNERSTEIN, M., AND CHURG, J., 1972, Pathology of carcinoma of the lung associated with asbestos exposure, *Cancer* **30:**14–21.

KANNERSTEIN, M., AND CHURG, J., 1977, Peritoneal mesothelioma, *Hum. Pathol.* **8:**83–94.

KOURI, J., AND ANCHETA, O., 1972, Transformation of macrophages into fibroblasts, *Exp. Cell Res.* **71:**168–176.

KUNTZ, R. E., CHEEVER, A. W., BRYAN, G. T., MOORE, J. A., AND HUANG, T., 1978, Natural history of papillary lesions of the urinary bladder in schistosomiasis, *Cancer Res.* **38:**3836–3839.

LEIBOVICH, S. J., AND ROSS, R., 1975, The role of the macrophage in wound repair. A study with hydrocortisone and antimacrophage serum, *Am. J. Pathol.* **78:**71–100.

LEIBOVICH, S. J., AND ROSS, R., 1976, A macrophage-dependent factor that stimulates the proliferation of fibroblasts *in vitro*, *Am. J. Pathol.* **84:**501–513.

LICHTENBERG, F. V., SMITH, T. M., LUCIA, H. L., AND DOUGHTY, B. L., 1971, New model for *Schistosoma* granuloma formation using a soluble egg antigen and bentonite particles, *Nature (London)* **229:**199.

LOEWENSTEIN, W. R., 1979, Junctional intercellular communication and the control of growth, *Biochim. Biophys. Acta* **560:**1–65.

MARTISCHNIG, K. M., NEWELL, D. J., BARNSLEY, W. C., COWAN, W. K., FEINMANN, E. L., AND OLIVER, E., 1977, Unsuspected exposure to asbestos and bronchogenic carcinoma, *Br. Med. J.* **1:**746–749.

MAXIMOW, A. A., 1927, Morphology of the mesenchymal reactions, *Arch. Pathol.* **4:**557–606.

MCDOUGAL, J. S., AND AZAR, H. A., 1972, Tritiated proline in macrophages: *In vivo* and *in vitro* uptake by foreign-body granulomas, *Arch. Pathol.* **93:**13–17.

MICHELICH, V. J., AND BRAND, K. G., 1980, Effects of gonadectomy on foreign body tumorigenesis in CBA/H mice, *J. Natl. Cancer. Inst.* **64:**807–808.

MICHELICH, V. J., BUOEN, L. C., AND BRAND, K. G., 1977, Immunosuppression studies in foreign body tumorigenesis: No evidence for tumor-specific antigenicity, *J. Natl. Cancer Inst.* **58:**757–761.

MILLER, K., 1978, The effects of asbestos on macrophages, *CRC Crit. Rev. Toxicol.* **5:**319–354.

NEWHOUSE, M. L., AND THOMPSON, H., 1965, Mesothelioma of pleura and peritoneum following exposure to asbestos in the London area, *Br. J. Ind. Med.* **22:**261–269.

691

ASBESTOSIS,
SCHISTO-
SOMIASIS,
FOREIGN
BODIES,
AND SCARS

O'CONNELL, T. X., FEE, H. J., AND GOLDING, A., 1976, Sarcoma associated with Dacron prosthetic material, *J. Thorac. Cardiovasc. Surg.* **72:**94–96.

OTT, G., 1970, Fremdkörpersarkome, *Exp. Med. Path. Klin.* **32**.

POTT, F., AND FRIEDRICHS, K. H., 1972, Tumoren der Ratte nach i.p.-Injection faserförmiger Stäube, *Naturwissenschaften* **59:**318.

POTT, F., FRIEDRICHS, K. H., AND HUTH, F., 1976, Ergebnisse aus Tierversuchen zur kanzerogenen Wirkung faserförmiger Stäube und ihre Deutung im Hinblick auf die Tumorentstehung beim Menschen, *Zentralbl. Bakteriol. Parasitenkd. Infektionskr. Hyg. Abt. 1 Orig. Reihe B* **162:**467–505.

RAEBURN, C., AND SPENCER, H., 1957, Lung scar cancers, *Br. J. Tuberc.* **51:**237–245.

RICHARDS, R. J., HEXT, P. M., BLUNDELL, G., HENDERSON, W. J., AND VOLCANI, B. E., 1974, Ultrastructural changes in lung fibroblast cultures exposed to chrysotile asbestos, *Br. J. Exp. Pathol.* **55:**275.

RIPSTEIN, C. B., SPAIN, D. M., AND BLUTH, I., 1968, Scar cancer of the lung, *J. Thorac. Cardiovasc. Surg.* **56:**362–370.

SCARANO, E., 1971, The control of gene function in cell differentiation and in embryogenesis, *Adv. Cytopharmacol.* **1:**13–24.

SELIKOFF, I. J., 1974, Epidemiology of gastrointestinal cancer, *Environ. Health Perspect.* **9:**299–305.

SELIKOFF, I. J., HAMMOND, E. C., AND CHURG, J., 1968, Asbestos exposure, smoking, and neoplasia, *J. Am. Med. Assoc.* **204:**106–112.

SHELTON, E., EVANS, V. J., AND PARKER, G. A., 1963, Malignant transformation of mouse connective tissue grown in diffusion chambers, *J. Natl. Cancer Inst.* **30:**377–391.

SHETTIGARA, P. T., AND MORGAN, R. W., 1975, Asbestos, smoking, and laryngeal carcinoma, *Arch. Environ. Health* **30:**517–519.

SHURGIN, A., AND BECKER, F. F., 1974, Sequential events in induction of sarcomas by 4-hydroxyaminoquinoline 1-oxide: Fibroplasia, a premalignant phase, *J. Natl. Cancer Inst.* **53:**159–164.

SIDDONS, A. H. M., AND McARTHUR, A. M., 1952, Carcinomata developing at the site of foreign bodies in the lung, *Br. J. Surg.* **39:**542–545.

SPAIN, D. M., 1957, The association of terminal bronchiolar carcinoma with chronic interstitial inflammation and fibrosis of the lungs, *Am. Rev. Tuberc.* **76:**559–567.

STANTON, M. F., 1973, Tumors of the pleura induced with asbestos and fibrous glass, *J. Natl. Cancer Inst.* **51:**317–319.

STANTON, M. F., AND WRENCH, C., 1972, Mechanisms of mesothelioma induction with asbestos and fibrous glass, *J. Natl. Cancer Inst.* **48:**797–821.

STANTON, M. F., LAYARD, M., TEGERIS, A., MILLER, E., MAY, M., AND KENT, E., 1977, Carcinogenicity of fibrous glass: Pleural response in the rat in relation to fiber dimension, *J. Natl. Cancer Inst.* **58:**587–603.

STELL, P. M., AND McGILL, T., 1973, Asbestos and laryngeal carcinoma, *Lancet* **2:**416–417.

STRAUSS, F. H., DORDAL, E., AND KAPPAS, A., 1963, The problem of pulmonary scar tumors, *Arch. Pathol.* **76:**693–699.

TETLEY, T. D., HEXT, P. M., RICHARDS, R. J., AND McDERMOTT, M., 1976, Chrysotile-induced asbestosis: Changes in the free cell population. Pulmonary surfactant and whole lung tissue of rats, *Br. J. Exp. Pathol.* **57:**505–514.

THOMPSON, J. R., AND ENTIN, S. D., 1969, Primary extraskeletal chondrosarcoma. Report of a case arising in conjunction with extrapleural Lucite ball plombage, *Cancer* **23:**936–939.

TIMBRELL, V., GRIFFITHS, D. M., AND POOLEY, F. D., 1971, Possible biological importance of fibre diameters of South African amphiboles, *Nature (London)* **232:**55–56.

TREVES, N., AND PACK, G. T., 1930, The development of cancer in burn scars: Analysis and report of 34 cases, *Surg. Gynecol. Obstet.* **51:**749–782.

TURUSOV, V., DAY, N., ANDRIANOV, L., AND JAIN, D., 1971, Influence of dose on skin tumors induced in mice by single application of 7,12-dimethylbenz[a]anthracene, *J. Natl. Cancer Inst.* **47:**105–111.

VIANNA, N. J., AND POLAN, A. K., 1978, Non-occupational exposure to asbestos and malignant mesothelioma in females, *Lancet* **1:**1061–1063.

VOLKMAN, A., AND GOWANS, J. L., 1965, The origin of macrophages from the bone marrow in the rat, *Br. J. Exp. Pathol.* **46:**62–70.

WAGNER, J. C., 1963, Asbestosis in experimental animals, *Br. J. Ind. Med.* **20:**1–12.

WAGNER, J. C., AND BERRY, G., 1969, Mesotheliomas in rats following inoculation with asbestos, *Br. J. Cancer* **23:**567–581.

692

K. GERHARD
BRAND

WAGNER, J. C., BERRY, G., SKIDMORE, J. W., AND TIMBRELL, V., 1974, The effects of the inhalation of asbestos in rats, *Br. J. Cancer* **29:**252–269.

WARNOCK, M. L., AND CHURG, A. M., 1975, Association of asbestos and bronchogenic carcinoma in a population with low asbestos exposure, *Cancer* **35:**1236–1242.

WARREN, L., 1974, The malignant cell and its membranes, *Am. J. Pathol.* **77:**69–76.

WEBSTER, I., 1973, Asbestos and malignancy, *S. Afr. Med. J.* **47:**165–171.

ZAFIRACOPOULOS, P., AND ROUSKAS, A., 1974, Breast cancer at site of implantation of pacemaker generator, *Lancet* **1:**1114.

Index